FOR REFERENCE

Do Not Take From This Room

VITAL STATISTICS OF THE UNITED STATES

VITAL STATISTICS OF THE UNITED STATES

Births, Life Expectancy, Deaths, and Selected Health Data

Ninth Edition
2020

Edited by Shana Hertz Hattis

Lanham • Boulder • New York • London

Published by Bernan Press
An imprint of The Rowman & Littlefield Publishing Group, Inc.
4501 Forbes Boulevard, Suite 200, Lanham, Maryland 20706
www.rowman.com
800-462-6420

6 Tinworth Street, London SE11 5AL, United Kingdom

ISBN: 978-1-64143-404-1
E-ISBN: 978-1-64143-405-8
ISSN: 1549-8603

CONTENTS

LIST OF TABLES

PART II: MORTALITY

PART III: HEALTH

Determinants and Measures of Health

Use of Addictive Substances

Ambulatory Care

Inpatient Care

Health Personnel

Health Expenditures

Health Insurance

Part 4: Marriage and Divorce

LIST OF FIGURES

INTRODUCTION

Bernan Press is pleased to present a comprehensive collection of birth, mortality, and health data in the ninth edition of *Vital Statistics of the United States: Births, Life Expectancy, Deaths, and Selected Health Data*. This volume provides valuable information compiled by various government agencies including the Centers for Disease Control (CDC) and its National Center for Health Statistics (NCHS) and National Vital Statistics System (NVSS), the U.S. Census Bureau, and the Bureau of Labor Statistics (BLS).

Until 1993, the federal government published *Vital Statistics of the United States* in several thick-bound volumes. However, between the last publication of the federal volume and the first *Vital Statistics* edition from Bernan Press, nothing comparable was offered. During this time, the CDC continued to compile its information as periodical reports and news releases, and Bernan took this opportunity to streamline this information into a cohesive, inclusive volume.

This edition builds upon the groundwork laid by previous editions in the areas of birth, mortality, health, and marriage and divorce. Each part is preceded by highlights of salient data. These sections also contain a diverse array of information about their tables and figures. Notes and definitions and source information are also provided for all four parts.

The Birth section, in many instances, provides final data through 2018. This section covers many aspects of natality, including birth and fertility rates, number of children, births to unmarried women, methods of delivery, and demographic characteristics of mothers.

The Mortality section focuses on deaths and death rates as told through various medical, demographic, and social characteristics. Especially detailed are the tables on causes of death, which are shown by leading causes of death, age, sex, Hispanic origin, race, and (to a lesser extent) state of residence. Death rates are also given by marital status and level of educational attainment, and special tables are provided for infant mortality.

The Health section, the largest in the book, offers a collection of statistics concerning health and disease. While health is not a traditional component of vital statistics, its importance to this volume cannot be overstated. Health data provides the user with an even deeper picture of births and deaths in the United States. For example, a user interested in cerebrovascular disease mortality may glean useful information from tables about incidence and survival rates. This chapter shows selected data on several topics, including determinants and measures of health, use of addictive substances, ambulatory care, inpatient care, health personnel, health expenditures, and health insurance.

The Marriage and Divorce section provides marriage and divorce rates by state and demographic characteristics. This chapter also provides statistics on multiple marriages, marriages ending in widowhood, and number of marriages for U.S. residents.

About the Editor

Shana Hertz Hattis is an editor with over a decade of experience in statistical and government research publications. Past titles include *State Profiles: The Population and Economy of Each U.S. State, Housing Statistics of the United States*, and *Justice Statistics: An Extended Look at Crime in the United States*. She earned her bachelor of science in journalism and master of science in education degrees from Northwestern University.

PART I: BIRTHS

PART I: BIRTHS

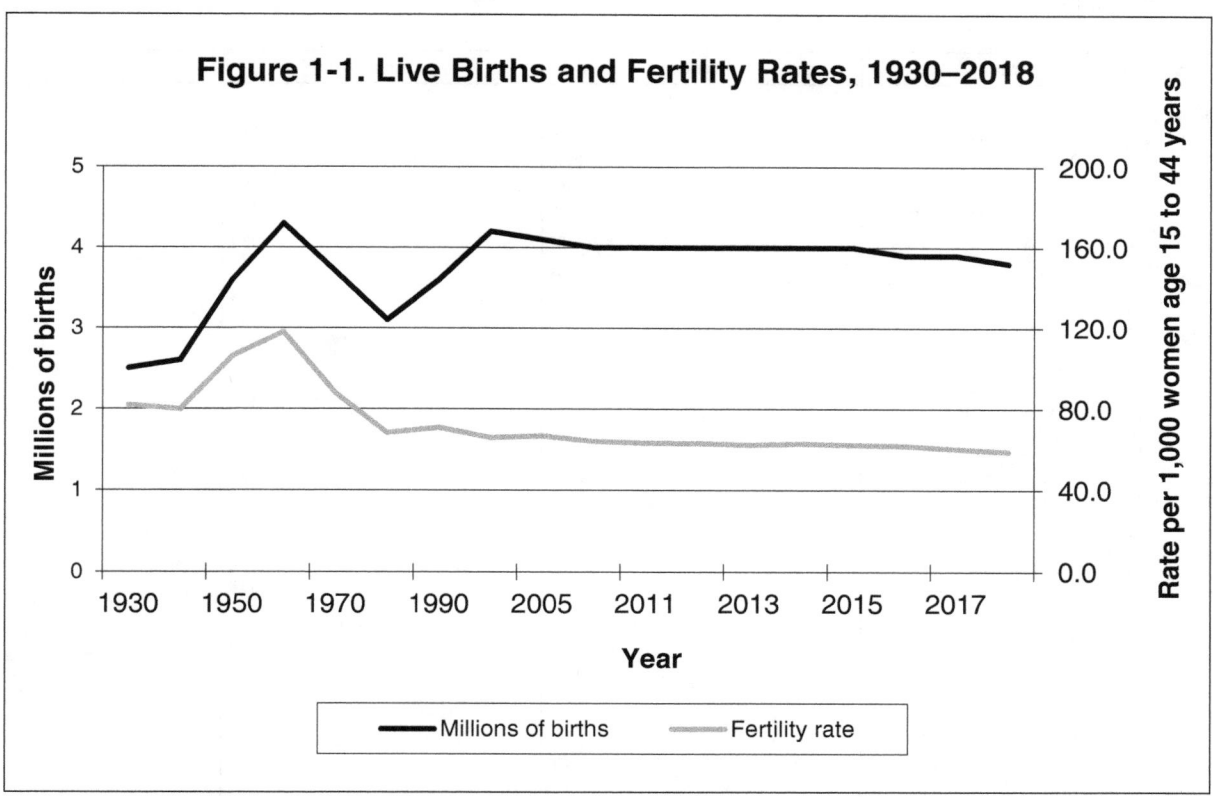

Figure 1-1. Live Births and Fertility Rates, 1930–2018

HIGHLIGHTS

- There were 3,791,712 births in the United States in 2018, down from 3,855,500 in 2017. Births declined for all racial and ethnic groups, except for the Native Hawaiian or Other Pacific Islander groups, which experienced an increase of 0.5 percent.

- The U.S. general fertility rate (births per 1,000 women aged 15–44) declined 2 percent between 2017 and 2018; fertility rates declined for most racial groups including non-Hispanic white, non-Hispanic black, and Hispanic women.

- The birth rate for teenagers age 15 to 19 years fell 7 percent from 2017 to 2018, reaching 17.4 births per 1,000 females age 15 to 19 years. Rates fell for each race and Hispanic-origin group.

- The proportion of vaginal births after previous cesarean (VBAC) rose to 13.3 percent in 2018 with increases in VBAC deliveries for the three race and Hispanic-origin groups.

- Percentages of births delivered preterm and early term increased from 2017 to 2018, whereas full-term and late- and post-term deliveries declined. These patterns were consistent across race and Hispanic-origin groups.

Table 1-1. Births and Birth Rates: United States, 2010–2018, and by Race and Hispanic Origin, United States, 2016–2018

(Number, rate.)

Race and Hispanic origin of mother	Number	Birth rate	Fertility rate
All Races and Origins[1]			
2010	3,999,386	13.0	64.1
2011	3,953,590	12.7	63.2
2012	3,952,841	12.6	63.0
2013	3,932,181	12.4	62.5
2014	3,988,076	12.5	62.9
2015	3,978,497	12.4	62.5
2016	3,945,875	12.2	62.0
2017	3,855,500	11.8	60.3
2018	3,791,712	11.6	59.1
Non-Hispanic, Single Race[2]			
White			
2016	2,056,332	10.5	58.8
2017	1,992,461	10.2	57.2
2018	1,956,413	10.0	56.3
Black			
2016	558,622	14.0	63.3
2017	560,715	13.9	63.1
2018	552,029	13.6	62.0
American Indian or Alaska Native			
2016	31,452	13.3	62.7
2017	29,957	12.6	59.5
2018	29,092	12.2	57.7
Asian			
2016	254,471	14.6	61.1
2017	249,250	13.8	58.0
2018	240,798	13.2	55.6
Native Hawaiian or Other Pacific Islander			
2016	9,342	16.8	72.9
2017	9,426	16.7	72.8
2018	9,476	16.6	73.0
Hispanic[3]			
2016	918,447	16.0	70.6
2017	898,764	15.2	67.6
2018	886,210	14.8	65.9

NOTE: Birth rates are births per 1,000 population in specified group. Fertility rates are births per 1,000 women aged 15–44 years in specified group. Populations based on counts enumerated as of April 1 for census years and estimated as of July 1 for all other years.

[1] Includes births to race and origin groups not shown separately, such as Hispanic single-race white, Hispanic single-race black, and non-Hispanic multiple-race women, and births with origin not stated.

[2] Race and Hispanic origin are reported separately on birth certificates; persons of Hispanic origin may be of any race. In this table, non-Hispanic women are classified by race. Race categories are consistent with the 1997 Office of Management and Budget standards. Single race is defined as only one race reported on the birth certificate.

[3] Includes all persons of Hispanic origin of any race.

Table 1-2. Birth Rates, by Age of Mother: United States, 2010–2018, and by Age and Race and Hispanic Origin of Mother, United States, 2016–2018

(Number, rate per 1,000 women in specified age group.)

Race and Hispanic origin of mother	Total fertility rate	10–14 years	Age of mother 15–19 years Total	15–17 years	18–19 years	20–24 years	25–29 years	30–34 years	35–39 years	40–44 years	45–49 years[1]
All Races and Origins[2]											
2010	1,931.0	0.4	34.2	17.3	58.2	90.0	108.3	96.5	45.9	10.2	0.7
2011	1,894.5	0.4	31.3	15.4	54.1	85.3	107.2	96.5	47.2	10.3	0.7
2012	1,880.5	0.4	29.4	14.1	51.4	83.1	106.5	97.3	48.3	10.4	0.7
2013	1,857.5	0.3	26.5	12.3	47.1	80.7	105.5	98.0	49.3	10.4	0.8
2014	1,862.5	0.3	24.2	10.9	43.8	79.0	105.8	100.8	51.0	10.6	0.8
2015	1,843.5	0.2	22.3	9.9	40.7	76.8	104.3	101.5	51.8	11.0	0.8
2016	1,820.5	0.2	20.3	8.8	37.5	73.8	102.1	102.7	52.7	11.4	0.9
2017	1,765.5	0.2	18.8	7.9	35.1	71.0	98.0	100.3	52.3	11.6	0.9
2018	1,729.5	0.2	17.4	7.2	32.3	68.0	95.3	99.7	52.6	11.8	0.9
Non-Hispanic, Single Race[3]											
White											
2016	1,719.0	0.1	14.3	5.2	27.7	62.4	99.3	106.2	51.1	9.7	0.7
2017	1,666.5	0.1	13.2	4.6	26.0	59.8	95.3	103.7	50.6	9.9	0.7
2018	1,640.0	0.1	12.1	4.1	23.6	57.8	92.9	103.1	51.1	10.2	0.7
Black											
2016	1,832.5	0.5	29.3	13.7	52.5	95.8	100.8	83.0	45.0	11.1	1.0
2017	1,824.5	0.4	27.5	12.5	49.8	94.2	99.5	84.5	46.1	11.7	1.0
2018	1,792.0	0.4	26.3	11.9	46.9	90.0	97.1	84.1	47.1	12.3	1.1
American Indian or Alaska Native											
2016	1,794.5	0.5	35.1	16.8	62.6	97.2	103.4	77.1	37.1	8.2	0.3
2017	1,702.0	0.5	32.9	15.7	58.1	93.6	96.4	72.1	36.3	8.2	0.4
2018	1,650.5	0.2	29.7	13.5	52.9	87.7	94.4	73.2	36.1	8.3	0.5
Asian											
2016	1,690.5	*	3.9	1.4	7.5	28.9	87.0	127.4	72.8	16.4	1.7
2017	1,597.0	*	3.3	1.1	6.5	26.6	79.6	120.1	71.5	16.5	1.8
2018	1,525.0	*	2.8	1.0	5.4	24.1	73.0	116.5	70.7	16.1	1.8
Native Hawaiian or Other Pacific Islander											
2016	2,076.5	*	28.6	11.0	55.3	109.5	115.5	96.0	49.9	14.7	*
2017	2,085.5	*	25.5	8.7	50.6	113.3	115.7	94.0	54.6	13.1	*
2018	2,106.5	*	26.5	8.2	53.7	118.5	118.9	91.9	49.2	15.4	*
Hispanic[4]											
2016	2,092.5	0.4	31.9	15.6	57.3	98.4	117.4	99.2	55.8	14.5	0.9
2017	2,006.5	0.3	28.9	13.6	52.7	93.8	111.8	96.4	54.6	14.5	1.0
2018	1,959.0	0.3	26.7	12.4	48.5	89.3	108.9	96.6	54.5	14.5	1.0

NOTE: Total fertility rates are sums of birth rates for 5-year age groups multiplied by 5. Birth rates are births per 1,000 women in specified group. Populations based on counts enumerated as of April 1 for census years and estimated as of July 1 for all other years.
* = Estimate does not meet NCHS standards of reliability.
[1]Birth rates computed by relating births to women aged 45 and over to women aged 45–49 years.
[2]Includes births to race and origin groups not shown separately, such as Hispanic single-race White, Hispanic single-race Black, and non-Hispanic multiple-race women, and births with origin not stated.
[3]Race and Hispanic origin are reported separately on birth certificates; persons of Hispanic origin may be of any race. In this table, non-Hispanic women are classified by race. Race categories are consistent with the 1997 Office of Management and Budget standards. Single race is defined as only one race reported on the birth certificate.
[4]Includes all persons of Hispanic origin of any race.

Table 1-3. Births, by Age of Mother, Live-Birth Order, and Race and Hispanic Origin of Mother, 2018

(Number.)

Live-birth order and race and Hispanic origin of mother	All ages	Under 15 years	15 to 19 years						20 to 24 years	25 to 29 years	30 to 34 years	35 to 39 years	40 to 44 years	45 to 49 years	50 to 54 years
			Total	15 years	16 years	17 years	18 years	19 years							
All Races and Origins[1]	3,791,712	1,736	179,871	4,953	13,088	26,250	50,088	85,492	726,175	1,099,491	1,090,697	566,786	117,381	8,616	959
1st child	1,433,915	1,712	151,440	4,842	12,458	23,863	42,670	67,607	383,388	409,940	332,492	127,893	24,364	2,375	311
2nd child	1,208,762	16	24,506	91	586	2,196	6,535	15,098	231,051	362,863	370,337	185,345	32,257	2,154	233
3rd child	651,049	1	3,122	4	18	136	714	2,250	81,852	200,639	214,401	125,246	24,191	1,457	140
4th child	283,877	–	332	–	4	7	45	276	21,454	81,158	99,793	64,469	15,597	957	117
5th child	111,885	–	42	–	–	1	14	27	4,966	27,694	39,788	30,271	8,481	573	70
6th child	47,066	–	12	–	1	–	1	10	1,061	9,304	17,144	14,609	4,557	343	36
7th child	21,456	–	4	–	–	–	–	4	248	3,034	7,649	7,646	2,644	208	23
8th child and over	23,095	–	13	–	–	–	2	11	237	1,695	6,061	9,687	4,869	505	28
Not stated	10,607	7	400	16	21	47	107	209	1,918	3,164	3,032	1,620	421	44	1
Non-Hispanic, Single Race[2]															
White	1,956,413	337	64,917	1,244	3,555	8,237	17,848	34,033	326,575	576,811	624,015	304,062	55,417	3,875	404
1st child	768,672	330	55,599	1,224	3,433	7,619	15,560	27,763	179,304	238,135	205,709	74,987	13,255	1,203	150
2nd child	651,254	4	8,189	19	109	573	2,063	5,425	103,311	192,901	223,283	105,807	16,587	1,053	119
3rd child	320,395	–	880	1	4	28	172	675	33,444	94,689	115,044	65,194	10,494	596	54
4th child	125,198	–	82	–	–	4	9	69	7,643	34,360	47,303	29,496	5,981	300	33
5th child	45,494	–	17	–	–	1	7	9	1,441	10,600	17,486	12,635	3,094	201	20
6th child	18,970	–	2	–	–	–	–	2	274	3,105	7,456	6,294	1,709	117	13
7th child	9,173	–	1	–	–	–	–	1	61	904	3,380	3,583	1,146	89	9
8th child and over	11,599	–	3	–	–	–	1	2	94	524	2,555	5,186	2,943	288	6
Not stated	5,658	3	144	–	9	12	36	87	1,003	1,593	1,799	880	208	28	–
Black	552,029	554	37,715	1,276	3,013	5,709	10,523	17,194	137,974	166,802	124,206	67,268	15,988	1,348	174
1st child	194,089	546	31,512	1,234	2,856	5,172	8,918	13,332	70,246	48,551	27,559	12,438	2,832	337	68
2nd child	157,412	4	5,166	31	146	488	1,375	3,126	42,064	52,505	35,953	17,664	3,726	299	31
3rd child	101,714	–	816	1	5	36	184	590	17,514	35,129	28,655	15,835	3,503	238	24
4th child	52,115	–	109	–	–	1	18	90	5,666	17,876	16,225	9,566	2,490	167	16
5th child	23,576	–	9	–	–	–	3	6	1,606	7,477	7,858	5,172	1,354	90	10
6th child	10,948	–	3	–	–	–	1	2	396	3,024	3,916	2,739	796	68	6
7th child	5,139	–	2	–	–	–	–	2	87	1,099	1,931	1,508	460	43	9
8th child and over	5,504	–	5	–	–	–	–	5	67	664	1,746	2,140	772	100	10
Not stated	1,532	4	93	10	6	12	24	41	328	477	363	206	55	6	–
American Indian or Alaska Native	29,092	19	2,578	103	229	362	743	1,141	7,841	9,146	6,105	2,787	585	29	2
1st child	8,684	19	2,107	99	215	328	603	862	3,454	1,931	815	291	60	6	1
2nd child	7,575	–	406	4	12	31	126	233	2,678	2,605	1,318	481	79	8	–
3rd child	5,586	–	50	–	1	3	12	34	1,183	2,261	1,411	572	107	2	–
4th child	3,422	–	9	–	–	–	1	8	374	1,302	1,113	527	92	5	–
5th child	1,838	–	1	–	–	–	–	1	108	635	688	322	82	2	–
6th child	972	–	1	–	–	–	–	1	19	246	407	235	63	–	1
7th child	475	–	–	–	–	–	–	–	3	87	170	164	49	2	–
8th child and over	462	–	1	–	–	–	–	1	3	49	170	183	52	4	–
Not stated	78	–	3	–	1	–	1	1	19	30	13	12	1	–	–
Asian	240,798	18	1,444	34	92	182	393	743	14,876	57,810	96,385	57,136	11,951	1,055	123
1st child	109,429	16	1,220	34	84	165	329	608	9,807	34,162	43,369	17,113	3,319	383	40
2nd child	90,179	2	190	–	7	14	57	112	3,749	17,094	38,592	25,573	4,603	335	41
3rd child	28,123	–	26	–	–	2	5	19	1,015	4,552	10,088	9,844	2,413	171	14
4th child	8,367	–	5	–	1	–	1	3	211	1,328	2,836	2,925	958	91	13
5th child	2,595	–	–	–	–	–	–	–	60	398	820	937	346	28	6
6th child	994	–	–	–	–	–	–	–	10	134	342	349	133	21	5
7th child	378	–	–	–	–	–	–	–	4	32	119	143	68	10	2
8th child and over	448	–	–	–	–	–	–	–	3	28	116	188	95	16	2
Not stated	285	–	3	–	–	1	1	1	17	82	103	64	16	–	–
Native Hawaiian or Other Pacific Islander	9,476	3	516	10	23	62	159	262	2,482	2,887	2,189	1,097	290	12	–
1st child	2,791	3	424	10	22	57	135	200	1,151	712	336	124	39	2	–
2nd child	2,264	–	72	–	1	4	21	46	797	762	419	178	35	1	–
3rd child	1,773	–	14	–	–	–	3	11	349	666	488	207	47	2	–
4th child	1,196	–	1	–	–	–	–	1	124	426	394	193	56	2	–
5th child	672	–	1	–	–	–	–	1	30	190	272	137	41	1	–
6th child	364	–	–	–	–	–	–	–	10	84	136	109	25	–	–
7th child	180	–	–	–	–	–	–	–	–	31	80	50	17	2	–
8th child and over	184	–	–	–	–	–	–	–	–	11	50	91	30	2	–
Not stated	52	–	4	–	–	1	–	3	21	5	14	8	–	–	–
Hispanic[3]	886,210	730	65,122	2,044	5,574	10,567	18,369	28,568	209,701	253,977	208,193	117,383	29,192	1,787	125
1st child	303,049	724	54,158	2,003	5,283	9,490	15,360	22,022	105,410	75,046	44,923	18,465	3,936	350	37
2nd child	264,775	5	9,498	35	278	1,000	2,635	5,550	70,061	86,821	61,610	30,255	6,164	341	20
3rd child	174,777	1	1,225	1	7	61	316	840	25,259	57,438	53,376	30,248	6,881	331	18
4th child	84,987	–	112	–	2	2	14	94	6,660	23,209	29,120	20,017	5,535	312	22
5th child	33,963	–	12	–	–	–	4	8	1,518	7,414	11,388	10,142	3,274	201	14
6th child	13,213	–	4	–	1	–	–	3	315	2,350	4,327	4,425	1,672	117	3
7th child	5,392	–	1	–	–	–	–	1	78	771	1,719	1,960	810	50	3
8th child and over	4,152	–	3	–	–	–	1	2	62	371	1,223	1,578	830	78	7
Not stated	1,902	–	109	5	3	14	39	48	338	557	507	293	90	7	1

NOTE: Live-birth order refers to number of children born alive to mother.
– = Quantity zero.
[1]Includes births to race and origin groups not shown separately, such as Hispanic single-race White, Hispanic single-race Black, and non-Hispanic multiple-race women, and births with origin not stated.
[2]Race and Hispanic origin are reported separately on birth certificates; persons of Hispanic origin may be of any race. In this table, non-Hispanic women are classified by race. Race categories are consistent with the 1997 Office of Management and Budget standards. Single race is defined as only one race reported on the birth certificate.
[3]Includes all persons of Hispanic origin of any race.

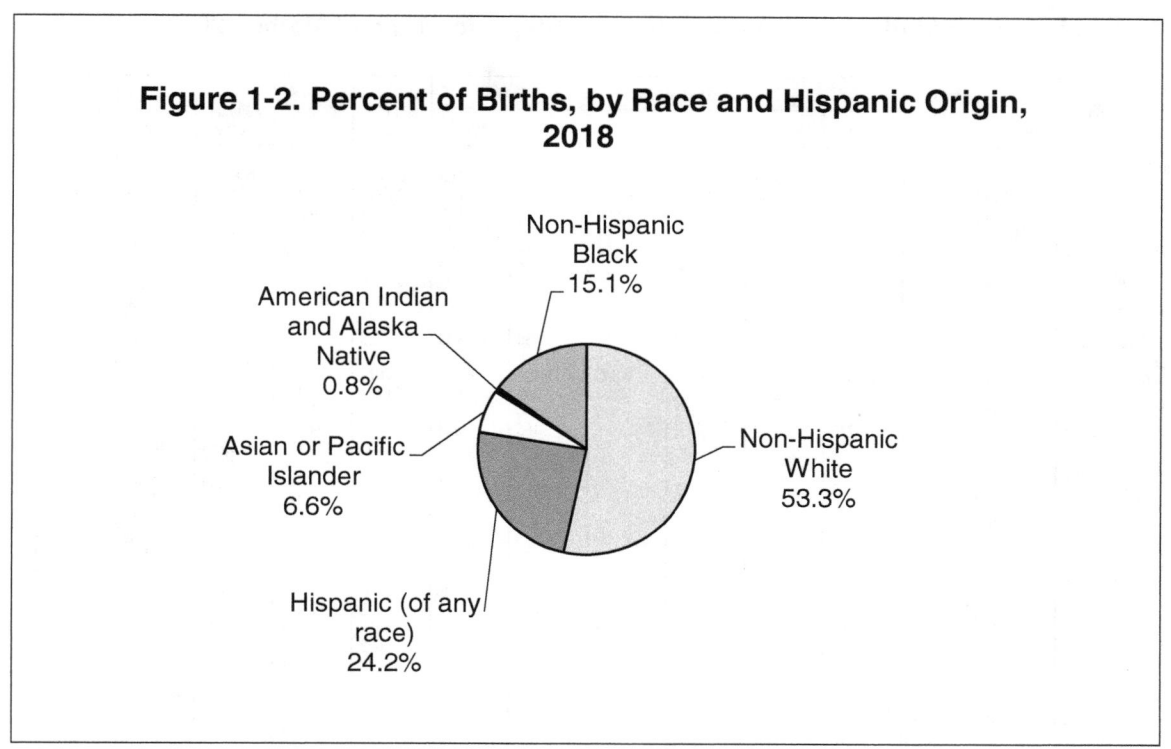

Figure 1-2. Percent of Births, by Race and Hispanic Origin, 2018

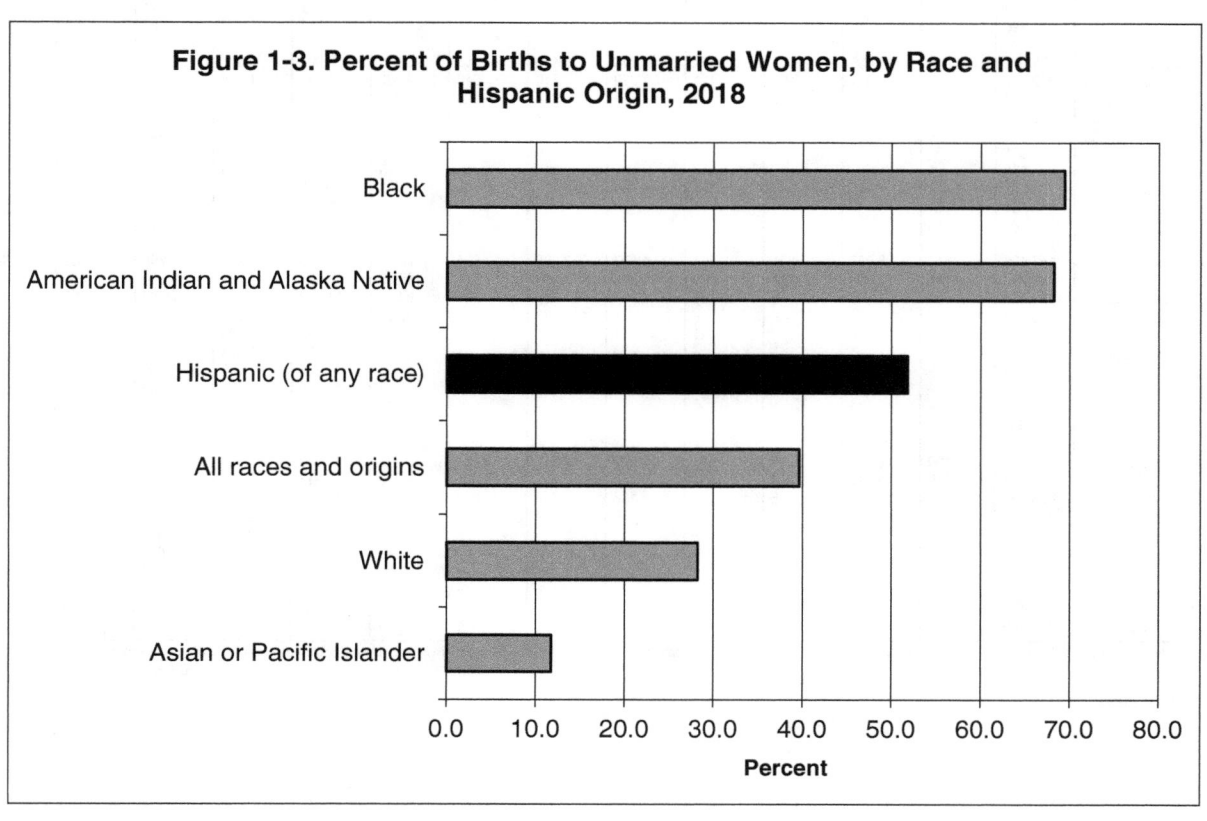

Figure 1-3. Percent of Births to Unmarried Women, by Race and Hispanic Origin, 2018

Table 1-4. Births, by Age of Mother, Live-Birth Order, and Hispanic Origin of Mother, 2018

(Number.)

Live-birth order and race and Hispanic origin of mother	All ages	Under 15 years	15 to 19 years						20 to 24 years	25 to 29 years	30 to 34 years	35 to 39 years	40 to 44 years	45 to 49 years	50 to 54 years
			Total	15 years	16 years	17 years	18 years	19 years							
Total	886,210	730	65,122	2,044	5,574	10,567	18,369	28,568	209,701	253,977	208,193	117,383	29,192	1,787	125
1st child	303,049	724	54,158	2,003	5,283	9,490	15,360	22,022	105,410	75,046	44,923	18,465	3,936	350	37
2nd child	264,775	5	9,498	35	278	1,000	2,635	5,550	70,061	86,821	61,610	30,255	6,164	341	20
3rd child	174,777	1	1,225	1	7	61	316	840	25,259	57,438	53,376	30,248	6,881	331	18
4th child	84,987	–	112	–	2	2	14	94	6,660	23,209	29,120	20,017	5,535	312	22
5th child	33,963	–	12	–	–	–	4	8	1,518	7,414	11,388	10,142	3,274	201	14
6th child	13,213	–	4	–	1	–	–	3	315	2,350	4,327	4,425	1,672	117	3
7th child	5,392	–	1	–	–	–	–	1	78	771	1,719	1,960	810	50	3
8th child and over	4,152	–	3	–	–	–	1	2	62	371	1,223	1,578	830	78	7
Not stated	1,902	–	109	5	3	14	39	48	338	557	507	293	90	7	1
Mexican	495,831	401	38,396	1,224	3,276	6,333	10,753	16,810	122,074	143,052	112,535	62,578	15,845	917	33
1st child	160,303	396	31,850	1,201	3,101	5,692	8,999	12,857	59,784	38,468	20,125	7,862	1,671	137	10
2nd child	141,295	5	5,679	20	171	598	1,556	3,334	41,533	47,795	30,176	13,345	2,616	139	7
3rd child	102,882	–	747	1	4	39	180	523	15,295	34,999	31,313	16,686	3,669	169	4
4th child	54,104	–	76	–	–	1	9	66	4,138	14,721	18,713	12,760	3,515	177	4
5th child	22,025	–	4	–	–	–	–	4	935	4,724	7,411	6,637	2,173	137	4
6th child	8,518	–	1	–	–	–	–	1	192	1,434	2,805	2,881	1,123	81	1
7th child	3,499	–	1	–	–	–	–	1	51	488	1,106	1,293	531	29	–
8th child and over	2,586	–	1	–	–	–	-	1	25	236	739	1,018	519	45	3
Not stated	619	–	37	2	–	3	9	23	121	187	147	96	28	3	–
Puerto Rican	71,614	51	5,511	136	419	785	1,534	2,637	19,577	21,578	15,055	7,910	1,824	91	17
1st child	27,045	51	4,636	134	400	718	1,288	2,096	10,207	6,553	3,697	1,542	331	22	6
2nd child	22,147	–	770	2	17	63	217	471	6,218	7,443	4,742	2,461	489	21	3
3rd child	12,705	–	86	–	–	2	21	63	2,286	4,653	3,467	1,794	400	17	2
4th child	5,553	–	3	–	1	–	–	2	623	1,864	1,734	1,038	265	20	6
5th child	2,265	–	3	–	–	–	3	–	149	651	771	533	154	4	–
6th child	954	–	1	–	1	–	–	–	36	242	325	273	75	2	–
7th child	394	–	–	–	–	–	–	–	8	79	141	123	43	–	–
8th child and over	361	–	–	–	–	–	–	–	9	32	135	122	58	5	–
Not stated	190	–	12	–	–	2	5	5	41	61	43	24	9	–	–
Cuban	23,471	2	725	11	48	101	207	358	3,878	7,331	7,426	3,280	770	56	3
1st child	10,976	2	643	11	47	97	187	301	2,623	3,624	2,920	953	186	23	2
2nd child	8,249	–	70	–	1	4	15	50	948	2,553	2,992	1,365	307	14	–
3rd child	2,789	–	9	–	–	–	3	6	216	761	1,022	606	167	8	–
4th child	801	–	–	–	–	–	–	–	46	221	274	205	49	6	–
5th child	260	–	–	–	–	–	–	–	15	62	82	78	22	1	–
6th child	102	–	–	–	–	–	–	–	3	19	39	28	13	–	–
7th child	50	–	–	–	–	–	–	–	–	13	18	12	7	–	–
8th child and over	54	–	–	–	–	–	–	–	4	7	19	11	11	2	–
Not stated	190	–	3	–	–	–	2	1	23	71	60	22	8	2	1
Dominican	32,072	9	1,655	52	127	248	470	758	6,891	9,990	7,837	4,512	1,073	94	11
1st child	12,726	9	1,459	50	121	229	419	640	4,338	3,931	1,998	791	172	25	3
2nd child	10,861	–	172	2	5	16	44	105	1,921	3,811	3,005	1,600	323	26	3
3rd child	5,826	–	23	–	1	3	7	12	505	1,689	1,896	1,360	327	24	2
4th child	1,794	–	–	–	–	–	–	–	96	391	666	475	150	15	1
5th child	512	–	–	–	–	–	–	–	14	100	157	171	67	3	–
6th child	159	–	–	–	–	–	–	–	5	27	49	60	18	–	–
7th child	63	–	–	–	–	–	–	–	1	13	16	27	6	–	–
8th child and over	51	–	–	–	–	–	–	–	–	4	18	18	8	1	2
Not stated	80	–	1	–	–	–	–	1	11	24	32	10	2	–	–
Central and South American	147,430	147	8,837	301	801	1,473	2,588	3,674	27,040	38,213	40,173	25,755	6,789	441	35
1st child	50,072	147	7,358	293	766	1,298	2,180	2,821	13,735	12,557	10,224	4,860	1,076	102	13
2nd child	47,566	–	1,286	6	33	161	358	728	9,343	13,978	13,290	7,786	1,787	91	5
3rd child	28,914	–	140	–	–	7	31	102	3,105	7,784	9,565	6,567	1,666	82	5
4th child	12,451	–	8	–	1	1	–	6	600	2,722	4,420	3,588	1,044	66	3
5th child	4,832	–	1	–	–	–	–	1	113	730	1,663	1,701	581	38	5
6th child	1,788	–	1	–	–	–	–	1	17	208	535	700	301	25	1
7th child	651	–	–	–	–	–	–	–	5	44	190	250	147	14	1
8th child and over	522	–	1	–	–	–	–	1	14	31	107	191	155	21	2
Not stated	634	–	42	2	1	6	19	14	108	159	179	112	32	2	–
Other and Unknown Hispanic	115,792	120	9,998	320	903	1,627	2,817	4,331	30,241	33,813	25,167	13,348	2,891	188	26
1st child	41,927	119	8,212	314	848	1,456	2,287	3,307	14,723	9,913	5,959	2,457	500	41	3
2nd child	34,657	–	1,521	5	51	158	445	862	10,098	11,241	7,405	3,698	642	50	2
3rd child	21,661	1	220	–	2	10	74	134	3,852	7,552	6,113	3,235	652	31	5
4th child	10,284	–	25	–	–	–	5	20	1,157	3,290	3,313	1,951	512	28	8
5th child	4,069	–	4	–	–	–	–	3	292	1,147	1,304	1,022	277	18	5
6th child	1,692	–	1	–	–	–	–	1	62	420	574	483	142	9	1
7th child	735	–	–	–	–	–	–	–	13	134	248	255	76	7	2
8th child and over	578	–	1	–	–	–	1	–	10	61	205	218	79	4	–
Not stated	189	–	14	1	2	3	4	4	34	55	46	29	11	–	–

NOTE: Live-birth order refers to number of children born alive to mother. Includes births with stated origin of mother only. In this table, Hispanic women are classified only by place of origin; non–Hispanic women are not shown.
– = Quantity zero.

Table 1-5. Birth Rates, by Age of Mother, Live-Birth Order, and Race and Hispanic Origin of Mother, 2018

(Rates per 1,000 women in specified age and race and Hispanic-origin groups.)

Live-birth order and race and Hispanic origin of mother	15 to 44 years[1]	10 to 14 years	15 to 19 years			20 to 24 years	25 to 29 years	30 to 34 years	35 to 39 years	40 to 44 years	45 to 49 years[1]
			Total	15 to 17 years	18 to 19 years						
All Races and Origins[2]	59.1	0.2	17.4	7.2	32.3	68.0	95.3	99.7	52.6	11.8	0.9
1st child	22.4	0.2	14.7	6.7	26.4	36.0	35.6	30.5	11.9	2.5	0.3
2nd child	18.9	*	2.4	0.5	5.2	21.7	31.5	33.9	17.3	3.3	0.2
3rd child	10.2	*	0.3	0.0	0.7	7.7	17.4	19.6	11.7	2.4	0.2
4th child	4.4	*	0.0	*	0.1	2.0	7.1	9.1	6.0	1.6	0.1
5th child	1.7	*	0.0	*	0.0	0.5	2.4	3.6	2.8	0.9	0.1
6th and 7th child	1.1	*	*	*	*	0.1	1.1	2.3	2.1	0.7	0.1
8th child and over	0.4	*	*	*	*	0.0	0.1	0.6	0.9	0.5	0.1
Non-Hispanic, Single Race[3]											
White	56.3	0.1	12.1	4.1	23.6	57.8	92.9	103.1	51.1	10.2	0.7
1st child	22.2	0.1	10.4	3.9	19.7	31.8	38.5	34.1	12.7	2.4	0.2
2nd child	18.8	*	1.5	0.2	3.4	18.3	31.2	36.9	17.8	3.0	0.2
3rd child	9.2	*	0.2	0.0	0.4	5.9	15.3	19.0	11.0	1.9	0.1
4th child	3.6	*	0.0	*	0.0	1.4	5.6	7.8	5.0	1.1	0.1
5th child	1.3	*	*	*	*	0.3	1.7	2.9	2.1	0.6	0.0
6th and 7th child	0.8	*	*	*	*	0.1	0.7	1.8	1.7	0.5	0.0
8th child and over	0.3	*	*	*	*	0.0	0.1	0.4	0.9	0.5	0.0
Black	62.0	0.4	26.3	11.9	46.9	90.0	97.1	84.1	47.1	12.3	1.1
1st child	21.9	0.4	22.0	11.0	37.7	45.9	28.4	18.8	8.8	2.2	0.3
2nd child	17.7	*	3.6	0.8	7.6	27.5	30.7	24.4	12.4	2.9	0.2
3rd child	11.5	*	0.6	0.0	1.3	11.4	20.5	19.4	11.1	2.7	0.2
4th child	5.9	*	0.1	*	0.2	3.7	10.4	11.0	6.7	1.9	0.1
5th child	2.7	*	*	*	*	1.0	4.4	5.3	3.6	1.0	0.1
6th and 7th child	1.8	*	*	*	*	0.3	2.4	4.0	3.0	1.0	0.1
8th child and over	0.6	*	*	*	*	0.0	0.4	1.2	1.5	0.6	0.1
American Indian or Alaska Native	57.7	0.2	29.7	13.5	52.9	87.7	94.4	73.2	36.1	8.3	0.5
1st child	17.3	0.2	24.3	12.6	41.1	38.7	20.0	9.9	3.8	0.9	*
2nd child	15.1	*	4.7	0.9	10.2	30.0	27.0	15.8	6.2	1.1	*
3rd child	11.1	*	0.6	*	1.3	13.3	23.4	16.9	7.4	1.5	*
4th child	6.8	*	*	*	*	4.2	13.4	13.3	6.9	1.3	*
5th child	3.7	*	*	*	*	1.2	6.5	8.3	4.2	1.1	*
6th and 7th child	2.9	*	*	*	*	0.2	3.5	6.9	5.2	1.6	*
8th child and over	0.9	*	*	*	*	*	0.5	2.0	2.4	0.7	*
Asian	55.6	*	2.8	1.0	5.4	24.1	73.0	116.5	70.7	16.1	1.8
1st child	25.2	*	2.4	1.0	4.5	15.9	43.0	52.4	21.2	4.5	0.6
2nd child	20.8	*	0.4	0.1	0.8	6.1	21.6	46.6	31.5	6.1	0.6
3rd child	6.5	*	0.1	*	0.1	1.7	5.8	12.3	12.2	3.3	0.3
4th child	2.0	*	*	*	*	0.3	1.7	3.5	3.7	1.3	0.2
5th child	0.6	*	*	*	*	0.1	0.5	1.0	1.2	0.5	0.1
6th and 7th child	0.3	*	*	*	*	*	0.2	0.6	0.6	0.3	0.1
8th child and over	0.1	*	*	*	*	*	0.0	0.1	0.2	0.1	0.0
Native Hawaiian or Other Pacific Islander	73.0	*	26.5	8.2	53.7	118.5	118.9	91.9	49.2	15.4	*
1st child	21.7	*	21.9	7.8	42.9	55.4	29.7	14.3	5.8	2.1	*
2nd child	17.7	*	3.8	*	8.7	38.4	31.5	18.2	8.2	2.0	*
3rd child	13.7	*	*	*	*	16.8	27.5	20.6	9.5	2.4	*
4th child	9.2	*	*	*	*	6.0	17.4	16.6	8.5	3.0	*
5th child	5.2	*	*	*	*	1.4	7.7	11.3	6.1	2.2	*
6th and 7th child	4.2	*	*	*	*	*	4.7	8.8	7.1	2.2	*
8th child and over	1.4	*	*	*	*	*	*	2.1	4.1	1.6	*
Hispanic[4]	65.9	0.3	26.7	12.4	48.5	89.3	108.9	96.6	54.5	14.5	1.0
1st child	22.6	0.3	22.3	11.4	38.7	45.0	32.2	20.9	8.6	2.0	0.2
2nd child	19.7	*	3.9	0.9	8.5	29.9	37.3	28.6	14.1	3.1	0.2
3rd child	13.0	*	0.5	0.0	1.2	10.8	24.7	24.8	14.1	3.4	0.2
4th child	6.3	*	0.0	*	0.1	2.8	10.0	13.5	9.3	2.8	0.2
5th child	2.5	*	*	*	*	0.6	3.2	5.3	4.7	1.6	0.1
6th and 7th child	1.4	*	*	*	*	0.2	1.3	2.8	3.0	1.2	0.1
8th child and over	0.3	*	*	*	*	0.0	0.2	0.6	0.7	0.4	0.0

NOTE: Fertility rate computed by relating total births, regardless of age of mother, to women aged 15–44 years. Populations estimated as of July 1. Live-birth order refers to number of children born alive to mother. Figures for live-birth order not stated are distributed.
* = Estimate does not meet NCHS standards of reliability.
0.0 = Quantity more than zero but less than 0.05.
[1] Birth rates computed by relating births to women aged 45 years and over to women aged 45–49 years.
[2] Includes births to race and origin groups not shown separately, such as Hispanic single-race White, Hispanic single-race Black, and non-Hispanic multiple-race women, and births with origin not stated.
[3] Race and Hispanic origin are reported separately on birth certificates; persons of Hispanic origin may be of any race. In this table, non-Hispanic women are classified by race. Race categories are consistent with the 1997 Office of Management and Budget standards. Single race is defined as only one race reported on the birth certificate.
[4] Includes all persons of Hispanic origin of any race.

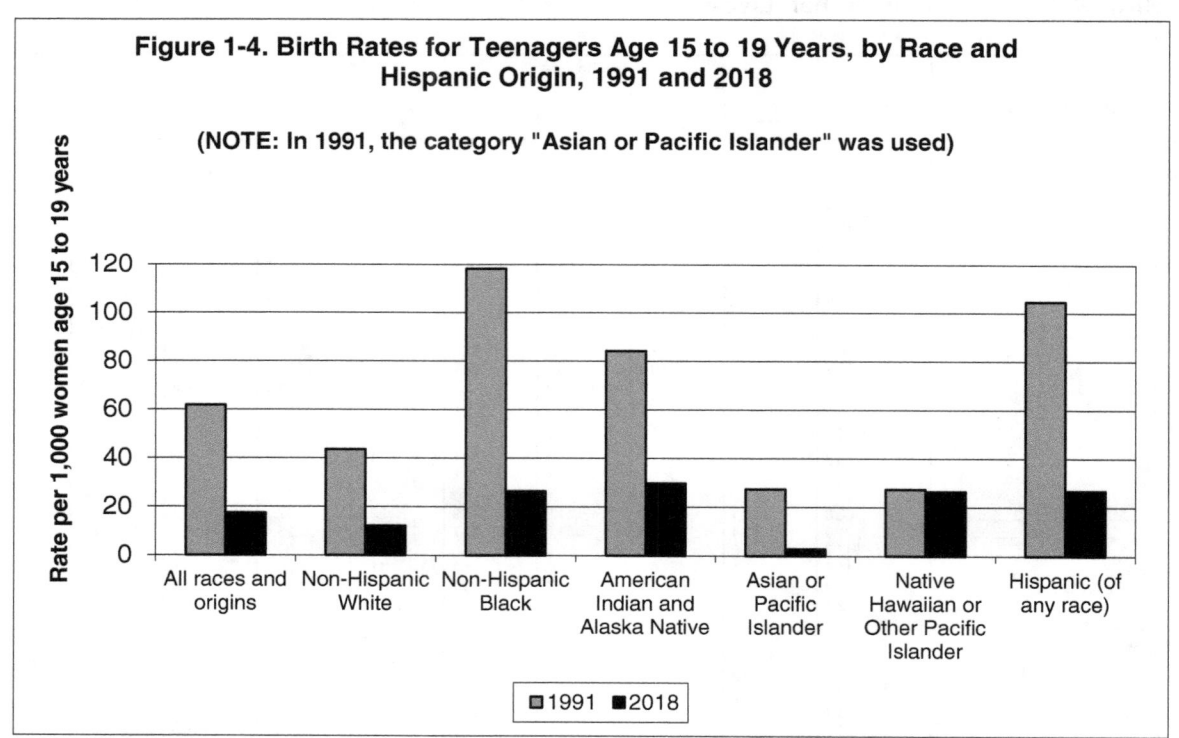

Figure 1-4. Birth Rates for Teenagers Age 15 to 19 Years, by Race and Hispanic Origin, 1991 and 2018

(NOTE: In 1991, the category "Asian or Pacific Islander" was used)

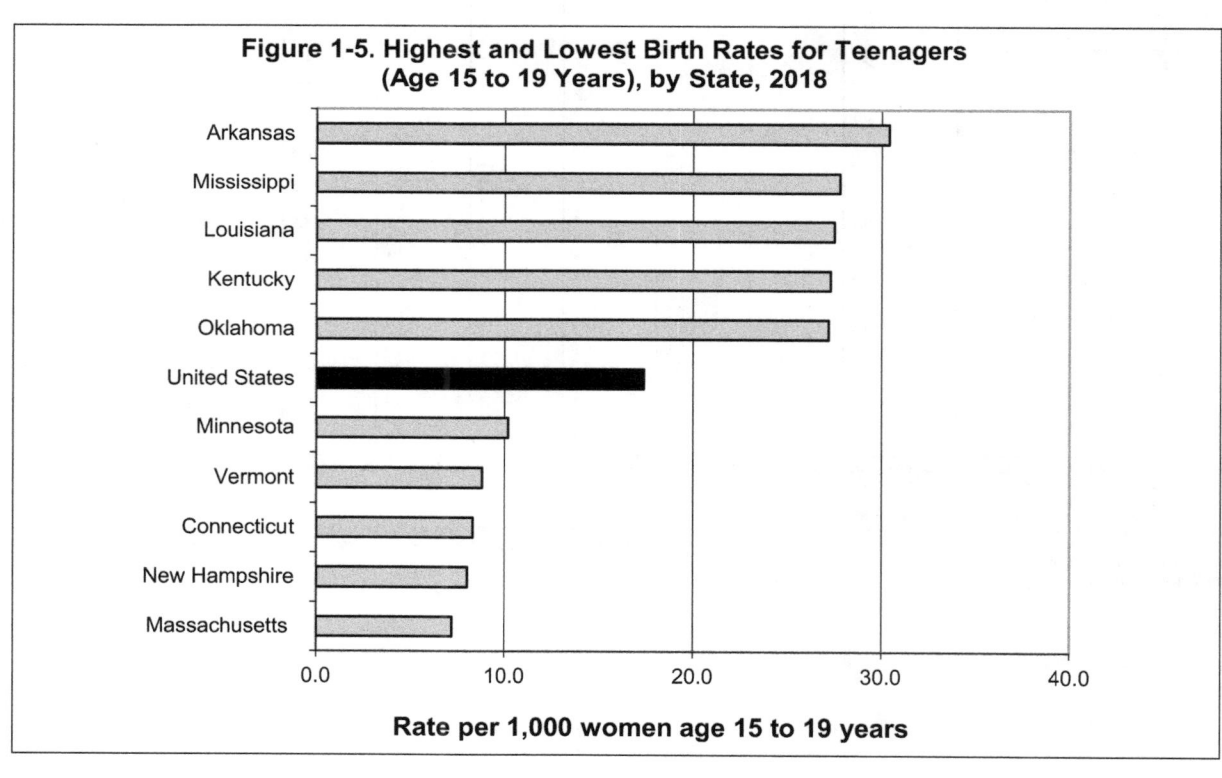

Figure 1-5. Highest and Lowest Birth Rates for Teenagers (Age 15 to 19 Years), by State, 2018

Table 1-6. Births, by Race and Hispanic Origin of Mother, by State and Territory, 2018

(Number by place of residence.)

Area	All races and origins[1]	Non-Hispanic, single race[2]					Hispanic[3]
		White	Black	American Indian or Alaska Native	Asian	Native Hawaiian or Other Pacific Islander	
United States[4]	3,791,712	1,956,413	552,029	29,092	240,798	9,476	886,210
Alabama..	57,761	33,776	17,597	148	903	46	4,403
Alaska..	10,086	5,057	280	1,873	641	299	807
Arizona...	80,723	32,805	4,305	4,155	2,908	248	34,084
Arkansas.......................................	37,018	23,609	6,966	220	775	498	4,099
California.......................................	454,920	123,139	22,380	1,411	68,444	1,732	211,271
Colorado	62,885	36,466	3,032	352	2,496	155	17,817
Connecticut....................................	34,725	18,488	4,423	38	2,232	5	8,762
Delaware	10,621	5,171	2,773	10	634	4	1,710
District of Columbia	9,212	3,040	4,252	15	444	2	1,296
Florida..	221,542	95,868	48,174	261	6,996	152	67,201
Georgia...	126,172	55,676	43,746	102	5,768	104	17,432
Hawaii..	16,972	3,288	424	33	4,366	1,706	2,580
Idaho	21,403	16,574	233	220	348	65	3,549
Illinois..	144,815	77,244	24,482	97	9,452	32	30,362
Indiana...	81,646	59,520	10,242	73	2,382	59	7,867
Iowa	37,785	29,327	2,615	152	1,176	149	3,694
Kansas	36,261	25,323	2,575	151	1,228	66	5,977
Kentucky.......................................	53,922	43,317	4,950	68	1,144	79	3,226
Louisiana.......................................	59,615	30,458	22,119	299	1,156	32	4,717
Maine	12,311	11,022	546	96	202	3	224
Maryland..	71,080	29,585	21,893	83	4,928	31	12,470
Massachusetts................................	69,109	39,663	6,826	53	6,183	23	13,810
Michigan..	110,032	74,777	20,558	412	4,395	34	7,139
Minnesota......................................	67,344	46,014	8,207	983	5,298	57	4,991
Mississippi.....................................	37,000	18,597	15,797	221	411	17	1,666
Missouri..	73,269	53,697	10,589	140	1,698	199	4,409
Montana..	11,513	9,224	58	1,162	112	15	558
Nebraska.......................................	25,488	17,645	1,739	318	925	24	4,155
Nevada...	35,682	13,021	4,564	280	2,613	340	13,307
New Hampshire................................	11,995	10,317	241	7	472	6	745
New Jersey.....................................	101,223	45,500	13,886	40	11,452	27	27,597
New Mexico	23,039	6,450	387	2,590	409	13	12,783
New York.......................................	226,238	110,840	33,145	395	24,383	50	51,755
North Carolina.................................	118,954	63,514	27,670	1,448	4,834	151	18,360
North Dakota..................................	10,636	7,816	609	828	250	16	635
Ohio	135,134	97,423	22,201	96	4,285	73	7,432
Oklahoma......................................	49,800	28,444	4,136	4,557	1,306	214	7,545
Oregon...	42,188	28,265	959	388	2,260	309	7,993
Pennsylvania...................................	135,673	90,862	17,779	74	6,207	54	15,826
Rhode Island..................................	10,506	6,008	783	36	519	5	2,756
South Carolina	56,669	31,890	16,681	106	1,172	50	5,255
South Dakota..................................	11,893	8,481	416	1,645	224	7	661
Tennessee......................................	80,751	53,256	15,921	79	1,877	69	7,824
Texas...	378,624	125,549	48,144	721	19,850	487	179,142
Utah	47,209	34,303	521	418	1,131	468	8,133
Vermont..	5,432	4,934	118	11	152	1	121
Virginia...	99,843	54,798	20,860	157	7,625	103	14,397
Washington....................................	86,085	49,019	3,922	1,166	8,729	1,159	16,073
West Virginia..................................	18,248	16,621	626	14	176	2	378
Wisconsin......................................	64,098	45,654	6,622	678	3,155	29	6,365
Wyoming	6,562	5,078	57	212	72	7	851
Puerto Rico....................................	21,424	480	49	3	30	–	20,837
Virgin Islands..................................	NA	NA	NA	NA	NA	NA	NA
Guam...	3,165	170	23	6	719	2,096	25
American Samoa..............................	NA	NA	NA	NA	NA	NA	NA
Northern Marianas............................	566	13	–	–	162	377	–

– = Quantity zero.
NA = Not available.
[1] Includes births to race and origin groups not shown separately, such as Hispanic single-race White, Hispanic single-race Black, and non-Hispanic multiple-race women, and births with origin not stated.
[2] Race and Hispanic origin are reported separately on birth certificates; persons of Hispanic origin may be of any race. In this table, non-Hispanic women are classified by race. Race categories are consistent with the 1997 Office of Management and Budget standards Single race is defined as only one race reported on the birth certificate.
[3] Includes all persons of Hispanic origin of any race.
[4] Excludes data for the territories.

Table 1-7. Births, by Hispanic Origin of Mother, by State and Territory, 2018

(Number by place of residence.)

Area	Total	Mexican	Puerto Rican	Cuban	Dominican	Central and South American	Other and unknown Hispanic
United States[1]	886,210	495,831	71,614	23,471	32,072	147,430	115,792
Alabama	4,403	2,517	243	50	38	1,440	115
Alaska	807	427	117	15	41	93	114
Arizona	34,084	29,499	639	218	68	1,389	2,271
Arkansas	4,099	2,893	148	31	17	669	341
California	211,271	155,578	1,951	795	160	17,538	35,249
Colorado	17,817	11,135	522	191	43	1,393	4,533
Connecticut	8,762	715	4,261	114	837	2,354	481
Delaware	1,710	605	441	18	62	494	90
District of Columbia	1,296	160	38	13	47	820	218
Florida	67,201	10,931	13,649	14,833	3,085	22,981	1,722
Georgia	17,432	10,082	1,296	337	325	4,540	852
Hawaii	2,580	753	871	25	19	174	738
Idaho	3,549	2,718	76	15	7	223	510
Illinois	30,362	24,549	2,219	255	123	2,541	675
Indiana	7,867	5,483	515	71	62	1,161	575
Iowa	3,694	2,726	137	44	15	612	160
Kansas	5,977	4,331	196	50	15	785	600
Kentucky	3,226	1,497	257	362	27	765	318
Louisiana	4,717	1,181	202	132	138	2,317	747
Maine	224	72	60	11	12	55	14
Maryland	12,470	1,688	721	126	400	8,535	1,000
Massachusetts	13,810	484	4,548	146	2,978	3,972	1,682
Michigan	7,139	4,121	526	127	106	820	1,439
Minnesota	4,991	3,319	219	60	30	1,105	258
Mississippi	1,666	861	115	19	26	513	132
Missouri	4,409	2,575	263	119	45	844	563
Montana	558	342	27	6	2	40	141
Nebraska	4,155	2,742	80	121	9	996	207
Nevada	13,307	9,849	418	457	62	1,578	943
New Hampshire	745	94	219	24	121	151	136
New Jersey	27,597	4,251	6,179	710	5,194	9,968	1,295
New Mexico	12,783	6,605	102	58	14	185	5,819
New York	51,755	7,020	11,090	667	12,786	16,534	3,658
North Carolina	18,360	9,637	1,734	352	506	5,114	1,017
North Dakota	635	400	69	12	6	68	80
Ohio	7,432	3,025	1,900	126	195	1,651	535
Oklahoma	7,545	5,726	249	54	19	849	648
Oregon	7,993	6,760	196	74	13	679	271
Pennsylvania	15,826	2,181	7,444	278	2,506	2,226	1,191
Rhode Island	2,756	135	691	19	943	829	139
South Carolina	5,255	2,499	605	122	121	1,518	390
South Dakota	661	354	58	12	9	151	77
Tennessee	7,824	4,188	448	142	76	2,448	522
Texas	179,142	124,114	2,725	1,571	375	16,160	34,197
Utah	8,133	5,033	174	35	66	1,552	1,273
Vermont	121	27	27	3	5	37	22
Virginia	14,397	3,024	1,276	223	210	4,439	5,225
Washington	16,073	12,045	521	143	45	1,459	1,860
West Virginia	378	149	63	12	8	80	66
Wisconsin	6,365	4,208	1,059	69	50	523	456
Wyoming	851	523	30	4	5	62	227
Puerto Rico	20,837	33	20,261	11	413	108	11
Virgin Islands	NA	NA	NA	NA	NA	NA	NA
Guam	25	12	2	–	2	4	5
American Samoa	NA	NA	NA	NA	NA	NA	NA
Northern Marianas	–	–	–	–	–	–	–

NOTE: In this table, Hispanic women are classified only by place of origin; non-Hispanic women are not shown.
– = Quantity zero.
NA = Not available.
[1]Excludes data for the territories.

Table 1-8. Birth Rates, by Age of Mother, by State and Territory, 2018

(Rate by place of residence.)

Area	Birth rate	Fertility rate	Total fertility rate	10 to 14 years	15 to 19 years			20 to 24 years	25 to 29 years	30 to 34 years	35 to 39 years	40 to 44 years	45 to 49 years[1]
					Total	15 to 17 years	18 to 19 years						
United States[2]	11.6	59.1	1,729.5	0.2	17.4	7.2	32.3	68.0	95.3	99.7	52.6	11.8	0.9
Alabama	11.8	60.9	1,786.5	0.2	25.2	10.6	46.7	94.5	107.5	86.3	36.3	6.9	0.4
Alaska	13.7	69.3	1,965.5	*	19.3	5.6	43.9	96.4	109.9	101.7	52.7	12.5	*
Arizona	11.3	58.6	1,722.0	0.1	20.1	8.9	36.2	75.7	97.9	92.1	46.8	10.9	0.8
Arkansas	12.3	64.0	1,879.5	0.3	30.4	12.1	57.7	106.5	112.4	83.9	35.3	6.8	0.3
California	11.5	56.2	1,632.0	0.1	13.6	5.7	25.2	53.6	78.8	98.8	63.8	16.1	1.6
Colorado	11.0	54.1	1,557.0	*	14.3	6.1	26.4	58.2	81.1	93.5	52.1	11.3	0.8
Connecticut	9.7	51.8	1,570.5	*	8.3	3.1	15.2	37.1	82.3	109.1	62.4	13.9	0.9
Delaware	11.0	59.1	1,724.0	*	16.7	7.1	29.4	68.5	93.9	102.9	51.0	10.8	0.8
District of Columbia	13.1	48.8	1,346.5	*	19.3	16.0	21.5	43.0	40.9	71.3	69.6	21.7	3.1
Florida	10.4	57.2	1,674.0	0.2	16.7	6.7	31.8	66.6	92.2	95.1	51.3	11.9	0.8
Georgia	12.0	58.3	1,729.0	0.2	20.6	8.8	38.3	78.3	97.2	92.1	46.3	10.4	0.7
Hawaii	11.9	64.2	1,847.0	*	17.2	7.0	33.5	76.4	95.9	97.9	63.0	17.3	1.5
Idaho	12.2	63.4	1,899.0	*	16.0	5.6	32.5	93.3	120.4	96.3	44.5	8.6	0.6
Illinois	11.4	57.5	1,690.0	0.1	15.8	6.5	30.1	58.8	89.4	104.7	56.3	12.1	0.8
Indiana	12.2	62.8	1,853.5	0.2	21.8	8.3	41.6	84.0	115.8	98.9	41.0	8.5	0.5
Iowa	12.0	63.5	1,897.5	*	15.3	6.6	27.1	65.6	131.2	113.9	44.7	8.2	0.5
Kansas	12.5	64.7	1,915.0	*	20.0	8.0	37.7	77.0	122.1	108.5	45.9	8.9	0.5
Kentucky	12.1	63.5	1,871.5	0.2	27.3	10.6	51.9	97.5	110.5	92.8	38.8	6.8	0.4
Louisiana	12.8	64.3	1,862.5	0.4	27.5	11.2	52.8	99.6	108.5	87.6	40.2	8.3	0.4
Maine	9.2	53.3	1,577.5	*	11.1	4.3	20.9	62.2	94.5	94.9	43.5	8.8	*
Maryland	11.8	59.9	1,745.0	0.2	14.1	6.0	26.0	55.5	91.3	109.3	62.5	14.8	1.3
Massachusetts	10.0	49.5	1,449.5	*	7.2	3.0	12.1	30.4	64.1	105.1	67.0	15.1	0.9
Michigan	11.0	58.5	1,725.0	0.1	15.8	5.9	30.1	63.6	104.0	105.6	45.9	9.4	0.6
Minnesota	12.0	62.7	1,829.0	0.1	10.2	3.8	20.0	51.4	110.9	123.6	57.4	11.2	1.0
Mississippi	12.4	62.8	1,842.0	0.5	27.8	12.1	50.1	105.6	114.6	80.0	33.4	6.2	0.3
Missouri	12.0	62.4	1,818.5	0.2	21.6	8.6	41.0	81.9	110.2	97.7	42.8	8.8	0.5
Montana	10.8	59.6	1,733.0	*	17.2	6.7	33.5	70.3	106.1	99.9	44.1	8.4	*
Nebraska	13.2	68.4	2,031.0	*	16.7	6.7	31.3	68.4	133.6	123.8	52.6	10.3	0.7
Nevada	11.8	60.0	1,752.5	*	20.5	8.2	42.1	85.6	94.4	87.6	49.2	12.1	1.0
New Hampshire	8.8	49.1	1,465.5	*	8.0	2.8	14.8	38.8	84.4	101.9	50.0	9.2	0.7
New Jersey	11.4	60.1	1,784.5	0.1	10.3	4.2	20.2	47.5	87.4	122.6	71.1	16.6	1.3
New Mexico	11.0	58.0	1,700.0	*	25.3	11.1	46.7	83.3	101.0	80.2	40.4	9.0	0.5
New York	11.6	57.9	1,666.5	0.1	11.7	4.8	21.2	52.2	78.2	102.9	68.4	18.1	1.7
North Carolina	11.5	58.4	1,728.5	0.2	18.7	7.9	33.8	75.1	97.9	96.5	47.1	9.6	0.6
North Dakota	14.0	72.2	2,033.5	*	16.4	7.5	28.0	67.9	134.1	125.7	52.1	9.6	*
Ohio	11.6	61.1	1,791.5	0.2	18.9	7.5	35.7	77.6	105.8	101.9	44.7	8.6	0.6
Oklahoma	12.6	64.6	1,884.5	0.2	27.2	10.7	52.4	98.6	114.9	90.8	37.2	7.6	0.4
Oregon	10.1	51.4	1,490.0	*	13.3	5.0	25.7	56.7	81.2	87.8	47.1	11.1	0.7
Pennsylvania	10.6	56.9	1,665.0	0.2	14.1	6.4	24.3	59.3	93.7	103.5	51.3	10.2	0.7
Rhode Island	9.9	50.5	1,493.0	*	11.5	6.1	17.0	42.5	79.3	97.0	54.7	13.1	*
South Carolina	11.1	58.1	1,705.0	0.2	22.0	9.1	40.1	79.1	98.6	90.0	42.3	8.3	0.5
South Dakota	13.5	73.6	2,154.5	*	20.4	9.9	35.6	81.5	144.8	125.6	49.6	8.1	*
Tennessee	11.9	61.1	1,781.0	0.3	25.3	9.5	49.7	88.7	101.7	90.1	41.6	8.0	0.5
Texas	13.2	63.4	1,870.0	0.3	25.3	11.4	47.1	86.0	104.7	96.7	49.1	11.1	0.8
Utah	14.9	68.4	2,026.5	*	13.1	4.9	26.2	78.3	132.7	117.3	51.6	11.4	0.8
Vermont	8.7	47.2	1,443.5	*	8.8	2.5	15.2	37.8	85.5	96.9	49.6	9.4	*
Virginia	11.7	59.1	1,733.5	0.2	14.3	5.7	26.2	61.4	93.8	105.4	57.7	12.8	1.1
Washington	11.4	57.5	1,642.5	*	12.7	4.8	25.0	61.3	86.5	98.6	55.5	12.8	1.0
West Virginia	10.1	57.2	1,709.5	*	25.4	8.4	50.4	94.3	105.0	79.4	31.4	5.7	0.5
Wisconsin	11.0	58.9	1,757.0	0.1	13.0	5.0	24.4	56.1	109.4	113.7	49.2	9.4	0.5
Wyoming	11.4	61.0	1,787.5	*	20.8	6.3	43.6	83.8	113.7	91.5	37.8	9.1	*
Puerto Rico	6.7	34.8	1,035.0	*	19.3	9.8	32.4	62.2	56.8	42.8	21.0	4.5	0.3
Virgin Islands	NA	NA	NA	NA	NA	NA	NA	NA	NA	NA	NA	NA	NA
Guam	18.9	96.1	2,846.5	*	34.4	15.1	64.0	135.7	157.9	137.1	82.5	19.8	*
American Samoa	NA	NA	NA	NA	NA	NA	NA	NA	NA	NA	NA	NA	NA
Northern Marianas	10.9	63.0	2,104.0	*	28.3	*	58.4	87.1	87.1	131.5	47.8	*	*

NOTE: Fertility rates are births per 1,000 women aged 15–44 years; total fertility rates are sums of birth rates for 5-year age groups multiplied by 5; birth rates by age are births per 1,000 women in specified age group estimated in each area. Populations estimated as of July 1.

* = Estimate does not meet NCHS standards of reliability.

NA = Not available.

[1]Birth rates computed by relating births to women aged 45 years and over to women aged 45–49 years.

[2]Excludes data for the territories.

Table 1-9. Births and Percentage of Births to Unmarried Women, by Age and Race and Hispanic Origin of Mother, 2018

(Number; percent.)

Age of mother	All races and origins[1]	Non-Hispanic, single race[2]					Hispanic[3]
		White	Black	American Indian or Alaska Native	Asian	Native Hawaiian or Other Pacific Islander	
NUMBER							
All Ages	1,503,361	551,217	383,364	19,853	28,191	4,776	459,242
Under 15 years............................	1,733	336	554	19	17	3	729
15 to 19 years............................	161,547	55,719	36,839	2,429	1,008	465	58,055
15 to 17 years	42,974	12,443	9,950	683	263	89	17,599
18 and 19 years	118,573	43,276	26,889	1,746	745	376	40,456
20 to 24 years............................	479,425	182,007	122,286	6,172	5,103	1,639	142,699
25 to 29 years............................	437,867	160,778	120,229	6,024	8,351	1,372	125,361
30 to 34 years............................	261,055	94,865	66,381	3,475	7,532	821	79,267
35 to 39 years............................	128,958	46,157	30,209	1,418	4,690	384	41,704
40 years and over	32,776	11,355	6,866	316	1,490	92	11,427
PERCENT							
All Ages	39.6	28.2	69.4	68.2	11.7	50.4	51.8
Under 15 years............................	99.8	99.7	100.0	*	*	*	99.9
15 to 19 years............................	89.8	85.8	97.7	94.2	69.8	90.1	89.1
15 to 17 years	97.0	95.5	99.5	98.4	85.4	93.7	96.8
18 and 19 years	87.5	83.4	97.0	92.7	65.6	89.3	86.2
20 to 24 years............................	66.0	55.7	88.6	78.7	34.3	66.0	68.0
25 to 29 years............................	39.8	27.9	72.1	65.9	14.4	47.5	49.4
30 to 34 years............................	23.9	15.2	53.4	56.9	7.8	37.5	38.1
35 to 39 years............................	22.8	15.2	44.9	50.9	8.2	35.0	35.5
40 years and over	25.8	19.0	39.2	51.3	11.3	30.5	36.7

NOTE: For New York, mother's marital status is inferred.
* = Estimate does not meet NCHS standards of reliability.
[1]Includes births to race and origin groups not shown separately, such as Hispanic single-race White, Hispanic single-race Black, and non-Hispanic multiple-race women, and births with origin not stated.
[2]Race and Hispanic origin are reported separately on birth certificates; persons of Hispanic origin may be of any race. In this table, non-Hispanic women are classified by race. Race categories are consistent with the 1997 Office of Management and Budget standards
Single race is defined as only one race reported on the birth certificate.
[3]Includes all persons of Hispanic origin of any race.

Table 1-10. Birth Rates for Unmarried Women, United States, 2010–2018, and Rates by Selected Age, Race, and Hispanic Origin of Mother, United States, 2016–2018

(Rate by year.)

Year and race and Hispanic origin	Fertility rate[1]	15 to 19 years			20 to 24 years	25 to 29 years	30 to 34 years	35 to 39 years	40 to 44 years[2]
		Total	15 to 17 years	18 to 19 years					
All races and origins[3]									
2010	47.5	31.1	16.8	52.0	70.0	69.2	56.3	29.6	8.0
2011	46.0	28.4	14.9	48.2	66.7	67.8	56.2	29.9	8.2
2012	45.3	26.7	13.7	45.8	64.7	67.2	56.3	30.9	8.5
2013	44.3	24.0	11.9	42.1	63.1	66.7	56.6	31.8	8.3
2014	43.9	22.0	10.6	39.4	61.6	67.6	58.1	33.4	8.5
2015	43.4	20.2	9.6	36.5	59.7	66.9	60.3	34.1	9.0
2016	42.4	18.5	8.6	33.5	56.6	65.8	59.2	35.6	10.0
2017	41.0	17.1	7.7	31.4	54.2	64.4	57.9	36.0	10.1
2018	40.1	16.0	7.1	29.2	52.2	62.8	59.5	35.2	10.6
Non-Hispanic, single race[4]									
White									
2016	30.3	12.4	5.0	23.5	40.9	47.3	43.0	25.2	6.8
2017	29.2	11.5	4.4	22.1	38.9	46.2	41.9	25.3	7.2
2018	28.8	10.6	4.0	20.3	37.6	45.7	43.9	25.9	7.5
Black									
2016	57.9	29.0	13.9	51.2	90.0	89.6	64.4	33.8	8.9
2017	57.5	27.3	12.6	48.7	88.8	89.3	66.2	35.1	8.9
2018	56.4	26.1	12.0	46.1	85.0	85.9	68.2	35.6	9.7
Hispanic[5]									
2016	66.0	29.2	15.1	51.2	83.1	106.4	103.6	65.0	19.3
2017	62.5	26.3	13.3	47.0	78.6	102.3	98.7	64.2	18.7
2018	59.5	24.4	12.2	43.4	74.6	95.7	96.1	57.4	20.0

NOTE: Rates are births to unmarried women per 1,000 unmarried women. Populations estimated as of July 1 for all years.
[1]Rates computed by relating total births to unmarried mothers, regardless of age of mother, to unmarried women aged 15–44 years.
[2]Rates computed by relating births to unmarried women aged 40 years and over to unmarried women aged 40–44 years.
[3]Includes births to race and origin groups not shown separately, such as Hispanic single-race White, Hispanic single-race Black, and non-Hispanic multiple-race women, and births with origin not stated.
[4]Race and Hispanic origin are reported separately on birth certificates; persons of Hispanic origin may be of any race. In this table, non-Hispanic women are classified by race. Race categories are consistent with the 1997 Office of Management and Budget standards. Single race is defined as only one race reported on the birth certificate.
[5]Includes all persons of Hispanic origin of any race.

Table 1-11. Selected Demographic Characteristics of Births, by Race and Hispanic Origin of Mother, 2018

(Number; rate; percent.)

Characteristic	All races and origins[1]	Non-Hispanic, single race[2]					Hispanic[3]
		White	Black	American Indian or Alaska Native	Asian	Native Hawaiian or Other Pacific Islander	
NUMBER							
Total births..................................	3,791,712	1,956,413	552,029	29,092	240,798	9,476	886,210
Birth rate....................................	11.6	10.0	13.6	12.2	13.2	16.6	14.8
Fertility rate................................	59.1	56.3	62.0	57.7	55.6	73.0	65.9
Total fertility rate	1,729.5	1,640.0	1,792.0	1,650.5	1,525.0	2,106.5	1,959.0
Unmarried rate............................	40.1	28.8	56.4	58.2	14.3	82.1	59.5
RATIO							
Sex ratio[4]..................................	1,046	1,052	1,029	1,036	1,063	1,022	1,036
PERCENT							
Births to mothers under age 20	4.8	3.3	6.9	8.9	0.6	5.5	7.4
4th and higher-order births[5].......................	12.9	10.8	17.7	24.7	5.3	27.5	16.0
Births to unmarried mothers......................	39.6	28.2	69.4	68.2	11.7	50.4	51.8
Mothers born in the 50 states or							
District of Columbia	77.2	93.2	83.1	98.9	19.0	35.9	52.9
Educational attainment of mother							
High school diploma or higher................	87.3	93.0	86.8	79.5	93.6	77.3	73.6
Bachelor's degree or higher	33.0	42.5	17.8	9.0	65.1	8.8	14.4
Mean age (years) of mother at first birth	26.9	27.7	25.1	23.5	30.5	24.7	25.0

NOTE: Birth rates are births per 1,000 population. Fertility rates are computed by relating total births, regardless of age of mother, to women aged 15–44 years. Total fertility rates are sums of birth rates for 5-year age groups multiplied by 5. Unmarried rates are births to unmarried women per 1,000 unmarried women. Populations estimated as of July 1. Mean age at first birth is the arithmetic average of the age of mothers at the time of birth, computed directly from the frequency of first births by age of mother.
[1]Includes births to race and origin groups not shown separately, such as Hispanic single-race White, Hispanic single-race Black, and non-Hispanic multiple-race women, and births with origin not stated.
[2]Race and Hispanic origin are reported separately on birth certificates; persons of Hispanic origin may be of any race. In this table, non-Hispanic women are classified by race. Race categories are consistent with the 1997 Office of Management and Budget standards. Single race is defined as only one race reported on the birth certificate.
[3]Includes all persons of Hispanic origin of any race.
[4]Male births per 1,000 female births.
[5]Based on live-birth order.

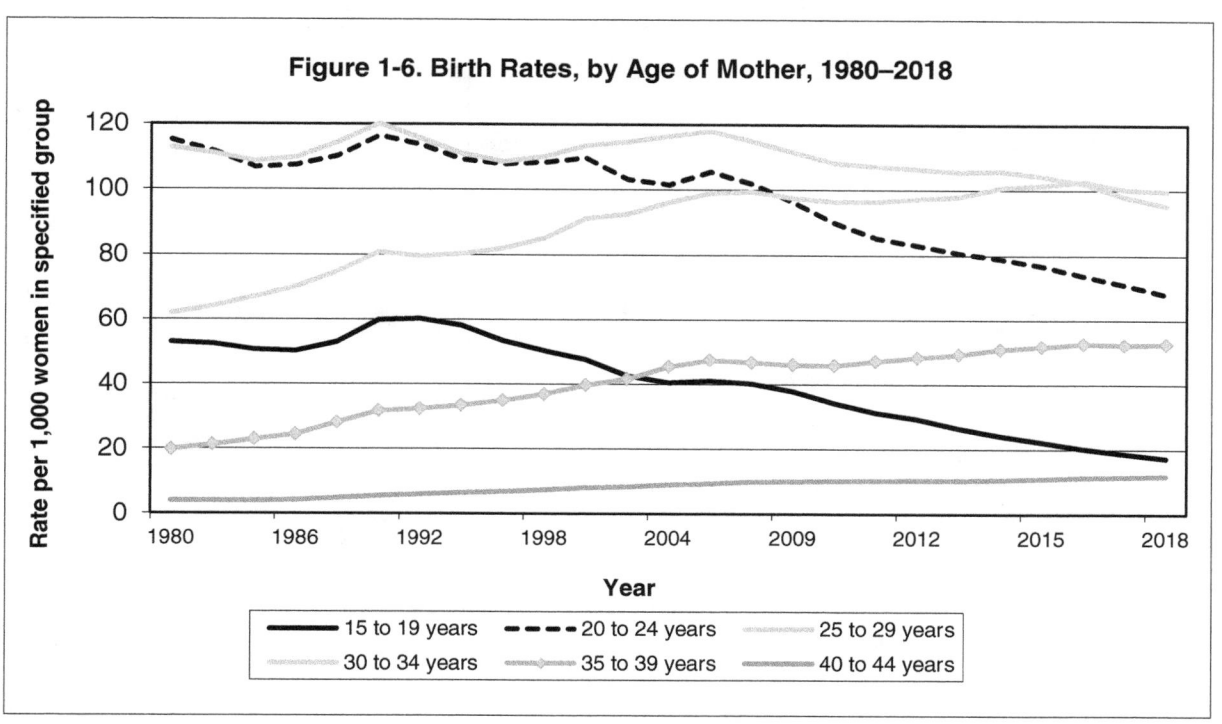

Figure 1-6. Birth Rates, by Age of Mother, 1980–2018

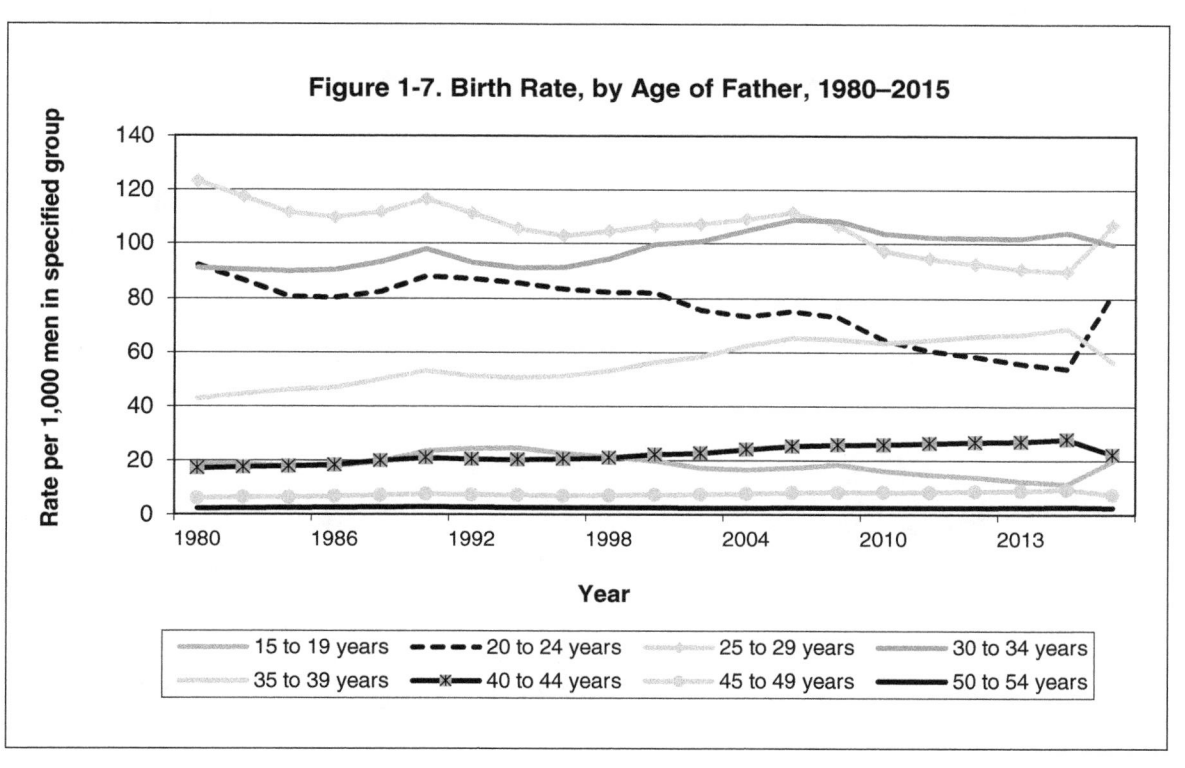

Figure 1-7. Birth Rate, by Age of Father, 1980–2015

Table 1-12. Selected Demographic Characteristics of Births, by Hispanic Origin of Mother, 2018

(Number; rate; percent.)

Characteristic	Total[1]	Mexican	Puerto Rican	Cuban	Dominican	Central and South American	Other and unknown Hispanic
NUMBER							
Total births..	886,210	495,831	71,614	23,471	32,072	147,430	115,792
RATIO							
Sex ratio[2]..	1,036	1,034	1,046	1,062	1,033	1,032	1,038
PERCENT							
Births to mothers under age 20	7.4	7.8	7.8	3.1	5.2	6.1	8.7
4th and higher-order births[3].............................	16.0	18.3	13.3	5.4	8.1	13.8	15.0
Mothers born in the 50 states or District of Columbia	52.9	56.9	70.1	43.5	28.3	17.0	79.5
Educational attainment of mother							
High school diploma or higher.........................	73.6	72.5	84.1	91.8	83.1	61.9	80.1
Bachelor's degree or higher	14.4	11.2	17.0	29.8	20.8	19.1	15.2
Mean age (years) of mother at first birth	25.0	24.4	24.8	27.7	25.8	26.5	24.7

NOTE: In this table, Hispanic women are classified only by place of origin; non-Hispanic women are not shown.
[1]Includes origin not stated.
[2]Male births per 1,000 female births.
[3]Based on live-birth order.

Table 1-13. Selected Medical and Health Characteristics of Births, by Race and Hispanic Origin of Mother, 2018

(Percent; rate.)

Characteristic	All races and origins[1]	Non-Hispanic, single race[2]					Hispanic[3]
		White	Black	American Indian or Alaska Native	Asian	Native Hawaiian or Other Pacific Islander	
MOTHER							
Prenatal care initiation							
First trimester	77.5	82.5	67.1	62.6	81.8	51.0	72.7
Late or no care	6.2	4.5	9.9	13.1	4.9	20.2	7.7
Smoked during pregnancy	6.5	9.5	5.2	15.5	0.5	4.4	1.7
Pregnancy resulted from infertility treatment	1.9	2.7	0.7	0.4	3.4	0.5	0.7
Mother received WIC food for herself during this pregnancy[4]	36.0	23.6	54.6	55.3	20.3	42.1	55.5
Diabetes							
Prepregnancy (diagnosis prior to this pregnancy)	0.9	0.8	1.2	2.4	1.0	1.8	1.1
Gestational (diagnosis in this pregnancy)	6.7	6.0	5.2	9.9	12.8	8.6	7.2
Overweight or obese (BMI of 25.0 or over)[5]	54.7	51.1	64.9	67.5	33.1	73.9	61.7
Induction of labor	27.1	30.3	25.2	29.0	21.7	18.5	22.8
CNM delivery[6]	9.4	10.0	8.0	20.1	7.5	9.7	9.0
Home birth	1.0	1.5	0.5	0.6	0.3	0.3	0.4
Cesarean delivery (total)	31.9	30.8	36.1	28.7	33.0	31.1	31.6
Low-risk[7]	25.9	24.9	30.3	22.3	27.6	26.5	25.4
Source of payment for the delivery							
Medicaid	42.3	30.0	65.3	66.2	24.1	58.9	58.9
Private	49.6	63.3	28.4	20.4	67.0	27.0	29.5
Self-pay	4.2	3.2	2.9	1.9	5.9	6.2	6.8
Other[8]	3.9	3.5	3.3	11.6	3.0	7.9	4.7
Infant was being breastfed at discharge[9]	83.5	84.9	72.3	75.2	90.9	79.3	87.1
INFANT							
Gestational age							
Preterm[10]	10.0	9.1	14.1	11.5	8.6	11.8	9.7
Early preterm[11]	2.8	2.3	4.9	3.2	2.1	3.6	2.6
Late preterm[12]	7.3	6.8	9.2	8.4	6.5	8.2	7.2
Birthweight[13]							
Very low birthweight[14]	1.4	1.0	2.9	1.4	1.1	1.5	1.2
Low birthweight[15]	8.3	6.9	14.1	8.0	8.6	9.0	7.5
Twin births[16]	32.6	34.4	40.8	26.1	28.2	26.4	24.4
Triplet or higher-order births[17]	93.0	102.0	119.2	20.6	59.0	158.3	64.7

[1]Includes births to race and origin groups not shown separately, such as Hispanic single-race White, Hispanic single-race Black, and non-Hispanic multiple-race women, and births with origin not stated.
[2]Race and Hispanic origin are reported separately on birth certificates; persons of Hispanic origin may be of any race. In this table, non-Hispanic women are classified by race. Race categories are consistent with the 1997 Office of Management and Budget standards Single race is defined as only one race reported on the birth certificate.
[3]Includes all persons of Hispanic origin of any race.
[4]WIC is Special Supplemental Nutrition Program for Women, Infants, and Children.
[5]BMI is body mass index.
[6]Births delivered by certified nurse midwives.
[7]Low-risk cesarean rate is the number of singleton, term (37 or more weeks of gestation based on the obstetric estimate), cephalic, cesarean deliveries to women having a first birth per 100 women delivering singleton, term, cephalic births.
[8]Other includes Indian Health Service, CHAMPUS or TRICARE, other government (federal, state, or local), or charity.
[9]Excludes data for California which did not report if infant was being breastfed at discharge. Also excludes Michigan, for which item wording is not consistent with national standard.
[10]Born before 37 completed weeks of gestation based on the obstetric estimate.
[11]Born before 34 completed weeks of gestation based on the obstetric estimate.
[12]Born between 34 and 36 completed weeks of gestation based on the obstetric estimate.
[13]Equivalents of the gram weights in pounds are shown subsequently.
[14]Less than 1,500 grams (3 lb 4 oz).
[15]Less than 2,500 grams (5 lb 8 oz).
[16]Live births in twin deliveries per 1,000 live births.
[17]Live births in triplet and other higher-order multiple deliveries per 100,000 live births.

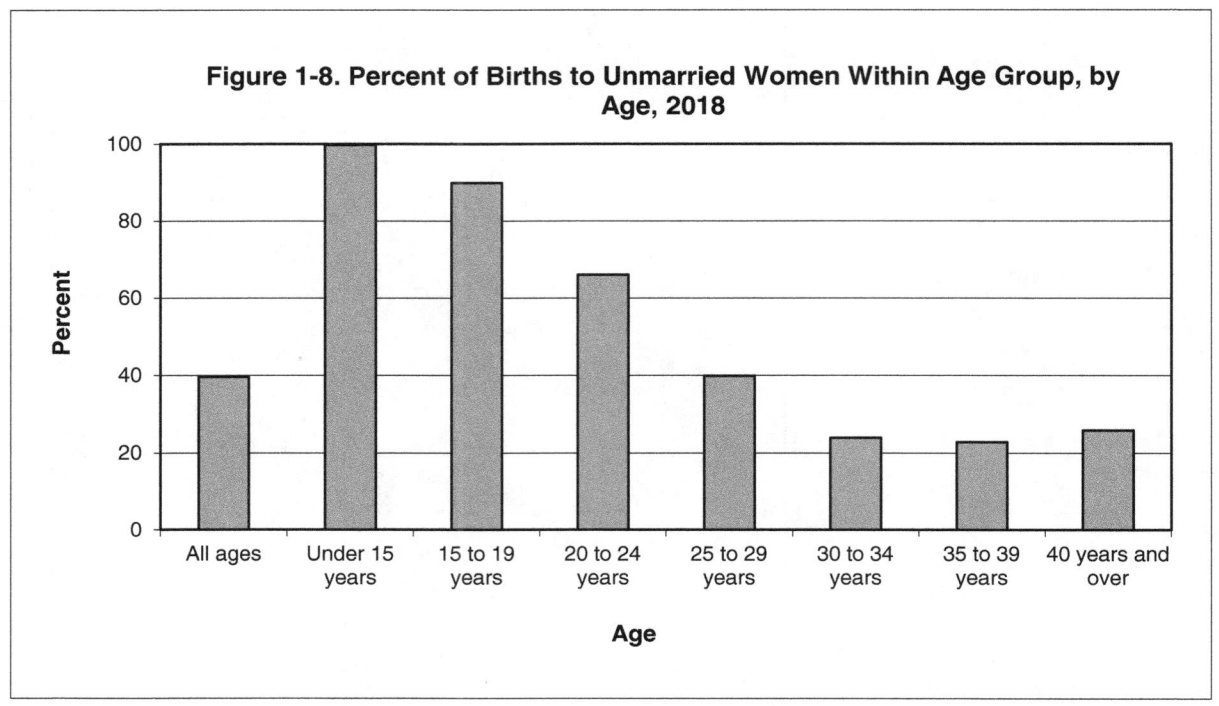

Figure 1-8. Percent of Births to Unmarried Women Within Age Group, by Age, 2018

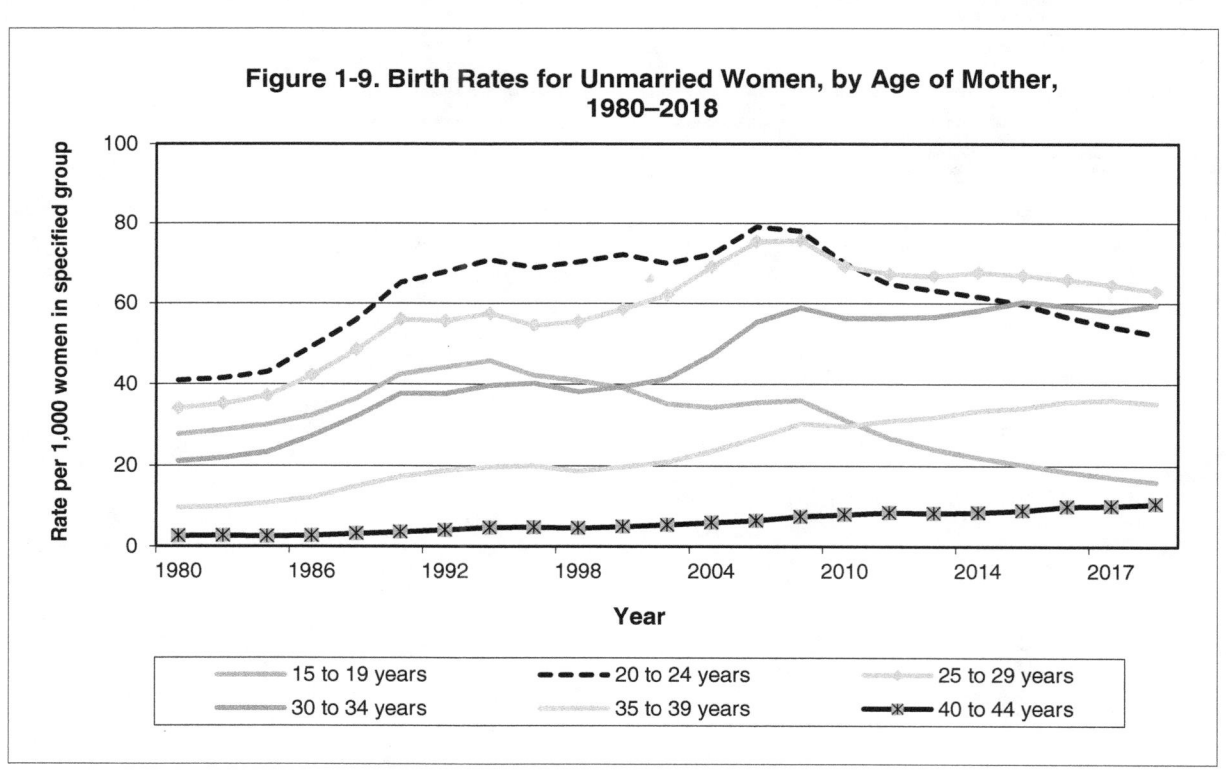

Figure 1-9. Birth Rates for Unmarried Women, by Age of Mother, 1980–2018

Table 1-14. Selected Medical and Health Characteristics of Births, by Hispanic Origin of Mother, 2018

(Percent; rate.)

Characteristic	Total	Mexican	Puerto Rican	Cuban	Dominican	Central and South American	Other and unknown Hispanic
MOTHER							
Prenatal care initiation							
First trimester	72.7	72.8	75.4	81.7	73.0	67.7	75.1
Late or no care	7.7	7.7	6.2	4.0	7.2	9.6	7.0
Smoked during pregnancy	1.7	1.4	5.3	1.8	0.9	0.5	2.3
Pregnancy resulted from infertility treatment	0.7	0.5	1.1	1.1	1.0	0.9	0.8
Mother received WIC food for herself during this pregnancy[1]	55.5	56.4	54.8	49.1	58.1	54.2	54.9
Diabetes							
Prepregnancy (diagnosis prior to this pregnancy)	1.1	1.2	1.2	0.6	0.8	0.8	1.0
Gestational (diagnosis in this pregnancy)	7.2	7.7	7.1	6.5	6.5	6.7	6.2
Overweight or obese (BMI of 25.0 or over)[2]	61.7	63.9	61.0	51.8	56.5	56.2	62.8
Induction of labor	22.8	22.4	25.5	23.3	24.5	21.4	24.2
CNM delivery[3]	9.0	8.7	11.4	5.3	8.3	10.3	8.1
Home birth	0.4	0.3	0.5	0.5	0.3	0.4	0.5
Cesarean delivery (total)	31.6	30.2	33.6	45.7	41.1	31.2	31.6
Low-risk[4]	25.4	23.8	27.2	38.8	29.6	25.9	24.9
Source of payment for the delivery							
Medicaid	58.9	59.9	60.3	51.2	66.1	54.1	59.9
Private	29.5	28.5	34.0	44.3	28.3	27.6	30.8
Self-pay	6.8	7.0	1.4	1.9	3.2	12.9	3.9
Other[5]	4.7	4.6	4.3	2.6	2.4	5.4	5.4
Infant was being breastfed at discharge[6]	87.1	87.2	82.0	90.0	88.8	89.5	85.7
INFANT							
Gestational age							
Preterm[7]	9.7	9.6	10.9	9.2	9.3	9.3	10.6
Early preterm[8]	2.6	2.5	3.2	2.6	2.8	2.3	2.8
Late preterm[9]	7.2	7.1	7.7	6.6	6.5	6.9	7.8
Birthweight[10]							
Very low birthweight[11]	1.2	1.2	1.7	1.3	1.5	1.2	1.4
Low birthweight[12]	7.5	7.1	9.4	7.1	8.3	7.0	8.4
Twin births[13]	24.4	23.0	30.6	28.8	30.0	22.3	27.1
Triplet or higher-order births[14]	64.7	56.9	58.6	25.6	102.9	90.2	66.5

NOTE: Race and Hispanic origin are reported separately on birth certificates; persons of Hispanic origin may be of any race. In this table, Hispanic women are classified only by place of origin.
[1] WIC is Special Supplemental Nutrition Program for Women, Infants, and Children.
[2] BMI is body mass index.
[3] Births delivered by certified nurse midwives.
[4] Low-risk cesarean rate is the number of singleton, term (37 or more weeks of gestation based on the obstetric estimate), cephalic, cesarean deliveries to women having a first birth per 100 women delivering singleton, term, cephalic births.
[5] Other includes Indian Health Service, CHAMPUS or TRICARE, other government (federal, state, or local), or charity.
[6] Excludes data for California which did not report if infant was being breastfed at discharge. Also excludes Michigan, for which item wording is not consistent with national standard.
[7] Born before 37 completed weeks of gestation based on the obstetric estimate.
[8] Born before 34 completed weeks of gestation based on the obstetric estimate.
[9] Born between 34 and 36 completed weeks of gestation based on the obstetric estimate.
[10] Equivalents of the gram weights in pounds are shown subsequently.
[11] Less than 1,500 grams (3 lb 4 oz).
[12] Less than 2,500 grams (5 lb 8 oz).
[13] Live births in twin deliveries per 1,000 live births.
[14] Live births in triplet and other higher-order multiple deliveries per 100,000 live births.

Table 1-15. Mothers Who Smoked for the 3 Months Before and Anytime During Pregnancy and Those Who Quit Before and During Pregnancy, by Age and Race and Hispanic Origin of Mother, 2018

(Number; percent.)

Tobacco use and race and Hispanic origin	Number							Percent						
	All ages	Under 20 years	20 to 24 years	25 to 29 years	30 to 34 years	35 to 39 years	40 to 54 years	All ages	Under 20 years	20 to 24 years	25 to 29 years	30 to 34 years	35 to 39 years	40 to 54 years
All races and origins[1]														
3 months before	X	X	X	X	X	X	X	8.4	10.2	12.2	9.7	6.4	5.5	4.4
Anytime during pregnancy	X	X	X	X	X	X	X	6.5	7.6	9.2	7.5	5.0	4.3	3.5
First trimester	X	X	X	X	X	X	X	6.3	7.3	9.0	7.3	4.9	4.2	3.4
Second trimester	X	X	X	X	X	X	X	5.4	5.9	7.5	6.3	4.3	3.7	3.0
Third trimester	X	X	X	X	X	X	X	5.2	5.5	7.1	6.1	4.1	3.5	2.8
Quit before pregnancy[2]	X	X	X	X	X	X	X	24.2	27.5	25.4	23.5	23.2	23.4	22.0
Quit during pregnancy[3]	X	X	X	X	X	X	X	20.2	27.4	23.0	19.2	18.0	17.6	17.9
Non-Hispanic, single race[4]														
White														
3 months before	X	X	X	X	X	X	X	12.1	21.6	20.4	13.6	8.2	7.4	6.4
Anytime during pregnancy	X	X	X	X	X	X	X	9.5	16.5	15.9	10.8	6.5	5.8	5.2
First trimester	X	X	X	X	X	X	X	9.3	16.0	15.6	10.6	6.4	5.7	5.1
Second trimester	X	X	X	X	X	X	X	8.1	13.1	13.3	9.3	5.6	5.1	4.5
Third trimester	X	X	X	X	X	X	X	7.7	12.3	12.6	8.9	5.4	4.9	4.3
Quit before pregnancy[2]	X	X	X	X	X	X	X	22.3	25.2	22.9	21.5	22.1	22.2	20.7
Quit during pregnancy[3]	X	X	X	X	X	X	X	18.4	25.3	20.8	17.2	16.3	15.9	16.4
Black														
3 months before	X	X	X	X	X	X	X	6.8	3.4	6.4	8.0	7.2	6.3	4.7
Anytime during pregnancy	X	X	X	X	X	X	X	5.2	2.5	4.6	6.1	5.8	5.1	3.7
First trimester	X	X	X	X	X	X	X	5.0	2.3	4.5	5.9	5.6	5.0	3.7
Second trimester	X	X	X	X	X	X	X	4.2	1.8	3.5	4.9	4.8	4.2	3.2
Third trimester	X	X	X	X	X	X	X	3.9	1.6	3.2	4.6	4.5	4.0	3.1
Quit before pregnancy[2]	X	X	X	X	X	X	X	25.8	30.9	29.9	26.2	22.7	21.9	22.9
Quit during pregnancy[3]	X	X	X	X	X	X	X	24.6	32.8	29.5	24.7	21.3	21.0	18.3
Hispanic[5]														
3 months before	X	X	X	X	X	X	X	2.6	2.4	3.2	2.9	2.3	1.9	1.4
Anytime during pregnancy	X	X	X	X	X	X	X	1.7	1.4	1.9	1.9	1.6	1.3	1.0
First trimester	X	X	X	X	X	X	X	1.6	1.4	1.8	1.8	1.5	1.3	1.0
Second trimester	X	X	X	X	X	X	X	1.2	0.9	1.3	1.4	1.2	1.0	0.8
Third trimester	X	X	X	X	X	X	X	1.1	0.8	1.2	1.3	1.1	1.0	0.7
Quit before pregnancy[2]	X	X	X	X	X	X	X	38.7	42.9	42.1	38.3	35.6	35.0	30.5
Quit during pregnancy[3]	X	X	X	X	X	X	X	31.2	40.9	35.7	29.2	28.1	26.3	30.3
FURTHER CHARACTERISTICS														
All races and origins[1]														
Total	3,791,712	181,607	726,175	1,099,491	1,090,697	566,786	126,956	X	X	X	X	X	X	X
Not stated 3 months before	18,048	1,122	3,982	5,457	4,389	2,492	606	X	X	X	X	X	X	X
Not stated during pregnancy	17,013	991	3,711	5,154	4,206	2,380	571	X	X	X	X	X	X	X
Quit before pregnancy[2]														
Smokers	317,730	18,386	87,784	105,599	69,562	30,878	5,521	X	X	X	X	X	X	X
Unknown if quit	587	35	143	195	140	61	13	X	X	X	X	X	X	X
Quit during pregnancy[3]														
Smokers	245,290	13,663	66,630	82,155	54,324	24,121	4,397	X	X	X	X	X	X	X
Unknown if quit	425	38	113	127	102	42	3	X	X	X	X	X	X	X
Non-Hispanic, single race[4]														
White														
Total	1,956,413	65,254	326,575	576,811	624,015	304,062	59,696	X	X	X	X	X	X	X
Not stated 3 months before	7,417	382	1,581	2,180	1,969	1,079	226	X	X	X	X	X	X	X
Not stated during pregnancy	7,003	336	1,452	2,055	1,880	1,061	219	X	X	X	X	X	X	X
Quit before pregnancy[2]														
Smokers	235,717	14,024	66,228	78,086	51,248	22,303	3,828	X	X	X	X	X	X	X
Unknown if quit	331	24	78	111	74	35	9	X	X	X	X	X	X	X
Quit during pregnancy[3]														
Smokers	185,707	10,693	51,774	62,108	40,449	17,605	3,078	X	X	X	X	X	X	X
Unknown if quit	276	25	77	85	59	28	2	X	X	X	X	X	X	X
Black														
Total	552,029	38,269	137,974	166,802	124,206	67,268	17,510	X	X	X	X	X	X	X
Not stated 3 months before	3,321	234	803	1,068	721	391	104	X	X	X	X	X	X	X
Not stated during pregnancy	3,209	225	780	1,029	708	368	99	X	X	X	X	X	X	X
Quit before pregnancy[2]														
Smokers	37,188	1,277	8,727	13,222	8,925	4,221	816	X	X	X	X	X	X	X
Unknown if quit	94	5	21	27	29	10	2	X	X	X	X	X	X	X
Quit during pregnancy[3]														
Smokers	28,549	933	6,341	10,102	7,109	3,415	649	X	X	X	X	X	X	X
Unknown if quit	72	4	12	23	27	6	–	X	X	X	X	X	X	X
Hispanic[5]														
Total	886,210	65,852	209,701	253,977	208,193	117,383	31,104	X	X	X	X	X	X	X
Not stated 3 months before	4,156	368	1,026	1,210	857	542	153	X	X	X	X	X	X	X
Not stated during pregnancy	3,718	298	913	1,099	791	483	134	X	X	X	X	X	X	X
Quit before pregnancy[2]														
Smokers	23,214	1,590	6,613	7,442	4,860	2,269	440	X	X	X	X	X	X	X
Unknown if quit	79	6	19	30	16	8	–	X	X	X	X	X	X	X
Quit during pregnancy[3]														
Smokers	14,740	944	3,961	4,751	3,233	1,528	323	X	X	X	X	X	X	X
Unknown if quit	28	4	9	9	5	1	–	X	X	X	X	X	X	X

– = Quantity zero.
X = Not applicable.
[1]Includes births to race and origin groups not shown separately, such as Hispanic single-race White, Hispanic single-race Black, and non-Hispanic multiple-race women, and births with origin not stated.
[2]Quit in the 3 months before pregnancy: births to women not reporting smoking during pregnancy per 100 women who smoked in the 3 months before pregnancy.
[3]Quit during pregnancy: births to women not reporting smoking in the third trimester of pregnancy per 100 women who smoked in either the first or second trimester.
[4]Race and Hispanic origin are reported separately on birth certificates; persons of Hispanic origin may be of any race. In this table, non-Hispanic women are classified by race. Race categories are consistent with the 1997 Office of Management and Budget standards. Single race is defined as only one race reported on the birth certificate.
[5]Includes all persons of Hispanic origin of any race.

Table 1-16. Trimester Prenatal Care Began, by Age and Race and Hispanic Origin of Mother, 2018

(Percent; number.)

Trimester care began and race and Hispanic origin of mother	All ages	Under 20 years	20 to 24 years	25 to 29 years	30 to 34 years	35 to 39 years	40 to 54 years
All races and origins[1]							
First trimester	77.5	61.2	70.9	77.7	82.1	81.7	78.2
Second trimester	16.3	27.1	21.0	16.2	13.0	13.4	16.0
Late or no care	6.2	11.7	8.1	6.1	4.9	4.9	5.8
Third trimester	4.5	8.4	5.9	4.4	3.5	3.6	4.2
No care	1.7	3.3	2.3	1.7	1.3	1.4	1.6
Total	3,791,712	181,607	726,175	1,099,491	1,090,697	566,786	126,956
Not stated	95,362	5,343	19,977	27,209	25,633	13,934	3,266
Non-Hispanic, single race[2]							
White							
First trimester	82.5	68.5	75.8	82.3	86.1	85.5	82.3
Second trimester	13.1	23.3	18.1	13.2	10.4	10.8	13.1
Late or no care	4.5	8.2	6.1	4.5	3.5	3.7	4.5
Third trimester	3.3	6.3	4.7	3.4	2.6	2.7	3.3
No care	1.1	1.9	1.4	1.1	0.9	1.0	1.2
Total	1,956,413	65,254	326,575	576,811	624,015	304,062	59,696
Not stated	41,224	1,481	7,203	11,561	13,007	6,559	1,413
Black							
First trimester	67.1	54.7	63.7	68.1	70.6	71.6	69.2
Second trimester	23.0	31.1	25.5	22.5	20.4	19.6	21.1
Late or no care	9.9	14.2	10.7	9.4	9.0	8.8	9.7
Third trimester	6.8	9.5	7.1	6.4	6.4	6.1	7.1
No care	3.1	4.7	3.6	3.0	2.7	2.6	2.6
Total	552,029	38,269	137,974	166,802	124,206	67,268	17,510
Not stated	21,500	1,585	5,585	6,539	4,531	2,605	655
Hispanic[3]							
First trimester	72.7	58.3	68.7	74.4	76.8	76.5	73.9
Second trimester	19.6	28.3	22.1	18.6	17.0	17.4	19.5
Late or no care	7.7	13.4	9.2	7.1	6.2	6.1	6.5
Third trimester	5.4	9.5	6.6	5.0	4.3	4.2	4.7
No care	2.2	3.8	2.6	2.0	1.8	1.9	1.9
Total	886,210	65,852	209,701	253,977	208,193	117,383	31,104
Not stated	22,096	1,895	5,449	6,175	4,955	2,880	742

[1]Includes births to race and origin groups not shown separately, such as Hispanic single-race White, Hispanic single-race Black, and non-Hispanic multiple-race women, and births with origin not stated.
[2]Race and Hispanic origin are reported separately on birth certificates; persons of Hispanic origin may be of any race. In this table, non-Hispanic women are classified by race. Race categories are consistent with the 1997 Office of Management and Budget standards. Single race is defined as only one race reported on the birth certificate.
[3]Includes all persons of Hispanic origin of any race.

Table 1-17. Births, by Method of Delivery, United States, 2010–2018, and by Selected Race and Hispanic Origin of Mother, 2016–2018

(Number; percent.)

Year and race and Hispanic origin of mother	All births	Vaginal (number)		Cesarean (number)			Not stated	Cesarean (percent)			Vaginal birth after previous cesarean delivery (percent)[7]
		Total[1]	After previous cesarean	Total[2]	Primary	Low-risk[3]		Total[4]	Primary[5]	Low-risk[6]	
All Races and Origins[8]											
2010	3,999,386	2,680,947	NA	1,309,182	NA	368,523	9,257	32.8	NA	27.5	NA
2011	3,953,590	2,651,428	NA	1,293,267	NA	359,669	8,895	32.8	NA	27.2	NA
2012	3,952,841	2,650,744	NA	1,296,070	NA	355,942	6,027	32.8	NA	27.2	NA
2013	3,932,181	2,642,892	NA	1,284,339	NA	344,405	4,950	32.7	NA	26.8	NA
2014	3,988,076	2,699,951	NA	1,284,551	NA	337,086	3,574	32.2	NA	26.0	NA
2015	3,978,497	2,703,504	NA	1,272,503	NA	331,982	2,490	32.0	NA	25.8	NA
2016	3,945,875	2,684,803	75,244	1,258,581	728,500	329,614	2,491	31.9	21.8	25.7	12.4
2017	3,855,500	2,621,010	76,301	1,232,339	710,963	325,086	2,151	32.0	21.9	26.0	12.8
2018	3,791,712	2,581,992	78,842	1,208,176	693,276	319,022	1,544	31.9	21.7	25.9	13.3
Non-Hispanic, Single Race[9]											
White											
2016	2,056,332	1,419,788	37,442	635,588	379,240	172,006	956	30.9	21.5	24.7	12.8
2017	1,992,461	1,375,702	37,295	615,830	366,505	167,434	929	30.9	21.5	24.9	13.0
2018	1,956,413	1,353,424	38,345	602,361	356,796	164,087	628	30.8	21.4	24.9	13.5
Black											
2016	558,622	357,859	11,763	200,460	117,410	50,287	303	35.9	25.4	30.3	12.4
2017	560,715	358,467	12,457	201,991	117,054	50,217	257	36.0	25.3	30.4	12.8
2018	552,029	352,750	12,702	199,117	114,150	49,481	162	36.1	25.2	30.3	13.0
Hispanic[10]											
2016	918,447	627,095	17,847	290,832	153,462	67,278	520	31.7	20.1	25.1	11.5
2017	898,764	613,101	18,423	285,379	150,592	67,860	284	31.8	20.2	25.6	12.0
2018	886,210	605,674	19,371	280,386	147,149	67,040	150	31.6	20.1	25.4	12.7

NA = Comparable data were not available for the 50 states and the District of Columbia for 2010–2015 because not all reporting areas had adopted the 2003 U.S. Certificate of Live Birth.
[1]Includes unknown type of vaginal delivery.
[2]Includes unknown type of cesarean delivery.
[3]Low-risk cesarean is defined as singleton, term (37 or more completed weeks of gestation based on the obstetric estimate), cephalic, cesarean deliveries to women having a first birth.
[4]Percentage of all live births delivered by cesarean.
[5]Primary cesarean rate is the number of births to women having a cesarean delivery per 100 births to women without a previous cesarean.
[6]Low-risk cesarean is defined as singleton, term (37 or more completed weeks of gestation based on the obstetric estimate), cephalic, cesarean deliveries to women having a first birth per 100 women delivering singleton, term, cephalic, first births.
[7]Vaginal birth after cesarean delivery rate is the number of births to women having a vaginal delivery per 100 births to women with a previous cesarean delivery.
[8]Includes births to race and origin groups not shown separately, such as Hispanic single-race White, Hispanic single-race Black, and non-Hispanic multiple-race women, and births with origin not stated.
[9]Race and Hispanic origin are reported separately on birth certificates. Persons of Hispanic origin may be of any race. Multiple-race data, when reported, were bridged to single-race categories in order to maintain comparability among all reported areas. Forty-nine states and the District of Columbia reported multiple-race data for 2015 that were bridged to single-race categories for comparability with other states. Multiple-race reporting areas vary for 2003–2015.
[10]Includes all persons of Hispanic origin of any race.

Table 1-18. Births, by Method of Delivery, by Age and Selected Race and Hispanic Origin of Mother, 2018

(Number; percent.)

Year and race and Hispanic origin of mother	All births	Vaginal (number)		Cesarean (number)			Not stated	Cesarean (percent)			Vaginal birth after previous cesarean delivery (percent)[7]
		Total[1]	After previous cesarean	Total[2]	Primary	Low-risk[3]		Total[4]	Primary[5]	Low-risk[6]	
All Races and Origins[8]											
Total	3,791,712	2,581,992	78,842	1,208,176	693,276	319,022	1,544	31.9	21.7	25.9	13.3
Under 20 years	181,607	145,667	561	35,877	32,264	21,678	63	19.8	18.2	16.1	13.5
20 to 24 years	726,175	540,586	8,665	185,252	127,269	72,690	337	25.5	19.3	21.6	13.0
25 to 29 years	1,099,491	769,495	22,256	329,512	190,914	90,763	484	30.0	20.4	25.5	13.8
30 to 34 years	1,090,697	721,045	27,500	369,271	197,717	82,938	381	33.9	22.2	29.5	13.8
35 to 39 years	566,786	339,252	16,337	227,331	112,599	40,160	203	40.1	25.9	38.8	12.5
40 years or over	126,956	65,947	3,523	60,933	32,513	10,793	76	48.0	34.3	53.0	11.0
Non-Hispanic, Single Race[9]											
White											
Total	1,956,413	1,353,424	38,345	602,361	356,796	164,087	628	30.8	21.4	24.9	13.5
Under 20 years	65,254	52,167	136	13,058	11,886	7,789	29	20.0	18.6	15.9	10.4
20 to 24 years	326,575	245,152	3,048	81,289	57,174	31,790	134	24.9	19.1	20.2	11.2
25 to 29 years	576,811	411,907	9,921	164,709	101,506	48,801	195	28.6	20.2	23.6	13.6
30 to 34 years	624,015	424,241	14,753	199,603	111,895	47,858	171	32.0	21.5	27.5	14.4
35 to 39 years	304,062	187,866	8,733	116,125	59,158	22,268	71	38.2	24.8	36.6	13.3
40 years or over	59,696	32,091	1,754	27,577	15,177	5,581	28	46.2	33.4	50.3	12.4
Black											
Total	552,029	352,750	12,702	199,117	114,150	49,481	162	36.1	25.2	30.3	13.0
Under 20 years	38,269	29,707	140	8,552	7,692	5,181	10	22.4	20.7	18.8	14.0
20 to 24 years	137,974	97,638	1,990	40,300	27,891	15,649	36	29.2	22.6	25.9	13.8
25 to 29 years	166,802	107,994	4,357	58,760	32,119	13,624	48	35.2	23.7	33.3	14.1
30 to 34 years	124,206	73,762	3,746	50,407	25,420	8,914	37	40.6	26.7	39.9	13.0
35 to 39 years	67,268	35,593	1,984	31,651	15,928	4,704	24	47.1	32.2	49.4	11.2
40 years or over	17,510	8,056	485	9,447	5,100	1,409	7	54.0	40.3	61.9	10.0
Hispanic[10]											
Total	886,210	605,674	19,371	280,386	147,149	67,040	150	31.6	20.1	25.4	12.7
Under 20 years	65,852	53,847	248	11,989	10,610	7,354	16	18.2	16.5	15.1	15.3
20 to 24 years	209,701	157,962	2,957	51,706	33,760	20,301	33	24.7	17.9	21.7	14.2
25 to 29 years	253,977	175,985	6,038	77,951	39,196	18,263	41	30.7	18.7	27.9	13.5
30 to 34 years	208,193	133,067	5,844	75,093	34,613	12,854	33	36.1	21.4	33.8	12.6
35 to 39 years	117,383	68,554	3,455	48,813	21,727	6,463	16	41.6	25.0	43.3	11.3
40 years or over	31,104	16,259	829	14,834	7,243	1,805	11	47.7	32.0	55.7	9.8

[1]Includes unknown type of vaginal delivery.
[2]Includes unknown type of cesarean delivery.
[3]Low-risk cesarean is defined as singleton, term (37 or more completed weeks of gestation based on the obstetric estimate), cephalic, cesarean deliveries to women having a first birth.
[4]Percentage of all live births delivered by cesarean.
[5]Primary cesarean rate is the number of births to women having a cesarean delivery per 100 births to women without a previous cesarean.
[6]Low-risk cesarean is defined as singleton, term (37 or more completed weeks of gestation based on the obstetric estimate), cephalic, cesarean deliveries to women having a first birth per 100 women delivering singleton, term, cephalic, first births.
[7]Vaginal birth after cesarean delivery rate is the number of births to women having a vaginal delivery per 100 births to women with a previous cesarean delivery.
[8]Includes births to race and origin groups not shown separately, such as Hispanic single-race White, Hispanic single-race Black, and non-Hispanic multiple-race women, and births with origin not stated.
[9]Race and Hispanic origin are reported separately on birth certificates. Persons of Hispanic origin may be of any race. Multiple-race data, when reported, were bridged to single-race categories in order to maintain comparability among all reported areas. Forty-nine states and the District of Columbia reported multiple-race data for 2015 that were bridged to single-race categories for comparability with other states. Multiple-race reporting areas vary for 2003–2015.
[10]Includes all persons of Hispanic origin of any race.

Table 1-19. Principal Source of Payment for the Delivery, by Age and Selected Race and Hispanic Origin of Mother, 2018

(Percent; number.)

Trimester care began and race and Hispanic origin of mother	All ages	Under 20 years	20 to 24 years	25 to 29 years	30 to 34 years	35 to 39 years	40 to 54 years
All races and origins[1]							
Total	100.0	100.0	100.0	100.0	100.0	100.0	100.0
Medicaid	42.3	77.3	63.1	44.8	29.4	27.4	29.9
Private insurance	49.6	15.1	28.2	47.0	63.0	64.8	61.2
Self-pay	4.2	3.8	3.8	4.0	4.2	4.6	5.7
Other[2]	3.9	3.8	4.9	4.1	3.4	3.2	3.1
Total	3,791,712	181,607	726,175	1,099,491	1,090,697	566,786	126,956
Not stated	22,595	1,144	4,305	6,801	6,396	3,184	765
Non-Hispanic, single race[3]							
White							
Total	100.0	100.0	100.0	100.0	100.0	100.0	100.0
Medicaid	30.0	72.3	53.5	32.4	18.6	16.8	18.3
Private insurance	63.3	22.2	38.6	60.4	75.4	77.2	74.7
Self-pay	3.2	2.0	3.2	3.3	3.1	3.4	4.4
Other[2]	3.5	3.5	4.8	3.9	3.0	2.6	2.6
Total	1,956,413	65,254	326,575	576,811	624,015	304,062	59,696
Not stated	12,651	447	2,154	3,852	3,983	1,830	385
Black							
Total	100.0	100.0	100.0	100.0	100.0	100.0	100.0
Medicaid	65.3	84.2	76.4	68.4	55.6	47.5	43.6
Private insurance	28.4	11.2	18.0	25.7	37.3	45.0	48.2
Self-pay	2.9	2.3	2.0	2.6	3.7	4.1	5.1
Other[2]	3.3	2.3	3.6	3.4	3.3	3.4	3.1
Total	552,029	38,269	137,974	166,802	124,206	67,268	17,510
Not stated	2,832	187	615	841	705	367	117
Hispanic[4]							
Total	100.0	100.0	100.0	100.0	100.0	100.0	100.0
Medicaid	58.9	78.5	69.4	58.9	49.9	48.0	49.5
Private insurance	29.5	10.0	19.2	30.0	38.5	39.9	37.8
Self-pay	6.8	6.8	6.0	6.3	7.4	8.0	8.5
Other[2]	4.7	4.7	5.3	4.8	4.3	4.2	4.3
Total	886,210	65,852	209,701	253,977	208,193	117,383	31,104
Not stated	4,177	384	1,030	1,160	904	539	160

[1]Includes births to race and origin groups not shown separately, such as Hispanic single-race White, Hispanic single-race Black, and non-Hispanic multiple-race women, and births with origin not stated.
[2]Other includes Indian Health Service, CHAMPUS or TRICARE, other government (federal, state, or local), or charity.
[3]Race and Hispanic origin are reported separately on birth certificates; persons of Hispanic origin may be of any race. In this table, non-Hispanic women are classified by race. Race categories are consistent with the 1997 Office of Management and Budget standards. Single race is defined as only one race reported on the birth certificate.
[4]Includes all persons of Hispanic origin of any race.

Table 1-20. Births, by Gestational Age (Weeks), 2010–2018, and by Selected Race and Hispanic Origin of Mother, 2016–2018

(Percent; number.)

Race and Hispanic origin of mother and year	All births	Preterm[1] Total under 37 weeks	Preterm Total under 34 weeks	Preterm Early Under 28 weeks	Preterm Early 28 to 31 weeks	Preterm Early 32 and 33 weeks	Preterm Late 34 to 36 weeks	Term Total 37 to 41 weeks	Term Early 37 to 38 weeks	Term Full 39 and 40 weeks	Term Late 41 weeks	Postterm 42 weeks and over	Not stated
PERCENT													
All Races and Origins[2]													
2010	3,999,386	9.98	2.84	0.71	0.94	1.18	7.15	90.01	27.29	56.08	6.19	0.46	10,538
2011	3,953,590	9.81	2.81	0.70	0.93	1.18	6.99	90.19	26.09	57.51	6.16	0.43	9,290
2012	3,952,841	9.76	2.80	0.71	0.92	1.17	6.96	90.24	25.47	58.30	6.06	0.40	8,380
2013	3,932,181	9.62	2.79	0.70	0.92	1.17	6.83	90.38	24.81	58.85	6.31	0.41	7,467
2014	3,988,076	9.57	2.75	0.69	0.91	1.15	6.82	90.43	24.76	58.72	6.53	0.42	3,246
2015	3,978,497	9.63	2.76	0.68	0.91	1.17	6.87	89.98	24.99	58.47	6.51	0.40	2,926
2016	3,945,875	9.85	2.76	0.68	0.92	1.17	7.09	89.80	25.47	57.94	6.38	0.35	3,454
2017	3,855,500	9.93	2.76	0.67	0.92	1.17	7.17	89.74	26.00	57.49	6.25	0.33	2,759
2018	3,791,712	10.02	2.75	0.66	0.91	1.18	7.28	89.68	26.53	57.24	5.90	0.30	2,507
Non-Hispanic, Single Race[3]													
White													
2016	2,056,332	9.04	2.33	0.48	0.78	1.07	6.72	90.53	23.64	59.61	7.28	0.43	1,409
2017	1,992,461	9.05	2.30	0.46	0.77	1.06	6.76	90.54	24.16	59.27	7.11	0.40	1,051
2018	1,956,413	9.09	2.26	0.44	0.76	1.07	6.83	90.53	24.68	59.16	6.70	0.37	924
Black													
2016	558,622	13.77	4.93	1.56	1.61	1.75	8.84	85.94	28.48	52.42	5.04	0.30	506
2017	560,715	13.93	4.87	1.53	1.62	1.72	9.06	85.79	28.93	51.90	4.96	0.28	445
2018	552,029	14.13	4.90	1.51	1.60	1.79	9.23	85.62	29.64	51.34	4.64	0.25	384
Hispanic[4]													
2016	918,447	9.45	2.98	0.62	0.84	1.09	6.92	90.30	27.02	57.85	5.43	0.25	676
2017	898,764	9.62	2.56	0.62	0.85	1.09	7.05	90.16	27.58	57.15	5.43	0.23	455
2018	886,210	9.73	2.56	0.62	0.84	1.09	7.17	90.07	28.05	56.83	5.19	0.20	382
NUMBER													
All Races and Origins[2]													
2010	3,999,386	398,402	113,131	28,437	37,435	47,259	285,271	3,325,476	1,088,564	2,236,912	246,768	18,413	10,538
2011	3,953,590	386,855	111,002	27,737	36,758	46,507	275,853	3,297,649	1,029,157	2,268,492	242,999	16,797	9,290
2012	3,952,841	385,082	110,444	28,004	36,366	46,074	274,638	3,304,365	1,004,750	2,299,615	239,148	15,866	8,380
2013	3,932,181	377,655	109,435	27,550	36,096	45,789	268,220	3,283,457	973,569	2,309,888	247,476	16,126	7,467
2014	3,988,076	381,321	109,474	27,320	36,245	45,909	271,847	3,586,933	986,745	2,339,796	260,392	19,822	3,246
2015	3,978,497	382,786	109,660	26,996	36,149	46,515	273,126	3,577,072	993,599	2,324,474	258,999	15,713	2,926
2016	3,945,875	388,218	108,836	26,618	36,239	45,979	279,382	3,540,290	1,004,224	2,284,399	251,667	13,913	3,454
2017	3,855,500	382,726	106,417	25,913	35,476	45,028	276,309	3,457,455	1,001,601	2,214,983	240,871	12,560	2,759
2018	3,791,712	379,777	104,031	24,945	34,386	44,700	275,746	3,398,110	1,005,405	2,169,016	223,689	11,318	2,507
Non-Hispanic, Single Race[3]													
White													
2016	2,056,332	185,854	47,823	9,766	16,101	21,956	138,031	1,860,243	485,846	1,224,872	149,525	8,826	1,409
2017	1,992,461	180,322	45,761	9,200	15,429	21,132	134,561	1,803,063	481,048	1,180,394	141,621	8,025	1,051
2018	1,956,413	177,842	44,287	8,665	14,764	20,858	133,555	1,770,366	482,550	1,156,775	131,041	7,281	924
Black													
2016	558,622	76,834	27,501	8,729	8,987	9,785	49,333	479,630	158,937	292,539	28,154	1,652	506
2017	560,715	78,024	27,274	8,548	9,070	9,656	50,750	480,661	162,072	290,803	27,786	1,585	445
2018	552,029	77,939	27,008	8,348	8,804	9,856	50,931	472,316	163,530	283,202	25,584	1,390	384
Hispanic[4]													
2016	918,447	86,691	23,195	5,649	7,665	9,881	63,496	828,783	247,999	530,951	49,833	2,297	676
2017	898,764	86,393	23,025	5,605	7,635	9,785	63,368	809,882	247,788	513,342	48,752	2,034	455
2018	886,210	86,186	22,637	5,490	7,467	9,680	63,549	797,905	248,463	503,429	46,013	1,737	382

[1]Expressed in completed weeks based on the obstetric estimate of gestation.
[2]Includes births to race and origin groups not shown separately, such as Hispanic single-race White, Hispanic single-race Black, and non-Hispanic multiple-race women, and births with origin not stated.
[3]Race and Hispanic origin are reported separately on birth certificates. Persons of Hispanic origin may be of any race. Multiple-race data, when reported, were bridged to single-race categories in order to maintain comparability among all reported areas. Forty-nine states and the District of Columbia reported multiple-race data for 2015 that were bridged to single-race categories for comparability with other states.
[4]Includes all persons of Hispanic origin of any race.

Table 1-21. Births, by Gestational Age (Weeks) and by Age and Selected Race and Hispanic Origin of Mother, 2018

(Number; percent.)

Race and Hispanic origin of mother and year	All births	Period of gestation										
		Preterm[1]					Term				Postterm	
		Total under 37 weeks	Early			Late	Total	Early	Full	Late		
			Under 28 weeks	28 to 31 weeks	32 and 33 weeks	34 to 36 weeks	37 to 41 weeks	37 to 38 weeks	39 and 40 weeks	41 weeks	42 weeks and over	Not stated
All Races and Origins[2]												
Total	3,791,712	10.02	0.66	0.91	1.18	7.28	89.68	26.53	57.24	5.90	0.30	2,507
Under 15 years	1,736	15.40	1.33	1.74	1.51	10.83	84.42	27.97	50.32	6.14	0.17	9
15 to 19 years	179,871	10.41	0.90	1.01	1.23	7.27	89.37	26.40	56.31	6.65	0.22	157
20 to 24 years	726,175	9.65	0.70	0.90	1.11	6.95	90.10	26.65	57.43	6.01	0.26	524
25 to 29 years	1,099,491	9.38	0.63	0.84	1.06	6.85	90.34	25.95	58.26	6.12	0.28	805
30 to 34 years	1,090,697	9.62	0.59	0.85	1.16	7.03	90.04	25.84	57.90	6.31	0.34	580
35 to 39 years	566,786	11.39	0.67	1.03	1.39	8.30	88.27	27.83	55.43	5.01	0.33	334
40 to 44 years	117,381	13.80	0.83	1.25	1.70	10.02	85.91	31.10	51.89	2.92	0.29	90
45 to 54 years	9,575	22.12	1.33	2.54	3.44	14.81	77.58	33.18	42.09	2.31	0.30	8
Non-Hispanic, Single Race[3]												
White												
Total	1,956,413	9.09	0.44	0.76	1.07	6.83	90.53	24.68	59.16	6.70	0.37	924
Under 15 years	337	14.93	1.49	0.90	0.60	11.94	85.07	24.78	53.43	6.87	*	2
15 to 19 years	64,917	10.11	0.79	0.97	1.17	7.18	89.65	25.09	57.73	6.82	0.25	49
20 to 24 years	326,575	9.00	0.48	0.78	1.04	6.70	90.69	25.17	59.08	6.44	0.31	181
25 to 29 years	576,811	8.55	0.44	0.71	0.97	6.43	91.12	24.25	59.98	6.89	0.33	293
30 to 34 years	624,015	8.64	0.38	0.70	1.03	6.52	90.95	23.88	59.77	7.29	0.42	249
35 to 39 years	304,062	10.19	0.43	0.80	1.22	7.74	89.37	25.61	57.75	6.01	0.44	114
40 to 44 years	55,417	12.47	0.59	1.07	1.51	9.29	87.12	29.00	54.49	3.63	0.40	32
45 to 54 years	4,279	19.58	0.89	2.15	3.37	13.17	80.07	32.23	45.15	2.69	0.35	4
Black												
Total	552,029	14.13	1.51	1.60	1.79	9.23	85.62	29.64	51.34	4.64	0.25	384
Under 15 years	554	16.67	1.63	1.45	2.17	11.41	82.97	28.26	49.28	5.43	0.36	2
15 to 19 years	37,715	12.96	1.48	1.43	1.71	8.33	86.90	28.01	52.99	5.91	0.14	40
20 to 24 years	137,974	13.03	1.38	1.49	1.58	8.57	86.77	29.26	52.73	4.78	0.20	96
25 to 29 years	166,802	13.57	1.46	1.51	1.67	8.93	86.18	29.18	52.31	4.69	0.25	105
30 to 34 years	124,206	14.38	1.57	1.60	1.86	9.35	85.29	29.58	50.91	4.80	0.33	80
35 to 39 years	67,268	16.60	1.74	1.97	2.16	10.73	83.13	31.36	47.96	3.81	0.27	53
40 to 44 years	15,988	18.55	1.76	2.05	2.54	12.21	81.20	34.55	44.36	2.29	0.24	8
45 to 54 years	1,522	26.94	2.43	2.89	4.40	17.21	72.40	34.03	35.74	2.63	0.66	–
Hispanic[4]												
Total	886,210	9.73	0.62	0.84	1.09	7.17	90.07	28.05	56.83	5.19	0.20	382
Under 15 years	730	14.62	0.69	2.34	1.24	10.34	85.24	28.00	50.90	6.34	0.14	5
15 to 19 years	65,122	9.23	0.68	0.81	1.00	6.74	90.54	26.77	56.94	6.83	0.23	43
20 to 24 years	209,701	8.47	0.58	0.71	0.93	6.25	91.33	27.10	58.17	6.05	0.20	107
25 to 29 years	253,977	8.86	0.56	0.75	0.93	6.63	90.94	27.32	58.21	5.41	0.20	92
30 to 34 years	208,193	10.15	0.62	0.87	1.18	7.48	89.66	28.24	56.57	4.85	0.19	69
35 to 39 years	117,383	12.05	0.73	1.13	1.46	8.74	87.77	30.40	53.65	3.72	0.18	51
40 to 44 years	29,192	14.08	0.81	1.18	1.68	10.41	85.76	32.72	50.90	2.14	0.16	14
45 to 54 years	1,912	23.02	1.31	2.93	2.83	15.96	76.87	35.95	39.46	1.47	0.10	1

* = Estimate does not meet NCHS standards of reliability.
– = Quantity zero.
[1]Expressed in completed weeks based on the obstetric estimate of gestation.
[2]Includes births to race and origin groups not shown separately, such as Hispanic single-race White, Hispanic single-race Black, and non-Hispanic multiple-race women, and births with origin not stated.
[3]Race and Hispanic origin are reported separately on birth certificates. Persons of Hispanic origin may be of any race. Multiple-race data, when reported, were bridged to single-race categories in order to maintain comparability among all reported areas. Forty-nine states and the District of Columbia reported multiple-race data for 2015 that were bridged to single-race categories for comparability with other states.
[4]Includes all persons of Hispanic origin of any race.

Table 1-22. Births, by Birthweight (Grams), 2010–2018, and by Selected Race and Hispanic Origin of Mother, 2016–2018

(Percent; number.)

Year and race and Hispanic origin of mother and year	All births	Birthweight (grams)													Not stated
		Low birthweight													
		Very low birthweight													
		Total under 2,500 grams	Total under 1,500 grams	Less than 500 grams	500 to 999 grams	1,000 to 1,499 grams	1,500 to 1,999 grams	2,000 to 2,400 grams	2,500 to 2,999 grams	3,000 to 3,499 grams	3,500 to 3,999 grams	4,000 to 4,499 grams	4,500 to 4,999 grams	5,000 grams or more	

PERCENT

All Races and Origins[1]

2010	3,999,386	8.15	1.45	0.15	0.55	0.75	1.59	5.11	18.63	39.21	26.41	6.58	0.92	0.11	3,964
2011	3,953,590	8.10	1.44	0.15	0.54	0.75	1.58	5.08	18.44	39.13	26.56	6.71	0.95	0.11	4,570
2012	3,952,841	7.99	1.42	0.15	0.54	0.73	1.56	5.01	18.28	39.00	26.81	6.83	0.97	0.12	4,008
2013	3,932,181	8.02	1.41	0.15	0.53	0.73	1.56	5.05	18.22	38.93	26.85	6.86	0.99	0.11	4,452
2014	3,988,076	8.00	1.40	0.15	0.52	0.74	1.56	5.04	18.27	38.80	26.88	6.94	0.99	0.12	3,270
2015	3,978,497	8.07	1.40	0.15	0.52	0.73	1.58	5.09	18.36	38.84	26.73	6.90	0.98	0.12	3,621
2016	3,945,875	8.17	1.40	0.14	0.52	0.74	1.59	5.17	18.54	38.76	26.60	6.85	0.97	0.11	4,518
2017	3,855,500	8.28	1.41	0.14	0.52	0.74	1.63	5.25	18.72	38.76	26.44	6.75	0.95	0.11	3,002
2018	3,791,712	8.28	1.38	0.14	0.50	0.74	1.62	5.28	18.75	38.76	26.44	6.72	0.94	0.11	2,932

Non-Hispanic, Single Race[2]
White

2016	2,056,332	6.97	1.07	0.09	0.37	0.61	1.39	4.51	15.88	37.59	29.82	8.39	1.21	0.12	2,212
2017	1,992,461	7.00	1.05	0.09	0.36	0.60	1.40	4.54	16.05	37.68	29.70	8.28	1.17	0.12	1,211
2018	1,956,413	6.91	1.02	0.09	0.34	0.58	1.38	4.52	16.01	37.80	29.74	8.25	1.16	0.12	1,259

Black

2016	558,622	13.68	2.95	0.37	1.20	1.38	2.67	8.06	25.38	38.24	18.42	3.69	0.52	0.07	936
2017	560,715	13.89	2.95	0.36	1.18	1.41	2.72	8.22	25.44	37.96	18.37	3.76	0.51	0.07	642
2018	552,029	14.07	2.92	0.35	1.16	1.41	2.79	8.35	25.44	37.90	18.33	3.68	0.51	0.07	571

Hispanic[3]

2016	918,447	7.32	1.24	0.13	0.46	0.65	1.41	4.68	18.76	40.79	26.06	6.10	0.85	0.12	556
2017	898,764	7.43	1.26	0.13	0.47	0.66	1.42	4.76	18.86	40.76	25.95	6.02	0.85	0.11	428
2018	886,210	7.49	1.24	0.12	0.46	0.66	1.43	4.81	19.01	40.64	25.90	6.02	0.83	0.11	381

NUMBER

All Races and Origins[1]

2010	3,999,386	325,563	57,841	5,980	22,015	29,846	63,427	204,295	744,181	1,566,755	1,055,004	262,997	36,706	4,216	3,964
2011	3,953,590	319,711	56,754	5,942	21,289	29,523	62,504	200,453	728,201	1,545,355	1,048,902	265,040	37,475	4,336	4,570
2012	3,952,841	315,709	56,252	5,947	21,432	28,873	61,499	197,958	721,840	1,540,161	1,058,604	269,581	38,288	4,650	4,008
2013	3,932,181	315,099	55,458	5,945	20,866	28,647	61,238	198,403	715,764	1,529,258	1,054,767	269,594	38,834	4,413	4,452
2014	3,988,076	318,847	55,947	5,936	20,721	29,290	61,992	200,908	727,987	1,546,274	1,071,007	276,592	39,353	4,746	3,270
2015	3,978,497	320,869	55,592	5,863	20,689	29,040	62,862	202,415	729,673	1,544,024	1,062,456	274,404	38,796	4,654	3,621
2016	3,945,875	321,839	55,110	5,710	20,323	29,077	62,863	203,866	730,710	1,527,707	1,048,476	269,865	38,264	4,496	4,518
2017	3,855,500	318,873	54,135	5,470	19,979	28,686	62,605	202,133	721,165	1,493,081	1,018,613	260,042	36,493	4,231	3,002
2018	3,791,712	313,752	52,171	5,303	18,970	27,898	61,509	200,072	710,444	1,468,639	1,001,803	254,704	35,435	4,003	2,932

Non-Hispanic, Single Race[2]
White

2016	2,056,332	143,254	21,979	1,888	7,565	12,526	28,578	92,697	326,279	772,165	612,641	172,434	24,781	2,566	2,212
2017	1,992,461	139,358	20,981	1,752	7,233	11,996	27,968	90,409	319,523	750,331	591,376	164,898	23,299	2,465	1,211
2018	1,956,413	135,185	19,872	1,721	6,719	11,432	26,964	88,349	313,105	739,031	581,499	161,395	22,645	2,294	1,259

Black

2016	558,622	76,299	16,465	2,083	6,675	7,707	14,885	44,949	141,557	213,260	102,702	20,571	2,880	417	936
2017	560,715	77,815	16,544	2,024	6,597	7,923	15,228	46,043	142,459	212,599	102,878	21,065	2,854	403	642
2018	552,029	77,584	16,127	1,941	6,406	7,780	15,411	46,046	140,295	209,028	101,089	20,285	2,806	371	571

Hispanic[3]

2016	918,447	67,210	11,378	1,175	4,237	5,966	12,910	42,922	172,171	374,434	239,210	55,983	7,770	1,113	556
2017	898,764	66,766	11,275	1,137	4,229	5,909	12,772	42,719	169,467	366,198	233,157	54,096	7,631	1,021	428
2018	886,210	66,310	11,006	1,084	4,040	5,882	12,706	42,598	168,418	359,966	229,450	53,359	7,358	968	381

[1]Includes births to race and origin groups not shown separately, such as Hispanic single-race White, Hispanic single-race Black, and non-Hispanic multiple-race women, and births with origin not stated.
[2]Race and Hispanic origin are reported separately on birth certificates. Persons of Hispanic origin may be of any race. Multiple-race data, when reported, were bridged to single-race categories in order to maintain comparability among all reported areas. Forty-nine states and the District of Columbia reported multiple-race data for 2015 that were bridged to single-race categories for comparability with other states.
[3]Includes all persons of Hispanic origin of any race.

Table 1-23. Births, by Birthweight (Grams), by Age and Selected Race and Hispanic Origin of Mother, 2018
(Number; percent.)

Age (years) and race and Hispanic origin of mother and year	All births	Total under 2,500 grams	Total under 1,500 grams	Less than 500 grams	500 to 999 grams	1,000 to 1,499 grams	1,500 to 1,999 grams	2,000 to 2,400 grams	2,500 to 2,999 grams	3,000 to 3,499 grams	3,500 to 3,999 grams	4,000 to 4,499 grams	4,500 to 4,999 grams	5,000 grams or more	Not stated
PERCENT															
All Races and Origins[1]															
Total	3,791,712	8.28	1.38	0.14	0.50	0.74	1.62	5.28	18.75	38.76	26.44	6.72	0.94	0.11	2,932
Under 15 years	1,736	12.73	2.59	0.40	0.75	1.44	2.36	7.78	26.84	41.65	16.19	2.48	0.12	*	–
15 to 19 years	179,871	10.09	1.74	0.17	0.68	0.89	1.82	6.53	23.78	41.12	20.76	3.82	0.39	0.04	127
20 to 24 years	726,175	8.59	1.41	0.15	0.52	0.73	1.60	5.58	20.91	40.51	24.08	5.22	0.63	0.06	520
25 to 29 years	1,099,491	7.78	1.29	0.14	0.47	0.68	1.50	4.99	18.37	39.20	26.91	6.74	0.90	0.10	877
30 to 34 years	1,090,697	7.63	1.24	0.12	0.44	0.68	1.53	4.87	17.24	37.99	28.22	7.66	1.13	0.12	843
35 to 39 years	566,786	8.83	1.50	0.13	0.54	0.82	1.83	5.50	17.80	36.94	27.37	7.73	1.18	0.15	457
40 to 44 years	117,381	10.77	1.88	0.17	0.67	1.04	2.32	6.57	19.58	36.51	25.04	6.91	1.05	0.14	100
45 to 54 years	9,575	18.39	3.42	0.17	1.20	2.05	4.35	10.62	21.71	33.89	20.04	5.14	0.77	0.06	8
Non-Hispanic, Single Race[2]															
White															
Total	1,956,413	6.91	1.02	0.09	0.34	0.58	1.38	4.52	16.01	37.80	29.74	8.25	1.16	0.12	1,259
Under 15 years	337	10.39	2.37	0.30	1.19	0.89	0.89	7.12	21.96	41.54	21.36	4.75	*	*	–
15 to 19 years	64,917	8.97	1.57	0.12	0.63	0.82	1.60	5.79	20.14	40.43	24.67	5.15	0.59	0.04	44
20 to 24 years	326,575	7.21	1.08	0.09	0.38	0.61	1.36	4.77	18.01	39.81	27.49	6.59	0.81	0.08	193
25 to 29 years	576,811	6.52	0.98	0.09	0.33	0.56	1.28	4.27	15.71	38.30	30.07	8.18	1.09	0.11	347
30 to 34 years	624,015	6.40	0.90	0.08	0.29	0.53	1.31	4.19	14.85	37.06	31.15	9.07	1.33	0.13	417
35 to 39 years	304,062	7.39	1.05	0.09	0.35	0.61	1.54	4.80	15.59	36.03	30.22	9.21	1.40	0.16	211
40 to 44 years	55,417	9.27	1.45	0.12	0.46	0.88	1.99	5.83	17.67	35.84	27.58	8.22	1.25	0.17	43
45 to 54 years	4,279	15.98	2.78	0.12	0.80	1.87	3.53	9.66	19.53	34.69	22.13	6.60	0.96	0.12	4
Black															
Total	552,029	14.07	2.92	0.35	1.16	1.41	2.79	8.35	25.44	37.90	18.33	3.68	0.51	0.07	571
Under 15 years	554	14.62	3.25	0.54	0.90	1.81	2.71	8.66	31.05	39.17	13.36	1.62	0.18	*	–
15 to 19 years	37,715	14.91	2.84	0.35	1.13	1.36	2.85	9.22	30.48	38.79	13.86	1.77	0.16	0.02	34
20 to 24 years	137,974	14.06	2.71	0.33	1.05	1.33	2.68	8.67	28.02	39.02	16.01	2.55	0.30	0.03	136
25 to 29 years	166,802	13.54	2.75	0.37	1.08	1.30	2.66	8.14	25.28	38.54	18.53	3.61	0.44	0.06	173
30 to 34 years	124,206	13.49	2.96	0.34	1.20	1.42	2.74	7.79	23.17	37.11	20.65	4.76	0.70	0.11	146
35 to 39 years	67,268	15.13	3.51	0.37	1.43	1.71	3.15	8.47	22.37	35.84	20.65	5.03	0.88	0.10	66
40 to 44 years	15,988	16.63	3.77	0.38	1.51	1.87	3.63	9.23	23.44	35.11	19.34	4.63	0.74	0.11	13
45 to 54 years	1,522	24.16	5.00	0.26	2.11	2.63	6.85	12.31	23.90	30.35	17.12	3.88	0.59	*	3
Hispanic[3]															
Total	886,210	7.49	1.24	0.12	0.46	0.66	1.43	4.81	19.01	40.64	25.90	6.02	0.83	0.11	381
Under 15 years	730	12.19	1.78	0.41	0.14	1.23	2.60	7.81	25.48	43.56	16.85	1.78	0.14	*	–
15 to 19 years	65,122	8.40	1.28	0.11	0.48	0.69	1.43	5.69	23.53	43.36	20.80	3.57	0.31	0.04	35
20 to 24 years	209,701	7.13	1.11	0.13	0.41	0.57	1.25	4.77	20.46	42.54	24.35	4.89	0.57	0.06	76
25 to 29 years	253,977	6.78	1.11	0.11	0.41	0.58	1.28	4.40	18.28	40.96	26.82	6.22	0.83	0.11	106
30 to 34 years	208,193	7.32	1.27	0.13	0.45	0.69	1.44	4.61	17.49	39.43	27.60	6.97	1.06	0.14	93
35 to 39 years	117,383	8.55	1.56	0.12	0.58	0.86	1.84	5.16	18.08	37.99	26.91	7.17	1.12	0.18	57
40 to 44 years	29,192	10.19	1.69	0.15	0.66	0.88	2.30	6.20	19.24	37.67	24.94	6.77	1.08	0.12	13
45 to 54 years	1,912	18.32	3.72	0.26	1.41	2.04	3.35	11.25	22.29	34.59	19.73	4.19	0.84	0.05	1

* = Estimate does not meet NCHS standards of reliability.
– = Quantity zero.
[1]Includes births to race and origin groups not shown separately, such as Hispanic single-race White, Hispanic single-race Black, and non-Hispanic multiple-race women, and births with origin not stated.
[2]Race and Hispanic origin are reported separately on birth certificates. Persons of Hispanic origin may be of any race. Multiple-race data, when reported, were bridged to single-race categories in order to maintain comparability among all reported areas. Forty-nine states and the District of Columbia reported multiple-race data for 2015 that were bridged to single-race categories for comparability with other states.
[3]Includes all persons of Hispanic origin of any race.

Table 1-24. Twin, Triplet, and Higher-Order Multiple Births, 2010–2018, and by Selected Race and Hispanic Origin of Mother, 2016–2018

(Number; rate.)

Year and race and Hispanic origin of mother and year	Total births	Twin births	Triplet and higher-order births	Multiple birth rate	Twin birth rate	Triplet and higher-order birth rate
All Races and Origins[1]						
2010	3,999,386	132,562	5,503	34.5	33.1	137.6
2011	3,953,590	131,269	5,417	34.6	33.2	137.0
2012	3,952,841	131,024	4,919	34.4	33.1	124.4
2013	3,932,181	132,324	4,700	34.8	33.7	119.5
2014	3,988,076	135,336	4,526	35.1	33.9	113.5
2015	3,978,497	133,155	4,123	34.5	33.5	103.6
2016	3,945,875	131,723	4,003	34.4	33.4	101.4
2017	3,855,500	128,310	3,917	34.3	33.3	101.6
2018	3,791,712	123,536	3,525	33.5	32.6	93.0
Non-Hispanic, Single Race[2]						
White						
2016	2,056,332	73,425	2,502	36.9	35.7	121.7
2017	1,992,461	70,704	2,324	36.7	35.5	116.6
2018	1,956,413	67,203	1,996	35.4	34.4	102.0
Black						
2016	558,622	22,267	628	41.0	39.9	112.4
2017	560,715	22,982	671	42.2	41.0	119.7
2018	552,029	22,502	658	42.0	40.8	119.2
Hispanic[3]						
2016	918,447	22,625	538	25.2	24.6	58.6
2017	898,764	22,041	614	25.2	24.5	68.3
2018	886,210	21,654	573	25.1	24.4	64.7

NOTE: "Higher-order births" includes quadruplet, quintuplet, and higher-order multiple deliveries. The multiple and twin birth rates are per 1,000 births; the triplet and higher-order birth rates are per 100,000 births.
[1]Includes births to race and origin groups not shown separately, such as Hispanic single-race White, Hispanic single-race Black, and non-Hispanic multiple-race women, and births with origin not stated.
[2]Race and Hispanic origin are reported separately on birth certificates. Persons of Hispanic origin may be of any race. Multiple-race data, when reported, were bridged to single-race categories in order to maintain comparability among all reported areas. Forty-nine states and the District of Columbia reported multiple-race data for 2015 that were bridged to single-race categories for comparability with other states.
[3]Includes all persons of Hispanic origin of any race.

Table 1-25. Births, by Plurality and Age and Selected Race and Hispanic Origin of Mother, 2018

(Number; rate.)

Year and race and Hispanic origin of mother and year	Live births				Rates		
	Total	Singleton	Twin	Triplet and higher-order multiple	Multiple birth	Twin birth	Triplet and higher-order multiple birth
All Races and Origins[1]							
Total	3,791,712	3,664,651	123,536	3,525	33.5	32.6	93.0
Under 15 years	1,736	1,715	21	–	12.1	12.1	0.0
15 to 19 years	179,871	176,756	3,084	31	17.3	17.1	17.2
15 to 17 years	44,291	43,658	624	9	14.3	14.1	20.3
18 and 19 years	135,580	133,098	2,460	22	18.3	18.1	16.2
20 to 24 years	726,175	709,046	16,835	294	23.6	23.2	40.5
25 to 29 years	1,099,491	1,065,264	33,394	833	31.1	30.4	75.8
30 to 34 years	1,090,697	1,050,006	39,441	1,250	37.3	36.2	114.6
35 to 39 years	566,786	541,686	24,268	832	44.3	42.8	146.8
40 to 44 years	117,381	111,902	5,269	210	46.7	44.9	178.9
45 to 54 years	9,575	8,276	1,224	75	135.7	127.8	783.3
Non-Hispanic, Single Race[2]							
Total	1,956,413	1,887,214	67,203	1,996	35.4	34.4	102.0
Under 15 years	337	327	10	–	29.7	29.7	0.0
15 to 19 years	64,917	63,840	1,068	9	16.6	16.5	13.9
15 to 17 years	13,036	12,858	175	3	13.7	13.4	23.0
18 and 19 years	51,881	50,982	893	6	17.3	17.2	11.6
20 to 24 years	326,575	319,134	7,314	127	22.8	22.4	38.9
25 to 29 years	576,811	558,625	17,709	477	31.5	30.7	82.7
30 to 34 years	624,015	599,564	23,656	795	39.2	37.9	127.4
35 to 39 years	304,062	289,438	14,123	501	48.1	46.4	164.8
40 to 44 years	55,417	52,542	2,792	83	51.9	50.4	149.8
45 to 54 years	4,279	3,744	531	4	125.0	124.1	93.5
Black							
Total	552,029	528,869	22,502	658	42.0	40.8	119.2
Under 15 years	554	552	2	–	3.6	3.6	0.0
15 to 19 years	37,715	36,790	912	13	24.5	24.2	34.5
15 to 17 years	9,998	9,814	181	3	18.4	18.1	30.0
18 and 19 years	27,717	26,976	731	10	26.7	26.4	36.1
20 to 24 years	137,974	133,230	4,654	90	34.4	33.7	65.2
25 to 29 years	166,802	159,426	7,198	178	44.2	43.2	106.7
30 to 34 years	124,206	118,410	5,626	170	46.7	45.3	136.9
35 to 39 years	67,268	63,932	3,230	106	49.6	48.0	157.6
40 to 44 years	15,988	15,245	685	58	46.5	42.8	362.8
45 to 54 years	1,522	1,284	195	43	156.4	128.1	2,825.2
Hispanic[3]							
Total	886,210	863,983	21,654	573	25.1	24.4	64.7
Under 15 years	730	723	7	–	9.6	9.6	0.0
15 to 19 years	65,122	64,226	890	6	13.8	13.7	9.2
15 to 17 years	18,185	17,968	214	3	11.9	11.8	16.5
18 and 19 years	46,937	46,258	676	3	14.5	14.4	6.4
20 to 24 years	209,701	205,889	3,752	60	18.2	17.9	28.6
25 to 29 years	253,977	247,961	5,891	125	23.7	23.2	49.2
30 to 34 years	208,193	201,987	6,001	205	29.8	28.8	98.5
35 to 39 years	117,383	113,358	3,906	119	34.3	33.3	101.4
40 to 44 years	29,192	28,164	985	43	35.2	33.7	147.3
45 to 54 years	1,912	1,675	222	15	124.0	116.1	784.5

– = Quantity zero.

NOTE: "Higher-order births" includes quadruplet, quintuplet, and higher-order multiple deliveries. The multiple and twin birth rates are per 1,000 births; the triplet and higher-order birth rates are per 100,000 births.

[1]Includes births to race and origin groups not shown separately, such as Hispanic single-race White, Hispanic single-race Black, and non-Hispanic multiple-race women, and births with origin not stated.

[2]Race and Hispanic origin are reported separately on birth certificates. Persons of Hispanic origin may be of any race. Multiple-race data, when reported, were bridged to single-race categories in order to maintain comparability among all reported areas. Forty-nine states and the District of Columbia reported multiple-race data for 2015 that were bridged to single-race categories for comparability with other states.

[3]Includes all persons of Hispanic origin of any race.

Table 1-26. Gestational Age and Birthweight Characteristics, by Plurality, 2018

(Number; percent.)

Plurality	Number of births	Early preterm	Preterm	Very low birthweight	Low birthweight
All births	3,791,712	2.75	10.02	1.38	8.28
Singleton	3,664,651	2.12	8.24	1.09	6.60
Twin	123,536	19.52	60.32	9.07	55.62
Triplet	3,400	63.09	98.32	33.60	94.77
Quadruplet	115	82.61	97.39	50.44	98.23
Quintuplet and higher-order	10	100.00	100.00	100.00	100.00

NOTE: "Early preterm" is less than 34 completed weeks of gestation. "Preterm" indicates less than 37 completed weeks of gestation. "Very low birthweight " is less then 1,500 grams. "Low birthweight" is less than 2,500 grams.

Table 1-27. Time of Birth by Day of Week of Birth and Race and Hispanic Origin of Mother: United States, 2018

(Number; percent.)

Time of birth and race and Hispanic origin of mother	All births	Sunday	Monday	Tuesday	Wednesday	Thursday	Friday	Saturday
All races and origins[1]								
Total (percent)	100.0	100.0	100.0	100.0	100.0	100.0	100.0	100.0
12:00 a.m.–5:59 a.m.	17.7	22.4	14.3	16.4	17.0	16.8	17.3	23.4
6:00 a.m.–11:59 a.m.	28.9	27.1	29.9	29.4	28.9	28.7	29.9	26.9
12:00 p.m.–5:59 p.m.	30.6	27.1	32.4	31.5	31.3	31.4	30.9	27.0
6:00 p.m.–11:59 p.m.	22.9	23.4	23.5	22.7	22.8	23.1	22.0	22.8
Total (number)	3,791,712	366,243	575,544	607,836	605,916	611,806	602,388	421,979
Not stated[2]	271	36	39	40	29	34	40	53
Non-Hispanic, single race[3]								
White								
Total (percent)	100.0	100.0	100.0	100.0	100.0	100.0	100.0	100.0
12:00 a.m.–5:59 a.m.	17,2	22.8	13.4	15.8	16.4	16.2	16.7	23.7
6:00 a.m.–11:59 a.m.	28.9	26.6	30.0	29.4	28.9	28.7	30.2	26.4
12:00 p.m.–5:59 p.m.	31.0	26.9	33.0	32.0	31.8	32.0	31.3	26.9
6:00 p.m.–11:59 p.m.	22.9	23.7	23.6	22.8	22.9	23.1	21.8	23.0
Total (number)	1,956,413	178,034	300,657	318,056	317,046	321,098	314,708	206,814
Not stated[2]	103	14	18	14	11	15	12	19
Black								
Total (percent)	100.0	100.0	100.0	100.0	100.0	100.0	100.0	100.0
12:00 a.m.–5:59 a.m.	18.2	22.6	14.9	16.8	17.6	17.4	17.8	23.4
6:00 a.m.–11:59 a.m.	28,5	27.1	29.4	29.1	28.8	28.2	29.2	26.8
12:00 p.m.–5:59 p.m.	30.4	26.9	32.3	31.4	30.8	31.4	30.8	26.8
6:00 p.m.–11:59 p.m.	22.9	23.4	23.4	22.6	22.9	23.0	22.2	22.9
Total (number)	552,029	54,421	83,231	88,174	87,833	87,998	86,778	63,594
Not stated[2]	19	3	3	4	1	2	4	2
Hispanic[4]								
Total (percent)	100.0	100.0	100.0	100.0	100.0	100.0	100.0	100.0
12:00 a.m.–5:59 a.m.	18.1	21.8	15.2	16.9	17.4	17.2	17.7	22.7
6:00 a.m.–11:59 a.m.	29.2	27.9	29.9	29.8	29.2	29.2	29.9	27.8
12:00 p.m.–5:59 p.m.	30.1	27.5	31.7	30.8	30.8	30.7	30.5	27.3
6:00 p.m.–11:59 p.m.	22.6	22.8	23.2	22.4	22.6	23.0	21.9	22.3
Total (number)	886,210	91,349	132,817	139,739	139,583	139,747	138,584	104,391
Not stated[2]	23	2	2	3	4	4	1	7

NOTE: Percentages are numbers of live births with specified time of birth per 100 live births in specified group.
[1]Includes births to race and origin groups not shown separately, such as Hispanic single-race White, Hispanic single-race Black, and non-Hispanic multiple-race women, and births with origin not stated.
[2]No response recorded for time of birth.
[3]Race and Hispanic origin are reported separately on birth certificates. Persons of Hispanic origin may be of any race. Multiple-race data, when reported, were bridged to single-race categories in order to maintain comparability among all reported areas. Forty-nine states and the District of Columbia reported multiple-race data for 2015 that were bridged to single-race categories for comparability with other states.
[4]Includes all persons of Hispanic origin of any race.

Table 1-28. Births and Seasonally Adjusted Birth Rates, by Month, 2018
(Number; rate.)

Month	Number	Observed		Seasonally adjusted[1]	
		Birth rate	Fertility rate	Birth rate	Fertility rate
Total...	3,791,712	11.6	59.1	X	X
January...	314,808	11.4	57.9	12.8	64.4
February...	284,250	11.4	57.9	12.7	64.3
March...	316,044	11.4	58.1	12.7	64.2
April...	298,394	11.1	56.7	12.7	63.9
May...	320,622	11.6	58.9	12.7	64.1
June...	314,816	11.7	59.7	12.6	64.0
July...	329,009	11.8	60.4	12.6	63.8
August...	344,750	12.4	63.2	12.6	63.9
September...	322,772	12.0	61.1	12.5	63.3
October...	326,778	11.7	59.9	12.5	63.5
November...	308,703	11.5	58.4	12.4	63.1
December...	310,766	11.2	56.9	12.5	63.1

NOTE: Rates are on an annual basis per 1,000 population for specified month. Birth rates are births per 1,000 total population. Fertility rates are births per 1,000 women aged 15–44 years. Monthly populations estimated as of the first of each month. Monthly population estimates for 2018 were provided by the U.S. Census Bureau (U.S. Census Bureau, Population Division, Monthly national population estimates by age, sex, race, and Hispanic origin, and population Universe for the United States: April 1, 2010 to December 1, 2018, monthly postcensal resident population: https://www.census.gov/data/tables/time- series/demo/popest/2010s-national-detail.html).
X = Not applicable.
[1]Method of seasonal adjustment developed by the U.S. Census Bureau (Shiskin J, Young AH, Musgrave JC. The X11 variant of the census method II seasonal adjustment program. Technical Paper no. 15. U.S. Census Bureau: Washington, DC. 1967. Available from: http://www.census.gov/ts/papers/ShiskinYoungMusgrave1967.pdf).

Table 1-29. Births, by Day of Week and Method of Delivery, 2018
(Number; ratio.)

Day of the week	Average number of births	Index of occurrence[1]		
		Total[2]	Method of delivery	
			Vaginal	Cesarean
Total...	10,388	100.0	100.0	100.0
Sunday...	7,043	67.8	76.5	49.3
Monday...	10,859	104.5	98.9	116.7
Tuesday...	11,689	112.5	109.0	119.9
Wednesday...	11,652	112.2	110.1	116.6
Thursday...	11,766	113.3	111.1	117.9
Friday...	11,584	111.5	107.1	120.9
Saturday...	8,115	78.1	87.4	58.3

[1]Index is the ratio of the average number of births by a specified method of delivery on a given day of the week to the average daily number of births by a specified method of delivery for the year, multiplied by 100.
[2]Includes method of delivery not stated.

Table 1-30. Births, by Attendant, Place of Delivery, and Selected Race and Hispanic Origin of Mother, 2018
(Number.)

Place of delivery and race and Hispanic origin of mother	All births	Physician			Midwife			Other	Unspecified
		Total	Doctor of medicine	Doctor of osteopathy	Total	Certified nurse midwife	Other midwife		
All races and origins[1]									
Total	3,791,712	3,369,567	3,066,477	303,090	387,519	357,297	30,222	32,185	2,441
In hospital[2]	3,729,199	3,366,916	3,064,153	302,763	341,657	336,267	5,390	19,364	1,262
Not in hospital	62,266	2,615	2,289	326	45,786	21,008	24,778	12,759	1,106
Freestanding birthing center	19,871	531	404	127	18,266	11,139	7,127	958	116
Clinic or doctor's office	596	140	125	15	426	305	121	23	7
Residence	38,512	1,416	1,296	120	26,222	9,399	16,823	10,089	785
Other	3,287	528	464	64	872	165	707	1,689	198
Not specified	247	36	35	1	76	22	54	62	73
Non-Hispanic, single race[3]									
White									
Total	1,956,413	1,718,149	1,534,961	183,188	218,770	195,495	23,275	18,265	1,229
In hospital[2]	1,908,350	1,716,594	1,533,646	182,948	181,405	178,319	3,086	9,754	597
Not in hospital	47,957	1,537	1,298	239	37,315	17,163	20,152	8,489	616
Freestanding birthing center	15,547	475	357	118	14,203	8,885	5,318	780	89
Clinic or doctor's office	502	88	79	9	400	282	118	10	4
Residence	29,994	712	642	70	21,927	7,881	14,046	6,925	430
Other	1,914	262	220	42	785	115	670	774	93
Not specified	106	18	17	1	50	13	37	22	16
Black									
Total	552,029	501,224	469,168	32,056	45,851	44,163	1,688	4,570	384
In hospital[2]	547,810	500,688	468,661	32,027	43,946	43,218	728	2,951	225
Not in hospital	4,190	529	500	29	1,901	944	957	1,606	154
Freestanding birthing center	1,110	17	16	1	1,037	595	442	41	15
Clinic or doctor's office	23	17	17	–	4	4	–	2	–
Residence	2,652	364	345	19	840	334	506	1,336	112
Other	405	131	122	9	20	11	9	227	27
Not specified	29	7	7	–	4	1	3	13	5
Hispanic[4]									
Total	886,210	796,921	735,728	61,193	82,999	79,560	3,439	5,815	475
In hospital[2]	880,488	796,598	735,434	61,164	79,154	77,969	1,185	4,497	239
Not in hospital	5,671	317	288	29	3,837	1,587	2,250	1,304	213
Freestanding birthing center	2,030	25	23	2	1,923	981	942	76	6
Clinic or doctor's office	31	15	13	2	11	9	2	2	3
Residence	3,142	192	173	19	1,867	578	1,289	932	151
Other	468	85	79	6	36	19	17	294	53
Not specified	51	6	6	–	8	4	4	14	23

– = Quantity zero.
[1]Includes births to race and origin groups not shown separately, such as Hispanic single-race White, Hispanic single-race Black, and non-Hispanic multiple-race women, and births with origin not stated.
[2]Includes births occurring en route to or on arrival at hospital.
[3]Race and Hispanic origin are reported separately on birth certificates. Persons of Hispanic origin may be of any race. Multiple-race data, when reported, were bridged to single-race categories in order to maintain comparability among all reported areas. Forty-nine states and the District of Columbia reported multiple-race data for 2015 that were bridged to single-race categories for comparability with other states.
[4]Includes all persons of Hispanic origin of any race.

Table 1-31. Births Occurring at Home, by State, 2018

(Number; percent.)

Area	Number	Percent
United States	38,512	1.0
Alabama	218	0.4
Alaska	194	1.9
Arizona	667	0.8
Arkansas	326	0.9
California	3,269	0.7
Colorado	1,001	1.6
Connecticut	222	0.6
Delaware	78	0.7
District of Columbia	41	0.4
Florida	2,081	0.9
Georgia	792	0.6
Hawaii	256	1.5
Idaho	475	2.2
Illinois	855	0.6
Indiana	1,255	1.5
Iowa	557	1.5
Kansas	530	1.5
Kentucky	721	1.3
Louisiana	164	0.3
Maine	228	1.9
Maryland	521	0.7
Massachusetts	379	0.5
Michigan	1,487	1.4
Minnesota	826	1.2
Mississippi	184	0.5
Missouri	1,183	1.6
Montana	275	2.4
Nebraska	81	0.3
Nevada	480	1.3
New Hampshire	166	1.4
New Jersey	443	0.4
New Mexico	291	1.3
New York	2,477	1.1
North Carolina	624	0.5
North Dakota	107	1.0
Ohio	1,529	1.1
Oklahoma	516	1.0
Oregon	845	2.0
Pennsylvania	2,638	1.9
Rhode Island	59	0.6
South Carolina	393	0.7
South Dakota	98	0.8
Tennessee	896	1.1
Texas	2,428	0.6
Utah	1,043	2.2
Vermont	109	2.0
Virginia	968	1.0
Washington	1,822	2.1
West Virginia	130	0.7
Wisconsin	1,458	2.3
Wyoming	126	1.9

Table 1-32. Mean Age of Mother, by Live-Birth Order, 2010–2018, and by Race and Hispanic Origin of Mother, 2016–2018

(Number.)

Year and race and Hispanic origin of mother	Total	Live-birth order								
		1	2	3	4	5	6 and 7	8 and over	Unknown or not stated
All races and origins[1]									
2010	27.7	25.4	28.2	29.6	30.7	31.7	33.0	35.7	27.7
2011	27.9	25.6	28.3	29.7	30.8	31.8	33.1	35.5	28.2
2012	28.0	25.8	28.4	29.8	30.9	31.9	33.2	35.7	27.9
2013	28.2	26.0	28.6	29.9	31.0	32.0	33.3	35.7	28.3
2014	28.3	26.3	28.7	30.0	31.1	32.0	33.4	35.7	28.7
2015	28.5	26.4	28.8	30.1	31.2	32.2	33.4	35.8	29.3
2016	28.7	26.6	29.0	30.2	31.3	32.3	33.5	35.9	28.7
2017	28.8	26.8	29.2	30.3	31.4	32.4	33.7	36.0	29.1
2018	29	26.9	29.3	30.5	31.5	32.5	33.7	36.1	29.3
Non-Hispanic, single race[2]									
White									
2016	29.2	27.4	29.5	30.6	31.5	32.5	33.9	36.7	29.4
2017	29.3	27.6	29.7	30.7	31.6	32.6	34.0	36.8	29.5
2018	29.4	27.7	29.8	30.8	31.7	32.7	34.1	36.8	29.6
Black									
2016	27.4	24.8	27.6	29.1	30.2	31.1	32.3	34.6	27.1
2017	27.7	24.9	27.7	29.3	30.4	31.3	32.5	34.9	28.0
2018	27.9	25.1	28.0	29.6	30.6	31.5	32.6	34.9	28.4
American Indian or Alaska Native									
2016	26.7	23.2	26.1	28.0	29.6	31.1	32.0	34.8	28.1
2017	26.8	23.3	26.1	28.1	29.6	31.3	32.6	34.4	27.8
2018	27.1	23.5	26.4	28.4	30.0	31.1	32.8	34.8	27.6
Asian									
2016	31.5	30.1	32.3	33.3	33.6	34.1	34.9	36.3	31.4
2017	31.7	30.3	32.5	33.4	33.9	34.4	35.2	36.3	32.0
2018	31.8	30.5	32.6	33.5	34.0	34.4	35.0	36.5	31.6
Native Hawaiian or Other Pacific Islander									
2016	27.9	24.8	27.0	28.9	30.1	31.7	33.2	35.3	27.6
2017	28.0	24.9	27.2	28.9	30.5	31.4	33.0	35.4	26.8
2018	27.9	24.7	26.9	28.9	30.5	31.7	33.0	35.8	27.2
Hispanic[3]									
2016	27.8	24.7	27.6	29.8	31.5	32.7	34.0	35.3	28.3
2017	28.0	24.8	27.8	29.9	31.6	32.9	34.1	35.5	29.0
2018	28.1	25.0	28.0	30.1	31.7	33.0	34.1	35.6	29.2

NOTE: Mean age at birth is the arithmetic average of the age of mothers at time of birth, computed directly from the frequency of births by age of mother and live-birth order. Live-birth order refers to number of children born alive to mother.
[1]Includes births to race and origin groups not shown separately, such as Hispanic single-race White, Hispanic single-race Black, and non-Hispanic multiple-race women, and births with origin not stated.
[2]Race and Hispanic origin are reported separately on birth certificates. Persons of Hispanic origin may be of any race. Multiple-race data, when reported, were bridged to single-race categories in order to maintain comparability among all reported areas. Forty-nine states and the District of Columbia reported multiple-race data for 2015 that were bridged to single-race categories for comparability with other states.
[3]Includes all persons of Hispanic origin of any race.

Table 1-33. Births to Unmarried Women, by Selected Race and Hispanic Origin of Mother, by State and Territory of Residence, 2018

(Number, percent.)

Area	Births to unmarried women				Percent unmarried			
	All races and origins[1]	Non-Hispanic, single race		Hispanic[3]	All races[1]	Non-Hispanic		Hispanic[3]
		White[2]	Black[2]			White[2]	Black[2]	
United States[4]	1,503,361	551,217	383,364	459,242	39.6	28.2	69.4	51.8
Alabama	27,014	10,590	13,812	1,933	46.8	31.4	78.5	43.9
Alaska	3,559	998	104	261	35.3	19.7	37.1	32.3
Arizona	36,235	9,957	2,575	18,876	44.9	30.4	59.8	55.4
Arkansas	16,795	8,053	5,613	2,057	45.4	34.1	80.6	50.2
California	168,892	26,320	14,260	108,337	37.1	21.4	63.7	51.3
Colorado	14,598	6,013	1,222	6,116	23.2	16.5	40.3	34.3
Connecticut	12,878	4,117	2,817	5,360	37.1	22.3	63.7	61.2
Delaware	4,987	1,806	1,942	1,003	47.0	34.9	70.0	58.7
District of Columbia	4,283	172	3,287	714	46.5	5.7	77.3	55.1
Florida	102,751	34,714	31,773	33,448	46.4	36.2	66.0	49.8
Georgia	56,966	15,467	30,712	8,503	45.1	27.8	70.2	48.8
Hawaii	6,468	567	58	1,227	38.1	17.2	13.7	47.6
Idaho	5,777	3,782	85	1,557	27.0	22.8	36.5	43.9
Illinois	56,946	19,710	19,204	15,835	39.3	25.5	78.4	52.2
Indiana	35,303	21,705	7,862	4,387	43.2	36.5	76.8	55.8
Iowa	13,191	8,729	1,684	1,929	34.9	29.8	64.4	52.2
Kansas	13,187	7,529	1,760	3,102	36.4	29.7	68.3	51.9
Kentucky	22,616	16,371	3,557	1,741	41.9	37.8	71.9	54.0
Louisiana	31,775	10,544	17,664	2,648	53.3	34.6	79.9	56.1
Maine	4,780	4,285	158	109	38.8	38.9	28.9	48.7
Maryland	27,895	6,899	12,926	6,672	39.2	23.3	59.0	53.5
Massachusetts	22,453	9,281	3,431	8,005	32.5	23.4	50.3	58.0
Michigan	44,882	22,645	16,420	3,637	40.8	30.3	79.9	50.9
Minnesota	21,463	10,690	4,096	2,684	31.9	23.2	49.9	53.8
Mississippi	20,003	6,094	12,656	854	54.1	32.8	80.1	51.3
Missouri	29,511	17,340	8,048	2,247	40.3	32.3	76.0	51.0
Montana	4,016	2,620	18	253	34.9	28.4	31.0	45.3
Nebraska	8,289	4,277	1,056	2,163	32.5	24.2	60.7	52.1
Nevada	17,231	4,596	3,381	7,324	48.3	35.3	74.1	55.0
New Hampshire	3,946	3,374	80	361	32.9	32.7	33.2	48.5
New Jersey	34,204	7,924	9,073	15,527	33.8	17.4	65.3	56.3
New Mexico	11,785	2,046	207	7,274	51.2	31.7	53.5	56.9
New York	84,767	26,290	21,794	31,143	37.5	23.7	65.8	60.2
North Carolina	48,632	16,685	19,756	9,010	40.9	26.3	71.4	49.1
North Dakota	3,392	1,873	257	297	31.9	24.0	42.2	46.8
Ohio	58,331	34,244	16,769	4,366	43.2	35.1	75.5	58.7
Oklahoma	21,010	9,663	3,016	3,667	42.2	34.0	72.9	48.6
Oregon	15,303	9,085	513	4,020	36.3	32.1	53.5	50.3
Pennsylvania	55,324	27,910	13,428	10,167	40.8	30.7	75.5	64.2
Rhode Island	4,582	2,050	439	1,652	43.6	34.1	56.1	59.9
South Carolina	26,157	9,547	12,827	2,659	46.2	29.9	76.9	50.6
South Dakota	4,290	2,009	159	357	36.1	23.7	38.2	54.0
Tennessee	35,160	17,706	12,168	4,021	43.5	33.2	76.4	51.4
Texas	154,645	31,755	29,458	89,525	40.8	25.3	61.2	50.0
Utah	9,076	4,600	190	3,155	19.2	13.4	36.5	38.8
Vermont	2,093	1,942	42	37	38.5	39.4	35.6	30.6
Virginia	34,665	12,875	13,343	7,086	34.7	23.5	64.0	49.2
Washington	26,760	12,516	1,675	7,671	31.1	25.5	42.7	47.7
West Virginia	8,340	7,403	454	174	45.7	44.5	72.5	46.0
Wisconsin	23,972	12,397	5,510	3,670	37.4	27.2	83.2	57.7
Wyoming	2,183	1,452	25	421	33.3	28.6	*	49.5
Puerto Rico	14,790	311	36	14,418	*	64.8	73.5	69.2
Virgin Islands	NA	NA	NA	NA	NA	NA	NA	NA
Guam	1,951	27	1	3	*	15.9	*	*
American Samoa	NA	NA	NA	NA	NA	NA	NA	NA
Northern Marianas	380	1	–	–	*	*	*	*

NA = Not available.
– = Quantity zero.
* = Estimate does not meet NCHS standards of reliability.
[1]Includes births to race and origin groups not shown separately, such as Hispanic single-race White, Hispanic single-race Black, and non-Hispanic multiple-race women, and births with origin not stated.
[2]Race and Hispanic origin are reported separately on birth certificates; persons of Hispanic origin may be of any race. In this table, non-Hispanic women are classified by race. Race categories are consistent with the 1997 Office of Management and Budget standards. Single race is defined as only one race reported on the birth certificate.
[3]Includes all persons of Hispanic origin of any race.
[4]Excludes data for the territories.

Table 1-34. Educational Attainment of Mother, by Age (Years) and Race and Hispanic Origin of Mother, 2018

(Number; percent.)

Educational attainment and race and Hispanic origin of mother	All ages	Under 20 years	20 to 24 years	25 to 29 years	30 to 34 years	35 to 39 years	40 to 54 years
All races and origins[1]							
Total	100.0	100.0	100.0	100.0	100.0	100.0	100.0
12th grade or less with no diploma	12.7	48.1	16.5	10.4	8.2	9.6	13.2
8th grade or less	3.1	4.3	2.7	2.6	2.9	4.1	6.7
9th–12th grade with no diploma	9.6	43.8	13.8	7.8	5.3	5.5	6.5
High school graduate[2]	25.8	42.0	45.1	27.0	16.2	14.4	15.4
Some college credit, but no degree	20.1	9.5	27.1	24.1	16.6	14.5	14.3
Associate's degree[3]	8.4	0.4	5.8	10.3	9.4	8.6	8.2
Bachelor's degree[4]	20.7	0.0	5.1	21.2	29.4	28.5	25.9
Master's degree[5]	9.6	0.0	0.4	6.0	15.7	18.0	16.4
Doctorate or professional degree[6]	2.8	0.0	0.0	1.1	4.5	6.4	6.6
All births	3,791,712	181,607	726,175	1,099,491	1,090,697	566,786	126,956
Not stated[7]	48,987	2,039	7,309	12,522	14,397	9,481	3,239
Non-Hispanic, single race[8]							
White							
Total	100.0	100.0	100.0	100.0	100.0	100.0	100.0
12th grade or less with no diploma	7.0	42.5	13.4	5.9	3.2	3.1	4.1
8th grade or less	1.3	2.7	2.0	1.3	0.9	1.0	1.9
9th–12th grade with no diploma	5.7	39.9	11.4	4.6	2.3	2.0	2.1
High school graduate[2]	21.4	45.9	43.7	22.7	12.1	10.6	11.5
Some college credit, but no degree	19.4	11.1	28.3	23.3	15.3	13.8	14.4
Associate's degree[3]	9.6	0.5	7.3	12.0	10.0	9.0	8.8
Bachelor's degree[4]	26.6	0.0	6.7	27.2	35.2	33.8	31.9
Master's degree[5]	12.4	0.0	0.5	7.6	18.9	22.2	21.1
Doctorate or professional degree[6]	3.5	0.0	0.0	1.4	5.3	7.6	8.2
All births	1,956,413	65,254	326,575	576,811	624,015	304,062	59,696
Not stated[7]	10,180	375	1,585	2,752	3,040	1,917	511
Black							
Total	100.0	100.0	100.0	100.0	100.0	100.0	100.0
12th grade or less with no diploma	13.2	46.6	13.3	10.3	9.3	9.4	10.7
8th grade or less	1.5	2.4	0.8	1.1	1.8	2.2	3.6
9th–12th grade with no diploma	11.7	44.1	12.5	9.1	7.5	7.2	7.1
High school graduate[2]	35.6	43.4	49.9	35.8	26.0	22.3	21.5
Some college credit, but no degree	25.6	9.7	28.8	29.6	24.8	21.6	19.2
Associate's degree[3]	7.8	0.3	4.2	8.7	10.9	10.9	10.5
Bachelor's degree[4]	11.7	0.0	3.7	12.2	18.1	19.8	19.5
Master's degree[5]	5.0	0.0	0.2	3.2	9.0	12.7	14.4
Doctorate or professional degree[6]	1.1	0.0	0.0	0.4	1.9	3.3	4.2
All births	552,029	38,269	137,974	166,802	124,206	67,268	17,510
Not stated[7]	4,672	307	946	1,310	1,143	725	241
Hispanic[9]							
Total	100.0	100.0	100.0	100.0	100.0	100.0	100.0
12th grade or less with no diploma	26.4	54.2	23.4	21.0	24.2	29.5	35.9
8th grade or less	8.7	7.2	5.2	6.5	10.3	14.7	19.7
9th–12th grade with no diploma	17.8	47.0	18.2	14.5	13.9	14.8	16.2
High school graduate[2]	32.7	37.6	44.8	33.4	25.6	22.6	21.8
Some college credit, but no degree	19.9	7.8	24.0	23.9	18.6	15.1	13.0
Associate's degree[3]	6.6	0.4	4.7	8.3	8.1	7.1	6.3
Bachelor's degree[4]	10.3	0.0	2.9	11.1	16.1	16.1	13.9
Master's degree[5]	3.2	0.0	0.2	2.0	5.9	7.4	6.8
Doctorate or professional degree[6]	0.9	0.0	0.0	0.4	1.5	2.3	2.4
All births	886,210	65,852	209,701	253,977	208,193	117,383	31,104
Not stated[7]	10,965	779	2,136	2,893	2,699	1,856	602

0.0 = Zero events in the numerator or percentage of less than 0.05 percent.
[1]Includes births to race and origin groups not shown separately, such as Hispanic single-race White, Hispanic single-race Black, and non-Hispanic multiple-race women, and births with origin not stated.
[2]Includes GED.
[3]Includes Associate in Arts and Associate in Science.
[4]Includes Bachelor in Arts and Bachelor in Science.
[5]Includes Master in Arts, Master in Science, Master of Engineering, Master of Education, Master of Social Work, and Master of Business Administration.
[6]Includes Doctor of Philosophy, Doctor of Education, Doctor of Medicine, Doctor of Dental Surgery, Doctor of Veterinary Medicine, Doctor of Laws, and Juris Doctor.
[7]No response reported for education attainment of mother item.
[8]Race and Hispanic origin are reported separately on birth certificates; persons of Hispanic origin may be of any race. In this table, non-Hispanic women are classified by race. Race categories are consistent with the 1997 Office of Management and Budget standards. Single race is defined as only one race reported on the birth certificate.
[9]Includes all persons of Hispanic origin of any race.

Table 1-35. Maternal Prepregnancy Body Mass Index, by Age (Years) and Selected Race and Hispanic Origin of Mother, 2018

(Number; percent.)

BMI category and race and Hispanic origin of mother	All ages	Under 20 years	20 to 24 years	25 to 29 years	30 to 34 years	35 to 39 years	40 to 54 years
All races and origins[1]							
Total	100.0	100.0	100.0	100.0	100.0	100.0	100.0
Underweight (BMI less than 18.5)	3.2	6.9	4.7	3.1	2.4	2.0	1.8
Normal weight (BMI of 18.5 to 24.9)	42.1	49.4	41.2	40.4	43.7	42.1	39.0
Overweight (BMI of 25.0 to 29.9)	26.6	23.8	25.4	26.6	26.9	27.8	29.5
Obese (BMI of 30.0 and over)	28.1	19.8	28.7	29.9	27.0	28.1	29.8
Total	3,791,712	181,607	726,175	1,099,491	1,090,697	566,786	126,956
Not stated[2]	85,897	4,754	16,024	23,614	24,052	13,921	3,532
Non-Hispanic, single race[3]							
White							
Total	100.0	100.0	100.0	100.0	100.0	100.0	100.0
Underweight (BMI less than 18.5)	3.1	8.2	5.1	3.0	2.3	2.0	1.8
Normal weight (BMI of 18.5 to 24.9)	45.8	48.7	43.0	44.2	48.0	46.8	44.4
Overweight (BMI of 25.0 to 29.9)	25.3	22.9	24.0	25.4	25.5	26.0	26.9
Obese (BMI of 30.0 and over)	25.8	20.2	27.8	27.3	24.2	25.2	26.8
Total	1,956,413	65,254	326,575	576,811	624,015	304,062	59,696
Not stated[2]	34,730	1,045	5,147	9,500	11,279	6,327	1,432
Black							
Total	100.0	100.0	100.0	100.0	100.0	100.0	100.0
Underweight (BMI less than 18.5)	3.0	6.5	4.6	2.9	1.8	1.2	1.0
Normal weight (BMI of 18.5 to 24.9)	32.1	48.5	38.7	30.9	26.9	23.8	22.6
Overweight (BMI of 25.0 to 29.9)	26.9	23.2	24.6	26.5	28.6	30.2	31.4
Obese (BMI of 30.0 and over)	38.0	21.9	32.1	39.7	42.7	44.7	45.1
Total	552,029	38,269	137,974	166,802	124,206	67,268	17,510
Not stated[2]	17,437	1,409	4,198	4,950	3,956	2,313	611
Hispanic[4]							
Total	100.0	100.0	100.0	100.0	100.0	100.0	100.0
Underweight (BMI less than 18.5)	2.4	5.9	3.7	2.0	1.3	1.0	0.8
Normal weight (BMI of 18.5 to 24.9)	35.9	50.7	39.3	34.4	33.4	31.5	28.8
Overweight (BMI of 25.0 to 29.9)	30.4	25.1	28.3	30.3	31.9	33.1	35.3
Obese (BMI of 30.0 and over)	31.3	18.2	28.7	33.2	33.5	34.4	35.2
Total	886,210	65,852	209,701	253,977	208,193	117,383	31,104
Not stated[2]	22,592	1,882	4,971	6,046	5,491	3,269	933

[1]Includes births to race and origin groups not shown separately, such as Hispanic single-race White, Hispanic single-race Black, and non-Hispanic multiple-race women, and births with origin not stated.
[2]No response reported for component measures for pre-pregnancy BMI.
[3]Race and Hispanic origin are reported separately on birth certificates; persons of Hispanic origin may be of any race. In this table, non-Hispanic women are classified by race. Race categories are consistent with the 1997 Office of Management and Budget standards. Single race is defined as only one race reported on the birth certificate.
[4]Includes all persons of Hispanic origin of any race.

Table 1-36. Live Births by Interval Since Last Birth, by Age (Years) and Selected Race and Hispanic Origin of Mother, 2018

(Number; percent.)

Interval since last live birth and race and Hispanic origin of mother	All ages	Under 20 years	20 to 24 years	25 to 29 years	30 to 34 years	35 to 39 years	40 to 54 years
All races and origins[1]							
Total	100.0	100.0	100.0	100.0	100.0	100.0	100.0
0 to 3 months (plural deliveries)	2.2	4.6	2.0	2.0	2.2	2.4	2.9
4 to 11 months	1.4	7.7	3.1	1.4	0.8	0.6	0.5
12 to 17 months	8.1	27.6	16.1	8.8	5.7	4.5	3.3
18 to 23 months	12.5	21.8	17.7	13.3	11.7	9.3	6.8
24 to 35 months	23.4	23.7	25.7	23.2	24.9	21.2	15.5
36 to 47 months	15.0	9.9	15.7	14.9	15.5	14.7	11.8
48 to 59 months	10.0	3.6	9.7	10.9	9.7	9.9	8.9
60 to 71 months	7.0	0.9	5.4	8.2	6.8	7.1	6.8
72 months and over	20.4	0.3	4.6	17.3	22.5	30.3	43.4
All births	2,357,797	28,455	342,787	689,551	758,205	438,893	99,906
Not stated[2]	121,828	1,585	15,572	32,813	39,053	25,712	7,093
Median interval (months)	37	20	28	36	38	45	60
Non-Hispanic, single race[3]							
White							
Total	100.0	100.0	100.0	100.0	100.0	100.0	100.0
0 to 3 months (plural deliveries)	2.4	4.5	2.0	2.1	2.4	2.6	3.2
4 to 11 months	1.1	7.1	2.6	1.1	0.7	0.6	0.5
12 to 17 months	7.6	28.9	16.4	8.6	5.4	4.4	3.5
18 to 23 months	14.3	23.1	20.0	15.6	13.5	10.8	8.4
24 to 35 months	27.9	23.7	27.9	27.7	30.3	25.7	19.6
36 to 47 months	16.3	8.9	15.4	15.5	17.3	16.8	13.9
48 to 59 months	9.4	2.8	8.5	9.8	9.2	10.3	9.7
60 to 71 months	5.9	0.7	4.2	6.8	5.6	6.5	6.7
72 months and over	15.1	0.2	3.0	12.8	15.7	22.2	34.7
All births	1,187,741	9,325	147,271	338,676	418,306	229,075	45,088
Not stated[2]	55,462	472	6,259	14,268	19,338	12,139	2,986
Median interval (months)	34	20	27	33	34	39	49
Black							
Total	100.0	100.0	100.0	100.0	100.0	100.0	100.0
0 to 3 months (plural deliveries)	2.6	6.2	2.8	2.5	2.5	2.5	3.0
4 to 11 months	2.3	8.5	4.2	2.3	1.4	1.0	0.6
12 to 17 months	10.5	27.8	18.4	10.3	7.6	5.8	3.7
18 to 23 months	11.2	19.8	16.5	11.2	9.5	7.9	5.6
24 to 35 months	17.8	22.1	23.5	17.7	16.2	14.6	11.9
36 to 47 months	12.8	10.1	14.8	13.5	12.0	11.0	10.3
48 to 59 months	10.0	4.0	9.3	11.5	9.7	9.1	8.4
60 to 71 months	7.7	1.1	5.4	9.4	7.9	7.3	7.2
72 months and over	25.2	0.4	5.1	21.7	33.2	41.0	49.3
All births	357,940	6,211	67,728	118,251	96,647	54,830	14,273
Not stated[2]	22,515	349	3,372	6,769	6,381	4,319	1,325
Median interval (months)	40	20	27	41	48	57	70
Hispanic[4]							
Total	100.0	100.0	100.0	100.0	100.0	100.0	100.0
0 to 3 months (plural deliveries)	1.7	3.7	1.6	1.5	1.7	1.8	2.1
4 to 11 months	1.5	7.4	2.8	1.4	0.9	0.7	0.5
12 to 17 months	7.8	26.1	13.6	7.8	5.5	4.5	2.8
18 to 23 months	10.1	21.8	15.2	10.2	8.5	7.0	4.9
24 to 35 months	17.9	24.8	24.2	18.2	16.6	14.1	10.7
36 to 47 months	13.5	10.8	16.8	14.5	12.6	11.1	8.8
48 to 59 months	10.7	4.2	11.8	12.4	10.3	8.8	7.5
60 to 71 months	8.4	0.9	7.2	10.1	8.6	7.5	6.4
72 months and over	28.5	0.4	6.7	24.0	35.2	44.6	56.3
All births	583,161	10,970	104,291	178,931	163,270	98,918	26,781
Not stated[2]	29,703	594	4,659	8,612	8,487	5,592	1,759
Median interval (months)	45	21	31	44	52	63	85

[1]Includes births to race and origin groups not shown separately, such as Hispanic single-race White, Hispanic single-race Black, and non-Hispanic multiple-race women, and births with origin not stated.
[2]No response reported for interval since last live birth.
[3]Race and Hispanic origin are reported separately on birth certificates; persons of Hispanic origin may be of any race. In this table, non-Hispanic women are classified by race. Race categories are consistent with the 1997 Office of Management and Budget standards. Single race is defined as only one race reported on the birth certificate.
[4]Includes all persons of Hispanic origin of any race.

Table 1-37. Mother Received WIC food for Herself During This Pregnancy and Infant Was Being Breastfed at Discharge, by Age (Years) and Selected Race and Hispanic Origin of Mother, 2018

(Number; percent.)

Selected characteristic and race and Hispanic origin of mother	All births	Characteristic reported	All ages	Under 20 years	20 to 24 years	25 to 29 years	30 to 34 years	35 to 39 years	40 to 54 years	Not stated[1]
All races and origins[2]										
Mother received WIC food for herself during this pregnancy................	3,791,712	1,351,158	36.0	70.5	55.5	36.5	24.5	23.6	26.2	42,078
Infant was being breastfed at discharge[3]..	3,226,760	2,671,835	83.5	72.6	78.4	83.2	87.2	87.2	86.0	27,979
Non-Hispanic, single race[4]										
White										
Mother received WIC food for herself during this pregnancy.............	1,956,413	457,170	23.6	67.5	46.3	24.0	13.4	12.1	13.0	17,742
Infant was being breastfed at discharge[3]...	1,758,497	1,481,074	84.9	70.5	78.8	84.6	88.4	88.2	86.9	14,763
Black										
Mother received WIC food for herself during this pregnancy.............	552,029	297,866	54.6	72.4	64.3	54.7	46.9	42.6	40.4	6,970
Infant was being breastfed at discharge[3]...	509,091	364,257	72.3	60.4	67.5	71.9	77.1	79.0	80.3	5,182
Hispanic[5]										
Mother received WIC food for herself during this pregnancy................	886,210	487,752	55.5	73.1	64.4	54.2	48.0	47.9	49.2	8,130
Infant was being breastfed at discharge[3]..	667,800	577,212	87.1	83.2	85.9	87.4	88.5	88.3	87.2	4,941

NOTE: WIC is Special Supplemental Nutrition Program for Women, Infants, and Children.

[1]No response reported for selected characteristic.

[2]Includes births to race and origin groups not shown separately, such as Hispanic single-race White, Hispanic single-race Black, and non-Hispanic multiple-race women, and births with origin not stated.

[3]Excludes data for California which did not report infant was being breastfed at discharge. Also excludes Michigan, for which item wording is not consistent with national standard.

[4]Race and Hispanic origin are reported separately on birth certificates; persons of Hispanic origin may be of any race. In this table, non-Hispanic women are classified by race. Race categories are consistent with the 1997 Office of Management and Budget standards. Single race is defined as only one race reported on the birth certificate.

[5]Includes all persons of Hispanic origin of any race.

Table 1-38. Pregnancy Risk Factors, by Age (Years) and Selected Race and Hispanic Origin of Mother, 2018

(Number; rate per 1,000 live births in group.)

Risk factor and race and Hispanic origin of mother	All births	Factor reported	All ages	Under 20 years	20 to 24 years	25 to 29 years	30 to 34 years	35 to 39 years	40 to 54 years	Not stated[1]
All races and origins[2]										
Diabetes										
Prepregnancy (diagnosis prior to this pregnancy)	3,791,712	35,735	9.4	4.0	6.1	7.7	9.9	15.0	22.1	2,882
Gestational (diagnosis in this pregnancy)	3,791,712	252,522	66.6	21.8	36.6	56.1	76.9	104.3	137.9	2,882
Hypertension										
Prepregnancy (chronic)	3,791,712	78,310	20.7	7.4	12.6	17.0	22.1	33.0	49.3	2,882
Gestational (PIH[3], preeclampsia)	3,791,712	271,596	71.7	77.1	72.1	69.3	68.9	74.7	92.6	2,882
Eclampsia[4]	3,654,292	9,449	2.6	3.4	2.8	2.3	2.3	2.9	3.8	2,837
Previous preterm birth	3,791,712	134,038	35.4	8.3	26.3	35.7	38.3	46.1	51.1	2,882
Pregnancy resulted from infertility treatment	3,791,712	73,709	19.5	0.3	2.3	9.3	23.6	42.0	96.4	2,882
Mother had a previous cesarean delivery[5]	2,611,486	591,618	226.7	102.4	165.4	210.5	240.4	276.5	291.7	1,426
Non-Hispanic, single race[6]										
White										
Diabetes										
Prepregnancy (diagnosis prior to this pregnancy)	1,956,413	14,863	7.6	4.5	6.2	6.6	7.5	10.5	14.4	1,224
Gestational (diagnosis in this pregnancy)	1,956,413	117,673	60.2	25.4	38.3	52.4	64.5	86.3	115.1	1,224
Hypertension										
Prepregnancy (chronic)	1,956,413	37,880	19.4	8.3	13.1	16.2	20.1	28.4	42.4	1,224
Gestational (PIH[3], preeclampsia)	1,956,413	149,415	76.4	83.1	79.5	76.5	72.7	75.9	93.2	1,224
Eclampsia[4]	1,871,267	4,588	2.5	3.4	2.9	2.3	2.2	2.6	3.2	1,210
Previous preterm birth	1,956,413	64,270	32.9	8.1	24.8	31.3	34.6	43.0	49.6	1,224
Pregnancy resulted from infertility treatment	1,956,413	52,164	26.7	0.4	3.6	13.7	30.8	53.8	125.7	1,224
Mother had a previous cesarean delivery[5]	1,325,823	282,921	213.5	91.1	155.2	192.6	222.4	263.0	280.6	751
Black										
Diabetes										
Prepregnancy (diagnosis prior to this pregnancy)	552,029	6,876	12.5	3.9	6.8	10.1	15.6	24.0	31.2	495
Gestational (diagnosis in this pregnancy)	552,029	28,915	52.4	16.0	26.8	44.5	70.5	95.2	116.6	495
Hypertension										
Prepregnancy (chronic)	552,029	22,601	41.0	11.2	20.4	33.5	52.3	80.8	106.5	495
Gestational (PIH[3], preeclampsia)	552,029	47,737	86.6	92.7	82.7	80.5	88.0	97.1	110.2	495
Eclampsia[4]	519,427	1,731	3.3	4.3	3.0	2.8	3.4	4.2	4.9	484
Previous preterm birth	552,029	28,604	51.9	10.6	34.5	56.7	64.8	70.1	70.4	495
Pregnancy resulted from infertility treatment	552,029	3,879	7.0	0.3	0.9	2.9	8.6	18.5	54.7	495
Mother had a previous cesarean delivery[5]	398,918	97,252	244.0	112.7	177.1	236.6	274.7	300.0	311.5	273
Hispanic[7]										
Diabetes										
Prepregnancy (diagnosis prior to this pregnancy)	886,210	9,749	11.0	3.6	5.4	8.5	13.3	21.0	31.6	392
Gestational (diagnosis in this pregnancy)	886,210	63,931	72.2	20.7	37.5	60.8	91.2	127.7	170.7	392
Hypertension										
Prepregnancy (chronic)	886,210	11,961	13.5	4.5	7.5	10.4	15.7	25.3	39.3	392
Gestational (PIH[3], preeclampsia)	886,210	52,650	59.4	62.6	55.9	53.7	59.1	69.2	89.3	392
Eclampsia[4]	873,131	1,841	2.1	2.5	2.2	1.9	1.9	2.4	3.2	385
Previous preterm birth	886,210	29,579	33.4	7.3	23.2	34.4	40.1	47.8	50.1	392
Pregnancy resulted from infertility treatment	886,210	6,350	7.2	0.1	1.0	3.5	9.0	17.6	41.7	392
Mother had a previous cesarean delivery[5]	629,539	152,073	241.6	110.4	175.6	232.5	267.7	294.0	298.6	223

NOTE: Rates are number of live births with specified risk factor per 1,000 live births in specified group.
[1]No response reported for pregnancy risk factor item.
[2]Includes births to race and origin groups not shown separately, such as Hispanic single-race White, Hispanic single-race Black, and non-Hispanic multiple-race women, and births with origin not stated.
[3]PIH is pregnancy-induced hypertension.
[4]Excludes data for South Carolina and Tennessee.
[5]Excludes women who have not had a previous pregnancy and for whom total birth order is unknown.
[6]Race and Hispanic origin are reported separately on birth certificates; persons of Hispanic origin may be of any race. In this table, non-Hispanic women are classified by race. Race categories are consistent with the 1997 Office of Management and Budget standards. Single race is defined as only one race reported on the birth certificate.
[7]Includes all persons of Hispanic origin of any race.

Table 1-39. Infections Present or Treated During This Pregnancy, by Age (Years) and Selected Race and Hispanic Origin of Mother, 2018

(Number; rate per 100,000 live births in group.)

Infection and race and Hispanic origin of mother	All births	Factor reported	All ages	Under 20 years	20 to 24 years	25 to 29 years	30 to 34 years	35 to 39 years	40 to 54 years	Not stated[1]
All races and origins[2]										
Gonorrhea	3,791,712	11,734	310.2	1,151.5	631.5	279.5	128.6	92.1	67.9	8,460
Syphilis	3,791,712	4,416	116.7	152.9	166.3	122.7	85.4	90.9	113.8	8,460
Chlamydia	3,791,712	69,758	1,843.9	7,288.4	4,062.2	1,549.1	659.3	438.9	375.2	8,460
Hepatitis B	3,791,712	8,192	216.5	67.9	106.7	181.2	262.7	332.1	450.3	8,460
Hepatitis C	3,791,712	18,927	500.3	157.9	433.7	659.1	495.8	431.3	341.3	8,460
Non-Hispanic, single race[3]										
White										
Gonorrhea	1,956,413	3,317	169.9	654.3	370.4	168.7	80.3	60.6	48.7	3,831
Syphilis	1,956,413	1,029	52.7	84.5	83.5	51.6	41.4	37.9	53.7	3,831
Chlamydia	1,956,413	21,816	1,117.3	5,368.0	2,882.0	966.0	389.5	264.3	236.7	3,831
Hepatitis B	1,956,413	1,609	82.4	46.1	60.2	75.2	94.2	97.2	114.2	3,831
Hepatitis C	1,956,413	15,282	782.7	290.3	768.5	1,044.7	704.9	620.4	505.3	3,831
Black										
Gonorrhea	552,029	5,494	998.2	2,915.5	1,640.2	846.9	418.2	247.6	189.4	1,636
Syphilis	552,029	1,809	328.7	291.0	378.8	360.6	281.0	261.0	310.0	1,636
Chlamydia	552,029	23,207	4,216.4	12,556.0	7,124.2	3,453.8	1,703.5	948.5	729.0	1,636
Hepatitis B	552,029	2,133	387.5	112.7	169.4	336.0	557.9	662.1	935.7	1,636
Hepatitis C	552,029	798	145.0	62.9	101.1	151.5	166.3	207.3	218.1	1,636
Hispanic[4]										
Gonorrhea	886,210	1,874	211.9	531.2	343.5	170.0	118.9	93.1	61.3	1,885
Syphilis	886,210	1,197	135.4	137.0	157.2	132.9	112.6	143.5	125.8	1,885
Chlamydia	886,210	19,025	2,151.4	5,870.8	3,835.9	1,715.2	909.8	638.9	493.5	1,885
Hepatitis B	886,210	684	77.3	33.5	64.0	77.3	84.7	99.9	125.8	1,885
Hepatitis C	886,210	1,380	156.1	71.5	122.8	181.9	173.8	181.9	132.2	1,885

NOTE: Rates are number of live births with specified infection per 100,000 live births in specified group.

[1]No response reported for infection item.

[2]Includes births to race and origin groups not shown separately, such as Hispanic single-race White, Hispanic single-race Black, and non-Hispanic multiple-race women, and births with origin not stated.

[3]Race and Hispanic origin are reported separately on birth certificates; persons of Hispanic origin may be of any race. In this table, non-Hispanic women are classified by race. Race categories are consistent with the 1997 Office of Management and Budget standards. Single race is defined as only one race reported on the birth certificate.

[4]Includes all persons of Hispanic origin of any race.

Table 1-40. External Cephalic Version, by Age (Years) and Selected Race and Hispanic Origin of Mother, 2018

(Number; rate per 1,000 live births in group; percent.)

Characteristic and race and Hispanic origin of mother	All births[1]	Procedure reported	All ages	Under 20 years	20 to 24 years	25 to 29 years	30 to 34 years	35 to 39 years	40 to 54 years	Not stated[2]
All races and origins[3]										
External cephalic version	3,791,712	10,934	2.9	1.6	2.1	2.7	3.3	3.6	4.1	3,511
Percent successful[4]	10,934	5,645	51.6	46.6	47.0	49.4	52.1	55.6	61.5	–
Non-Hispanic, single race[5]										
White										
External cephalic version	1,956,413	6,843	3.5	1.7	2.5	3.3	3.9	4.3	4.9	1,469
Percent successful[4]	6,843	3,322	48.5	33.6	39.8	46.3	50.1	53.2	59.3	–
Black										
External cephalic version	552,029	974	1.8	1.3	1.5	1.5	2.1	2.3	2.7	698
Percent successful[4]	974	584	60.0	60.0	60.1	56.7	59.4	63.2	68.8	–
Hispanic[6]										
External cephalic version	886,210	1,861	2.1	1.6	1.6	1.9	2.4	2.7	3.4	509
Percent successful[4]	1,861	1,071	57.5	51.9	54.4	55.8	59.0	60.9	64.5	–

NOTE: Rates are number of live births with specified obstetric procedure per 1,000 live births in specified group.
– = Quantity zero.
[1]Number for percent successful is women with an external cephalic version (ECV) in specified group.
[2]No response reported for obstetric procedure item.
[3]Includes births to race and origin groups not shown separately, such as Hispanic single-race White, Hispanic single-race Black, and non-Hispanic multiple-race women, and births with origin not stated.
[4]Percent successful ECV is the number of successful ECVs per 100 live births to women with an ECV in specified group.
[5]Race and Hispanic origin are reported separately on birth certificates; persons of Hispanic origin may be of any race. In this table, non-Hispanic women are classified by race. Race categories are consistent with the 1997 Office of Management and Budget standards. Single race is defined as only one race reported on the birth certificate.
[6]Includes all persons of Hispanic origin of any race.

Table 1-41. Characteristics of Labor and Delivery, by Age (Years) and Selected Race and Hispanic Origin of Mother, 2018

(Number; rate per 1,000 live births in group.)

Labor and delivery characteristic and race and Hispanic origin of mother	All births	Procedure reported	All ages	Under 20 years	20 to 24 years	25 to 29 years	30 to 34 years	35 to 39 years	40 to 54 years	Not stated[1]
All races and origins[2]										
Induction of labor	3,791,712	1,025,834	270.8	308.4	294.7	274.7	255.6	250.1	271.1	4,151
Augmentation of labor	3,791,712	816,748	215.5	269.0	244.0	223.2	205.6	179.2	154.9	1,369
Steroids (glucocorticoids) for fetal lung maturation	3,791,712	131,900	34.8	37.8	34.1	32.9	33.4	38.2	47.7	1,369
Antibiotics received by mother during labor	3,791,712	956,104	252.2	261.8	251.7	244.3	250.8	262.3	278.0	1,369
Clinical chorioamnionitis during labor	3,791,712	60,805	16.0	24.9	19.4	16.3	14.7	12.1	11.0	1,369
Epidural or spinal anesthesia during labor	3,791,712	2,846,929	751.1	783.0	762.8	748.5	746.5	741.7	741.7	1,369
Non-Hispanic, single race[3]										
White										
Induction of labor	1,956,413	592,611	303.4	374.5	344.2	311.6	282.1	273.8	297.9	3,240
Augmentation of labor	1,956,413	423,055	216.3	267.9	242.7	227.5	209.2	182.1	155.3	716
Steroids (glucocorticoids) for fetal lung maturation	1,956,413	67,522	34.5	40.9	35.3	32.8	32.8	36.8	46.9	716
Antibiotics received by mother during labor	1,956,413	480,567	245.7	253.2	240.3	236.8	245.9	260.1	278.1	716
Clinical chorioamnionitis during labor	1,956,413	24,191	12.4	16.1	14.0	12.9	12.0	10.0	9.5	716
Epidural or spinal anesthesia during labor	1,956,413	1,495,272	764.6	820.4	786.1	764.2	756.5	749.9	748.4	716
Black										
Induction of labor	552,029	138,976	251.9	290.9	266.1	246.1	236.7	242.7	254.1	327
Augmentation of labor	552,029	110,329	199.9	248.5	231.0	200.7	180.8	157.5	140.4	211
Steroids (glucocorticoids) for fetal lung maturation	552,029	26,375	47.8	47.0	44.4	46.3	47.7	55.5	61.5	211
Antibiotics received by mother during labor	552,029	156,419	283.5	308.9	294.2	278.0	275.9	274.3	284.2	211
Clinical chorioamnionitis during labor	552,029	8,570	15.5	22.1	18.3	15.8	13.1	11.5	9.8	211
Epidural or spinal anesthesia during labor	552,029	412,447	747.4	779.0	761.9	741.8	734.8	737.4	746.3	211
Hispanic[4]										
Induction of labor	886,210	202,135	228.1	256.2	244.0	224.0	211.4	217.9	247.1	232
Augmentation of labor	886,210	190,136	214.6	278.2	249.7	215.9	191.4	170.8	152.3	179
Steroids (glucocorticoids) for fetal lung maturation	886,210	25,750	29.1	29.5	25.6	26.5	29.9	35.4	42.9	179
Antibiotics received by mother during labor	886,210	213,614	241.1	239.1	238.9	234.8	242.2	251.9	263.4	179
Clinical chorioamnionitis during labor	886,210	17,666	19.9	35.0	27.2	19.3	14.8	11.5	10.6	179
Epidural or spinal anesthesia during labor	886,210	640,099	722.4	753.1	734.9	719.6	711.9	710.0	713.9	179

NOTE: Rates are number of live births with characteristic per 1,000 live births in specified group.
[1]No response reported for selected characteristic.
[2]Includes births to race and origin groups not shown separately, such as Hispanic single-race White, Hispanic single-race Black, and non-Hispanic multiple-race women, and births with origin not stated.
[3]Race and Hispanic origin are reported separately on birth certificates; persons of Hispanic origin may be of any race. In this table, non-Hispanic women are classified by race. Race categories are consistent with the 1997 Office of Management and Budget standards. Single race is defined as only one race reported on the birth certificate.
[4]Includes all persons of Hispanic origin of any race.

Table 1-42. Total Cesarean Delivery and Low-Risk Cesarean Delivery, by Selected Race and Hispanic Origin of Mother, by State and Territory of Residence, 2018

(Percent.)

State and territory	Total cesarean delivery rate[1]				Low-risk cesarean delivery rate[2]			
	All races and origins[3]	Non-Hispanic, single race[4]		Hispanic[5]	All races and origins[3]	Non-Hispanic, single race[4]		Hispanic[5]
		White	Black			White[4]	Black[4]	
United States[6]	31.9	30.8	36.1	31.6	25.9	24.9	30.3	25.4
Alabama............................	34.7	34.1	37.9	26.5	28.6	27.9	31.3	22.5
Alaska..............................	22.4	24.6	26.8	25.7	16.7	18.4	16.5	15.6
Arizona.............................	27.5	27.4	34.2	26.7	21.3	21.1	27.7	20.8
Arkansas...........................	34.8	35.0	37.1	31.1	28.4	27.8	31.8	25.0
California...........................	30.9	29.8	35.7	30.6	24.0	23.3	28.5	23.3
Colorado	26.1	26.3	29.5	24.1	21.2	21.3	27.4	18.8
Connecticut........................	34.8	34.4	39.0	33.8	29.4	29.1	34.2	27.9
Delaware...........................	31.3	30.6	33.4	28.6	24.1	24.4	26.0	18.7
District of Columbia	31.5	29.1	33.9	28.7	28.0	24.1	31.6	27.8
Florida..............................	36.8	33.9	38.4	40.2	30.4	27.6	31.7	33.8
Georgia	34.0	33.5	36.2	30.0	27.9	27.3	30.2	23.7
Hawaii..............................	26.9	25.0	33.3	26.4	22.4	20.4	24.8	21.7
Idaho...............................	24.0	23.6	32.6	24.7	18.5	17.9	34.9	18.0
Illinois..............................	31.2	31.2	32.9	28.9	25.2	24.6	27.5	23.8
Indiana.............................	29.8	29.5	32.8	28.5	23.5	23.3	25.6	21.7
Iowa................................	29.8	29.6	32.1	28.8	23.4	22.9	31.6	22.0
Kansas.............................	29.7	30.1	31.9	26.9	24.2	24.3	25.2	22.2
Kentucky...........................	34.3	34.6	35.9	29.8	27.8	27.9	29.5	25.2
Louisiana	37.0	37.1	37.9	33.9	29.3	29.3	30.4	25.0
Maine...............................	30.4	30.1	33.0	29.0	25.0	24.6	29.5	26.1
Maryland...........................	33.9	31.9	39.3	28.4	28.2	26.2	33.1	22.7
Massachusetts.....................	31.5	31.1	37.0	31.0	25.4	25.1	32.3	23.8
Michigan	32.1	31.5	34.4	30.9	27.3	26.2	31.5	25.8
Minnesota..........................	27.0	27.0	29.4	26.3	22.9	22.5	28.2	21.4
Mississippi.........................	38.3	37.6	40.1	30.1	31.2	30.2	32.9	24.4
Missouri............................	30.0	29.9	30.6	27.4	23.9	23.3	26.4	22.9
Montana............................	28.1	27.5	25.9	30.5	22.7	22.1	*	28.6
Nebraska...........................	29.9	30.5	32.4	26.7	22.5	22.1	26.0	22.1
Nevada.............................	33.8	32.8	40.9	31.8	28.0	27.1	34.2	26.2
New Hampshire....................	31.6	31.4	39.0	32.0	27.0	26.6	42.3	25.1
New Jersey	34.9	32.6	38.4	35.9	27.8	26.3	31.3	27.3
New Mexico	25.3	25.0	32.3	25.7	19.6	18.9	28.3	19.7
New York...........................	33.9	31.3	38.9	36.0	28.9	27.2	33.6	29.9
North Carolina.....................	29.4	29.5	32.2	24.9	23.3	22.8	26.3	20.2
North Dakota......................	26.5	25.6	30.5	23.5	19.3	18.6	29.9	11.7
Ohio................................	30.8	30.4	32.3	29.0	25.4	24.8	28.4	23.4
Oklahoma..........................	32.8	32.9	37.1	29.6	24.6	24.5	29.6	21.3
Oregon.............................	28.0	27.5	35.5	27.8	23.8	23.0	34.5	23.8
Pennsylvania.......................	30.1	29.6	31.8	30.6	25.1	24.8	27.8	23.2
Rhode Island.......................	32.2	32.9	34.2	30.8	27.8	28.3	30.0	24.9
South Carolina	33.5	32.9	36.5	28.4	26.9	25.7	30.6	23.9
South Dakota	24.6	24.2	27.9	23.4	18.7	17.8	34.3	18.7
Tennessee	32.4	32.1	34.9	28.9	26.4	26.0	28.7	23.6
Texas...............................	35.0	33.9	40.3	34.3	28.7	27.3	33.4	28.2
Utah................................	22.7	21.6	28.8	24.7	18.3	17.0	31.3	19.8
Vermont............................	25.9	25.6	37.3	24.0	20.3	20.0	*	*
Virginia.............................	32.4	31.0	36.1	29.9	25.8	24.7	29.0	22.9
Washington.........................	27.9	26.8	33.7	26.6	23.1	22.4	28.1	21.2
West Virginia.......................	34.1	34.0	38.7	34.5	27.3	27.2	27.6	31.6
Wisconsin	26.6	26.7	27.6	26.5	22.3	22.0	25.6	21.4
Wyoming	27.4	27.5	36.8	26.9	20.4	20.7	*	19.2
Puerto Rico.........................	46.3	46.0	46.9	46.4	41.9	42.3	*	41.8
Virgin Islands......................	NA	NA	NA	NA	NA	NA	NA	NA
Guam...............................	25.4	21.9	*	*	23.1	28.6	*	*
American Samoa...................	NA	NA	NA	NA	NA	NA	NA	NA
Northern Marianas.................	31.5	*	*	*	32.3	*	*	*

NA = Not available.
* = Estimate does not meet NCHS standards of reliability.
[1]Percent of all live births by cesarean delivery.
[2]Low-risk cesarean is defined as singleton, term (37 or more weeks of gestation), vertex (not breech) cesarean deliveries to women having a first birth per 100 women delivering singleton, term, vertex first births.
[3]Includes births to race and origin groups not shown separately, such as Hispanic single-race White, Hispanic single-race Black, and non-Hispanic multiple-race women, and births with origin not stated.
[4]Race and Hispanic origin are reported separately on birth certificates; persons of Hispanic origin may be of any race. In this table, non-Hispanic women are classified by race. Race categories are consistent with the 1997 Office of Management and Budget standard. Single race is defined as only one race reported on the birth certificate.
[5]Includes all persons of Hispanic origin of any race.
[6]Excludes data for the territories.

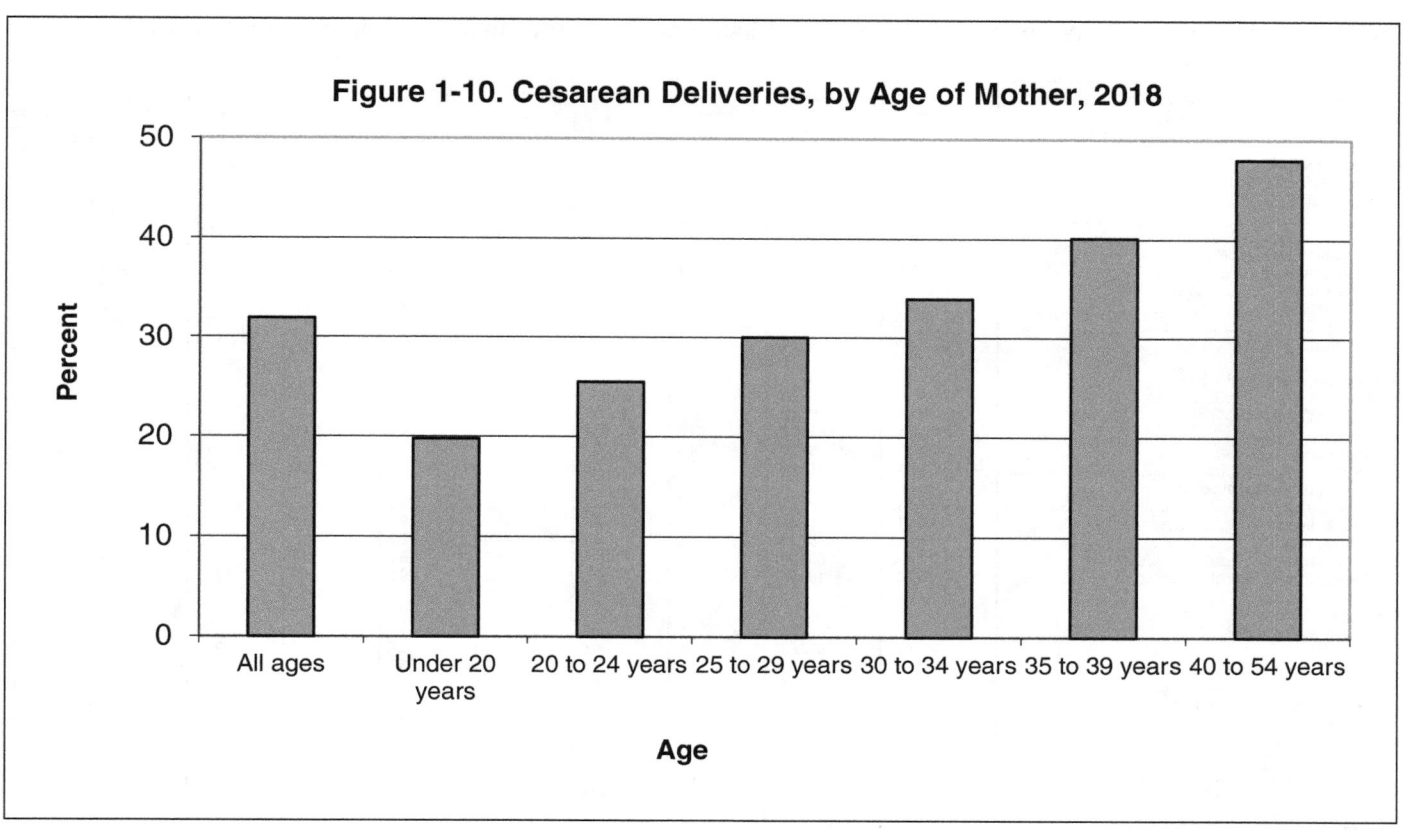

Figure 1-10. Cesarean Deliveries, by Age of Mother, 2018

Table 1-43. Method of Delivery, by Age (Years) and Selected Race and Hispanic Origin of Mother, 2018

(Number; rate per 100 live births in group.)

Method of delivery characteristic and race and Hispanic origin of mother	All births[1]	Method reported	All ages	Under 20 years	20 to 24 years	25 to 29 years	30 to 34 years	35 to 39 years	40 to 54 years	Not stated[2]
All races and origins[3]										
Fetal presentation at birth										
Cephalic	3,791,712	3,596,499	95.2	96.7	96.3	95.6	94.8	93.9	92.3	12,637
Breech	3,791,712	150,057	4.0	2.6	2.9	3.6	4.4	5.1	6.5	12,637
Other	3,791,712	32,519	0.9	0.8	0.8	0.8	0.9	1.0	1.2	12,637
Final route and method of delivery										
Vaginal, spontaneous	3,791,712	2,466,372	65.1	75.9	71.2	67.0	63.1	57.2	49.6	1,544
Vaginal, forceps	3,791,712	19,439	0.5	0.6	0.5	0.5	0.5	0.5	0.5	1,544
Vaginal, vacuum	3,791,712	96,181	2.5	3.8	2.7	2.5	2.5	2.2	1.9	1,544
Cesarean	3,791,712	1,208,176	31.9	19.8	25.5	30.0	33.9	40.1	48.0	1,544
Cesarean, trial of labor attempted[4]	1,208,176	317,704	26.4	49.4	35.6	27.8	23.5	19.9	19.8	6,203
Non-Hispanic, single race[5]										
White										
Fetal presentation at birth										
Cephalic	1,956,413	1,849,663	94.8	96.2	95.9	95.2	94.5	93.8	92.1	5,743
Breech	1,956,413	84,776	4.3	3.1	3.4	4.0	4.6	5.3	6.7	5,743
Other	1,956,413	16,231	0.8	0.7	0.8	0.8	0.8	0.9	1.2	5,743
Final route and method of delivery										
Vaginal, spontaneous	1,956,413	1,290,705	66.0	75.1	71.5	68.2	64.9	59.1	51.3	628
Vaginal, forceps	1,956,413	11,525	0.6	0.7	0.6	0.6	0.6	0.5	0.5	628
Vaginal, vacuum	1,956,413	51,194	2.6	4.2	3.0	2.7	2.5	2.2	2.0	628
Cesarean	1,956,413	602,361	30.8	20.0	24.9	28.6	32.0	38.2	46.2	628
Cesarean, trial of labor attempted[4]	602,361	163,947	27.3	52.2	36.9	29.6	24.6	20.9	21.0	2,630
Black										
Fetal presentation at birth										
Cephalic	552,029	525,630	95.5	96.9	96.5	95.8	95.0	93.7	92.2	1,648
Breech	552,029	19,602	3.6	2.2	2.6	3.3	4.1	5.2	6.7	1,648
Other	552,029	5,149	0.9	0.8	0.9	0.9	1.0	1.1	1.1	1,648
Final route and method of delivery										
Vaginal, spontaneous	552,029	339,161	61.5	73.2	67.8	62.5	57.3	51.1	44.6	162
Vaginal, forceps	552,029	2,065	0.4	0.6	0.4	0.3	0.3	0.3	0.3	162
Vaginal, vacuum	552,029	11,524	2.1	3.8	2.5	1.9	1.7	1.5	1.1	162
Cesarean	552,029	199,117	36.1	22.4	29.2	35.2	40.6	47.1	54.0	162
Cesarean, trial of labor attempted[4]	199,117	55,339	27.9	49.6	36.4	27.5	23.7	21.0	20.8	1,088
Hispanic[6]										
Fetal presentation at birth										
Cephalic	886,210	845,165	95.7	97.0	96.7	96.1	95.1	94.1	92.7	3,202
Breech	886,210	29,973	3.4	2.2	2.5	3.0	4.0	4.8	5.9	3,202
Other	886,210	7,870	0.9	0.8	0.8	0.8	0.9	1.1	1.4	3,202
Final route and method of delivery										
Vaginal, spontaneous	886,210	583,866	65.9	78.0	72.6	67.0	61.7	56.4	50.3	150
Vaginal, forceps	886,210	3,258	0.4	0.5	0.4	0.3	0.3	0.3	0.3	150
Vaginal, vacuum	886,210	18,550	2.1	3.3	2.4	1.9	1.9	1.7	1.7	150
Cesarean	886,210	280,386	31.6	18.2	24.7	30.7	36.1	41.6	47.7	150
Cesarean, trial of labor attempted[4]	280,386	64,674	23.2	45.7	32.3	22.9	18.9	17.0	17.3	1,979

NOTE: Percentages are number of live births with specified method of delivery per 100 live births in specified group.
[1] Total for vaginal birth after cesarean delivery is the number of births to women delivering after a previous cesarean. Total for primary cesarean is the number of births to women delivering without a previous cesarean. Total for "cesarean, trial of labor attempted" is the number of women delivering by cesarean.
[2] No response reported for selected characteristic.
[3] Includes births to race and origin groups not shown separately, such as Hispanic single-race White, Hispanic single-race Black, and non-Hispanic multiple-race women, and births with origin not stated.
[4] Number of women who attempted a trial of labor before cesarean delivery per 100 cesarean births.
[5] Race and Hispanic origin are reported separately on birth certificates; persons of Hispanic origin may be of any race. In this table, non-Hispanic women are classified by race. Race categories are consistent with the 1997 Office of Management and Budget standards. Single race is defined as only one race reported on the birth certificate.
[6] Includes all persons of Hispanic origin of any race.

Table 1-44. Maternal Morbidity, by Age (Years) and Selected Race and Hispanic Origin of Mother, 2018

(Number; rate per 100 live births in group.)

Maternal morbidity characteristic and race and Hispanic origin of mother	All births	Method reported	All ages	Under 20 years	20 to 24 years	25 to 29 years	30 to 34 years	35 to 39 years	40 to 54 years	Not stated[1]
All races and origins[2]										
Maternal transfusion	3,791,712	15,646	413.0	572.6	415.7	376.2	377.1	456.7	601.7	3,464
Third- or fourth-degree perineal laceration	3,791,712	31,532	832.4	929.7	784.1	894.2	920.4	655.8	465.2	3,464
Ruptured uterus	3,791,712	1,315	34.7	17.6	24.4	29.9	39.5	46.4	67.0	3,464
Unplanned hysterectomy	3,791,712	1,773	46.8	7.7	15.4	33.9	54.8	84.8	156.1	3,464
Admission to the intensive care unit	3,791,712	6,309	166.5	147.1	125.3	140.8	165.0	233.5	367.5	3,464
Non-Hispanic, single race[3]										
White										
Maternal transfusion	1,956,413	7,538	385.6	552.2	390.1	353.3	357.5	439.5	511.5	1,617
Third- or fourth-degree perineal laceration	1,956,413	18,467	944.7	966.4	894.9	1,048.2	1,011.4	740.7	534.9	1,617
Ruptured uterus	1,956,413	637	32.6	10.7	21.1	25.3	39.1	45.1	57.0	1,617
Unplanned hysterectomy	1,956,413	829	42.4	9.2	16.9	28.1	47.8	73.1	144.2	1,617
Admission to the intensive care unit	1,956,413	2,806	143.5	135.0	115.8	126.0	138.6	191.6	281.7	1,617
Black										
Maternal transfusion	552,029	2,872	520.7	536.1	465.7	490.9	511.7	620.6	886.2	506
Third- or fourth-degree perineal laceration	552,029	2,383	432.1	771.4	476.6	399.6	419.9	303.6	228.7	506
Ruptured uterus	552,029	249	45.1	26.1	38.4	45.6	49.2	46.1	102.9	506
Unplanned hysterectomy	552,029	302	54.8	10.5	9.4	45.6	76.6	122.0	183.0	506
Admission to the intensive care unit	552,029	1,329	241.0	170.0	164.7	201.6	268.4	385.4	623.2	506
Hispanic[4]										
Maternal transfusion	886,210	3,526	398.1	582.0	402.7	349.9	359.5	419.5	550.1	598
Third- or fourth-degree perineal laceration	886,210	5,320	600.7	984.7	731.0	576.4	529.2	405.9	321.7	598
Ruptured uterus	886,210	261	29.5	15.2	21.0	29.5	32.7	38.4	61.1	598
Unplanned hysterectomy	886,210	401	45.3	6.1	13.8	38.2	54.8	99.8	128.7	598
Admission to the intensive care unit	886,210	1,326	149.7	138.3	108.8	120.2	161.5	231.9	302.4	598

NOTE: Rates are number of live births with morbidity per 100,000 live births in specified group.
[1]No response reported for selected characteristic.
[2]Includes births to race and origin groups not shown separately, such as Hispanic single-race White, Hispanic single-race Black, and non-Hispanic multiple-race women, and births with origin not stated.
[3]Race and Hispanic origin are reported separately on birth certificates; persons of Hispanic origin may be of any race. In this table, non-Hispanic women are classified by race. Race categories are consistent with the 1997 Office of Management and Budget standards. Single race is defined as only one race reported on the birth certificate.
[4]Includes all persons of Hispanic origin of any race.

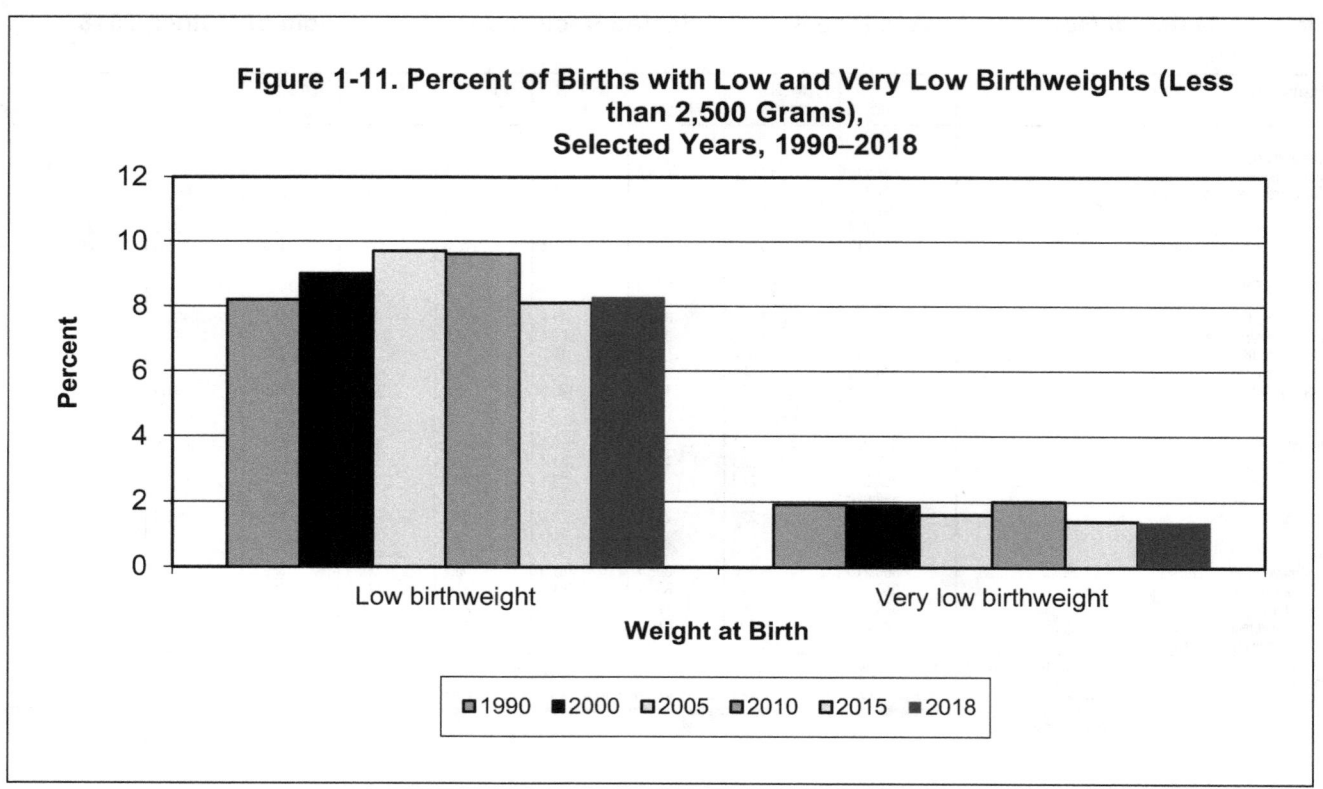

Figure 1-11. Percent of Births with Low and Very Low Birthweights (Less than 2,500 Grams), Selected Years, 1990–2018

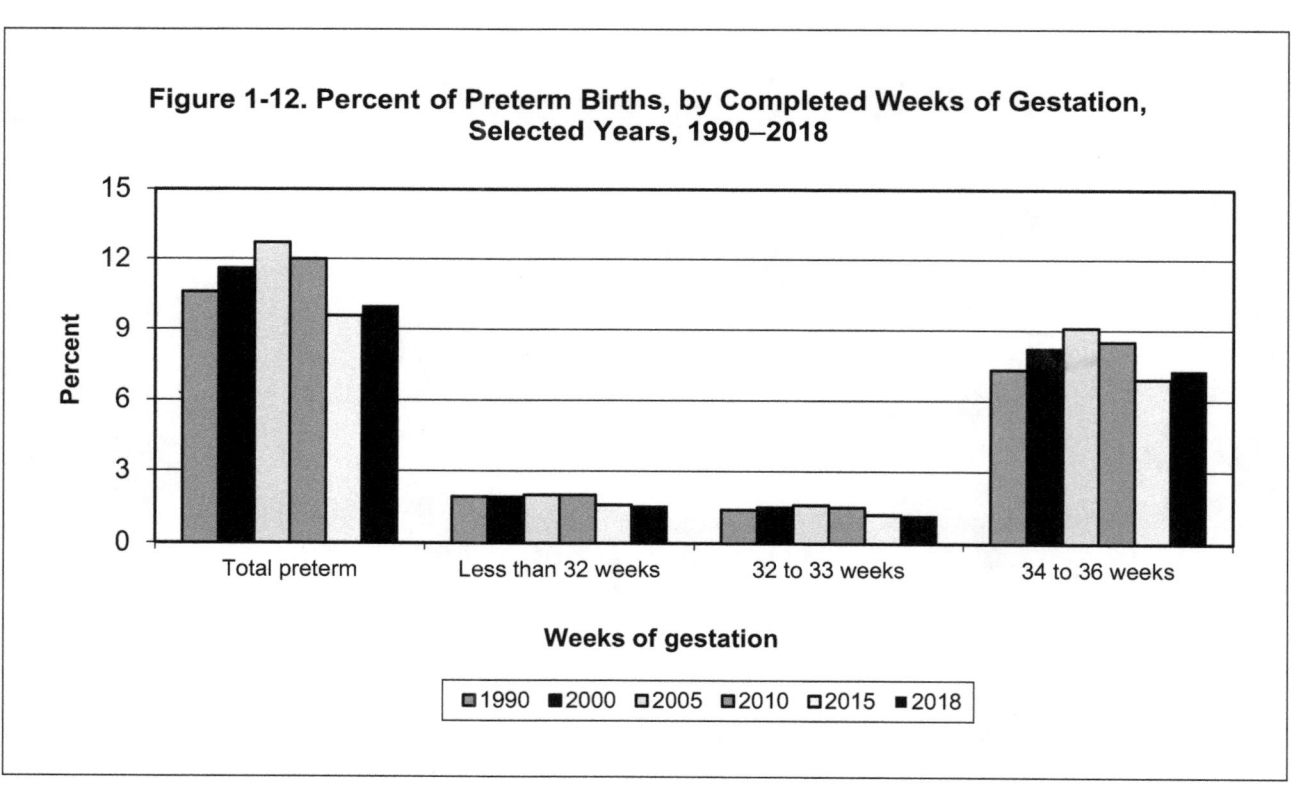

Figure 1-12. Percent of Preterm Births, by Completed Weeks of Gestation, Selected Years, 1990–2018

Table 1-45. Preterm Births (Less Than 37 Completed Weeks of Gestation), by Selected Race and Hispanic Origin of Mother, by State and Territory of Residence, 2018

(Number, percent.)

State and territory	Number				Percent			
	All races and origins[1]	Non-Hispanic, single race[2]		Hispanic[3]	All races and origins[1]	Non-Hispanic, single race[2]		Hispanic[3]
		White	Black			White	Black	
United States[4]	379,777	177,842	77,939	86,186	10.02	9.09	14.13	9.73
Alabama	7,204	3,671	2,903	413	12.48	10.87	16.51	9.40
Alaska	933	383	30	77	9.26	7.58	10.75	9.54
Arizona	7,673	2,911	543	3,257	9.52	8.88	12.61	9.56
Arkansas	4,299	2,465	1,153	418	11.62	10.45	16.57	10.20
California	39,964	9,449	2,751	19,142	8.79	7.68	12.30	9.07
Colorado	5,795	3,171	323	1,728	9.22	8.70	10.66	9.70
Connecticut	3,251	1,504	586	893	9.36	8.14	13.25	10.20
Delaware	1,015	450	359	142	9.56	8.70	12.95	8.30
District of Columbia	930	191	573	122	10.10	6.28	13.49	9.41
Florida	22,701	8,834	6,750	6,136	10.25	9.22	14.02	9.13
Georgia	14,509	5,559	6,365	1,715	11.50	9.99	14.56	9.84
Hawaii	1,744	249	56	230	10.28	7.58	13.21	8.92
Idaho	1,933	1,458	22	340	9.03	8.80	9.44	9.58
Illinois	15,445	7,369	3,643	3,146	10.67	9.54	14.89	10.37
Indiana	8,351	5,671	1,464	790	10.23	9.53	14.30	10.04
Iowa	3,745	2,802	293	409	9.91	9.56	11.21	11.07
Kansas	3,440	2,321	349	556	9.49	9.17	13.56	9.31
Kentucky	6,109	4,865	701	303	11.33	11.24	14.17	9.39
Louisiana	7,743	3,224	3,755	510	12.99	10.59	16.98	10.81
Maine	1,054	939	51	13	8.56	8.52	9.36	5.80
Maryland	7,231	2,573	2,821	1,139	10.18	8.70	12.89	9.14
Massachusetts	6,172	3,309	761	1,355	8.94	8.34	11.15	9.81
Michigan	11,039	6,579	3,069	706	10.04	8.80	14.94	9.90
Minnesota	6,004	3,953	783	487	8.92	8.59	9.54	9.76
Mississippi	5,269	2,269	2,727	182	14.25	12.20	17.27	10.93
Missouri	7,849	5,239	1,603	456	10.72	9.77	15.16	10.35
Montana	1,047	761	4	60	9.10	8.25	*	10.75
Nebraska	2,664	1,792	235	409	10.45	10.16	13.51	9.85
Nevada	3,616	1,214	594	1,245	10.14	9.33	13.02	9.36
New Hampshire	995	835	22	68	8.30	8.10	9.13	9.13
New Jersey	9,618	3,736	1,860	2,717	9.50	8.21	13.40	9.85
New Mexico	2,254	584	52	1,285	9.79	9.06	13.44	10.06
New York	20,281	8,447	4,225	4,993	8.98	7.62	12.75	9.65
North Carolina	12,340	5,950	3,809	1,675	10.38	9.37	13.78	9.13
North Dakota	1,018	700	60	64	9.57	8.96	9.85	10.09
Ohio	13,845	9,213	3,110	711	10.25	9.46	14.02	9.57
Oklahoma	5,670	3,148	651	807	11.39	11.07	15.75	10.70
Oregon	3,304	2,044	102	733	7.83	7.23	10.65	9.17
Pennsylvania	12,915	7,830	2,431	1,583	9.54	8.63	13.70	10.01
Rhode Island	943	494	88	269	8.98	8.22	11.25	9.76
South Carolina	6,426	3,080	2,531	495	11.34	9.66	15.18	9.42
South Dakota	1,122	719	32	68	9.44	8.48	7.71	10.29
Tennessee	8,911	5,460	2,332	734	11.06	10.27	14.69	9.41
Texas	40,799	12,054	7,023	19,276	10.78	9.60	14.60	10.76
Utah	4,445	3,030	57	904	9.42	8.83	10.96	11.12
Vermont	462	427	10	10	8.51	8.66	8.47	8.26
Virginia	9,401	4,577	2,757	1,267	9.42	8.36	13.23	8.80
Washington	7,147	3,751	398	1,400	8.31	7.66	10.17	8.72
West Virginia	2,158	1,954	89	37	11.83	11.76	14.22	9.79
Wisconsin	6,348	4,124	1,030	638	9.91	9.04	15.57	10.04
Wyoming	646	510	3	73	9.85	10.05	*	8.58
Puerto Rico	2,549	69	5	2,466	11.90	14.38	*	11.84
Virgin Islands	NA	NA	NA	NA	NA	NA	NA	NA
Guam	315	9	–	2	9.98	*	*	*
American Samoa	NA	NA	NA	NA	NA	NA	NA	NA
Northern Marianas	59	1	–	–	10.44	*	*	*

NA = Not available.
* = Estimate does not meet NCHS standards of reliability.
– = Quantity zero.
[1]Includes births to race and origin groups not shown separately, such as Hispanic single-race White, Hispanic single-race Black, and non-Hispanic multiple-race women, and births with origin not stated.
[2]Race and Hispanic origin are reported separately on birth certificates; persons of Hispanic origin may be of any race. In this table, non-Hispanic women are classified by race. Race categories are consistent with the 1997 Office of Management and Budget standard. Single race is defined as only one race reported on the birth certificate.
[3]Includes all persons of Hispanic origin of any race.
[4]Excludes data for the territories.

Table 1-46. Late Preterm Births (34 to 36 Completed Weeks of Gestation), by Selected Race and Hispanic Origin of Mother, by State and Territory of Residence, 2018

(Number, percent.)

State and territory	Number				Percent			
	All races and origins[1]	Non-Hispanic, single race[2]		Hispanic[3]	All races and origins[1]	Non-Hispanic, single race[2]		Hispanic[3]
		White	Black			White	Black	
United States[4]	275,746	133,555	50,931	63,549	7.28	6.83	9.23	7.17
Alabama	5,116	2,747	1,903	324	8.86	8.14	10.82	7.38
Alaska	697	299	17	55	6.91	5.91	6.09	6.82
Arizona	5,705	2,189	383	2,425	7.08	6.68	8.90	7.12
Arkansas	3,145	1,870	779	309	8.50	7.93	11.19	7.54
California	29,526	7,183	1,839	14,151	6.49	5.84	8.22	6.70
Colorado	4,244	2,363	234	1,242	6.75	6.48	7.72	6.97
Connecticut	2,346	1,131	382	633	6.76	6.12	8.64	7.23
Delaware	722	346	221	105	6.80	6.69	7.97	6.14
District of Columbia	619	158	348	83	6.72	5.20	8.19	6.40
Florida	16,244	6,629	4,363	4,524	7.34	6.92	9.06	6.73
Georgia	10,169	4,173	4,125	1,260	8.06	7.50	9.43	7.23
Hawaii	1,285	191	36	176	7.58	5.81	8.49	6.83
Idaho	1,470	1,107	14	258	6.87	6.68	6.01	7.27
Illinois	11,153	5,492	2,394	2,330	7.71	7.11	9.79	7.68
Indiana	6,097	4,246	953	579	7.47	7.14	9.31	7.36
Iowa	2,752	2,075	196	308	7.29	7.08	7.50	8.34
Kansas	2,518	1,722	236	410	6.95	6.80	9.17	6.86
Kentucky	4,502	3,664	458	206	8.35	8.46	9.26	6.39
Louisiana	5,576	2,478	2,533	376	9.36	8.14	11.46	7.97
Maine	788	706	35	10	6.40	6.41	6.42	*
Maryland	5,042	1,891	1,824	830	7.10	6.40	8.34	6.66
Massachusetts	4,490	2,504	472	944	6.50	6.31	6.92	6.84
Michigan	8,066	4,976	2,042	526	7.33	6.66	9.94	7.37
Minnesota	4,453	3,003	529	355	6.62	6.53	6.45	7.12
Mississippi	3,733	1,721	1,803	138	10.09	9.26	11.42	8.29
Missouri	5,777	3,957	1,062	350	7.89	7.38	10.04	7.95
Montana	790	575	3	45	6.87	6.24	*	8.06
Nebraska	1,999	1,382	155	285	7.84	7.83	8.91	6.86
Nevada	2,654	913	406	925	7.44	7.02	8.90	6.95
New Hampshire	719	610	12	48	6.00	5.92	4.98	6.44
New Jersey	6,963	2,848	1,162	1,997	6.88	6.26	8.37	7.24
New Mexico	1,674	459	39	949	7.27	7.12	10.08	7.43
New York	14,482	6,262	2,669	3,593	6.41	5.65	8.05	6.94
North Carolina	8,759	4,462	2,446	1,216	7.37	7.03	8.85	6.62
North Dakota	756	531	42	45	7.11	6.79	6.90	7.10
Ohio	9,949	6,825	2,013	532	7.37	7.01	9.08	7.16
Oklahoma	4,192	2,375	433	618	8.42	8.35	10.48	8.20
Oregon	2,491	1,522	70	564	5.91	5.39	7.31	7.06
Pennsylvania	9,227	5,807	1,563	1,110	6.81	6.40	8.81	7.02
Rhode Island	667	366	56	186	6.35	6.09	7.16	6.75
South Carolina	4,571	2,295	1,652	384	8.07	7.20	9.91	7.31
South Dakota	868	570	21	50	7.31	6.72	5.06	7.56
Tennessee	6,380	4,056	1,496	547	7.92	7.63	9.42	7.01
Texas	29,816	9,057	4,641	14,325	7.88	7.21	9.65	8.00
Utah	3,392	2,331	42	680	7.19	6.80	8.08	8.36
Vermont	346	325	7	6	6.38	6.59	*	*
Virginia	6,758	3,424	1,805	952	6.77	6.25	8.66	6.61
Washington	5,293	2,806	261	1,035	6.16	5.73	6.67	6.45
West Virginia	1,592	1,453	62	24	8.73	8.75	9.90	6.35
Wisconsin	4,684	3,097	694	470	7.31	6.79	10.49	7.39
Wyoming	489	383	–	56	7.45	7.54	*	6.58
Puerto Rico	1,897	46	4	1,842	8.86	9.58	*	8.84
Virgin Islands	NA	NA	NA	NA	NA	NA	NA	NA
Guam	252	9	–	2	7.98	*	*	*
American Samoa	NA	NA	NA	NA	NA	NA	NA	NA
Northern Marianas	39	1	–	–	6.90	*	*	*

NA = Not available.
* = Estimate does not meet NCHS standards of reliability.
– = Quantity zero.
[1]Includes births to race and origin groups not shown separately, such as Hispanic single-race White, Hispanic single-race Black, and non-Hispanic multiple-race women, and births with origin not stated.
[2]Race and Hispanic origin are reported separately on birth certificates; persons of Hispanic origin may be of any race. In this table, non-Hispanic women are classified by race. Race categories are consistent with the 1997 Office of Management and Budget standard. Single race is defined as only one race reported on the birth certificate.
[3]Includes all persons of Hispanic origin of any race.
[4]Excludes data for the territories.

Table 1-47. Low Birthweight Babies (Less Than 2,500 Grams), by Selected Race and Hispanic Origin of Mother, by State and Territory of Residence, 2018

(Number, percent.)

State and territory	Number All races and origins[1]	Number Non-Hispanic, single race[2] White	Number Non-Hispanic, single race[2] Black	Number Hispanic[3]	Percent All races and origins[1]	Percent Non-Hispanic, single race[2] White	Percent Non-Hispanic, single race[2] Black	Percent Hispanic[3]
United States[4]	313,752	135,185	77,584	66,310	8.3	6.9	14.1	7.5
Alabama	6,184	2,748	2,886	334	10.7	8.1	16.4	7.6
Alaska	590	245	35	47	5.9	4.8	12.5	5.8
Arizona	6,116	2,285	532	2,479	7.6	7.0	12.4	7.3
Arkansas	3,465	1,823	1,115	305	9.4	7.7	16.0	7.4
California	31,745	7,116	2,704	14,188	7.0	5.8	12.1	6.7
Colorado	5,906	3,135	407	1,704	9.4	8.6	13.4	9.6
Connecticut	2,641	1,114	557	705	7.6	6.0	12.6	8.1
Delaware	948	379	380	120	8.9	7.3	13.7	7.0
District of Columbia	918	157	620	88	10.0	5.2	14.6	6.8
Florida	19,217	6,838	6,675	4,781	8.7	7.1	13.9	7.1
Georgia	12,733	4,062	6,472	1,271	10.1	7.3	14.8	7.3
Hawaii	1,416	185	50	168	8.3	5.6	11.8	6.5
Idaho	1,553	1,166	26	268	7.3	7.0	11.2	7.6
Illinois	12,370	5,352	3,538	2,280	8.5	6.9	14.5	7.5
Indiana	6,572	4,218	1,416	561	8.1	7.1	13.8	7.1
Iowa	2,608	1,837	295	279	6.9	6.3	11.3	7.6
Kansas	2,676	1,702	344	434	7.4	6.7	13.4	7.3
Kentucky	4,782	3,588	717	231	8.9	8.3	14.5	7.2
Louisiana	6,428	2,269	3,537	413	10.8	7.5	16.0	8.8
Maine	885	778	51	18	7.2	7.1	9.3	8.1
Maryland	6,266	1,980	2,760	863	8.8	6.7	12.6	6.9
Massachusetts	5,237	2,575	746	1,181	7.6	6.5	11.0	8.6
Michigan	9,302	5,069	3,063	519	8.5	6.8	14.9	7.3
Minnesota	4,617	2,702	836	378	6.9	5.9	10.2	7.6
Mississippi	4,484	1,602	2,685	118	12.1	8.6	17.0	7.1
Missouri	6,389	3,905	1,684	320	8.7	7.3	15.9	7.3
Montana	855	637	5	58	7.4	6.9	*	10.4
Nebraska	1,927	1,208	242	320	7.6	6.8	13.9	7.7
Nevada	3,097	998	578	1,027	8.7	7.7	12.7	7.7
New Hampshire	812	652	30	59	6.8	6.3	12.4	7.9
New Jersey	8,001	2,822	1,796	2,075	7.9	6.2	12.9	7.5
New Mexico	2,084	526	53	1,203	9.0	8.2	13.7	9.4
New York	18,208	7,030	4,273	4,254	8.1	6.3	12.9	8.2
North Carolina	10,970	4,728	3,969	1,374	9.2	7.4	14.4	7.5
North Dakota	698	469	55	49	6.6	6.0	9.0	7.7
Ohio	11,471	7,033	3,103	559	8.5	7.2	14.0	7.5
Oklahoma	4,115	2,215	631	531	8.3	7.8	15.3	7.0
Oregon	2,826	1,744	110	587	6.7	6.2	11.5	7.3
Pennsylvania	11,222	6,253	2,462	1,419	8.3	6.9	13.9	9.0
Rhode Island	801	394	92	217	7.6	6.6	11.7	7.9
South Carolina	5,432	2,235	2,532	384	9.6	7.0	15.2	7.3
South Dakota	789	514	35	49	6.6	6.1	8.4	7.4
Tennessee	7,471	4,143	2,393	562	9.3	7.8	15.1	7.2
Texas	32,037	8,815	6,707	14,172	8.5	7.0	13.9	7.9
Utah	3,385	2,258	55	695	7.2	6.6	10.6	8.6
Vermont	381	339	9	12	7.0	6.9	*	9.9
Virginia	8,175	3,600	2,781	1,000	8.2	6.6	13.3	6.9
Washington	5,690	2,816	384	1,076	6.6	5.7	9.8	6.7
West Virginia	1,708	1,525	85	30	9.4	9.2	13.6	7.9
Wisconsin	4,935	2,910	1,066	478	7.7	6.4	16.1	7.5
Wyoming	614	491	7	67	9.4	9.7	*	7.9
Puerto Rico	2,212	55	5	2,143	10.3	11.5	*	10.3
Virgin Islands	NA	NA	NA	NA	NA	NA	NA	NA
Guam	317	8	1	2	10.1	*	*	*
American Samoa	–	NA	NA	NA	NA	NA	NA	NA
Northern Marianas	61	1	–	–	10.9	*	*	*

NA = Not available.
* = Estimate does not meet NCHS standards of reliability.
– = Quantity zero.
[1]Includes births to race and origin groups not shown separately, such as Hispanic single-race White, Hispanic single-race Black, and non-Hispanic multiple-race women, and births with origin not stated.
[2]Race and Hispanic origin are reported separately on birth certificates; persons of Hispanic origin may be of any race. In this table, non-Hispanic women are classified by race. Race categories are consistent with the 1997 Office of Management and Budget standard. Single race is defined as only one race reported on the birth certificate.
[3]Includes all persons of Hispanic origin of any race.
[4]Excludes data for the territories.

Table 1-48. Very Low Birthweight Babies (Less Than 1,500 Grams), by Selected Race and Hispanic Origin of Mother, by State and Territory of Residence, 2018

(Number, percent.)

State and territory	Number				Percent			
	All races and origins[1]	Non-Hispanic, single race[2]		Hispanic[3]	All races and origins[1]	Non-Hispanic, single race[2]		Hispanic[3]
		White	Black			White	Black	
United States[4]	52,171	19,872	16,127	11,006	1.4	1.0	2.9	1.2
Alabama	1,084	413	584	47	1.9	1.2	3.3	1.1
Alaska	98	34	7	7	1.0	0.7	2.5	0.9
Arizona	977	336	91	421	1.2	1.0	2.1	1.2
Arkansas	565	285	198	54	1.5	1.2	2.8	1.3
California	5,039	985	544	2,387	1.1	0.8	2.4	1.1
Colorado	761	365	55	252	1.2	1.0	1.8	1.4
Connecticut	459	154	123	139	1.3	0.8	2.8	1.6
Delaware	161	42	88	23	1.5	0.8	3.2	1.3
District of Columbia	165	10	128	17	1.8	0.3	3.0	1.3
Florida	3,482	1,026	1,473	836	1.6	1.1	3.1	1.2
Georgia	2,259	585	1,337	203	1.8	1.1	3.1	1.2
Hawaii	240	23	15	36	1.4	0.7	3.5	1.4
Idaho	224	172	5	33	1.0	1.0	2.1	0.9
Illinois	2,132	839	715	377	1.5	1.1	2.9	1.2
Indiana	1,111	636	324	99	1.4	1.1	3.2	1.3
Iowa	425	291	54	44	1.1	1.0	2.1	1.2
Kansas	459	277	65	85	1.3	1.1	2.5	1.4
Kentucky	756	523	152	40	1.4	1.2	3.1	1.2
Louisiana	1,145	329	711	72	1.9	1.1	3.2	1.5
Maine	121	103	9	2	1.0	0.9	1.6	0.9
Maryland	1,175	300	606	146	1.7	1.0	2.8	1.2
Massachusetts	822	355	168	211	1.2	0.9	2.5	1.5
Michigan	1,485	731	595	77	1.4	1.0	2.9	1.1
Minnesota	786	439	153	75	1.2	1.0	1.9	1.5
Mississippi	794	228	541	17	2.1	1.2	3.4	1.0
Missouri	991	559	318	47	1.4	1.0	3.0	1.1
Montana	108	84	–	5	0.9	0.9	*	0.9
Nebraska	287	155	54	57	1.1	0.9	3.1	1.4
Nevada	459	130	112	147	1.3	1.0	2.5	1.1
New Hampshire	131	100	6	13	1.1	1.0	2.5	1.7
New Jersey	1,401	401	414	376	1.4	0.9	3.0	1.4
New Mexico	294	62	8	178	1.3	1.0	2.1	1.4
New York	2,968	953	953	729	1.3	0.9	2.9	1.4
North Carolina	1,887	704	839	212	1.6	1.1	3.0	1.2
North Dakota	121	73	10	11	1.1	0.9	1.6	1.7
Ohio	1,995	1,144	632	94	1.5	1.2	2.9	1.3
Oklahoma	721	359	127	89	1.4	1.3	3.1	1.2
Oregon	370	227	19	76	0.9	0.8	2.0	1.0
Pennsylvania	1,869	923	534	222	1.4	1.0	3.0	1.4
Rhode Island	136	56	23	37	1.3	0.9	2.9	1.3
South Carolina	965	342	535	50	1.7	1.1	3.2	1.0
South Dakota	104	64	6	4	0.9	0.8	1.4	0.6
Tennessee	1,303	623	521	106	1.6	1.2	3.3	1.4
Texas	5,345	1,332	1,378	2,307	1.4	1.1	2.9	1.3
Utah	495	328	9	106	1.0	1.0	1.7	1.3
Vermont	58	53	2	2	1.1	1.1	*	*
Virginia	1,453	569	590	176	1.5	1.0	2.8	1.2
Washington	865	415	91	160	1.0	0.8	2.3	1.0
West Virginia	285	250	15	12	1.6	1.5	2.4	3.2
Wisconsin	765	425	187	85	1.2	0.9	2.8	1.3
Wyoming	70	60	3	5	1.1	1.2	*	0.6
Puerto Rico	302	14	1	284	1.4	2.9	*	1.4
Virgin Islands	NA	NA	NA	NA	NA	NA	NA	NA
Guam	34	–	–	–	1.1	0.0	*	*
American Samoa	–	NA	NA	NA	NA	NA	NA	NA
Northern Marianas	5	–	–	–	0.9	*	*	*

NA = Not available.
* = Estimate does not meet NCHS standards of reliability.
– = Quantity zero.
0.0 = Equals zero events in the numerator or percentage of less than 0.05 percent.
[1]Includes births to race and origin groups not shown separately, such as Hispanic single-race White, Hispanic single-race Black, and non-Hispanic multiple-race women, and births with origin not stated.
[2]Race and Hispanic origin are reported separately on birth certificates; persons of Hispanic origin may be of any race. In this table, non-Hispanic women are classified by race. Race categories are consistent with the 1997 Office of Management and Budget standard. Single race is defined as only one race reported on the birth certificate.
[3]Includes all persons of Hispanic origin of any race.
[4]Excludes data for the territories.

Table 1-49. Twin and Triplet or Higher-Order Multiple Births, by State, 2018
(Number, rate.)

State	Twin Number	Twin Rate per 1,000 live births	Triplet/higher-order[1] Number	Triplet/higher-order[1] Rate per 100,000 live births
United States	383,569	33.1	11,445	98.7
Alabama	6,265	35.6	285	162.1
Alaska	1,001	31.5	24	75.6
Arizona	7,709	31.2	260	105.2
Arkansas	3,410	30.2	88	78.0
California	43,414	30.7	1,180	83.4
Colorado	6,021	31.1	147	75.8
Connecticut	4,202	39.7	108	101.9
Delaware	999	30.8	6	18.5
District of Columbia	1,060	37.0	13	45.4
Florida	21,356	31.9	490	73.1
Georgia	13,008	33.7	383	99.4
Hawaii	1,698	32.3	64	121.8
Idaho	2,107	31.9	52	78.7
Illinois	16,211	36.1	505	112.6
Indiana	8,103	32.8	314	127.2
Iowa	3,864	33.4	120	103.8
Kansas	3,479	31.4	67	60.5
Kentucky	5,571	33.9	146	89.0
Louisiana	6,285	34.2	218	118.6
Maine	1,170	31.4	43	115.2
Maryland	7,329	34.0	248	114.9
Massachusetts	7,467	35.4	209	99.0
Michigan	12,351	36.9	386	115.3
Minnesota	7,018	34.1	182	88.5
Mississippi	3,713	33.1	125	111.3
Missouri	7,802	35.3	254	114.9
Montana	1,081	30.4	18	50.6
Nebraska	2,745	35.2	143	183.6
Nevada	3,241	30.1	73	67.8
New Hampshire	1,204	33.1	37	101.7
New Jersey	10,999	36.0	313	102.6
New Mexico	1,815	25.4	53	74.1
New York	24,404	35.4	756	109.5
North Carolina	12,240	34.0	378	105.0
North Dakota	1,081	33.0	38	116.0
Ohio	14,147	34.5	471	114.9
Oklahoma	4,806	31.5	106	69.5
Oregon	4,480	34.1	117	89.1
Pennsylvania	13,842	33.5	380	92.0
Rhode Island	1,121	35.1	42	131.5
South Carolina	5,873	34.3	151	88.3
South Dakota	1,280	35.3	38	104.7
Tennessee	7,803	32.2	260	107.2
Texas	36,034	31.1	1,148	99.1
Utah	5,124	35.0	176	120.3
Vermont	541	32.1	11	65.3
Virginia	10,312	34.1	307	101.4
Washington	7,757	29.4	233	88.2
West Virginia	1,726	30.8	52	92.9
Wisconsin	6,703	34.3	201	102.7
Wyoming	597	28.6	26	124.7

[1]Includes triplet, quadruplet, and other higher-order multiple births.

Table 1-50. Abnormal Conditions of the Newborn, by Age (Years) and Selected Race and Hispanic Origin of Mother, 2018

(Number; rate.)

Abnormal condition and race and Hispanic origin of mother	All births	Condition reported	All ages	Under 20 years	20 to 24 years	25 to 29 years	30 to 34 years	35 to 39 years	40 to 54 years	Not stated[1]
All races and origins[2]										
Assisted ventilation required immediately following delivery	3,791,712	170,764	45.1	47.9	44.8	43.5	43.8	47.8	55.4	3,394
Assisted ventilation required for more than 6 hours	3,791,712	58,503	15.4	15.7	15.1	14.8	14.9	16.8	21.1	3,394
NICU admission[3]	3,791,712	346,812	91.5	94.4	87.9	86.7	88.9	101.6	127.8	3,394
Surfactant replacement therapy given to newborn	3,791,712	17,703	4.7	5.0	4.8	4.5	4.4	4.9	6.3	3,394
Antibiotics received by newborn for suspected neonatal sepsis	3,791,712	81,016	21.4	27.1	23.2	21.0	19.8	20.7	23.0	3,394
Seizure or serious neurologic dysfunction	3,791,712	1,325	0.3	0.5	0.4	0.3	0.3	0.4	0.4	3,394
Non-Hispanic, single race[4]										
White										
Assisted ventilation required immediately following delivery	1,956,413	94,591	48.4	55.8	49.4	46.9	46.2	50.8	59.3	1,503
Assisted ventilation required for more than 6 hours	1,956,413	32,300	16.5	18.4	16.7	15.9	15.6	17.7	22.7	1,503
NICU admission[3]	1,956,413	166,985	85.4	87.7	81.7	81.3	83.1	94.6	121.4	1,503
Surfactant replacement therapy given to newborn	1,956,413	9,405	4.8	6.0	5.0	4.7	4.4	5.0	6.5	1,503
Antibiotics received by newborn for suspected neonatal sepsis	1,956,413	39,997	20.5	24.5	22.1	20.3	19.3	20.1	23.0	1,503
Seizure or serious neurologic dysfunction	1,956,413	801	0.4	0.8	0.4	0.4	0.4	0.4	0.6	1,503
Black										
Assisted ventilation required immediately following delivery	552,029	30,256	54.9	52.7	51.0	52.5	56.3	62.2	73.4	438
Assisted ventilation required for more than 6 hours	552,029	10,760	19.5	17.5	17.8	18.6	20.6	22.3	27.6	438
NICU admission[3]	552,029	67,728	122.8	115.7	112.6	116.1	126.4	145.8	168.8	438
Surfactant replacement therapy given to newborn	552,029	3,777	6.8	6.0	6.8	6.5	6.7	7.9	9.3	438
Antibiotics received by newborn for suspected neonatal sepsis	552,029	14,753	26.7	29.8	26.5	26.3	25.4	28.6	29.1	438
Seizure or serious neurologic dysfunction	552,029	205	0.4	0.5	0.4	0.3	0.3	0.4	0.7	438
Hispanic[5]										
Assisted ventilation required immediately following delivery	886,210	30,281	34.2	36.0	33.0	32.0	33.9	38.2	43.2	751
Assisted ventilation required for more than 6 hours	886,210	10,402	11.7	11.8	11.1	11.0	11.5	13.5	17.3	751
NICU admission[3]	886,210	77,000	87.0	88.6	81.3	80.5	87.0	100.5	123.3	751
Surfactant replacement therapy given to newborn	886,210	3,074	3.5	3.3	3.4	3.1	3.5	3.9	5.2	751
Antibiotics received by newborn for suspected neonatal sepsis	886,210	17,798	20.1	27.5	22.2	18.6	18.0	18.9	21.3	751
Seizure or serious neurologic dysfunction	886,210	200	0.2	0.3	0.3	0.2	0.2	0.2	0.1	751

NOTE: Rates are number of live births with specified condition per 1,000 live births in specified group.
[1] No response reported for selected characteristic.
[2] Includes births to race and origin groups not shown separately, such as Hispanic single-race White, Hispanic single-race Black, and non-Hispanic multiple-race women, and births with origin not stated.
[3] NICU is newborn intensive care unit.
[4] Race and Hispanic origin are reported separately on birth certificates; persons of Hispanic origin may be of any race. In this table, non-Hispanic women are classified by race. Race categories are consistent with the 1997 Office of Management and Budget standards. Single race is defined as only one race reported on the birth certificate.
[5] Includes all persons of Hispanic origin of any race.

Table 1-51. Congenital Abnormalities of the Newborn, by Age (Years) of Mother, 2018

(Number; rate.)

Congenital abnormality	All births	Condition reported	All ages	Under 20 years	20 to 24 years	25 to 29 years	30 to 34 years	35 to 39 years	40 to 54 years	Not stated[1]
Anencephaly	3,791,712	354	9.4	10.5	11.7	9.8	8.2	7.6	7.9	6,044
Menigomyelocele or spina bifida	3,791,712	555	14.7	14.3	15.4	16.0	12.5	15.0	15.8	6,044
Cyanotic congenital heart disease	3,791,712	2,213	58.5	56.3	57.8	55.3	55.3	65.2	90.0	6,044
Congenital diaphragmatic hernia	3,791,712	471	12.4	12.7	12.3	12.7	11.9	13.6	10.3	6,044
Omphalocele	3,791,712	406	10.7	12.1	11.9	9.8	9.8	9.7	22.1	6,044
Gastroschisis	3,791,712	830	21.9	82.7	46.2	20.9	7.7	4.9	3.2	6,044
Limb reduction defect	3,791,712	487	12.9	14.9	13.7	12.3	11.7	13.6	17.4	6,044
Cleft lip with or without cleft palate	3,791,712	2,050	54.2	54.6	59.7	54.9	48.8	53.5	63.1	6,044
Cleft palate alone	3,791,712	920	24.3	22.6	27.3	26.9	22.5	19.8	22.9	6,044
Down syndrome	3,791,712	2,106	55.6	28.7	25.9	29.1	38.5	111.2	393.8	6,044
Suspected chromosomal disorder	3,791,712	1,724	45.5	36.4	38.3	35.4	39.8	61.9	164.1	6,044
Hypospadias[2]	3,791,712	2,235	59.0	46.3	55.9	56.3	63.4	62.9	63.9	6,044
Males only[3]	1,938,177	2,235	115.5	90.4	109.4	110.1	124.2	122.9	125.8	3,083

NOTE: Rates are number of live births with specified anomalies per 100,000 live births in specified group.
[1] No response reported for selected characteristic.
[2] Denominator includes both male and female births.
[3] Denominator includes male births only.

Table 1-52. Total Fertility Rate, by Urbanization Level, 2007–2017

(Rate.)

Year	Rural counties	Small or medium metro counties	Large metro counties
2007	2,206.5	2,110.0	2,096.0
2008	2,174.5	2,061.0	2,044.0
2009	2,111.5	1,998.0	1,969.0
2010	2,037.5	1,938.0	1,894.5
2011	1,999.0	1,902.5	1,856.5
2012			
2013	1,997.5	1,892.0	1,811.5
2014	2,000.0	1,872.0	1,814.0
2015	2,006.5	1,880.0	1,793.0
2016	1,988.5	1,860.5	1,770.5
2017	1,950.0	1,778.0	1,712.0

NOTE: Total fertility rate is based on births per 1,000 women in a specified area. County designation is based on mother's county of residence. County classification is based on the 2006 and 2013 NCHS Urban–Rural Classification Scheme for Counties.

Table 1-53. Total Fertility Rate, by Race and Hispanic Origin and Urbanization Level, 2007 and 2017

(Rate.)

Race and Hispanic origin	2007	2017
Non-Hispanic White		
Rural counties	2,088.5	1,907.5
Small or medium metro counties	1,910.0	1,663.5
Large metro counties	1,820.5	1,575.5
Non-Hispanic Black		
Rural counties	2,194.5	1,851.5
Small or medium metro counties	2,123.5	1,880.5
Large metro counties	2,131.5	1,789.0
Hispanic		
Rural counties	3,126.5	2,320.0
Small or medium metro counties	2,978.0	2,124.0
Large metro counties	2,754.0	1,929.5

NOTE: Total fertility rate is based on births per 1,000 women in a specified area. County designation is based on mother's county of residence. County classification is based on the 2006 and 2013 NCHS Urban–Rural Classification Scheme for Counties. Race and Hispanic origin are reported separately on birth certificates. Persons of Hispanic origin may be of any race. Persons of non-Hispanic ancestry are further classified by race because of differences in fertility and maternal characteristics between Hispanic and non-Hispanic persons. Multiple-race data reported were bridged to single-race categories for comparability with earlier years. Multiple-race reporting areas vary in 2007 and 2017, with all states and the District of Columbia reporting multiple race data in 2017.

Table 1-54. Trends in Fertility and Mother's Age at First Birth Among Rural and Metropolitan Counties, by Urbanization Level, 2007–2017

(Years.)

Year	Rural counties	Small or medium metro counties	Large metro counties
2007	23.2	24.3	25.9
2008	23.2	24.4	26.0
2009	23.3	24.4	26.1
2010	23.4	24.6	26.3
2011	23.6	24.9	26.6
2012	23.7	25.0	26.7
2013	23.8	25.1	27.0
2014	24.0	25.4	27.2
2015	24.2	25.5	27.4
2016	24.4	25.7	27.6
2017	24.5	25.8	27.7

NOTE: County designation is based on mother's county of residence. County classification is based on the 2006 and 2013 NCHS Urban–Rural Classification Scheme for Counties. Age in years.

Table 1-55. Mean Age at First Birth, by Race and Hispanic Origin and Urbanization Level, 2007 and 2017

(Years.)

Race and Hispanic origin	2007	2017
Non-Hispanic White		
Rural counties	23.7	24.9
Small or medium metro counties	25.2	26.6
Large metro counties	27.5	29.0
Non-Hispanic Black		
Rural counties	21.0	22.7
Small or medium metro counties	21.9	23.8
Large metro counties	23.2	25.6
Hispanic		
Rural counties	21.7	23.0
Small or medium metro counties	22.4	23.9
Large metro counties	23.5	25.4

NOTE: County designation is based on mother's county of residence. County classification is based on the 2006 and 2013 NCHS Urban–Rural Classification Scheme for Counties. Race and Hispanic origin are reported separately on birth certificates. Persons of Hispanic origin may be of any race. Persons of non-Hispanic ancestry are further classified by race because of differences in fertility and maternal characteristics between Hispanic and non-Hispanic persons. Multiple-race data reported were bridged to single-race categories for comparability with earlier years. Multiple-race reporting areas vary in 2007 and 2017, with all states and the District of Columbia reporting multiple race data in 2017.

NOTES AND DEFINITIONS

Sources of Data

The tables in Part 1 are from the National Center for Health Statistics (NCHS), a component of the Centers for Disease Control and Prevention (CDC).

Most of the tables found in Part 1 were obtained from Martin JA, Hamilton BE, Osterman MJK, Driscoll AK. *Births: Final Data for 2018*. National Vital Statistics Reports; vol 68, no 13. Hyattsville, MD: National Center for Health Statistics. 2019.

Some data for the year 2017 was derived from Martin JA, Hamilton BE, Osterman MJK, Driscoll AK, Drake P. *Births: Final Data for 2017*. National Vital Statistics Reports; vol 67 no 8. Hyattsville, MD: National Center for Health Statistics. 2018.

Notes on the Data

Race and Hispanic origin are noted separately on birth certificates. Some rates for 2001 through 2009 have been revised using new population estimates that are based on the 2010 census; thus, these rates may differ from those previously published. Population estimates are generally for July 1 of the year shown.

2003 revision of U.S. Standard Certificate of Live Birth

Starting in 2016, all 50 states, D.C., Puerto Rico, Guam, Commonwealth of the Northern Marianas, and U.S. Virgin Islands reported data based on the 2003 U.S. Certificate of Live Birth. American Samoa continued to report based on the 1989 birth certificate revision. For information on data quality, see reports that assessed the quality of selected medical and health data from the 2003 revised birth certificate and the "User Guide to the 2018 Natality Public Use File."

The 2003 revision of the U.S. Standard Certificate of Live Birth allows the reporting of more than one race (multiple races) for each parent in accordance with the revised standards issued by OMB in 1997. Starting in 2016, all 50 states, D.C., Puerto Rico, Guam, Northern Marianas, and U.S. Virgin Islands reported race data in accordance with these 1997 OMB standards that allow for the reporting of a minimum of five race categories either by single race (i.e., reported alone) or in combination (i.e., more than one race or multiple races). The race and Hispanic-origin groups shown in this report follow the 1997 standards and differ from the bridged-race categories shown in most previous reports that are based on data from 2015 and earlier. The new categories are non-Hispanic single-race White, non-Hispanic single-race Black or African American, non-Hispanic single-race AIAN,

non-Hispanic single-race Asian, non-Hispanic single-race NHOPI, and Hispanic. Because single-race data are not available for the entire United States prior to 2016, this report only makes comparisons by race for 2016–2018.

Race and Hispanic origin are reported independently on the birth certificate. Most tables in this report show data for the categories of non-Hispanic single-race white, non-Hispanic single-race black, and Hispanic. Selected tables also include data for non-Hispanic single-race AIAN, non-Hispanic single-race Asian, and non-Hispanic single-race NHOPI. Data are also presented in some tables for specific Hispanic groups: Mexican, Puerto Rican, Cuban, Central and South American, and other and unknown Hispanic. Beginning with 2018, data are presented for an additional Hispanic group, Dominican.

Concepts and Definitions

Anencephaly—A congenital anomaly that consists of a partial or complete absence of the brain and skull.

Apgar score—This has been employed for over 50 years to assess the physical condition and short-term prognosis of newborns. Historically, the score has been measured at 1 minute, 5 minutes, and if needed, at additional 5-minute intervals after delivery. Information on the 5-minute score is included in national birth certificate data. The Apgar score measures five easily identifiable characteristics of newborns. A 5-minute score of 0 to 3 indicates an infant in immediate need of resuscitation; 4 to 6 is considered intermediate, and 7 to 10 is considered normal. The Apgar score is a useful clinical indicator for reporting overall status of the neonate and need for, and response to resuscitation efforts.

Birth cohort—Consists of all persons born within a given period of time, such as a calendar year.

Birthweight—The first weight of the newborn obtained after birth. Low birthweight is defined as less than 2,500 grams or 5 pounds 8 ounces. Very low birthweight is defined as less than 1,500 grams or 3 pounds 4 ounces. Before 1979, low birthweight was defined as weighing 2,500 grams or less, and very low birthweight was defined as 1,500 grams or less. Equivalents of the gram weights in terms of pounds and ounces are as follows:

Less than 500 grams = 1 lb 1 oz or less
500–999 grams = 1 lb 2 oz–2 lb 3 oz
1,000–1,499 grams = 2 lb 4 oz–3 lb 4 oz
1,500–1,999 grams = 3 lb 5 oz–4 lb 6 oz
2,000–2,499 grams = 4 lb 7 oz–5 lb 8 oz
2,500–2,999 grams = 5 lb 9 oz–6 lb 9 oz

3,000–3,499 grams = 6 lb 10 oz–7 lb 11 oz
3,500–3,999 grams = 7 lb 12 oz–8 lb 13 oz
4,000–4,499 grams = 8 lb 14 oz–9 lb 14 oz
4,500–4,999 grams = 9 lb 15 oz–11 lb 0 oz
5,000 grams or more = 11 lb 1 oz or more

Birth rate—Calculated by dividing the number of live births in a population in a year by the midyear resident population. Birth rates are expressed as the number of live births per 1,000 population. The rate may be restricted to births to women of specific age, race, marital status, or geographic location (specific rate), or it may be related to the entire population (crude rate).

Breech/malpresentation—Presenting part of the fetus listed as breech, complete breech, frank breech, footling breech.

Cervical cerclage—Circumferential banding or suture of the cervix to prevent or treat early dilation of the cervix (e.g., incompetent cervix) in an attempt to avoid premature delivery.

Cleft lip/palate—Incomplete closure of the lip. May be unilateral, bilateral, or median. Cleft palate is incomplete fusion of the palatal shelves. May be limited to the soft palate, or may extend into the hard palate.

Contraception—The National Survey of Family Growth collects information on contraceptive use reported by women 15–44 years old. For current contraceptive use, women were asked about contraceptive use during the month of interview. Women were classified by whether they reported using any of the 19 methods of contraception at any time in the month of interview.

Cyanotic heart disease—Congenital heart defects resulting in lack of oxygen that cause cyanosis.

Down syndrome—The most common chromosomal defect (trisomy 21).

Fertility rate—Total number of live births per 1,000 women of reproductive age (defined as women age 15 to 44 years).

Gestation—The time period between the first day of the last normal menstrual period and the day of birth or day of termination of pregnancy according to the National Vital Statistics System and the CDC's Abortion Surveillance.

Hispanic origin—Includes persons of Mexican, Puerto Rican, Cuban, Central and South American, and other or unknown Latin American or Spanish origins. Persons of Hispanic origin may be of any race.

Hypertension, chronic—Diagnosis prior to the onset of this pregnancy of elevated blood pressure above normal for age, gender, and physiological condition.

Hypertension, pregnancy-associated—Diagnosis in pregnancy of elevated blood pressure above normal for age, gender, and physiological condition.

Induction of labor—Initiation of uterine contractions by medical and/or surgical means for the purpose of delivery before the spontaneous onset of labor.

Maternal morbidities—Information on six maternal morbidities is collected on the 2003 revised birth certificate: maternal transfusion, third-or fourth-degree perineal laceration, ruptured uterus, unplanned hysterectomy, admission to intensive care unit, and unplanned operating room procedure. More than one morbidity may be reported. Maternal morbidity data are not available for Delaware for 2011 because of concerns with data quality.

Meconium, moderate/heavy—Staining of the amniotic fluid caused by passage of fetal bowel contents during labor and/or at delivery that is more than enough to cause a greenish color change of an otherwise clear fluid.

Meningomyecele/Spina bifida—Meningomyelocele is herniation of meninges and spinal cord tissue. Meningocele (herniation of meninges without spinal cord tissue) should also be included in this category. Both open and closed (covered with skin) lesions should be included. Spina bifida is herniation of the meninges and/or spinal cord tissue through a bony defect of spine closure.

Nonvertex presentation—Includes any nonvertex fetal presentation, that is, presentation of a part of the infant's body other than the upper and back part of the infant's head.

Omphalocele/Gastroschisis—Omphalocele is a defect in the anterior abdominal wall, accompanied by herniation of some abdominal organs through a widened umbilical ring into the umbilical stalk. Gastroschisis is an abnormality of the anterior abdominal wall, lateral to the umbilicus, resulting in herniation of the abdominal contents directly into the amniotic cavity.

Precipitous labor—Labor lasting less than 3 hours.

Prenatal care—Medical care provided to a pregnant woman to prevent complications and decrease the incidence of maternal and prenatal mortality. Information on when pregnancy care began is recorded on the birth certificate. Between 1970 and 1980, the reporting area for prenatal care expanded. In 1970, 39 states and the District of Columbia (D.C.) reported prenatal care on the birth certificate. Data were not available from Alabama, Alaska, Arkansas, Connecticut, Delaware, Georgia, Idaho, Massachusetts, New Mexico, Pennsylvania, and Virginia. In 1975, these data were available from three additional states—Connecticut, Delaware, and Georgia—increasing the number of states reporting prenatal care to 42 and D.C. During 1980–2002, prenatal care information was available for the entire United States.

Prepregnancy BMI—The 2003 Standard Certificate of Live Birth includes the components needed to compute both prepregnancy BMI and maternal weight gain (i.e., maternal height, prepregnancy weight, and weight at delivery). BMI is calculated as weight in kilograms divided by height in meters squared (kg/m^2) (4).

Suspected chromosomal disorder—Includes any constellation of congenital malformations resulting from, or compatible with, known syndromes caused by detectable defects in chromosome structure.

Tocolysis—Administration of any agent with the intent to inhibit preterm uterine contractions to extend the length of the pregnancy.

WIC Program—The WIC program is run by the U.S. Department of Agriculture. It is intended to help low-income pregnant women, infants, and children through age 5 years receive proper nutrition by providing vouchers for food, nutrition counseling, health care screenings, and referrals.

PART II:
MORTALITY

PART II: MORTALITY

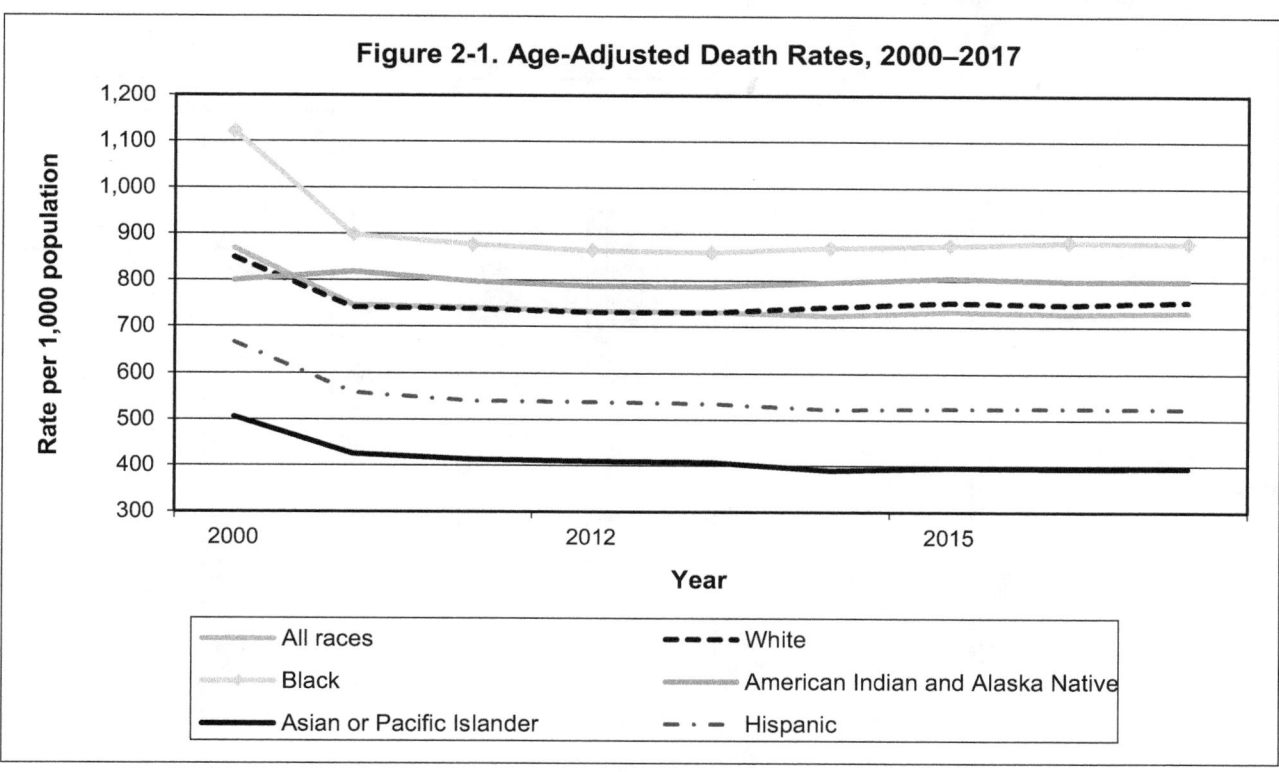

Figure 2-1. Age-Adjusted Death Rates, 2000–2017

Legend:
- All races
- Black
- Asian or Pacific Islander
- White
- American Indian and Alaska Native
- Hispanic

HIGHLIGHTS

- In 2017, 2,813,530 deaths were registered in the United States. The age-adjusted death rate increased 0.4 percent to 731.9 deaths per 100,000 population in 2017 after a decrease in 2016. Among all states, West Virginia had the highest age-adjusted death rate at 957.1, while Hawaii had the lowest age-adjusted death rate at 584.9.

- Hispanic females had the highest life expectancy of all races and ethnic origins at 84.3 years in 2017. Life expectancy was 78.6 years for the population as a whole.

- The five leading causes of death in 2017 were diseases of heart (heart disease), malignant neoplasms (cancer), accidents (unintentional injuries), chronic lower respiratory diseases, and cerebrovascular diseases (stroke).

- The infant mortality rate was 5.7 deaths per 1,000 live births in 2017, down from rates of 6.6 in 2008 and 6.4 in 2009. This number did not represent a significant change from 2016. The neonatal mortality rate also declined, falling from 4.3 in 2008 to 3.8 in 2017. The postneonatal mortality rate declined from 2.3 in 2008 to 2.0 in 2017.

Table 2-1. Number of Deaths, Death Rates, and Age-Adjusted Death Rates, by Race, Hispanic Origin, and Sex, Selected Years, 1940–2017

(Number, rate per 100,000 population.)

Year	Total[1]			Non-Hispanic White[2]			Non-Hispanic Black[2]		
	Both sexes	Male	Female	Both sexes	Male	Female	Both sexes	Male	Female
Number									
1940	1,417,269	781,003	626,266	NA	NA	NA	NA	NA	NA
1950	1,452,454	827,749	624,705	NA	NA	NA	NA	NA	NA
1960	1,711,982	975,648	736,334	NA	NA	NA	NA	NA	NA
1970	1,921,031	1,078,478	842,553	NA	NA	NA	NA	NA	NA
1980	1,989,841	1,075,078	914,763	NA	NA	NA	NA	NA	NA
1990	2,148,463	1,113,417	1,035,046	NA	NA	NA	NA	NA	NA
2000	2,403,351	177,578	1,225,773	1,959,919	944,781	1,015,138	282,676	143,297	139,379
2010	2,468,435	1,232,432	1,236,003	1,969,916	971,604	998,312	283,438	143,824	139,614
2011	2,515,458	1,254,978	1,260,480	2,006,319	989,835	1,016,484	286,797	145,052	141,745
2012	2,543,279	1,273,722	1,269,557	2,016,896	998,832	1,018,064	291,179	148,344	142,835
2013	2,596,993	1,306,034	1,290,959	2,052,660	1,021,135	1,031,525	299,227	152,661	146,566
2014	2,626,418	1,328,241	1,298,177	2,066,949	1,035,345	1,031,604	303,844	154,836	149,008
2015	2,712,630	1,373,404	1,339,226	2,123,631	1,063,705	1,059,926	315,254	161,850	153,404
2016	2,744,248	1,400,232	1,344,016	2,133,463	1,077,362	1,056,101	326,810	168,750	158,060
2017	2,813,503	1,439,111	1,374,392	2,179,857	1,102,838	1,077,019	335,667	174,403	161,264
Crude Death Rate[5]									
1940	1,076.4	1,197.4	954.6	NA	NA	NA	NA	NA	NA
1950	963.8	1,106.1	823.5	NA	NA	NA	NA	NA	NA
1960	954.7	1,104.5	809.2	NA	NA	NA	NA	NA	NA
1970	945.3	1,090.3	807.8	NA	NA	NA	NA	NA	NA
1980	878.3	976.9	785.3	NA	NA	NA	NA	NA	NA
1990	863.8	918.4	812.0	NA	NA	NA	NA	NA	NA
2000	854.0	853.0	855.0	993.2	978.5	1,007.3	805.5	859.5	756.7
2010	799.5	812.0	787.4	984.3	987.5	981.2	718.7	764.5	676.9
2011	807.3	818.7	796.3	1,001.0	1,004.1	998.1	718.0	760.4	679.2
2012	810.2	824.5	796.4	1,004.9	1,011.2	998.8	720.9	768.5	677.3
2013	821.5	839.1	804.4	1,021.6	1,032.1	1,011.5	733.4	782.5	688.4
2014	823.7	846.4	801.7	1,028.1	1,045.4	1,011.3	735.4	783.3	691.4
2015	844.0	868.0	820.7	1,055.3	1,072.5	1,038.5	754.6	809.4	704.3
2016	849.3	880.2	819.3	1,059.7	1,085.6	1,034.6	775.5	836.2	719.7
2017	863.8	897.2	831.4	1,083.2	1,111.4	1,055.8	787.5	854.2	726.1
Age-Adjusted Death Rate[6]									
1940	1,785.0	1,976.0	1,599.4	NA	NA	NA	NA	NA	NA
1950	1,446.0	1,674.2	1,236.0	NA	NA	NA	NA	NA	NA
1960	1,339.2	1,609.0	1,105.3	NA	NA	NA	NA	NA	NA
1970	1,222.6	1,542.1	971.4	NA	NA	NA	NA	NA	NA
1980	1,039.1	1,348.1	817.9	NA	NA	NA	NA	NA	NA
1990	938.7	1,202.8	750.9	NA	NA	NA	NA	NA	NA
2000	869.0	1,053.8	731.4	855.5	1,035.4	721.5	1,137.0	1,422.0	941.2
2010	747.0	887.1	634.9	755.0	892.5	643.3	920.4	1,131.7	770.8
2011	741.3	875.3	632.4	754.3	887.2	644.6	901.6	1,098.3	759.8
2012	732.8	865.1	624.7	745.8	876.2	637.6	887.1	1,086.4	742.1
2013	731.9	863.6	623.5	747.1	876.8	638.4	885.2	1,083.3	740.6
2014	724.6	855.1	616.7	742.8	872.3	633.8	870.7	1,060.3	731.2
2015	733.1	863.2	624.2	753.2	881.3	644.1	876.1	1,070.1	731.0
2016	728.8	861.0	617.5	749.0	879.5	637.2	882.8	1,081.2	734.1
2017	731.9	864.5	619.7	755.0	885.1	642.8	881.0	1,083.3	728.0

NOTE: Beginning in 1970, excludes deaths of nonresidents of the United States. Race and Hispanic-origin categories are consistent with 1977 Office of Management and Budget (OMB) standards. Data for specified race or Hispanic- origin groups other than non-Hispanic White and non-Hispanic Black should be interpreted with caution because of inconsistencies in reporting these items on death certificates and surveys, although misclassification is very minor for the Hispanic and non-Hispanic Asian or Pacific Islander populations.
NA= Not available.
[1]Includes deaths for origin not stated.
[2]Multiple-race data reported according to 1997 OMB standards were bridged to the single-race categories of 1977 OMB standards.
[5]Rates are based on populations enumerated as of April 1 for census years and estimated as of July 1 for all other years.
[6]Age-adjusted rates are per 100,000 U.S. standard population.

Table 2-1. Number of Deaths, Death Rates, and Age-Adjusted Death Rates, by Race, Hispanic Origin, and Sex, Selected Years, 1940–2017—*Continued*

(Number, rate per 100,000 population.)

Year	Non-Hispanic American Indian or Alaska Native[2,3]			Non-Hispanic Asian or Pacific Islander[2,4]			Hispanic		
	Both sexes	Male	Female	Both sexes	Male	Female	Both sexes	Male	Female
Number									
1940	NA	NA	NA	NA	NA	NA	NA	NA	NA
1950	NA	NA	NA	NA	NA	NA	NA	NA	NA
1960	NA	NA	NA	NA	NA	NA	NA	NA	NA
1970	NA	NA	NA	NA	NA	NA	NA	NA	NA
1980	NA	NA	NA	NA	NA	NA	NA	NA	NA
1990	NA	NA	NA	NA	NA	NA	NA	NA	NA
2000	11,025	5,973	5,052	34,226	18,653	15,573	107,254	60,172	47,082
2010	14,846	8,072	6,774	50,018	25,938	24,080	144,490	79,622	64,868
2011	15,181	8,175	7,006	52,346	26,909	25,437	149,635	81,887	67,748
2012	15,705	8,598	7,107	55,298	28,214	27,084	156,419	85,238	71,181
2013	16,219	8,840	7,379	58,702	30,343	28,359	163,241	88,880	74,361
2014	17,138	9,338	7,800	60,424	31,039	29,385	169,387	92,474	76,913
2015	18,039	9,869	8,170	65,277	33,306	31,971	179,457	98,170	81,287
2016	18,595	10,280	8,315	68,235	34,892	33,343	188,254	103,532	84,722
2017	19,198	10,502	8,696	72,598	37,236	35,362	197,249	108,579	88,670
Crude Death Rate[5]									
1940	NA	NA	NA	NA	NA	NA	NA	NA	NA
1950	NA	NA	NA	NA	NA	NA	NA	NA	NA
1960	NA	NA	NA	NA	NA	NA	NA	NA	NA
1970	NA	NA	NA	NA	NA	NA	NA	NA	NA
1980	NA	NA	NA	NA	NA	NA	NA	NA	NA
1990	NA	NA	NA	NA	NA	NA	NA	NA	NA
2000	470.3	517.0	425.0	301.4	338.3	266.5	303.8	331.3	274.6
2010	577.8	640.1	517.7	310.0	336.7	285.6	286.2	310.8	260.9
2011	584.2	640.9	529.5	315.7	339.9	293.7	287.5	309.7	264.6
2012	599.3	668.7	532.5	322.0	344.1	301.7	295.0	316.5	272.7
2013	613.7	681.4	548.3	331.8	359.2	306.7	301.9	323.7	279.4
2014	642.5	713.4	574.2	327.7	352.7	305.0	305.8	330.1	281.0
2015	670.7	747.4	596.7	341.5	364.9	320.1	317.1	343.2	290.4
2016	685.9	772.8	602.2	350.3	374.9	327.8	327.6	356.8	297.7
2017	703.4	784.4	625.5	359.8	386.2	335.6	334.6	364.6	304.0
Age-Adjusted Death Rate[6]									
1940	NA	NA	NA	NA	NA	NA	NA	NA	NA
1950	NA	NA	NA	NA	NA	NA	NA	NA	NA
1960	NA	NA	NA	NA	NA	NA	NA	NA	NA
1970	NA	NA	NA	NA	NA	NA	NA	NA	NA
1980	NA	NA	NA	NA	NA	NA	NA	NA	NA
1990	NA	NA	NA	NA	NA	NA	NA	NA	NA
2000	800.5	955.6	679.1	507.0	624.9	417.3	665.7	818.1	546.0
2010	818.8	965.8	696.8	425.6	513.0	360.6	558.6	677.7	463.4
2011	798.1	933.8	684.7	413.2	493.4	352.8	540.7	647.3	452.8
2012	787.8	929.9	666.3	409.6	486.3	351.4	539.1	643.9	452.5
2013	787.5	930.6	666.4	407.5	490.2	344.8	535.4	639.8	448.6
2014	796.9	935.0	677.4	390.5	464.2	333.3	523.3	626.8	437.5
2015	805.7	950.2	679.5	396.2	468.9	339.6	525.3	628.9	438.3
2016	800.3	954.0	668.0	394.4	466.6	337.4	525.8	631.8	436.4
2017	800.2	943.9	674.0	395.3	470.1	336.4	524.7	631.8	434.2

NOTE: Beginning in 1970, excludes deaths of nonresidents of the United States. Race and Hispanic-origin categories are consistent with 1977 Office of Management and Budget (OMB) standards. Data for specified race or Hispanic-origin groups other than non-Hispanic White and non-Hispanic Black should be interpreted with caution because of inconsistencies in reporting these items on death certificates and surveys, although misclassification is very minor for the Hispanic and non-Hispanic Asian or Pacific Islander populations.

NA= Not available.

[2] Multiple-race data reported according to 1997 OMB standards were bridged to the single-race categories of 1977 OMB standards.

[3] Includes Aleuts and Eskimo persons.

[4] Includes Chinese, Filipino, Hawaiian, Japanese, and other Asian or Pacific Islander persons.

[5] Rates are based on populations enumerated as of April 1 for census years and estimated as of July 1 for all other years.

[6] Age-adjusted rates are per 100,000 U.S. standard population.

Table 2-2. Number of Deaths and Death Rates, by Age, Race, and Sex, 2017

(Number, rate per 100,000 population in specified group.)

Age (years)	Number								
	Total[1]			Non-Hispanic White[2]			Non-Hispanic Black[2]		
	Both sexes	Male	Female	Both sexes	Male	Female	Both sexes	Male	Female
All ages	2,813,503	1,439,111	1,374,392	2,179,857	1,102,838	1,077,019	335,667	174,403	161,264
Under 1 year	22,335	12,468	9,867	9,359	5,281	4,078	6,730	3,760	2,970
1 to 4 years	3,880	2,232	1,648	1,858	1,107	751	985	535	450
5 to 9 years	2,354	1,299	1,055	1,115	623	492	573	319	254
10 to 14 years	3,217	1,970	1,247	1,667	1,005	662	723	465	258
15 to 19 years	10,886	7,849	3,037	5,592	3,894	1,698	2,560	2,019	541
20 to 24 years	21,139	15,654	5,485	11,615	8,391	3,224	4,804	3,692	1,112
25 to 29 years	28,276	20,385	7,891	16,736	11,865	4,871	6,066	4,454	1,612
30 to 34 years	31,939	21,764	10,175	20,028	13,495	6,533	6,018	4,098	1,920
35 to 39 years	36,901	24,105	12,796	22,872	14,806	8,066	7,251	4,663	2,588
40 to 44 years	42,895	26,687	16,208	26,524	16,468	10,056	8,475	5,058	3,417
45 to 49 years	65,698	40,223	25,475	42,453	25,965	16,488	12,288	7,229	5,059
50 to 54 years	104,444	63,581	40,863	70,312	42,816	27,496	18,938	10,952	7,986
55 to 59 years	162,098	98,387	63,711	114,084	69,506	44,578	28,790	16,723	12,067
60 to 64 years	209,908	126,948	82,960	150,915	91,792	59,123	35,708	20,829	14,879
65 to 69 years	248,087	145,258	102,829	184,996	108,920	76,076	37,568	21,346	16,222
70 to 74 years	283,523	158,673	124,850	223,431	125,660	97,771	33,453	18,050	15,403
75 to 79 years	307,498	163,505	143,993	245,250	131,567	113,683	32,828	16,251	16,577
80 to 84 years.....................	350,261	173,166	177,095	284,866	142,527	142,339	32,248	14,488	17,760
85 years and over	878,035	334,866	543,169	746,124	287,103	459,021	59,645	19,462	40,183
Not stated	129	91	38	60	47	13	16	10	6
Rate									
All ages	863.8	897.2	831.4	1,083.2	1,111.4	1,055.8	787.5	854.2	726.1
Under 1 year[5]	567.0	618.7	512.8	458.5	505.2	409.5	1,110.6	1,215.4	1,001.3
1 to 4 years	24.3	27.3	21.1	22.4	26.1	18.6	40.1	42.9	37.3
5 to 9 years	11.6	12.5	10.6	10.6	11.5	9.6	18.5	20.2	16.6
10 to 14 years	15.5	18.6	12.3	15.0	17.7	12.2	23.4	29.7	17.0
15 to 19 years	51.5	72.7	29.4	48.2	65.5	30.1	80.0	124.2	34.4
20 to 24 years	95.6	137.9	50.9	95.1	133.6	54.3	140.8	213.0	66.3
25 to 29 years	121.0	171.3	68.8	127.9	178.2	75.8	171.4	252.3	90.9
30 to 34 years	145.4	196.3	93.5	159.3	212.4	105.0	203.9	286.3	126.3
35 to 39 years	173.8	227.1	120.5	187.5	241.1	133.2	257.9	349.0	175.4
40 to 44 years	218.4	273.6	163.9	233.9	289.1	178.2	332.4	422.2	252.8
45 to 49 years	313.2	387.3	240.6	326.7	399.0	254.1	461.4	578.4	357.9
50 to 54 years	488.0	604.2	375.5	499.8	613.5	387.8	703.6	869.7	557.6
55 to 59 years	736.5	919.5	563.4	741.6	919.5	569.7	1,088.2	1,365.8	849.1
60 to 64 years	1,050.2	1,328.3	795.4	1,040.5	1,305.4	791.3	1,583.5	2,051.5	1,200.3
65 to 69 years	1,473.5	1,831.8	1,154.5	1,463.6	1,799.6	1,154.9	2,168.8	2,831.9	1,657.9
70 to 74 years	2,206.9	2,668.0	1,809.5	2,240.1	2,675.8	1,852.4	2,899.5	3,717.9	2,305.0
75 to 79 years	3,517.8	4,193.7	2,973.6	3,603.5	4,259.2	3,058.6	4,258.0	5,298.3	3,570.7
80 to 84 years.....................	5,871.7	6,901.6	5,123.9	6,078.8	7,102.6	5,312.1	6,363.6	7,821.4	5,523.7
85 years and over	13,573.6	14,689.2	12,966.5	14,336.0	15,521.8	13,682.1	12,101.9	13,164.9	11,646.4

NOTE: Rates are per 100,000 population in specified group. Race and Hispanic-origin categories are consistent with 1977 Office of Management and Budget (OMB) standards. Data for specified race or Hispanic-origin groups other than non-Hispanic white and non-Hispanic black should be interpreted with caution because of inconsistencies in reporting these items on death certificates and surveys, although misclassification is very minor for the Hispanic and non-Hispanic Asian or Pacific Islander populations

– = Quantity zero.
* = Rate does not meet NCHS standards of reliability.
[1]Includes deaths for origin not stated.
[2]Multiple-race data reported according to 1997 OMB standards were bridged to single-race categories of 1977 OMB standards.
[5]Death rates for "Under 1 year" (based on population estimates) differ from infant mortality rates (based on live births).

Table 2-2. Number of Deaths and Death Rates, by Age, Race, and Sex, 2017—*Continued*

(Number, rate per 100,000 population in specified group.)

Age (years)	Number								
	Non-Hispanic American Indian or Alaska Native[2,3]			Non-Hispanic Asian or Pacific Islander[2,4]			Hispanic		
	Both sexes	Male	Female	Both sexes	Male	Female	Both sexes	Male	Female
All ages	19,198	10,502	8,696	72,598	37,236	35,362	197,249	108,579	88,670
Under 1 year	284	151	133	957	528	429	4,808	2,635	2,173
1 to 4 years	72	33	39	148	96	52	805	455	350
5 to 9 years	38	19	19	100	52	48	521	282	239
10 to 14 years	64	36	28	108	62	46	644	395	249
15 to 19 years	208	148	60	325	222	103	2,175	1,547	628
20 to 24 years	354	244	110	635	445	190	3,679	2,840	839
25 to 29 years	547	348	199	680	477	203	4,166	3,181	985
30 to 34 years	647	431	216	820	536	284	4,326	3,128	1,198
35 to 39 years	680	441	239	944	584	360	5,014	3,516	1,498
40 to 44 years	729	430	299	1,283	790	493	5,724	3,842	1,882
45 to 49 years	948	592	356	2,007	1,181	826	7,738	5,072	2,666
50 to 54 years	1,338	775	563	2,678	1,613	1,065	10,671	7,073	3,598
55 to 59 years	1,686	1,000	686	3,611	2,133	1,478	13,056	8,392	4,664
60 to 64 years	1,857	1,068	789	4,891	2,898	1,993	15,477	9,582	5,895
65 to 69 years	1,889	1,087	802	6,260	3,600	2,660	16,280	9,533	6,747
70 to 74 years	1,855	997	858	6,633	3,752	2,881	17,088	9,499	7,589
75 to 79 years	1,798	933	865	8,035	4,393	3,642	18,699	9,834	8,865
80 to 84 years.....................	1,731	829	902	9,495	4,705	4,790	21,131	10,177	10,954
85 years and over	2,473	940	1,533	22,988	9,169	13,819	45,236	17,588	27,648
Not stated	–	–	–	–	–	–	11	8	3
Rate									
All ages	703.4	784.4	625.5	359.8	386.2	335.6	334.6	364.6	304.0
Under 1 year[5]	723.8	755.9	690.6	431.2	464.0	396.7	466.4	500.3	431.0
1 to 4 years	45.3	40.8	50.0	15.6	19.6	11.3	19.4	21.5	17.2
5 to 9 years	18.6	*	*	8.4	8.6	8.3	9.9	10.5	9.3
10 to 14 years	31.1	34.7	27.5	8.9	10.1	7.6	12.5	15.0	9.8
15 to 19 years	99.5	139.8	58.2	26.5	35.9	16.9	44.4	61.8	26.2
20 to 24 years	163.3	221.7	103.0	44.2	61.2	26.8	76.1	113.7	35.9
25 to 29 years	245.7	307.8	181.7	39.2	55.8	23.1	86.9	126.7	43.2
30 to 34 years	343.2	459.6	227.9	47.4	64.5	31.6	95.5	131.5	55.7
35 to 39 years	394.3	518.1	273.6	57.8	76.3	41.5	113.5	153.7	70.3
40 to 44 years	465.5	561.2	373.8	83.2	109.4	60.1	141.2	186.5	94.4
45 to 49 years	584.1	748.4	427.9	137.6	173.3	106.4	209.4	271.5	146.0
50 to 54 years	784.4	945.4	635.5	210.9	272.4	157.1	333.4	439.8	225.9
55 to 59 years	969.7	1,219.9	746.4	313.1	402.2	237.2	492.5	643.2	346.5
60 to 64 years	1,251.2	1,549.5	992.5	475.1	625.4	352.0	754.5	979.9	549.2
65 to 69 years	1,649.4	2,037.6	1,310.8	736.9	957.5	561.7	1,085.1	1,372.9	837.1
70 to 74 years	2,355.3	2,739.0	2,025.5	1,122.0	1,426.1	878.2	1,628.5	2,037.5	1,301.5
75 to 79 years	3,598.9	4,166.7	3,137.7	1,962.4	2,418.3	1,598.9	2,652.3	3,288.8	2,183.5
80 to 84 years.....................	5,805.8	6,639.4	5,205.1	3,529.8	4,126.1	3,091.0	4,462.8	5,338.6	3,872.5
85 years and over	9,157.2	9,649.9	8,879.2	8,567.8	9,252.7	8,166.7	9,504.4	10,147.1	9,136.3

NOTE: Rates are per 100,000 population in specified group. Race and Hispanic-origin categories are consistent with 1977 Office of Management and Budget (OMB) standards. Data for specified race or Hispanic-origin groups other than non-Hispanic white and non-Hispanic black should be interpreted with caution because of inconsistencies in reporting these items on death certificates and surveys, although misclassification is very minor for the Hispanic and non-Hispanic Asian or Pacific Islander populations.
– = Quantity zero.
* = Rate does not meet NCHS standards of reliability.
[2]Multiple-race data reported according to 1997 OMB standards were bridged to single-race categories of 1977 OMB standards.
[3]Includes Aleut and Eskimo persons.
[4]Includes Chinese, Filipino, Hawaiian, Japanese, and other Asian or Pacific Islander persons.
[5]Death rates for "Under 1 year" (based on population estimates) differ from infant mortality rates (based on live births).

Table 2-3. Number of Deaths and Death Rates, by Age, and Age-Adjusted Death Rates, by Specified Hispanic Origin, Race for Non-Hispanic Group, and Sex, 2017

(Number, rate per 100,000 population in specified group.)

Hispanic origin, race for non-Hispanic population, and sex	All ages	Under 1 year[1]	1 to 4 years	5 to 14 years	15 to 24 years	25 to 34 years	35 to 44 years	45 to 54 years	55 to 64 years	65 to 74 years	75 to 84 years	85 years and over	Age not stated	Age-adjusted rate[2]
NUMBER														
All origins	2,813,503	22,335	3,880	5,571	32,025	60,215	79,796	170,142	372,006	531,610	657,759	878,035	129	X
Male	1,439,111	12,468	2,232	3,269	23,503	42,149	50,792	103,804	225,335	303,931	336,671	334,866	91	X
Female	1,374,392	9,867	1,648	2,302	8,522	18,066	29,004	66,338	146,671	227,679	321,088	543,169	38	X
														X
Hispanic	197,249	4,808	805	1,165	5,854	8,492	10,738	18,409	28,533	33,368	39,830	45,236	11	X
Male	108,579	2,635	455	677	4,387	6,309	7,358	12,145	17,974	19,032	20,011	17,588	8	X
Female	88,670	2,173	350	488	1,467	2,183	3,380	6,264	10,559	14,336	19,819	27,648	3	X
Mexican	105,392	2,917	506	725	3,626	4,830	6,264	10,649	16,076	18,370	20,076	21,350	3	X
Male	59,793	1,600	280	431	2,730	3,597	4,255	7,072	10,254	10,588	10,252	8,733	1	X
Female	45,599	1,317	226	294	896	1,233	2,009	3,577	5,822	7,782	9,824	12,617	2	X
Puerto Rican	25,077	463	65	96	497	982	1,379	2,412	3,751	4,634	5,406	5,388	4	X
Male	13,592	260	42	51	360	722	983	1,568	2,333	2,599	2,709	1,961	4	X
Female	11,485	203	23	45	137	260	396	844	1,418	2,035	2,697	3,427	–	X
Cuban	16,899	91	18	15	148	217	267	720	1,473	2,368	4,575	7,007	–	X
Male	8,636	49	13	11	111	167	178	497	1,020	1,463	2,348	2,779	–	X
Female	8,263	42	5	4	37	50	89	223	453	905	2,227	4,228	–	X
Central American	10,706	359	52	88	450	737	875	1,182	1,648	1,585	1,746	1,983	1	X
Male	5,689	186	29	51	360	591	649	793	964	795	733	537	1	X
Female	5,017	173	23	37	90	146	226	389	684	790	1,013	1,446	–	X
South American	8,309	109	22	29	154	239	299	557	974	1,442	2,050	2,434	–	X
Male	4,081	45	12	11	113	167	194	334	566	773	984	882	–	X
Female	4,228	64	10	18	41	72	105	223	408	669	1,066	1,552	–	X
Dominican	4,865	103	11	21	140	225	255	389	690	836	1,079	1,116	–	X
Male	2,476	59	6	11	108	161	174	223	388	473	484	389	–	X
Female	2,389	44	5	10	32	64	81	166	302	363	595	727	–	X
Other and unknown Hispanic	26,001	766	131	191	839	1,262	1,399	2,500	3,921	4,133	4,898	5,958	3	X
Male	14,312	436	73	111	605	904	925	1,658	2,449	2,341	2,501	2,307	2	X
Female	11,689	330	58	80	234	358	474	842	1,472	1,792	2,397	3,651	1	X
Non-Hispanic[3]	2,607,320	17,330	3,063	4,388	26,093	51,542	68,758	150,962	341,542	496,085	616,251	831,230	76	X
Male	1,324,979	9,720	1,771	2,581	19,055	35,704	43,240	91,123	205,949	283,412	315,693	316,674	57	X
Female	1,282,341	7,610	1,292	1,807	7,038	15,838	25,518	59,839	135,593	212,673	300,558	514,556	19	X
White[4]	2,179,857	9,359	1,858	2,782	17,207	36,764	49,396	112,765	264,999	408,427	530,116	746,124	60	X
Male	1,102,838	5,281	1,107	1,628	12,285	25,360	31,274	68,781	161,298	234,580	274,094	287,103	47	X
Female	1,077,019	4,078	751	1,154	4,922	11,404	18,122	43,984	103,701	173,847	256,022	459,021	13	X
Black[4]	335,667	6,730	985	1,296	7,364	12,084	15,726	31,226	64,498	71,021	65,076	59,645	16	X
Male	174,403	3,760	535	784	5,711	8,552	9,721	18,181	37,552	39,396	30,739	19,462	10	X
Female	161,264	2,970	450	512	1,653	3,532	6,005	13,045	26,946	31,625	34,337	40,183	6	X
Origin not stated[5]	8,934	197	12	18	78	181	300	771	1,931	2,157	1,678	1,569	42	X
Male	5,553	113	6	11	61	136	194	536	1,412	1,487	967	604	26	X
Female	3,381	84	6	7	17	45	106	235	519	670	711	965	16	X
RATE[6]														
All origins[7]	863.8	567.0	24.3	13.6	74.0	132.8	195.2	401.5	885.8	1,790.9	4,472.6	13,573.6	X	731.9
Male	897.2	618.7	27.3	15.6	106.1	183.3	249.4	496.5	1,112.3	2,190.2	5,254.0	14,689.2	X	864.5
Female	831.4	512.8	21.1	11.4	40.4	80.8	141.4	309.0	674.7	1,440.4	3,869.1	12,966.5	X	619.7
Hispanic	334.6	466.4	19.4	11.2	60.1	91.1	126.7	267.0	606.8	1,308.7	3,379.7	9,504.4	X	524.7
Male	364.6	500.3	21.5	12.7	87.7	129.0	169.2	349.4	787.4	1,639.9	4,086.8	10,147.1	X	631.8
Female	304.0	431.0	17.2	9.5	31.0	49.3	81.9	183.2	436.4	1,032.1	2,877.0	9,136.3	X	434.2
Mexican	287.4	473.9	18.3	10.2	56.6	84.4	120.0	261.7	614.0	1,351.9	3,402.6	9,910.4	X	532.3
Male	320.2	512.9	19.9	11.9	83.2	120.0	157.7	339.9	783.5	1,656.1	4,067.8	10,841.7	X	637.5
Female	253.4	433.8	16.7	8.4	28.6	45.3	79.7	179.9	444.6	1,081.5	2,906.6	9,354.2	X	441.1
Puerto Rican	448.7	526.0	17.0	10.2	54.2	113.4	183.7	368.4	756.0	1,551.0	3,710.0	11,446.8	X	624.4
Male	489.3	584.7	21.6	10.6	75.5	163.1	261.2	490.9	995.5	1,955.8	4,740.6	11,823.9	X	764.0
Female	408.6	466.2	12.3	9.8	31.2	61.5	105.8	251.7	541.7	1,226.7	3,045.0	11,241.6	X	511.5
Cuban	729.7	306.1	*	*	52.9	64.7	88.4	199.5	546.5	1,318.9	3,374.9	11,805.2	X	532.6
Male	740.7	386.7	*	*	76.9	97.8	111.1	256.2	748.2	1,752.8	4,114.2	13,077.6	X	652.7
Female	718.5	246.3	*	*	27.3	30.3	62.7	133.6	340.0	941.9	2,837.3	11,095.7	X	431.6
Central American	192.5	402.1	12.9	9.5	51.6	74.1	93.4	181.7	402.0	871.4	2,457.3	7,558.6	X	384.6
Male	199.8	420.3	14.1	10.7	78.1	108.7	131.6	238.3	511.0	1,096.2	3,098.7	8,738.8	X	478.7
Female	184.8	384.2	11.6	8.2	21.9	32.3	51.0	122.4	309.1	722.4	2,137.1	7,197.6	X	321.5

NOTE: Rates are per 100,000 population in specified group; age-adjusted rates are per 100,000 U.S. standard population. Populations used for computing death rates for "All Origins," Hispanic, non-Hispanic, non-Hispanic white, and non-Hispanic black are postcensal estimates based on the 2010 census estimated as of July 1, 2017; populations used for computing death rates for Mexican, Puerto Rican, Cuban, Central American, South American, Dominican, and Other and Unknown Hispanic are estimates based on the 2017 1-year American Community Survey adjusted to control totals. The control totals are 2010-based postcensal estimates for the United States for July 1, 2017. Race and Hispanic origin are reported separately on the death certificate. Persons of Hispanic origin may be of any race. Data for Hispanic persons are not tabulated separately by race; data for non-Hispanic persons are tabulated by race. Data for Hispanic origin should be interpreted with caution because of inconsistencies between reporting Hispanic origin on death certificates and on censuses and surveys.

X = Not applicable.

– = Quantity zero.

* = Rate does not meet NCHS standards of reliability.

[1]Death rates for "Under 1" (based on population estimates) differ from infant mortality rates (based on live births).

[2]For method of computation, see chapter notes.

[3]Includes races other than White and Black.

[4]Race categories are consistent with 1977 Office of Management and Budget (OMB) standards. In 2017, multiple-race data were reported by 50 states and the District of Columbia. Multiple-race data for these reporting areas were bridged to the single-race categories of 1977 OMB standards for comparability with other reporting areas.

[5]Includes deaths for which Hispanic origin was not reported on the death certificate.

[6]Figures for age not stated are included in "All ages" but not distributed among age groups.

[7]Figures for origin not stated are included in "All origins" but not distributed among specified origins.

Table 2-3. Number of Deaths and Death Rates, by Age, and Age-Adjusted Death Rates, by Specified Hispanic Origin, Race for Non-Hispanic Group, and Sex, 2017—*Continued*

(Number, rate per 100,000 population in specified group.)

Hispanic origin, race for non-Hispanic population, and sex	All ages	Under 1 year[1]	1 to 4 years	5 to 14 years	15 to 24 years	25 to 34 years	35 to 44 years	45 to 54 years	55 to 64 years	65 to 74 years	75 to 84 years	85 years and over	Age not stated	Age-adjusted rate[2]
South American	223.3	236.9	11.3	6.2	30.9	42.1	49.2	102.3	234.3	643.8	1,836.8	6,390.1	X	281.0
Male	229.2	196.7	*	*	45.0	58.8	66.7	134.0	302.3	794.4	2,175.5	7,124.4	X	334.0
Female	217.9	276.6	*	*	16.5	25.3	33.1	75.6	178.6	528.1	1,606.0	6,036.6	X	242.9
Dominican	233.7	266.6	*	6.6	41.2	64.8	88.0	155.4	373.9	757.0	2,957.4	6,266.1	X	367.2
Male	248.5	265.0	*	*	60.5	95.5	132.6	206.3	470.0	1,056.9	3,470.8	7,150.7	X	453.1
Female	220.1	268.8	*	*	19.9	35.8	51.0	116.7	296.1	552.6	2,639.8	5,877.1	X	308.5
Other and unknown Hispanic	893.9	2,084.9	73.6	41.7	177.3	308.1	381.3	719.0	1,289.5	2,137.5	4,862.7	14,795.1	X	965.4
Male	967.4	2,273.2	81.7	45.7	241.7	403.6	485.2	940.7	1,731.4	2,639.5	5,781.3	17,082.6	X	1,186.1
Female	817.8	1,879.3	65.4	37.2	104.9	192.8	269.0	491.1	905.2	1,712.1	4,171.2	13,640.9	X	776.3
Non-Hispanic[3]	977.4	595.8	25.8	14.3	77.9	143.1	212.2	425.5	915.8	1,828.3	4,555.4	13,870.6	X	753.8
Male	1,014.3	653.0	29.2	16.5	111.1	197.2	269.9	522.8	1,145.7	2,228.7	5,334.2	15,034.3	X	889.0
Female	941.9	535.9	22.3	12.1	43.0	88.4	155.8	331.5	701.9	1,475.1	3,949.6	13,239.9	X	639.5
White[4]	1,083.2	458.5	22.4	12.9	72.3	143.3	209.8	416.7	886.6	1,806.1	4,612.9	14,336.0	X	755.0
Male	1,111.4	505.2	26.1	14.7	100.5	194.9	264.2	510.0	1,105.5	2,182.5	5,378.9	15,521.8	X	885.1
Female	1,055.8	409.5	18.6	10.9	42.5	90.2	154.9	323.9	677.9	1,465.2	4,002.6	13,682.1	X	642.8
Black[4]	787.5	1,110.6	40.1	20.9	111.4	186.2	293.4	583.2	1,316.1	2,460.9	5,093.1	12,101.9	X	881.0
Male	854.2	1,215.4	42.9	24.9	170.0	267.5	383.6	724.6	1,676.6	3,179.0	6,248.3	13,164.9	X	1,083.3
Female	726.1	1,001.3	37.3	16.8	50.8	107.3	212.4	458.4	1,012.7	1,920.5	4,369.8	11,646.4	X	728.0

NOTE: Rates are per 100,000 population in specified group; age-adjusted rates are per 100,000 U.S. standard population. Populations used for computing death rates for "All Origins," Hispanic, non-Hispanic, non-Hispanic white, and non-Hispanic black are postcensal estimates based on the 2010 census estimated as of July 1, 2017; populations used for computing death rates for Mexican, Puerto Rican, Cuban, Central American, South American, Dominican, and Other and Unknown Hispanic are estimates based on the 2017 1-year American Community Survey adjusted to control totals. The control totals are 2010-based postcensal estimates for the United States for July 1, 2017. Race and Hispanic origin are reported separately on the death certificate. Persons of Hispanic origin may be of any race. Data for Hispanic persons are not tabulated separately by race; data for non-Hispanic persons are tabulated by race. Data for Hispanic origin should be interpreted with caution because of inconsistencies between reporting Hispanic origin on death certificates and on censuses and surveys.

X = Not applicable.

– = Quantity zero.

* = Rate does not meet NCHS standards of reliability.

[1]Death rates for "Under 1" (based on population estimates) differ from infant mortality rates (based on live births).

[2]For method of computation, see chapter notes.

[3]Includes races other than White and Black.

[4]Race categories are consistent with 1977 Office of Management and Budget (OMB) standards. In 2017, multiple-race data were reported by 50 states and the District of Columbia. Multiple-race data for these reporting areas were bridged to the single-race categories of 1977 OMB standards for comparability with other reporting areas.

Table 2-4. Life Table for the Total Population, 2017
(Number.)

Age	Probability of dying between ages x and x + 1 q_x	Number surviving to age x l_x	Number dying between ages x and x + 1 d_x	Person-years lived between ages x and x + 1 L_x	Total number of person-years lived above age x T_x	Expectancy of life at age x e_x
0 to 1	0.005777	100,000	578	99,493	7,860,752	78.6
1 to 2	0.000382	99,422	38	99,403	7,761,259	78.1
2 to 3	0.000248	99,384	25	99,372	7,661,855	77.1
3 to 4	0.000193	99,360	19	99,350	7,562,483	76.1
4 to 5	0.000149	99,341	15	99,333	7,463,133	75.1
5 to 6	0.000141	99,326	14	99,319	7,363,800	74.1
6 to 7	0.000126	99,312	13	99,305	7,264,481	73.1
7 to 8	0.000114	99,299	11	99,294	7,165,176	72.2
8 to 9	0.000104	99,288	10	99,283	7,065,882	71.2
9 to 10	0.000095	99,278	9	99,273	6,966,600	70.2
10 to 11	0.000093	99,268	9	99,264	6,867,327	69.2
11 to 12	0.000103	99,259	10	99,254	6,768,063	68.2
12 to 13	0.000133	99,249	13	99,242	6,668,809	67.2
13 to 14	0.000186	99,236	18	99,226	6,569,567	66.2
14 to 15	0.000258	99,217	26	99,204	6,470,341	65.2
15 to 16	0.000338	99,191	34	99,175	6,371,137	64.2
16 to 17	0.000421	99,158	42	99,137	6,271,962	63.3
17 to 18	0.000510	99,116	51	99,091	6,172,825	62.3
18 to 19	0.000603	99,066	60	99,036	6,073,734	61.3
19 to 20	0.000698	99,006	69	98,971	5,974,699	60.3
20 to 21	0.000795	98,937	79	98,897	5,875,727	59.4
21 to 22	0.000889	98,858	88	98,814	5,776,830	58.4
22 to 23	0.000970	98,770	96	98,722	5,678,016	57.5
23 to 24	0.001032	98,674	102	98,623	5,579,293	56.5
24 to 25	0.001080	98,573	106	98,519	5,480,670	55.6
25 to 26	0.001123	98,466	111	98,411	5,382,151	54.7
26 to 27	0.001165	98,355	115	98,298	5,283,740	53.7
27 to 28	0.001207	98,241	119	98,182	5,185,442	52.8
28 to 29	0.001252	98,122	123	98,061	5,087,260	51.8
29 to 30	0.001300	97,999	127	97,936	4,989,199	50.9
30 to 31	0.001351	97,872	132	97,806	4,891,263	50.0
31 to 32	0.001402	97,740	137	97,671	4,793,457	49.0
32 to 33	0.001454	97,603	142	97,532	4,695,786	48.1
33 to 34	0.001506	97,461	147	97,388	4,598,254	47.2
34 to 35	0.001556	97,314	151	97,238	4,500,867	46.3
35 to 36	0.001615	97,163	157	97,084	4,403,628	45.3
36 to 37	0.001679	97,006	163	96,924	4,306,544	44.4
37 to 38	0.001740	96,843	168	96,759	4,209,619	43.5
38 to 39	0.001798	96,674	174	96,588	4,112,861	42.5
39 to 40	0.001860	96,501	179	96,411	4,016,273	41.6
40 to 41	0.001936	96,321	186	96,228	3,919,862	40.7
41 to 42	0.002036	96,135	196	96,037	3,823,634	39.8
42 to 43	0.002160	95,939	207	95,835	3,727,597	38.9
43 to 44	0.002306	95,732	221	95,621	3,631,762	37.9
44 to 45	0.002470	95,511	236	95,393	3,536,140	37.0
45 to 46	0.002647	95,275	252	95,149	3,440,747	36.1
46 to 47	0.002846	95,023	270	94,888	3,345,598	35.2
47 to 48	0.003079	94,753	292	94,607	3,250,710	34.3
48 to 49	0.003357	94,461	317	94,302	3,156,104	33.4
49 to 50	0.003682	94,144	347	93,970	3,061,801	32.5
50 to 51	0.004030	93,797	378	93,608	2,967,831	31.6
51 to 52	0.004401	93,419	411	93,214	2,874,223	30.8
52 to 53	0.004820	93,008	448	92,784	2,781,009	29.9
53 to 54	0.005285	92,560	489	92,315	2,688,226	29.0
54 to 55	0.005778	92,070	532	91,804	2,595,911	28.2
55 to 56	0.006284	91,538	575	91,251	2,504,106	27.4
56 to 57	0.006794	90,963	618	90,654	2,412,855	26.5
57 to 58	0.007319	90,345	661	90,015	2,322,201	25.7
58 to 59	0.007869	89,684	706	89,331	2,232,186	24.9
59 to 60	0.008456	88,978	752	88,602	2,142,855	24.1
60 to 61	0.009093	88,226	802	87,825	2,054,253	23.3
61 to 62	0.009768	87,424	854	86,997	1,966,428	22.5
62 to 63	0.010467	86,570	906	86,117	1,879,431	21.7
63 to 64	0.011181	85,664	958	85,185	1,793,315	20.9
64 to 65	0.011922	84,706	1,010	84,201	1,708,130	20.2
65 to 66	0.012710	83,696	1,064	83,164	1,623,929	19.4
66 to 67	0.013621	82,632	1,126	82,069	1,540,765	18.6
67 to 68	0.014620	81,507	1,192	80,911	1,458,695	17.9
68 to 69	0.015770	80,315	1,267	79,682	1,377,785	17.2
69 to 70	0.017100	79,048	1,352	78,373	1,298,103	16.4

Table 2-4. Life Table for the Total Population, 2017—*Continued*

(Number.)

Age	Probability of dying between ages x and $x+1$ q_x	Number surviving to age x l_x	Number dying between ages x and $x+1$ d_x	Person-years lived between ages x and $x+1$ L_x	Total number of person-years lived above age x T_x	Expectancy of life at age x e_x
70 to 71	0.018428	77,697	1,432	76,981	1,219,730	15.7
71 to 72	0.020317	76,265	1,549	75,490	1,142,750	15.0
72 to 73	0.022102	74,715	1,651	73,890	1,067,259	14.3
73 to 74	0.024194	73,064	1,768	72,180	993,370	13.6
74 to 75	0.026342	71,296	1,878	70,357	921,190	12.9
75 to 76	0.029042	69,418	2,016	68,410	850,832	12.3
76 to 77	0.032001	67,402	2,157	66,324	782,422	11.6
77 to 78	0.035443	65,245	2,313	64,089	716,098	11.0
78 to 79	0.039257	62,933	2,471	61,698	652,009	10.4
79 to 80	0.043393	60,462	2,624	59,150	590,312	9.8
80 to 81	0.048163	57,839	2,786	56,446	531,161	9.2
81 to 82	0.053216	55,053	2,930	53,588	474,715	8.6
82 to 83	0.059240	52,123	3,088	50,579	421,127	8.1
83 to 84	0.066564	49,035	3,264	47,403	370,548	7.6
84 to 85	0.074045	45,771	3,389	44,077	323,145	7.1
85 to 86	0.081954	42,382	3,473	40,646	279,068	6.6
86 to 87	0.090879	38,909	3,536	37,141	238,422	6.1
87 to 88	0.101938	35,373	3,606	33,570	201,281	5.7
88 to 89	0.114075	31,767	3,624	29,955	167,711	5.3
89 to 90	0.127331	28,143	3,584	26,352	137,756	4.9
90 to 91	0.141733	24,560	3,481	22,819	111,405	4.5
91 to 92	0.157289	21,079	3,315	19,421	88,585	4.2
92 to 93	0.173986	17,763	3,091	16,218	69,164	3.9
93 to 94	0.191788	14,673	2,814	13,266	52,946	3.6
94 to 95	0.210633	11,859	2,498	10,610	39,680	3.3
95 to 96	0.230432	9,361	2,157	8,282	29,071	3.1
96 to 97	0.251066	7,204	1,809	6,300	20,788	2.9
97 to 98	0.272395	5,395	1,470	4,660	14,489	2.7
98 to 99	0.294253	3,926	1,155	3,348	9,828	2.5
99 to 100	0.316456	2,770	877	2,332	6,480	2.3
100 and over	1.000000	1,894	1,894	4,148	4,148	2.2

Table 2-4a. Life Table for the Male Population, 2017

(Number.)

Age	Probability of dying between ages x and x + 1 q_x	Number surviving to age x l_x	Number dying between ages x and x + 1 d_x	Person-years lived between ages x and x + 1 L_x	Total number of person-years lived above age x T_x	Expectancy of life at age x e_x
0 to 1	0.006302	100,000	630	99,449	7,610,075	76.1
1 to 2	0.000423	99,370	42	99,349	7,510,627	75.6
2 to 3	0.000287	99,328	29	99,313	7,411,278	74.6
3 to 4	0.000225	99,299	22	99,288	7,311,964	73.6
4 to 5	0.000158	99,277	16	99,269	7,212,676	72.7
5 to 6	0.000156	99,261	15	99,253	7,113,407	71.7
6 to 7	0.000138	99,246	14	99,239	7,014,154	70.7
7 to 8	0.000124	99,232	12	99,226	6,914,915	69.7
8 to 9	0.000110	99,220	11	99,214	6,815,689	68.7
9 to 10	0.000098	99,209	10	99,204	6,716,475	67.7
10 to 11	0.000094	99,199	9	99,194	6,617,271	66.7
11 to 12	0.000108	99,190	11	99,184	6,518,077	65.7
12 to 13	0.000152	99,179	15	99,171	6,418,893	64.7
13 to 14	0.000232	99,164	23	99,152	6,319,721	63.7
14 to 15	0.000341	99,141	34	99,124	6,220,569	62.7
15 to 16	0.000461	99,107	46	99,084	6,121,445	61.8
16 to 17	0.000584	99,061	58	99,032	6,022,360	60.8
17 to 18	0.000718	99,003	71	98,968	5,923,328	59.8
18 to 19	0.000859	98,932	85	98,890	5,824,360	58.9
19 to 20	0.001001	98,848	99	98,798	5,725,470	57.9
20 to 21	0.001147	98,749	113	98,692	5,626,672	57.0
21 to 22	0.001286	98,635	127	98,572	5,527,980	56.0
22 to 23	0.001403	98,508	138	98,439	5,429,408	55.1
23 to 24	0.001490	98,370	147	98,297	5,330,969	54.2
24 to 25	0.001554	98,224	153	98,147	5,232,672	53.3
25 to 26	0.001609	98,071	158	97,992	5,134,525	52.4
26 to 27	0.001664	97,913	163	97,832	5,036,533	51.4
27 to 28	0.001713	97,750	167	97,667	4,938,701	50.5
28 to 29	0.001762	97,583	172	97,497	4,841,034	49.6
29 to 30	0.001810	97,411	176	97,323	4,743,537	48.7
30 to 31	0.001859	97,235	181	97,144	4,646,215	47.8
31 to 32	0.001907	97,054	185	96,961	4,549,070	46.9
32 to 33	0.001959	96,869	190	96,774	4,452,109	46.0
33 to 34	0.002014	96,679	195	96,582	4,355,335	45.0
34 to 35	0.002072	96,484	200	96,384	4,258,754	44.1
35 to 36	0.002139	96,284	206	96,181	4,162,369	43.2
36 to 37	0.002211	96,078	212	95,972	4,066,188	42.3
37 to 38	0.002277	95,866	218	95,757	3,970,216	41.4
38 to 39	0.002333	95,648	223	95,536	3,874,459	40.5
39 to 40	0.002390	95,425	228	95,311	3,778,923	39.6
40 to 41	0.002463	95,196	234	95,079	3,683,612	38.7
41 to 42	0.002566	94,962	244	94,840	3,588,533	37.8
42 to 43	0.002701	94,718	256	94,591	3,493,693	36.9
43 to 44	0.002870	94,463	271	94,327	3,399,102	36.0
44 to 45	0.003066	94,192	289	94,047	3,304,775	35.1
45 to 46	0.003280	93,903	308	93,749	3,210,728	34.2
46 to 47	0.003520	93,595	329	93,430	3,116,979	33.3
47 to 48	0.003804	93,265	355	93,088	3,023,549	32.4
48 to 49	0.004146	92,910	385	92,718	2,930,462	31.5
49 to 50	0.004547	92,525	421	92,315	2,837,744	30.7
50 to 51	0.004978	92,105	459	91,875	2,745,429	29.8
51 to 52	0.005441	91,646	499	91,397	2,653,554	29.0
52 to 53	0.005965	91,147	544	90,876	2,562,157	28.1
53 to 54	0.006549	90,604	593	90,307	2,471,281	27.3
54 to 55	0.007170	90,010	645	89,688	2,380,974	26.5
55 to 56	0.007803	89,365	697	89,016	2,291,287	25.6
56 to 57	0.008445	88,668	749	88,293	2,202,270	24.8
57 to 58	0.009116	87,919	801	87,518	2,113,977	24.0
58 to 59	0.009838	87,117	857	86,689	2,026,459	23.3
59 to 60	0.010619	86,260	916	85,802	1,939,770	22.5
60 to 61	0.011470	85,344	979	84,855	1,853,967	21.7
61 to 62	0.012361	84,365	1,043	83,844	1,769,113	21.0
62 to 63	0.013260	83,323	1,105	82,770	1,685,269	20.2
63 to 64	0.014140	82,218	1,163	81,636	1,602,498	19.5
64 to 65	0.015019	81,055	1,217	80,446	1,520,862	18.8
65 to 66	0.015942	79,838	1,273	79,201	1,440,416	18.0
66 to 67	0.017026	78,565	1,338	77,896	1,361,214	17.3
67 to 68	0.018189	77,227	1,405	76,525	1,283,318	16.6
68 to 69	0.019483	75,823	1,477	75,084	1,206,793	15.9
69 to 70	0.020990	74,345	1,561	73,565	1,131,709	15.2

Table 2-4a. Life Table for the Male Population, 2017—*Continued*

(Number.)

Age	Probability of dying between ages x and $x + 1$ q_x	Number surviving to age x l_x	Number dying between ages x and $x + 1$ d_x	Person-years lived between ages x and $x + 1$ L_x	Total number of person-years lived above age x T_x	Expectancy of life at age x e_x
70 to 71	0.022448	72,785	1,634	71,968	1,058,144	14.5
71 to 72	0.024631	71,151	1,753	70,275	986,176	13.9
72 to 73	0.026570	69,399	1,844	68,477	915,901	13.2
73 to 74	0.029040	67,555	1,962	66,574	847,424	12.5
74 to 75	0.031539	65,593	2,069	64,558	780,851	11.9
75 to 76	0.034644	63,524	2,201	62,424	716,292	11.3
76 to 77	0.038148	61,323	2,339	60,154	653,869	10.7
77 to 78	0.042250	58,984	2,492	57,738	593,715	10.1
78 to 79	0.046522	56,492	2,628	55,178	535,977	9.5
79 to 80	0.051401	53,864	2,769	52,479	480,799	8.9
80 to 81	0.056783	51,095	2,901	49,644	428,320	8.4
81 to 82	0.062514	48,194	3,013	46,687	378,675	7.9
82 to 83	0.069452	45,181	3,138	43,612	331,988	7.3
83 to 84	0.077622	42,043	3,263	40,411	288,376	6.9
84 to 85	0.086155	38,780	3,341	37,109	247,965	6.4
85 to 86	0.095450	35,439	3,383	33,747	210,855	5.9
86 to 87	0.105788	32,056	3,391	30,360	177,108	5.5
87 to 88	0.118527	28,665	3,398	26,966	146,748	5.1
88 to 89	0.132437	25,267	3,346	23,594	119,782	4.7
89 to 90	0.147541	21,921	3,234	20,304	96,188	4.4
90 to 91	0.163839	18,687	3,062	17,156	75,884	4.1
91 to 92	0.181308	15,625	2,833	14,209	58,728	3.8
92 to 93	0.199900	12,792	2,557	11,514	44,519	3.5
93 to 94	0.219535	10,235	2,247	9,112	33,006	3.2
94 to 95	0.240108	7,988	1,918	7,029	23,894	3.0
95 to 96	0.261480	6,070	1,587	5,276	16,865	2.8
96 to 97	0.283491	4,483	1,271	3,847	11,589	2.6
97 to 98	0.305955	3,212	983	2,721	7,741	2.4
98 to 99	0.328673	2,229	733	1,863	5,021	2.3
99 to 100	0.351434	1,497	526	1,234	3,158	2.1
100 and over	1.000000	971	971	1,924	1,924	2.0

Table 2-4b. Life Table for the Female Population, 2017

(Number.)

Age	Probability of dying between ages x and x + 1 q_x	Number surviving to age x l_x	Number dying between ages x and x + 1 d_x	Person-years lived between ages x and x + 1 L_x	Total number of person-years lived above age x T_x	Expectancy of life at age x e_x
0 to 1	0.005226	100,000	523	99,541	8,110,475	81.1
1 to 2	0.000339	99,477	34	99,461	8,010,934	80.5
2 to 3	0.000208	99,444	21	99,433	7,911,474	79.6
3 to 4	0.000159	99,423	16	99,415	7,812,040	78.6
4 to 5	0.000139	99,407	14	99,400	7,712,625	77.6
5 to 6	0.000126	99,393	12	99,387	7,613,225	76.6
6 to 7	0.000113	99,381	11	99,375	7,513,838	75.6
7 to 8	0.000104	99,370	10	99,365	7,414,463	74.6
8 to 9	0.000097	99,359	10	99,355	7,315,098	73.6
9 to 10	0.000092	99,350	9	99,345	7,215,744	72.6
10 to 11	0.000092	99,341	9	99,336	7,116,398	71.6
11 to 12	0.000098	99,331	10	99,327	7,017,062	70.6
12 to 13	0.000113	99,322	11	99,316	6,917,736	69.6
13 to 14	0.000138	99,311	14	99,304	6,818,420	68.7
14 to 15	0.000172	99,297	17	99,288	6,719,116	67.7
15 to 16	0.000210	99,280	21	99,269	6,619,828	66.7
16 to 17	0.000250	99,259	25	99,247	6,520,559	65.7
17 to 18	0.000293	99,234	29	99,220	6,421,312	64.7
18 to 19	0.000336	99,205	33	99,188	6,322,092	63.7
19 to 20	0.000379	99,172	38	99,153	6,222,904	62.7
20 to 21	0.000424	99,134	42	99,113	6,123,751	61.8
21 to 22	0.000471	99,092	47	99,069	6,024,638	60.8
22 to 23	0.000513	99,045	51	99,020	5,925,569	59.8
23 to 24	0.000550	98,995	54	98,967	5,826,549	58.9
24 to 25	0.000583	98,940	58	98,911	5,727,582	57.9
25 to 26	0.000613	98,883	61	98,852	5,628,670	56.9
26 to 27	0.000646	98,822	64	98,790	5,529,818	56.0
27 to 28	0.000682	98,758	67	98,724	5,431,028	55.0
28 to 29	0.000724	98,691	72	98,655	5,332,304	54.0
29 to 30	0.000774	98,619	76	98,581	5,233,649	53.1
30 to 31	0.000828	98,543	82	98,502	5,135,068	52.1
31 to 32	0.000885	98,461	87	98,418	5,036,566	51.2
32 to 33	0.000940	98,374	92	98,328	4,938,148	50.2
33 to 34	0.000989	98,282	97	98,233	4,839,820	49.2
34 to 35	0.001036	98,185	102	98,134	4,741,587	48.3
35 to 36	0.001087	98,083	107	98,030	4,643,453	47.3
36 to 37	0.001144	97,976	112	97,920	4,545,423	46.4
37 to 38	0.001203	97,864	118	97,805	4,447,503	45.4
38 to 39	0.001264	97,746	124	97,685	4,349,698	44.5
39 to 40	0.001332	97,623	130	97,558	4,252,013	43.6
40 to 41	0.001414	97,493	138	97,424	4,154,455	42.6
41 to 42	0.001513	97,355	147	97,281	4,057,031	41.7
42 to 43	0.001626	97,208	158	97,129	3,959,750	40.7
43 to 44	0.001750	97,050	170	96,965	3,862,621	39.8
44 to 45	0.001883	96,880	182	96,788	3,765,657	38.9
45 to 46	0.002025	96,697	196	96,599	3,668,868	37.9
46 to 47	0.002183	96,501	211	96,396	3,572,269	37.0
47 to 48	0.002366	96,291	228	96,177	3,475,873	36.1
48 to 49	0.002584	96,063	248	95,939	3,379,696	35.2
49 to 50	0.002836	95,815	272	95,679	3,283,757	34.3
50 to 51	0.003105	95,543	297	95,395	3,188,078	33.4
51 to 52	0.003391	95,246	323	95,085	3,092,683	32.5
52 to 53	0.003711	94,923	352	94,747	2,997,598	31.6
53 to 54	0.004066	94,571	385	94,379	2,902,851	30.7
54 to 55	0.004441	94,187	418	93,977	2,808,472	29.8
55 to 56	0.004829	93,768	453	93,542	2,714,495	28.9
56 to 57	0.005221	93,315	487	93,072	2,620,953	28.1
57 to 58	0.005613	92,828	521	92,568	2,527,881	27.2
58 to 59	0.006011	92,307	555	92,030	2,435,313	26.4
59 to 60	0.006429	91,752	590	91,457	2,343,284	25.5
60 to 61	0.006880	91,162	627	90,849	2,251,826	24.7
61 to 62	0.007371	90,535	667	90,202	2,160,977	23.9
62 to 63	0.007903	89,868	710	89,513	2,070,776	23.0
63 to 64	0.008481	89,158	756	88,780	1,981,263	22.2
64 to 65	0.009111	88,401	805	87,999	1,892,484	21.4
65 to 66	0.009793	87,596	858	87,167	1,804,485	20.6
66 to 67	0.010568	86,738	917	86,280	1,717,318	19.8
67 to 68	0.011436	85,822	981	85,331	1,631,038	19.0
68 to 69	0.012474	84,840	1,058	84,311	1,545,707	18.2
69 to 70	0.013659	83,782	1,144	83,210	1,461,396	17.4

Table 2-4b. Life Table for the Female Population, 2017—*Continued*

(Number.)

Age	Probability of dying between ages x and $x + 1$ q_x	Number surviving to age x l_x	Number dying between ages x and $x + 1$ d_x	Person-years lived between ages x and $x + 1$ L_x	Total number of person-years lived above age x T_x	Expectancy of life at age x e_x
70 to 71	0.014881	82,637	1,230	82,023	1,378,187	16.7
71 to 72	0.016529	81,408	1,346	80,735	1,296,164	15.9
72 to 73	0.018210	80,062	1,458	79,333	1,215,429	15.2
73 to 74	0.020011	78,604	1,573	77,818	1,136,096	14.5
74 to 75	0.021903	77,031	1,687	76,188	1,058,278	13.7
75 to 76	0.024322	75,344	1,833	74,428	982,091	13.0
76 to 77	0.026899	73,511	1,977	72,523	907,663	12.3
77 to 78	0.029886	71,534	2,138	70,465	835,141	11.7
78 to 79	0.033413	69,396	2,319	68,237	764,675	11.0
79 to 80	0.037065	67,078	2,486	65,834	696,439	10.4
80 to 81	0.041478	64,591	2,679	63,252	630,604	9.8
81 to 82	0.046150	61,912	2,857	60,484	567,352	9.2
82 to 83	0.051681	59,055	3,052	57,529	506,869	8.6
83 to 84	0.058587	56,003	3,281	54,362	449,340	8.0
84 to 85	0.065586	52,722	3,458	50,993	394,978	7.5
85 to 86	0.072855	49,264	3,589	47,469	343,985	7.0
86 to 87	0.081115	45,675	3,705	43,822	296,515	6.5
87 to 88	0.091618	41,970	3,845	40,047	252,693	6.0
88 to 89	0.103241	38,125	3,936	36,157	212,645	5.6
89 to 90	0.116041	34,189	3,967	32,205	176,488	5.2
90 to 91	0.130061	30,222	3,931	28,256	144,283	4.8
91 to 92	0.145329	26,291	3,821	24,380	116,027	4.4
92 to 93	0.161848	22,470	3,637	20,652	91,647	4.1
93 to 94	0.179598	18,833	3,382	17,142	70,995	3.8
94 to 95	0.198530	15,451	3,067	13,917	53,853	3.5
95 to 96	0.218561	12,383	2,707	11,030	39,936	3.2
96 to 97	0.239579	9,677	2,318	8,518	28,906	3.0
97 to 98	0.261439	7,359	1,924	6,397	20,388	2.8
98 to 99	0.283967	5,435	1,543	4,663	13,991	2.6
99 to 100	0.306967	3,891	1,195	3,294	9,328	2.4
100 and over	1.000000	2,697	2,697	6,034	6,034	2.2

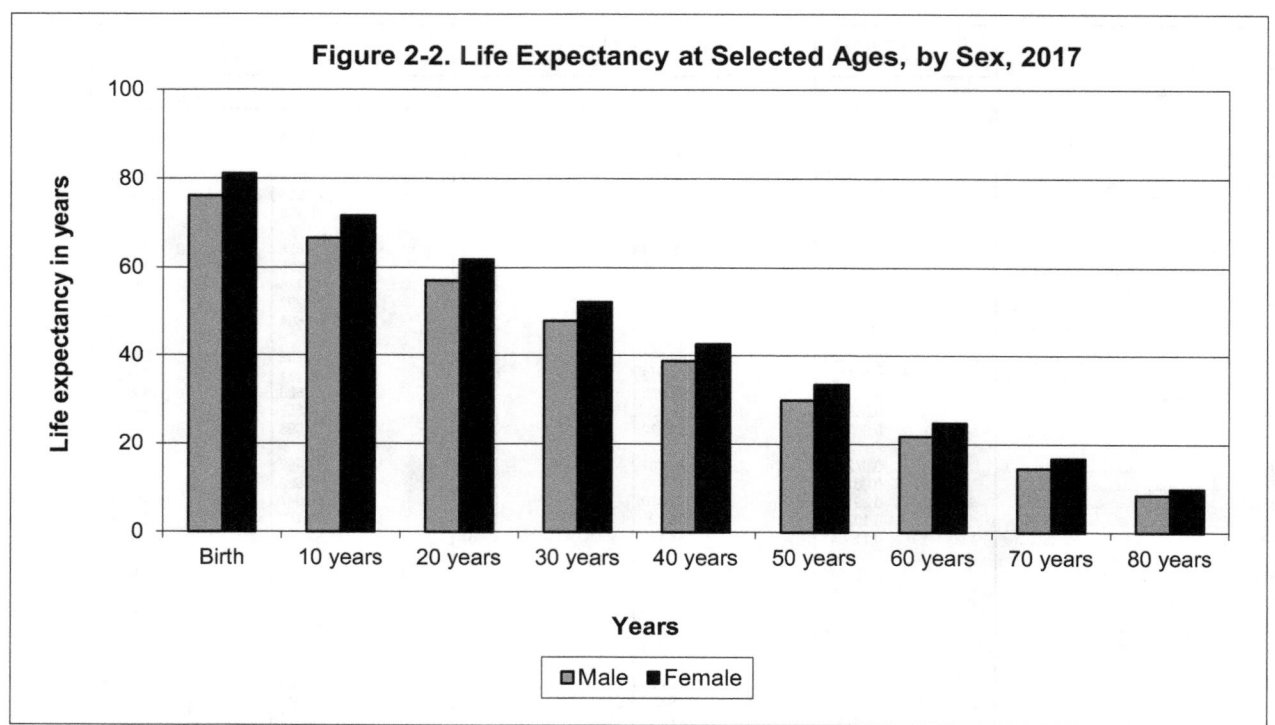

Figure 2-2. Life Expectancy at Selected Ages, by Sex, 2017

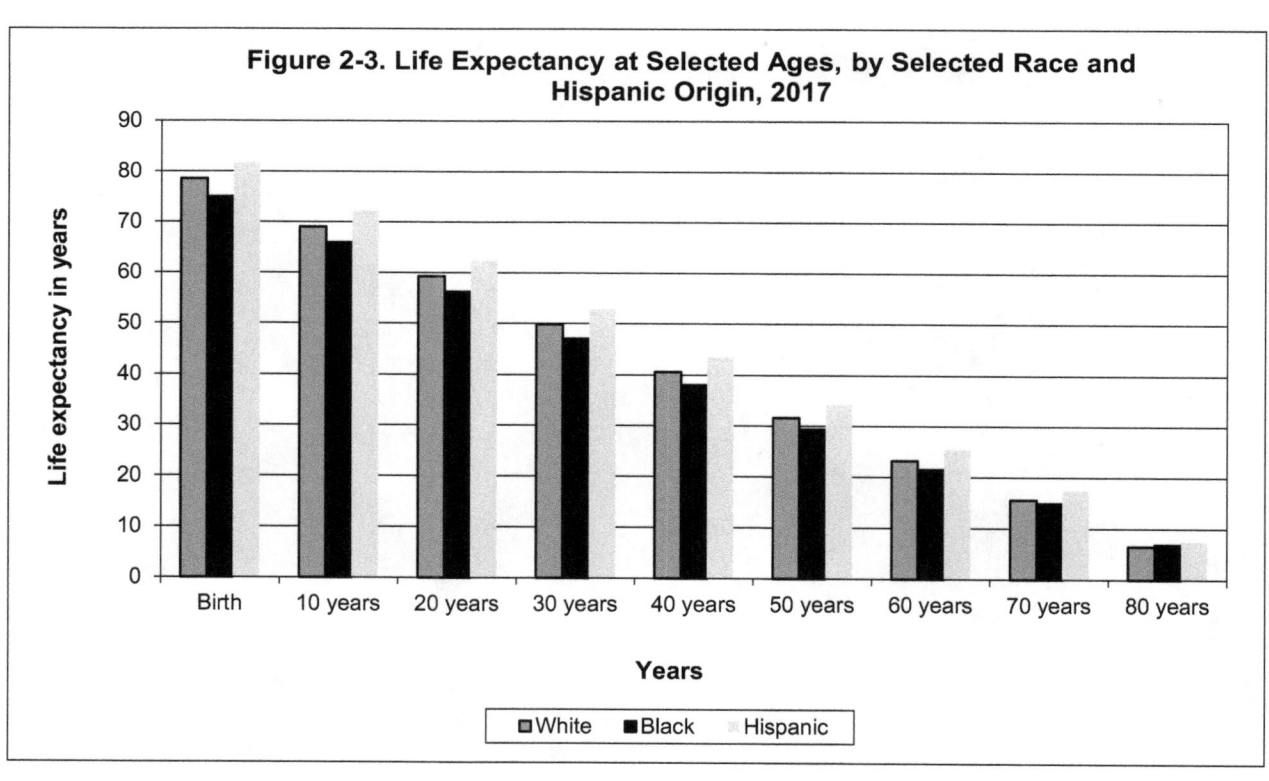

Figure 2-3. Life Expectancy at Selected Ages, by Selected Race and Hispanic Origin, 2017

Table 2-5. Life Expectancy at Birth by Race and Hispanic Origin and Sex, Selected Years, 1940–2017

(Years.)

Year	All races and origins[1]			Non-Hispanic White[2]			Non-Hispanic Black[2]			Hispanic[3]		
	Both sexes	Male	Female	Both sexes	Male	Female	Both sexes	Male	Female	Both sexes	Male	Female
1940	62.9	60.8	65.2	NA	NA	NA	NA	NA	NA	NA	NA	NA
1950	68.2	65.6	71.1	NA	NA	NA	NA	NA	NA	NA	NA	NA
1960	69.7	66.6	73.1	NA	NA	NA	NA	NA	NA	NA	NA	NA
1970	70.8	67.1	74.7	NA	NA	NA	NA	NA	NA	NA	NA	NA
1980	73.7	70.0	77.4	NA	NA	NA	NA	NA	NA	NA	NA	NA
1990	75.4	71.8	78.8	NA	NA	NA	NA	NA	NA	NA	NA	NA
2000	76.8	74.1	79.3	NA	NA	NA	NA	NA	NA	NA	NA	NA
2001[4]	77.0	74.3	79.5	NA	NA	NA	NA	NA	NA	NA	NA	NA
2002[4]	77.0	74.4	79.6	NA	NA	NA	NA	NA	NA	NA	NA	NA
2003[4]	77.2	74.5	79.7	NA	NA	NA	NA	NA	NA	NA	NA	NA
2004[4]	77.6	75.0	80.1	NA	NA	NA	NA	NA	NA	NA	NA	NA
2005[4]	77.6	75.0	80.1	NA	NA	NA	NA	NA	NA	NA	NA	NA
2006[4]	77.8	75.2	80.3	78.2	75.7	80.6	73.1	69.5	76.4	80.3	77.5	82.9
2007[4]	78.1	75.5	80.6	78.4	75.9	80.8	73.5	69.9	76.7	80.7	77.8	83.2
2008[4]	78.2	75.6	80.6	78.4	76.0	80.7	73.9	70.5	77.0	80.8	78.0	83.3
2009[4]	78.5	76.0	80.9	78.7	76.3	81.0	74.4	71.0	77.4	81.1	78.4	83.5
2010[4,5]	78.7	76.2	81.0	78.8	76.4	81.1	74.7	71.5	77.7	81.7	78.8	84.3
2011[4,5]	78.7	76.3	81.1	78.7	76.4	81.1	75.0	71.8	77.8	81.8	79.2	84.2
2012[4,5]	78.8	76.4	81.2	78.9	76.5	81.2	75.1	71.9	78.1	81.9	79.3	84.3
2013[4,5]	78.8	76.4	81.2	78.8	76.5	81.2	75.1	71.9	78.1	81.9	79.2	84.2
2014[4,5,6]	78.9	76.5	81.3	78.8	76.5	81.2	75.3	72.2	78.2	82.1	79.4	84.5
2015[4,5]	78.7	76.3	81.1	78.7	76.3	81.0	75.1	71.9	78.1	82.0	79.3	84.3
2016[4,5,6]	78.7	76.2	81.1	78.6	76.2	81.0	74.9	71.6	78.0	81.8	79.1	84.3
2017[4,5]	78.6	76.1	81.1	78.5	76.1	81.0	74.9	71.5	78.1	81.8	79.1	84.3

NA = Not available.
[1]Includes races and origins not shown separately.
[2]Multiple-race data reported according to 1997 OMB standards were bridged to the single-race categories of 1977 OMB standards.
[3]Based on death rates adjusted for misclassification.
[4]Life table data for 2001–2017 are based on revised life table methodology.
[5]Life expectancies by Hispanic origin were revised using updated adjustment factors to correct for race and Hispanic-origin misclassification.
[6]Life expectancies were revised using updated Medicare data; therefore, data may differ from those previously published.

Table 2-6. Life Expectancy at Selected Ages, by Race and Hispanic Origin and Sex, 2017

(Years.)

Exact age in years	All races and origins[1]			Non-Hispanic White[2]			Non-Hispanic Black[2]			Hispanic[3]		
	Both sexes	Male	Female	Both sexes	Male	Female	Both sexes	Male	Female	Both sexes	Male	Female
0 years	78.6	76.1	81.1	78.5	76.1	81.0	74.9	71.5	78.1	81.8	79.1	84.3
1 year	78.1	75.6	80.5	77.9	75.5	80.3	74.7	71.4	77.9	81.2	78.5	83.7
5 years	74.1	71.7	76.6	74.0	71.6	76.4	70.8	67.5	74.0	77.3	74.6	79.8
10 years	69.2	66.7	71.6	69.0	66.6	71.4	65.9	62.5	69.0	72.3	69.6	74.8
15 years	64.2	61.8	66.7	64.0	61.7	66.4	61.0	57.6	64.1	67.4	64.7	69.8
20 years	59.4	57.0	61.8	59.2	56.9	61.5	56.2	53.0	59.2	62.5	59.9	64.9
25 years	54.7	52.4	56.9	54.5	52.2	56.7	51.6	48.5	54.4	57.7	55.2	60.1
30 years	50.0	47.8	52.1	49.8	47.7	51.9	47.0	44.1	49.6	53.0	50.5	55.2
35 years	45.3	43.2	47.3	45.2	43.2	47.2	42.5	39.7	44.9	48.2	45.8	50.3
40 years	40.7	38.7	42.6	40.6	38.6	42.5	38.0	35.3	40.3	43.5	41.2	45.5
45 years	36.1	34.2	37.9	36.0	34.2	37.8	33.6	31.0	35.8	38.8	36.6	40.7
50 years	31.6	29.8	33.4	31.6	29.8	33.3	29.3	26.9	31.4	34.2	32.1	36.0
55 years	27.4	25.6	28.9	27.3	25.6	28.8	25.2	23.0	27.2	29.8	27.7	31.4
60 years	23.3	21.7	24.7	23.2	21.7	24.6	21.5	19.4	23.3	25.5	23.6	27.0
65 years	19.4	18.0	20.6	19.3	18.0	20.5	18.1	16.2	19.5	21.4	19.7	22.7
70 years	15.7	14.5	16.7	15.6	14.5	16.6	14.9	13.3	16.0	17.5	16.0	18.6
75 years	12.3	11.3	13.0	12.2	11.2	12.9	11.9	10.6	12.7	13.8	12.6	14.7
80 years	9.2	8.4	9.8	9.1	8.3	9.7	9.2	8.1	9.8	10.5	9.4	11.1
85 years	6.6	5.9	7.0	6.5	5.9	6.9	6.9	6.1	7.3	7.6	6.7	8.0
90 years	4.5	4.1	4.8	4.5	4.0	4.7	5.0	4.5	5.2	5.3	4.6	5.5
95 years	3.1	2.8	3.2	3.0	2.7	3.2	3.6	3.3	3.7	3.6	3.2	3.7
100 years	2.2	2.0	2.2	2.1	1.9	2.2	2.7	2.5	2.7	2.6	2.2	2.6

[1]Includes races and origins not shown separately.
[2]Multiple-race data reported according to 1997 OMB standards were bridged to the single-race categories of 1977 OMB standards.
[3]Life expectancies by Hispanic origin are based on death rates adjusted for misclassification.

Table 2-7. Percent Distribution of Deaths by Educational Attainment: Alabama, Alaska, Arizona, Arkansas, California, Colorado, Connecticut, Delaware, District of Columbia, Florida, Hawaii, Idaho, Illinois, Indiana, Iowa, Kansas, Kentucky, Louisiana, Maine, Maryland, Massachusetts, Michigan, Minnesota, Mississippi, Missouri, Montana, Nebraska, Nevada, New Hampshire, New Jersey, New Mexico, New York, North Carolina, North Dakota, Ohio, Oklahoma, Oregon, Pennsylvania, South Carolina, Tennessee, Texas, Utah, Vermont, Virginia, Washington, Wisconsin, and Wyoming, 2002 and 2017

(Percent.)

2002		2017	
Years of school completed	Percent distribution	Educational attainment	Percent distribution
Total	100.0	Total	100.0
Under 12 years	21.1	Less than a high school diploma or GED	17.8
12 years	43.9	High school diploma or GED	43.9
13 years or more	32.0	Some college or collegiate degree	36.1
Not stated	3.0	Not stated	2.2

NOTE: By state of occurrence. Excludes nonresidents of the United States. Because of rounding, the sum of the subgroups may not add to total. GED is General Educational Development high school equivalency diploma.

Table 2-8. Death Rates by Age and Age-Adjusted Death Rates for the 10 Leading Causes of Death in 2017 and Drug-Induced Deaths, Alcohol-Induced Deaths, and Injury by Firearm, 1999–2017

(Rate per 100,000 population in specified group; age-adjusted rates per 100,000 U.S. standard population.)

Cause of death (based on International Classification of Diseases, 10th Revision) and year	All ages[1]	Under 1 year[2]	1 to 4 years	5 to 14 years	15 to 24 years	25 to 34 years	35 to 44 years	45 to 54 years	55 to 64 years	65 to 74 years	75 to 84 years	85 years and over	Age-adjusted rate[3]
All causes													
1999	857.0	736.0	34.2	18.6	79.3	102.2	198.0	418.2	1,005.0	2,457.3	5,714.5	15,554.6	875.6
2000	854.0	736.7	32.4	18.0	79.9	101.4	198.9	425.6	992.2	2,399.1	5,666.5	15,524.4	869.0
2001	848.0	687.0	33.4	17.2	80.2	105.6	203.5	426.7	972.5	2,344.2	5,573.7	15,432.6	858.8
2002	849.5	709.5	31.4	17.4	80.9	105.1	204.2	431.0	948.7	2,300.3	5,543.8	15,589.5	855.9
2003	843.9	704.9	31.8	16.9	81.1	105.2	202.6	433.1	937.3	2,235.0	5,451.3	15,401.4	843.5
2004	818.8	695.9	30.3	16.7	79.7	104.1	194.9	426.8	903.2	2,141.0	5,267.4	14,777.6	813.7
2005	828.4	710.2	29.9	16.3	80.7	106.8	194.9	431.9	898.5	2,109.7	5,251.8	14,982.4	815.0
2006	813.1	705.8	29.1	15.2	81.4	109.0	192.0	427.5	881.3	2,031.4	5,096.1	14,426.7	791.8
2007	804.6	702.5	29.4	15.2	78.8	107.2	186.0	420.3	866.7	1,976.0	4,987.1	14,160.9	775.3
2008	812.9	678.9	29.3	13.9	74.2	105.1	181.0	419.6	867.1	1,958.4	4,998.1	14,332.4	774.9
2009	794.5	659.7	27.4	13.8	69.8	104.4	180.0	418.1	856.7	1,888.7	4,820.2	13,660.1	749.6
2010	799.5	623.4	26.5	12.9	67.7	102.9	170.5	407.1	851.9	1,875.1	4,790.2	13,934.3	747.0
2011	807.3	600.1	26.3	13.2	67.7	104.7	172.0	409.8	849.4	1,846.2	4,753.0	13,779.3	741.3
2012	810.2	599.3	26.3	12.6	66.4	105.4	170.7	405.4	854.2	1,802.5	4,674.5	13,678.6	732.8
2013	821.5	594.7	25.5	13.0	64.8	106.1	172.0	406.1	860.0	1,802.1	4,648.1	13,660.4	731.9
2014	823.7	588.0	24.0	12.7	65.5	108.4	175.2	404.8	870.3	1,786.3	4,564.2	13,407.9	724.6
2015	844.0	589.6	24.9	13.2	69.5	116.7	180.1	404.0	875.3	1,796.8	4,579.2	13,673.9	733.1
2016	849.3	583.4	25.3	13.4	74.9	129.0	192.2	405.5	883.8	1,788.6	4,474.8	13,392.1	728.8
2017	863.8	567.0	24.3	13.6	74.0	132.8	195.2	401.5	885.8	1,790.9	4,472.6	13,573.6	731.9
Diseases of heart (I00–I09,I11,I13,I20–I51)													
1999	259.9	13.8	1.2	0.7	2.8	7.6	30.2	95.7	269.9	701.7	1,849.9	6,063.0	266.5
2000	252.6	13.0	1.2	0.7	2.6	7.4	29.2	94.2	261.2	665.6	1,780.3	5,926.1	257.6
2001	245.7	11.9	1.5	0.7	2.5	8.0	29.6	92.4	248.9	632.6	1,723.0	5,784.1	249.5
2002	242.3	12.7	1.1	0.6	2.5	8.0	30.7	93.9	240.5	612.0	1,673.2	5,726.3	244.6
2003	236.1	11.0	1.2	0.6	2.7	8.3	30.8	92.4	232.3	579.8	1,607.7	5,570.7	236.3
2004	222.8	10.5	1.2	0.6	2.5	8.1	29.5	90.2	217.1	535.7	1,504.1	5,233.8	221.6
2005	220.7	8.9	0.9	0.6	2.6	8.3	29.2	89.7	212.8	512.3	1,458.5	5,188.3	216.8
2006	211.7	8.6	1.0	0.6	2.5	8.4	28.5	88.0	205.1	483.0	1,378.0	4,877.6	205.5
2007	204.5	10.2	1.1	0.6	2.5	8.1	27.7	85.2	197.8	454.8	1,308.6	4,668.1	196.1
2008	202.8	9.6	1.2	0.6	2.5	8.1	26.9	85.2	195.3	441.4	1,271.7	4,598.4	192.1
2009	195.4	9.6	0.9	0.5	2.4	7.8	26.7	82.3	190.0	422.8	1,210.8	4,316.9	182.8
2010	193.6	8.3	1.0	0.5	2.4	7.8	25.8	81.6	186.6	409.2	1,172.0	4,285.2	179.1
2011	191.5	7.7	1.0	0.5	2.3	7.9	26.2	80.7	183.2	399.0	1,134.7	4,111.6	173.7
2012	191.0	8.5	1.0	0.4	2.2	7.6	25.9	79.7	184.6	388.3	1,103.7	4,046.1	170.5
2013	193.3	7.8	1.1	0.4	2.1	7.6	25.6	80.3	184.6	390.3	1,095.1	4,013.9	169.8
2014	192.7	8.0	0.9	0.5	2.2	7.7	25.6	80.1	185.8	385.2	1,070.2	3,920.9	167.0
2015	197.2	7.3	0.9	0.5	2.3	8.0	25.6	79.3	188.1	389.5	1,071.6	3,986.5	168.5
2016	196.6	7.4	0.7	0.5	2.2	7.7	25.9	79.5	189.6	392.5	1,037.1	3,873.4	165.5
2017	198.8	7.7	0.8	0.4	2.1	8.1	25.4	77.1	190.7	392.9	1,028.4	3,882.9	165.0
Malignant neoplasms (C00–C97)													
1999	197.0	1.8	2.7	2.5	4.5	10.0	37.1	127.6	374.6	827.1	1,331.5	1,805.8	200.8
2000	196.5	2.4	2.7	2.5	4.4	9.8	36.6	127.5	366.7	816.3	1,335.6	1,819.4	199.6
2001	194.3	1.6	2.7	2.4	4.2	10.1	36.8	125.8	359.4	799.7	1,313.7	1,802.9	196.5
2002	193.7	1.9	2.6	2.6	4.2	9.8	36.0	124.1	349.7	787.2	1,308.8	1,812.4	194.3
2003	192.0	1.9	2.5	2.6	4.0	9.5	35.1	122.1	341.6	763.5	1,299.7	1,792.3	190.9
2004	189.2	1.8	2.5	2.5	4.1	9.3	33.6	119.0	330.8	746.8	1,278.6	1,767.4	186.8
2005	189.3	1.9	2.4	2.5	4.0	9.2	33.5	118.6	323.9	733.2	1,272.8	1,778.2	185.1
2006	187.6	1.9	2.4	2.2	3.8	9.3	32.2	116.3	317.7	716.3	1,259.2	1,748.3	181.8
2007	186.9	1.7	2.3	2.4	3.8	8.7	31.0	114.2	311.4	702.9	1,250.1	1,739.4	179.3
2008	186.0	1.7	2.4	2.2	3.8	8.8	30.1	113.4	304.7	688.4	1,230.9	1,724.6	176.4
2009	185.0	1.8	2.2	2.2	3.8	9.0	30.2	112.8	301.7	668.2	1,213.0	1,699.3	173.5
2010	186.2	1.6	2.1	2.2	3.7	8.8	28.8	111.6	300.1	666.1	1,202.2	1,729.5	172.8
2011	185.1	1.8	2.2	2.1	3.7	8.4	28.8	109.3	295.8	647.6	1,179.1	1,676.2	169.0
2012	185.6	1.6	2.4	2.2	3.6	8.7	28.0	108.5	293.2	632.2	1,161.7	1,658.9	166.5
2013	185.0	1.6	2.1	2.2	3.4	8.6	28.1	105.5	288.2	616.9	1,139.4	1,635.4	163.2
2014	185.6	1.3	2.0	2.1	3.6	8.3	27.8	103.2	287.6	603.1	1,125.9	1,632.9	161.2
2015	185.4	1.3	2.2	2.1	3.4	8.4	26.9	99.7	284.1	594.3	1,100.8	1,628.6	158.5
2016	185.1	1.7	2.4	2.1	3.3	8.5	26.9	96.5	280.6	578.3	1,081.7	1,620.3	155.8
2017	183.9	1.4	2.0	2.1	3.2	8.0	26.7	92.7	273.4	567.5	1,060.2	1,600.3	152.5

NOTE: Rates are on an annual basis per 100,000 population in specified group; age-adjusted rates are per 100,000 U.S. standard population.

X = Not applicable.

* = Rate does not meet NCHS standards of reliability.

[1] Figures for age not stated included in "All ages" but not distributed among age groups.

[2] Death rates for "Under 1 year" (based on population estimates) differ from infant mortality rates (based on live births); please see chapter notes for more information.

[3] For method of computation, please see chapter notes.

Table 2-8. Death Rates by Age and Age-Adjusted Death Rates for the 10 Leading Causes of Death in 2017 and Drug-Induced Deaths, Alcohol-Induced Deaths, and Injury by Firearm, 1999–2017—*Continued*

(Rate per 100,000 population in specified group; age-adjusted rates per 100,000 U.S. standard population.)

Cause of death (based on International Classification of Diseases, 10th Revision) and year	All ages[1]	Under 1 year[2]	1 to 4 years	5 to 14 years	15 to 24 years	25 to 34 years	35 to 44 years	45 to 54 years	55 to 64 years	65 to 74 years	75 to 84 years	85 years and over	Age-adjusted rate[3]
Accidents (unintentional injuries) (V01–X59,Y85–Y86)													
1999	35.1	22.3	12.4	7.6	35.3	29.6	33.8	31.8	30.6	44.6	100.5	282.4	35.3
2000	34.8	23.1	11.9	7.3	36.0	29.5	34.1	32.6	30.9	41.9	95.1	273.5	34.9
2001	35.6	24.3	11.2	6.9	35.8	30.0	35.4	33.9	30.5	42.6	100.7	282.2	35.7
2002	37.1	23.9	10.6	6.6	37.7	31.9	37.4	36.7	31.3	44.0	101.1	289.6	37.1
2003	37.7	23.8	11.0	6.4	36.9	32.0	38.0	38.8	32.7	43.7	101.6	294.3	37.6
2004	38.3	26.2	10.4	6.5	36.8	33.2	37.6	40.7	32.9	43.5	103.6	295.8	38.1
2005	39.9	27.0	10.5	5.9	37.1	35.7	38.9	43.2	35.4	45.7	106.0	303.5	39.5
2006	40.8	28.4	10.1	5.6	37.9	38.0	40.5	45.5	35.8	43.8	104.7	299.2	40.2
2007	41.1	31.0	9.9	5.4	36.8	37.7	39.6	46.2	36.8	44.4	105.0	313.6	40.4
2008	40.1	31.8	9.1	4.6	32.5	36.3	38.1	45.8	37.4	43.9	105.7	318.3	39.2
2009	38.5	29.5	9.0	4.1	28.6	34.5	36.4	44.5	36.5	42.1	103.5	310.9	37.5
2010	39.1	28.1	8.6	4.0	28.3	35.5	36.0	43.7	38.4	43.3	106.1	328.4	38.0
2011	40.6	29.1	8.5	4.0	28.2	37.1	37.5	46.4	39.8	44.5	107.0	333.8	39.1
2012	40.7	29.6	8.4	3.8	27.1	37.5	37.1	46.1	41.0	44.0	107.8	336.9	39.1
2013	41.3	29.3	8.3	3.7	26.4	37.8	38.0	46.5	43.4	43.5	107.4	340.0	39.4
2014	42.6	29.4	7.6	3.6	26.8	39.8	39.6	47.4	44.9	45.1	108.7	349.1	40.5
2015	45.6	32.5	7.8	3.7	28.5	44.8	43.9	49.8	47.7	47.0	111.5	364.5	43.2
2016	49.9	30.7	7.9	4.0	31.9	53.7	51.8	54.6	52.7	49.1	110.7	365.7	47.4
2017	52.2	33.4	7.9	3.8	31.1	56.6	55.8	57.7	55.7	50.7	113.3	374.9	49.4
												273.5	34.9
Chronic lower respiratory diseases (J40–J47)												282.2	35.7
1999	44.5	0.9	0.4	0.3	0.5	0.8	2.0	8.5	47.5	177.2	397.8	646.0	45.4
2000	43.4	0.9	0.3	0.3	0.5	0.7	2.1	8.6	44.2	169.4	386.1	648.6	44.2
2001	43.2	1.0	0.3	0.3	0.4	0.7	2.2	8.4	44.5	167.3	379.3	658.3	43.9
2002	43.4	1.0	0.4	0.3	0.5	0.8	2.3	8.7	42.2	162.0	385.8	670.3	43.9
2003	43.6	0.8	0.4	0.3	0.5	0.7	2.2	8.7	43.1	161.7	382.2	670.2	43.7
2004	41.7	0.9	0.3	0.3	0.4	0.6	2.0	8.4	40.1	152.1	366.2	643.2	41.6
2005	44.3	0.8	0.4	0.3	0.3	0.7	2.0	9.4	41.6	158.4	385.0	691.9	43.9
2006	41.8	0.7	0.3	0.3	0.4	0.6	1.9	9.1	38.8	147.0	362.0	641.3	41.0
2007	42.5	1.0	0.4	0.3	0.3	0.7	1.9	9.5	38.6	145.5	367.1	652.0	41.4
2008	46.4	0.8	0.3	0.3	0.4	0.6	1.9	9.9	41.1	155.9	395.4	722.7	44.7
2009	44.8	0.7	0.4	0.3	0.4	0.7	1.8	10.4	40.0	147.5	376.4	684.9	42.7
2010	44.7	0.9	0.3	0.3	0.3	0.7	1.7	9.9	39.0	146.3	369.9	690.7	42.2
2011	45.9	0.8	0.3	0.3	0.4	0.6	1.8	10.4	39.5	144.3	374.9	697.9	42.5
2012	45.7	0.5	0.3	0.3	0.3	0.7	1.8	10.2	39.4	140.0	364.0	687.8	41.5
2013	47.2	0.6	0.4	0.4	0.4	0.7	1.9	10.6	40.5	141.2	367.0	699.3	42.1
2014	46.1	*	0.3	0.3	0.4	0.8	1.9	10.1	41.2	134.9	349.0	670.5	40.5
2015	48.2	0.7	0.3	0.4	0.5	0.7	1.7	10.1	42.7	136.6	357.9	705.1	41.6
2016	47.8	0.7	0.3	0.3	0.5	0.8	1.7	10.1	43.0	134.1	347.2	676.9	40.6
2017	49.2	*	0.2	0.3	0.4	0.7	1.7	9.4	44.4	133.8	347.6	700.6	40.9
Cerebrovascular diseases (I60–I69)													
1999	60.0	2.7	0.3	0.2	0.5	1.4	5.7	15.2	40.6	130.8	469.8	1,614.8	61.6
2000	59.6	3.3	0.3	0.2	0.5	1.5	5.8	16.0	41.0	128.6	461.3	1,589.2	60.9
2001	57.4	2.7	0.4	0.2	0.5	1.5	5.5	15.0	38.3	122.9	443.3	1,532.0	58.4
2002	56.6	3.0	0.3	0.2	0.4	1.4	5.4	15.1	37.1	119.6	430.0	1,520.1	57.2
2003	54.4	2.5	0.3	0.2	0.5	1.5	5.6	15.0	35.5	111.9	409.8	1,446.0	54.6
2004	51.3	3.2	0.3	0.2	0.5	1.4	5.4	14.8	34.0	106.6	385.6	1,331.9	51.2
2005	48.6	3.1	0.4	0.2	0.5	1.4	5.2	15.0	32.7	99.8	358.4	1,239.7	48.0
2006	46.0	3.5	0.3	0.2	0.5	1.3	5.1	14.6	32.9	94.9	333.9	1,131.7	44.8
2007	45.1	3.2	0.3	0.2	0.5	1.3	5.0	14.5	31.7	91.4	320.8	1,110.7	43.5
2008	44.1	3.4	0.4	0.2	0.4	1.3	4.8	13.7	30.6	87.3	313.3	1,071.0	42.1
2009	42.0	3.7	0.3	0.2	0.4	1.3	4.6	13.7	29.7	82.8	294.9	992.2	39.6
2010	41.9	3.3	0.3	0.2	0.4	1.3	4.6	13.1	29.3	81.7	288.3	993.8	39.1
2011	41.4	3.4	0.3	0.2	0.4	1.3	4.2	12.8	29.4	78.2	285.4	943.7	37.9
2012	40.9	2.6	0.3	0.2	0.4	1.3	4.3	12.8	28.7	75.7	272.2	931.2	36.9
2013	40.8	2.7	0.2	0.2	0.3	1.2	4.2	12.4	28.9	74.2	268.9	906.0	36.2
2014	41.7	2.4	0.2	0.2	0.4	1.3	4.3	12.3	29.3	74.5	265.7	929.7	36.5
2015	43.7	2.2	0.3	0.2	0.4	1.3	4.4	12.3	29.6	75.5	273.0	975.8	37.6
2016	44.0	3.1	0.3	0.2	0.3	1.3	4.6	12.5	29.7	76.0	265.5	972.9	37.3
2017	44.9	2.5	0.4	0.2	0.4	1.3	4.4	12.3	30.3	76.4	263.1	993.5	37.6

NOTE: Rates are on an annual basis per 100,000 population in specified group; age-adjusted rates are per 100,000 U.S. standard population.
X = Not applicable.
* = Rate does not meet NCHS standards of reliability.
[1]Figures for age not stated included in "All ages" but not distributed among age groups.
[2]Death rates for "Under 1 year" (based on population estimates) differ from infant mortality rates (based on live births); please see chapter notes for more information.
[3]For method of computation, please see chapter notes.

Table 2-8. Death Rates by Age and Age-Adjusted Death Rates for the 10 Leading Causes of Death in 2017 and Drug-Induced Deaths, Alcohol-Induced Deaths, and Injury by Firearm, 1999–2017—*Continued*

(Rate per 100,000 population in specified group; age-adjusted rates per 100,000 U.S. standard population.)

Cause of death (based on International Classification of Diseases, 10th Revision) and year	All ages[1]	Under 1 year[2]	1 to 4 years	5 to 14 years	15 to 24 years	25 to 34 years	35 to 44 years	45 to 54 years	55 to 64 years	65 to 74 years	75 to 84 years	85 years and over	Age-adjusted rate[3]
Alzheimer's Disease (G30)													
1999	16.0	*	*	*	*	*	*	0.2	1.9	17.4	129.5	601.3	16.5
2000	17.6	*	*	*	*	*	*	0.2	2.0	18.7	139.6	667.7	18.1
2001	18.9	*	*	*	*	*	*	0.2	2.1	18.6	147.2	725.4	19.3
2002	20.5	*	*	*	*	*	*	0.1	1.9	19.6	157.7	790.9	20.8
2003	21.9	*	*	*	*	*	*	0.2	2.0	20.7	164.1	846.8	22.1
2004	22.5	*	*	*	*	*	*	0.2	1.8	19.5	168.5	875.3	22.6
2005	24.2	*	*	*	*	*	*	0.2	2.1	20.2	177.0	935.5	24.0
2006	24.3	*	*	*	*	*	*	0.2	2.1	19.9	175.0	923.4	23.7
2007	24.8	*	*	*	*	*	*	0.2	2.2	20.2	175.8	928.7	23.8
2008	27.1	*	*	*	*	*	*	0.2	2.2	21.1	192.5	1,002.2	25.8
2009	25.8	*	*	*	*	*	*	0.2	2.0	19.4	179.1	945.3	24.2
2010	27.0	*	*	*	*	*	*	0.3	2.1	19.8	184.5	987.1	25.1
2011	27.3	*	*	*	*	*	*	0.2	2.2	19.2	183.9	967.1	24.7
2012	26.6	*	*	*	*	*	*	0.2	2.2	17.9	175.4	936.1	23.8
2013	26.8	*	*	*	*	*	*	0.2	2.2	18.1	171.6	929.5	23.5
2014	29.3	*	*	*	*	*	*	0.2	2.1	19.6	185.6	1,006.8	25.4
2015	34.4	*	*	*	*	*	*	0.2	2.4	22.4	211.9	1,174.2	29.4
2016	35.9	*	*	*	*	*	*	0.2	2.7	23.6	214.1	1,216.9	30.3
2017	37.3	*	*	*	*	*	*	0.2	2.8	24.5	219.7	1,244.7	31.0
Diabetes Mellitus (E10–E14)													
1999	24.5	*	*	0.1	0.4	1.4	4.3	12.9	38.3	91.8	178.0	317.2	25.0
2000	24.6	*	*	0.1	0.4	1.6	4.3	13.1	37.8	90.7	179.5	319.7	25.0
2001	25.0	*	*	0.1	0.4	1.5	4.3	13.6	38.1	91.0	181.1	328.6	25.4
2002	25.5	*	*	0.1	0.4	1.6	4.8	13.7	37.5	90.9	182.4	337.0	25.6
2003	25.6	*	*	0.1	0.4	1.7	4.6	13.9	38.3	90.0	180.7	335.1	25.5
2004	25.0	*	*	0.1	0.4	1.5	4.6	13.4	36.8	86.2	176.6	328.2	24.7
2005	25.4	*	*	0.1	0.5	1.6	4.7	13.4	36.9	85.7	177.0	338.8	24.9
2006	24.3	*	*	0.1	0.4	1.7	4.8	13.1	35.8	80.6	166.2	310.4	23.6
2007	23.7	*	*	0.1	0.4	1.5	4.6	13.1	34.1	76.7	161.9	302.2	22.8
2008	23.2	*	*	0.1	0.5	1.4	4.4	12.6	33.3	74.7	153.2	298.9	22.0
2009	22.4	*	*	0.1	0.4	1.5	4.5	12.8	32.1	69.6	145.8	282.6	21.0
2010	22.4	*	*	0.1	0.4	1.5	4.4	12.5	32.0	67.6	144.1	285.5	20.8
2011	23.7	*	*	0.1	0.4	1.6	4.5	13.4	33.3	72.0	148.8	289.5	21.6
2012	23.6	*	*	0.1	0.4	1.5	4.6	13.0	32.5	69.7	145.8	285.7	21.2
2013	23.9	*	*	0.1	0.4	1.6	4.8	13.5	33.2	68.5	145.7	279.5	21.2
2014	24.0	*	*	0.1	0.4	1.6	4.9	13.9	33.3	69.0	141.8	268.6	20.9
2015	24.7	*	*	0.1	0.4	1.8	4.9	14.4	34.7	70.6	143.0	267.0	21.3
2016	24.8	*	*	0.1	0.5	1.8	5.1	14.6	34.4	69.9	137.9	263.6	21.0
2017	25.7	*	*	0.1	0.6	1.8	5.2	15.1	35.5	71.9	140.8	262.4	21.5
Influenza and pneumonia (J09–J18)													
1999	22.8	8.4	0.8	0.2	0.5	0.8	2.4	4.6	11.0	37.2	157.0	751.8	23.5
2000	23.2	7.6	0.7	0.2	0.5	0.9	2.4	4.7	11.9	39.1	160.3	744.1	23.7
2001	21.8	7.5	0.7	0.2	0.5	0.9	2.2	4.6	10.8	36.2	148.3	700.1	22.2
2002	22.8	6.7	0.7	0.2	0.4	0.9	2.2	4.8	11.2	37.2	156.6	732.4	23.2
2003	22.5	8.1	1.0	0.4	0.5	1.0	2.2	5.2	11.2	36.9	150.8	703.0	22.6
2004	20.4	6.8	0.8	0.2	0.4	0.8	2.0	4.6	10.8	34.2	139.1	622.8	20.4
2005	21.3	6.6	0.7	0.3	0.4	0.9	2.1	5.1	11.2	35.1	142.0	644.9	21.0
2006	18.9	6.5	0.8	0.2	0.4	0.9	1.9	4.6	9.9	31.6	127.3	547.0	18.4
2007	17.5	5.4	0.7	0.3	0.4	0.8	1.8	4.3	9.5	28.2	113.5	506.7	16.8
2008	18.5	5.5	0.9	0.2	0.5	0.9	2.1	5.1	10.9	30.5	118.6	512.3	17.6
2009	17.5	6.3	0.9	0.6	1.0	2.0	3.2	6.5	11.7	29.5	107.0	433.8	16.5
2010	16.2	4.9	0.6	0.2	0.4	0.9	1.9	4.3	9.9	27.9	102.4	426.2	15.1
2011	17.3	5.2	0.7	0.3	0.5	1.2	2.1	5.0	11.0	28.9	104.0	439.2	15.7
2012	16.1	4.0	0.6	0.2	0.3	0.8	1.7	4.1	10.2	26.1	98.2	408.4	14.4
2013	18.0	4.5	0.6	0.3	0.4	1.0	2.2	5.1	12.2	29.5	103.7	441.0	15.9
2014	17.3	4.7	0.7	0.2	0.5	1.3	2.8	6.3	13.4	29.8	96.4	385.9	15.1
2015	17.8	4.4	0.6	0.2	0.4	0.9	1.7	4.7	11.3	29.5	101.6	421.4	15.2
2016	15.9	4.2	0.6	0.2	0.4	1.0	2.2	5.0	12.1	28.5	88.5	340.3	13.5
2017	17.1	4.0	0.7	0.3	0.4	0.9	1.9	4.8	12.0	29.6	93.8	375.3	14.3

NOTE: Rates are on an annual basis per 100,000 population in specified group; age-adjusted rates are per 100,000 U.S. standard population.
X = Not applicable.
* = Rate does not meet NCHS standards of reliability.
[1]Figures for age not stated included in "All ages" but not distributed among age groups.
[2]Death rates for "Under 1 year" (based on population estimates) differ from infant mortality rates (based on live births); please see chapter notes for more information.
[3]For method of computation, please see chapter notes.

Table 2-8. Death Rates by Age and Age-Adjusted Death Rates for the 10 Leading Causes of Death in 2017 and Drug-Induced Deaths, Alcohol-Induced Deaths, and Injury by Firearm, 1999–2017—Continued

(Rate per 100,000 population in specified group; age-adjusted rates per 100,000 U.S. standard population.)

Cause of death (based on *International Classification of Diseases, 10th Revision*) and year	All ages[1]	Under 1 year[2]	1 to 4 years	5 to 14 years	15 to 24 years	25 to 34 years	35 to 44 years	45 to 54 years	55 to 64 years	65 to 74 years	75 to 84 years	85 years and over	Age-adjusted rate[3]
Nephritis, nephrotic syndrome and nephrosis (N00–N07,N17–N19, N25–N27)													
1999	12.7	4.4	*	0.1	0.2	0.6	1.6	4.0	12.0	37.1	97.6	268.9	13.0
2000	13.2	4.3	*	0.1	0.2	0.6	1.6	4.4	12.8	38.0	100.8	277.8	13.5
2001	13.9	3.3	*	*	0.2	0.6	1.7	4.6	13.1	40.0	104.0	293.8	14.1
2002	14.2	4.4	*	0.1	0.2	0.7	1.7	4.7	12.9	39.0	108.9	303.4	14.4
2003	14.6	4.6	*	0.1	0.2	0.7	1.8	4.9	13.6	39.7	109.3	309.3	14.7
2004	14.5	4.3	*	0.1	0.2	0.6	1.8	5.0	13.5	38.1	108.2	306.4	14.5
2005	14.9	4.0	*	0.1	0.2	0.7	1.7	4.8	13.5	38.8	110.2	313.1	14.7
2006	15.2	4.0	*	*	0.2	0.7	1.8	5.2	13.7	38.8	111.0	316.2	14.8
2007	15.4	3.5	0.1	0.1	0.2	0.7	1.8	5.1	13.4	39.4	112.4	317.9	14.9
2008	15.9	3.5	*	*	0.2	0.6	1.8	5.0	14.1	39.9	113.3	325.6	15.1
2009	16.0	2.8	*	*	0.2	0.7	2.0	5.2	13.5	38.7	115.1	321.4	15.1
2010	16.3	2.7	*	0.1	0.2	0.6	1.8	4.9	13.9	39.3	115.7	333.8	15.3
2011	14.6	1.9	*	*	0.2	0.5	1.6	4.4	12.5	34.2	101.4	292.1	13.4
2012	14.5	2.1	*	*	0.2	0.5	1.6	4.7	12.3	33.3	99.9	280.0	13.1
2013	14.9	2.2	*	*	0.1	0.6	1.5	4.6	12.6	33.8	99.0	285.4	13.2
2014	15.1	2.3	*	*	0.2	0.5	1.7	4.7	12.6	34.3	98.6	282.4	13.2
2015	15.5	2.1	*	*	0.1	0.6	1.7	4.9	13.3	35.1	99.7	281.8	13.4
2016	15.5	1.6	*	*	0.1	0.6	1.8	5.0	13.6	34.6	98.1	270.1	13.1
2017	15.5	2.0	*	*	0.1	0.6	1.7	5.2	13.5	34.7	95.8	267.1	13.0
Intentional self-harm (suicide) (*U03,X60–X84,Y87.0)[4]													
1999	10.5	X	X	0.6	10.1	12.7	14.3	13.9	12.2	13.4	18.1	19.3	10.5
2000	10.4	X	X	0.7	10.2	12.0	14.5	14.4	12.1	12.5	17.6	19.6	10.4
2001[5]	10.7	X	X	0.7	9.9	12.8	14.7	15.1	13.2	13.2	17.4	17.8	10.7
2002	11.0	X	X	0.6	9.8	12.8	15.3	15.8	13.5	13.4	17.7	18.9	10.9
2003	10.9	X	X	0.6	9.6	12.9	15.0	15.9	13.7	12.6	16.4	17.9	10.8
2004	11.1	X	X	0.7	10.3	12.9	15.2	16.6	13.7	12.2	16.3	17.6	11.0
2005	11.0	X	X	0.7	9.9	12.7	15.1	16.5	13.7	12.4	16.8	18.3	10.9
2006	11.2	X	X	0.5	9.8	12.7	15.2	17.2	14.4	12.4	15.8	17.3	11.0
2007	11.5	X	X	0.5	9.6	13.3	15.7	17.7	15.3	12.4	16.2	17.0	11.3
2008	11.8	X	X	0.5	9.9	13.2	15.9	18.6	16.0	13.6	16.1	16.4	11.6
2009	12.0	X	X	0.6	10.0	13.1	16.1	19.2	16.4	13.7	15.8	16.4	11.8
2010	12.4	X	X	0.7	10.5	14.0	16.0	19.6	17.5	13.7	15.7	17.6	12.1
2011	12.7	X	X	0.7	11.0	14.6	16.2	19.8	17.1	14.1	16.5	16.9	12.3
2012	12.9	X	X	0.8	11.1	14.7	16.7	20.0	18.0	14.0	16.8	17.8	12.6
2013	13.0	X	X	1.0	11.1	14.8	16.2	19.7	18.1	15.0	17.1	18.6	12.6
2014	13.4	X	X	1.0	11.6	15.1	16.6	20.2	18.8	15.6	17.5	19.3	13.0
2015	13.7	X	X	1.0	12.5	15.7	17.1	20.3	18.9	15.2	17.9	19.4	13.3
2016	13.9	X	X	1.1	13.2	16.5	17.4	19.7	18.7	15.4	18.2	19.0	13.5
2017	14.5	X	X	1.3	14.5	17.5	17.9	20.2	19.0	15.6	18.0	20.1	14.0
Drug-Induced Causes[6]													
1999	6.9	0.6	0.2	0.1	3.5	8.9	15.7	12.6	4.9	3.0	3.8	4.8	6.8
2000	7.0	*	*	0.1	4.0	8.8	16.0	13.2	4.9	2.6	3.5	5.7	7.0
2001	7.6	0.5	0.2	0.1	4.5	9.5	17.0	14.7	5.4	3.0	3.5	5.2	7.6
2002	9.1	0.7	0.2	0.1	5.4	11.3	19.8	18.0	6.8	3.6	3.8	6.0	9.1
2003	9.9	0.6	0.2	0.1	6.3	12.3	20.7	20.0	8.0	4.1	4.2	6.3	9.9
2004	10.5	0.7	0.2	0.2	6.9	12.9	21.1	21.7	9.0	4.2	4.8	6.7	10.5
2005	11.3	0.9	0.2	0.1	7.3	14.6	21.5	23.6	10.6	4.7	5.4	8.3	11.3
2006	12.9	1.1	0.2	0.1	8.5	17.2	23.5	26.7	12.1	5.2	6.0	8.8	12.8
2007	12.7	0.8	0.3	0.2	8.5	17.5	22.6	26.8	13.4	4.6	3.9	5.2	12.6
2008	12.7	0.5	0.3	0.1	8.3	17.4	22.2	26.8	14.0	5.2	4.0	5.0	12.6
2009	12.8	0.8	0.2	0.1	8.0	17.8	21.5	26.9	14.9	5.4	4.5	5.1	12.6
2010	13.1	0.6	0.3	0.2	8.4	19.2	21.7	26.5	16.2	5.2	4.0	5.5	12.9
2011	14.0	0.6	0.2	0.1	8.9	20.9	23.4	28.2	17.1	6.0	4.0	4.9	13.9
2012	14.0	0.8	0.2	0.1	8.3	20.9	23.1	28.3	17.9	6.5	4.0	5.1	13.8
2013	14.7	0.8	0.3	0.1	8.6	21.7	24.1	29.0	20.6	7.1	4.4	5.3	14.6
2014	15.6	0.6	0.3	0.1	8.9	24.0	26.2	29.8	21.7	7.6	4.4	5.0	15.5
2015	17.2	0.7	0.4	0.1	10.0	28.0	29.6	31.9	23.3	8.1	4.4	5.6	17.2
2016	20.8	0.9	0.3	0.1	12.8	35.9	36.6	36.5	27.7	9.2	4.1	5.3	20.8
2017	22.7	0.9	0.2	0.2	13.0	39.8	40.6	39.8	30.0	10.5	4.5	5.3	22.8

NOTE: Rates are on an annual basis per 100,000 population in specified group; age-adjusted rates are per 100,000 U.S. standard population.

X = Not applicable.

* = Rate does not meet NCHS standards of reliability.

[1]Figures for age not stated included in "All ages" but not distributed among age groups.

[2]Death rates for "Under 1 year" (based on population estimates) differ from infant mortality rates (based on live births); please see chapter notes for more information.

[3]For method of computation, please see chapter notes.

[4]Asterisks (*) preceding cause-of-death codes indicate they are not part of the *International Classification of Diseases, Tenth Revision* (*ICD–10*).

[5]Data include September 11, 2001-related deaths for which death certificates were filed as of October 24, 2002; see Technical Notes for National Vital Statistics Reports vol 52 no 3, "Deaths: Final Data for 2001."

[6]For the list of *ICD–10* codes included, see chapter notes.

Table 2-8. Death Rates by Age and Age-Adjusted Death Rates for the 10 Leading Causes of Death in 2017 and Drug-Induced Deaths, Alcohol-Induced Deaths, and Injury by Firearm, 1999–2017—Continued

(Rate per 100,000 population in specified group; age-adjusted rates per 100,000 U.S. standard population.)

Cause of death (based on International Classification of Diseases, 10th Revision) and year	All ages[1]	Age group (years)											Age-adjusted rate[3]
		Under 1 year[2]	1 to 4 years	5 to 14 years	15 to 24 years	25 to 34 years	35 to 44 years	45 to 54 years	55 to 64 years	65 to 74 years	75 to 84 years	85 years and over	
Alcohol-Induced Causes[6]													
1999	7.0	*	*	*	0.3	1.6	8.5	16.4	18.7	15.9	10.6	5.5	7.1
2000	7.0	*	*	*	0.2	1.6	8.5	16.3	18.7	15.8	9.9	5.4	7.0
2001	7.1	*	*	*	0.3	1.6	8.3	17.1	18.3	15.5	9.6	5.1	7.0
2002	7.0	*	*	*	0.3	1.5	8.1	16.9	18.3	15.4	9.3	4.6	6.9
2003	7.1	*	*	*	0.3	1.5	8.1	17.3	18.5	15.0	9.2	4.3	7.0
2004	7.2	*	*	*	0.3	1.6	7.7	17.3	18.6	15.5	9.2	4.6	7.0
2005	7.3	*	*	*	0.4	1.4	7.5	17.6	19.4	14.9	9.2	5.0	7.0
2006	7.4	*	*	*	0.3	1.6	7.5	17.5	19.2	14.5	9.7	5.3	7.0
2007	7.7	*	*	*	0.4	1.9	7.3	18.2	19.9	15.2	9.6	5.0	7.2
2008	8.0	*	*	*	0.4	2.0	7.6	18.6	20.7	15.3	9.4	5.2	7.4
2009	8.0	*	*	*	0.4	1.8	7.6	18.7	20.8	15.1	9.2	4.8	7.4
2010	8.3	*	*	*	0.3	2.2	7.5	19.1	21.9	15.8	9.6	5.3	7.6
2011	8.6	*	*	*	0.4	2.1	7.6	19.8	22.7	15.2	9.6	5.1	7.7
2012	8.8	*	*	*	0.4	2.4	7.4	20.0	24.1	15.8	10.3	5.0	8.0
2013	9.2	*	*	*	0.3	2.5	7.7	20.1	25.3	16.6	10.3	4.9	8.2
2014	9.6	*	*	*	0.3	2.8	8.0	20.4	26.8	17.6	10.5	5.6	8.5
2015	10.3	*	*	*	0.4	3.2	8.7	21.6	28.2	19.1	11.2	5.8	9.1
2016	10.8	*	*	*	0.4	3.6	9.2	21.4	29.7	20.3	11.8	6.3	9.5
2017	11.0	*	*	*	0.3	3.4	9.4	21.8	30.2	20.9	11.7	6.4	9.6
Injury by Firearm[6]													
1999	10.3	*	0.4	1.0	17.6	14.9	11.6	10.2	9.7	11.0	14.2	13.5	10.3
2000	10.2	*	0.3	0.9	16.8	14.5	11.9	10.5	9.4	10.6	13.9	14.2	10.2
2001	10.4	*	0.5	0.8	16.6	15.5	11.7	10.5	10.1	10.9	14.3	13.1	10.3
2002	10.5	*	0.4	0.8	16.6	15.6	12.2	10.8	10.2	10.8	14.4	13.2	10.5
2003	10.4	*	0.3	0.8	16.5	15.8	11.6	11.1	10.0	10.3	13.4	13.2	10.3
2004	10.1	*	0.3	0.7	15.6	15.3	11.4	11.0	9.8	10.1	13.3	12.7	10.0
2005	10.4	*	0.4	0.8	16.1	16.1	11.7	11.2	9.7	10.2	13.6	13.0	10.3
2006	10.4	*	0.4	0.9	16.7	15.7	11.6	11.2	9.7	9.9	12.9	12.5	10.3
2007	10.4	*	0.4	0.8	16.0	15.9	12.0	11.1	10.1	9.8	13.1	12.7	10.3
2008	10.4	*	0.5	0.7	15.4	15.4	11.8	11.5	10.8	10.7	13.2	12.5	10.3
2009	10.2	*	0.4	0.7	14.4	14.5	11.9	11.8	10.8	10.9	13.3	12.5	10.1
2010	10.3	*	0.4	0.7	14.2	15.0	11.7	12.0	11.1	10.7	12.7	13.2	10.1
2011	10.4	*	0.5	0.8	14.4	15.0	11.7	12.2	11.0	10.9	13.7	13.1	10.2
2012	10.7	*	0.4	0.8	14.7	15.3	12.4	12.4	11.6	10.8	14.1	13.6	10.5
2013	10.6	*	0.4	0.8	14.1	15.3	12.3	12.3	11.5	11.3	14.1	13.9	10.4
2014	10.5	*	0.4	0.9	14.0	14.7	12.1	12.2	11.4	11.5	13.9	15.0	10.3
2015	11.3	*	0.5	0.9	15.7	16.8	13.1	12.4	11.7	11.3	14.5	14.5	11.1
2016	12.0	*	0.6	0.9	17.2	18.2	14.5	12.8	11.9	11.4	14.7	14.3	11.8
2017	12.2	*	0.5	1.1	17.7	18.5	14.4	13.1	12.3	11.4	14.8	15.6	12.0

NOTE: Rates are on an annual basis per 100,000 population in specified group; age-adjusted rates are per 100,000 U.S. standard population.
X = Not applicable.
* = Rate does not meet NCHS standards of reliability.
[1]Figures for age not stated included in "All ages" but not distributed among age groups.
[2]Death rates for "Under 1 year" (based on population estimates) differ from infant mortality rates (based on live births); please see chapter notes for more information.
[3]For method of computation, please see chapter notes.
[6]For the list of ICD–10 codes included, see chapter notes.

Table 2-9. Number of Deaths from Selected Causes, by Age, 2017

(Number.)

Cause of death (based on *International Classification of Diseases, 10th Revision*)	All ages	Under 1 year	1 to 4 years	5 to 14 years	15 to 24 years	25 to 34 years	35 to 44 years	45 to 54 years	55 to 64 years	65 to 74 years	75 to 84 years	85 years and over	Not stated
All causes	2,813,503	22,335	3,880	5,571	32,025	60,215	79,796	170,142	372,006	531,610	657,759	878,035	129
Enterocolitis due to Clostridium difficile (A04.7).................	6,118	2	–	4	7	20	48	178	529	1,192	1,834	2,304	–
Septicemia (A40–A41)	40,922	147	48	57	123	392	854	2,441	5,838	9,164	10,648	11,210	–
Viral hepatitis (B15–B19)	5,611	1	–	1	1	42	201	927	2,517	1,314	426	177	4
Human immunodeficiency virus (HIV) disease (B20–B24)	5,698	–	–	–	69	513	831	1,609	1,737	685	220	34	–
Malignant neoplasms (C00–C97)..................	599,108	57	325	855	1,374	3,616	10,900	39,266	114,810	168,458	155,917	103,521	9
Malignant neoplasms of lip, oral cavity and pharynx (C00–C14) ...	10,126	–	–	4	14	54	189	962	2,638	2,969	1,987	1,309	–
Malignant neoplasm of esophagus (C15).................	15,321	–	–	–	12	35	206	1,137	3,821	4,948	3,443	1,719	–
Malignant neoplasm of stomach (C16).................	11,158	–	–	3	24	145	422	1,020	2,197	2,772	2,727	1,848	–
Malignant neoplasms of colon, rectum and anus (C18–C21)......	53,447	–	–	1	40	342	1,453	4,976	10,398	13,011	12,447	10,779	–
Malignant neoplasms of liver and intrahepatic bile ducts (C22)......	27,106	–	14	21	21	110	338	1,847	7,754	8,580	5,657	2,762	2
Malignant neoplasm of pancreas (C25)	44,012	–	–	1	3	56	470	2,556	8,633	13,692	11,839	6,761	1
Malignant neoplasms of trachea, bronchus and lung (C33–C34)......	145,932	–	6	6	17	112	843	6,989	29,505	47,654	41,701	19,099	–
Malignant melanoma of skin (C43)	8,056	1	2	–	15	129	313	705	1,512	2,040	1,952	1,387	–
Malignant neoplasm of breast (C50)	42,510	–	–	–	13	385	1,873	4,978	9,024	10,272	8,472	7,493	–
Malignant neoplasm of cervix uteri (C53)	4,208	–	–	–	8	226	576	869	1,007	776	462	283	1
Malignant neoplasm of ovary (C56)	14,193	–	–	1	20	82	290	1,215	3,113	4,077	3,488	1,907	–
Malignant neoplasm of prostate (C61).................	30,488	–	–	1	1	1	8	399	2,743	7,280	10,143	9,910	2
Malignant neoplasms of kidney and renal pelvis (C64–C65)..........	13,960	3	16	19	26	58	247	980	2,743	4,000	3,538	2,329	1
Malignant neoplasm of bladder (C67).................	16,657	–	–	2	–	12	78	430	1,848	3,733	5,207	5,347	–
Malignant neoplasms of meninges, brain and other parts of central nervous system (C70–C72).................	16,804	13	73	336	232	421	803	1,846	4,040	4,603	3,126	1,311	–
Non-Hodgkin lymphoma (C82–C85).................	20,460	1	4	29	69	167	332	947	2,678	5,069	6,356	4,807	1
Multiple myeloma and immunoproliferative neoplasms (C88,C90).................	12,809	–	–	–	2	8	94	556	1,870	3,613	4,124	2,542	–
Leukemia (C91–C95).................	23,359	19	110	186	310	367	541	1,115	2,839	5,481	7,036	5,355	–
In situ neoplasms, benign neoplasms and neoplasms of uncertain or unknown behavior (D00–D48).................	15,824	41	44	62	80	143	204	567	1,528	3,108	4,735	5,312	–
Anemias (D50–D64).................	5,382	15	24	24	69	159	177	250	523	867	1,245	2,029	–
Diabetes mellitus (E10–E14)	83,564	1	6	34	248	823	2,118	6,409	14,904	21,344	20,703	16,973	1
Nutritional deficiencies (E40–E64).................	7,846	6	1	3	5	23	48	139	501	1,042	1,784	4,294	–
Obesity (E66)	7,740	–	1	5	65	438	904	1,478	2,124	1,726	762	236	1
Parkinson disease (G20–G21)	31,963	–	–	–	1	4	7	60	714	4,661	13,172	13,344	–
Alzheimer's disease (G30).................	121,404	–	–	–	–	–	11	95	1,189	7,281	32,309	80,517	–
Major cardiovascular diseases (I00–I78)	854,390	421	195	288	1,126	4,596	13,179	40,643	99,610	150,078	204,614	339,597	43
Diseases of heart (I00–I09,I11,I13,I20–I51)	647,457	304	127	179	913	3,681	10,401	32,658	80,102	116,633	151,249	251,170	40
Essential hypertension and hypertensive renal disease (I10,I12,I15).................	35,316	1	1	1	10	119	514	1,642	3,991	5,856	8,211	14,969	1
Cerebrovascular diseases (I60–I69).................	146,383	100	66	97	155	593	1,811	5,198	12,708	22,690	38,697	64,266	2
Atherosclerosis (I70).................	5,547	3	–	–	3	5	15	108	381	711	1,320	3,001	–
Aortic aneurysm and dissection (I71).................	9,928	1	–	1	28	141	308	650	1,323	2,127	2,709	2,640	–
Influenza and pneumonia (J09–J18).................	55,672	157	104	113	190	405	782	2,013	5,045	8,784	13,802	24,276	1
Chronic lower respiratory diseases (J40–J47).................	160,201	14	31	134	188	332	713	3,975	18,667	39,704	51,116	45,319	8
Pneumonitis due to solids and liquids (J69).................	20,108	6	6	12	42	96	162	585	1,610	2,992	5,236	9,361	–
Chronic liver disease and cirrhosis (K70,K73–K74).................	41,743	2	1	2	23	918	3,000	8,312	13,737	9,400	4,610	1,736	2
Alcoholic liver disease (K70).................	22,246	–	–	–	14	753	2,266	5,786	8,126	3,976	1,097	227	1
Cholelithiasis and other disorders of gallbladder (K80–K82).................	3,793	–	–	–	10	21	43	128	338	652	1,052	1,549	–
Nephritis, nephrotic syndrome and nephrosis (N00–N07, N17–N19,N25–N27).................	50,633	79	7	10	52	255	692	2,197	5,671	10,302	14,093	17,275	–
Pregnancy, childbirth and the puerperium (O00–O99).................	1,208	...	...	1	168	512	328	192	4	1	1	1	–
Certain conditions originating in the perinatal period (P00–P96).......	11,108	11,000	42	21	18	3	4	8	5	3	1	2	1
Congenital malformations, deformations and chromosomal abnormalities (Q00–Q99).................	9,902	4,580	424	379	355	437	419	735	1,228	650	367	327	1
Symptoms, signs and abnormal clinical and laboratory findings, not elsewhere classified (R00–R99).................	32,750	2,692	274	108	501	1,189	1,326	1,938	3,216	3,927	5,269	12,292	18
Accidents (unintentional injuries) (V01–X59,Y85–Y86).................	169,936	1,317	1,267	1,578	13,441	25,669	22,828	24,461	23,408	15,038	16,661	24,252	16
Motor vehicle accidents (V02–V04,V09.0,V09.2, V12–V14, V19.0–V19.2,V19.4–V19.6,V20–V79, V80.3–V80.5, V81.0–V81.1,V82.0–V82.1,V83–V86, V87.0–V87.8,V88.0–V88.8,V89.0,V89.2)	40,231	91	453	855	6,864	7,024	5,324	5,660	5,828	3,823	2,836	1,473	–
Falls (W00–W19).................	36,338	13	12	30	212	351	522	1,248	2,760	4,752	9,218	17,220	–
Accidental discharge of firearms (W32–W34).................	486	1	31	30	117	93	64	50	47	30	18	5	–
Accidental drowning and submersion (W65–W74).................	3,709	43	424	235	469	479	397	451	510	381	226	93	1
Accidental hanging, strangulation and suffocation (W75–W84)	6,946	1,106	110	71	101	175	211	441	811	1,048	1,246	1,626	–

NOTE: Only selected causes of deaths are shown; therefore, subcategories do not add to totals.
X = Not applicable.
– = Quantity zero.

Table 2-9. Number of Deaths from Selected Causes, by Age, 2017—*Continued*

(Number.)

Cause of death (based on *International Classification of Diseases, 10th Revision*)	All ages	Under 1 year	1 to 4 years	5 to 14 years	15 to 24 years	25 to 34 years	35 to 44 years	45 to 54 years	55 to 64 years	65 to 74 years	75 to 84 years	85 years and over	Not stated
Accidental exposure to smoke, fire and flames (X00–X09)	2,812	15	89	149	83	154	202	311	585	567	413	244	–
Accidental poisoning and exposure to noxious substances (X40–X49)	64,795	9	29	45	5,030	16,478	15,032	14,707	10,581	2,241	406	224	13
Intentional self-harm (suicide) (*U03,X60–X84,Y87.0)[1]	47,173	X	X	522	6,252	7,948	7,335	8,561	7,982	4,620	2,648	1,300	5
Intentional self-harm (suicide) by poisoning (X60–X69)	6,554	X	X	39	463	788	1,089	1,604	1,459	724	252	135	1
Intentional self-harm (suicide) by hanging, strangulation and suffocation (X70)	13,075	X	X	284	2,321	3,063	2,562	2,294	1,631	572	227	120	1
Intentional self-harm (suicide) by discharge of firearms (X72–X74)	23,854	X	X	186	2,959	3,458	3,098	3,937	4,219	2,989	2,040	967	1
Assault (homicide) (*U01–*U02,X85–Y09,Y87.1)[1]	19,510	302	303	332	4,905	5,488	3,351	2,275	1,552	633	252	116	1
Assault (homicide) by discharge of firearms (*U01.4,X93–X95)[1]	14,542	12	44	204	4,391	4,594	2,561	1,447	824	322	109	34	–
Legal intervention (Y35,Y89.0)	616	–	–	1	97	192	148	114	41	18	3	2	–
Complications of medical and surgical care (Y40–Y84,Y88)	4,459	14	24	25	52	97	191	380	773	1,153	1,044	705	1
Drug-induced deaths[2]	73,990	36	38	73	5,606	18,061	16,592	16,859	12,607	3,106	657	340	15
Alcohol-induced deaths[2]	35,823	–	1	4	136	1,548	3,859	9,234	12,695	6,216	1,714	413	3
Injury by firearms[2]	39,773	13	80	438	7,656	8,381	5,899	5,558	5,174	3,379	2,182	1,011	2

NOTE: Only selected causes of deaths are shown; therefore, subcategories do not add to totals.

X = Not applicable.

– = Quantity zero.

[1]Asterisks (*) preceding cause-of-death codes indicate they are not part of the *International Classification of Diseases, Tenth Revision* (*ICD–10*).

[2]Included in selected categories above.

Table 2-10. Death Rates for Selected Causes, by Age, 2017

(Rate; Rates are on an annual basis per 100,000 population in specified group.)

Cause of death (based on *International Classification of Diseases, 10th Revision*)	All ages[1]	Under 1 year[2]	1 to 4 years	5 to 14 years	15 to 24 years	25 to 34 years	35 to 44 years	45 to 54 years	55 to 64 years	65 to 74 years	75 to 84 years	85 years and over
All causes	863.8	567.0	24.3	13.6	74.0	132.8	195.2	401.5	885.8	1,790.9	4,472.6	13,573.6
Enterocolitis due to Clostridium difficile (A04.7)	1.9	*	*	*	*	0.0	0.1	0.4	1.3	4.0	12.5	35.6
Septicemia (A40–A41)	12.6	3.7	0.3	0.1	0.3	0.9	2.1	5.8	13.9	30.9	72.4	173.3
Viral hepatitis (B15–B19)	1.7	*	*	*	*	0.1	0.5	2.2	6.0	4.4	2.9	2.7
Human immunodeficiency virus (HIV) disease (B20–B24)	1.7	*	*	*	0.2	1.1	2.0	3.8	4.1	2.3	1.5	0.5
Malignant neoplasms (C00–C97)	183.9	1.4	2.0	2.1	3.2	8.0	26.7	92.7	273.4	567.5	1,060.2	1,600.3
Malignant neoplasms of lip, oral cavity and pharynx (C00–C14)	3.1	*	*	*	*	0.1	0.5	2.3	6.3	10.0	13.5	20.2
Malignant neoplasm of esophagus (C15)	4.7	*	*	*	*	0.1	0.5	2.7	9.1	16.7	23.4	26.6
Malignant neoplasm of stomach (C16)	3.4	*	*	*	0.1	0.3	1.0	2.4	5.2	9.3	18.5	28.6
Malignant neoplasms of colon, rectum and anus (C18–C21)	16.4	*	*	*	0.1	0.8	3.6	11.7	24.8	43.8	84.6	166.6
Malignant neoplasms of liver and intrahepatic bile ducts (C22)	8.3	*	*	0.1	0.0	0.2	0.8	4.4	18.5	28.9	38.5	42.7
Malignant neoplasm of pancreas (C25)	13.5	*	*	*	*	0.1	1.1	6.0	20.6	46.1	80.5	104.5
Malignant neoplasms of trachea, bronchus and lung (C33–C34)	44.8	*	*	*	*	0.2	2.1	16.5	70.3	160.5	283.6	295.3
Malignant melanoma of skin (C43)	2.5	*	*	*	*	0.3	0.8	1.7	3.6	6.9	13.3	21.4
Malignant neoplasm of breast (C50)	13.1	*	*	*	*	0.8	4.6	11.7	21.5	34.6	57.6	115.8
Malignant neoplasm of cervix uteri (C53)	1.3	*	*	*	*	0.5	1.4	2.1	2.4	2.6	3.1	4.4
Malignant neoplasm of ovary (C56)	4.4	*	*	*	0.0	0.2	0.7	2.9	7.4	13.7	23.7	29.5
Malignant neoplasm of prostate (C61)	9.4	*	*	*	*	*	*	0.9	6.5	24.5	69.0	153.2
Malignant neoplasms of kidney and renal pelvis (C64–C65)	4.3	*	*	*	0.1	0.1	0.6	2.3	6.5	13.5	24.1	36.0
Malignant neoplasm of bladder (C67)	5.1	*	*	*	*	*	0.2	1.0	4.4	12.6	35.4	82.7
Malignant neoplasms of meninges, brain and other parts of central nervous system (C70–C72)	5.2	*	0.5	0.8	0.5	0.9	2.0	4.4	9.6	15.5	21.3	20.3
Non-Hodgkin lymphoma (C82–C85)	6.3	*	*	0.1	0.2	0.4	0.8	2.2	6.4	17.1	43.2	74.3
Multiple myeloma and immunoproliferative neoplasms (C88,C90)	3.9	*	*	*	*	*	0.2	1.3	4.5	12.2	28.0	39.3
Leukemia (C91–C95)	7.2	*	0.7	0.5	0.7	0.8	1.3	2.6	6.8	18.5	47.8	82.8
In situ neoplasms, benign neoplasms and neoplasms of uncertain or unknown behavior (D00–D48)	4.9	1.0	0.3	0.2	0.2	0.3	0.5	1.3	3.6	10.5	32.2	82.1
Anemias (D50–D64)	1.7	*	0.2	0.1	0.2	0.4	0.4	0.6	1.2	2.9	8.5	31.4
Diabetes mellitus (E10–E14)	25.7	*	*	0.1	0.6	1.8	5.2	15.1	35.5	71.9	140.8	262.4
Nutritional deficiencies (E40–E64)	2.4	*	*	*	*	0.1	0.1	0.3	1.2	3.5	12.1	66.4
Obesity (E66)	2.4	*	*	*	0.2	1.0	2.2	3.5	5.1	5.8	5.2	3.6
Parkinson disease (G20–G21)	9.8	*	*	*	*	*	*	0.1	1.7	15.7	89.6	206.3
Alzheimer disease (G30)	37.3	*	*	*	*	*	*	0.2	2.8	24.5	219.7	1,244.7
Major cardiovascular diseases (I00–I78)	262.3	10.7	1.2	0.7	2.6	10.1	32.2	95.9	237.2	505.6	1,391.3	5,249.9
Diseases of heart (I00–I09,I11,I13,I20–I51)	198.8	7.7	0.8	0.4	2.1	8.1	25.4	77.1	190.7	392.9	1,028.4	3,882.9
Essential hypertension and hypertensive renal disease (I10,I12,I15)	10.8	*	*	*	*	0.3	1.3	3.9	9.5	19.7	55.8	231.4
Cerebrovascular diseases (I60–I69)	44.9	2.5	0.4	0.2	0.4	1.3	4.4	12.3	30.3	76.4	263.1	993.5
Atherosclerosis (I70)	1.7	*	*	*	*	*	*	0.3	0.9	2.4	9.0	46.4
Aortic aneurysm and dissection (I71)	3.0	*	*	*	0.1	0.3	0.8	1.5	3.2	7.2	18.4	40.8
Influenza and pneumonia (J09–J18)	17.1	4.0	0.7	0.3	0.4	0.9	1.9	4.8	12.0	29.6	93.8	375.3
Chronic lower respiratory diseases (J40–J47)	49.2	*	0.2	0.3	0.4	0.7	1.7	9.4	44.4	133.8	347.6	700.6
Pneumonitis due to solids and liquids (J69)	6.2	*	*	*	0.1	0.2	0.4	1.4	3.8	10.1	35.6	144.7
Chronic liver disease and cirrhosis (K70,K73–K74)	12.8	*	*	*	0.1	2.0	7.3	19.6	32.7	31.7	31.3	26.8
Alcoholic liver disease (K70)	6.8	*	*	*	*	1.7	5.5	13.7	19.3	13.4	7.5	3.5
Cholelithiasis and other disorders of gallbladder (K80–K82)	1.2	*	*	*	*	0.0	0.1	0.3	0.8	2.2	7.2	23.9
Nephritis, nephrotic syndrome and nephrosis (N00–N07,N17–N19,N25–N27)	15.5	2.0	*	*	0.1	0.6	1.7	5.2	13.5	34.7	95.8	267.1
Pregnancy, childbirth and the puerperium (O00–O99)	0.4	X	X	*	0.4	1.1	0.8	0.5	*	*	*	*
Certain conditions originating in the perinatal period (P00–P96)	3.4	279.2	0.3	0.1	*	*	*	*	*	*	*	*
Congenital malformations, deformations and chromosomal abnormalities (Q00–Q99)	3.0	116.3	2.7	0.9	0.8	1.0	1.0	1.7	2.9	2.2	2.5	5.1
Symptoms, signs and abnormal clinical and laboratory findings, not elsewhere classified (R00–R99)	10.1	68.3	1.7	0.3	1.2	2.6	3.2	4.6	7.7	13.2	35.8	190.0
Accidents (unintentional injuries) (V01–X59,Y85–Y86)	52.2	33.4	7.9	3.8	31.1	56.6	55.8	57.7	55.7	50.7	113.3	374.9
Motor vehicle accidents (V02–V04,V09.0, V09.2,V12–V14,V19.0–V19.2,V19.4–V19.6, V20–V79,V80.3–V80.5,V81.0–V81.1,V82.0–V82.1, V83–V86,V87.0–V87.8,V88.0–V88.8,V89.0,V89.2)	12.4	2.3	2.8	2.1	15.9	15.5	13.0	13.4	13.9	12.9	19.3	22.8

X = Not applicable.
* = Rate does not meet NCHS standards of reliability.
0.0 = Quantity more than zero but less than 0.05.
[1]Figures for age not stated are included in "All ages" but are not distributed among age groups.
[2]Death rates for "Under 1 year" (based on population estimates) differ from infant mortality rates (based on live births); for more information, see chapter notes.

Table 2-10. Death Rates for Selected Causes, by Age, 2017—*Continued*

(Rate; Rates are on an annual basis per 100,000 population in specified group.)

Cause of death (based on *International Classification of Diseases, 10th Revision*)	All ages[1]	Under 1 year[2]	1 to 4 years	5 to 14 years	15 to 24 years	25 to 34 years	35 to 44 years	45 to 54 years	55 to 64 years	65 to 74 years	75 to 84 years	85 years and over
Falls (W00–W19)	11.2	*	*	0.1	0.5	0.8	1.3	2.9	6.6	16.0	62.7	266.2
Accidental discharge of firearms (W32–W34)	0.1	*	0.2	0.1	0.3	0.2	0.2	0.1	0.1	0.1	*	*
Accidental drowning and submersion (W65–W74)	1.1	1.1	2.7	0.6	1.1	1.1	1.0	1.1	1.2	1.3	1.5	1.4
Accidental hanging, strangulation and suffocation (W75–W84)	2.1	28.1	0.7	0.2	0.2	0.4	0.5	1.0	1.9	3.5	8.5	25.1
Accidental exposure to smoke, fire and flames (X00–X09)	0.9	*	0.6	0.4	0.2	0.3	0.5	0.7	1.4	1.9	2.8	3.8
Accidental poisoning and exposure to noxious substances (X40–X49)	19.9	*	0.2	0.1	11.6	36.3	36.8	34.7	25.2	7.5	2.8	3.5
Intentional self-harm (suicide) (*U03,X60–X84,Y87.0)3	14.5	X	X	1.3	14.5	17.5	17.9	20.2	19.0	15.6	18.0	20.1
Intentional self-harm (suicide) by poisoning (X60–X69)	2.0	X	X	0.1	1.1	1.7	2.7	3.8	3.5	2.4	1.7	2.1
Intentional self-harm (suicide) by hanging, strangulation and suffocation (X70)	4.0	X	X	0.7	5.4	6.8	6.3	5.4	3.9	1.9	1.5	1.9
Intentional self-harm (suicide) by discharge of firearms (X72–X74)	7.3	X	X	0.5	6.8	7.6	7.6	9.3	10.0	10.1	13.9	14.9
Assault (homicide) (*U01–*U02,X85–Y09,Y87.1)[3]	6.0	7.7	1.9	0.8	11.3	12.1	8.2	5.4	3.7	2.1	1.7	1.8
Assault (homicide) by discharge of firearms (*U01.4,X93–X95)[3]	4.5	*	0.3	0.5	10.2	10.1	6.3	3.4	2.0	1.1	0.7	0.5
Legal intervention (Y35,Y89.0)	0.2	*	*	*	0.2	0.4	0.4	0.3	0.1	*	*	*
Complications of medical and surgical care (Y40–Y84,Y88)	1.4	*	0.2	0.1	0.1	0.2	0.5	0.9	1.8	3.9	7.1	10.9
Drug-induced deaths[4]	22.7	0.9	0.2	0.2	13.0	39.8	40.6	39.8	30.0	10.5	4.5	5.3
Alcohol-induced deaths[4]	11.0	*	*	*	0.3	3.4	9.4	21.8	30.2	20.9	11.7	6.4
Injury by firearms[4]	12.2	*	0.5	1.1	17.7	18.5	14.4	13.1	12.3	11.4	14.8	15.6

X = Not applicable.
* = Rate does not meet NCHS standards of reliability.
[1]Figures for age not stated are included in "All ages" but are not distributed among age groups.
[2]Death rates for "Under 1 year" (based on population estimates) differ from infant mortality rates (based on live births); for more information, see chapter notes.
[3]Asterisks (*) preceding cause-of-death codes indicate they are not part of the *International Classification of Diseases, Tenth Revision* (*ICD–10*).
[4]Included in selected categories above.

Table 2-11. Number of Deaths from Selected Causes, by Race, Hispanic Origin, and Sex, 2017

(Number.)

Cause of death (based on *International Classification of Diseases, 10th Revision*)	Total[1]			Non-Hispanic White[2]			Non-Hispanic Black[2]		
	Both sexes	Male	Female	Both sexes	Male	Female	Both sexes	Male	Female
All causes	2,813,503	1,439,111	1,374,392	2,179,857	1,102,838	1,077,019	335,667	174,403	161,264
Enterocolitis due to Clostridium difficile (A04.7).................................	6,118	2,481	3,637	4,975	2,002	2,973	557	226	331
Septicemia (A40–A41)	40,922	19,603	21,319	30,198	14,419	15,779	6,568	3,052	3,516
Viral hepatitis (B15–B19)	5,611	3,685	1,926	3,528	2,290	1,238	818	555	263
Human immunodeficiency virus (HIV) disease (B20–B24)	5,698	4,207	1,491	1,750	1,461	289	2,965	1,963	1,002
Malignant neoplasms (C00–C97)...........................	599,108	315,147	283,961	465,679	247,022	218,657	69,872	35,261	34,611
Malignant neoplasms of lip, oral cavity and pharynx (C00–C14)	10,126	7,235	2,891	7,995	5,680	2,315	1,058	788	270
Malignant neoplasm of esophagus (C15)............	15,321	12,314	3,007	12,875	10,484	2,391	1,246	869	377
Malignant neoplasm of stomach (C16)....................	11,158	6,680	4,478	6,322	3,908	2,414	1,867	1,118	749
Malignant neoplasms of colon, rectum and anus (C18–C21)........	53,447	28,093	25,354	39,790	20,736	19,054	7,214	3,793	3,421
Malignant neoplasms of liver and intrahepatic bile ducts (C22)..........	27,106	18,246	8,860	17,862	12,025	5,837	3,714	2,561	1,153
Malignant neoplasms of pancreas (C25)................	44,012	22,919	21,093	33,940	18,027	15,913	5,305	2,574	2,731
Malignant neoplasms of trachea, bronchus and lung (C33–C34)........	145,932	78,743	67,189	120,048	63,989	56,059	15,392	8,727	6,665
Malignant melanoma of skin (C43).........................	8,056	5,312	2,744	7,582	5,055	2,527	132	56	76
Malignant neoplasm of breast (C50)......................	42,510	510	42,000	31,427	397	31,030	6,436	79	6,357
Malignant neoplasm of cervix uteri (C53)..............	4,208	X	4,208	2,560	X	2,560	793	X	793
Malignant neoplasm of ovary (C56).......................	14,193	X	14,193	11,101	X	11,101	1,389	X	1,389
Malignant neoplasm of prostate (C61)...................	30,488	30,488	X	22,660	22,660	X	5,000	5,000	X
Malignant neoplasms of kidney and renal pelvis (C64–C65)...............	13,960	9,037	4,923	10,881	7,064	3,817	1,386	886	500
Malignant neoplasm of bladder (C67).....................	16,657	11,888	4,769	14,207	10,337	3,870	1,257	736	521
Malignant neoplasms of meninges, brain and other parts of central nervous system (C70–C72)....................	16,804	9,389	7,415	13,883	7,815	6,068	1,105	581	524
Non-Hodgkin lymphoma (C82–C85).......................	20,460	11,648	8,812	16,548	9,442	7,106	1,564	890	674
Multiple myeloma and immunoproliferative neoplasms (C88,C90).....	12,809	7,142	5,667	9,171	5,237	3,934	2,340	1,198	1,142
Leukemia (C91–C95)...	23,359	13,520	9,839	18,832	11,034	7,798	1,959	1,017	942
In situ neoplasms, benign neoplasms and neoplasms of uncertain or unknown behavior (D00–D48)........................	15,824	8,502	7,322	13,071	7,067	6,004	1,344	682	662
Anemias (D50–D64)...	5,382	2,395	2,987	3,800	1,681	2,119	1,078	488	590
Diabetes mellitus (E10–E14)..................................	83,564	46,302	37,262	55,116	31,343	23,773	14,798	7,494	7,304
Nutritional deficiencies (E40–E64).........................	7,846	2,883	4,963	6,194	2,202	3,992	933	387	546
Obesity (E66)..	7,740	4,032	3,708	5,577	2,958	2,619	1,397	645	752
Parkinson disease (G20–G21)...............................	31,963	19,388	12,575	27,582	16,841	10,741	1,518	894	624
Alzheimer disease (G30).......................................	121,404	37,325	84,079	101,876	31,577	70,299	8,991	2,476	6,515
Major cardiovascular diseases (I00–I78)	854,390	438,041	416,349	663,092	338,319	324,773	106,397	54,323	52,074
Diseases of heart (I00–I09,I11,I13,I20–I51)..........	647,457	347,879	299,578	508,485	272,428	236,057	78,161	41,411	36,750
Essential hypertension and hypertensive renal disease (I10,I12,I15)..	35,316	15,749	19,567	24,465	10,696	13,769	6,273	2,874	3,399
Cerebrovascular diseases (I60–I69)......................	146,383	61,645	84,738	110,038	45,078	64,960	19,088	8,566	10,522
Atherosclerosis (I70)..	5,547	2,385	3,162	4,627	1,970	2,657	467	200	267
Aortic aneurysm and dissection (I71)....................	9,928	5,798	4,130	8,015	4,626	3,389	1,039	613	426
Influenza and pneumonia (J09–J18).......................	55,672	26,558	29,114	43,397	20,515	22,882	5,556	2,682	2,874
Chronic lower respiratory diseases (J40–J47).........	160,201	75,005	85,196	139,833	64,673	75,160	11,217	5,605	5,612
Pneumonitis due to solids and liquids (J69)...........	20,108	11,350	8,758	16,449	9,352	7,097	1,928	1,019	909
Chronic liver disease and cirrhosis (K70,K73–K74) ...	41,743	26,451	15,292	30,223	18,866	11,357	3,290	2,064	1,226
Alcoholic liver disease (K70)..................................	22,246	15,470	6,776	15,910	10,815	5,095	1,660	1,087	573
Cholelithiasis and other disorders of gallbladder (K80–K82)	3,793	1,898	1,895	2,866	1,429	1,437	344	160	184
Nephritis, nephrotic syndrome and nephrosis (N00–N07,N17–N19, N25–N27)	50,633	25,744	24,889	35,191	18,187	17,004	9,542	4,555	4,987
Pregnancy, childbirth and the puerperium (O00–O99)...........................	1,208	X	1,208	561	X	561	383	X	383
Certain conditions originating in the perinatal period (P00–P96)...........	11,108	6,303	4,805	4,264	2,422	1,842	3,637	2,080	1,557
Congenital malformations, deformations and chromosomal abnormalities (Q00–Q99)................................	9,902	5,198	4,704	6,044	3,198	2,846	1,597	834	763
Symptoms, signs and abnormal clinical and laboratory findings, not elsewhere classified (R00–R99)........................	32,750	15,391	17,359	24,949	11,184	13,765	4,510	2,302	2,208
Accidents (unintentional injuries) (V01–X59,Y85–Y86)	169,936	109,722	60,214	127,029	79,280	47,749	19,869	13,844	6,025
Motor vehicle accidents (V02–V04, V09.0,V09.2,V12–V14,V19.0–V19.2, V19.4–V19.6,V20–V79,V80.3–V80.5, V81.0–V81.1,V82.0–V82.1,V83–V86, V87.0–V87.8,V88.0–V88.8, V89.0,V89.2)	40,231	28,629	11,602	26,177	18,356	7,821	6,109	4,510	1,599

NOTE: Includes selected causes of deaths; therefore, subcategories do not add to totals. Race and Hispanic-origin categories are consistent with 1977 Office of Management and Budget (OMB) standards. Data for specified race or Hispanic-origin groups other than non-Hispanic White and non-Hispanic Black should be interpreted with caution because of inconsistencies in reporting these items on death certificates and surveys, although misclassification is very minor for the Hispanic and non-Hispanic Asian or Pacific Islander populations.
X = Not applicable.
[1]Includes deaths for origin not stated.
[2]Multiple-race data reported according to 1997 OMB standards were bridged to the single-race categories of 1977 OMB standards.

Table 2-11. Number of Deaths from Selected Causes, by Race, Hispanic Origin, and Sex, 2017—*Continued*

(Number.)

Cause of death (based on *International Classification of Diseases, 10th Revision*)	Non-Hispanic American Indian and Alaskan Native[2,3]			Non-Hispanic Asian or Pacific Islander[2,4]			Hispanic		
	Both sexes	Male	Female	Both sexes	Male	Female	Both sexes	Male	Female
All causes	19,198	10,502	8,696	72,598	37,236	35,362	197,249	108,579	88,670
Enterocolitis due to Clostridium difficile (A04.7)....................	49	18	31	116	47	69	405	178	227
Septicemia (A40–A41)...................................	295	130	165	879	460	419	2,869	1,473	1,396
Viral hepatitis (B15–B19)	71	45	26	262	161	101	876	591	285
Human immunodeficiency virus (HIV) disease (B20–B24)	35	27	8	64	56	8	816	645	171
Malignant neoplasms (C00–C97)............................	3,257	1,725	1,532	18,257	9,243	9,014	40,550	21,034	19,516
Malignant neoplasms of lip, oral cavity and pharynx (C00–C14)	57	43	14	386	276	110	596	425	171
Malignant neoplasm of esophagus (C15).................	79	59	20	311	242	69	762	619	143
Malignant neoplasm of stomach (C16).................	94	59	35	960	516	444	1,894	1,066	828
Malignant neoplasms of colon, rectum and anus (C18–C21)...........	358	204	154	1,801	959	842	4,146	2,318	1,828
Malignant neoplasms of liver and intrahepatic bile ducts (C22).........	259	174	85	1,643	1,079	564	3,528	2,332	1,196
Malignant neoplasm of pancreas (C25)..............	200	109	91	1,408	670	738	3,069	1,499	1,570
Malignant neoplasms of trachea, bronchus and lung (C33–C34).......	790	422	368	3,870	2,202	1,668	5,457	3,184	2,273
Malignant melanoma of skin (C43)	18	13	5	57	28	29	251	149	102
Malignant neoplasm of breast (C50)	202	1	201	1,345	12	1,333	3,000	17	2,983
Malignant neoplasm of cervix uteri (C53)	31	X	31	203	X	203	606	X	606
Malignant neoplasm of ovary (C56)	80	X	80	496	X	496	1,107	X	1,107
Malignant neoplasm of prostate (C61)	136	136	X	609	609	X	2,011	2,011	...
Malignant neoplasms of kidney and renal pelvis (C64–C65)...............	107	71	36	304	194	110	1,252	803	449
Malignant neoplasm of bladder (C67)	61	43	18	288	195	93	804	543	261
Malignant neoplasms of meninges, brain and other parts of central nervous system (C70–C72)	68	33	35	424	235	189	1,297	710	587
Non-Hodgkin lymphoma (C82–C85)	82	47	35	640	375	265	1,578	862	716
Multiple myeloma and immunoproliferative neoplasms (C88,C90).....	74	38	36	307	168	139	894	490	404
Leukemia (C91–C95)	92	55	37	661	397	264	1,755	979	776
In situ neoplasms, benign neoplasms and neoplasms of uncertain or unknown behavior (D00–D48)	61	32	29	434	230	204	882	466	416
Anemias (D50–D64)	26	10	16	132	59	73	330	151	179
Diabetes mellitus (E10–E14)............................	1,114	624	490	3,047	1,612	1,435	9,216	5,054	4,162
Nutritional deficiencies (E40–E64).......................	50	22	28	196	81	115	460	186	274
Obesity (E66)...	79	48	31	63	38	25	591	329	262
Parkinson disease (G20–G21)	114	68	46	869	489	380	1,818	1,060	758
Alzheimer disease (G30)	376	120	256	2,583	790	1,793	7,383	2,297	5,086
Major cardiovascular diseases (I00–I78)	4,524	2,501	2,023	23,065	11,861	11,204	54,352	29,171	25,181
Diseases of heart (I00–I09,I11,I13,I20–I51)	3,472	2,033	1,439	15,490	8,418	7,072	39,402	22,009	17,393
Essential hypertension and hypertensive renal disease (I10,I12,I15)..	190	97	93	1,472	654	818	2,799	1,354	1,445
Cerebrovascular diseases (I60–I69)..................	737	322	415	5,430	2,442	2,988	10,775	5,073	5,702
Atherosclerosis (I70).............................	15	5	10	126	55	71	293	148	145
Aortic aneurysm and dissection (I71)................	43	23	20	343	204	139	462	310	152
Influenza and pneumonia (J09–J18).....................	391	186	205	2,286	1,155	1,131	3,851	1,911	1,940
Chronic lower respiratory diseases (J40–J47).............	939	441	498	2,063	1,198	865	5,599	2,759	2,840
Pneumonitis due to solids and liquids (J69)..............	92	50	42	549	317	232	1,022	567	455
Chronic liver disease and cirrhosis (K70,K73–K74)..........	1,047	559	488	725	468	257	6,286	4,369	1,917
Alcoholic liver disease (K70)......................	782	445	337	302	243	59	3,489	2,804	685
Cholelithiasis and other disorders of gallbladder (K80–K82)	34	22	12	155	91	64	382	190	192
Nephritis, nephrotic syndrome and nephrosis (N00–N07,N17–N19, N25–N27)	333	154	179	1,534	789	745	3,928	1,988	1,940
Pregnancy, childbirth and the puerperium (O00–O99)...........	17	X	17	41	X	41	204	X	204
Certain conditions originating in the perinatal period (P00–P96)...........	117	61	56	536	308	228	2,409	1,356	1,053
Congenital malformations, deformations and chromosomal abnormalities (Q00–Q99).................................	93	47	46	333	175	158	1,791	918	873
Symptoms, signs and abnormal clinical and laboratory findings, not elsewhere classified (R00–R99).........................	269	149	120	629	328	301	2,237	1,327	910
Accidents (unintentional injuries) (V01–X59,Y85–Y86)	2,229	1,448	781	3,256	2,074	1,182	16,757	12,455	4,302
Motor vehicle accidents (V02–V04, V09.0,V09.2,V12–V14,V19.0–V19.2, V19.4–V19.6,V20–V79,V80.3–V80.5, V81.0–V81.1,V82.0–V82.1,V83–V86, V87.0–V87.8,V88.0–V88.8, V89.0,V89.2)	799	522	277	946	592	354	6,076	4,549	1,527

NOTE: Includes selected causes of deaths; therefore, subcategories do not add to totals. Race and Hispanic-origin categories are consistent with 1977 Office of Management and Budget (OMB) standards. Data for specified race or Hispanic-origin groups other than non-Hispanic White and non-Hispanic Black should be interpreted with caution because of inconsistencies in reporting these items on death certificates and surveys, although misclassification is very minor for the Hispanic and non-Hispanic Asian or Pacific Islander populations.

X = Not applicable.

[2] Multiple-race data reported according to 1997 OMB standards were bridged to the single-race categories of 1977 OMB standards.

[3] Includes Aleut and Eskimo persons.

[4] Includes Chinese, Filipino, Hawaiian, Japanese, and other Asian and Pacific Islander persons.

Table 2-11. Number of Deaths from Selected Causes, by Race, Hispanic Origin, and Sex, 2017—*Continued*

(Number.)

Cause of death (based on *International Classification of Diseases, 10th Revision*)	Total[1]			Non-Hispanic White[2]			Non-Hispanic Black[2]		
	Both sexes	Male	Female	Both sexes	Male	Female	Both sexes	Male	Female
Falls (W00–W19)	36,338	18,392	17,946	31,455	15,511	15,944	1,525	873	652
Accidental discharge of firearms (W32–W34)	486	423	63	312	263	49	105	97	8
Accidental drowning and submersion (W65–W74)	3,709	2,802	907	2,312	1,698	614	591	465	126
Accidental hanging, strangulation and suffocation (W75–W84)	6,946	3,966	2,980	5,027	2,870	2,157	1,125	616	509
Accidental exposure to smoke, fire and flames (X00–X09)	2,812	1,666	1,146	1,990	1,164	826	520	300	220
Accidental poisoning and exposure to noxious substances (X40–X49)	64,795	44,545	20,250	48,568	32,538	16,030	8,266	5,894	2,372
Intentional self-harm (suicide) (*U03,X60–X84,Y87.0)[5]	47,173	36,782	10,391	38,106	29,708	8,398	2,940	2,324	616
Intentional self-harm (suicide) by poisoning (X60–X69)	6,554	3,295	3,259	5,666	2,848	2,818	301	143	158
Intentional self-harm (suicide) by hanging, strangulation and suffocation (X70)	13,075	10,175	2,900	9,497	7,467	2,030	836	630	206
Intentional self-harm (suicide) by discharge of firearms (X72–X74)	23,854	20,615	3,239	20,328	17,516	2,812	1,444	1,282	162
Assault (homicide) (*U01–*U02, X85–Y09,Y87.1)[5]	19,510	15,524	3,986	5,747	3,815	1,932	9,908	8,643	1,265
Assault (homicide) by discharge of firearms (*U01.4,X93–X95)[5]	14,542	12,220	2,322	3,549	2,466	1,083	8,371	7,546	825
Legal intervention (Y35,Y89.0)	616	586	30	312	292	20	152	148	4
Complications of medical and surgical care (Y40–Y84,Y88)	4,459	2,303	2,156	3,333	1,727	1,606	650	330	320
Drug-induced deaths[6]	73,990	48,967	25,023	56,232	36,166	20,066	9,406	6,602	2,804
Alcohol-induced deaths[6]	35,823	25,911	9,912	26,064	18,486	7,578	3,022	2,172	850
Injury by firearms[6]	39,773	34,062	5,711	24,690	20,686	4,004	10,117	9,107	1,010

NOTE: Includes selected causes of deaths; therefore, subcategories do not add to totals. Race and Hispanic-origin categories are consistent with 1977 Office of Management and Budget (OMB) standards. Data for specified race or Hispanic-origin groups other than non-Hispanic White and non-Hispanic Black should be interpreted with caution because of inconsistencies in reporting these items on death certificates and surveys, although misclassification is very minor for the Hispanic and non-Hispanic Asian or Pacific Islander populations.

[1]Includes deaths for origin not stated.
[2]Multiple-race data reported according to 1997 OMB standards were bridged to the single-race categories of 1977 OMB standards.
[5]Asterisks (*) preceding cause-of-death codes indicate they are not part of the *ICD-10*.
[6]Included in selected categories above.

Table 2-11. Number of Deaths from Selected Causes, by Race, Hispanic Origin, and Sex, 2017—*Continued*

(Number.)

Cause of death (based on *International Classification of Diseases, 10th Revision*)	Non-Hispanic American Indian and Alaskan Native[2,3]			Non-Hispanic Asian or Pacific Islander[2,4]			Hispanic		
	Both sexes	Male	Female	Both sexes	Male	Female	Both sexes	Male	Female
Falls (W00–W19)	237	136	101	917	503	414	2,122	1,314	808
Accidental discharge of firearms (W32–W34)	10	7	3	7	7	–	50	48	2
Accidental drowning and submersion (W65–W74)	62	47	15	217	158	59	512	419	93
Accidental hanging, strangulation and suffocation (W75–W84)	79	50	29	153	90	63	539	326	213
Accidental exposure to smoke, fire and flames (X00–X09)	48	30	18	39	17	22	196	138	58
Accidental poisoning and exposure to noxious substances (X40–X49)	780	502	278	669	518	151	6,051	4,728	1,323
Intentional self-harm (suicide) (*U03,X60–X84,Y87.0)[5]	602	448	154	1,414	990	424	3,933	3,175	758
Intentional self-harm (suicide) by poisoning (X60–X69)	48	24	24	162	81	81	348	184	164
Intentional self-harm (suicide) by hanging, strangulation and suffocation (X70)	284	193	91	665	432	233	1,729	1,400	329
Intentional self-harm (suicide) by discharge of firearms (X72–X74)	229	197	32	367	312	55	1,423	1,252	171
Assault (homicide) (*U01–*U02, X85–Y09,Y87.1)[5]	266	199	67	347	234	113	3,186	2,588	598
Assault (homicide) by discharge of firearms (*U01.4,X93–X95)[5]	124	99	25	197	144	53	2,268	1,936	332
Legal intervention (Y35,Y89.0)	21	21	–	13	13	–	118	112	6
Complications of medical and surgical care (Y40–Y84,Y88)	43	21	22	113	56	57	311	164	147
Drug-induced deaths[6]	731	444	287	803	583	220	6,322	4,797	1,525
Alcohol-induced deaths[6]	1,206	753	453	498	398	100	4,817	3,934	883
Injury by firearms[6]	394	333	61	588	479	109	3,884	3,369	515

NOTE: Includes selected causes of deaths; therefore, subcategories do not add to totals. Race and Hispanic-origin categories are consistent with 1977 Office of Management and Budget (OMB) standards. Data for specified race or Hispanic-origin groups other than non-Hispanic White and non-Hispanic Black should be interpreted with caution because of inconsistencies in reporting these items on death certificates and surveys, although misclassification is very minor for the Hispanic and non-Hispanic Asian or Pacific Islander populations.

– = Quantity zero.

[2]Multiple-race data reported according to 1997 OMB standards were bridged to the single-race categories of 1977 OMB standards.

[3]Includes Aleut and Eskimo persons.

[4]Includes Chinese, Filipino, Hawaiian, Japanese, and other Asian and Pacific Islander persons.

[5]Asterisks (*) preceding cause-of-death codes indicate they are not part of the *ICD-10*.

[6]Included in selected categories above.

Table 2-12. Death Rates for Selected Causes, by Race, Hispanic Origin, and Sex, 2017

(Rate; rates are on an annual basis per 100,000 population in specified group.)

Cause of death (based on *International Classification of Diseases, 10th Revision*)	All races[1]			Non-Hispanic White[2]			Non-Hispanic Black[2]		
	Both sexes	Male	Female	Both sexes	Male	Female	Both sexes	Male	Female
All causes	863.8	897.2	831.4	1,083.2	1,111.4	1,055.8	787.5	854.2	726.1
Enterocolitis due to Clostridium difficile (A04.7).................................	1.9	1.5	2.2	2.5	2.0	2.9	1.3	1.1	1.5
Septicemia (A40–A41)	12.6	12.2	12.9	15.0	14.5	15.5	15.4	14.9	15.8
Viral hepatitis (B15–B19)	1.7	2.3	1.2	1.8	2.3	1.2	1.9	2.7	1.2
Human immunodeficiency virus (HIV) disease (B20–B24)	1.7	2.6	0.9	0.9	1.5	0.3	7.0	9.6	4.5
Malignant neoplasms (C00–C97)...	183.9	196.5	171.8	231.4	248.9	214.3	163.9	172.7	155.8
Malignant neoplasms of lip, oral cavity and pharynx (C00–C14)	3.1	4.5	1.7	4.0	5.7	2.3	2.5	3.9	1.2
Malignant neoplasm of esophagus (C15)	4.7	7.7	1.8	6.4	10.6	2.3	2.9	4.3	1.7
Malignant neoplasm of stomach (C16)	3.4	4.2	2.7	3.1	3.9	2.4	4.4	5.5	3.4
Malignant neoplasms of colon, rectum and anus (C18–C21)............	16.4	17.5	15.3	19.8	20.9	18.7	16.9	18.6	15.4
Malignant neoplasms of liver and intrahepatic bile ducts (C22)........	8.3	11.4	5.4	8.9	12.1	5.7	8.7	12.5	5.2
Malignant neoplasms of pancreas (C25)	13.5	14.3	12.8	16.9	18.2	15.6	12.4	12.6	12.3
Malignant neoplasms of trachea, bronchus and lung (C33–C34)......	44.8	49.1	40.6	59.7	64.5	55.0	36.1	42.7	30.0
Malignant melanoma of skin (C43)	2.5	3.3	1.7	3.8	5.1	2.5	0.3	0.3	0.3
Malignant neoplasm of breast (C50)	13.1	0.3	25.4	15.6	0.4	30.4	15.1	0.4	28.6
Malignant neoplasm of cervix uteri (C53)	1.3	X	2.5	1.3	X	2.5	1.9	X	3.6
Malignant neoplasm of ovary (C56)	4.4	X	8.6	5.5	X	10.9	3.3	X	6.3
Malignant neoplasm of prostate (C61)	9.4	19.0	X	11.3	22.8	X	11.7	24.5	X
Malignant neoplasms of kidney and renal pelvis (C64–C65).............	4.3	5.6	3.0	5.4	7.1	3.7	3.3	4.3	2.3
Malignant neoplasm of bladder (C67)	5.1	7.4	2.9	7.1	10.4	3.8	2.9	3.6	2.3
Malignant neoplasms of meninges, brain and other parts of central nervous system (C70–C72)	5.2	5.9	4.5	6.9	7.9	5.9	2.6	2.8	2.4
Non-Hodgkin lymphoma (C82–C85)	6.3	7.3	5.3	8.2	9.5	7.0	3.7	4.4	3.0
Multiple myeloma and immunoproliferative neoplasms (C88,C90)...	3.9	4.5	3.4	4.6	5.3	3.9	5.5	5.9	5.1
Leukemia (C91–C95)	7.2	8.4	6.0	9.4	11.1	7.6	4.6	5.0	4.2
In situ neoplasms, benign neoplasms and neoplasms of uncertain or unknown behavior (D00–D48)	4.9	5.3	4.4	6.5	7.1	5.9	3.2	3.3	3.0
Anemias (D50–D64)	1.7	1.5	1.8	1.9	1.7	2.1	2.5	2.4	2.7
Diabetes mellitus (E10–E14)...	25.7	28.9	22.5	27.4	31.6	23.3	34.7	36.7	32.9
Nutritional deficiencies (E40–E64)	2.4	1.8	3.0	3.1	2.2	3.9	2.2	1.9	2.5
Obesity (E66)	2.4	2.5	2.2	2.8	3.0	2.6	3.3	3.2	3.4
Parkinson disease (G20–G21)	9.8	12.1	7.6	13.7	17.0	10.5	3.6	4.4	2.8
Alzheimer disease (G30)	37.3	23.3	50.9	50.6	31.8	68.9	21.1	12.1	29.3
Major cardiovascular diseases (I00–I78)	262.3	273.1	251.9	329.5	340.9	318.4	249.6	266.1	234.5
Diseases of heart (I00–I09,I11,I13,I20–I51)	198.8	216.9	181.2	252.7	274.5	231.4	183.4	202.8	165.5
Essential hypertension and hypertensive renal disease (I10,I12,I15)	10.8	9.8	11.8	12.2	10.8	13.5	14.7	14.1	15.3
Cerebrovascular diseases (I60–I69)...................................	44.9	38.4	51.3	54.7	45.4	63.7	44.8	42.0	47.4
Atherosclerosis (I70)	1.7	1.5	1.9	2.3	2.0	2.6	1.1	1.0	1.2
Aortic aneurysm and dissection (I71)	3.0	3.6	2.5	4.0	4.7	3.3	2.4	3.0	1.9
Influenza and pneumonia (J09–J18)......................................	17.1	16.6	17.6	21.6	20.7	22.4	13.0	13.1	12.9
Chronic lower respiratory diseases (J40–J47).........................	49.2	46.8	51.5	69.5	65.2	73.7	26.3	27.5	25.3
Pneumonitis due to solids and liquids (J69)..........................	6.2	7.1	5.3	8.2	9.4	7.0	4.5	5.0	4.1
Chronic liver disease and cirrhosis (K70,K73–K74)	12.8	16.5	9.3	15.0	19.0	11.1	7.7	10.1	5.5
Alcoholic liver disease (K70)	6.8	9.6	4.1	7.9	10.9	5.0	3.9	5.3	2.6
Cholelithiasis and other disorders of gallbladder (K80–K82)	1.2	1.2	1.1	1.4	1.4	1.4	0.8	0.8	0.8
Nephritis, nephrotic syndrome and nephrosis (N00–N07,N17–N19,N25–N27)	15.5	16.0	15.1	17.5	18.3	16.7	22.4	22.3	22.5
Pregnancy, childbirth and the puerperium (O00–O99)...........................	0.4	X	0.7	0.3	X	0.5	0.9	X	1.7
Certain conditions originating in the perinatal period (P00–P96)..........	3.4	3.9	2.9	2.1	2.4	1.8	8.5	10.2	7.0
Congenital malformations, deformations and chromosomal abnormalities (Q00–Q99)...	3.0	3.2	2.8	3.0	3.2	2.8	3.7	4.1	3.4
Symptoms, signs and abnormal clinical and laboratory findings, not elsewhere classified (R00–R99)..	10.1	9.6	10.5	12.4	11.3	13.5	10.6	11.3	9.9
Accidents (unintentional injuries) (V01–X59,Y85–Y86)	52.2	68.4	36.4	63.1	79.9	46.8	46.6	67.8	27.1
Motor vehicle accidents (V02–V04, V09.0,V09.2,V12–V14, V19.0–V19.2, V19.4–V19.6,V20–V79,V80.3–V80.5, V81.0–V81.1,V82.0–V82.1,V83–V86, V87.0–V87.8,V88.0–V88.8, V89.0,V89.2)...	12.4	17.8	7.0	13.0	18.5	7.7	14.3	22.1	7.2

NOTE: Race and Hispanic-origin categories are consistent with 1977 Office of Management and Budget (OMB) standards. Data for specified race or Hispanic-origin groups other than non-Hispanic White and non-Hispanic Black should be interpreted with caution because of inconsistencies in reporting these items on death certificates and surveys, although misclassification is very minor for the Hispanic and non-Hispanic Asian or Pacific Islander populations.
X = Not applicable.
[1]Includes deaths for origin not stated.
[2]Multiple-race data reported according to 1997 OMB standards were bridged to the single-race categories of 1977 OMB standards.

Table 2-12. Death Rates for Selected Causes, by Race, Hispanic Origin, and Sex, 2017—Continued

(Rate; rates are on an annual basis per 100,000 population in specified group.)

Cause of death (based on *International Classification of Diseases, 10th Revision*)	Non-Hispanic American Indian and Alaskan Native[2,3]			Non-Hispanic Asian or Pacific Islander[2,4]			Hispanic		
	Both sexes	Male	Female	Both sexes	Male	Female	Both sexes	Male	Female
All causes..	703.4	784.4	625.5	359.8	386.2	335.6	334.6	364.6	304.0
Enterocolitis due to Clostridium difficile (A04.7)................	1.8	*	2.2	0.6	0.5	0.7	0.7	0.6	0.8
Septicemia (A40–A41)...	10.8	9.7	11.9	4.4	4.8	4.0	4.9	4.9	4.8
Viral hepatitis (B15–B19)...	2.6	3.4	1.9	1.3	1.7	1.0	1.5	2.0	1.0
Human immunodeficiency virus (HIV) disease (B20–B24)	1.3	2.0	*	0.3	0.6	*	1.4	2.2	0.6
Malignant neoplasms (C00–C97).................................	119.3	128.8	110.2	90.5	95.9	85.6	68.8	70.6	66.9
Malignant neoplasms of lip, oral cavity and pharynx (C00–C14)	2.1	3.2	*	1.9	2.9	1.0	1.0	1.4	0.6
Malignant neoplasm of esophagus (C15)........................	2.9	4.4	1.4	1.5	2.5	0.7	1.3	2.1	0.5
Malignant neoplasm of stomach (C16)...........................	3.4	4.4	2.5	4.8	5.4	4.2	3.2	3.6	2.8
Malignant neoplasms of colon, rectum and anus (C18–C21)........	13.1	15.2	11.1	8.9	9.9	8.0	7.0	7.8	6.3
Malignant neoplasms of liver and intrahepatic bile ducts (C22).......	9.5	13.0	6.1	8.1	11.2	5.4	6.0	7.8	4.1
Malignant neoplasm of pancreas (C25).........................	7.3	8.1	6.5	7.0	6.9	7.0	5.2	5.0	5.4
Malignant neoplasms of trachea, bronchus and lung (C33–C34)......	28.9	31.5	26.5	19.2	22.8	15.8	9.3	10.7	7.8
Malignant melanoma of skin (C43)	*	*	*	0.3	0.3	0.3	0.4	0.5	0.3
Malignant neoplasm of breast (C50).............................	7.4	*	14.5	6.7	*	12.7	5.1	*	10.2
Malignant neoplasm of cervix uteri (C53).......................	1.1	X	2.2	1.0	X	1.9	1.0	X	2.1
Malignant neoplasm of ovary (C56)..............................	2.9	X	5.8	2.5	X	4.7	1.9	X	3.8
Malignant neoplasm of prostate (C61)...........................	5.0	10.2	X	3.0	6.3	X	3.4	6.8	X
Malignant neoplasms of kidney and renal pelvis (C64–C65)...........	3.9	5.3	2.6	1.5	2.0	1.0	2.1	2.7	1.5
Malignant neoplasm of bladder (C67)...........................	2.2	3.2	*	1.4	2.0	0.9	1.4	1.8	0.9
Malignant neoplasms of meninges, brain and other parts of central nervous system (C70–C72)	2.5	2.5	2.5	2.1	2.4	1.8	2.2	2.4	2.0
Non-Hodgkin lymphoma (C82–C85).............................	3.0	3.5	2.5	3.2	3.9	2.5	2.7	2.9	2.5
Multiple myeloma and immunoproliferative neoplasms (C88,C90)...	2.7	2.8	2.6	1.5	1.7	1.3	1.5	1.6	1.4
Leukemia (C91–C95)...	3.4	4.1	2.7	3.3	4.1	2.5	3.0	3.3	2.7
In situ neoplasms, benign neoplasms and neoplasms of uncertain or unknown behavior (D00–D48)	2.2	2.4	2.1	2.2	2.4	1.9	1.5	1.6	1.4
Anemias (D50–D64)	1.0	*	*	0.7	0.6	0.7	0.6	0.5	0.6
Diabetes mellitus (E10–E14)......................................	40.8	46.6	35.2	15.1	16.7	13.6	15.6	17.0	14.3
Nutritional deficiencies (E40–E64)...............................	1.8	1.6	2.0	1.0	0.8	1.1	0.8	0.6	0.9
Obesity (E66)...	2.9	3.6	2.2	0.3	0.4	0.2	1.0	1.1	0.9
Parkinson disease (G20–G21).....................................	4.2	5.1	3.3	4.3	5.1	3.6	3.1	3.6	2.6
Alzheimer disease (G30)..	13.8	9.0	18.4	12.8	8.2	17.0	12.5	7.7	17.4
Major cardiovascular diseases (I00–I78).........................	165.8	186.8	145.5	114.3	123.0	106.3	92.2	98.0	86.3
Diseases of heart (I00–I09,I11,I13,I20–I51)	127.2	151.8	103.5	76.8	87.3	67.1	66.8	73.9	59.6
Essential hypertension and hypertensive renal disease (I10,I12,I15)	7.0	7.2	6.7	7.3	6.8	7.8	4.7	4.5	5.0
Cerebrovascular diseases (I60–I69).............................	27.0	24.0	29.9	26.9	25.3	28.4	18.3	17.0	19.5
Atherosclerosis (I70)...	*	*	*	0.6	0.6	0.7	0.5	0.5	0.5
Aortic aneurysm and dissection (I71)...........................	1.6	1.7	1.4	1.7	2.1	1.3	0.8	1.0	0.5
Influenza and pneumonia (J09–J18).............................	14.3	13.9	14.7	11.3	12.0	10.7	6.5	6.4	6.7
Chronic lower respiratory diseases (J40–J47)...................	34.4	32.9	35.8	10.2	12.4	8.2	9.5	9.3	9.7
Pneumonitis due to solids and liquids (J69)....................	3.4	3.7	3.0	2.7	3.3	2.2	1.7	1.9	1.6
Chronic liver disease and cirrhosis (K70,K73–K74).............	38.4	41.8	35.1	3.6	4.9	2.4	10.7	14.7	6.6
Alcoholic liver disease (K70).....................................	28.7	33.2	24.2	1.5	2.5	0.6	5.9	9.4	2.3
Cholelithiasis and other disorders of gallbladder (K80–K82).....	1.2	1.6	*	0.8	0.9	0.6	0.6	0.6	0.7
Nephritis, nephrotic syndrome and nephrosis (N00–N07,N17–N19,N25–N27)...	12.2	11.5	12.9	7.6	8.2	7.1	6.7	6.7	6.7
Pregnancy, childbirth and the puerperium (O00–O99)............	*	X	*	0.2	X	0.4	0.3	X	0.7
Certain conditions originating in the perinatal period (P00–P96)..........	4.3	4.6	4.0	2.7	3.2	2.2	4.1	4.6	3.6
Congenital malformations, deformations and chromosomal abnormalities (Q00–Q99)....................................	3.4	3.5	3.3	1.7	1.8	1.5	3.0	3.1	3.0
Symptoms, signs and abnormal clinical and laboratory findings, not elsewhere classified (R00–R99)........................	9.9	11.1	8.6	3.1	3.4	2.9	3.8	4.5	3.1
Accidents (unintentional injuries) (V01–X59,Y85–Y86).......................	81.7	108.1	56.2	16.1	21.5	11.2	28.4	41.8	14.7
Motor vehicle accidents (V02–V04, V09.0,V09.2,V12–V14, V19.0–V19.2, V19.4–V19.6,V20–V79,V80.3–V80.5, V81.0–V81.1,V82.0–V82.1,V83–V86, V87.0–V87.8,V88.0–V88.8, V89.0,V89.2)...	29.3	39.0	19.9	4.7	6.1	3.4	10.3	15.3	5.2

NOTE: Race and Hispanic-origin categories are consistent with 1977 Office of Management and Budget (OMB) standards. Data for specified race or Hispanic-origin groups other than non-Hispanic White and non-Hispanic Black should be interpreted with caution because of inconsistencies in reporting these items on death certificates and surveys, although misclassification is very minor for the Hispanic and non-Hispanic Asian or Pacific Islander populations.
* = Rate does not meet NCHS standards of reliability.
X = Not applicable.
[2]Multiple-race data reported according to 1997 OMB standards were bridged to the single-race categories of 1977 OMB standards.
[3]Includes Aleut and Eskimo persons.
[4]Includes Chinese, Filipino, Hawaiian, Japanese, and other Asian and Pacific Islander persons.

Table 2-12. Death Rates for Selected Causes, by Race, Hispanic Origin, and Sex, 2017—*Continued*

(Rate; rates are on an annual basis per 100,000 population in specified group.)

Cause of death (based on *International Classification of Diseases, 10th Revision*)	All races[1]			Non-Hispanic White[2]			Non-Hispanic Black[2]		
	Both sexes	Male	Female	Both sexes	Male	Female	Both sexes	Male	Female
Falls (W00–W19)	11.2	11.5	10.9	15.6	15.6	15.6	3.6	4.3	2.9
Accidental discharge of firearms (W32–W34)	0.1	0.3	0.0	0.2	0.3	0.0	0.2	0.5	*
Accidental drowning and submersion (W65–W74)	1.1	1.7	0.5	1.1	1.7	0.6	1.4	2.3	0.6
Accidental hanging, strangulation and suffocation (W75–W84)	2.1	2.5	1.8	2.5	2.9	2.1	2.6	3.0	2.3
Accidental exposure to smoke, fire and flames (X00–X09)	0.9	1.0	0.7	1.0	1.2	0.8	1.2	1.5	1.0
Accidental poisoning and exposure to noxious substances (X40–X49)	19.9	27.8	12.2	24.1	32.8	15.7	19.4	28.9	10.7
Intentional self-harm (suicide) (*U03, X60–X84,Y87.0)[5]	14.5	22.9	6.3	18.9	29.9	8.2	6.9	11.4	2.8
Intentional self-harm (suicide) by poisoning (X60–X69)	2.0	2.1	2.0	2.8	2.9	2.8	0.7	0.7	0.7
Intentional self-harm (suicide) by hanging, strangulation and suffocation (X70)	4.0	6.3	1.8	4.7	7.5	2.0	2.0	3.1	0.9
Intentional self-harm (suicide) by discharge of firearms (X72–X74)	7.3	12.9	2.0	10.1	17.7	2.8	3.4	6.3	0.7
Assault (homicide) (*U01–*U02, X85–Y09,Y87.1)[5]	6.0	9.7	2.4	2.9	3.8	1.9	23.2	42.3	5.7
Assault (homicide) by discharge of firearms (*U01.4,X93–X95)[5]	4.5	7.6	1.4	1.8	2.5	1.1	19.6	37.0	3.7
Legal intervention (Y35,Y89.0)	0.2	0.4	0.0	0.2	0.3	0.0	0.4	0.7	*
Complications of medical and surgical care (Y40–Y84,Y88)	1.4	1.4	1.3	1.7	1.7	1.6	1.5	1.6	1.4
Drug-induced deaths[6]	22.7	30.5	15.1	27.9	36.4	19.7	22.1	32.3	12.6
Alcohol-induced deaths[6]	11.0	16.2	6.0	13.0	18.6	7.4	7.1	10.6	3.8
Injury by firearms[6]	12.2	21.2	3.5	12.3	20.8	3.9	23.7	44.6	4.5

NOTE: Race and Hispanic-origin categories are consistent with 1977 Office of Management and Budget (OMB) standards. Data for specified race or Hispanic-origin groups other than non-Hispanic White and non-Hispanic Black should be interpreted with caution because of inconsistencies in reporting these items on death certificates and surveys, although misclassification is very minor for the Hispanic and non-Hispanic Asian or Pacific Islander populations.
* = Rate does not meet NCHS standards of reliability.
0.0 = Quantity more than zero but less than 0.05.
[1]Includes deaths for origin not stated.
[2]Multiple-race data reported according to 1997 OMB standards were bridged to the single-race categories of 1977 OMB standards.
[5]Asterisks (*) preceding cause-of-death codes indicate they are not part of the *ICD-10.*
[6]Included in selected categories above.

Table 2-12. Death Rates for Selected Causes, by Race, Hispanic Origin, and Sex, 2017—*Continued*

(Rate; rates are on an annual basis per 100,000 population in specified group.)

Cause of death (based on *International Classification of Diseases, 10th Revision*)	Non-Hispanic American Indian and Alaskan Native[2,3]			Non-Hispanic Asian or Pacific Islander[2,4]			Hispanic		
	Both sexes	Male	Female	Both sexes	Male	Female	Both sexes	Male	Female
Falls (W00–W19)	8.7	10.2	7.3	4.5	5.2	3.9	3.6	4.4	2.8
Accidental discharge of firearms (W32–W34)	*	*	*	*	*	*	0.1	0.2	*
Accidental drowning and submersion (W65–W74)	2.3	3.5	*	1.1	1.6	0.6	0.9	1.4	0.3
Accidental hanging, strangulation and suffocation (W75–W84)	2.9	3.7	2.1	0.8	0.9	0.6	0.9	1.1	0.7
Accidental exposure to smoke, fire and flames (X00–X09)	1.8	2.2	*	0.2	*	0.2	0.3	0.5	0.2
Accidental poisoning and exposure to noxious substances (X40–X49)	28.6	37.5	20.0	3.3	5.4	1.4	10.3	15.9	4.5
Intentional self-harm (suicide) (*U03, X60–X84,Y87.0)[5]	22.1	33.5	11.1	7.0	10.3	4.0	6.7	10.7	2.6
Intentional self-harm (suicide) by poisoning (X60–X69)	1.8	1.8	1.7	0.8	0.8	0.8	0.6	0.6	0.6
Intentional self-harm (suicide) by hanging, strangulation and suffocation (X70)	10.4	14.4	6.5	3.3	4.5	2.2	2.9	4.7	1.1
Intentional self-harm (suicide) by discharge of firearms (X72–X74)	8.4	14.7	2.3	1.8	3.2	0.5	2.4	4.2	0.6
Assault (homicide) (*U01–*U02, X85–Y09,Y87.1)[5]	9.7	14.9	4.8	1.7	2.4	1.1	5.4	8.7	2.1
Assault (homicide) by discharge of firearms (*U01.4,X93–X95)[5]	4.5	7.4	1.8	1.0	1.5	0.5	3.8	6.5	1.1
Legal intervention (Y35,Y89.0)	0.8	1.6	*	*	*	*	0.2	0.4	*
Complications of medical and surgical care (Y40–Y84,Y88)	1.6	1.6	1.6	0.6	0.6	0.5	0.5	0.6	0.5
Drug-induced deaths[6]	26.8	33.2	20.6	4.0	6.0	2.1	10.7	16.1	5.2
Alcohol-induced deaths[6]	44.2	56.2	32.6	2.5	4.1	0.9	8.2	13.2	3.0
Injury by firearms[6]	14.4	24.9	4.4	2.9	5.0	1.0	6.6	11.3	1.8

NOTE: Race and Hispanic-origin categories are consistent with 1977 Office of Management and Budget (OMB) standards. Data for specified race or Hispanic-origin groups other than non-Hispanic White and non-Hispanic Black should be interpreted with caution because of inconsistencies in reporting these items on death certificates and surveys, although misclassification is very minor for the Hispanic and non-Hispanic Asian or Pacific Islander populations.
* = Rate does not meet NCHS standards of reliability.
[2]Multiple-race data reported according to 1997 OMB standards were bridged to the single-race categories of 1977 OMB standards.
[3]Includes Aleut and Eskimo persons.
[4]Includes Chinese, Filipino, Hawaiian, Japanese, and other Asian and Pacific Islander persons.
[5]Asterisks (*) preceding cause-of-death codes indicate they are not part of the *ICD-10.*
[6]Included in selected categories above.

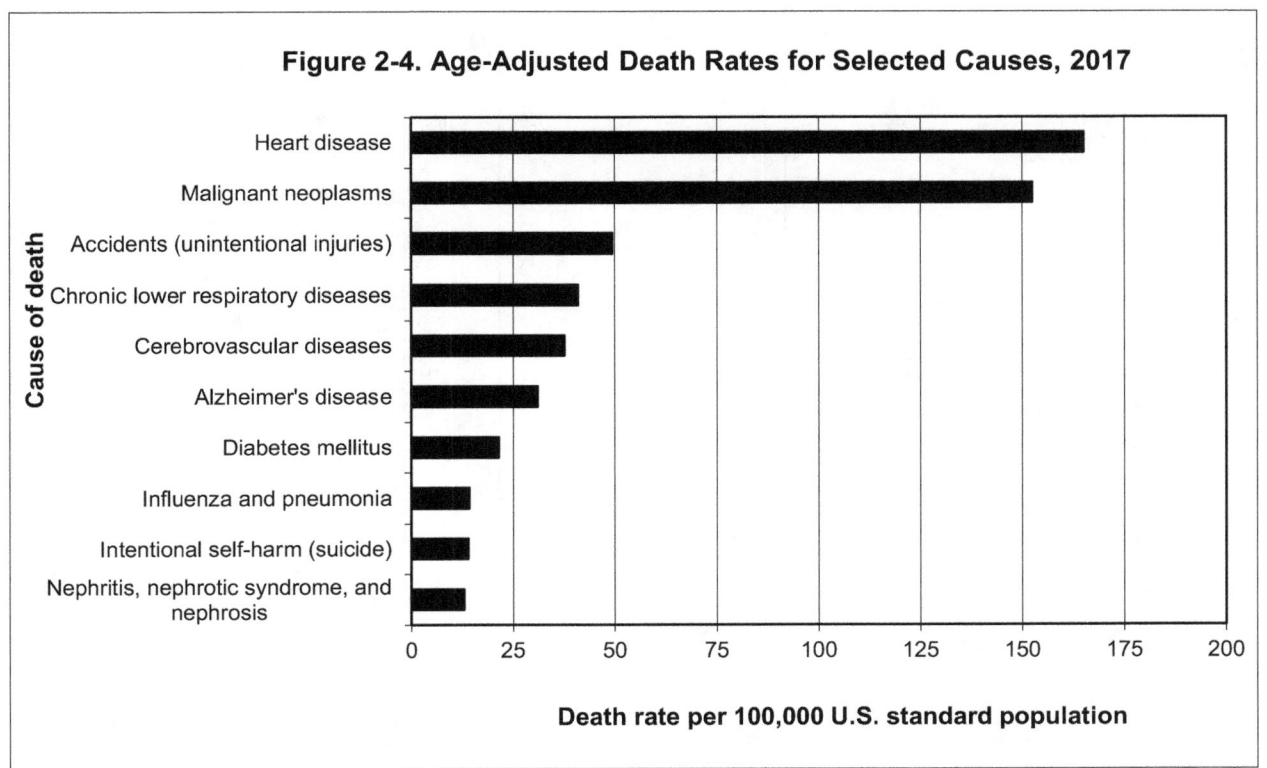

Figure 2-4. Age-Adjusted Death Rates for Selected Causes, 2017

Table 2-13. Age-Adjusted Death Rates from Selected Causes, by Race and Hispanic Origin and Sex, 2017

(Age-adjusted rates per 100,000 U.S. standard population.)

Cause of death (based on *International Classification of Diseases, 10th Revision*)	All races[1]			Non-Hispanic White[2]			Non-Hispanic Black[2]		
	Both sexes	Male	Female	Both sexes	Male	Female	Both sexes	Male	Female
All causes	731.9	864.5	619.7	755.0	885.1	642.8	881.0	1,083.3	728.0
Enterocolitis due to Clostridium difficile (A04.7).............................	1.6	1.5	1.6	1.6	1.6	1.7	1.5	1.5	1.5
Septicemia (A40–A41)	10.6	11.7	9.7	10.3	11.3	9.5	17.4	19.8	15.8
Viral hepatitis (B15–B19)	1.4	1.9	0.9	1.2	1.6	0.9	1.8	2.7	1.0
Human immunodeficiency virus (HIV) disease (B20–B24)	1.6	2.4	0.8	0.7	1.2	0.3	6.9	9.9	4.4
Malignant neoplasms (C00–C97)................................	152.5	181.1	131.4	157.9	186.6	136.2	178.0	219.8	151.9
Malignant neoplasms of lip, oral cavity and pharynx (C00–C14) ...	2.5	4.0	1.3	2.7	4.2	1.4	2.5	4.4	1.2
Malignant neoplasm of esophagus (C15)	3.8	6.8	1.4	4.3	7.7	1.5	3.0	5.1	1.6
Malignant neoplasm of stomach (C16)	2.9	3.8	2.1	2.2	3.0	1.5	4.9	7.1	3.4
Malignant neoplasms of colon, rectum and anus (C18–C21)........	13.7	16.2	11.7	13.7	15.9	11.8	18.4	23.0	15.1
Malignant neoplasms of liver and intrahepatic bile ducts (C22).....	6.7	9.8	4.1	5.9	8.6	3.6	8.7	13.6	4.9
Malignant neoplasm of pancreas (C25)	11.1	12.9	9.6	11.3	13.3	9.6	13.5	15.3	12.0
Malignant neoplasms of trachea, bronchus and lung (C33–C34).....	36.6	44.4	30.6	39.9	47.1	34.3	38.8	53.4	28.9
Malignant melanoma of skin (C43)	2.1	3.1	1.3	2.7	3.9	1.7	0.3	0.3	0.4
Malignant neoplasm of breast (C50)	11.0	0.3	19.9	10.9	0.3	20.0	16.2	0.5	27.8
Malignant neoplasm of cervix uteri (C53)	1.2	X	2.2	1.0	X	2.0	1.9	X	3.5
Malignant neoplasm of ovary (C56)	3.6	X	6.6	3.8	X	7.0	3.5	X	6.0
Malignant neoplasm of prostate (C61)	7.8	18.7	X	7.5	17.8	X	13.9	36.8	X
Malignant neoplasms of kidney and renal pelvis (C64–C65)	3.5	5.1	2.2	3.7	5.3	2.3	3.6	5.4	2.3
Malignant neoplasm of bladder (C67)............................	4.3	7.2	2.1	4.7	8.0	2.2	3.5	5.2	2.4
Malignant neoplasms of meninges, brain and other parts of central nervous system (C70–C72)....................................	4.4	5.3	3.6	5.1	6.1	4.2	2.7	3.2	2.3
Non-Hodgkin lymphoma (C82–C85).............................	5.3	6.9	4.0	5.6	7.3	4.3	4.1	5.5	3.1
Multiple myeloma and immunoproliferative neoplasms (C88,C90)....	3.3	4.2	2.6	3.1	4.0	2.3	6.2	7.9	5.2
Leukemia (C91–C95)..	6.1	8.1	4.6	6.5	8.7	4.9	5.2	6.5	4.2
In situ neoplasms, benign neoplasms and neoplasms of uncertain or unknown behavior (D00–D48)..	4.1	5.2	3.3	4.4	5.6	3.5	3.7	4.6	3.1
Anemias (D50–D64)	1.4	1.5	1.3	1.3	1.4	1.2	2.8	2.9	2.7
Diabetes mellitus (E10–E14)....................................	21.5	26.8	17.1	18.8	24.0	14.6	38.7	46.6	32.8
Nutritional deficiencies (E40–E64)	2.0	1.8	2.1	2.0	1.8	2.2	2.7	2.9	2.5
Obesity (E66)	2.1	2.3	1.9	2.2	2.4	1.9	3.3	3.3	3.3
Parkinson disease (G20–G21)	8.4	12.6	5.5	9.2	13.7	6.1	4.6	7.5	3.0
Alzheimer disease (G30)	31.0	24.9	34.8	32.8	26.2	36.9	28.5	22.7	31.2
Major cardiovascular diseases (I00–I78).........................	218.1	264.1	180.1	220.1	266.4	181.1	285.5	351.3	236.5
Diseases of heart (I00–I09,I11,I13,I20–I51)	165.0	209.0	129.6	168.9	214.0	131.9	208.0	264.8	166.3
Essential hypertension and hypertensive renal disease (I10,I12,I15)...	9.0	9.5	8.4	8.0	8.4	7.6	17.1	19.1	15.5
Cerebrovascular diseases (I60–I69).............................	37.6	38.0	36.6	36.4	36.0	36.0	52.7	57.9	48.3
Atherosclerosis (I70)	1.4	1.5	1.3	1.5	1.6	1.4	1.3	1.5	1.2
Aortic aneurysm and dissection (I71)	2.6	3.4	1.9	2.8	3.6	2.0	2.7	3.7	1.9
Influenza and pneumonia (J09–J18).............................	14.3	16.5	12.7	14.4	16.5	13.0	15.2	18.4	13.1
Chronic lower respiratory diseases (J40–J47).....................	40.9	45.0	38.1	46.4	49.7	44.2	30.2	38.5	25.2
Pneumonitis due to solids and liquids (J69).......................	5.1	7.1	3.8	5.4	7.5	4.0	5.4	7.4	4.2
Chronic liver disease and cirrhosis (K70,K73–K74)	10.9	14.5	7.6	11.3	14.6	8.2	7.5	10.4	5.2
Alcoholic liver disease (K70)	5.9	8.5	3.6	6.2	8.5	4.1	3.7	5.4	2.4
Cholelithiasis and other disorders of gallbladder (K80–K82)	1.0	1.2	0.8	0.9	1.1	0.8	0.9	1.0	0.8
Nephritis, nephrotic syndrome and nephrosis (N00–N07,N17–N19,N25–N27)	13.0	15.7	11.1	11.7	14.4	9.8	25.8	30.6	22.6
Pregnancy, childbirth and the puerperium (O00–O99)	0.4	X	0.8	0.3	X	0.6	0.9	X	1.8
Certain conditions originating in the perinatal period (P00–P96).....	3.9	4.3	3.4	2.9	3.2	2.5	8.3	9.3	7.3
Congenital malformations, deformations and chromosomal abnormalities (Q00–Q99)	3.1	3.3	2.9	3.1	3.4	2.9	3.7	3.9	3.5
Symptoms, signs and abnormal clinical and laboratory findings, not elsewhere classified (R00–R99)	8.8	9.5	8.0	9.1	9.7	8.5	11.6	13.1	10.1
Accidents (unintentional injuries) (V01–X59,Y85–Y86)..............	49.4	67.8	32.0	56.2	75.3	37.8	47.6	71.6	27.1
Motor vehicle accidents (V02–V04, V09.0,V09.2,V12–V14,V19.0–V19.2, V19.4–V19.6,V20–V79,V80.3–V80.5, V81.0–V81.1,V82.0–V82.1,V83–V86, V87.0–V87.8,V88.0–V88.8, V89.0,V89.2)	12.0	17.5	6.7	12.3	17.5	7.2	14.3	22.5	7.1
Falls (W00–W19)	9.4	11.5	7.7	10.5	12.6	8.8	4.2	5.9	3.0
Accidental discharge of firearms (W32–W34)	0.2	0.3	0.0	0.2	0.3	0.1	0.3	0.5	*

NOTE: Age-adjusted rates are per 100,000 U.S. standard population. Race and Hispanic-origin categories are consistent with 1977 Office of Management and Budget (OMB) standards. Data for specified race or Hispanic-origin groups other than non-Hispanic White and non-Hispanic Black should be interpreted with caution because of inconsistencies in reporting these items on death certificates and surveys, although misclassification is very minor for the Hispanic and non-Hispanic Asian or Pacific Islander populations.
X = Not applicable.
0.0 = Quantity more than zero but less than 0.05.
* = Rate does not meet NCHS standards of reliability.
[1]Includes deaths for origin not stated.
[2]Multiple-race data reported according to 1997 OMB standards were bridged to the single-race categories of 1977 OMB standards.

Table 2-13. Age-Adjusted Death Rates from Selected Causes, by Race and Hispanic Origin and Sex, 2017—*Continued*

(Age-adjusted rates per 100,000 U.S. standard population.)

Cause of death (based on *International Classification of Diseases, 10th Revision*)	Non-Hispanic American Indian and Alaskan Native[2,3]			Non-Hispanic Asian or Pacific Islander[2,4]			Hispanic		
	Both sexes	Male	Female	Both sexes	Male	Female	Both sexes	Male	Female
All causes	800.2	943.9	674.0	395.3	470.1	336.4	524.7	631.8	434.2
Enterocolitis due to Clostridium difficile (A04.7)................	2.3	*	2.6	0.6	0.7	0.6	1.2	1.3	1.2
Septicemia (A40–A41)..	12.1	11.4	12.5	4.8	5.9	4.0	7.9	9.1	6.9
Viral hepatitis (B15–B19)..	2.5	3.3	1.7	1.3	1.8	0.9	2.0	2.7	1.3
Human immunodeficiency virus (HIV) disease (B20–B24)	1.3	2.1	*	0.3	0.6	*	1.7	2.7	0.7
Malignant neoplasms (C00–C97)..	130.0	152.2	112.5	95.2	112.2	82.9	108.1	129.5	93.0
Malignant neoplasms of lip, oral cavity and pharynx (C00–C14)	2.0	3.2	*	1.9	3.1	1.0	1.6	2.5	0.8
Malignant neoplasm of esophagus (C15)........................	2.7	4.4	1.3	1.6	2.8	0.7	2.0	3.6	0.7
Malignant neoplasm of stomach (C16)...........................	4.0	5.7	2.6	5.0	6.3	4.1	4.9	6.2	3.9
Malignant neoplasms of colon, rectum and anus (C18–C21)......	14.5	17.2	12.0	9.4	11.4	7.8	10.9	13.7	8.7
Malignant neoplasms of liver and intrahepatic bile ducts (C22)......	9.7	14.0	6.2	8.4	12.4	5.3	9.2	13.0	5.9
Malignant neoplasm of pancreas (C25)..........................	7.9	9.3	6.8	7.4	8.0	7.0	8.4	9.0	7.9
Malignant neoplasms of trachea, bronchus and lung (C33–C34)......	31.3	37.7	26.2	20.4	27.0	15.5	15.6	21.2	11.5
Malignant melanoma of skin (C43).................................	*	*	*	0.3	0.4	0.2	0.6	0.8	0.5
Malignant neoplasm of breast (C50)..............................	8.1	*	14.8	6.6	*	11.8	7.3	*	13.4
Malignant neoplasm of cervix uteri (C53)......................	1.2	X	2.3	1.0	X	1.8	1.3	X	2.5
Malignant neoplasm of ovary (C56)...............................	2.9	X	5.4	2.4	X	4.4	2.8	X	5.2
Malignant neoplasm of prostate (C61)...........................	6.2	14.4	...	3.4	8.4	X	6.3	15.4	X
Malignant neoplasms of kidney and renal pelvis (C64–C65)......	4.3	6.1	2.8	1.6	2.3	1.0	3.3	4.7	2.2
Malignant neoplasm of bladder (C67)............................	2.7	4.4	*	1.6	2.7	0.9	2.4	4.0	1.4
Malignant neoplasms of meninges, brain and other parts of central nervous system (C70–C72)	2.5	2.7	2.4	2.1	2.6	1.7	3.1	3.6	2.6
Non-Hodgkin lymphoma (C82–C85)...............................	3.3	4.3	2.5	3.5	4.7	2.5	4.4	5.4	3.6
Multiple myeloma and immunoproliferative neoplasms (C88,C90)......	3.1	3.5	2.8	1.7	2.1	1.3	2.5	3.1	2.1
Leukemia (C91–C95)...	3.7	4.6	3.0	3.5	5.0	2.5	4.4	5.3	3.6
In situ neoplasms, benign neoplasms and neoplasms of uncertain or unknown behavior (D00–D48)	2.6	3.1	2.3	2.4	3.0	1.9	2.5	3.1	2.1
Anemias (D50–D64)..	1.3	*	*	0.7	0.8	0.7	0.9	1.0	0.9
Diabetes mellitus (E10–E14)...	46.1	55.0	38.3	16.5	20.1	13.7	25.5	31.3	20.9
Nutritional deficiencies (E40–E64)....................................	2.4	2.5	2.3	1.1	1.2	1.1	1.4	1.4	1.4
Obesity (E66)..	3.1	3.9	2.2	0.3	0.4	0.2	1.2	1.3	1.1
Parkinson disease (G20–G21)	6.0	8.7	4.2	5.1	7.1	3.8	6.1	8.8	4.2
Alzheimer disease (G30)...	20.6	16.2	23.5	15.3	12.0	17.2	24.7	19.8	27.7
Major cardiovascular diseases (I00–I78)...........................	199.6	244.2	162.8	127.7	153.3	107.4	158.2	191.9	130.5
Diseases of heart (I00–I09,I11,I13,I20–I51)......................	151.4	196.0	115.2	85.5	108.1	67.7	114.1	143.9	90.1
Essential hypertension and hypertensive renal disease (I10,I12,I15)......	8.5	9.8	7.5	8.3	8.7	7.9	8.3	9.1	7.5
Cerebrovascular diseases (I60–I69).................................	34.1	33.3	34.4	30.3	32.1	28.7	31.8	34.0	29.6
Atherosclerosis (I70)...	*	*	*	0.7	0.8	0.7	0.9	1.1	0.8
Aortic aneurysm and dissection (I71)...............................	1.8	2.3	1.5	1.8	2.4	1.3	1.2	1.8	0.7
Influenza and pneumonia (J09–J18).................................	17.3	18.3	16.4	13.0	16.1	10.8	11.3	13.1	9.9
Chronic lower respiratory diseases (J40–J47)..................	40.7	44.3	38.2	11.8	16.7	8.5	17.2	20.6	14.9
Pneumonitis due to solids and liquids (J69)......................	4.0	5.1	3.3	3.2	4.5	2.2	3.1	4.2	2.4
Chronic liver disease and cirrhosis (K70,K73–K74)...........	39.5	43.3	35.9	3.6	5.2	2.3	14.3	20.4	8.7
Alcoholic liver disease (K70)..	29.5	34.5	24.9	1.4	2.5	0.5	7.3	12.3	2.7
Cholelithiasis and other disorders of gallbladder (K80–K82)......	1.6	2.6	*	0.9	1.2	0.6	1.2	1.4	1.0
Nephritis, nephrotic syndrome and nephrosis (N00–N07,N17–N19,N25–N27)	14.3	14.3	14.0	8.5	10.3	7.2	11.3	13.1	9.9
Pregnancy, childbirth and the puerperium (O00–O99)........	*	X	*	0.2	X	0.4	0.3	X	0.7
Certain conditions originating in the perinatal period (P00–P96)........	4.1	4.2	4.0	3.3	3.7	2.9	3.2	3.5	2.9
Congenital malformations, deformations and chromosomal abnormalities (Q00–Q99)	3.5	3.6	3.3	1.9	2.0	1.8	2.6	2.7	2.6
Symptoms, signs and abnormal clinical and laboratory findings, not elsewhere classified (R00–R99)	10.8	11.9	9.5	3.5	4.0	3.0	5.0	6.2	3.9
Accidents (unintentional injuries) (V01–X59,Y85–Y86)......	86.3	115.5	59.1	16.7	23.1	11.2	32.5	48.3	17.2
Motor vehicle accidents (V02–V04, V09.0,V09.2,V12–V14,V19.0–V19.2, V19.4–V19.6,V20–V79,V80.3–V80.5, V81.0–V81.1,V82.0–V82.1,V83–V86, V87.0–V87.8,V88.0–V88.8, V89.0,V89.2)........	29.9	39.8	20.5	4.6	6.2	3.3	10.8	16.1	5.5

NOTE: Age-adjusted rates are per 100,000 U.S. standard population. Race and Hispanic-origin categories are consistent with 1977 Office of Management and Budget (OMB) standards. Data for specified race or Hispanic-origin groups other than non-Hispanic White and non-Hispanic Black should be interpreted with caution because of inconsistencies in reporting these items on death certificates and surveys, although misclassification is very minor for the Hispanic and non-Hispanic Asian or Pacific Islander populations.
X = Not applicable.
* = Rate does not meet NCHS standards of reliability.
[2]Multiple-race data reported according to 1997 OMB standards were bridged to the single-race categories of 1977 OMB standards.
[3]Includes Aleut and Eskimo persons.
[4]Includes Chinese, Filipino, Hawaiian, Japanese, and other Asian and Pacific Islander persons.

Table 2-13. Age-Adjusted Death Rates from Selected Causes, by Race and Hispanic Origin and Sex, 2017—Continued

(Age-adjusted rates per 100,000 U.S. standard population.)

Cause of death (based on *International Classification of Diseases, 10th Revision*)	All races[1]			Non-Hispanic White[2]			Non-Hispanic Black[2]		
	Both sexes	Male	Female	Both sexes	Male	Female	Both sexes	Male	Female
Accidental drowning and submersion (W65–W74)	1.1	1.7	0.5	1.1	1.6	0.6	1.4	2.2	0.6
Accidental hanging, strangulation and suffocation (W75–W84)	1.9	2.5	1.5	2.0	2.5	1.5	2.8	3.5	2.3
Accidental exposure to smoke, fire and flames (X00–X09)	0.8	1.0	0.6	0.8	1.0	0.6	1.3	1.7	1.0
Accidental poisoning and exposure to noxious substances (X40–X49)	20.1	27.9	12.4	25.2	33.9	16.3	19.3	29.3	10.6
Intentional self-harm (suicide) (*U03, X60–X84,Y87.0)[5]	14.0	22.4	6.1	17.8	28.2	7.9	6.9	11.4	2.8
Intentional self-harm (suicide) by poisoning (X60–X69)	1.9	2.0	1.9	2.6	2.7	2.5	0.7	0.7	0.7
Intentional self-harm (suicide) by hanging, strangulation and suffocation (X70)	4.1	6.4	1.8	4.9	7.7	2.1	1.9	3.0	0.9
Intentional self-harm (suicide) by discharge of firearms (X72–X74)	6.9	12.4	1.9	9.1	16.0	2.6	3.4	6.3	0.7
Assault (homicide) (*U01–*U02, X85–Y09,Y87.1)[5]	6.2	9.8	2.5	2.9	3.9	1.9	22.7	40.6	5.7
Assault (homicide) by discharge of firearms (*U01.4,X93–X95)[5]	4.6	7.8	1.4	1.8	2.6	1.1	19.1	35.2	3.7
Legal intervention (Y35,Y89.0)	0.2	0.4	0.0	0.2	0.3	0.0	0.4	0.7	*
Complications of medical and surgical care (Y40–Y84,Y88)	1.2	1.4	1.0	1.2	1.4	1.1	1.6	2.0	1.4
Drug-induced deaths[6]	22.8	30.5	15.2	28.8	37.4	20.1	21.9	32.7	12.5
Alcohol-induced deaths[6]	9.6	14.3	5.3	10.3	14.8	6.1	6.9	10.9	3.6
Injury by firearms[6]	12.0	20.9	3.4	11.4	19.3	3.8	23.2	42.8	4.5

NOTE: Age-adjusted rates are per 100,000 U.S. standard population. Race and Hispanic-origin categories are consistent with 1977 Office of Management and Budget (OMB) standards. Data for specified race or Hispanic-origin groups other than non-Hispanic White and non-Hispanic Black should be interpreted with caution because of inconsistencies in reporting these items on death certificates and surveys, although misclassification is very minor for the Hispanic and non-Hispanic Asian or Pacific Islander populations.
0.0 = Quantity more than zero but less than 0.05.
* = Rate does not meet NCHS standards of reliability.
[1]Includes deaths for origin not stated.
[2]Multiple-race data reported according to 1997 OMB standards were bridged to the single-race categories of 1977 OMB standards.
[5]Asterisks (*) preceding cause-of-death codes indicate they are not part of the *ICD-10*.
[6]Included in selected categories above.

Table 2-13. Age-Adjusted Death Rates from Selected Causes, by Race and Hispanic Origin and Sex, 2017—*Continued*

(Age-adjusted rates per 100,000 U.S. standard population.)

Cause of death (based on *International Classification of Diseases, 10th Revision*)	Non-Hispanic American Indian and Alaskan Native[2,3]			Non-Hispanic Asian or Pacific Islander[2,4]			Hispanic		
	Both sexes	Male	Female	Both sexes	Male	Female	Both sexes	Male	Female
Falls (W00–W19)	10.4	13.0	8.2	5.2	6.8	4.0	5.9	7.9	4.2
Accidental discharge of firearms (W32–W34)	*	*	*	*	*	*	0.1	0.1	*
Accidental drowning and submersion (W65–W74)	2.2	3.4	*	1.1	1.6	0.6	0.8	1.4	0.3
Accidental hanging, strangulation and suffocation (W75–W84)	3.0	4.3	2.0	0.9	1.1	0.7	1.2	1.6	0.8
Accidental exposure to smoke, fire and flames (X00–X09)	1.9	2.6	*	0.2	*	0.2	0.4	0.7	0.2
Accidental poisoning and exposure to noxious substances (X40–X49)	30.0	39.3	21.1	3.1	5.0	1.3	10.7	16.6	4.7
Intentional self-harm (suicide) (*U03, X60–X84,Y87.0)[5]	22.1	33.8	11.0	6.8	9.9	3.9	6.9	11.2	2.6
Intentional self-harm (suicide) by poisoning (X60–X69)	1.9	1.9	1.9	0.8	0.8	0.7	0.6	0.7	0.6
Intentional self-harm (suicide) by hanging, strangulation and suffocation (X70)	10.2	14.1	6.5	3.2	4.4	2.1	2.9	4.8	1.1
Intentional self-harm (suicide) by discharge of firearms (X72–X74)	8.5	15.1	2.2	1.7	3.1	0.5	2.5	4.6	0.6
Assault (homicide) (*U01–*U02, X85–Y09,Y87.1)[5]	9.9	15.1	4.9	1.6	2.3	1.0	5.2	8.2	2.0
Assault (homicide) by discharge of firearms (*U01.4,X93–X95)[5]	4.5	7.2	1.8	0.9	1.4	0.5	3.6	6.0	1.1
Legal intervention (Y35,Y89.0)	0.7	1.5	*	*	*	*	0.2	0.4	*
Complications of medical and surgical care (Y40–Y84,Y88)	1.7	1.9	1.5	0.6	0.6	0.5	0.8	0.9	0.7
Drug-induced deaths[6]	27.9	34.4	21.6	3.7	5.6	2.0	11.2	16.8	5.5
Alcohol-induced deaths[6]	45.7	58.9	33.6	2.4	4.1	0.9	9.9	16.9	3.5
Injury by firearms[6]	14.4	24.9	4.3	2.8	4.7	1.0	6.5	11.1	1.8

NOTE: Age-adjusted rates are per 100,000 U.S. standard population. Race and Hispanic-origin categories are consistent with 1977 Office of Management and Budget (OMB) standards. Data for specified race or Hispanic-origin groups other than non-Hispanic White and non-Hispanic Black should be interpreted with caution because of inconsistencies in reporting these items on death certificates and surveys, although misclassification is very minor for the Hispanic and non-Hispanic Asian or Pacific Islander populations.
* = Rate does not meet NCHS standards of reliability.
[2]Multiple-race data reported according to 1997 OMB standards were bridged to the single-race categories of 1977 OMB standards.
[3]Includes Aleut and Eskimo persons.
[4]Includes Chinese, Filipino, Hawaiian, Japanese, and other Asian and Pacific Islander persons.
[5]Asterisks (*) preceding cause-of-death codes indicate they are not part of the *ICD*-10.
[6]Included in selected categories above.

Table 2-14. Age-Adjusted Death Rates, by Race, Hispanic Origin, Average Annual, 1979–1981, 1989–1991, 2009–2011, 2010–2012, 2011–2013, 2012–2014, 2013–2015, and 2014–2016

(Age-adjusted death rate per 100,000 population.[1])

Area	All persons								White					
	1979–1981	1989–1991	2009–2011	2010–2012	2011–2013	2012–2014	2013–2015	2014–2016	2009–2011	2010–2012	2011–2013	2012–2014	2013–2015	2014–2016
United States[3]	1,022.8	942.2	745.9	740.2	735.3	729.7	729.9	728.8	741.1	737.1	733.5	729.1	730.5	730.1
Alabama	1,091.2	1,037.9	937.8	933.2	928.4	920.2	919.5	918.0	913.7	913.4	910.6	905.9	906.1	905.6
Alaska	1,087.4	944.6	760.8	749.3	734.0	730.5	736.2	743.3	709.0	699.3	682.6	678.5	680.9	684.9
Arizona	951.5	873.5	691.9	688.1	681.8	672.6	669.2	669.9	685.8	682.4	676.8	667.4	663.9	663.4
Arkansas	1,017.0	996.3	894.9	895.2	895.6	891.6	893.1	892.9	877.1	881.3	883.4	881.8	885.0	884.9
California	975.5	911.0	647.7	639.3	633.8	621.8	619.1	614.8	674.3	667.1	663.4	652.8	651.4	647.9
Colorado	941.1	856.1	683.3	675.1	666.0	661.8	661.7	666.3	687.7	679.4	670.7	667.0	667.6	672.5
Connecticut	961.5	857.5	657.6	653.8	651.7	647.0	649.6	652.2	656.8	654.6	654.1	651.0	655.2	657.9
Delaware	1,069.7	1,001.9	767.3	759.6	745.0	735.4	734.2	740.6	761.4	752.3	740.6	727.8	733.2	740.0
District of Columbia	1,243.1	1,255.3	793.4	768.2	755.1	751.0	748.1	753.0	495.9	483.5	468.1	467.3	463.6	448.5
Florida	960.8	870.9	692.5	682.3	670.0	665.0	662.7	663.8	684.1	675.3	663.7	659.4	657.8	659.9
Georgia	1,094.3	1,037.4	834.2	822.8	810.0	805.4	805.4	803.4	815.7	808.4	797.9	793.9	795.0	794.4
Hawaii	801.2	752.2	598.4	587.1	587.4	588.6	589.2	582.8	645.3	637.9	632.6	649.7	652.8	655.8
Idaho	936.7	856.6	734.1	734.3	733.9	726.9	727.4	725.5	735.5	736.1	736.5	730.2	731.7	731.0
Illinois	1,063.7	973.8	740.4	734.3	729.9	726.3	726.1	726.1	721.6	716.6	713.6	711.2	712.9	712.3
Indiana	1,048.3	962.0	822.2	824.4	828.3	827.3	829.5	830.4	815.1	817.9	821.9	821.6	824.6	825.4
Iowa	919.9	848.2	722.5	720.8	721.5	721.7	723.8	722.8	720.6	718.6	719.0	719.5	722.7	721.6
Kansas	940.1	867.2	762.4	763.4	761.9	759.3	763.8	763.4	754.1	756.5	754.9	752.0	756.2	756.8
Kentucky	1,088.9	1,024.5	912.5	913.8	908.7	907.4	910.3	923.2	912.3	915.5	911.7	911.8	915.8	928.3
Louisiana	1,132.6	1,074.6	899.3	896.3	894.3	896.7	888.5	879.5	854.7	855.8	854.3	855.3	844.7	836.4
Maine	1,002.9	918.7	751.6	744.0	745.7	741.2	758.9	760.5	753.4	746.3	748.6	744.6	762.4	764.0
Maryland	1,063.3	985.2	731.4	717.6	711.7	706.3	705.1	707.6	706.7	696.7	695.6	693.3	692.6	695.4
Massachusetts	982.6	884.8	677.6	669.5	665.8	661.5	670.5	672.2	689.4	682.4	680.4	677.7	689.5	693.0
Michigan	1,050.2	966.0	784.5	781.5	780.2	780.1	783.5	784.5	761.0	758.9	758.2	759.0	763.8	765.4
Minnesota	892.9	825.2	657.6	656.5	653.1	649.1	650.6	649.6	652.2	651.1	647.1	642.2	643.3	642.4
Mississippi	1,108.7	1,071.4	956.2	953.5	952.9	946.6	953.6	950.1	911.9	912.7	914.0	908.1	919.5	918.1
Missouri	1,033.7	952.4	815.6	811.4	807.5	805.9	810.6	810.7	805.5	800.1	796.9	794.5	799.6	798.6
Montana	1,013.6	890.2	757.7	748.9	751.5	742.0	751.9	746.0	738.1	728.0	729.3	718.0	726.0	719.7
Nebraska	930.6	867.9	716.3	718.9	717.7	717.2	724.1	721.5	708.6	710.7	710.3	711.1	719.5	715.7
Nevada	1,077.4	1,017.4	793.2	786.3	777.8	764.1	758.5	756.5	820.3	812.1	805.0	793.2	788.5	784.9
New Hampshire	982.3	891.7	697.6	696.0	692.0	690.9	702.1	716.0	703.1	702.1	699.1	698.9	711.2	725.3
New Jersey	1,047.5	956.0	690.4	686.4	681.5	673.2	669.3	666.7	688.3	686.5	685.0	679.7	677.4	676.5
New Mexico	967.1	891.9	749.2	747.3	741.6	741.9	740.8	748.1	747.4	745.6	740.9	739.6	736.5	740.6
New York	1,051.8	973.7	668.5	660.9	655.5	645.9	643.2	640.4	681.9	675.8	672.7	663.7	663.9	663.4
North Carolina	1,050.4	986.0	799.9	793.9	784.8	779.8	781.2	782.7	778.3	774.0	765.6	760.3	761.8	763.6
North Dakota	922.4	818.4	704.6	700.8	702.9	701.2	699.7	692.7	681.0	677.6	681.1	678.8	677.8	669.4
Ohio	1,070.6	967.4	817.4	818.4	816.9	813.0	816.6	823.6	804.5	807.8	807.0	804.3	808.3	815.8
Oklahoma	1,025.6	961.4	910.2	905.7	904.3	900.0	904.2	896.7	896.8	893.5	893.8	888.6	890.9	882.1
Oregon	953.9	893.0	725.2	717.8	716.0	710.3	715.5	711.6	732.4	724.7	723.5	718.2	724.5	721.0
Pennsylvania	1,076.4	963.4	772.5	767.0	765.4	756.9	760.0	762.9	759.6	754.9	754.8	746.8	751.9	755.4
Rhode Island	990.8	889.6	713.4	705.2	701.1	699.0	710.8	704.3	720.5	715.5	714.9	715.0	726.9	720.0
South Carolina	1,104.6	1,030.0	847.0	843.0	837.5	833.9	835.6	832.9	811.6	811.3	807.3	805.7	808.2	806.1
South Dakota	941.9	846.4	714.1	715.9	703.7	700.3	701.7	715.2	679.1	678.7	666.9	664.6	664.1	676.1
Tennessee	1,045.5	1,011.8	885.1	883.4	880.3	880.6	882.5	884.2	870.2	872.4	871.1	872.8	875.4	877.4
Texas	1,014.9	947.6	765.2	758.8	752.1	750.0	747.2	740.2	761.5	756.5	750.9	750.4	748.5	741.7
Utah	924.9	823.2	696.4	700.7	703.4	706.7	710.7	712.2	698.6	703.2	706.3	709.6	714.5	716.8
Vermont	990.2	908.6	704.2	709.8	707.2	701.6	706.7	707.4	708.0	713.3	710.7	705.2	711.1	712.0
Virginia	1,054.0	963.1	744.6	737.6	732.0	724.1	721.3	718.1	729.1	724.7	721.5	714.7	714.6	712.4
Washington	947.7	869.4	696.9	687.9	683.6	677.8	679.9	677.4	706.1	698.4	695.5	691.2	694.1	692.3
West Virginia	1,100.3	1,031.5	944.7	941.9	938.6	930.7	932.0	938.5	946.0	943.6	940.3	933.4	935.3	941.8
Wisconsin	956.4	879.1	714.5	715.9	716.2	713.3	716.0	715.2	701.5	702.5	702.7	699.7	702.9	701.6
Wyoming	1,016.1	897.4	767.4	760.3	744.5	740.6	740.8	737.2	762.7	754.4	742.7	739.8	742.9	738.2
American Samoa[4]	NA	NA	1,063.0	1,054.4	1,080.6	1,029.4	1,042.0	1,016.8	NA	NA	NA	NA	NA	NA
Guam[4]	NA	NA	729.0	780.9	767.3	787.5	793.4	825.4	NA	NA	NA	NA	NA	NA
Northern Marianas[4]	NA	NA	816.2	770.4	746.1	811.2	861.3	878.5	NA	NA	NA	NA	NA	NA
Puerto Rico[4]	NA	NA	708.8	707.1	692.0	680.7	656.4	651.9	NA	NA	NA	NA	NA	NA
Virgin Islands[4]	NA	NA	628.1	644.0	NA	NA	NA	NA	NA	NA	NA	NA	NA	NA

NOTE: Data are based on death certificates. Age-adjusted average annual death rates are calculated using the year 2000. Prior to 2001, age-adjusted rates were calculated using standard million proportions based on rounded population numbers. Starting with 2001 data, unrounded population numbers are used to calculate age-adjusted rates. Age-adjusted rates for Puerto Rico, Virgin Islands, Guam, American Samoa, and Northern Marianas were computed by applying the age-specific death rates to the U.S. standard population combining the age groups for age 75 and over. For the territories, age groups were not available for those age 75 and over by age. Prior to 2009–2011, denominators for rates are resident population estimates for the middle year of each 3-year period, multiplied by 3. Starting with 2009–2011 estimates, denominators for rates are the 3-year average population. The race groups, White, Black, American Indian or Alaska Native, and Asian or Pacific Islander, include persons of Hispanic and non-Hispanic origin. Persons of Hispanic origin may be of any race. United States, state, and territory rates for 2011 and beyond were calculated using 2010-based postcensal population estimates. Starting with 2003 data, some states began to collect information on more than one race on the death certificate, according to 1997 Office of Management and Budget (OMB) standards. The multiple-race data for these states were bridged to the single-race categories of the 1977 OMB standards, for comparability with other states. Rates are rounded at the end of the calculation process. They may differ from rates based on the same data presented elsewhere if rounding is done earlier in the calculation process. Data for additional years are available.
NA = Not available.
[1]Death rates for Hispanic, American Indian or Alaska Native, and Asian or Pacific Islander persons should be interpreted with caution because of inconsistencies in reporting Hispanic origin or race on the death certificate (death rate numerators) compared with population figures (death rate denominators). The net effect of misclassification is an underestimation of deaths and death rates for races other than White and Black.
[3]Excludes data for American Samoa, Guam, Northern Marianas, Puerto Rico, and Virgin Islands.
[4]Comparable population data were not available for all time periods and for all racial and ethnicity groups. Therefore, only selected rates are presented for the territories.

Table 2-14. Age-Adjusted Death Rates, by Race, Hispanic Origin, Average Annual, 1979–1981, 1989–1991, 2009–2011, 2010–2012, 2011–2013, 2012–2014, 2013–2015, and 2014–2016—Continued

(Age-adjusted death rate per 100,000 population.[1])

Area	Black or African American						American Indian or Alaska Native[2]					
	2009–2011	2010–2012	2011–2013	2012–2014	2013–2015	2014–2016	2009–2011	2010–2012	2011–2013	2012–2014	2013–2015	2014–2016
United States[3]	895.8	879.7	867.4	858.1	853.9	852.9	614.7	607.2	595.8	593.6	594.1	593.8
Alabama	1,045.7	1,025.9	1,016.5	998.2	994.8	986.7	315.3	332.5	325.7	332.2	326.9	310.3
Alaska	675.1	692.2	664.9	651.2	657.1	631.3	1,162.6	1,133.8	1,129.2	1,138.2	1,169.7	1,196.2
Arizona	785.2	783.7	783.7	769.5	763.4	767.6	867.9	848.5	828.6	837.6	843.4	856.0
Arkansas	1,059.1	1,036.7	1,026.9	1,005.4	992.6	995.1	364.2	311.9	288.7	235.2	250.2	275.5
California	853.2	833.5	825.8	808.4	807.6	806.9	363.2	366.2	371.7	371.0	380.2	379.0
Colorado	785.5	786.7	765.2	745.6	741.6	735.0	450.5	448.0	449.7	468.5	462.4	489.3
Connecticut	725.3	704.1	691.6	681.5	683.2	690.6	213.2	229.9	210.1	214.2	194.9	167.2
Delaware	845.6	846.8	813.3	816.7	790.5	804.3	*	*	*	*	*	*
District of Columbia	1,010.3	978.1	967.9	966.1	969.7	994.6	*	*	*	*	*	*
Florida	798.3	776.6	758.7	748.7	741.2	738.2	300.7	290.8	277.6	283.7	285.2	291.5
Georgia	920.6	897.2	879.2	872.7	869.3	863.1	185.1	184.4	185.9	190.9	205.7	191.3
Hawaii	536.6	514.2	492.6	516.8	532.6	523.3	*	*	*	*	*	*
Idaho	577.9	613.1	554.1	532.0	413.7	389.6	798.5	727.5	711.1	733.4	716.4	670.2
Illinois	943.3	932.3	923.9	918.8	915.0	925.5	177.1	180.4	178.2	153.5	127.1	124.1
Indiana	964.3	960.5	963.1	952.6	951.2	956.8	162.8	185.1	180.6	190.6	192.3	204.0
Iowa	926.5	936.4	922.2	912.3	877.9	891.2	719.7	705.6	623.7	542.5	540.7	558.4
Kansas	953.6	932.9	926.0	928.1	936.0	939.5	1,157.0	1,123.3	1,079.3	1,100.1	1,127.3	1,068.1
Kentucky	986.3	963.3	935.2	916.7	914.6	936.5	290.8	249.6	229.6	186.1	161.2	172.9
Louisiana	1,033.9	1,018.3	1,013.4	1,019.9	1,019.3	1,008.5	439.3	453.1	451.8	390.6	367.4	348.2
Maine	451.6	419.9	467.0	454.3	464.6	442.5	1,070.5	896.0	731.1	693.5	793.4	868.4
Maryland	849.5	827.1	810.2	800.4	799.8	803.3	180.0	205.7	217.5	241.6	253.5	262.6
Massachusetts	640.6	622.7	612.3	595.1	583.9	585.1	240.4	251.9	272.4	312.1	289.7	297.1
Michigan	975.9	969.9	966.6	963.9	961.9	963.6	851.5	827.2	829.6	820.8	819.5	821.2
Minnesota	681.2	699.8	718.1	727.9	736.0	727.3	1,074.5	1,040.8	1,009.4	1,048.3	1,066.6	1,098.5
Mississippi	1,061.5	1,050.0	1,045.3	1,037.1	1,029.8	1,017.6	783.2	771.9	769.5	716.8	740.6	745.6
Missouri	948.6	952.1	942.2	952.9	956.7	967.7	409.8	421.4	387.5	396.5	376.2	341.8
Montana	*	*	*	*	*	*	1,172.2	1,184.2	1,209.1	1,229.0	1,268.9	1,246.8
Nebraska	961.3	957.4	937.1	912.4	892.9	909.9	881.5	904.2	886.4	868.3	823.8	841.7
Nevada	840.8	846.9	836.3	817.8	815.1	829.6	570.4	539.0	551.1	531.4	525.1	537.1
New Hampshire	532.4	504.7	376.6	383.4	374.2	444.2	*	*	*	*	*	*
New Jersey	843.9	833.0	813.5	793.5	791.2	789.1	206.4	190.9	181.2	167.6	148.2	141.0
New Mexico	726.2	720.8	706.6	707.7	707.7	687.2	789.7	786.1	781.0	802.8	826.1	862.5
New York	696.7	685.8	674.4	666.9	654.8	647.8	192.1	188.0	179.7	178.0	180.0	173.5
North Carolina	913.9	900.4	888.6	884.2	884.9	886.5	781.0	784.9	777.7	765.8	759.9	753.0
North Dakota	*	*	370.2	337.4	397.1	413.8	1,364.4	1,378.4	1,319.9	1,353.8	1,278.2	1,322.0
Ohio	962.0	944.8	940.6	928.6	932.6	937.4	268.5	250.4	235.4	262.2	249.8	277.9
Oklahoma	1,051.6	1,042.5	1,020.0	1,017.9	1,014.5	1,000.1	987.6	984.2	978.3	981.6	1,015.8	1,028.0
Oregon	797.8	813.3	809.6	785.9	761.3	740.8	679.5	663.2	658.1	666.7	674.7	677.2
Pennsylvania	960.3	942.9	926.4	915.7	908.1	914.5	236.7	258.4	285.5	274.1	280.3	242.0
Rhode Island	596.8	548.0	486.0	453.2	474.7	488.3	549.3	457.0	477.3	507.0	560.3	605.8
South Carolina	972.3	955.9	948.7	942.7	942.6	938.4	457.4	448.5	437.4	377.1	351.4	336.8
South Dakota	364.8	406.3	320.4	266.9	273.7	307.6	1,278.9	1,291.3	1,280.2	1,274.7	1,283.2	1,319.9
Tennessee	1,021.0	993.9	976.8	966.9	967.1	968.7	253.7	264.3	247.2	257.1	229.2	245.9
Texas	934.7	915.6	901.2	891.5	889.8	887.4	156.7	159.6	148.1	150.3	150.7	151.5
Utah	760.2	696.9	660.9	615.2	600.7	615.9	752.6	746.8	723.3	731.5	713.0	725.3
Vermont	*	*	*	*	497.0	522.2	*	*	*	*	*	*
Virginia	892.7	875.9	864.3	856.6	847.4	844.3	387.3	359.4	315.0	263.0	283.7	290.9
Washington	776.6	758.9	738.4	727.4	734.4	733.8	901.6	879.4	856.3	852.2	856.5	838.3
West Virginia	1,027.5	1,019.4	1,026.8	983.6	981.0	1,002.0	*	*	*	*	*	*
Wisconsin	977.9	984.9	973.3	964.6	948.6	962.2	985.9	999.2	990.5	1,015.3	958.6	903.7
Wyoming	*	*	356.7	331.6	333.2	364.8	1,093.8	1,174.8	1,155.3	1,158.6	1,042.5	1,006.2
American Samoa[4]	NA	NA	NA	NA	NA	NA	NA	NA	NA	NA	NA	NA
Guam[4]	NA	NA	NA	NA	NA	NA	NA	NA	NA	NA	NA	NA
Northern Marianas[4]	NA	NA	NA	NA	NA	NA	NA	NA	NA	NA	NA	NA
Puerto Rico[4]	NA	NA	NA	NA	NA	NA	NA	NA	NA	NA	NA	NA
Virgin Islands[4]	NA	NA	NA	NA	NA	NA	NA	NA	NA	NA	NA	NA

NOTE: Data are based on death certificates. Age-adjusted average annual death rates are calculated using the year 2000. Prior to 2001, age-adjusted rates were calculated using standard million proportions based on rounded population numbers. Starting with 2001 data, unrounded population numbers are used to calculate age-adjusted rates. Age-adjusted rates for Puerto Rico, Virgin Islands, Guam, American Samoa, and Northern Marianas were computed by applying the age-specific death rates to the U.S. standard population combining the age groups for age 75 and over. For the territories, age groups were not available for those age 75 and over by age. Prior to 2009–2011, denominators for rates are resident population estimates for the middle year of each 3-year period, multiplied by 3. Starting with 2009–2011 estimates, denominators for rates are the 3-year average population. The race groups, White, Black, American Indian or Alaska Native, and Asian or Pacific Islander, include persons of Hispanic and non-Hispanic origin. Persons of Hispanic origin may be of any race. United States, state, and territory rates for 2011 and beyond were calculated using 2010-based postcensal population estimates. Starting with 2003 data, some states began to collect information on more than one race on the death certificate, according to 1997 Office of Management and Budget (OMB) standards. The multiple-race data for these states were bridged to the single-race categories of the 1977 OMB standards, for comparability with other states. Rates are rounded at the end of the calculation process. They may differ from rates based on the same data presented elsewhere if rounding is done earlier in the calculation process. Data for additional years are available.
* = Prior to 2009–2011 (shown in spreadsheet version), data for states with populations under 10,000 in the middle year of a 3-year period, or fewer than 50 deaths for the 3-year period, are considered unreliable and are not shown. Starting with 2009–2011 estimates (shown in spreadsheet version), data for states with an average population for the 3-year period of under 10,000, or fewer than 50 deaths for the 3-year period, are considered unreliable and are not shown.
NA = Not available.
[1]Death rates for Hispanic, American Indian or Alaska Native, and Asian or Pacific Islander persons should be interpreted with caution because of inconsistencies in reporting Hispanic origin or race on the death certificate (death rate numerators) compared with population figures (death rate denominators). The net effect of misclassification is an underestimation of deaths and death rates for races other than White and Black.
[2]Age-adjusted average annual death rates are calculated using the year 2000 standard population. Prior to 2001, age-adjusted rates were calculated using standard million proportions based on rounded population numbers. Starting with 2001 data, unrounded population numbers are used to calculate age-adjusted rates. Age-adjusted rates for Puerto Rico, Virgin Islands, Guam, American Samoa, and Northern Marianas were computed by applying the age-specific death rates to the U.S. standard population combining the age groups for age 75 and over. For the territories, age groups were not available for those aged 75 and over by age. Prior to 2009–2011 (shown in spreadsheet version), denominators for rates are resident population estimates for the middle year of each 3-year period, multiplied by 3. Starting with 2009–2011 estimates (shown in spreadsheet version), denominators for rates are the 3-year average population.
[3]Excludes data for American Samoa, Guam, Northern Marianas, Puerto Rico, and Virgin Islands.
[4]Comparable population data were not available for all time periods and for all racial and ethnicity groups. Therefore, only selected rates are presented for the territories.

Table 2-14. Age-Adjusted Death Rates, by Race, Hispanic Origin, Average Annual, 1979–1981, 1989–1991, 2009–2011, 2010–2012, 2011–2013, 2012–2014, 2013–2015, and 2014–2016—*Continued*

(Age-adjusted death rate per 100,000 population.[1])

Area	Asian or Pacific Islander[2]						Hispanic or Latino[2]					
	2009–2011	2010–2012	2011–2013	2012–2014	2013–2015	2014–2016	2009–2011	2010–2012	2011–2013	2012–2014	2013–2015	2014–2016
United States[3]	419.4	413.5	407.5	399.8	395.9	391.9	552.6	545.6	538.3	532.2	527.8	524.8
Alabama	411.2	349.5	296.6	253.0	219.6	281.3	366.0	343.1	346.7	336.2	346.2	323.0
Alaska	475.9	476.7	486.6	486.1	479.3	494.8	454.8	457.6	385.6	352.1	356.7	387.5
Arizona	413.1	410.7	394.8	382.2	376.0	387.0	616.4	607.7	604.6	598.5	590.1	587.6
Arkansas	554.7	508.5	507.3	508.4	519.6	494.6	386.8	367.6	354.7	318.3	303.2	297.1
California	422.6	416.4	408.8	398.1	394.5	391.4	540.5	532.2	527.9	517.2	514.4	511.0
Colorado	404.7	403.8	404.8	392.8	389.0	395.9	671.8	658.8	657.1	655.0	652.5	657.6
Connecticut	357.9	356.9	334.0	325.0	311.7	320.5	532.3	522.2	511.2	517.2	519.8	518.6
Delaware	288.3	330.2	338.2	374.4	329.3	308.9	446.9	405.8	415.5	405.5	403.9	435.1
District of Columbia	340.2	337.6	365.3	319.0	345.4	338.2	396.3	379.4	378.9	385.2	362.8	374.9
Florida	347.0	329.0	316.3	324.6	331.9	331.3	540.7	533.7	520.1	513.6	507.4	509.8
Georgia	424.0	413.4	392.5	394.0	394.4	395.3	313.9	324.9	298.0	299.0	316.2	338.8
Hawaii	582.6	570.5	572.9	568.5	568.5	559.6	776.3	752.3	769.7	802.7	828.2	851.8
Idaho	476.7	524.9	500.1	457.1	411.6	393.9	508.7	497.2	491.5	485.4	486.7	494.5
Illinois	392.5	387.9	385.2	376.9	370.6	363.0	470.4	468.7	465.1	456.8	451.2	448.8
Indiana	391.8	383.6	379.2	380.0	384.2	397.7	447.9	470.3	466.3	476.8	461.3	455.1
Iowa	444.5	485.1	506.8	496.5	447.3	422.1	410.4	381.4	398.6	396.6	382.9	375.8
Kansas	437.6	434.1	465.3	455.7	445.5	419.9	557.3	564.2	550.4	534.4	528.0	520.6
Kentucky	399.8	389.4	420.1	428.3	390.9	382.0	330.7	333.4	302.4	314.1	319.9	344.3
Louisiana	431.6	414.1	414.3	421.9	423.5	392.1	349.7	361.1	362.8	387.8	393.5	393.7
Maine	334.2	359.3	355.6	327.7	292.6	276.2	363.1	343.3	269.9	270.1	243.3	252.2
Maryland	373.0	366.3	351.2	342.1	338.3	337.7	315.2	339.2	330.1	323.6	312.2	320.5
Massachusetts	360.1	357.0	342.5	345.6	353.1	349.9	453.1	452.4	453.1	447.8	446.0	453.2
Michigan	348.4	345.1	348.1	345.3	341.1	334.2	641.0	615.3	608.5	617.8	623.9	627.9
Minnesota	512.1	489.1	485.3	483.4	480.1	459.0	400.8	401.5	391.1	394.9	402.4	406.4
Mississippi	476.1	473.5	504.4	485.5	494.2	476.2	296.1	300.3	296.1	260.4	243.4	222.7
Missouri	376.7	437.5	446.1	417.4	399.9	384.8	333.9	370.6	400.7	424.7	417.0	404.2
Montana	*	*	*	*	413.6	414.8	487.9	473.6	484.4	457.7	511.8	536.9
Nebraska	410.6	433.4	405.9	407.9	365.9	403.7	434.5	436.3	439.9	436.5	450.7	458.4
Nevada	434.7	447.2	439.9	429.7	429.9	436.2	492.7	482.3	470.9	461.9	462.1	458.5
New Hampshire	301.8	285.4	315.5	320.2	331.4	352.4	349.3	324.0	285.6	256.2	243.6	266.0
New Jersey	347.1	340.8	334.0	325.5	317.1	310.2	483.2	473.6	469.4	463.4	460.0	454.4
New Mexico	370.4	385.9	344.5	342.7	339.0	377.4	721.9	722.0	720.8	714.8	709.4	716.7
New York	361.6	360.0	359.2	355.5	354.6	351.5	530.6	521.1	510.4	501.6	492.2	486.7
North Carolina	349.6	352.5	347.8	360.2	374.2	386.2	295.8	294.0	276.1	301.2	321.2	344.8
North Dakota	*	*	*	*	504.2	479.2	545.9	534.6	454.8	518.0	527.9	501.6
Ohio	401.9	389.2	369.6	369.0	368.1	375.6	481.4	468.3	466.8	459.3	468.6	459.3
Oklahoma	525.4	496.8	468.7	464.0	478.2	482.8	518.7	524.8	533.4	536.6	522.3	523.1
Oregon	433.0	444.1	435.7	436.2	424.7	428.6	456.2	444.1	437.9	454.2	450.3	449.4
Pennsylvania	380.1	394.3	393.5	396.7	390.2	386.1	507.8	527.7	547.3	562.9	563.2	552.0
Rhode Island	475.1	444.6	414.2	389.6	402.8	395.0	419.0	418.6	413.6	390.7	404.2	406.9
South Carolina	430.3	425.4	399.6	376.4	365.6	371.2	404.9	375.3	357.4	356.5	368.2	370.7
South Dakota	*	*	498.7	395.2	375.5	366.0	349.5	317.0	284.1	258.0	254.1	284.2
Tennessee	448.1	426.5	414.3	404.8	394.1	386.0	295.3	302.8	298.4	330.6	338.4	355.9
Texas	382.3	392.6	399.6	393.4	383.6	374.3	643.4	638.8	633.3	631.6	626.6	616.6
Utah	529.0	531.4	534.4	549.0	543.3	526.4	540.1	524.1	528.1	533.0	538.9	538.1
Vermont	*	*	*	*	375.3	402.4	*	*	359.9	344.2	329.3	348.2
Virginia	390.2	382.1	377.1	374.2	364.3	358.9	387.1	380.0	354.8	353.6	350.1	348.1
Washington	458.2	440.3	431.3	417.5	418.6	414.7	479.0	463.8	448.8	448.1	454.0	460.2
West Virginia	338.2	253.7	279.4	281.3	276.2	214.5	239.3	248.9	232.4	215.8	226.6	242.6
Wisconsin	430.4	452.8	491.9	494.8	499.8	476.5	449.0	439.0	445.0	451.0	449.4	451.6
Wyoming	*	*	*	*	*	*	661.8	649.4	588.4	551.0	533.9	548.7
American Samoa[4]	NA	NA	NA	NA	NA	NA	NA	NA	NA	NA	NA	NA
Guam[4]	NA	NA	NA	NA	NA	NA	NA	NA	NA	NA	NA	NA
Northern Marianas[4]	NA	NA	NA	NA	NA	NA	NA	NA	NA	NA	NA	NA
Puerto Rico[4]	NA	NA	NA	NA	NA	NA	NA	NA	NA	NA	NA	NA
Virgin Islands[4]	NA	NA	NA	NA	NA	NA	NA	NA	NA	NA	NA	NA

NOTE: Data are based on death certificates. Age-adjusted average annual death rates are calculated using the year 2000. Prior to 2001, age-adjusted rates were calculated using standard million proportions based on rounded population numbers. Starting with 2001 data, unrounded population numbers are used to calculate age-adjusted rates. Age-adjusted rates for Puerto Rico, Virgin Islands, Guam, American Samoa, and Northern Marianas were computed by applying the age-specific death rates to the U.S. standard population combining the age groups for age 75 and over. For the territories, age groups were not available for those age 75 and over by age. Prior to 2009–2011, denominators for rates are resident population estimates for the middle year of each 3-year period, multiplied by 3. Starting with 2009–2011 estimates, denominators for rates are the 3-year average population. The race groups, White, Black, American Indian or Alaska Native, and Asian or Pacific Islander, include persons of Hispanic and non-Hispanic origin. Persons of Hispanic origin may be of any race. United States, state, and territory rates for 2011 and beyond were calculated using 2010-based postcensal population estimates. Starting with 2003 data, some states began to collect information on more than one race on the death certificate, according to 1997 Office of Management and Budget (OMB) standards. The multiple-race data for these states were bridged to the single-race categories of the 1977 OMB standards, for comparability with other states. Rates are rounded at the end of the calculation process. They may differ from rates based on the same data presented elsewhere if rounding is done earlier in the calculation process. Data for additional years are available.
* = Prior to 2009–2011 (shown in spreadsheet version), data for states with populations under 10,000 in the middle year of a 3-year period, or fewer than 50 deaths for the 3-year period, are considered unreliable and are not shown. Starting with 2009–2011 estimates (shown in spreadsheet version), data for states with an average population for the 3-year period of under 10,000, or fewer than 50 deaths for the 3-year period, are considered unreliable and are not shown.
NA = Not available.
[1]Death rates for Hispanic, American Indian or Alaska Native, and Asian or Pacific Islander persons should be interpreted with caution because of inconsistencies in reporting Hispanic origin or race on the death certificate (death rate numerators) compared with population figures (death rate denominators). The net effect of misclassification is an underestimate of deaths and death rates for races other than White and Black.
[2]Age-adjusted average annual death rates are calculated using the year 2000 standard population. Prior to 2001, age-adjusted rates were calculated using standard million proportions based on rounded population numbers. Starting with 2001 data, unrounded population numbers are used to calculate age-adjusted rates. Age-adjusted rates for Puerto Rico, Virgin Islands, Guam, American Samoa, and Northern Marianas were computed by applying the age-specific death rates to the U.S. standard population combining the age groups for age 75 and over. For the territories, age groups were not available for those aged 75 and over by age. Prior to 2009–2011 (shown in spreadsheet version), denominators for rates are resident population estimates for the middle year of each 3-year period, multiplied by 3. Starting with 2009–2011 estimates (shown in spreadsheet version), denominators for rates are the 3-year average population.
[3]Excludes data for American Samoa, Guam, Northern Marianas, Puerto Rico, and Virgin Islands.
[4]Comparable population data were not available for all time periods and for all racial and ethnicity groups. Therefore, only selected rates are presented for the territories.

Table 2-14. Age-Adjusted Death Rates, by Race, Hispanic Origin, Average Annual, 1979–1981, 1989–1991, 2009–2011, 2010–2012, 2011–2013, 2012–2014, 2013–2015, and 2014–2016—*Continued*

(Age-adjusted death rate per 100,000 population.[1])

Area	White, not Hispanic or Latino[2]						Black, not Hispanic or Latino[2]					
	2009–2011	2010–2012	2011–2013	2012–2014	2013–2015	2014–2016	2009–2011	2010–2012	2011–2013	2012–2014	2013–2015	2014–2016
United States[3]	754.8	751.6	749.0	745.2	747.7	748.3	918.6	902.7	891.1	880.8	877.2	876.6
Alabama	920.5	921.2	919.0	914.4	914.8	915.5	1,050.0	1,031.0	1,021.4	1,002.9	998.8	991.2
Alaska	714.2	704.9	690.6	688.3	690.3	692.9	689.7	714.6	692.0	689.5	693.9	663.7
Arizona	694.9	692.3	686.4	675.2	672.1	670.5	824.0	821.8	823.9	803.2	794.8	795.1
Arkansas	888.7	893.5	893.3	891.2	894.6	897.6	1,061.8	1,038.9	1,026.9	1,003.9	988.9	991.4
California	704.5	698.9	696.3	686.6	686.4	683.5	896.5	877.8	871.0	853.5	853.6	854.0
Colorado	682.5	675.4	665.6	662.5	663.1	668.2	816.4	817.7	795.6	776.4	772.8	766.6
Connecticut	656.5	654.8	655.4	652.2	657.0	660.1	763.6	743.3	733.4	721.9	724.7	733.5
Delaware	764.2	758.5	746.7	734.2	739.9	747.3	848.0	852.0	820.9	825.2	799.3	814.3
District of Columbia	492.7	481.2	462.8	459.0	458.7	440.2	1,011.9	982.0	970.6	966.2	971.4	997.4
Florida	715.7	707.2	696.8	694.0	694.7	699.3	828.3	806.2	787.7	776.0	767.5	764.5
Georgia	831.9	824.8	816.6	813.9	816.0	815.5	928.6	904.7	888.9	883.3	880.0	873.9
Hawaii	651.5	640.8	631.2	640.7	638.3	634.9	542.2	503.2	502.9	519.0	542.4	524.3
Idaho	742.9	743.9	745.1	738.7	741.0	740.4	633.6	681.4	629.4	611.6	470.7	439.4
Illinois	735.7	731.3	728.9	727.7	730.9	731.6	951.4	941.8	932.3	926.2	922.8	934.8
Indiana	820.0	823.9	829.9	829.5	833.2	834.7	971.9	969.0	972.5	962.9	962.8	968.9
Iowa	723.5	722.0	722.4	723.4	727.3	726.6	941.3	952.0	937.5	928.1	894.2	909.2
Kansas	759.4	762.4	761.5	758.9	763.2	764.0	965.9	940.6	934.8	937.8	948.6	952.5
Kentucky	917.6	921.3	918.1	917.5	921.2	934.0	993.5	970.6	943.0	924.3	922.1	944.8
Louisiana	869.0	870.7	869.9	870.6	859.9	851.7	1,041.0	1,025.5	1,021.2	1,027.8	1,027.0	1,015.6
Maine	752.5	743.1	744.9	741.5	762.2	764.8	459.3	425.2	488.7	476.1	487.5	464.8
Maryland	718.3	708.2	708.7	707.7	708.3	712.7	859.2	834.4	817.2	806.1	806.9	811.3
Massachusetts	690.2	683.4	682.1	678.0	684.3	682.9	712.8	695.3	685.3	662.9	639.8	632.3
Michigan	761.4	759.7	758.9	759.6	763.8	765.3	981.0	975.6	971.6	968.5	966.0	966.6
Minnesota	653.9	653.1	649.3	644.6	645.5	644.3	691.2	710.5	731.8	740.3	749.5	738.9
Mississippi	917.7	919.2	921.1	916.6	929.7	929.1	1,065.0	1,053.6	1,049.7	1,041.8	1,035.6	1,023.7
Missouri	811.9	806.2	802.5	799.6	804.9	804.3	954.7	958.3	948.4	958.4	961.6	972.8
Montana	732.5	723.6	727.0	715.8	721.6	716.0	*	*	*	*	*	*
Nebraska	713.8	716.3	716.2	717.5	726.7	723.4	984.9	983.5	962.7	939.2	919.8	937.8
Nevada	866.9	862.2	859.2	848.8	845.3	843.4	868.9	875.4	865.4	847.3	844.6	861.9
New Hampshire	705.0	704.5	702.1	702.3	715.3	729.8	567.3	516.7	386.1	392.6	396.0	466.6
New Jersey	702.5	702.2	702.2	698.3	697.3	697.4	899.5	889.3	870.9	850.7	851.1	852.0
New Mexico	738.9	735.6	727.4	728.9	729.0	730.1	801.7	793.1	783.2	784.9	795.5	778.2
New York	678.0	671.5	669.4	662.6	663.4	664.0	761.8	744.9	735.4	720.9	711.3	703.1
North Carolina	788.0	785.1	778.5	772.9	774.4	775.3	923.6	910.6	899.5	892.8	892.3	892.7
North Dakota	679.8	675.9	679.6	677.5	677.3	669.5	*	*	386.3	329.1	392.2	407.7
Ohio	806.6	810.3	809.6	807.2	811.4	819.9	969.7	952.5	948.8	937.0	941.5	946.9
Oklahoma	909.3	905.7	905.5	900.5	903.6	895.3	1,062.2	1,051.6	1,030.2	1,027.8	1,026.3	1,011.5
Oregon	740.5	733.4	733.0	727.1	734.3	730.7	830.7	848.9	845.3	823.7	798.1	780.5
Pennsylvania	760.8	751.7	750.5	740.8	748.5	752.6	984.7	958.1	939.6	926.0	925.4	936.1
Rhode Island	724.8	720.1	720.0	722.7	733.9	728.3	704.4	656.6	584.4	547.0	573.1	585.7
South Carolina	813.6	816.4	815.1	816.0	818.9	817.6	953.6	954.9	950.7	947.1	947.2	943.2
South Dakota	680.3	680.8	669.9	668.0	667.9	679.5	387.7	428.6	338.2	283.7	291.7	329.0
Tennessee	877.6	880.1	879.1	879.5	882.4	885.0	1,028.6	999.8	981.7	968.5	968.9	970.4
Texas	793.4	791.4	786.9	787.3	787.0	782.5	947.3	932.5	919.6	910.1	908.4	906.4
Utah	705.4	711.5	715.0	718.7	724.0	726.4	847.1	779.3	736.1	689.9	680.7	704.6
Vermont	707.2	714.0	712.9	707.1	713.2	713.5	*	*	*	*	*	*
Virginia	736.1	732.5	731.1	724.8	725.5	724.4	893.1	875.1	864.7	855.4	844.6	841.7
Washington	713.1	706.0	703.8	699.6	702.5	700.3	791.1	774.8	756.4	746.2	752.4	749.0
West Virginia	949.4	947.3	944.7	938.2	940.2	946.6	1,036.5	1,027.5	1,035.3	993.4	990.9	1,011.8
Wisconsin	704.9	706.3	706.6	703.4	706.6	705.6	996.5	1,004.0	993.3	984.3	969.4	983.5
Wyoming	764.5	756.8	749.3	748.1	752.0	746.0	*	*	*	350.1	347.5	*
American Samoa[4]	NA	NA	NA	NA	NA	NA	NA	NA	NA	NA	NA	NA
Guam[4]	NA	NA	NA	NA	NA	NA	NA	NA	NA	NA	NA	NA
Northern Marianas[4]	NA	NA	NA	NA	NA	NA	NA	.	NA	NA	NA	NA
Puerto Rico[4]	NA	NA	NA	NA	NA	NA	NA	NA	NA	NA	NA	NA
Virgin Islands[4]	NA	NA	NA	NA	NA	NA	NA	NA	NA	NA	NA	NA

NOTE: Data are based on death certificates. Age-adjusted average annual death rates are calculated using the year 2000. Prior to 2001, age-adjusted rates were calculated using standard million proportions based on rounded population numbers. Starting with 2001 data, unrounded population numbers are used to calculate age-adjusted rates. Age-adjusted rates for Puerto Rico, Virgin Islands, Guam, American Samoa, and Northern Marianas were computed by applying the age-specific death rates to the U.S. standard population combining the age groups for age 75 and over. For the territories, age groups were not available for those age 75 and over by age. Prior to 2009–2011, denominators for rates are resident population estimates for the middle year of each 3-year period, multiplied by 3. Starting with 2009–2011 estimates, denominators for rates are the 3-year average population. The race groups, White, Black, American Indian or Alaska Native, and Asian or Pacific Islander, include persons of Hispanic and non-Hispanic origin. Persons of Hispanic origin may be of any race. United States, state, and territory rates for 2011 and beyond were calculated using 2010-based postcensal population estimates. Starting with 2003 data, some states began to collect information on more than one race on the death certificate, according to 1997 Office of Management and Budget (OMB) standards. The multiple-race data for these states were bridged to the single-race categories of the 1977 OMB standards, for comparability with other states. Rates are rounded at the end of the calculation process. They may differ from rates based on the same data presented elsewhere if rounding is done earlier in the calculation process. Data for additional years are available.

* = Prior to 2009–2011 (shown in spreadsheet version), data for states with populations under 10,000 in the middle year of a 3-year period, or fewer than 50 deaths for the 3-year period, are considered unreliable and are not shown. Starting with 2009–2011 estimates (shown in spreadsheet version), data for states with an average population for the 3-year period of under 10,000, or fewer than 50 deaths for the 3-year period, are considered unreliable and are not shown.

NA = Not available.

[1]Death rates for Hispanic, American Indian or Alaska Native, and Asian or Pacific Islander persons should be interpreted with caution because of inconsistencies in reporting Hispanic origin or race on the death certificate (death rate numerators) compared with population figures (death rate denominators). The net effect of misclassification is an underestimate of deaths and death rates for races other than White and Black.

[2]Age-adjusted average annual death rates are calculated using the year 2000 standard population. Starting with 2001 data, unrounded population numbers are used to calculate age-adjusted rates. Age-adjusted rates for Puerto Rico, Virgin Islands, Guam, American Samoa, and Northern Marianas were computed by applying the age-specific death rates to the U.S. standard population combining the age groups for age 75 and over. For the territories, age groups were not available for those aged 75 and over by age. Prior to 2009–2011 (shown in spreadsheet version), denominators for rates are resident population estimates for the middle year of each 3-year period, multiplied by 3. Starting with 2009–2011 estimates (shown in spreadsheet version), denominators for rates are the 3-year average population.

[3]Excludes data for American Samoa, Guam, Northern Marianas, Puerto Rico, and Virgin Islands.

[4]Comparable population data were not available for all time periods and for all racial and ethnicity groups. Therefore, only selected rates are presented for the territories.

Table 2-15. Age-Adjusted Death Rates for Selected Causes of Death, by Sex, Race, and Hispanic Origin, Selected Years, 1950–2016

(Age-adjusted rate per 100,000 population; data based on death certificates.)

Sex, race, Hispanic origin, and cause of death[1]	1950[2,3]	1960[2,3]	1970[3]	1980[3]	1985[3]	1990[3]	1995[3]	2000[4]	2005[4]	2006[4]	2007[4]	2008[4]	2009[4]	2010[4]	2011[4]	2012[4]	2013[4]	2014[4]	2015[4]	2016[4]
All Persons									Age-adjusted death rate per 100,000 population[5]											
All causes	1,446.0	1,339.2	1,222.6	1,039.1	988.1	938.7	909.8	869.0	815.0	791.8	775.3	774.9	749.6	747.0	741.3	732.8	731.9	724.6	733.1	728.8
Diseases of heart	588.8	559.0	492.7	412.1	375.0	321.8	293.4	257.6	216.8	205.5	196.1	192.1	182.8	179.1	173.7	170.5	169.8	167.0	168.5	165.5
Ischemic heart disease	NA	NA	NA	345.2	296.2	249.6	219.7	186.8	148.2	138.3	129.2	126.1	117.7	113.6	109.2	105.4	102.6	98.8	97.2	94.3
Cerebrovascular diseases	180.7	177.9	147.7	96.2	76.4	65.3	63.1	60.9	48.0	44.8	43.5	42.1	39.6	39.1	37.9	36.9	36.2	36.5	37.6	37.3
Malignant neoplasms	193.9	193.9	198.6	207.9	211.3	216.0	209.9	199.6	185.1	181.8	179.3	176.4	173.5	172.8	169.0	166.5	163.2	161.2	158.5	155.8
Trachea, bronchus, and lung	15.0	24.1	37.1	49.9	54.6	59.3	58.4	56.1	52.7	51.5	50.6	49.5	48.4	47.6	46.0	44.9	43.4	42.1	40.5	38.4
Colon, rectum, and anus	NA	30.3	28.9	27.4	26.3	24.5	22.5	20.8	17.7	17.4	17.0	16.6	16.0	15.8	15.3	14.9	14.6	14.3	14.2	13.9
Chronic lower respiratory diseases[6,7]	NA	NA	NA	28.3	34.5	37.2	40.1	44.2	43.9	41.0	41.4	44.7	42.7	42.2	42.5	41.5	42.1	40.5	41.6	40.6
Influenza and pneumonia[7]	48.1	53.7	41.7	31.4	34.5	36.8	33.4	23.7	21.0	18.4	16.8	17.6	16.5	15.1	15.7	14.4	15.9	15.1	15.2	13.5
Chronic liver disease and cirrhosis	11.3	13.3	17.8	15.1	12.3	11.1	9.9	9.5	8.9	8.8	9.1	9.2	9.1	9.4	9.7	9.9	10.2	10.4	10.8	10.7
Diabetes mellitus[8]	23.1	22.5	24.3	18.1	17.4	20.7	23.2	25.0	24.9	23.6	22.8	22.0	21.0	20.8	21.6	21.2	21.2	20.9	21.3	21.0
Alzheimer's disease[9]	NA	NA	NA	NA	NA	NA	NA	18.1	24.0	23.7	23.8	25.8	24.2	25.1	24.7	23.8	23.5	25.4	29.4	30.3
Human immunodeficiency virus (HIV) disease	X	X	X	X	NA	10.2	16.2	5.2	4.2	4.0	3.7	3.3	3.0	2.6	2.4	2.2	2.1	2.0	1.9	1.8
Unintentional injuries	78.0	62.3	60.1	46.4	38.5	36.3	34.4	34.9	39.5	40.2	40.4	39.2	37.5	38.0	39.1	39.1	39.4	40.5	43.2	47.4
Motor vehicle-related injuries	24.6	23.1	27.6	22.3	18.6	18.5	16.3	15.4	15.2	15.0	14.4	12.9	11.6	11.3	11.1	11.4	10.9	10.8	11.4	12.1
Drug overdose	2.5	1.7	2.8	1.9	2.2	2.3	3.4	4.5	8.0	9.2	9.9	10.2	10.3	10.6	11.6	11.5	12.2	13.1	14.8	18.2
Nephritis, nephrotic syndrome, and nephrosis[9]	NA	NA	NA	9.1	10.4	9.3	9.4	13.5	14.7	14.8	14.9	15.1	15.1	15.3	13.4	13.1	13.2	13.2	13.4	13.1
Suicide[10]	13.2	12.5	13.1	12.2	12.5	12.5	11.8	10.4	10.9	11.0	11.3	11.6	11.8	12.1	12.3	12.6	12.6	13.0	13.3	13.5
Homicide[10]	5.1	5.0	8.8	10.4	7.9	9.4	8.3	5.9	6.1	6.2	6.1	5.9	5.5	5.3	5.3	5.4	5.2	5.1	5.7	6.2
Male																				
All causes	1,674.2	1,609.0	1,542.1	1,348.1	1,278.1	1,202.8	1,143.9	1,053.8	971.9	943.5	922.9	918.8	890.9	887.1	875.3	865.1	863.6	855.1	863.2	861.0
Diseases of heart	699.0	687.6	634.0	538.9	488.0	412.4	371.0	320.0	268.2	254.9	243.7	238.5	229.4	225.1	218.1	214.7	214.5	210.9	211.8	209.1
Ischemic heart disease	NA	NA	NA	459.7	393.7	328.2	286.5	241.4	192.3	180.7	169.2	165.1	156.2	151.3	145.6	141.1	138.2	133.5	131.2	128.3
Cerebrovascular diseases	186.4	186.1	157.4	102.2	79.9	68.5	65.9	62.4	48.4	45.2	43.7	42.2	39.9	39.3	37.9	37.1	36.7	36.9	37.8	37.5
Malignant neoplasms	208.1	225.1	247.6	271.2	274.4	280.4	267.5	248.9	227.2	221.7	218.8	214.9	210.9	209.9	204.0	200.3	196.0	192.9	189.2	185.4
Trachea, bronchus, and lung	24.6	43.6	67.5	85.2	88.6	91.1	84.2	76.7	69.1	67.0	64.9	63.5	61.4	60.3	57.7	56.1	53.7	51.7	49.5	46.7
Colon, rectum, and anus	NA	31.8	32.3	32.8	31.8	30.4	27.4	25.1	21.2	20.7	20.3	19.7	19.1	19.0	18.1	17.7	17.4	16.9	16.8	16.4
Prostate	28.6	28.7	28.8	32.8	33.4	38.4	37.0	30.4	25.3	24.2	24.2	23.0	22.1	21.9	20.7	19.5	19.2	19.0	18.8	19.3
Chronic lower respiratory diseases[6,7]	NA	NA	NA	49.9	56.2	55.4	54.8	55.8	52.2	48.4	48.8	52.3	49.5	48.7	48.6	47.2	47.5	45.4	46.0	45.1
Influenza and pneumonia[7]	55.0	65.8	54.0	42.1	46.8	47.8	42.8	28.9	24.9	22.1	20.2	20.7	19.6	18.2	18.8	17.3	18.6	17.8	17.7	15.9
Chronic liver disease and cirrhosis	15.0	18.5	24.8	21.3	17.4	15.9	14.2	13.4	12.4	12.1	12.7	12.7	12.5	12.9	13.1	13.4	13.8	14.1	14.5	14.3
Diabetes mellitus[8]	18.8	19.9	23.0	18.1	17.7	21.7	25.0	27.8	28.8	27.7	26.6	25.9	25.0	24.9	26.0	25.5	25.6	25.6	26.2	26.0
Alzheimer's disease[9]	NA	NA	NA	NA	NA	NA	NA	15.2	19.5	19.4	19.5	21.3	20.2	21.0	20.4	19.8	19.3	20.6	23.7	24.3
Human immunodeficiency virus (HIV) disease	X	X	X	X	NA	18.5	27.3	7.9	6.3	5.9	5.4	4.8	4.4	3.8	3.4	3.2	3.1	3.0	2.8	2.7
Unintentional injuries	101.8	85.5	87.4	69.0	57.1	52.9	49.6	49.3	55.0	56.0	55.9	54.3	51.4	51.5	52.8	52.6	53.1	54.6	58.7	65.0
Motor vehicle-related injuries	38.5	35.4	41.5	33.6	27.2	26.5	22.8	21.7	21.9	21.5	21.0	18.9	16.8	16.2	16.1	16.5	15.9	15.8	16.7	17.6
Drug overdose	3.3	2.3	3.9	2.7	3.2	3.5	5.3	6.6	10.8	12.6	13.1	13.6	13.5	13.8	15.1	15.0	16.0	17.3	19.8	25.1
Nephritis, nephrotic syndrome, and nephrosis[9]	NA	NA	NA	12.2	13.8	12.1	12.2	16.9	18.1	18.3	18.3	18.6	18.4	18.7	16.5	16.0	16.1	16.2	16.3	15.9
Suicide[10]	21.2	20.0	19.8	19.9	21.1	21.5	20.3	17.7	18.1	18.1	18.5	19.0	19.2	19.8	20.0	20.4	20.3	20.7	21.1	21.4
Homicide[10]	7.9	7.5	14.3	16.6	12.2	14.8	12.8	9.0	9.7	9.8	9.7	9.3	8.6	8.4	8.3	8.5	8.2	8.0	9.1	9.9
Female																				
All causes	1,236.0	1,105.3	971.4	817.9	784.5	750.9	739.4	731.4	692.3	672.2	658.1	659.9	636.8	634.9	632.4	624.7	623.5	616.7	624.2	617.5
Diseases of heart	486.6	447.0	381.6	320.8	294.5	257.0	236.6	210.9	177.5	167.2	159.0	155.9	146.6	143.3	138.7	135.5	134.3	131.8	133.6	130.4
Ischemic heart disease	NA	NA	NA	263.1	227.0	193.9	171.3	146.5	115.0	106.3	98.8	96.3	88.4	84.9	81.0	77.8	74.9	71.6	70.5	67.5
Cerebrovascular diseases	175.8	170.7	140.0	91.7	73.3	62.6	60.5	59.1	47.0	43.9	42.7	41.4	38.8	38.3	37.2	36.1	35.2	35.6	36.9	36.5
Malignant neoplasms	182.3	168.7	163.2	166.7	171.2	175.7	173.6	167.6	156.7	154.7	152.3	149.6	147.4	146.7	144.0	142.1	139.5	138.1	135.9	134.0
Trachea, bronchus, and lung	5.8	7.5	13.1	24.4	30.6	37.1	40.4	41.3	40.6	40.1	40.1	39.1	38.6	38.1	37.1	36.4	35.5	34.7	33.5	31.9
Colon, rectum, and anus	NA	29.1	26.5	23.8	22.7	20.6	19.1	17.7	15.0	14.9	14.6	14.2	13.5	13.3	13.0	12.6	12.3	12.1	12.1	11.8
Breast	31.9	31.7	32.1	31.9	33.0	33.3	30.5	26.8	24.2	23.6	23.0	22.6	22.3	22.1	21.6	21.3	20.8	20.6	20.3	20.1
Chronic lower respiratory diseases[6,7]	NA	NA	NA	14.9	21.7	26.6	31.8	37.4	38.7	36.4	36.6	39.8	38.3	38.0	38.5	37.8	38.5	37.1	38.6	37.4
Influenza and pneumonia[7]	41.9	43.8	32.7	25.1	27.6	30.5	28.1	20.7	18.6	16.1	14.7	15.6	14.5	13.1	13.7	12.5	14.0	13.2	13.5	11.8
Chronic liver disease and cirrhosis	7.8	8.7	11.9	9.9	7.9	7.1	6.2	6.2	5.8	5.8	5.9	6.0	6.1	6.2	6.6	6.7	6.8	7.1	7.6	7.5
Diabetes mellitus[8]	27.0	24.7	25.1	18.0	17.0	19.9	21.8	23.0	21.9	20.4	19.8	19.1	17.9	17.6	18.2	17.7	17.6	17.2	17.3	16.9
Alzheimer's disease[9]	NA	NA	NA	NA	NA	NA	NA	19.3	26.2	25.9	26.2	28.2	26.3	27.3	27.1	26.1	25.9	28.3	32.8	33.9
Human immunodeficiency virus (HIV) disease	X	X	X	X	NA	2.2	5.3	2.5	2.3	2.2	2.1	1.9	1.7	1.4	1.3	1.2	1.1	1.1	1.0	0.9

NA = Not available.
X = Not applicable.

[1] Underlying cause-of-death code numbers are based on the applicable *International Classification of Diseases* (*ICD*) revision for data years shown.
[2] Includes deaths of persons who were not residents of the 50 states and the District of Columbia.
[3] Underlying cause of death was coded according to the 6th revision of the *ICD* in 1950, 7th revision in 1960, 8th revision in 1970, and 9th revision in 1980–1998.
[4] Starting with 1999 data, cause of death is coded according to *ICD-10*.
[5] Age-adjusted rates are calculated using the year 2000 standard population. Prior to 2001, age-adjusted rates were calculated using standard million proportions based on rounded population numbers. Starting with 2001 data, unrounded population numbers are used to calculate age-adjusted rates.
[6] Between 1998 and 1999, the cause of death title for Chronic obstructive pulmonary diseases in the *ICD–9* was renamed to Chronic lower respiratory diseases (CLRD) in *ICD–10*.
[7] Starting with 1999 data, the rules for selecting CLRD and Pneumonia as the underlying cause of death changed, resulting in an increase in the number of deaths for CLRD and a decrease in the number of deaths for pneumonia. Therefore, trend data for these two causes of death should be interpreted with caution.
[8] Starting with 2011 data, the rules for selecting Renal failure as the underlying cause of death were changed, affecting the number of deaths in the Nephritis, nephrotic syndrome and nephrosis and Diabetes categories. These changes directly affect deaths with mention of Renal failure and other associated conditions, such as Diabetes mellitus with renal complications. The result is a decrease in the number of deaths for Nephritis, nephrotic syndrome and nephrosis and an increase in the number of deaths for Diabetes mellitus. Therefore, trend data for these two causes of death should be interpreted with caution.`
[9] Data for Alzheimer's disease are only presented for data years 1999 and beyond due to large differences in death rates caused by changes in the *ICD* coding of the causes of death between *ICD–9* and *ICD–10*.
[10] Rates for 2001 include September 11-related deaths for which death certificates were filed as of October 24, 2002.

Table 2-15. Age-Adjusted Death Rates for Selected Causes of Death, by Sex, Race, and Hispanic Origin, Selected Years, 1950–2016—Continued

(Age-adjusted rate per 100,000 population; data based on death certificates.)

Sex, race, Hispanic origin, and cause of death[1]	1950[2,3]	1960[2,3]	1970[3]	1980[3]	1985[3]	1990[3]	1995[3]	2000[4]	2005[4]	2006[4]	2007[4]	2008[4]	2009[4]	2010[4]	2011[4]	2012[4]	2013[4]	2014[4]	2015[4]	2016[4]
All Persons	Age-adjusted death rate per 100,000 population[5]																			
Unintentional injuries	54.0	40.0	35.1	26.1	22.2	21.5	21.0	22.0	25.3	25.8	26.1	25.4	24.8	25.6	26.5	26.4	26.6	27.3	28.7	30.8
Motor vehicle-related injuries	11.5	11.7	14.9	11.8	10.7	11.0	10.3	9.5	8.9	8.8	8.2	7.2	6.7	6.3	6.5	6.2	6.1	6.2	6.4	6.9
Drug overdose	1.7	1.1	1.8	1.3	1.2	1.2	1.6	2.5	5.1	5.9	6.6	6.8	7.1	7.5	8.2	8.1	8.5	9.1	9.8	11.4
Nephritis, nephrotic syndrome, and nephrosis[9]	NA	NA	NA	7.3	8.5	7.7	7.8	11.5	12.6	12.6	12.8	13.0	13.0	13.0	11.4	11.1	11.3	11.1	11.3	11.2
Suicide[10]	5.6	5.6	7.4	5.7	5.2	4.8	4.3	4.0	4.4	4.5	4.6	4.8	4.9	5.0	5.2	5.4	5.5	5.8	6.0	6.0
Homicide[10]	2.4	2.6	3.7	4.4	3.8	4.0	3.7	2.8	2.5	2.6	2.5	2.4	2.4	2.3	2.2	2.2	2.1	2.1	2.2	2.5
White[11]																				
All causes	1,410.8	1,311.3	1,193.3	1,012.7	963.6	909.8	882.3	849.8	801.1	779.3	764.3	767.2	742.8	741.8	738.8	730.9	731.0	725.4	735.0	729.9
Diseases of heart	586.0	559.0	492.2	409.4	371.4	317.0	288.6	253.4	213.2	202.0	192.8	189.3	180.1	176.9	172.2	168.9	168.2	165.9	167.9	164.5
Ischemic heart disease	NA	NA	NA	347.6	298.0	249.7	219.1	185.6	147.3	137.4	128.5	125.8	117.4	113.5	109.3	105.6	102.9	99.3	98.0	94.8
Cerebrovascular diseases	175.5	172.7	143.5	93.2	73.7	62.8	60.7	58.8	46.0	42.9	41.6	40.4	38.1	37.7	36.5	35.6	34.9	35.2	36.4	36.1
Malignant neoplasms	194.6	193.1	196.7	204.2	207.3	211.6	206.2	197.2	183.9	181.0	178.5	175.9	173.3	172.4	168.8	166.6	163.7	161.9	159.4	156.6
Trachea, bronchus, and lung	15.2	24.0	36.7	49.2	53.9	58.6	58.1	56.2	53.2	52.1	51.2	50.2	49.1	48.3	46.7	45.6	44.1	42.9	41.4	39.2
Colon, rectum, and anus	NA	30.9	29.2	27.4	26.1	24.1	22.0	20.3	17.1	16.9	16.6	16.1	15.6	15.3	14.8	14.5	14.3	14.0	13.9	13.6
Chronic lower respiratory diseases[6,7]	NA	NA	NA	29.3	35.6	38.3	41.5	46.0	46.0	43.1	43.5	47.1	45.1	44.6	45.1	44.1	44.8	43.1	44.5	43.3
Influenza and pneumonia[7]	44.8	50.4	39.8	30.9	34.3	36.4	33.0	23.5	20.9	18.2	16.6	17.4	16.3	14.9	15.6	14.3	15.8	15.1	15.2	13.4
Chronic liver disease and cirrhosis	11.5	13.2	16.6	13.9	11.4	10.5	9.7	9.6	9.2	9.1	9.5	9.6	9.9	10.2	10.5	10.7	11.2	11.7	11.9	11.6
Diabetes mellitus[8]	22.9	21.7	22.9	16.7	15.9	18.8	20.9	22.8	22.8	21.4	20.7	20.2	19.2	19.0	19.0	19.8	19.4	19.4	19.3	19.3
Alzheimer's disease[9]	NA	NA	NA	NA	NA	NA	NA	18.8	24.7	24.5	24.6	26.7	25.0	26.0	25.7	24.7	24.4	26.4	30.5	31.4
Human immunodeficiency virus (HIV) disease	X	X	X	X	NA	8.3	11.4	2.8	2.2	2.1	1.9	1.7	1.5	1.4	1.3	1.2	1.2	1.1	1.1	1.0
Unintentional injuries	77.0	60.4	57.8	45.3	37.7	35.5	33.9	35.1	40.7	41.7	42.1	41.4	39.5	40.3	41.6	41.5	41.9	43.1	46.0	50.4
Motor vehicle-related injuries	24.4	22.9	27.1	22.6	18.8	18.5	16.3	15.6	15.7	15.5	14.9	13.4	12.0	11.7	11.5	11.8	11.3	11.1	11.7	12.4
Drug overdose	2.4	1.6	2.4	1.8	2.0	2.1	3.1	4.5	8.5	9.8	10.7	11.3	11.4	11.9	13.0	12.9	13.7	14.8	16.7	20.3
Nephritis, nephrotic syndrome, and nephrosis[9]	NA	NA	NA	8.0	9.3	8.3	8.5	12.1	13.2	13.3	13.5	13.8	13.7	14.0	12.2	12.0	12.1	12.1	12.2	12.0
Suicide[10]	13.9	13.1	13.8	13.0	13.4	13.4	12.6	11.3	12.1	12.2	12.6	13.0	13.2	13.6	13.9	14.1	14.2	14.7	15.1	15.2
Homicide[10]	2.6	2.7	4.7	6.7	5.3	5.5	5.0	3.6	3.7	3.7	3.7	3.7	3.4	3.3	3.2	3.2	3.1	3.0	3.3	3.5
Black or African American[11]																				
All causes	1,722.1	1,577.5	1,518.1	1,314.8	1,261.2	1,250.3	1,213.9	1,121.4	1,035.1	997.9	972.0	947.7	912.8	898.2	877.1	864.8	860.8	849.3	851.9	857.2
Diseases of heart	588.7	548.3	512.0	455.3	430.6	391.5	363.8	324.8	278.0	263.5	252.5	243.4	231.8	224.9	214.1	211.7	210.4	206.3	205.1	205.3
Ischemic heart disease	NA	NA	NA	334.5	293.4	267.0	244.9	218.3	175.7	165.4	154.0	146.8	137.4	131.2	125.3	121.3	117.5	112.8	108.9	108.3
Cerebrovascular diseases	233.6	235.2	197.1	129.1	105.2	91.6	86.9	81.9	67.0	63.1	61.7	58.8	54.0	53.0	50.9	49.3	49.0	49.7	50.8	50.5
Malignant neoplasms	176.4	199.1	225.3	256.4	266.5	279.5	267.7	248.5	223.5	217.6	215.1	208.5	204.5	203.8	198.8	193.8	189.2	185.6	180.1	177.9
Trachea, bronchus, and lung	11.1	23.7	41.3	59.7	65.8	72.4	69.0	64.0	58.1	56.3	55.1	52.9	51.3	51.4	49.2	48.3	46.8	44.5	42.0	40.0
Colon, rectum, and anus	NA	22.8	26.1	28.3	30.0	30.6	29.3	28.2	25.1	24.4	23.6	22.9	22.0	21.8	21.2	20.0	19.4	18.6	18.8	18.5
Chronic lower respiratory diseases[6,7]	NA	NA	NA	19.2	24.6	28.1	30.1	31.6	31.1	28.5	28.5	30.8	28.9	29.0	29.2	29.0	29.5	28.4	28.9	29.3
Influenza and pneumonia[7]	76.7	81.1	57.2	34.4	35.8	39.4	36.4	25.6	22.6	20.4	19.2	19.5	18.0	16.8	16.8	15.7	16.7	16.1	15.9	15.0
Chronic liver disease and cirrhosis	9.0	13.6	28.1	25.0	19.3	16.5	12.0	9.4	7.6	6.8	7.2	6.8	6.7	7.0	6.9	7.3	7.2	7.4	7.2	7.1
Diabetes mellitus[8]	23.5	30.9	38.8	32.7	33.0	40.5	46.7	49.5	47.5	45.5	43.1	40.8	39.1	38.7	39.6	38.7	38.4	37.3	37.0	36.8
Alzheimer's disease[9]	NA	NA	NA	NA	NA	NA	NA	13.0	20.8	19.7	20.5	21.2	20.6	20.6	20.8	19.9	20.1	22.3	26.6	27.5
Human immunodeficiency virus (HIV) disease	X	X	X	X	NA	26.7	54.2	23.3	19.2	18.3	17.0	14.9	13.7	11.6	10.3	9.5	8.9	8.3	7.9	7.2
Unintentional injuries	79.9	74.0	78.3	57.6	47.1	43.8	41.0	37.7	38.8	38.2	36.5	33.1	31.6	31.3	31.6	31.4	32.6	33.7	36.8	42.7
Motor vehicle-related injuries	26.0	24.2	31.1	20.2	17.8	18.8	16.7	15.7	14.4	14.5	14.0	12.1	11.5	10.9	10.7	11.3	10.9	11.1	12.2	13.5
Drug overdose	2.8	2.9	5.8	3.1	3.6	4.1	6.2	6.0	8.1	9.3	8.4	7.7	7.4	7.3	8.0	8.1	8.9	9.6	11.1	15.4
Nephritis, nephrotic syndrome, and nephrosis[9]	NA	NA	NA	20.9	22.7	19.8	19.3	28.7	30.3	30.8	29.9	29.9	29.9	29.3	25.9	25.2	25.0	24.6	25.4	25.1
Suicide[10]	4.5	5.0	6.2	6.5	6.6	7.1	6.8	5.5	5.2	5.0	4.9	5.2	5.1	5.2	5.4	5.6	5.4	5.5	5.6	6.1
Homicide[10]	28.3	26.0	44.0	39.0	28.1	36.3	29.7	20.5	21.1	21.5	20.9	19.3	18.1	17.7	17.6	18.4	17.8	17.2	19.8	21.4
American Indian or Alaska Native[11]																				
All causes	NA	NA	NA	867.0	731.7	716.3	771.2	709.3	701.1	676.6	661.3	644.0	616.0	628.3	600.9	595.3	591.7	594.1	596.9	591.2
Diseases of heart	NA	NA	NA	240.6	219.0	200.6	204.6	178.2	156.6	153.2	140.5	132.6	130.7	128.6	124.2	119.6	120.6	119.1	118.5	115.4
Ischemic heart disease	NA	NA	NA	173.6	158.3	139.1	141.4	129.1	106.1	107.2	95.9	88.0	86.5	84.9	81.4	79.2	78.2	76.4	73.4	71.3
Cerebrovascular diseases	NA	NA	NA	57.8	46.2	40.7	48.6	45.0	38.8	33.4	34.2	27.7	29.2	28.1	27.1	25.2	24.6	25.4	24.7	23.8
Malignant neoplasms	NA	NA	NA	113.7	113.5	121.8	138.2	127.8	128.8	125.4	124.1	125.0	114.9	122.4	109.4	111.4	110.2	106.7	107.9	103.4
Trachea, bronchus, and lung	NA	NA	NA	20.7	25.8	30.9	37.4	32.3	35.3	32.3	34.1	34.8	29.5	33.1	30.0	30.1	27.7	27.8	26.7	25.1
Colon, rectum, and anus	NA	NA	NA	9.5	10.5	12.0	14.9	13.4	12.6	11.7	12.1	14.6	13.0	11.7	12.3	11.1	12.8	10.9	11.1	9.9

NA = Not available.
X = Not applicable.

[1] Underlying cause-of-death code numbers are based on the applicable *International Classification of Diseases* (*ICD*) revision for data years shown.
[2] Includes deaths of persons who were not residents of the 50 states and the District of Columbia.
[3] Underlying cause of death was coded according to the 6th revision of the *ICD* in 1950, 7th revision in 1960, 8th revision in 1970, and 9th revision in 1980–1998.
[4] Starting with 1999 data, cause of death is coded according to *ICD-10*.
[5] Age-adjusted rates are calculated using the year 2000 standard population. Prior to 2001, age-adjusted rates were calculated using standard million proportions based on rounded population numbers. Starting with 2001 data, unrounded population numbers are used to calculate age-adjusted rates.
[6] Between 1998 and 1999, the cause of death title for Chronic obstructive pulmonary diseases in the *ICD–9* was renamed to Chronic lower respiratory diseases (CLRD) in *ICD–10*.
[7] Starting with 1999 data, the rules for selecting CLRD and Pneumonia as the underlying cause of death changed, resulting in an increase in the number of deaths for CLRD and a decrease in the number of deaths for pneumonia. Therefore, trend data for these two causes of death should be interpreted with caution.
[8] Starting with 2011 data, the rules for selecting Renal failure as the underlying cause of death were changed, affecting the number of deaths in the Nephritis, nephrotic syndrome and nephrosis and Diabetes categories. These changes directly affect deaths with mention of Renal failure and other associated conditions, such as Diabetes mellitus with renal complications. The result is a decrease in the number of deaths for Nephritis, nephrotic syndrome and nephrosis and an increase in the number of deaths for Diabetes mellitus. Therefore, trend data for these two causes of death should be interpreted with caution.'
[9] Data for Alzheimer's disease are only presented for data years 1999 and beyond due to large differences in death rates caused by changes in the *ICD* coding of the causes of death between *ICD–9* and *ICD–10*.
[10] Rates for 2001 include September 11-related deaths for which death certificates were filed as of October 24, 2002.
[11] The race groups White, Black, Asian or Pacific Islander, and American Indian or Alaska Native, include persons of Hispanic and non-Hispanic origin. Persons of Hispanic origin may be of any race. Death rates for Hispanic, American Indian or Alaska Native, and Asian or Pacific Islander persons should be interpreted with caution because of inconsistencies in reporting Hispanic origin or race on the death certificate (death rate numerators) compared with population figures (death rate denominators). The net effect of misclassification is an underestimation of deaths and death rates for races other than White and Black.

Table 2-15. Age-Adjusted Death Rates for Selected Causes of Death, by Sex, Race, and Hispanic Origin, Selected Years, 1950–2016—*Continued*

(Age-adjusted rate per 100,000 population; data based on death certificates.)

Sex, race, Hispanic origin, and cause of death[1]	1950[2,3]	1960[2,3]	1970[3]	1980[3]	1985[3]	1990[3]	1995[3]	2000[4]	2005[4]	2006[4]	2007[4]	2008[4]	2009[4]	2010[4]	2011[4]	2012[4]	2013[4]	2014[4]	2015[4]	2016[4]
All Persons								Age-adjusted death rate per 100,000 population[5]												
Chronic lower respiratory diseases[6,7]	NA	NA	NA	14.2	17.6	25.4	27.6	32.8	31.6	29.8	33.9	31.9	30.7	33.8	28.7	29.8	30.8	29.9	30.9	29.7
Influenza and pneumonia[7]	NA	NA	NA	44.4	33.6	36.1	36.1	22.3	23.6	16.3	15.9	19.6	17.9	15.9	15.5	13.1	15.0	15.1	12.5	12.7
Chronic liver disease and cirrhosis	NA	NA	NA	45.3	27.9	24.1	27.4	24.3	21.6	20.9	23.1	23.6	21.3	22.8	22.9	25.3	24.8	24.2	26.4	26.7
Diabetes mellitus[8]	NA	NA	NA	29.6	29.0	34.1	45.9	41.5	44.1	42.2	40.0	36.3	34.9	36.4	36.5	36.9	34.1	31.3	34.2	34.3
Alzheimer's disease[9]	NA	NA	NA	NA	NA	NA	NA	9.1	15.0	13.6	14.3	15.1	13.1	17.2	13.4	12.3	12.7	15.2	15.4	17.3
Human immunodeficiency virus (HIV) disease	X	X	X	X	NA	1.8	6.5	2.2	2.5	2.1	2.3	1.8	1.7	1.6	1.2	1.0	1.3	1.2	1.4	1.0
Unintentional injuries	NA	NA	NA	99.0	67.4	62.6	55.3	51.3	51.3	52.6	50.8	49.0	48.7	46.9	48.3	49.5	47.1	49.5	50.7	53.9
Motor vehicle-related injuries	NA	NA	NA	54.5	34.8	32.5	29.1	27.3	22.6	24.1	20.8	18.4	17.2	15.7	16.6	16.3	15.4	16.6	16.9	17.8
Drug overdose	NA	NA	NA	2.3	3.1	3.2	4.6	4.7	8.6	9.4	10.3	12.4	13.8	13.0	14.0	15.1	14.2	15.5	16.1	18.1
Nephritis, nephrotic syndrome, and nephrosis[9]	NA	NA	NA	12.2	10.7	11.6	10.6	15.0	15.6	15.1	15.9	17.2	14.4	16.4	12.5	12.6	11.4	12.4	12.2	11.6
Suicide[10]	NA	NA	NA	11.9	10.9	11.7	10.6	9.8	10.7	10.4	10.1	10.1	10.0	10.8	10.6	10.8	11.7	10.9	12.6	13.5
Homicide[10]	NA	NA	NA	15.5	11.7	10.4	9.9	6.8	6.8	6.6	5.6	6.2	5.9	5.7	5.9	5.8	5.3	5.8	6.2	6.7
Asian or Pacific Islander[11]																				
All causes	NA	NA	NA	589.9	586.5	582.0	554.8	506.4	459.6	450.7	436.2	435.1	424.6	424.3	410.3	407.1	405.4	388.3	394.8	392.6
Diseases of heart	NA	NA	NA	202.1	196.7	181.7	171.3	146.0	119.7	115.8	108.3	107.7	103.8	100.9	93.2	92.2	92.8	86.1	86.5	85.2
Ischemic heart disease	NA	NA	NA	168.2	153.3	139.6	128.0	109.6	85.6	82.2	75.9	75.9	70.7	68.7	62.7	60.5	59.9	55.1	54.9	53.0
Cerebrovascular diseases	NA	NA	NA	66.1	58.7	56.9	55.2	52.9	40.8	39.3	36.6	35.2	33.0	33.2	31.6	30.8	29.4	28.3	29.8	30.7
Malignant neoplasms	NA	NA	NA	126.1	132.3	134.2	131.8	121.9	113.2	109.6	109.5	108.8	106.8	108.9	105.6	104.2	100.5	98.9	99.0	97.1
Trachea, bronchus, and lung	NA	NA	NA	28.4	27.2	30.2	29.9	28.1	26.3	25.9	26.0	25.6	25.2	24.8	24.6	24.0	23.3	22.7	22.2	21.5
Colon, rectum, and anus	NA	NA	NA	16.4	16.6	14.4	14.0	12.7	11.5	11.3	11.2	11.6	10.5	11.4	10.8	10.8	9.8	9.5	9.8	9.3
Chronic lower respiratory diseases[6,7]	NA	NA	NA	12.9	17.6	19.4	19.3	18.6	15.9	15.4	14.3	15.2	14.3	13.9	14.5	12.8	13.6	12.5	12.2	11.7
Influenza and pneumonia[7]	NA	NA	NA	24.0	26.1	31.4	29.1	19.7	16.8	16.1	14.9	15.7	15.0	14.4	14.2	14.0	15.0	12.9	14.0	12.9
Chronic liver disease and cirrhosis	NA	NA	NA	6.1	5.9	5.2	3.9	3.5	3.6	3.5	3.3	3.4	3.3	3.2	3.3	3.3	3.3	3.5	3.3	3.4
Diabetes mellitus[8]	NA	NA	NA	12.6	12.1	14.6	16.8	16.4	17.3	16.6	17.0	16.8	16.2	15.5	15.9	15.7	15.8	15.0	15.7	15.5
Alzheimer's disease[9]	NA	NA	NA	NA	NA	NA	NA	5.5	8.5	9.4	9.1	10.1	10.9	10.9	11.1	11.7	11.1	12.1	14.7	15.0
Human immunodeficiency virus (HIV) disease	X	X	X	X	NA	2.2	3.2	0.6	0.6	0.6	0.5	0.6	0.4	0.4	0.4	0.4	0.4	0.3	0.4	0.4
Unintentional injuries	NA	NA	NA	27.0	24.8	23.9	20.2	17.9	18.1	17.1	16.9	15.3	14.9	15.0	15.7	15.1	15.2	15.1	16.1	16.8
Motor vehicle-related injuries	NA	NA	NA	13.9	12.9	14.0	11.4	8.6	7.5	7.3	6.9	6.0	4.9	5.1	4.8	4.6	4.8	4.6	4.9	5.2
Drug overdose	NA	NA	NA	0.5	0.6	0.7	0.8	0.7	1.3	1.4	1.4	1.3	1.5	1.4	1.7	1.8	2.0	2.0	2.4	2.9
Nephritis, nephrotic syndrome, and nephrosis[9]	NA	NA	NA	7.2	7.2	7.1	6.5	8.4	8.7	9.4	9.2	8.9	9.8	9.6	7.7	8.0	8.1	8.2	8.3	8.1
Suicide[10]	NA	NA	NA	7.8	7.1	6.7	6.7	5.5	5.1	5.4	5.9	5.5	5.9	6.2	5.9	6.3	5.9	6.0	6.4	6.7
Homicide[10]	NA	NA	NA	5.9	4.1	5.0	4.7	3.0	2.8	2.7	2.2	2.1	2.0	1.8	2.0	1.9	1.5	1.5	1.6	1.8
Hispanic or Latino[11,12]																				
All causes	NA	NA	NA	NA	698.8	692.0	700.2	665.7	627.6	604.0	586.1	579.8	559.7	558.6	540.7	539.1	535.4	523.3	525.3	525.8
Diseases of heart	NA	NA	NA	NA	239.8	217.1	211.0	196.0	170.4	157.8	149.5	141.4	135.8	132.8	123.9	122.0	121.2	116.0	116.9	115.8
Ischemic heart disease	NA	NA	NA	NA	187.9	173.3	166.4	153.2	127.9	116.4	107.5	100.8	94.7	92.3	84.2	81.1	80.3	75.3	74.5	72.7
Cerebrovascular diseases	NA	NA	NA	NA	51.9	45.2	46.3	46.4	38.6	37.2	35.8	34.4	32.2	32.1	30.7	30.0	29.6	30.2	32.3	32.1
Malignant neoplasms	NA	NA	NA	NA	125.9	136.8	138.5	134.9	127.9	123.7	121.8	121.0	119.7	119.7	117.0	116.9	114.5	112.4	110.3	110.0
Trachea, bronchus, and lung	NA	NA	NA	NA	22.9	26.5	25.9	24.8	23.3	21.6	21.9	21.6	20.4	20.4	19.8	19.2	18.7	18.3	17.8	16.6
Colon, rectum, and anus	NA	NA	NA	NA	13.0	14.7	14.1	14.1	13.1	13.4	12.8	12.7	12.7	12.3	11.9	11.7	11.7	11.1	10.9	10.8
Chronic lower respiratory diseases[6,7]	NA	NA	NA	NA	17.4	19.3	22.6	21.1	20.9	19.0	19.3	20.5	19.8	19.6	19.1	18.5	18.7	17.5	17.7	17.1
Influenza and pneumonia[7]	NA	NA	NA	NA	30.2	29.7	26.2	20.6	18.5	16.7	14.7	15.9	15.6	13.7	13.6	12.0	13.2	12.8	11.4	11.1
Chronic liver disease and cirrhosis	NA	NA	NA	NA	20.3	18.3	17.4	16.5	14.1	13.6	14.0	14.0	14.0	13.7	14.1	14.1	14.0	14.5	14.9	14.7
Diabetes mellitus[8]	NA	NA	NA	NA	23.0	28.2	35.7	36.9	35.4	31.7	30.6	29.8	27.0	27.1	27.2	26.9	26.3	25.1	25.2	24.7
Alzheimer's disease[9]	NA	NA	NA	NA	NA	NA	NA	10.4	15.6	16.1	15.6	18.0	16.9	18.5	17.7	17.4	17.7	19.8	24.2	24.3
Human immunodeficiency virus (HIV) disease	X	X	X	X	NA	16.3	24.9	6.7	4.8	4.5	4.1	3.6	3.2	2.8	2.7	2.2	2.1	2.0	1.8	1.7
Unintentional injuries	NA	NA	NA	NA	34.3	34.6	32.2	30.1	31.8	32.0	30.5	28.4	26.3	25.8	26.3	26.5	26.9	26.8	28.6	31.4
Motor vehicle-related injuries	NA	NA	NA	NA	17.1	19.5	16.4	14.7	14.6	14.6	13.1	11.2	10.1	9.6	9.3	9.6	9.7	9.6	10.2	11.0
Drug overdose	NA	NA	NA	NA	3.2	3.2	4.9	4.1	5.2	5.7	5.8	5.9	5.8	5.6	6.2	6.2	6.7	6.8	7.7	9.5
Nephritis, nephrotic syndrome, and nephrosis[9]	NA	NA	NA	NA	10.3	8.4	6.9	11.8	12.8	13.5	13.3	13.6	13.8	14.1	11.2	11.3	11.1	11.1	11.4	11.4
Suicide[10]	NA	NA	NA	NA	6.3	7.8	7.2	5.9	5.6	5.3	6.0	5.5	5.8	5.9	5.7	5.8	5.7	6.3	6.2	6.7
Homicide[10]	NA	NA	NA	NA	14.6	16.2	12.5	7.5	7.4	7.2	6.8	6.4	6.0	5.3	5.0	4.9	4.5	4.5	4.9	5.3

NA = Not available.
X = Not applicable.
[1]Underlying cause-of-death code numbers are based on the applicable *International Classification of Diseases* (*ICD*) revision for data years shown.
[2]Includes deaths of persons who were not residents of the 50 states and the District of Columbia.
[3]Underlying cause of death was coded according to the 6th revision of the *ICD* in 1950, 7th revision in 1960, 8th revision in 1970, and 9th revision in 1980–1998.
[4]Starting with 1999 data, cause of death is coded according to *ICD*-10.
[5]Age-adjusted rates are calculated using the year 2000 standard population. Prior to 2001, age-adjusted rates were calculated using standard million proportions based on rounded population numbers. Starting with 2001 data, unrounded population numbers are used to calculate age-adjusted rates.
[6]Between 1998 and 1999, the cause of death title for Chronic obstructive pulmonary diseases in the *ICD*–9 was renamed to Chronic lower respiratory diseases (CLRD) in *ICD*–10.
[7]Starting with 1999 data, the rules for selecting CLRD and Pneumonia as the underlying cause of death changed, resulting in an increase in the number of deaths for CLRD and a decrease in the number of deaths for pneumonia. Therefore, trend data for these two causes of death should be interpreted with caution.
[8]Starting with 2011 data, the rules for selecting Renal failure as the underlying cause of death were changed, affecting the number of deaths in the Nephritis, nephrotic syndrome and nephrosis and Diabetes categories. These changes directly affect deaths with mention of Renal failure and other associated conditions, such as Diabetes mellitus with renal complications. The result is a decrease in the number of deaths for Nephritis, nephrotic syndrome and nephrosis and an increase in the number of deaths for Diabetes mellitus. Therefore, trend data for these two causes of death should be interpreted with caution.`
[9]Data for Alzheimer's disease are only presented for data years 1999 and beyond due to large differences in death rates caused by changes in the *ICD* coding of the causes of death between *ICD*–9 and *ICD*–10.
[10]Rates for 2001 include September 11-related deaths for which death certificates were filed as of October 24, 2002.
[11]The race groups White, Black, Asian or Pacific Islander, and American Indian or Alaska Native, include persons of Hispanic and non-Hispanic origin. Persons of Hispanic origin may be of any race. Death rates for Hispanic, American Indian or Alaska Native, and Asian or Pacific Islander persons should be interpreted with caution because of inconsistencies in reporting Hispanic origin or race on the death certificate (death rate numerators) compared with population figures (death rate denominators). The net effect of misclassification is an underestimation of deaths and death rates for races other than White and Black.
[12]Prior to 1997, data from states that did not report Hispanic origin on the death certificate were excluded.

Table 2-15. Age-Adjusted Death Rates for Selected Causes of Death, by Sex, Race, and Hispanic Origin, Selected Years, 1950–2016—*Continued*

(Age-adjusted rate per 100,000 population; data based on death certificates.)

Sex, race, Hispanic origin, and cause of death[1]	1950[2,3]	1960[2,3]	1970[3]	1980[3]	1985[3]	1990[3]	1995[3]	2000[4]	2005[4]	2006[4]	2007[4]	2008[4]	2009[4]	2010[4]	2011[4]	2012[4]	2013[4]	2014[4]	2015[4]	2016[4]
All Persons										Age-adjusted death rate per 100,000 population[5]									
White, not Hispanic or Latino[11, 12]																				
All causes	NA	NA	NA	NA	942.1	914.5	882.3	855.5	810.1	789.1	775.3	779.4	755.1	755.0	754.3	745.8	747.1	742.8	753.2	749.0
Diseases of heart	NA	NA	NA	NA	366.7	319.7	289.9	255.5	215.5	204.5	195.5	192.4	182.9	179.9	175.6	172.3	171.8	169.9	171.9	168.7
Ischemic heart disease	NA	NA	NA	NA	296.0	251.9	219.9	186.6	148.3	138.6	129.9	127.4	118.9	115.0	111.1	107.4	104.6	101.2	99.7	96.6
Cerebrovascular diseases	NA	NA	NA	NA	72.2	63.5	60.8	59.0	46.2	42.9	41.7	40.5	38.3	37.8	36.7	35.8	35.0	35.4	36.4	36.1
Malignant neoplasms	NA	NA	NA	NA	202.1	215.4	208.9	200.6	187.8	185.1	182.6	179.9	177.4	176.5	173.0	170.6	167.7	166.2	163.7	160.8
Trachea, bronchus, and lung	NA	NA	NA	NA	53.2	60.3	59.6	58.2	55.5	54.5	53.7	52.6	51.6	50.8	49.2	48.0	46.6	45.4	43.8	41.6
Colon, rectum, and anus	NA	NA	NA	NA	25.7	24.6	22.3	20.5	17.4	17.1	16.9	16.4	15.8	15.5	15.0	14.7	14.5	14.3	14.1	13.9
Chronic lower respiratory diseases[6,7]	NA	NA	NA	NA	36.3	39.2	42.1	47.2	47.7	44.8	45.3	49.1	47.1	46.6	47.2	46.3	47.0	45.4	46.9	45.8
Influenza and pneumonia[7]	NA	NA	NA	NA	35.2	36.5	33.0	23.5	21.0	18.3	16.7	17.4	16.2	14.9	15.7	14.4	15.9	15.1	15.4	13.5
Chronic liver disease and cirrhosis	NA	NA	NA	NA	10.9	9.9	9.0	9.0	8.7	8.6	8.9	9.1	9.1	9.4	9.7	10.0	10.3	10.6	11.1	11.0
Diabetes mellitus[8]	NA	NA	NA	NA	14.8	18.3	20.1	21.8	21.8	20.6	19.9	19.3	18.5	18.2	19.1	18.5	18.6	18.6	18.9	18.6
Alzheimer's disease[9]	NA	NA	NA	NA	NA	NA	NA	19.1	25.1	24.9	25.1	27.2	25.4	26.4	26.1	25.1	24.8	26.8	30.8	31.8
Human immunodeficiency virus (HIV) disease	X	X	X	X	NA	7.4	9.8	2.2	1.8	1.7	1.5	1.4	1.2	1.1	1.0	1.0	0.9	0.9	0.9	0.8
Unintentional injuries	NA	NA	NA	NA	35.2	35.0	33.4	35.3	41.5	42.7	43.6	43.2	41.3	42.4	44.0	43.9	44.2	45.8	49.0	53.9
Motor vehicle-related injuries	NA	NA	NA	NA	17.4	18.2	16.1	15.6	15.7	15.4	15.1	13.7	12.2	11.9	11.9	12.1	11.5	11.3	11.8	12.4
Drug overdose	NA	NA	NA	NA	2.2	2.0	2.9	4.6	9.1	10.6	11.8	12.4	12.6	13.3	14.6	14.4	15.3	16.7	18.8	23.0
Nephritis, nephrotic syndrome, and nephrosis[9]	NA	NA	NA	NA	8.8	8.1	8.4	12.0	13.1	13.2	13.4	13.6	13.5	13.8	12.2	11.9	12.1	12.1	12.2	11.9
Suicide[10]	NA	NA	NA	NA	13.8	13.8	13.1	12.0	13.0	13.3	13.7	14.3	14.5	15.0	15.5	15.7	15.9	16.4	17.0	17.0
Homicide[10]	NA	NA	NA	NA	4.4	4.0	3.6	2.8	2.7	2.7	2.8	2.9	2.6	2.5	2.6	2.6	2.5	2.5	2.6	2.9
Black, not Hispanic or Latino[11, 12]																				
All causes	NA	NA	NA	NA	NA	NA	NA	1,137.0	1,055.1	1,019.3	994.4	969.2	934.4	920.4	901.6	887.1	885.2	870.7	876.1	882.8
Diseases of heart	NA	NA	NA	NA	NA	NA	NA	328.4	282.4	268.2	257.4	248.1	236.4	229.5	219.3	216.3	215.5	210.8	210.1	210.7
Ischemic heart disease	NA	NA	NA	NA	NA	NA	NA	220.4	178.1	168.0	156.5	149.4	139.8	133.4	127.9	123.4	119.9	114.8	111.3	110.8
Cerebrovascular diseases	NA	NA	NA	NA	NA	NA	NA	82.9	68.2	64.3	63.0	59.9	55.2	54.3	52.3	50.4	50.3	50.9	52.2	51.9
Malignant neoplasms	NA	NA	NA	NA	NA	NA	NA	252.0	227.7	222.0	219.8	213.0	209.2	208.8	204.0	198.6	194.4	190.2	185.1	182.9
Trachea, bronchus, and lung	NA	NA	NA	NA	NA	NA	NA	64.9	59.4	57.5	56.3	54.1	52.6	52.6	50.5	49.6	48.2	45.7	43.1	41.2
Colon, rectum, and anus	NA	NA	NA	NA	NA	NA	NA	28.7	25.5	24.9	24.1	23.4	22.5	22.4	21.8	20.5	19.9	19.1	19.3	19.0
Chronic lower respiratory diseases[6,7]	NA	NA	NA	NA	NA	NA	NA	32.0	31.6	29.0	29.1	31.5	29.6	29.6	29.9	29.7	30.2	28.9	29.7	30.0
Influenza and pneumonia[7]	NA	NA	NA	NA	NA	NA	NA	25.9	22.9	20.7	19.5	19.9	18.3	17.1	17.2	16.1	17.1	16.3	16.3	15.4
Chronic liver disease and cirrhosis	NA	NA	NA	NA	NA	NA	NA	9.6	7.7	6.9	7.4	7.0	6.9	6.9	7.2	7.0	7.5	7.3	7.6	7.3
Diabetes mellitus[8]	NA	NA	NA	NA	NA	NA	NA	50.2	48.3	46.4	44.0	41.6	40.0	39.6	40.6	39.7	39.5	38.2	38.0	37.8
Alzheimer's disease[9]	NA	NA	NA	NA	NA	NA	NA	13.2	21.1	20.0	20.9	21.5	21.0	20.9	21.3	20.2	20.5	22.7	27.3	28.2
Human immunodeficiency virus (HIV) disease	X	X	X	X	NA	NA	NA	23.6	19.7	18.9	17.6	15.4	14.2	12.0	10.7	9.8	9.2	8.6	8.2	7.5
Unintentional injuries	NA	NA	NA	NA	NA	NA	NA	38.4	39.7	39.4	37.7	34.1	34.1	32.5	32.4	32.7	32.5	33.9	34.9	44.2
Motor vehicle-related injuries	NA	NA	NA	NA	NA	NA	NA	16.0	14.9	15.0	14.5	12.6	11.9	11.4	11.3	11.8	11.5	11.6	12.7	14.1
Drug overdose	NA	NA	NA	NA	NA	NA	NA	6.1	8.2	9.6	8.7	7.8	7.6	7.5	8.2	8.3	9.2	9.9	11.5	15.9
Nephritis, nephrotic syndrome, and nephrosis[9]	NA	NA	NA	NA	NA	NA	NA	29.1	30.9	31.5	30.6	30.6	30.6	30.1	26.6	25.9	25.8	25.3	26.2	25.8
Suicide[10]	NA	NA	NA	NA	NA	NA	NA	5.6	5.4	5.2	5.1	5.4	5.3	5.4	5.5	5.8	5.6	5.7	5.8	6.3
Homicide[10]	NA	NA	NA	NA	NA	NA	NA	21.1	21.9	22.5	21.9	20.3	19.0	18.6	18.6	19.4	18.8	18.2	20.9	22.8

NA = Not available.

X = Not applicable.

[1]Underlying cause-of-death code numbers are based on the applicable *International Classification of Diseases* (*ICD*) revision for data years shown.

[2]Includes deaths of persons who were not residents of the 50 states and the District of Columbia.

[3]Underlying cause of death was coded according to the 6th revision of the *ICD* in 1950, 7th revision in 1960, 8th revision in 1970, and 9th revision in 1980–1998.

[4]Starting with 1999 data, cause of death is coded according to *ICD-10*.

[5]Age-adjusted rates are calculated using the year 2000 standard population. Prior to 2001, age-adjusted rates were calculated using standard million proportions based on rounded population numbers. Starting with 2001 data, unrounded population numbers are used to calculate age-adjusted rates.

[6]Between 1998 and 1999, the cause of death title for Chronic obstructive pulmonary diseases in the *ICD–9* was renamed to Chronic lower respiratory diseases (CLRD) in *ICD–10*.

[7]Starting with 1999 data, the rules for selecting CLRD and Pneumonia as the underlying cause of death changed, resulting in an increase in the number of deaths for CLRD and a decrease in the number of deaths for pneumonia. Therefore, trend data for these two causes of death should be interpreted with caution.

[8]Starting with 2011 data, the rules for selecting Renal failure as the underlying cause of death were changed, affecting the number of deaths in the Nephritis, nephrotic syndrome and nephrosis and Diabetes categories. These changes directly affect deaths with mention of Renal failure and other associated conditions, such as Diabetes mellitus with renal complications. The result is a decrease in the number of deaths for Nephritis, nephrotic syndrome and nephrosis and an increase in the number of deaths for Diabetes mellitus. Therefore, trend data for these two causes of death should be interpreted with caution.`

[9]Data for Alzheimer's disease are only presented for data years 1999 and beyond due to large differences in death rates caused by changes in the *ICD* coding of the causes of death between *ICD–9* and *ICD–10*.

[10]Rates for 2001 include September 11-related deaths for which death certificates were filed as of October 24, 2002.

[11]The race groups White, Black, Asian or Pacific Islander, and American Indian or Alaska Native, include persons of Hispanic and non-Hispanic origin. Persons of Hispanic origin may be of any race. Death rates for Hispanic, American Indian or Alaska Native, and Asian or Pacific Islander persons should be interpreted with caution because of inconsistencies in reporting Hispanic origin or race on the death certificate (death rate numerators) compared with population figures (death rate denominators). The net effect of misclassification is an underestimation of deaths and death rates for races other than White and Black.

[12]Prior to 1997, data from states that did not report Hispanic origin on the death certificate were excluded.

Table 2-16. Number of Deaths, Death Rates, and Age-Adjusted Death Rates for Injury Deaths, by Mechanism and Intent of Death for All Injury Death and the Leading Causes of Injury Death, 2017

(Number; rates per 100,000 population; age-adjusted rates per 100,000 U.S. standard population.)

Mechanism and intent of death (based on the *ICD, Tenth Revision*)	Number	Rate	Age-adjusted rate[1]
All Injury (*U01'-*U03, V01'-Y36, Y85'-Y87, Y89)	243,039	74.6	71.5
Unintentional (V01'-X59, Y85'-Y86)	169,936	52.2	49.4
Suicide (*U03,X60'-X84, Y87.0)	47,173	14.5	14.0
Homicide (*U01'-*U02, X85'-Y09, Y87.1)	19,510	6.0	6.2
Undetermined (Y10'-Y34, Y87.2, Y89.9)	5,799	1.8	1.8
Legal intervention/war (Y35'-Y36, Y89[.0..1])	621	0.2	0.2
Poisoning (*U01[.6–.7],X40–X49,X60–X69,X85–X90,Y10–Y19,Y35.2)	75,354	23.1	23.2
Unintentional (W25'-W29, W45)	64,795	19.9	20.1
Suicide (X78)	6,554	2.0	1.9
Homicide (X99)	151	0.0	0.0
Undetermined (Y28)	3,854	1.2	1.2
Legal intervention/war (Y35.4)	–	*	*
Firearm (*U01.4, W32'-W34, X72'-X74, X93'-X95, Y22'-Y24, Y35.0)	39,773	12.2	12.0
Unintentional (W65'-W74)	486	0.1	0.2
Suicide (X71)	23,854	7.3	6.9
Homicide (X92)	14,542	4.5	4.6
Undetermined (Y21)	338	0.1	0.1
Legal intervention/war (Y35.4)	553	0.2	0.2
Motor vehicle traffic (V02'-V04[.1,.9], V09.2, V12'-V14[.3'-.9], V19[.4'-.6], V20'-V28[.3'-.9], V29'-V79[.4'-.9], V80[.3'- .5],V81.1, V82.1, V83'-V86[.0'-.3], V87[.0'-.8],V89.2)[2]	38,659	11.9	11.5
Occupant (V30'-V79[.4'-.9], V83'-V86[.0'-.3])[2]	9,463	2.9	2.8
Motorcyclist (V20'-V28[.3'-.9], V29[.4'-.9])[2]	4,777	1.5	1.4
Pedal cyclist (V12'-V14[.3'-.9], V19[.4'-.6])[2]	679	0.2	0.2
Pedestrian (V02'-V04[.1,.9], V09.2)[2]	6,480	2.0	1.9
Other (V80[.3'-.5], V81.1, V82.1)[2]	15	*	*
Unspecified (V87[.0'-.8], V89.2)[2]	17,245	5.3	5.2
Fall (W00'-W19, X80, Y01, Y30)	37,587	11.5	9.8
Unintentional (W00'-W19)	36,338	11.2	9.4
Suicide (X80)	1,124	0.3	0.3
Homicide (Y01)	6	*	*
Undetermined (Y30)	119	0.0	0.0

– = Quantity zero.
* = Rate does not meet NCHS standards of reliability.
0.0 = Quantity more than zero but less than 0.05.
[1]For method of computation, see chapter notes.
[2]Intent of death is unintentional.

Table 2-17. Leading Causes of Death and Numbers of Death, by Sex, Race, and Hispanic Origin, 1980 and 2016

(Number; data based on death certificates.)

Sex, race, Hispanic origin, and rank order	1980		Sex, race, Hispanic origin, and rank order	2016	
	Cause of death	Deaths		Cause of death	Deaths
All persons			**All persons**		
	All causes..	1,989,841		All causes..	2,744,248
1................................	Diseases of heart	761,085	1................................	Diseases of heart	635,260
2................................	Malignant neoplasms............................	416,509	2................................	Malignant neoplasms............................	598,038
3................................	Cerebrovascular diseases	170,225	3................................	Unintentional injuries	161,374
4................................	Unintentional injuries	105,718	4................................	Chronic lower respiratory diseases[1,2]........	154,596
5................................	Chronic obstructive pulmonary diseases[1]	56,050	5................................	Cerebrovascular diseases	142,142
6................................	Pneumonia and influenza[2]	54,619	6................................	Alzheimer's disease..............................	116,103
7................................	Diabetes mellitus..................................	34,851	7................................	Diabetes mellitus[3]................................	80,058
8................................	Chronic liver disease and cirrhosis	30,583	8................................	Influenza and pneumonia[2]......................	51,537
9................................	Atherosclerosis	29,449	9................................	Nephritis, nephrotic syndrome and nephrosis[3] ...	50,046
10................................	Suicide..	26,869	10................................	Suicide..	44,965
Male			**Male**		
	All causes..	1,075,078		All causes..	1,400,232
1................................	Diseases of heart	405,661	1................................	Diseases of heart	339,265
2................................	Malignant neoplasms............................	225,948	2................................	Malignant neoplasms............................	314,571
3................................	Unintentional injuries	74,180	3................................	Unintentional injuries	103,864
4................................	Cerebrovascular diseases	69,973	4................................	Chronic lower respiratory diseases[1,2]........	73,045
5................................	Chronic obstructive pulmonary diseases[1]	38,625	5................................	Cerebrovascular diseases	59,355
6................................	Pneumonia and influenza[2]	27,574	6................................	Diabetes mellitus[3]................................	43,763
7................................	Suicide..	20,505	7................................	Alzheimer's disease..............................	35,372
8................................	Chronic liver disease and cirrhosis	19,768	8................................	Suicide..	34,727
9................................	Homicide...	18,779	9................................	Chronic liver disease and cirrhosis	25,818
10................................	Diabetes mellitus..................................	14,325	10................................	Nephritis, nephrotic syndrome and nephrosis[3] ...	25,399
Female			**Female**		
	All causes..	914,763		All causes..	1,344,016
1................................	Diseases of heart	355,424	1................................	Diseases of heart	295,995
2................................	Malignant neoplasms............................	190,561	2................................	Malignant neoplasms............................	283,467
3................................	Cerebrovascular diseases	100,252	3................................	Cerebrovascular diseases	82,787
4................................	Unintentional injuries	31,538	4................................	Chronic lower respiratory diseases[1,2]........	81,551
5................................	Pneumonia and influenza[2]	27,045	5................................	Alzheimer's disease..............................	80,731
6................................	Diabetes mellitus..................................	20,526	6................................	Unintentional injuries	57,510
7................................	Atherosclerosis	17,848	7................................	Diabetes mellitus[3]................................	36,295
8................................	Chronic obstructive pulmonary diseases[1]	17,425	8................................	Influenza and pneumonia[2]......................	26,526
9................................	Chronic liver disease and cirrhosis	10,815	9................................	Nephritis, nephrotic syndrome and nephrosis[3] ...	24,647
10................................	Certain conditions originating in the perinatal period..................................	9,815	10................................	Septicemia	20,935
White			**White**		
	All causes..	1,738,607		All causes..	2,323,094
1................................	Diseases of heart	683,347	1................................	Diseases of heart	539,220
2................................	Malignant neoplasms............................	368,162	2................................	Malignant neoplasms............................	505,971
3................................	Cerebrovascular diseases	148,734	3................................	Chronic lower respiratory diseases[1,2]........	140,769
4................................	Unintentional injuries	90,122	4................................	Unintentional injuries	137,289
5................................	Chronic obstructive pulmonary diseases[1]	52,375	5................................	Cerebrovascular diseases	117,806
6................................	Pneumonia and influenza[2]	48,369	6................................	Alzheimer's disease..............................	104,638
7................................	Diabetes mellitus..................................	28,868	7................................	Diabetes mellitus[3]................................	61,934
8................................	Atherosclerosis	27,069	8................................	Influenza and pneumonia[2]......................	43,429
9................................	Chronic liver disease and cirrhosis	25,240	9................................	Suicide..	40,164
10................................	Suicide..	24,829	10................................	Nephritis, nephrotic syndrome and nephrosis[3] ...	39,005
Black or African American			**Black or African American**		
	All causes..	233,135		All causes..	331,788
1................................	Diseases of heart	72,956	1................................	Diseases of heart	77,729
2................................	Malignant neoplasms............................	45,037	2................................	Malignant neoplasms............................	70,628
3................................	Cerebrovascular diseases	20,135	3................................	Unintentional injuries	18,588
4................................	Unintentional injuries	13,480	4................................	Cerebrovascular diseases	18,382
5................................	Homicide...	10,172	5................................	Diabetes mellitus[3]................................	14,254
6................................	Certain conditions originating in the perinatal period..................................	6,961	6................................	Chronic lower respiratory diseases[1,2]........	10,989
7................................	Pneumonia and influenza[2]	5,648	7................................	Homicide...	9,995
8................................	Diabetes mellitus..................................	5,544	8................................	Nephritis, nephrotic syndrome and nephrosis[3] ...	9,305
9................................	Chronic liver disease and cirrhosis	4,790	9................................	Alzheimer's disease..............................	8,669
10................................	Nephritis, nephrotic syndrome and nephrosis	3,416	10................................	Septicemia	6,744

NOTE: Starting with 2003 data (shown in spreadsheet version), some states began to collect information on more than one race on the death certificate, according to 1997 Office of Management and Budget (OMB) standards. The multiple-race data for these states were bridged to the single-race categories of the 1977 OMB standards, for comparability with other states. The race groups White, Black, Asian or Pacific Islander, and American Indian or Alaska Native include persons of Hispanic and non-Hispanic origin. Persons of Hispanic origin may be of any race.

NA = Not available. Complete coverage of all states for the Hispanic origin variable began in 1997.

[1]Between 1998 and 1999, the cause of death title for Chronic obstructive pulmonary diseases (COPD) in the *International Classification of Diseases, 9th Revision* (*ICD–9*) was renamed Chronic lower respiratory diseases (CLRD) in *ICD–10*.

[2]Starting with 1999 data, the rules for selecting CLRD and Pneumonia as the underlying cause of death changed, resulting in an increase in the number of deaths for CLRD and a decrease in the number of deaths for Pneumonia. Therefore, trend data for these two causes of death should be interpreted with caution.

[3]Starting with 2011 data, the rules for selecting Renal failure as the underlying cause of death were changed, affecting the number of deaths in the Nephritis, nephrotic syndrome and nephrosis and Diabetes categories. These changes directly affect deaths with mention of Renal failure and other associated conditions, such as Diabetes mellitus with renal complications. The result is a decrease in the number of deaths for Nephritis, nephrotic syndrome and nephrosis and an increase in the number of deaths for Diabetes mellitus. Therefore, trend data for these two causes of death should be interpreted with caution. For more information, see Technical Notes in "Deaths: Final Data for 2011," available from: https://www.cdc.gov/nchs/data/nvsr/nvsr63/nvsr63_03.pdf.

Table 2-17. Leading Causes of Death and Numbers of Death, by Sex, Race, and Hispanic Origin, 1980 and 2016—*Continued*

(Number; data based on death certificates.)

Sex, race, Hispanic origin, and rank order	1980 Cause of death	Deaths	Sex, race, Hispanic origin, and rank order	2016 Cause of death	Deaths
American Indian or Alaska Native			**American Indian or Alaska Native**		
	All causes..........................	6,923		All causes..........................	19,708
1...................................	Diseases of heart	1,494	1...................................	Diseases of heart	3,508
2...................................	Unintentional injuries	1,290	2...................................	Malignant neoplasms...................	3,409
3...................................	Malignant neoplasms...................	770	3...................................	Unintentional injuries	2,265
4...................................	Chronic liver disease and cirrhosis	410	4...................................	Diabetes mellitus[3]	1,125
5...................................	Cerebrovascular diseases	322	5...................................	Chronic liver disease and cirrhosis	1,081
6...................................	Pneumonia and influenza[2]	257	6...................................	Chronic lower respiratory diseases[1,2]	888
7...................................	Homicide..............................	217	7...................................	Cerebrovascular diseases	664
8...................................	Diabetes mellitus......................	210	8...................................	Suicide................................	629
9...................................	Certain conditions originating in the perinatal period...................	199	9...................................	Alzheimer's disease	397
10..................................	Suicide................................	181	10..................................	Influenza and pneumonia[2]..............	377
Asian or Pacific Islander			**Asian or Pacific Islander**		
	All causes..........................	11,071		All causes..........................	69,658
1...................................	Diseases of heart	3,265	1...................................	Malignant neoplasms...................	18,030
2...................................	Malignant neoplasms...................	2,522	2...................................	Diseases of heart	14,803
3...................................	Cerebrovascular diseases	1,028	3...................................	Cerebrovascular diseases	5,290
4...................................	Unintentional injuries	810	4...................................	Unintentional injuries	3,232
5...................................	Pneumonia and influenza[2]	342	5...................................	Diabetes mellitus[3]...................	2,745
6...................................	Suicide................................	249	6...................................	Alzheimer's disease	2,399
7...................................	Certain conditions originating in the perinatal period...................	246	7...................................	Influenza and pneumonia[2].............	2,161
8...................................	Diabetes mellitus......................	227	8...................................	Chronic lower respiratory diseases[1,2]	1,950
9...................................	Homicide..............................	211	9...................................	Suicide................................	1,402
10..................................	Chronic obstructive pulmonary diseases[1]	207	10..................................	Nephritis, nephrotic syndrome and nephrosis[3] ...	1,378
Hispanic or Latino			**Hispanic or Latino**		
	NA	NA		All causes..........................	188,254
1...................................	NA	NA	1...................................	Malignant neoplasms...................	39,263
2...................................	NA	NA	2...................................	Diseases of heart	37,799
3...................................	NA	NA	3...................................	Unintentional injuries	15,711
4...................................	NA	NA	4...................................	Cerebrovascular diseases	10,283
5...................................	NA	NA	5...................................	Diabetes mellitus[3]...................	8,546
6...................................	NA	NA	6...................................	Alzheimer's disease	6,833
7...................................	NA	NA	7...................................	Chronic liver disease and cirrhosis	6,141
8...................................	NA	NA	8...................................	Chronic lower respiratory diseases[1,2]	5,287
9...................................	NA	NA	9...................................	Nephritis, nephrotic syndrome and nephrosis[3] ...	3,775
10..................................	NA	NA	10..................................	Suicide................................	3,668
White, not Hispanic or Latino			**White, not Hispanic or Latino**		
	NA	NA		All causes..........................	2,133,463
1...................................	NA	NA	1...................................	Diseases of heart	500,631
2...................................	NA	NA	2...................................	Malignant neoplasms...................	466,467
3...................................	NA	NA	3...................................	Chronic lower respiratory diseases[1,2]	135,268
4...................................	NA	NA	4...................................	Unintentional injuries	121,641
5...................................	NA	NA	5...................................	Cerebrovascular diseases	107,491
6...................................	NA	NA	6...................................	Alzheimer's disease	97,779
7...................................	NA	NA	7...................................	Diabetes mellitus[3]...................	53,399
8...................................	NA	NA	8...................................	Influenza and pneumonia[2].............	39,748
9...................................	NA	NA	9...................................	Suicide................................	36,531
10..................................	NA	NA	10..................................	Nephritis, nephrotic syndrome and nephrosis[3] ...	35,248
Black, not Hispanic or Latino			**Black, not Hispanic or Latino**		
	NA	NA		All causes..........................	326,810
1...................................	NA	NA	1...................................	Diseases of heart	76,608
2...................................	NA	NA	2...................................	Malignant neoplasms...................	69,725
3...................................	NA	NA	3...................................	Cerebrovascular diseases	18,189
4...................................	NA	NA	4...................................	Unintentional injuries	18,089
5...................................	NA	NA	5...................................	Diabetes mellitus[3]	14,053
6...................................	NA	NA	6...................................	Chronic lower respiratory diseases[1,2]	10,838
7...................................	NA	NA	7...................................	Homicide..............................	9,860
8...................................	NA	NA	8...................................	Nephritis, nephrotic syndrome and nephrosis[3] ...	9,200
9...................................	NA	NA	9...................................	Alzheimer's disease..................	8,577
10..................................	NA	NA	10..................................	Septicemia............................	6,684

NOTE: Starting with 2003 data (shown in spreadsheet version), some states began to collect information on more than one race on the death certificate, according to 1997 Office of Management and Budget (OMB) standards. The multiple-race data for these states were bridged to the single-race categories of the 1977 OMB standards, for comparability with other states. The race groups White, Black, Asian or Pacific Islander, and American Indian or Alaska Native include persons of Hispanic and non-Hispanic origin. Persons of Hispanic origin may be of any race.

NA = Not available. Complete coverage of all states for the Hispanic origin variable began in 1997.

[1]Between 1998 and 1999, the cause of death title for Chronic obstructive pulmonary diseases (COPD) in the *International Classification of Diseases, 9th Revision* (*ICD–9*) was renamed Chronic lower respiratory diseases (CLRD) in *ICD–10*.

[2]Starting with 1999 data, the rules for selecting CLRD and Pneumonia as the underlying cause of death changed, resulting in an increase in the number of deaths for CLRD and a decrease in the number of deaths for Pneumonia. Therefore, trend data for these two causes of death should be interpreted with caution.

[3]Starting with 2011 data, the rules for selecting Renal failure as the underlying cause of death were changed, affecting the number of deaths in the Nephritis, nephrotic syndrome and nephrosis and Diabetes categories. These changes directly affect deaths with mention of Renal failure and other associated conditions, such as Diabetes mellitus with renal complications. The result is a decrease in the number of deaths for Nephritis, nephrotic syndrome and nephrosis and an increase in the number of deaths for Diabetes mellitus. Therefore, trend data for these two causes of death should be interpreted with caution. For more information, see Technical Notes in "Deaths: Final Data for 2011," available from: https://www.cdc.gov/nchs/data/nvsr/nvsr63/nvsr63_03.pdf.

Table 2-17. Leading Causes of Death and Numbers of Death, by Sex, Race, and Hispanic Origin, 1980 and 2016—*Continued*

(Number; data based on death certificates.)

Sex, race, Hispanic origin, and rank order	1980		Sex, race, Hispanic origin, and rank order	2016	
	Cause of death	Deaths		Cause of death	Deaths
White male			**White male**		
	All causes............	933,878		All causes............	1,181,931
1............	Diseases of heart	364,679	1............	Diseases of heart	288,505
2............	Malignant neoplasms............	198,188	2............	Malignant neoplasms............	267,895
3............	Unintentional injuries............	62,963	3............	Unintentional injuries............	87,515
4............	Cerebrovascular diseases	60,095	4............	Chronic lower respiratory diseases[1,2]............	65,840
5............	Chronic obstructive pulmonary diseases[1]............	35,977	5............	Cerebrovascular diseases	48,523
6............	Pneumonia and influenza[2]............	23,810	6............	Diabetes mellitus[3]............	34,628
7............	Suicide............	18,901	7............	Alzheimer's disease............	32,046
8............	Chronic liver disease and cirrhosis	16,407	8............	Suicide............	31,032
9............	Diabetes mellitus............	12,125	9............	Chronic liver disease and cirrhosis	22,770
10............	Atherosclerosis............	10,543	10............	Influenza and pneumonia[2]............	20,930
Black or African American male			**Black or African American male**		
	All causes............	130,138		All causes............	171,674
1............	Diseases of heart	37,877	1............	Diseases of heart	40,708
2............	Malignant neoplasms............	25,861	2............	Malignant neoplasms............	35,709
3............	Unintentional injuries............	9,701	3............	Unintentional injuries............	12,817
4............	Cerebrovascular diseases	9,194	4............	Homicide............	8,650
5............	Homicide............	8,274	5............	Cerebrovascular diseases	8,225
6............	Certain conditions originating in the perinatal period............	3,869	6............	Diabetes mellitus[3]............	7,087
7............	Pneumonia and influenza[2]............	3,386	7............	Chronic lower respiratory diseases[1,2]............	5,599
8............	Chronic liver disease and cirrhosis	3,020	8............	Nephritis, nephrotic syndrome and nephrosis[3]...	4,405
9............	Chronic obstructive pulmonary diseases[1]............	2,429	9............	Septicemia............	3,110
10............	Diabetes mellitus............	2,010	10............	Essential hypertension and hypertensive renal disease............	2,851
American Indian or Alaska Native male			**American Indian or Alaska Native male**		
	All causes............	4,193		All causes............	10,945
1............	Unintentional injuries............	946	1............	Diseases of heart	2,054
2............	Diseases of heart	917	2............	Malignant neoplasms............	1,825
3............	Malignant neoplasms............	408	3............	Unintentional injuries............	1,516
4............	Chronic liver disease and cirrhosis	239	4............	Diabetes mellitus[3]............	605
5............	Cerebrovascular diseases	163	5............	Chronic liver disease and cirrhosis	594
6............	Homicide............	162	6............	Suicide............	482
7............	Pneumonia and influenza[2]............	148	7............	Chronic lower respiratory diseases[1,2]............	451
8............	Suicide............	147	8............	Cerebrovascular diseases	302
9............	Certain conditions originating in the perinatal period............	107	9............	Homicide............	233
10............	Diabetes mellitus............	86	10............	Influenza and pneumonia[2]............	186
Asian or Pacific Islander male			**Asian or Pacific Islander male**		
	All causes............	6,809		All causes............	35,682
1............	Diseases of heart	2,174	1............	Malignant neoplasms............	9,142
2............	Malignant neoplasms............	1,485	2............	Diseases of heart	7,998
3............	Unintentional injuries............	556	3............	Cerebrovascular diseases	2,305
4............	Cerebrovascular diseases	521	4............	Unintentional injuries............	2,016
5............	Pneumonia and influenza[2]............	227	5............	Diabetes mellitus[3]............	1,443
6............	Suicide............	159	6............	Chronic lower respiratory diseases[1,2]............	1,155
7............	Chronic obstructive pulmonary diseases[1]............	158	7............	Influenza and pneumonia[2]............	1,134
8............	Homicide............	151	8............	Suicide............	1,007
9............	Certain conditions originating in the perinatal period............	128	9............	Alzheimer's disease............	718
10............	Diabetes mellitus............	103	10............	Nephritis, nephrotic syndrome and nephrosis[3] ...	681
Hispanic or Latino male			**Hispanic or Latino male**		
	NA	NA		All causes............	103,532
1............	NA	NA	1............	Diseases of heart	20,945
2............	NA	NA	2............	Malignant neoplasms............	20,504
3............	NA	NA	3............	Unintentional injuries............	11,510
4............	NA	NA	4............	Cerebrovascular diseases	4,798
5............	NA	NA	5............	Diabetes mellitus[3]............	4,603
6............	NA	NA	6............	Chronic liver disease and cirrhosis	4,225
7............	NA	NA	7............	Suicide............	2,944
8............	NA	NA	8............	Chronic lower respiratory diseases[1,2]............	2,759
9............	NA	NA	9............	Homicide............	2,657
10............	NA	NA	10............	Alzheimer's disease............	2,151

NOTE: Starting with 2003 data (shown in spreadsheet version), some states began to collect information on more than one race on the death certificate, according to 1997 Office of Management and Budget (OMB) standards. The multiple-race data for these states were bridged to the single-race categories of the 1977 OMB standards, for comparability with other states. The race groups White, Black, Asian or Pacific Islander, and American Indian or Alaska Native include persons of Hispanic and non-Hispanic origin. Persons of Hispanic origin may be of any race.

NA = Not available. Complete coverage of all states for the Hispanic origin variable began in 1997.

[1] Between 1998 and 1999, the cause of death title for Chronic obstructive pulmonary diseases (COPD) in the *International Classification of Diseases, 9th Revision* (*ICD–9*) was renamed Chronic lower respiratory diseases (CLRD) in *ICD–10*.

[2] Starting with 1999 data, the rules for selecting CLRD and Pneumonia as the underlying cause of death changed, resulting in an increase in the number of deaths for CLRD and a decrease in the number of deaths for Pneumonia. Therefore, trend data for these two causes of death should be interpreted with caution.

[3] Starting with 2011 data, the rules for selecting Renal failure as the underlying cause of death were changed, affecting the number of deaths in the Nephritis, nephrotic syndrome and nephrosis and Diabetes categories. These changes directly affect deaths with mention of Renal failure and other associated conditions, such as Diabetes mellitus with renal complications. The result is a decrease in the number of deaths for Nephritis, nephrotic syndrome and nephrosis and an increase in the number of deaths for Diabetes mellitus. Therefore, trend data for these two causes of death should be interpreted with caution. For more information, see Technical Notes in "Deaths: Final Data for 2011," available from: https://www.cdc.gov/nchs/data/nvsr/nvsr63/nvsr63_03.pdf.

Table 2-17. Leading Causes of Death and Numbers of Death, by Sex, Race, and Hispanic Origin, 1980 and 2016—Continued

(Number; data based on death certificates.)

Sex, race, Hispanic origin, and rank order	1980		Sex, race, Hispanic origin, and rank order	2016	
	Cause of death	Deaths		Cause of death	Deaths
White, not Hispanic or Latino male	NA	NA	**White, not Hispanic or Latino male**	All causes	1,077,362
1	NA	NA	1	Diseases of heart	266,995
2	NA	NA	2	Malignant neoplasms	247,202
3	NA	NA	3	Unintentional injuries	76,033
4	NA	NA	4	Chronic lower respiratory diseases[1,2]	62,945
5	NA	NA	5	Cerebrovascular diseases	43,713
6	NA	NA	6	Diabetes mellitus[3]	30,010
7	NA	NA	7	Alzheimer's disease	29,886
8	NA	NA	8	Suicide	28,110
9	NA	NA	9	Influenza and pneumonia[2]	19,033
10	NA	NA	10	Chronic liver disease and cirrhosis	18,522
Black, not Hispanic or Latino male	NA	NA	**Black, not Hispanic or Latino male**	All causes	168,750
1	NA	NA	1	Diseases of heart	40,044
2	NA	NA	2	Malignant neoplasms	35,215
3	NA	NA	3	Unintentional injuries	12,453
4	NA	NA	4	Homicide	8,532
5	NA	NA	5	Cerebrovascular diseases	8,115
6	NA	NA	6	Diabetes mellitus[3]	6,976
7	NA	NA	7	Chronic lower respiratory diseases[1,2]	5,519
8	NA	NA	8	Nephritis, nephrotic syndrome and nephrosis[3]	4,348
9	NA	NA	9	Septicemia	3,074
10	NA	NA	10	Essential hypertension and hypertensive renal disease	2,805
White female	All causes	804,729	**White female**	All causes	1,141,163
1	Diseases of heart	318,668	1	Diseases of heart	250,715
2	Malignant neoplasms	169,974	2	Malignant neoplasms	238,076
3	Cerebrovascular diseases	88,639	3	Chronic lower respiratory diseases[1,2]	74,929
4	Unintentional injuries	27,159	4	Alzheimer's disease	72,592
5	Pneumonia and influenza[2]	24,559	5	Cerebrovascular diseases	69,283
6	Diabetes mellitus	16,743	6	Unintentional injuries	49,774
7	Atherosclerosis	16,526	7	Diabetes mellitus[3]	27,306
8	Chronic obstructive pulmonary diseases[1]	16,398	8	Influenza and pneumonia[2]	22,499
9	Chronic liver disease and cirrhosis	8,833	9	Nephritis, nephrotic syndrome and nephrosis[3]	18,868
10	Certain conditions originating in the perinatal period	6,512	10	Septicemia	16,726
Black or African American female	All causes	102,997	**Black or African American female**	All causes	160,114
1	Diseases of heart	35,079	1	Diseases of heart	37,021
2	Malignant neoplasms	19,176	2	Malignant neoplasms	34,919
3	Cerebrovascular diseases	10,941	3	Cerebrovascular diseases	10,157
4	Unintentional injuries	3,779	4	Diabetes mellitus[3]	7,167
5	Diabetes mellitus	3,534	5	Alzheimer's disease	6,186
6	Certain conditions originating in the perinatal period	3,092	6	Unintentional injuries	5,771
7	Pneumonia and influenza[2]	2,262	7	Chronic lower respiratory diseases[1,2]	5,390
8	Homicide	1,898	8	Nephritis, nephrotic syndrome and nephrosis[3]	4,900
9	Chronic liver disease and cirrhosis	1,770	9	Septicemia	3,634
10	Nephritis, nephrotic syndrome and nephrosis	1,722	10	Essential hypertension and hypertensive renal disease	3,154
American Indian or Alaska Native female	All causes	2,730	**American Indian or Alaska Native female**	All causes	8,763
1	Diseases of heart	577	1	Malignant neoplasms	1,584
2	Malignant neoplasms	362	2	Diseases of heart	1,454
3	Unintentional injuries	344	3	Unintentional injuries	749
4	Chronic liver disease and cirrhosis	171	4	Diabetes mellitus[3]	520
5	Cerebrovascular diseases	159	5	Chronic liver disease and cirrhosis	487
6	Diabetes mellitus	124	6	Chronic lower respiratory diseases[1,2]	437
7	Pneumonia and influenza[2]	109	7	Cerebrovascular diseases	362
8	Certain conditions originating in the perinatal period	92	8	Alzheimer's disease	272
9	Nephritis, nephrotic syndrome and nephrosis	56	9	Influenza and pneumonia[2]	191
10	Homicide	55	10	Nephritis, nephrotic syndrome and nephrosis[3]	182

NOTE: Starting with 2003 data (shown in spreadsheet version), some states began to collect information on more than one race on the death certificate, according to 1997 Office of Management and Budget (OMB) standards. The multiple-race data for these states were bridged to the single-race categories of the 1977 OMB standards, for comparability with other states. The race groups White, Black, Asian or Pacific Islander, and American Indian or Alaska Native include persons of Hispanic and non-Hispanic origin. Persons of Hispanic origin may be of any race.

NA = Not available. Complete coverage of all states for the Hispanic origin variable began in 1997.

[1]Between 1998 and 1999, the cause of death title for Chronic obstructive pulmonary diseases (COPD) in the *International Classification of Diseases, 9th Revision* (*ICD–9*) was renamed Chronic lower respiratory diseases (CLRD) in *ICD–10*.

[2]Starting with 1999 data, the rules for selecting CLRD and Pneumonia as the underlying cause of death changed, resulting in an increase in the number of deaths for CLRD and a decrease in the number of deaths for Pneumonia. Therefore, trend data for these two causes of death should be interpreted with caution.

[3]Starting with 2011 data, the rules for selecting Renal failure as the underlying cause of death were changed, affecting the number of deaths in the Nephritis, nephrotic syndrome and nephrosis and Diabetes categories. These changes directly affect deaths with mention of Renal failure and other associated conditions, such as Diabetes mellitus with renal complications. The result is a decrease in the number of deaths for Nephritis, nephrotic syndrome and nephrosis and an increase in the number of deaths for Diabetes mellitus. Therefore, trend data for these two causes of death should be interpreted with caution. For more information, see Technical Notes in "Deaths: Final Data for 2011," available from: https://www.cdc.gov/nchs/data/nvsr/nvsr63/nvsr63_03.pdf.

Table 2-17. Leading Causes of Death and Numbers of Death, by Sex, Race, and Hispanic Origin, 1980 and 2016—*Continued*

(Number; data based on death certificates.)

Sex, race, Hispanic origin, and rank order	1980		Sex, race, Hispanic origin, and rank order	2016	
	Cause of death	Deaths		Cause of death	Deaths
Asian or Pacific Islander female			**Asian or Pacific Islander female**		
	All causes	4,262		All causes	33,976
1	Diseases of heart	1,091	1	Malignant neoplasms	8,888
2	Malignant neoplasms	1,037	2	Diseases of heart	6,805
3	Cerebrovascular diseases	507	3	Cerebrovascular diseases	2,985
4	Unintentional injuries	254	4	Alzheimer's disease	1,681
5	Diabetes mellitus	124	5	Diabetes mellitus[3]	1,302
6	Certain conditions originating in the perinatal period.	118	6	Unintentional injuries	1,216
7	Pneumonia and influenza[2]	115	7	Influenza and pneumonia[2]	1,027
8	Congenital anomalies	104	8	Chronic lower respiratory diseases[1,2] ...	795
9	Suicide	90	9	Essential hypertension and hypertensive renal disease.	744
10	Homicide	60	10	Nephritis, nephrotic syndrome and nephrosis[3] ...	697
Hispanic or Latina female			**Hispanic or Latina female**		
	NA	NA		All causes	84,722
1	NA	NA	1	Malignant neoplasms	18,759
2	NA	NA	2	Diseases of heart	16,854
3	NA	NA	3	Cerebrovascular diseases	5,485
4	NA	NA	4	Alzheimer's disease	4,682
5	NA	NA	5	Unintentional injuries	4,201
6	NA	NA	6	Diabetes mellitus[3]	3,943
7	NA	NA	7	Chronic lower respiratory diseases[1,2]	2,528
8	NA	NA	8	Chronic liver disease and cirrhosis	1,916
9	NA	NA	9	Nephritis, nephrotic syndrome and nephrosis[3] ...	1,844
10	NA	NA	10	Influenza and pneumonia[2]	1,764
White, not Hispanic or Latina female			**White, not Hispanic or Latina female**		
	NA	NA		All causes	1,056,101
1	NA	NA	1	Diseases of heart	233,636
2	NA	NA	2	Malignant neoplasms	219,265
3	NA	NA	3	Chronic lower respiratory diseases[1,2] ...	72,323
4	NA	NA	4	Alzheimer's disease	67,893
5	NA	NA	5	Cerebrovascular diseases	63,778
6	NA	NA	6	Unintentional injuries	45,608
7	NA	NA	7	Diabetes mellitus[3]	23,389
8	NA	NA	8	Influenza and pneumonia[2]	20,715
9	NA	NA	9	Nephritis, nephrotic syndrome and nephrosis[3] ...	17,032
10	NA	NA	10	Septicemia	15,389
Black, not Hispanic or Latina female			**Black, not Hispanic or Latina female**		
	NA	NA		All causes	158,060
1	NA	NA	1	Diseases of heart	36,564
2	NA	NA	2	Malignant neoplasms	34,510
3	NA	NA	3	Cerebrovascular diseases	10,074
4	NA	NA	4	Diabetes mellitus[3]	7,077
5	NA	NA	5	Alzheimer's disease	6,126
6	NA	NA	6	Unintentional injuries	5,636
7	NA	NA	7	Chronic lower respiratory diseases[1,2] ...	5,319
8	NA	NA	8	Nephritis, nephrotic syndrome and nephrosis[3] ...	4,852
9	NA	NA	9	Septicemia	3,610
10	NA	NA	10	Essential hypertension and hypertensive renal disease.	3,119

NOTE: Starting with 2003 data (shown in spreadsheet version), some states began to collect information on more than one race on the death certificate, according to 1997 Office of Management and Budget (OMB) standards. The multiple-race data for these states were bridged to the single-race categories of the 1977 OMB standards, for comparability with other states. The race groups White, Black, Asian or Pacific Islander, and American Indian or Alaska Native include persons of Hispanic and non-Hispanic origin. Persons of Hispanic origin may be of any race.

NA = Not available. Complete coverage of all states for the Hispanic origin variable began in 1997.

[1]Between 1998 and 1999, the cause of death title for Chronic obstructive pulmonary diseases (COPD) in the *International Classification of Diseases, 9th Revision* (*ICD–9*) was renamed Chronic lower respiratory diseases (CLRD) in *ICD–10*.

[2]Starting with 1999 data, the rules for selecting CLRD and Pneumonia as the underlying cause of death changed, resulting in an increase in the number of deaths for CLRD and a decrease in the number of deaths for Pneumonia. Therefore, trend data for these two causes of death should be interpreted with caution.

[3]Starting with 2011 data, the rules for selecting Renal failure as the underlying cause of death were changed, affecting the number of deaths in the Nephritis, nephrotic syndrome and nephrosis and Diabetes categories. These changes directly affect deaths with mention of Renal failure and other associated conditions, such as Diabetes mellitus with renal complications. The result is a decrease in the number of deaths for Nephritis, nephrotic syndrome and nephrosis and an increase in the number of deaths for Diabetes mellitus. Therefore, trend data for these two causes of death should be interpreted with caution. For more information, see Technical Notes in "Deaths: Final Data for 2011," available from: https://www.cdc.gov/nchs/data/nvsr/nvsr63/nvsr63_03.pdf.

Table 2-18. Leading Causes of Death and Numbers of Deaths, by Age, 1980 and 2016

(Number; data are based on death certificates.)

	1980			2016	
Age and rank order	Cause of death	Deaths	Age and rank order	Cause of death	Deaths
Under 1 year			**Under 1 year**		
	All causes	45,526		All causes	23,161
1	Congenital anomalies	9,220	1	Congenital malformations, deformations and chromosomal abnormalities	4,816
2	Sudden infant death syndrome	5,510	2	Disorders related to short gestation and low birthweight	3,927
3	Respiratory distress syndrome	4,989	3	Sudden infant death syndrome	1,500
4	Disorders relating to short gestation and unspecified low birthweight	3,648	4	Newborn affected by maternal complications of pregnancy	1,402
5	Newborn affected by maternal complications of pregnancy	1,572	5	Unintentional injuries	1,219
6	Intrauterine hypoxia and birth asphyxia	1,497	6	Newborn affected by complications of placenta, cord, and membranes	841
7	Unintentional injuries	1,166	7	Bacterial sepsis of newborn	583
8	Birth trauma	1,058	8	Respiratory distress of newborn	488
9	Pneumonia and influenza[1]	1,012	9	Diseases of circulatory system	460
10	Newborn affected by complications of placenta, cord, and membranes	985	10	Neonatal hemorrhage	398
1 to 4 years			**1 to 4 years**		
	All causes	8,187		All causes	4,045
1	Unintentional injuries	3,313	1	Unintentional injuries	1,261
2	Congenital anomalies	1,026	2	Congenital malformations, deformations and chromosomal abnormalities	433
3	Malignant neoplasms	573	3	Malignant neoplasms	377
4	Diseases of heart	338	4	Homicide	339
5	Homicide	319	5	Diseases of heart	118
6	Pneumonia and influenza[1]	267	6	Influenza and pneumonia[1]	103
7	Meningitis	223	7	Septicemia	70
8	Meningococcal infection	110	8	Conditions originating in perinatal period	60
9	Certain conditions originating in the perinatal period	84	9	Cerebrovascular diseases	55
10	Septicemia	71	10	Chronic lower respiratory diseases[1,2]	51
5 to 14 years			**5 to 14 years**		
	All causes	10,689		All causes	5,503
1	Unintentional injuries	5,224	1	Unintentional injuries	1,634
2	Malignant neoplasms	1,497	2	Malignant neoplasms	880
3	Congenital anomalies	561	3	Suicide	443
4	Homicide	415	4	Congenital malformations, deformations and chromosomal abnormalities	349
5	Diseases of heart	330	5	Homicide	286
6	Pneumonia and influenza[1]	194	6	Diseases of heart	188
7	Suicide	142	7	Chronic lower respiratory diseases[1,2]	143
8	Benign neoplasms	104	8	Cerebrovascular diseases	88
9	Cerebrovascular diseases	95	9	Influenza and pneumonia[1]	87
10	Chronic obstructive pulmonary diseases[2]	85	10	Septicemia	71
15 to 24 years			**15 to 24 years**		
	All causes	49,027		All causes	32,575
1	Unintentional injuries	26,206	1	Unintentional injuries	13,895
2	Homicide	6,537	2	Suicide	5,723
3	Suicide	5,239	3	Homicide	5,172
4	Malignant neoplasms	2,683	4	Malignant neoplasms	1,431
5	Diseases of heart	1,223	5	Diseases of heart	949
6	Congenital anomalies	600	6	Congenital malformations, deformations and chromosomal abnormalities	388
7	Cerebrovascular diseases	418	7	Diabetes mellitus[3]	211
8	Pneumonia and influenza[1]	348	8	Chronic lower respiratory diseases[1,2]	206
9	Chronic obstructive pulmonary diseases[2]	141	9	Influenza and pneumonia[1]	189
10	Anemias	133	10	Pregnancy, childbirth and puerperium	184
25 to 44 years			**25 to 44 years**		
	All causes	108,658		All causes	135,408
1	Unintentional injuries	26,722	1	Unintentional injuries	44,959
2	Malignant neoplasms	17,551	2	Malignant neoplasms	14,694
3	Diseases of heart	14,513	3	Suicide	14,396
4	Homicide	10,983	4	Diseases of heart	13,922
5	Suicide	9,855	5	Homicide	8,745
6	Chronic liver disease and cirrhosis	4,782	6	Chronic liver disease and cirrhosis	3,776
7	Cerebrovascular diseases	3,154	7	Diabetes mellitus[3]	2,841
8	Diabetes mellitus	1,472	8	Cerebrovascular diseases	2,426
9	Pneumonia and influenza[1]	1,467	9	Human immunodeficiency virus (HIV) disease	1,517
10	Congenital anomalies	817	10	Influenza and pneumonia[1]	1,346

[1]Starting with 1999 data, the rules for selecting CLRD and Pneumonia as the underlying cause of death changed, resulting in an increase in the number of deaths for CLRD and a decrease in the number of deaths for pneumonia. Therefore, trend data for these two causes of death should be interpreted with caution.

[2]Between 1998 and 1999, the cause of death title for Chronic obstructive pulmonary diseases in the *ICD–9* was renamed to Chronic lower respiratory diseases (CLRD) in *ICD–10*.

[3]Starting with 2011 data, the rules for selecting Renal failure as the underlying cause of death were changed, affecting the number of deaths in the Nephritis, nephrotic syndrome and nephrosis and Diabetes categories. These changes directly affect deaths with mention of Renal failure and other associated conditions, such as Diabetes mellitus with renal complications. The result is a decrease in the number of deaths for Nephritis, nephrotic syndrome and nephrosis and an increase in the number of deaths for Diabetes mellitus. Therefore, trend data for these two causes of death should be interpreted with caution.

Table 2-18. Leading Causes of Death and Numbers of Deaths, by Age, 1980 and 2016—*Continued*

(Number; data are based on death certificates.)

	1980			2016	
Age and rank order	Cause of death	Deaths	Age and rank order	Cause of death	Deaths
45 to 64 years			**45 to 64 years**		
	All causes...	425,338		All causes..	539,961
1.............................	Diseases of heart..	148,322	1.............................	Malignant neoplasms.................................	157,655
2.............................	Malignant neoplasms..................................	135,675	2.............................	Diseases of heart......................................	112,637
3.............................	Cerebrovascular diseases...........................	19,909	3.............................	Unintentional injuries................................	45,237
4.............................	Unintentional injuries................................	18,140	4.............................	Chronic lower respiratory diseases[1,2].......	22,117
5.............................	Chronic liver disease and cirrhosis.............	16,089	5.............................	Chronic liver disease and cirrhosis.............	21,812
6.............................	Chronic obstructive pulmonary diseases[2]...	11,514	6.............................	Diabetes mellitus[3].....................................	20,518
7.............................	Diabetes mellitus.......................................	7,977	7.............................	Cerebrovascular diseases...........................	17,663
8.............................	Suicide...	7,079	8.............................	Suicide...	16,196
9.............................	Pneumonia and influenza[1]..........................	5,804	9.............................	Septicemia...	8,413
10...........................	Homicide..	4,019	10...........................	Nephritis, nephrotic syndrome and nephrosis[3]........	7,790
65 years and over			**65 years and over**		
	All causes	1,341,848		All causes..	2,003,458
1.............................	Diseases of heart..	595,406	1.............................	Diseases of heart......................................	507,118
2.............................	Malignant neoplasms..................................	258,389	2.............................	Malignant neoplasms.................................	422,927
3.............................	Cerebrovascular diseases...........................	146,417	3.............................	Chronic lower respiratory diseases[1,2].......	131,002
4.............................	Pneumonia and influenza[1]..........................	45,512	4.............................	Cerebrovascular diseases...........................	121,630
5.............................	Chronic obstructive pulmonary diseases[2]...	43,587	5.............................	Alzheimer's disease...................................	114,883
6.............................	Atherosclerosis..	28,081	6.............................	Diabetes mellitus[3].....................................	56,452
7.............................	Diabetes mellitus.......................................	25,216	7.............................	Unintentional injuries................................	53,141
8.............................	Unintentional injuries................................	24,844	8.............................	Influenza and pneumonia[1]..........................	42,479
9.............................	Nephritis, nephrotic syndrome and nephrosis......	12,968	9.............................	Nephritis, nephrotic syndrome and nephrosis[3]........	41,095
10...........................	Chronic liver disease and cirrhosis.............	9,519	10...........................	Septicemia...	30,405

[1]Starting with 1999 data, the rules for selecting CLRD and Pneumonia as the underlying cause of death changed, resulting in an increase in the number of deaths for CLRD and a decrease in the number of deaths for pneumonia. Therefore, trend data for these two causes of death should be interpreted with caution.
[2]Between 1998 and 1999, the cause of death title for Chronic obstructive pulmonary diseases in the *ICD–9* was renamed to Chronic lower respiratory diseases (CLRD) in *ICD–10*.
[3]Starting with 2011 data, the rules for selecting Renal failure as the underlying cause of death were changed, affecting the number of deaths in the Nephritis, nephrotic syndrome and nephrosis and Diabetes categories. These changes directly affect deaths with mention of Renal failure and other associated conditions, such as Diabetes mellitus with renal complications. The result is a decrease in the number of deaths for Nephritis, nephrotic syndrome and nephrosis and an increase in the number of deaths for Diabetes mellitus. Therefore, trend data for these two causes of death should be interpreted with caution.

Table 2-19. Deaths from Selected Occupational Diseases Among Persons 15 Years of Age and Over, Selected Years, 1980–2013

(Number of deaths.)

Cause of death	1980[1]	1985[1]	1990[1]	1995[1]	2000[2]	2005[2]	2006[2]	2007[2]	2008[2]	2009[2]	2010[2]	2011[2]	2012[2]	2013[2]
Multiple Cause of Death (Number of Death Certificates with Cause of Death Code(s) Mentioned)														
Angiosarcoma of liver[3]................................	NA	NA	NA	NA	16	26	23	22	17	27	29	22	29	22
Malignant mesothelioma[4]............................	699	715	874	897	2,531	2,704	2,588	2,606	2,709	2,753	2,744	2,832	2,874	2,686
Pneumoconiosis[5]...	4,151	3,783	3,644	3,151	2,859	2,425	2,308	2,189	2,155	1,993	2,028	1,890	1,850	1,859
Coal workers' pneumoconiosis....................	2,576	2,615	1,990	1,413	949	652	654	524	470	480	486	409	399	361
Asbestosis	339	534	948	1,169	1,486	1,416	1,340	1,393	1,341	1,255	1,308	1,243	1,208	1,229
Silicosis	448	334	308	242	151	160	126	122	146	121	101	88	103	111
Other (including unspecified)......................	814	321	413	343	290	222	206	163	215	158	146	166	153	170
Underlying Cause of Death														
Angiosarcoma of liver[3]................................	NA	NA	NA	NA	15	23	21	20	16	25	28	20	27	19
Malignant mesothelioma[4]............................	531	573	725	780	2,384	2,553	2,452	2,432	2,538	2,606	2,573	2,651	2,686	2,497
Pneumoconiosis	1,581	1,355	1,335	1,117	1,142	983	907	898	891	830	820	752	755	781
Coal workers' pneumoconiosis....................	982	958	734	533	389	270	266	209	183	206	213	160	158	151
Asbestosis	101	139	302	355	558	532	485	538	520	485	486	460	466	475
Silicosis	207	143	150	114	71	74	67	72	85	66	52	56	58	70
Other (including unspecified)......................	291	115	149	115	124	107	89	79	103	73	69	76	73	85

NA = Not available.
Note: Multiple cause of death includes underlying and nonunderlying causes of death. Cause-of-death titles for selected occupational diseases and corresponding code numbers according to the *International Classification of Diseases, 9th* and *10th Revisions*.
[1]For the period 1980-1998, underlying cause of death was coded according to the 9th Revision of the *International Classification of Diseases* (*ICD*).
[2]Starting with 1999 data, *ICD-10* was introduced for coding cause of death. Discontinuities exist between 1998 and 1999 due to *ICD-10* coding and classification changes.
[3]Prior to 1999, there was no discrete code for this condition.
[4]Prior to 1999, the combined *ICD-9* categories of malignant neoplasm of peritoneum and malignant neoplasm of pleura served as a crude surrogate for malignant mesothelioma category under *ICD-10*.
[5]For multiple cause of death, counts for pneumoconiosis subgroups may sum to slightly more than total pneumoconiosis due to the reporting of more than one type of pneumoconiosis on some death certificates. Multiple cause of death includes underlying and nonunderlying causes of death.

Table 2-20. Death Rates for Motor Vehicle–Related Injuries, by Sex and Age, Selected Years, 1950–2016

(Rate per 100,000 population; data are based on death certificates.)

Sex, race, Hispanic origin, and age	1950[1,2]	1960[1,2]	1970[2]	1980[2]	1985[2]	1990[2]	1995[2]	2000[3]	2005[3]	2006[3]	2007[3]	2008[3]	2009[3]	2010[3]	2011[3]	2012[3]	2013[3]	2014[3]	2015[3]	2016[3]
								Deaths per 100,000 resident population												
All Persons																				
All ages, age-adjusted[4]	24.6	23.1	27.6	22.3	18.6	18.5	16.3	15.4	15.2	15.0	14.4	12.9	11.6	11.3	11.1	11.4	10.9	10.8	11.4	12.1
All ages, crude	23.1	21.3	26.9	23.5	19.3	18.8	16.3	15.4	15.3	15.2	14.6	13.1	11.8	11.4	11.3	11.6	11.2	11.1	11.7	12.5
Under 1 year	8.4	8.1	9.8	7.0	4.9	4.9	4.7	4.4	3.6	3.5	3.0	2.5	2.4	2.0	2.4	1.8	1.7	1.7	1.8	2.3
1-14 years	9.8	8.6	10.5	8.2	7.0	6.0	5.3	4.3	3.7	3.4	3.2	2.6	2.5	2.3	2.3	2.2	2.2	2.2	2.2	2.4
1-4 years	11.5	10.0	11.5	9.2	7.2	6.3	5.2	4.2	3.9	3.7	3.4	2.9	2.9	2.8	2.6	2.9	2.7	2.5	2.6	2.6
5-14 years	8.8	7.9	10.2	7.9	6.9	5.9	5.3	4.3	3.6	3.3	3.2	2.5	2.4	2.2	2.1	2.0	2.1	2.0	2.1	2.3
15-24 years	34.4	38.0	47.2	44.8	35.7	34.1	28.9	26.9	25.7	25.7	24.5	20.6	17.6	16.6	16.2	16.1	15.2	15.3	15.9	16.6
15-19 years	29.6	33.9	43.6	43.0	33.5	33.1	28.1	26.0	23.1	22.6	21.4	17.4	15.2	13.6	13.2	12.6	11.4	11.9	12.4	12.7
20-24 years	38.8	42.9	51.3	46.6	37.6	35.0	29.7	28.0	28.3	28.9	27.7	24.0	20.2	19.7	19.1	19.3	18.8	18.3	19.2	20.2
25-34 years	24.6	24.3	30.9	29.1	23.0	23.6	19.2	17.3	18.4	18.7	17.8	16.3	14.5	14.0	13.7	14.5	13.9	13.9	14.7	16.1
35-44 years	20.3	19.3	24.9	20.9	17.2	16.9	15.3	15.3	15.5	15.4	14.9	13.4	12.2	11.6	11.3	11.8	11.4	11.1	11.9	12.9
45-64 years	25.2	23.0	26.5	18.0	15.4	15.7	14.1	14.3	14.8	14.8	14.1	13.3	12.2	11.9	11.9	12.4	12.1	12.0	12.8	13.5
45-54 years	22.2	21.4	25.5	18.6	15.2	15.6	13.8	14.2	15.1	15.3	14.9	13.7	12.7	12.0	12.3	12.6	12.2	12.1	12.8	13.4
55-64 years	29.0	25.1	27.9	17.4	15.6	15.9	14.5	14.4	14.5	14.1	13.2	12.8	11.5	11.9	11.5	12.2	11.9	11.9	12.7	13.6
65 years and over	43.1	34.7	36.2	22.5	21.7	23.1	22.6	21.4	20.1	19.0	18.7	16.9	15.8	16.0	15.9	15.7	15.1	14.8	15.3	16.0
65-74 years	39.1	31.4	32.8	19.2	17.9	18.6	17.5	16.5	16.5	15.2	14.9	13.8	12.7	12.3	13.0	13.0	12.2	11.9	12.8	13.3
75-84 years	52.7	41.8	43.5	28.1	27.4	29.1	28.4	25.7	22.9	22.2	21.7	19.2	18.6	18.8	18.3	17.9	17.8	17.5	17.5	18.9
85 years and over	45.1	37.9	34.2	27.6	26.5	31.2	31.0	30.4	27.3	25.5	25.3	23.2	20.9	23.8	21.8	22.1	21.0	20.9	21.7	21.8
Male																				
All ages, age-adjusted[4]	38.5	35.4	41.5	33.6	27.2	26.5	22.8	21.7	21.9	21.5	21.0	18.9	16.8	16.2	16.1	16.5	15.9	15.8	16.7	17.6
All ages, crude	35.4	31.8	39.7	35.3	28.0	26.7	22.4	21.3	21.8	21.6	21.0	18.9	16.9	16.3	16.3	16.6	16.1	16.0	17.0	18.0
Under 1 year	9.1	8.6	9.3	7.3	5.0	5.0	4.9	4.6	3.6	3.4	2.7	2.9	2.6	2.2	2.8	1.9	1.7	1.9	2.2	2.1
1-14 years	12.3	10.7	13.0	10.0	8.5	7.0	6.1	4.9	4.1	3.7	3.7	3.1	2.9	2.7	2.5	2.5	2.5	2.5	2.5	2.6
1-4 years	13.0	11.5	12.9	10.2	8.3	6.9	5.6	4.7	4.3	3.9	3.8	3.2	3.4	3.0	2.7	3.1	3.0	2.8	2.9	2.7
5-14 years	11.9	10.4	13.1	9.9	8.6	7.0	6.3	5.0	4.1	3.7	3.7	3.0	2.7	2.5	2.5	2.3	2.4	2.4	2.4	2.6
15-24 years	56.7	61.2	73.2	68.4	52.7	49.5	40.5	37.4	36.3	36.3	34.6	29.3	24.5	23.1	22.8	22.5	21.2	21.5	22.2	22.9
15-19 years	46.3	51.7	64.1	62.6	46.5	45.5	36.1	33.9	29.9	29.5	27.7	22.6	19.2	17.8	17.2	16.2	14.7	16.1	16.3	16.5
20-24 years	66.7	73.2	84.4	74.3	58.2	53.3	45.0	41.2	42.8	43.4	41.9	36.3	30.0	28.5	28.2	28.4	27.3	26.5	27.7	29.0
25-34 years	40.8	40.1	49.4	46.3	35.9	35.7	28.1	25.5	27.9	28.5	27.2	25.2	21.7	21.0	20.4	21.5	20.8	20.8	21.8	23.5
35-44 years	32.5	29.9	37.7	31.7	25.2	24.7	21.7	22.0	22.5	22.1	22.1	19.9	18.2	16.9	16.7	17.6	16.9	16.4	17.9	19.4
45-64 years	37.7	33.3	38.9	26.5	22.0	21.9	19.5	20.2	21.6	21.6	20.9	19.7	18.2	17.9	18.2	18.6	18.2	18.1	19.4	20.4
45-54 years	33.6	31.6	37.2	27.6	21.9	22.0	19.3	20.4	22.2	22.6	22.2	20.2	19.0	17.9	18.6	18.8	18.3	18.2	19.1	19.8
55-64 years	43.1	35.6	40.9	25.4	22.1	21.7	19.6	19.8	20.7	20.3	19.2	19.0	17.2	17.8	17.7	18.5	18.1	18.1	19.8	21.1
65 years and over	66.6	52.1	54.4	33.9	30.4	32.1	30.7	29.5	28.4	26.4	26.9	24.1	22.0	22.2	22.3	22.1	21.5	21.0	22.1	23.4
65-74 years	59.1	45.8	47.3	27.3	23.0	24.2	22.2	21.7	21.8	20.7	21.1	19.4	17.5	17.1	18.2	18.5	17.5	17.0	18.5	19.4
75-84 years	85.0	66.0	68.2	44.3	41.3	41.2	39.9	35.6	32.1	30.4	31.4	27.3	25.8	25.9	25.7	24.8	24.9	24.8	24.9	27.1
85 years and over	78.1	62.7	63.1	56.1	55.3	64.5	61.5	57.5	49.0	45.6	44.4	40.2	35.3	40.2	35.4	35.3	35.3	35.3	34.0	36.7
Female																				
All ages, age-adjusted[4]	11.5	11.7	14.9	11.8	10.7	11.0	10.3	9.5	8.9	8.8	8.2	7.2	6.7	6.5	6.3	6.5	6.2	6.1	6.4	6.9
All ages, crude	10.9	11.0	14.7	12.3	11.0	11.3	10.4	9.7	9.1	9.0	8.4	7.4	6.9	6.8	6.5	6.7	6.4	6.3	6.7	7.1
Under 1 year	7.6	7.5	10.4	6.7	4.7	4.9	4.5	4.2	3.7	3.5	3.3	2.0	2.1	1.8	1.9	1.8	1.8	1.5	1.3	2.5
1-14 years	7.2	6.3	7.9	6.3	5.4	4.9	4.4	3.7	3.1	3.1	2.8	2.2	2.2	2.0	2.0	1.9	1.9	1.8	1.9	2.1
1-4 years	10.0	8.4	10.0	8.1	6.0	5.6	4.8	3.8	3.4	3.5	3.1	2.5	2.5	2.5	2.6	2.6	2.3	2.3	2.3	2.5
5-14 years	5.7	5.4	7.2	5.7	5.1	4.7	4.2	3.6	3.0	2.9	2.6	2.0	2.0	1.8	1.8	1.7	1.8	1.6	1.8	2.0
15-24 years	12.6	15.1	21.6	20.8	18.2	17.9	16.8	15.9	14.5	14.5	13.8	11.5	10.5	9.9	9.4	9.3	8.9	8.7	9.3	9.9
15-19 years	12.9	16.0	22.7	22.8	20.1	20.0	19.7	17.5	15.9	15.4	14.8	11.8	10.9	9.2	9.0	8.9	7.9	7.6	8.4	8.8
20-24 years	12.2	14.0	20.4	18.9	16.7	16.0	13.8	14.2	13.2	13.6	12.8	11.2	10.0	10.5	9.7	9.8	9.9	9.7	10.2	10.8
25-34 years	9.3	9.2	13.0	12.2	10.1	11.5	10.2	8.8	8.9	8.8	8.5	7.4	7.2	6.9	7.0	7.4	6.9	6.8	7.5	8.5
35-44 years	8.5	9.1	12.9	10.4	9.4	9.2	9.0	8.8	8.6	8.8	7.8	7.0	6.2	6.2	6.0	6.2	5.9	5.8	6.1	6.5
45-64 years	12.6	13.1	15.3	10.3	9.5	10.1	9.0	8.7	8.4	8.3	7.7	7.2	6.5	6.3	5.9	6.4	6.3	6.2	6.4	6.9
45-54 years	10.9	11.6	14.5	10.2	9.0	9.6	8.4	8.2	8.2	8.2	7.8	7.4	6.6	6.3	6.1	6.5	6.3	6.2	6.7	7.1
55-64 years	14.9	15.2	16.2	10.5	9.9	10.8	9.9	9.5	8.8	8.5	7.5	6.9	6.3	6.3	5.7	6.4	6.2	6.1	6.1	6.6
65 years and over	21.9	20.3	23.1	15.0	15.8	17.2	17.0	15.8	14.1	13.6	12.6	11.5	11.1	11.3	10.9	10.8	10.0	9.9	10.0	10.2
65-74 years	20.6	19.0	21.6	13.0	14.0	14.1	13.7	12.3	11.1	10.5	9.6	8.9	8.5	8.2	8.4	8.2	7.5	7.5	7.8	8.0
75-84 years	25.2	23.0	27.2	18.5	19.2	21.9	21.2	19.2	16.5	16.5	15.0	13.5	13.5	13.7	12.8	12.9	12.5	12.0	11.9	12.6
85 years and over	22.1	22.0	18.0	15.2	15.0	18.3	19.3	19.3	17.6	16.4	16.5	15.3	14.0	15.9	15.1	15.5	13.7	14.1	14.4	13.8

NOTE: Starting with Health, United States, 2003, rates for 1991–1999 were revised using intercensal population estimates based on the 1990 and 2000 Censuses. For 2000, population estimates are bridged-race April 1 census counts. Starting with Health, United States, 2012, rates for 2001–2009 were revised using intercensal population estimates based on the 2000 and 2010 Censuses. For 2010, population estimates are bridged-race April 1 census counts. Rates for 2011 and beyond were computed using 2010-based postcensal estimates. Age groups were selected to minimize the presentation of unstable age-specific death rates based on small numbers of deaths and for consistency among comparison groups. For additional injury-related statistics, see Web-based Injury Statistics Query and Reporting System (WISQARS), available from: https://www.cdc.gov/injury/wisqars/index.html. Starting with 2003 data (shown in spreadsheet version), some states began to collect information on more than one race on the death certificate, according to 1997 Office of Management and Budget (OMB) standards. The multiple-race data for these states were bridged to the single-race categories of the 1977 OMB standards, for comparability with other states.
[1]Includes deaths of persons who were not residents of the 50 states and the District of Columbia.
[2]Underlying cause of death was coded according to the 6th Revision of the International Classification of Diseases (ICD) in 1950, 7th Revision in 1960, 8th Revision in 1970, and 9th Revision in 1980-1998.
[3]Starting with 1999 data, cause of death is coded according to ICD-10. Codes included were V02–V04, V09.0, V09.2, V12–V14, V19.0–V19.2, V19.4–V19.6, V20–V79, V80.3–V80.5, V81.0–V81.1, V82.0–V82.1, V83–V86, V87.0–V87.8, V88.0–V88.8, V89.0, and V89.2.
[4]Age-adjusted rates are calculated using the year 2000 standard population. Prior to 2001, age-adjusted rates were calculated using standard million proportions based on rounded population numbers. Starting with 2001 data, unrounded population numbers are used to calculate age-adjusted rates.

Table 2-20. Death Rates for Motor Vehicle–Related Injuries, by Sex and Age, Selected Years, 1950–2016—Continued

(Rate per 100,000 population; data are based on death certificates.)

Sex, race, Hispanic origin, and age	1950[1,2]	1960[1,2]	1970[2]	1980[2]	1985[2]	1990[2]	1995[2]	2000[3]	2005[3]	2006[3]	2007[3]	2008[3]	2009[3]	2010[3]	2011[3]	2012[3]	2013[3]	2014[3]	2015[3]	2016[3]
											Deaths per 100,000 resident population									
White Male[5]																				
All ages, age-adjusted[4]	37.9	34.8	40.4	33.8	27.2	26.3	22.6	21.8	22.4	22.1	21.6	19.6	17.3	16.7	16.6	17.0	16.3	16.1	17.0	17.8
All ages, crude	35.1	31.5	39.1	35.9	28.3	26.7	22.4	21.6	22.5	22.2	21.7	19.7	17.5	17.0	16.9	17.3	16.7	16.5	17.4	18.4
Under 1 year	9.1	8.8	9.1	7.0	4.6	4.8	4.3	4.2	3.4	3.3	2.9	2.9	2.5	2.0	2.5	1.9	1.7	1.8	1.9	1.6
1-14 years	12.4	10.6	12.5	9.8	8.3	6.6	5.9	4.8	4.1	3.6	3.8	3.1	2.8	2.7	2.6	2.4	2.4	2.4	2.5	2.5
15-24 years	58.3	62.7	75.2	73.8	56.5	52.5	42.4	39.6	39.2	39.3	37.4	31.7	26.6	24.6	24.6	24.5	22.9	23.0	23.3	23.9
25-34 years	39.1	38.6	47.0	46.6	35.8	35.4	27.9	25.1	28.4	28.8	27.8	26.2	21.8	21.4	20.9	22.0	21.1	20.8	22.1	23.7
35-44 years	30.9	28.4	35.2	30.7	24.3	23.7	21.1	21.8	22.8	22.6	22.2	20.3	18.5	17.4	17.0	18.0	17.3	16.6	18.0	19.2
45-64 years	36.2	31.7	36.5	25.2	20.8	20.6	18.7	19.7	21.7	21.6	21.1	20.1	18.7	18.3	18.5	19.0	18.5	18.3	19.5	20.7
65 years and over	67.1	52.1	54.2	32.7	29.9	31.4	30.1	29.4	28.7	26.6	27.0	24.5	22.3	22.7	22.8	22.6	22.1	21.5	22.7	23.7
Black or African American Male[5]																				
All ages, age-adjusted[4]	34.8	39.6	51.0	34.2	29.0	29.9	26.1	24.4	22.5	22.6	22.3	18.9	17.8	16.7	16.7	17.4	17.0	17.4	19.1	20.9
All ages, crude	37.2	33.1	44.3	31.1	27.1	28.1	24.1	22.5	21.1	21.4	21.0	18.0	16.7	15.9	15.8	16.6	16.4	16.8	18.7	20.3
Under 1 year	- - -	*	10.6	7.8	*	*	8.7	6.7	*	*	*	*	*	*	*	*	*	*	*	*
1-14 years[6]	10.4	11.2	16.3	11.4	9.7	8.9	7.5	5.5	4.4	4.8	4.0	3.1	3.5	3.0	2.7	3.2	3.3	2.9	3.2	3.3
15-24 years	42.5	46.4	58.1	34.9	32.0	36.1	33.9	30.2	27.8	26.9	26.9	22.4	18.5	19.4	17.7	17.5	17.6	18.7	21.8	23.0
25-34 years	54.4	51.0	70.4	44.9	37.7	39.5	32.2	32.6	32.1	34.4	32.0	27.0	26.9	24.9	22.4	25.6	25.1	25.7	26.7	30.2
35-44 years	46.7	43.6	59.5	41.2	34.7	33.5	28.7	27.2	25.8	25.1	27.2	23.0	21.9	19.4	20.8	20.8	20.5	21.2	23.7	27.2
45-64 years	54.6	47.8	61.7	39.5	32.9	33.3	26.2	27.1	24.1	25.2	24.0	21.5	19.3	19.1	20.2	20.8	21.1	21.1	24.5	23.8
65 years and over	52.6	48.2	53.4	42.4	35.2	36.3	36.9	32.1	29.1	26.1	27.4	22.9	22.8	20.0	21.3	21.8	18.5	19.8	19.6	24.7
American Indian or Alaska Native Male[5]																				
All ages, age-adjusted[4]	NA	NA	NA	78.9	50.9	48.3	40.7	35.8	31.5	33.5	28.6	24.1	22.7	21.1	22.5	22.2	20.0	23.4	22.8	24.5
All ages, crude	NA	NA	NA	74.6	51.7	47.6	40.1	33.6	31.3	32.2	27.3	23.5	22.0	19.8	21.8	22.2	19.0	22.2	22.1	23.5
1-14 years	NA	NA	NA	15.1	16.2	11.6	7.6	7.8	9.6	4.6	4.4	4.6	4.8	*	*	6.8	3.9	4.2	4.4	5.7
15-24 years	NA	NA	NA	126.1	77.3	75.2	69.0	56.8	44.1	47.9	40.0	37.5	35.2	31.9	30.9	27.3	26.8	27.3	24.9	29.2
25-34 years	NA	NA	NA	107.0	84.0	78.2	67.8	49.8	49.0	45.2	42.7	30.5	29.3	23.8	34.8	32.0	30.3	31.8	32.4	31.5
35-44 years	NA	NA	NA	82.8	55.8	57.0	45.2	36.3	36.9	34.3	32.0	29.3	28.5	24.5	21.9	30.4	19.8	24.2	30.3	29.7
45-64 years	NA	NA	NA	77.4	52.2	45.9	38.8	32.0	31.9	41.4	27.9	25.8	22.8	23.2	27.4	27.0	20.4	30.5	26.6	29.6
65 years and over	NA	NA	NA	97.0	*	43.0	*	48.5	27.8	37.4	38.5	24.5	22.2	26.6	23.7	*	25.8	26.8	26.3	26.0
Asian or Pacific Islander Male[5]																				
All ages, age-adjusted[4]	NA	NA	NA	19.0	17.3	17.9	14.5	10.6	9.5	9.3	9.1	7.9	6.2	6.5	6.6	5.9	6.4	6.2	6.3	6.9
All ages, crude	NA	NA	NA	17.1	16.0	15.8	12.6	9.8	8.7	8.6	8.3	7.5	5.8	6.2	6.2	5.6	5.9	6.0	6.1	6.6
1-14 years	NA	NA	NA	8.2	5.2	6.3	4.5	2.5	1.7	2.6	1.8	1.6	1.5	*	*	*	1.5	1.2	*	1.4
15-24 years	NA	NA	NA	27.2	28.1	25.7	18.5	17.0	14.5	14.9	15.7	11.6	8.8	9.6	9.3	8.9	8.1	8.6	9.7	9.1
25-34 years	NA	NA	NA	18.8	18.4	17.0	12.4	10.4	8.9	8.4	7.0	8.5	7.3	7.8	6.6	5.8	5.9	8.0	6.7	6.3
35-44 years	NA	NA	NA	13.1	12.0	12.2	9.9	6.9	6.6	6.0	6.1	6.4	4.5	4.1	4.8	3.5	5.3	4.1	3.8	5.9
45-64 years	NA	NA	NA	13.7	13.4	15.1	14.3	10.1	9.0	8.6	7.7	7.4	5.6	6.0	6.5	6.3	5.9	5.7	6.4	7.0
65 years and over	NA	NA	NA	37.3	37.3	33.6	32.1	21.1	20.8	19.7	20.9	16.1	11.9	14.6	14.9	12.5	14.3	13.1	13.5	14.5
Hispanic or Latino Male[5,7]																				
All ages, age-adjusted[4]	NA	NA	NA	NA	25.4	29.5	24.4	21.3	21.4	21.4	19.4	16.7	14.7	14.0	13.7	13.9	14.2	14.3	15.2	16.1
All ages, crude	NA	NA	NA	NA	25.6	29.2	22.4	20.1	20.8	20.9	18.6	16.1	14.2	12.8	12.9	13.1	13.3	13.5	14.4	15.3
1-14 years	NA	NA	NA	NA	7.7	7.2	5.7	4.4	4.6	4.4	4.1	2.9	3.0	2.5	2.3	2.5	2.5	2.5	2.6	2.3
15-24 years	NA	NA	NA	NA	44.9	48.2	37.1	34.7	37.6	38.1	32.8	26.9	24.1	20.2	20.7	20.3	20.5	22.0	22.8	23.7
25-34 years	NA	NA	NA	NA	31.2	41.0	28.8	24.9	28.0	27.6	25.9	24.7	20.1	18.0	17.4	19.9	18.2	19.6	21.2	23.9
35-44 years	NA	NA	NA	NA	26.3	28.0	23.2	21.6	20.9	21.6	18.6	16.4	15.5	13.9	13.9	13.9	14.5	13.4	14.8	15.4
45-64 years	NA	NA	NA	NA	25.9	28.9	23.0	21.7	20.2	21.6	18.8	16.9	14.4	14.3	15.2	14.7	15.9	14.9	15.9	17.5
65 years and over	NA	NA	NA	NA	22.9	35.3	37.0	28.9	27.6	24.8	25.6	19.7	16.9	20.7	18.0	17.5	18.8	19.5	20.1	20.5
White, not Hispanic or Latino Male[7]																				
All ages, age-adjusted[4]	NA	NA	NA	NA	24.9	25.7	22.1	21.7	22.2	21.8	21.6	19.8	17.4	17.1	17.0	17.3	16.5	16.2	17.0	17.9
All ages, crude	NA	NA	NA	NA	25.9	26.0	21.9	21.5	22.5	22.1	22.0	20.2	17.9	17.6	17.6	18.0	17.2	16.9	17.9	18.9
1-14 years	NA	NA	NA	NA	7.8	6.4	5.8	4.9	3.9	3.2	3.5	3.1	2.6	2.7	2.7	2.2	2.3	2.3	2.4	2.6
15-24 years	NA	NA	NA	NA	53.3	52.3	42.7	40.3	38.8	38.8	37.9	32.5	26.6	25.4	25.3	25.3	23.0	22.6	22.8	23.3
25-34 years	NA	NA	NA	NA	33.2	34.0	27.1	24.7	27.8	28.5	27.6	26.1	21.8	21.9	21.5	22.0	21.4	20.7	21.7	23.1
35-44 years	NA	NA	NA	NA	21.6	23.1	20.3	21.6	22.9	22.4	22.7	20.9	18.9	18.0	17.5	18.9	17.8	17.2	18.6	20.0
45-64 years	NA	NA	NA	NA	18.0	19.8	18.1	19.3	21.7	21.4	21.1	20.2	19.0	18.6	18.7	19.3	18.6	18.6	19.8	21.0
65 years and over	NA	NA	NA	NA	27.6	31.1	29.4	29.3	28.6	26.6	27.0	24.7	22.6	22.7	23.0	22.9	22.3	21.5	22.8	23.8

NOTE: Starting with Health, United States, 2003, rates for 1991–1999 were revised using intercensal population estimates based on the 1990 and 2000 Censuses. For 2000, population estimates are bridged-race April 1 census counts. Starting with Health, United States, 2012, rates for 2001–2009 were revised using intercensal population estimates based on the 2000 and 2010 Censuses. For 2010, population estimates are bridged-race April 1 census counts. Rates for 2011 and beyond were computed using 2010-based postcensal estimates. Age groups were selected to minimize the presentation of unstable age-specific death rates based on small numbers of deaths and for consistency among comparison groups. For additional injury-related statistics, see Web-based Injury Statistics Query and Reporting System (WISQARS), available from: https://www.cdc.gov/injury/wisqars/index.html. Starting with 2003 data (shown in spreadsheet version), some states began to collect information on more than one race on the death certificate, according to 1997 Office of Management and Budget (OMB) standards. The multiple-race data for these states were bridged to the single-race categories of the 1977 OMB standards, for comparability with other states.
NA = Not available.
*Rates based on fewer than 20 deaths are considered unreliable and are not shown.
[1]Includes deaths of persons who were not residents of the 50 states and the District of Columbia.
[2]Underlying cause of death was coded according to the 6th Revision of the *International Classification of Diseases* (*ICD*) in 1950, 7th Revision in 1960, 8th Revision in 1970, and 9th Revision in 1980-1998.
[3]Starting with 1999 data, cause of death is coded according to *ICD-10*. Codes included were V02–V04, V09.0, V09.2, V12–V14, V19.0–V19.2, V19.4–V19.6, V20–V79, V80.3–V80.5, V81.0–V81.1, V82.0–V82.1, V83–V86, V87.0–V87.8, V88.0–V88.8, V89.0, and V89.2.
[4]Age-adjusted rates are calculated using the year 2000 standard population. Prior to 2001, age-adjusted rates were calculated using standard million proportions based on rounded population numbers. Starting with 2001 data, unrounded population numbers are used to calculate age-adjusted rates.
[5]The race groups White, Black, Asian or Pacific Islander, and American Indian or Alaska Native include persons of Hispanic and non-Hispanic origin. Persons of Hispanic origin may be of any race. Death rates for Hispanic, American Indian or Alaska Native, and Asian or Pacific Islander persons should be interpreted with caution because of inconsistencies in reporting Hispanic origin or race on the death certificate (death rate numerators) compared with population figures (death rate denominators). The net effect of misclassification is an underestimation of deaths and death rates for races other than White and Black.
[6]In 1950, rate is for the age group under 15 years.
[7]Prior to 1997, data from states that did not report Hispanic origin on the death certificate were excluded.

Table 2-20. Death Rates for Motor Vehicle–Related Injuries, by Sex and Age, Selected Years, 1950–2016—*Continued*

(Rate per 100,000 population; data are based on death certificates.)

Sex, race, Hispanic origin, and age	1950[1,2]	1960[1,2]	1970[2]	1980[2]	1985[2]	1990[2]	1995[2]	2000[3]	2005[3]	2006[3]	2007[3]	2008[3]	2009[3]	2010[3]	2011[3]	2012[3]	2013[3]	2014[3]	2015[3]	2016[3]
								Deaths per 100,000 resident population												
Black, not Hispanic or Latino Male[7]																				
All ages, age-adjusted[4]	NA	NA	NA	NA	NA	NA	NA	24.9	23.2	23.3	23.1	19.6	18.4	17.4	17.5	18.2	17.8	18.2	19.9	21.8
All ages, crude	NA	NA	NA	NA	NA	NA	NA	23.1	21.9	22.2	21.8	18.8	17.4	16.7	16.7	17.4	17.3	17.7	19.7	21.2
1-14 years	NA	NA	NA	NA	NA	NA	NA	5.6	4.7	5.0	4.3	3.3	3.8	3.2	2.9	3.4	3.5	3.2	3.4	3.5
15-24 years	NA	NA	NA	NA	NA	NA	NA	31.1	28.8	27.7	27.7	23.3	19.3	20.6	18.5	18.2	18.6	19.6	22.7	24.0
25-34 years	NA	NA	NA	NA	NA	NA	NA	33.6	33.7	36.4	33.6	28.4	28.1	26.4	24.0	27.2	26.8	27.1	28.4	31.4
35-44 years	NA	NA	NA	NA	NA	NA	NA	27.9	26.6	26.1	28.3	24.1	22.7	20.3	22.0	21.9	21.6	22.3	25.0	28.8
45-64 years	NA	NA	NA	NA	NA	NA	NA	27.5	24.5	25.9	24.5	22.2	19.8	19.6	20.7	21.6	22.0	21.9	25.3	24.6
65 years and over	NA	NA	NA	NA	NA	NA	NA	32.4	29.5	26.5	27.8	23.4	22.8	20.2	21.9	22.2	18.8	20.3	19.9	25.2
White Female[5]																				
All ages, age-adjusted[4]	11.4	11.7	14.9	12.2	10.9	11.2	10.4	9.8	9.3	9.2	8.6	7.5	6.9	6.8	6.6	6.8	6.4	6.3	6.6	7.0
All ages, crude	10.9	11.2	14.8	12.8	11.4	11.6	10.7	10.0	9.6	9.4	8.8	7.8	7.2	7.1	6.9	7.1	6.7	6.6	6.9	7.3
Under 1 year	7.8	7.5	10.2	7.1	3.9	4.7	4.5	3.5	3.0	3.1	2.9	1.8	1.5	1.9	1.4	1.6	1.7	1.5	*	2.4
1-14 years	7.2	6.2	7.5	6.2	5.4	4.8	4.3	3.7	3.2	3.1	2.7	2.1	2.1	2.1	2.0	1.9	1.8	1.8	1.8	2.0
15-24 years	12.6	15.6	22.7	23.0	20.0	19.5	18.1	17.1	15.7	15.9	15.1	12.6	11.3	10.8	10.1	10.0	9.5	9.2	9.8	10.2
25-34 years	9.0	9.0	12.7	12.2	10.1	11.6	10.2	8.9	9.4	9.1	9.0	7.6	7.4	7.1	7.3	7.6	7.1	7.1	7.7	8.8
35-44 years	8.1	8.9	12.3	10.6	9.4	9.2	8.9	8.9	9.0	9.2	8.1	7.4	6.5	6.5	6.4	6.6	6.1	6.1	6.4	6.7
45-64 years	12.7	13.1	15.1	10.4	9.5	9.9	8.9	8.7	8.6	8.3	7.8	7.3	6.6	6.4	6.1	6.5	6.4	6.6	7.0	7.0
65 years and over	22.2	20.8	23.7	15.3	16.2	17.4	17.5	16.2	14.5	14.0	13.0	11.8	11.4	11.5	11.3	11.3	10.4	10.3	10.3	10.4
Black or African American Female[5]																				
All ages, age-adjusted[4]	9.3	10.4	14.1	8.5	8.5	9.6	9.0	8.4	7.6	7.7	7.0	6.4	6.2	5.9	5.7	5.9	5.7	5.6	6.1	7.1
All ages, crude	10.2	9.7	13.4	8.3	8.3	9.4	8.8	8.2	7.5	7.6	6.9	6.3	6.1	5.8	5.7	5.9	5.7	5.6	6.1	7.1
Under 1 year	NA	8.1	11.9	*	8.1	7.0	*	*	6.9	*	*	*	*	*	*	*	*	*	*	*
1-14 years[6]	7.2	6.9	10.2	6.3	5.1	5.3	4.9	3.9	3.4	3.4	3.3	2.5	2.6	2.0	2.3	2.4	2.3	2.3	2.6	3.1
15-24 years	11.6	9.9	13.4	8.0	9.1	9.9	10.5	11.7	10.5	9.8	9.5	8.4	8.1	7.8	7.6	7.7	7.7	7.7	8.9	10.3
25-34 years	10.8	9.8	13.3	10.6	9.3	11.1	10.3	9.4	7.6	8.7	7.5	7.1	7.6	6.8	7.1	7.4	7.2	6.9	7.8	9.0
35-44 years	11.1	11.0	16.1	8.3	9.1	9.4	9.7	8.2	7.7	8.0	7.0	6.7	6.0	5.8	5.4	5.7	6.4	5.7	6.1	7.3
45-64 years	11.8	12.7	16.7	9.2	9.0	10.7	9.3	9.0	8.2	8.8	7.4	7.0	6.5	6.3	5.9	6.5	6.2	6.2	6.3	7.1
65 years and over	14.3	13.2	15.7	9.5	11.2	13.5	11.4	10.4	9.9	9.5	8.7	8.4	7.9	8.6	7.6	7.7	5.9	6.4	6.8	7.6
American Indian or Alaska Native Female[5]																				
All ages, age-adjusted[4]	NA	NA	NA	32.0	19.8	17.5	18.2	19.5	14.0	15.1	13.5	12.8	11.8	10.6	10.8	10.2	11.0	10.1	11.2	11.3
All ages, crude	NA	NA	NA	32.0	20.6	17.3	18.8	18.6	13.8	14.9	13.5	12.4	11.7	10.0	10.5	10.1	10.7	10.0	11.2	11.0
1-14 years	NA	NA	NA	15.0	9.2	8.1	8.1	6.5	*	*	*	1.4	1.5	*	*	*	4.9	*	*	*
15-24 years	NA	NA	NA	42.3	29.5	31.4	30.4	30.3	22.0	24.5	21.4	17.4	19.8	13.4	14.7	16.2	13.6	16.5	13.8	15.5
25-34 years	NA	NA	NA	52.5	30.2	18.8	33.7	22.3	22.1	19.1	19.4	19.2	13.8	17.7	18.0	15.1	17.0	13.4	21.2	18.5
35-44 years	NA	NA	NA	38.1	27.0	18.2	17.2	22.0	15.7	17.7	18.8	15.3	16.9	13.1	11.3	11.6	14.2	12.0	12.6	14.5
45-64 years	NA	NA	NA	32.6	19.5	17.6	15.7	17.8	10.6	13.5	10.8	10.3	11.7	8.4	8.7	10.5	8.7	9.7	11.9	9.8
65 years and over	NA	NA	NA	*	*	*	*	24.0	*	17.1	*	17.8	*	*	14.8	14.4	*	*	*	11.6
Asian or Pacific Islander Female[5]																				
All ages, age-adjusted[4]	NA	NA	NA	9.3	8.8	10.4	8.6	6.7	5.7	5.4	5.0	4.2	3.8	3.9	3.3	3.3	3.4	3.2	3.6	3.7
All ages, crude	NA	NA	NA	8.2	7.9	9.0	7.7	5.9	5.3	5.1	4.6	3.9	3.5	3.6	3.1	3.3	3.4	3.2	3.6	3.7
1-14 years	NA	NA	NA	7.4	5.0	3.6	3.2	2.3	1.5	1.7	*	1.4	1.5	*	*	*	*	*	*	1.2
15-24 years	NA	NA	NA	7.4	7.4	11.4	11.5	6.0	7.0	6.3	6.7	4.5	4.3	3.3	3.7	3.0	3.0	3.0	3.4	3.4
25-34 years	NA	NA	NA	7.3	8.4	7.3	4.8	4.5	3.4	3.2	2.9	3.1	2.9	3.1	1.9	2.8	2.5	2.5	2.6	2.7
35-44 years	NA	NA	NA	8.6	7.0	7.5	5.9	4.9	4.3	4.1	2.7	2.2	2.1	2.0	2.3	1.7	*	2.0	1.7	1.6
45-64 years	NA	NA	NA	8.5	8.6	11.8	10.4	6.4	6.4	6.0	5.4	4.4	3.0	4.3	3.0	4.2	4.1	3.3	4.0	4.0
65 years and over	NA	NA	NA	18.6	20.5	24.3	18.9	18.5	13.9	13.6	13.4	12.1	11.4	12.2	10.2	8.7	10.8	9.4	11.2	11.6
Hispanic or Latina Female[5,7]																				
All ages, age-adjusted[4]	NA	NA	NA	NA	8.8	9.6	8.8	7.9	7.8	7.6	6.8	5.5	5.5	5.3	4.8	5.3	5.2	5.0	5.2	6.1
All ages, crude	NA	NA	NA	NA	7.9	8.9	8.0	7.2	7.3	7.0	6.3	5.0	5.1	4.9	4.5	4.9	4.8	4.7	5.0	5.8
1-14 years	NA	NA	NA	NA	4.8	4.8	4.3	3.9	3.3	3.1	2.7	2.1	2.3	2.0	1.7	1.9	1.7	1.9	1.8	2.0
15-24 years	NA	NA	NA	NA	10.1	11.6	11.8	10.6	12.7	10.9	10.1	7.8	7.8	7.7	6.3	7.2	7.4	7.5	7.7	9.4
25-34 years	NA	NA	NA	NA	7.5	9.4	7.2	6.5	7.1	6.8	6.6	5.4	5.5	5.0	5.1	5.4	5.1	5.3	6.1	7.5
35-44 years	NA	NA	NA	NA	8.8	8.0	7.9	7.3	7.3	7.1	6.7	4.8	4.6	4.5	4.6	4.5	4.7	4.1	4.6	4.8

NOTE: Starting with Health, United States, 2003, rates for 1991–1999 were revised using intercensal population estimates based on the 1990 and 2000 Censuses. For 2000, population estimates are bridged-race April 1 census counts. Starting with Health, United States, 2012, rates for 2001–2009 were revised using intercensal population estimates based on the 2000 and 2010 Censuses. For 2010, population estimates are bridged-race April 1 census counts. Rates for 2011 and beyond were computed using 2010-based postcensal estimates. Age groups were selected to minimize the presentation of unstable age-specific death rates based on small numbers of deaths and for consistency among comparison groups. For additional injury-related statistics, see Web-based Injury Statistics Query and Reporting System (WISQARS), available from: https://www.cdc.gov/injury/wisqars/index.html. Starting with 2003 data (shown in spreadsheet version), some states began to collect information on more than one race on the death certificate, according to 1997 Office of Management and Budget (OMB) standards. The multiple-race data for these states were bridged to the single-race categories of the 1977 OMB standards, for comparability with other states.

NA = Not available.

*Rates based on fewer than 20 deaths are considered unreliable and are not shown.

[1]Includes deaths of persons who were not residents of the 50 states and the District of Columbia.

[2]Underlying cause of death was coded according to the 6th Revision of the *International Classification of Diseases (ICD)* in 1950, 7th Revision in 1960, 8th Revision in 1970, and 9th Revision in 1980-1998.

[3]Starting with 1999 data, cause of death is coded according to *ICD-10.* Codes included were V02–V04, V09.0, V09.2, V12–V14, V19.0–V19.2, V19.4–V19.6, V20–V79, V80.3–V80.5, V81.0–V81.1, V82.0–V82.1, V83–V86, V87.0–V87.8, V88.0–V88.8, V89.0, and V89.2.

[4]Age-adjusted rates are calculated using the year 2000 standard population. Prior to 2001, age-adjusted rates were calculated using standard million proportions based on rounded population numbers. Starting with 2001 data, unrounded population numbers are used to calculate age-adjusted rates.

[5]The race groups White, Black, Asian or Pacific Islander, and American Indian or Alaska Native include persons of Hispanic and non-Hispanic origin. Persons of Hispanic origin may be of any race. Death rates for Hispanic, American Indian or Alaska Native, and Asian or Pacific Islander persons should be interpreted with caution because of inconsistencies in reporting Hispanic origin or race on the death certificate (death rate numerators) compared with population figures (death rate denominators). The net effect of misclassification is an underestimation of deaths and death rates for races other than White and Black.

[6]In 1950, rate is for the age group under 15 years.

[7]Prior to 1997, data from states that did not report Hispanic origin on the death certificate were excluded.

Table 2-20. Death Rates for Motor Vehicle–Related Injuries, by Sex and Age, Selected Years, 1950–2016—*Continued*

(Rate per 100,000 population; data are based on death certificates.)

Sex, race, Hispanic origin, and age	1950[1,2]	1960[1,2]	1970[2]	1980[2]	1985[2]	1990[2]	1995[2]	2000[3]	2005[3]	2006[3]	2007[3]	2008[3]	2009[3]	2010[3]	2011[3]	2012[3]	2013[3]	2014[3]	2015[3]	2016[3]
								Deaths per 100,000 resident population												
45-64 years	NA	NA	NA	NA	9.4	11.4	9.3	8.3	7.4	8.0	6.7	5.1	5.5	5.6	4.8	5.6	5.3	5.3	5.2	6.3
65 years and over	NA	NA	NA	NA	14.8	14.9	14.6	13.4	11.4	12.0	10.5	10.7	9.5	9.4	8.6	9.2	9.0	8.1	8.3	9.0
White, not Hispanic or Latina Female[7]																				
All ages, age-adjusted[4]	NA	NA	NA	NA	10.4	11.3	10.5	10.0	9.5	9.4	8.8	7.9	7.1	7.0	6.9	7.0	6.6	6.5	6.8	7.1
All ages, crude	NA	NA	NA	NA	10.9	11.7	10.9	10.3	9.9	9.8	9.2	8.3	7.5	7.5	7.3	7.5	7.1	7.0	7.3	7.6
1-14 years	NA	NA	NA	NA	4.9	4.7	4.2	3.5	3.0	3.0	2.6	2.1	1.9	2.0	2.1	1.8	1.8	1.7	1.8	1.9
15-24 years	NA	NA	NA	NA	20.2	20.4	19.0	18.4	16.3	16.9	16.2	13.7	12.0	11.4	11.0	10.7	10.0	9.6	10.3	10.2
25-34 years	NA	NA	NA	NA	9.8	11.7	10.5	9.3	9.9	9.6	9.5	8.1	7.7	7.6	7.7	8.2	7.5	7.5	8.0	9.0
35-44 years	NA	NA	NA	NA	8.6	9.3	8.9	9.0	9.2	9.4	8.3	7.9	6.8	6.9	6.7	7.0	6.4	6.6	6.8	7.2
45-64 years	NA	NA	NA	NA	8.6	9.7	8.6	8.7	8.6	8.3	7.9	7.6	6.7	6.4	6.2	6.6	6.5	6.4	6.7	7.0
65 years and over	NA	NA	NA	NA	15.3	17.5	17.5	16.3	14.7	14.1	13.1	11.8	11.5	11.6	11.5	11.4	10.5	10.4	10.5	10.5
Black, not Hispanic or Latina Female[7]																				
All ages, age-adjusted[4]	NA	NA	NA	NA	NA	NA	NA	8.7	7.8	8.0	7.2	6.6	6.4	6.1	5.9	6.2	6.0	5.8	6.3	7.4
All ages, crude	NA	NA	NA	NA	NA	NA	NA	8.5	7.7	7.9	7.2	6.6	6.4	6.1	5.9	6.3	6.0	5.9	6.4	7.4
1-14 years	NA	NA	NA	NA	NA	NA	NA	4.0	3.6	3.5	3.4	2.6	2.8	2.1	2.4	2.6	2.5	2.4	2.7	3.4
15-24 years	NA	NA	NA	NA	NA	NA	NA	12.3	10.8	10.2	10.0	8.8	8.4	8.2	8.0	8.2	8.0	8.0	9.1	10.8
25-34 years	NA	NA	NA	NA	NA	NA	NA	9.8	8.0	9.3	8.0	7.6	7.9	7.3	7.6	7.9	7.7	7.4	8.2	9.5
35-44 years	NA	NA	NA	NA	NA	NA	NA	8.5	7.9	8.3	7.3	6.9	6.2	6.2	5.7	6.1	6.9	6.1	6.4	7.6
45-64 years	NA	NA	NA	NA	NA	NA	NA	9.2	8.4	8.9	7.6	7.3	6.7	6.4	6.0	6.7	6.4	6.3	6.5	7.2
65 years and over	NA	NA	NA	NA	NA	NA	NA	10.4	10.2	9.5	8.9	8.5	8.0	8.7	7.8	7.8	5.9	6.4	7.0	7.7

NOTE: Starting with Health, United States, 2003, rates for 1991–1999 were revised using intercensal population estimates based on the 1990 and 2000 Censuses. For 2000, population estimates are bridged-race April 1 census counts. Starting with Health, United States, 2012, rates for 2001–2009 were revised using intercensal population estimates based on the 2000 and 2010 Censuses. For 2010, population estimates are bridged-race April 1 census counts. Rates for 2011 and beyond were computed using 2010-based postcensal estimates. Age groups were selected to minimize the presentation of unstable age-specific death rates based on small numbers of deaths and for consistency among comparison groups. For additional injury-related statistics, see Web-based Injury Statistics Query and Reporting System (WISQARS), available from: https://www.cdc.gov/injury/wisqars/index.html. Starting with 2003 data (shown in spreadsheet version), some states began to collect information on more than one race on the death certificate, according to 1997 Office of Management and Budget (OMB) standards. The multiple-race data for these states were bridged to the single-race categories of the 1977 OMB standards, for comparability with other states.
NA = Not available.
[1]Includes deaths of persons who were not residents of the 50 states and the District of Columbia.
[2]Underlying cause of death was coded according to the 6th Revision of the *International Classification of Diseases* (*ICD*) in 1950, 7th Revision in 1960, 8th Revision in 1970, and 9th Revision in 1980-1998.
[3]Starting with 1999 data, cause of death is coded according to *ICD-10*. Codes included were V02–V04, V09.0, V09.2, V12–V14, V19.0–V19.2, V19.4–V19.6, V20–V79, V80.3–V80.5, V81.0–V81.1, V82.0–V82.1, V83–V86, V87.0–V87.8, V88.0–V88.8, V89.0, and V89.2.
[4]Age-adjusted rates are calculated using the year 2000 standard population. Prior to 2001, age-adjusted rates were calculated using standard million proportions based on rounded population numbers. Starting with 2001 data, unrounded population numbers are used to calculate age-adjusted rates.
[7]Prior to 1997, data from states that did not report Hispanic origin on the death certificate were excluded.

Table 2-21. Occupational Fatal Injuries, by Industry, Sex, Age, Race, and Hispanic Origin, Selected Years, 2003–2016

(Number.)

Characteristic	2003	2004	2005	2006	2007	2008	2009	2010	2011	2012	2013	2014	2015	2016
Total workforce	5,575	5,764	5,734	5,840	5,657	5,214	4,551	4,690	4,693	4,628	4,585	4,821	4,836	5,190
Sex														
Male	5,129	5,349	5,328	5,396	5,228	4,827	4,216	4,322	4,308	4,277	4,265	4,454	4,492	4,803
Female	446	415	406	444	429	387	335	368	385	351	319	367	344	387
Unspecified	0	0	0	0	0	0	0	0	0	0	1	0	0	0
Age														
Under 16 years	25	13	23	11	18	11	13	16	10	19	5	8	12	13
16-17 years	28	25	31	21	20	23	14	18	13	10	9	14	12	17
18-19 years	84	103	111	106	97	66	57	56	61	59	57	42	50	43
20-24 years	462	421	403	390	424	353	275	245	292	287	279	292	329	310
25-34 years	1,018	996	1,017	1,041	991	850	704	785	714	736	777	753	758	834
35-44 years	1,329	1,342	1,243	1,288	1,168	1,113	908	868	875	829	853	860	864	979
45-54 years	1,301	1,384	1,389	1,417	1,425	1,292	1,173	1,169	1,222	1,161	1,115	1,161	1,130	1,145
55-64 years	802	907	933	963	934	920	853	948	936	936	933	1,007	1,031	1,160
65 years and over	523	569	578	599	574	580	551	582	569	588	557	684	650	688
Unspecified	3	4	6	4	6	6	3	3	1	3	0	0	0	1
Race and Hispanic origin														
Hispanic or Latino (may be of any race)	794	902	923	990	937	804	713	707	749	748	817	804	903	879
Not Hispanic or Latino	4,781	4,862	4,811	4,850	4,720	4,410	3,838	3,983	3,944	3,880	3,768	4,017	3,933	4,311
White	3,988	4,066	3,977	4,019	3,867	3,663	3,204	3,363	3,323	3,177	3,125	3,332	3,241	3,481
Black or African American	543	546	584	565	609	533	421	412	440	486	439	475	495	587
American Indian or Alaska Native	42	28	50	46	29	32	33	32	30	37	35	34	36	38
Asian	147	168	154	148	166	145	141	143	121	147	125	137	114	160
Native Hawaiian or Other Pacific Islander	11	12	9	11	6	7	7	6	3	7	7	5	9	7
Multiple races	3	4	*	11	10	6	7	8	15	5	12	20	12	15
Other races or not reported	47	38	35	50	33	24	25	19	12	21	25	14	26	23
Industry[1]														
Private sector	5,043	5,229	5,214	5,320	5,112	4,670	4,090	4,206	4,188	4,175	4,101	4,386	4,379	4,693
Agriculture, forestry, fishing, and hunting	709	669	715	655	585	672	575	621	566	509	500	584	570	593
Mining[2]	141	152	159	192	183	176	99	172	155	181	155	183	120	89
Utilities	32	51	30	53	34	37	16	26	39	23	24	17	22	30
Construction	1,131	1,234	1,192	1,239	1,204	975	834	774	738	806	828	899	937	991
Manufacturing	420	463	393	456	400	411	319	329	327	327	312	349	353	318
Wholesale trade	191	205	209	222	207	180	190	191	190	204	201	191	175	179
Retail trade	344	377	400	359	348	301	307	311	268	273	263	272	269	282
Transportation and warehousing	808	840	885	860	890	796	633	661	749	741	733	766	765	825
Information	64	55	65	66	79	47	33	43	56	42	40	35	42	46
Finance and insurance	45	46	42	44	46	24	33	24	36	21	21	29	19	26
Real estate and rental and leasing	84	70	57	82	73	82	75	89	62	64	66	88	64	91
Professional and technical services	97	77	83	78	77	69	85	76	74	57	87	80	76	100
Management, administrative, and waste services[3]	NA	NA	NA	NA	NA	NA	NA	NA	359	352	343	345	401	440
Educational services	41	44	46	49	34	28	27	30	37	34	32	40	30	42
Health care and social assistance	102	113	104	129	115	113	123	141	117	107	103	106	109	117
Arts, entertainment, and recreation	88	99	77	80	96	92	80	84	93	80	69	81	82	96
Accommodation and food services	187	148	136	185	164	146	151	154	138	152	138	135	143	202
Other services (except public administration)	194	207	210	183	175	178	173	192	183	199	186	186	202	223
Government[4]	532	535	520	520	545	544	461	484	505	453	484	435	457	497

NOTE: Fatal work injuries for years 2014 and prior are based on revised data and may differ from the preliminary data CFOI released during those years. In 2015, CFOI moved to a single release, and now releases only final data for each year. Private sector totals include injuries with unknown industry. Data for additional years are available. See https://www.cdc.gov/nchs/hus.htm. Data are compiled from various federal, state, and local administrative sources.
NA = Not available.
* = Estimates are unreliable or data do not meet publication criteria.
[1]Industry data from 2003 to 2008 are based on the North American Industry Classification System (NAICS), 2002. Industry data from 2009 to the present are based on NAICS 2007. NAICS replaces the Standard Industrial Classification (SIC) system. Because of substantial differences between these systems, industry data classified by these two systems are not comparable.
[2]Includes fatal injuries at all establishments categorized as Mining (Sector 21) in the NAICS, including establishments not governed by the Mine Safety and Health Administration (MSHA) rules and reporting, such as those in Oil and Gas Extraction.
[3]Starting with 2011 data, CFOI combined the categories "Management of companies and enterprises" and "Administrative and support and waste management and remediation services" into one category entitled "Management, administrative, and waste services."
[4]Includes fatal work injuries to workers employed by governmental organizations, regardless of industry.

Table 2-22. Number of Fatal Work Injuries, by Most Frequent Type, 1992–2018

(Number.)

Year	Total	Roadway incidents	Homicides	Falls, slips, trips	Struck by object
1992	6,217	1,158	1,044	600	557
1993	6,331	1,242	1,074	618	565
1994	6,632	1,343	1,080	665	591
1995	6,275	1,346	1,036	651	547
1996	6,202	1,346	927	691	582
1997	6,238	1,393	860	716	579
1998	6,055	1,442	714	706	520
1999	6,054	1,496	651	721	585
2000	5,920	1,365	677	734	571
2001	5,915	1,409	643	810	553
2002	5,534	1,373	609	719	505
2003	5,575	1,353	632	696	531
2004	5,764	1,398	559	822	602
2005	5,734	1,437	567	770	607
2006	5,840	1,356	540	827	589
2007	5,657	1,414	628	847	504
2008	5,214	1,215	526	700	520
2009	4,551	985	542	645	420
2010	4,690	1,044	518	646	404
2011	4,693	1,103	468	681	476
2012	4,383	1,044	463	668	519
2013	4,585	1,099	404	724	509
2014	4,821	1,157	409	818	503
2015	4,836	1,264	417	800	519
2016	5,190	1,252	500	849	533
2017	5,147	1,299	458	887	503
2018	5,250	1,276	451	791	566

Table 2-23. Number of Fatal Occupational Injuries, by Selected Industry Sector and Occupation, and Percentage of Fatal Incidents, 2018

(Number, percent.)

Characteristic	Count	Percent
Total	5,250	100.0
Industry		
Private industry	3,707	70.6
Government	471	9.1
Self-employed	1,072	20.7
Construction	1,038	20.0
Transportation and warehousing	909	17.5
Agriculture, forestry, fishing and hunting	574	11.1
Professional and business services	598	11.5
Manufacturing	343	6.6
Retail trade	275	5.3
Wholesale trade	196	3.8
Other services (exc. public administration)	223	4.3
Public administration	321	6.2
Real estate and rental and leasing	78	1.5
Mining[1]	130	2.5
Utilities	44	0.8
Educational and health services	218	4.2
Health care and social assistance	149	2.9
Arts, entertainment, and recreation	82	1.6
Financial activities	108	2.1
Information	31	0.6
Leisure and hospitality	258	5.0
Administrative and waste services	508	9.8
Occupation		
Fishers and related fishing workers	30	0.6
Logging workers	56	1.2
Aircraft pilots and flight engineers	70	1.5
Farmers, ranchers, and other agricultural managers	257	5.5
Extraction workers	64	1.4
Roofers	96	2.1
Refuse and recyclable material collectors	37	0.8
Driver/sales workers and truck drivers	966	20.6
Industrial machinery installation, repair, and maintenance workers	27	0.6
Police and sheriff's patrol officers	108	2.3

NA = Not available.

[1]CFOI has used several versions of the Standard Occupation Classification (SOC) system since 2003 to define occupation. For more information on the version of SOC used in this year, see the definitions page at http://www.bls.gov/iif/oshcfdef.htm.

Table 2-24. Number of Fatal Work Injuries, by State, 2010–2018
(Number.)

State	2010	2011	2012	2013	2014	2015	2016	2017	2018	Net change, 2010–2018	Net change, 2017–2018
Total	4,690	4,693	4,628	4,585	4,821	4,836	5,190	5,147	5,250	560	103
										0	0
Alabama	92	75	84	78	75	70	100	83	89	3	6
Alaska	39	39	31	32	30	14	35	33	32	7	1
Arizona	77	69	60	95	88	69	77	90	82	5	8
Arkansas	88	93	63	63	67	74	68	76	76	12	0
California	326	390	375	396	344	388	376	376	422	96	46
Colorado	85	92	82	65	84	75	81	77	72	13	5
Connecticut	49	37	36	29	35	44	28	35	48	1	13
Delaware	8	10	14	11	12	8	12	10	7	1	3
District of Columbia	16	9	11	25	11	8	5	13	10	6	3
Florida	225	226	218	239	228	272	309	299	332	107	33
Georgia	108	111	101	117	152	180	171	194	186	78	8
Hawaii	19	26	20	11	31	18	29	20	22	3	2
Idaho	33	37	19	30	34	36	30	37	45	12	8
Illinois	206	177	146	176	164	172	171	163	184	22	21
Indiana	118	125	115	127	130	115	137	138	173	55	35
Iowa	77	93	97	72	91	60	76	72	77	0	5
Kansas	85	78	76	55	73	60	74	72	61	24	11
Kentucky	69	93	91	86	82	99	92	70	83	14	13
Louisiana	111	111	116	114	120	112	95	117	98	13	19
Maine	20	26	19	19	19	15	18	18	17	3	1
Maryland	71	71	72	79	74	69	92	87	97	26	10
Massachusetts	54	68	44	57	55	69	109	108	97	43	11
Michigan	146	141	137	135	143	134	162	153	155	9	2
Minnesota	70	60	70	69	62	74	92	101	75	5	26
Mississippi	68	63	63	68	75	77	71	90	78	10	12
Missouri	106	132	88	118	106	117	124	125	145	39	20
Montana	36	49	34	28	28	36	38	32	28	8	4
Nebraska	54	39	48	39	55	50	60	35	44	10	9
Nevada	38	38	42	42	40	44	54	32	39	1	7
New Hampshire	6	9	14	14	17	18	22	11	20	14	9
New Jersey	81	99	92	102	87	97	101	69	83	2	14
New Mexico	38	52	39	54	53	35	41	44	43	5	1
New York (including NYC)	182	206	202	178	241	236	272	313	271	89	42
New York City	68	72	76	56	79	74	56	87	73	5	14
North Carolina	139	148	146	109	137	150	174	183	178	39	5
North Dakota	30	44	65	56	38	47	28	38	35	5	3
Ohio	161	155	161	149	185	202	164	174	158	3	16
Oklahoma	94	86	97	92	98	91	92	91	91	3	0
Oregon	47	58	43	49	69	44	72	60	62	15	2
Pennsylvania	221	186	194	183	179	173	163	172	177	44	5
Rhode Island	9	7	8	10	10	6	9	8	9	0	1
South Carolina	69	81	63	75	64	117	96	88	98	29	10
South Dakota	36	31	31	20	29	21	31	30	32	4	2
Tennessee	138	120	101	95	127	112	122	128	122	16	6
Texas	461	433	536	508	531	527	545	534	488	27	46
Utah	41	39	39	37	54	42	44	43	49	8	6
Vermont	12	8	11	7	10	9	10	22	11	1	11
Virginia	107	127	149	128	116	106	153	118	157	50	39
Washington	104	60	67	56	88	70	78	84	86	18	2
West Virginia	95	43	49	61	38	35	47	51	57	38	6
Wisconsin	91	89	114	97	99	104	105	106	114	23	8
Wyoming	33	32	35	26	37	34	34	20	31	2	11

NOTE: The Census of Fatal Occupational Injuries (CFOI) has published data on fatal occupational injuries for the United States since 1992. During this time, the classification systems and definitions of many data elements have changed. See the CFOI Definitions page (www.bls.gov/iif/oshcfdef.htm) for a more detailed description of each data element.

Table 2-25. Years of Potential Life Lost Before Age 75 for Selected Causes of Death, by Sex, Race, and Hispanic Origin, Selected Years, 1980–2016

(Years lost before 75 per 100,000 population; data are based on death certificates.)

Sex, race, Hispanic origin, and cause of death[1]	Crude 2016[3]	Age-adjusted[2] 1980[2]	1990[2]	1995[2]	2000[3]	2005[3]	2006[3]	2007[3]	2008[3]	2009[3]	2010[3]	2011[3]	2012[3]	2013[3]	2014[3]	2015[3]	2016[3]
ALL PERSONS																	
All causes	7,431.7	10,448.4	9,085.5	8,626.2	7,578.1	7,315.7	7,228.7	7,087.0	6,957.7	6,833.1	6,642.9	6,635.2	6,588.0	6,593.1	6,622.1	6,757.7	6,968.6
Diseases of heart	1,100.1	2,238.7	1,617.7	1,475.4	1,253.0	1,107.5	1,074.8	1,037.8	1,022.9	992.6	972.4	962.4	951.9	952.3	952.0	956.6	958.9
Ischemic heart disease	620.5	1,729.3	1,153.6	1,013.2	841.8	698.9	672.5	638.2	624.4	591.5	577.3	567.0	558.4	546.1	537.1	530.3	523.8
Cerebrovascular diseases	187.1	357.5	259.6	246.5	223.3	192.9	189.7	183.7	177.9	172.8	169.3	164.0	161.6	158.1	160.1	161.0	164.3
Malignant neoplasms	1,486.2	2,108.8	2,003.8	1,841.6	1,674.1	1,519.8	1,484.6	1,452.7	1,427.8	1,413.9	1,395.8	1,370.9	1,356.2	1,328.6	1,310.4	1,283.3	1,262.4
Trachea, bronchus, and lung	322.8	548.5	561.4	497.3	443.1	390.5	376.1	363.5	350.5	341.7	331.3	318.7	309.9	298.2	287.7	273.4	254.1
Colorectal	141.5	190.0	164.7	152.0	141.9	124.3	125.6	126.0	126.8	124.3	125.0	124.1	123.0	123.5	122.2	123.3	123.7
Prostate[4]	62.2	84.9	96.8	83.5	63.6	54.4	54.1	52.7	52.2	50.1	52.2	48.5	48.1	47.5	47.6	46.7	48.3
Breast[5]	269.3	463.2	451.6	398.6	332.6	295.4	285.9	274.0	269.2	269.6	262.4	259.4	256.0	250.0	245.9	241.9	241.0
Chronic lower respiratory diseases	219.6	169.1	187.4	190.4	188.1	180.1	169.7	170.5	179.8	177.2	172.4	174.7	171.6	176.6	174.1	175.9	175.8
Influenza and pneumonia	87.7	160.2	141.5	126.9	87.1	83.6	76.5	71.6	80.7	108.7	71.4	81.8	67.4	82.3	93.3	74.2	79.9
Chronic liver disease and cirrhosis	203.7	300.3	196.9	173.7	164.1	152.5	149.8	157.3	158.7	160.1	163.9	169.1	173.3	176.9	180.7	190.3	188.0
Diabetes mellitus[6]	202.8	134.4	155.9	174.7	178.4	179.4	176.0	169.3	164.4	161.2	158.2	167.6	164.3	168.3	170.8	176.2	177.7
Alzheimer's disease[7]	18.9	X	X	X	10.9	11.7	11.7	11.9	12.3	11.4	11.7	11.5	11.0	11.1	11.4	13.0	13.9
Human immunodeficiency virus (HIV) disease	46.9	X	383.8	595.3	174.6	134.5	126.9	115.8	100.2	89.2	76.6	68.0	61.8	58.1	55.0	50.4	47.0
Unintentional injuries	1,291.0	1,543.5	1,162.1	1,057.2	1,026.5	1,137.2	1,173.3	1,162.1	1,095.8	1,028.2	1,025.2	1,056.8	1,046.1	1,051.2	1,080.1	1,172.0	1,334.0
Motor vehicle-related injuries	418.3	912.9	716.4	616.3	574.3	565.9	563.0	538.4	473.2	421.7	400.6	394.8	402.4	386.6	383.0	404.9	431.2
Drug overdose	634.5	68.0	81.2	123.1	163.6	289.1	335.1	356.1	364.0	365.7	379.7	414.8	408.8	430.9	465.8	531.2	663.0
Nephritis, nephrotic syndrome and nephrosis[6]	80.9	NA	50.4	47.5	70.7	74.2	76.5	74.8	75.5	75.7	73.1	65.0	65.2	65.7	66.7	69.3	70.0
Suicide[8]	427.0	392.0	393.1	384.7	334.5	348.9	350.6	358.6	367.4	372.5	385.2	395.6	402.1	401.6	413.6	428.6	438.9
Homicide[8]	262.4	425.5	417.4	378.6	266.5	278.2	283.4	279.0	267.6	248.0	239.0	236.2	240.9	229.8	224.5	251.9	275.0
MALE																	
All causes	9,272.2	13,777.2	11,973.5	11,289.2	9,572.2	9,244.2	9,130.1	8,945.0	8,764.7	8,560.7	8,329.5	8,304.1	8,249.1	8,249.5	8,276.4	8,474.7	8,780.8
Diseases of heart	1,497.9	3,352.1	2,356.0	2,117.4	1,766.0	1,559.0	1,514.5	1,463.3	1,433.5	1,399.2	1,370.8	1,351.1	1,336.6	1,338.2	1,326.9	1,327.6	1,333.4
Ischemic heart disease	896.1	2,715.1	1,766.3	1,531.5	1,255.4	1,040.6	1,005.2	956.9	927.8	886.5	864.8	848.6	831.8	816.2	797.6	784.1	778.3
Cerebrovascular diseases	212.2	396.7	286.6	276.9	244.6	213.3	211.5	205.4	197.7	195.7	190.7	185.3	183.7	182.1	184.9	183.1	190.1
Malignant neoplasms	1,557.9	2,360.8	2,214.6	2,008.5	1,810.8	1,632.9	1,587.4	1,554.7	1,540.7	1,515.6	1,500.8	1,467.6	1,450.9	1,415.9	1,396.9	1,365.3	1,332.5
Trachea, bronchus, and lung	362.0	821.1	764.8	645.6	554.9	472.8	450.6	429.5	418.8	403.4	390.5	374.0	361.1	345.1	331.8	315.8	292.9
Colorectal	162.9	214.9	194.3	179.4	167.3	145.7	144.7	147.6	148.8	145.6	148.0	146.0	144.4	146.8	144.3	144.2	144.5
Prostate	62.2	84.9	96.8	83.5	63.6	54.4	54.1	52.7	52.2	50.1	52.2	48.5	48.1	47.5	47.6	46.7	48.3
Chronic lower respiratory diseases	223.4	235.1	224.8	213.1	206.0	194.3	180.8	185.6	192.2	186.9	182.8	185.5	179.7	185.2	182.8	184.5	184.1
Influenza and pneumonia	98.0	205.2	180.0	155.7	102.8	98.0	89.0	83.6	91.7	119.5	82.6	93.5	77.5	94.1	103.7	85.6	90.3
Chronic liver disease and cirrhosis	266.4	415.0	283.9	254.8	236.9	216.4	211.1	222.4	223.2	222.8	226.9	228.9	237.2	242.1	242.6	252.5	247.5
Diabetes mellitus[6]	248.5	140.4	170.4	194.6	203.8	216.1	212.8	206.3	200.7	201.2	194.8	206.4	203.5	208.6	214.0	220.7	222.2
Alzheimer's disease[7]	15.9	X	X	X	10.6	10.8	11.4	11.0	11.5	11.0	10.7	10.6	10.2	10.2	10.3	11.7	12.3
Human immunodeficiency virus (HIV) disease	67.8	X	686.2	991.2	258.9	194.0	180.3	162.6	141.0	126.7	109.5	94.8	87.0	84.3	79.0	72.7	67.7
Unintentional injuries	1,838.9	2,342.7	1,715.1	1,531.6	1,475.6	1,622.6	1,675.9	1,652.0	1,562.6	1,449.8	1,432.1	1,472.5	1,459.7	1,463.5	1,509.6	1,642.4	1,885.6
Motor vehicle-related injuries	601.1	1,359.7	1,018.4	851.1	796.4	802.0	797.8	771.0	683.8	600.5	569.2	563.5	574.3	552.2	550.4	579.7	612.1
Drug overdose	889.8	96.4	123.6	193.1	242.1	400.4	468.1	486.4	499.6	493.0	503.8	550.6	541.5	573.1	623.8	722.2	924.6
Nephritis, nephrotic syndrome and nephrosis[6]	91.1	NA	58.9	55.6	81.1	85.8	89.7	84.6	86.9	86.5	82.3	75.6	75.3	75.3	78.6	80.3	80.5
Suicide[8]	659.8	605.6	634.8	628.4	539.1	553.4	555.0	566.6	578.6	585.6	607.0	618.4	625.9	619.8	635.1	654.2	672.7
Homicide[8]	428.0	675.0	658.0	589.6	410.5	443.6	452.0	443.2	426.6	390.3	380.3	373.7	383.6	365.9	357.3	407.0	440.6
FEMALE																	
All causes	5,605.3	7,350.3	6,333.1	6,057.5	5,644.6	5,429.0	5,365.9	5,267.2	5,188.6	5,143.7	4,994.0	5,000.3	4,959.6	4,967.9	4,999.8	5,070.7	5,184.1
Diseases of heart	705.4	1,246.0	948.5	883.9	774.6	680.2	658.1	634.2	633.2	606.5	593.6	592.5	585.4	584.5	595.2	603.4	602.3
Ischemic heart disease	347.1	852.1	600.3	537.8	457.6	377.2	358.7	337.3	338.0	312.7	305.2	300.2	299.3	290.0	290.2	289.7	282.6
Cerebrovascular diseases	162.2	324.0	235.9	218.7	203.9	173.9	169.2	163.5	159.4	151.1	149.1	143.9	140.7	135.4	136.5	140.1	139.6
Malignant neoplasms	1,415.1	1,896.8	1,826.6	1,698.9	1,555.3	1,419.0	1,393.1	1,361.9	1,325.8	1,322.6	1,301.0	1,284.0	1,271.0	1,250.3	1,232.6	1,209.8	1,200.3
Trachea, bronchus, and lung	283.9	310.4	382.2	365.2	342.1	315.2	307.8	303.1	287.7	285.0	276.9	267.9	262.8	255.1	247.1	234.4	218.4
Colorectal	120.4	168.7	138.7	127.5	118.7	104.5	107.9	105.9	106.2	104.5	103.4	103.5	102.8	101.5	101.4	103.6	104.0
Breast	269.3	463.2	451.6	398.6	332.6	295.4	285.9	274.0	269.2	269.6	262.4	259.4	256.0	250.0	245.9	241.9	241.0
Chronic lower respiratory diseases	215.8	114.0	155.9	171.0	172.3	167.2	159.5	156.7	168.5	168.3	162.8	164.7	164.1	168.7	166.1	167.9	168.0
Influenza and pneumonia	77.5	122.0	106.2	100.2	72.3	69.9	64.7	60.1	70.3	98.4	60.7	70.7	57.8	70.9	83.4	63.1	69.9
Chronic liver disease and cirrhosis	141.6	194.5	115.1	96.6	94.5	91.4	91.1	95.0	96.9	99.9	103.5	111.9	111.9	114.4	121.5	130.6	130.9
Diabetes mellitus[6]	157.6	128.5	142.3	155.9	154.4	144.5	141.1	134.1	129.9	123.2	123.5	130.8	127.0	129.8	129.6	133.8	135.3
Alzheimer's disease[7]	21.9	X	X	X	11.1	12.5	11.9	12.7	13.0	11.8	12.6	12.4	11.8	12.0	12.5	14.1	15.4
Human immunodeficiency virus (HIV) disease	26.1	X	87.8	205.7	92.0	76.4	74.7	70.1	60.5	52.7	44.4	41.9	37.2	32.5	31.6	28.7	26.7
Unintentional injuries	747.3	755.3	607.4	580.1	573.2	647.9	666.3	668.5	625.8	604.6	616.4	638.5	629.6	635.7	647.5	698.3	778.3
Motor vehicle-related injuries	236.8	470.4	411.6	378.4	348.5	326.4	324.9	302.8	260.1	241.3	230.5	224.4	228.7	219.0	213.6	228.1	248.3

NA = Not available.

X = Not applicable.

[1]Underlying cause of death code was coded according to the 9th Revision of the *International Classification of Diseases* (*ICD*) in 1980-1998.

[2]Age-adjusted rates are calculated using the year 2000 standard population. Prior to 2001, age-adjusted rates were calculated using standard million proportions based on rounded population numbers. Starting with 2001 data, unrounded population numbers are used to calculate age-adjusted rates.

[3]Starting with 1999 data, cause of death is coded according to *ICD*-10.

[4]Rate for male population only.

[5]Rate for female population only.

[6]Starting with 2011 data, the rules for selecting Renal failure as the underlying cause of death were changed, affecting the number of deaths in the Nephritis, nephrotic syndrome and nephrosis and Diabetes categories. These changes directly affect deaths with mention of Renal failure and other associated conditions, such as Diabetes mellitus with renal complications. The result is a decrease in the number of deaths for Nephritis, nephrotic syndrome and nephrosis and an increase in the number of deaths for Diabetes mellitus. Therefore, trend data for these two causes of death should be interpreted with caution.

[7]Data for Alzheimer's disease are only presented for data years 1999 and beyond due to large differences in death rates caused by changes in the *ICD* coding of the causes of death between *ICD–9* and *ICD–10*.

[8]Figures for 2001 include September 11th-related deaths for which death certificates were filed as of October 24, 2002.

Table 2-25. Years of Potential Life Lost Before Age 75 for Selected Causes of Death, by Sex, Race, and Hispanic Origin, Selected Years, 1980–2016—*Continued*

(Years lost before 75 per 100,000 population; data are based on death certificates.)

Sex, race, Hispanic origin, and cause of death[1]	Crude 2016[3]	Age-adjusted[2]															
		1980[2]	1990[2]	1995[2]	2000[3]	2005[3]	2006[3]	2007[3]	2008[3]	2009[3]	2010[3]	2011[3]	2012[3]	2013[3]	2014[3]	2015[3]	2016[3]
Drug overdose	381.2	40.2	39.1	53.6	85.0	177.3	201.4	225.0	227.6	237.8	255.1	278.0	275.1	287.7	306.6	338.9	399.4
Nephritis, nephrotic syndrome and nephrosis[6]	70.8	NA	42.4	40.0	60.8	63.3	64.0	65.7	64.8	65.5	64.6	55.0	55.6	56.6	55.3	58.8	60.2
Suicide[8]	196.0	184.2	153.3	140.8	129.1	144.1	145.8	150.4	156.2	159.6	163.7	172.3	177.6	182.5	191.2	201.7	203.3
Homicide[8]	98.1	181.3	174.3	163.2	118.9	108.8	110.5	111.0	105.1	102.8	94.9	95.5	94.9	90.4	88.7	93.1	105.4
WHITE[9]																	
All causes	7,293.1	9,554.1	8,159.5	7,744.9	6,949.5	6,823.2	6,763.4	6,664.3	6,590.9	6,486.5	6,342.8	6,365.7	6,321.6	6,338.2	6,390.1	6,514.8	6,715.1
Diseases of heart	1,062.5	2,100.8	1,490.3	1,353.0	1,149.4	1,012.4	987.0	952.8	941.9	912.2	900.9	895.3	882.5	881.8	883.0	889.0	888.0
Ischemic heart disease	631.1	1,682.7	1,113.4	975.2	805.3	671.4	647.8	616.4	606.6	573.7	563.7	553.3	544.8	532.0	524.8	519.2	510.2
Cerebrovascular diseases	168.6	300.7	213.1	205.2	187.1	160.5	158.3	154.1	149.5	147.2	142.7	139.5	138.7	135.1	138.1	137.9	142.3
Malignant neoplasms	1,529.7	2,035.9	1,929.3	1,780.5	1,627.8	1,485.8	1,456.8	1,427.3	1,404.5	1,396.1	1,375.8	1,351.9	1,340.7	1,317.7	1,301.5	1,274.9	1,251.1
Trachea, bronchus, and lung	343.8	529.9	544.2	487.1	436.3	388.1	373.4	363.1	351.9	343.7	332.8	320.5	311.4	300.4	291.0	277.8	257.6
Colorectal	140.6	186.8	157.8	145.0	134.1	117.3	118.9	119.6	120.0	118.6	118.4	117.9	117.9	118.6	117.6	119.3	118.8
Prostate[4]	57.6	74.8	86.6	73.0	54.3	46.6	46.8	45.6	45.6	42.6	45.3	41.7	42.1	41.9	41.8	40.9	41.9
Breast[5]	261.3	460.2	441.7	381.5	315.6	275.2	269.3	256.9	253.5	255.7	245.0	241.6	239.3	236.0	230.3	226.7	226.2
Chronic lower respiratory diseases	239.3	165.4	182.3	185.7	185.3	181.5	171.2	173.1	182.9	180.4	176.1	178.3	175.3	180.1	178.7	180.1	180.2
Influenza and pneumonia	84.6	130.8	116.9	108.3	77.7	76.7	70.8	65.6	74.6	103.4	66.7	77.1	63.2	78.4	90.1	70.2	74.8
Chronic liver disease and cirrhosis	226.1	257.3	175.8	164.6	162.7	157.2	156.0	164.3	166.8	169.0	173.5	179.6	185.9	189.3	195.1	206.3	204.1
Diabetes mellitus[6]	187.4	115.7	133.7	149.4	155.6	156.3	153.0	147.7	145.6	142.7	139.0	148.7	145.4	149.2	152.6	157.5	157.9
Alzheimer's disease[7]	21.4	X	X	X	11.4	12.3	12.4	12.6	13.0	12.1	12.4	12.3	11.7	11.8	12.0	13.6	14.7
Human immunodeficiency virus (HIV) disease	26.4	X	309.0	422.6	94.7	70.5	65.4	58.8	51.8	44.5	39.9	36.1	32.8	31.5	30.2	27.3	26.1
Unintentional injuries	1,365.8	1,520.4	1,139.7	1,040.9	1,031.8	1,183.1	1,183.2	1,225.2	1,223.0	1,167.6	1,092.1	1,098.6	1,134.9	1,119.7	1,125.2	1,156.4	1,430.6
Motor vehicle-related injuries	419.5	939.9	726.7	623.6	586.1	591.1	587.2	563.4	497.3	438.5	419.0	413.1	420.1	401.2	395.9	415.4	438.8
Drug overdose	711.2	64.9	74.4	115.4	167.2	314.4	366.0	397.4	412.4	415.7	435.4	475.3	467.6	493.0	534.7	610.6	755.5
Nephritis, nephrotic syndrome and nephrosis[6]	67.9	NA	37.0	36.1	52.5	56.5	58.8	57.7	58.8	59.4	57.4	50.9	51.1	52.7	53.6	55.2	55.9
Suicide[8]	473.7	414.5	417.7	411.6	362.0	385.1	388.3	398.5	409.4	417.1	430.8	444.8	450.8	451.2	468.3	484.7	491.8
Homicide[8]	139.0	271.7	234.9	220.2	156.6	161.7	162.4	164.7	160.9	147.6	138.7	135.5	135.9	127.7	125.7	135.9	149.3
BLACK OR AFRICAN AMERICAN[9]																	
All causes	10,109.1	17,873.4	16,593.0	15,809.7	12,897.1	11,788.4	11,515.2	11,098.2	10,611.2	10,319.6	9,832.5	9,659.5	9,555.7	9,528.5	9,490.6	9,702.3	10,030.4
Diseases of heart	1,646.9	3,619.9	2,891.8	2,681.8	2,275.2	2,011.1	1,929.1	1,859.8	1,813.4	1,766.6	1,691.1	1,647.8	1,645.0	1,647.0	1,638.9	1,637.9	1,661.4
Ischemic heart disease	751.7	2,305.1	1,676.1	1,510.2	1,300.1	1,058.3	1,009.8	945.0	905.2	859.5	818.8	803.3	792.0	776.7	756.5	740.4	748.9
Cerebrovascular diseases	314.1	883.2	656.4	583.6	507.0	434.1	422.8	406.1	386.6	362.3	358.1	338.0	326.5	319.2	322.3	322.9	316.8
Malignant neoplasms	1,603.0	2,946.1	2,894.8	2,597.1	2,294.7	2,030.4	1,957.5	1,913.4	1,864.2	1,823.3	1,796.7	1,770.5	1,724.1	1,666.7	1,651.6	1,598.8	1,575.3
Trachea, bronchus, and lung	310.8	776.0	811.3	683.0	593.0	500.4	483.4	456.3	426.7	417.6	405.6	387.2	377.5	362.4	340.8	318.3	294.8
Colorectal	175.2	232.3	241.8	226.9	222.4	195.7	194.4	193.9	192.8	185.3	188.6	185.3	177.0	174.2	176.5	172.9	175.5
Prostate[4]	111.9	200.3	223.5	210.0	171.0	139.6	134.2	132.1	125.6	129.6	127.3	120.1	113.6	109.9	109.0	106.9	113.4
Breast[5]	373.3	524.2	592.9	577.4	500.0	480.1	444.0	437.7	421.6	415.1	420.8	420.2	406.2	389.8	386.7	379.2	375.5
Chronic lower respiratory diseases	206.6	203.7	240.6	244.0	232.7	207.4	193.6	188.0	197.9	195.9	187.7	192.7	192.8	200.1	193.6	198.3	200.4
Influenza and pneumonia	124.7	384.9	330.8	269.8	161.2	143.7	125.8	121.6	129.4	152.2	109.8	123.4	106.2	122.9	130.9	114.5	124.4
Chronic liver disease and cirrhosis	118.9	644.0	371.8	250.3	185.6	136.0	124.3	126.9	122.1	119.7	120.2	123.1	116.2	122.4	120.4	122.5	118.9
Diabetes mellitus[6]	330.3	305.3	361.5	400.8	383.4	373.1	367.6	349.6	323.2	317.0	316.4	324.1	316.6	323.8	321.4	329.6	333.5
Alzheimer's disease[7]	13.2	X	X	X	8.3	10.9	10.2	9.6	10.8	10.4	10.0	10.0	9.3	9.8	11.2	13.0	13.2
Human immunodeficiency virus (HIV) disease	176.3	X	1,014.7	1,945.4	763.3	590.3	561.1	514.8	435.4	397.3	329.5	287.8	259.0	238.4	222.9	203.5	185.8
Unintentional injuries	1,268.9	1,751.5	1,392.7	1,272.1	1,152.8	1,129.7	1,163.6	1,106.2	979.2	934.0	896.7	918.4	925.8	953.0	986.8	1,082.6	1,276.8
Motor vehicle-related injuries	503.8	750.2	699.5	621.8	580.8	530.4	538.7	516.7	443.6	420.0	393.4	386.6	404.0	402.6	404.6	450.7	498.8
Drug overdose	460.1	99.4	144.3	209.6	196.6	252.2	293.3	259.8	230.0	221.3	218.9	240.8	242.1	265.6	289.7	342.1	478.8
Nephritis, nephrotic syndrome and nephrosis[6]	174.1	NA	160.9	140.0	216.9	214.8	214.5	210.5	206.5	201.5	193.2	174.3	172.4	165.7	167.1	174.6	175.4
Suicide[8]	243.5	238.0	261.4	254.2	208.7	193.6	186.5	185.9	195.3	189.1	196.4	202.3	210.4	207.0	209.0	216.1	239.5
Homicide[8]	1,012.1	1,580.8	1,612.9	1,352.8	941.6	967.5	996.2	961.8	897.2	834.8	821.2	813.0	842.9	813.5	785.1	907.4	981.0
AMERICAN INDIAN OR ALASKA NATIVE[9]																	
All causes	7,119.7	13,390.9	9,506.2	9,332.5	7,758.2	7,705.7	7,449.2	7,233.7	7,121.7	7,000.8	6,771.3	6,712.5	6,842.6	6,698.8	6,954.0	7,176.2	7,360.2
Diseases of heart	747.2	1,819.9	1,391.0	1,296.3	1,030.1	945.6	927.9	887.0	853.9	839.3	820.6	796.0	797.4	807.4	822.2	850.0	821.5
Ischemic heart disease	413.7	1,208.2	901.8	877.3	709.3	591.1	572.7	536.8	510.2	502.3	487.6	484.2	486.4	484.4	492.0	487.5	457.3
Cerebrovascular diseases	112.7	269.3	223.3	255.3	198.1	195.8	161.9	153.5	137.3	130.6	129.7	144.3	121.5	124.1	123.2	138.6	123.1
Malignant neoplasms	777.0	1,101.3	1,141.1	1,099.5	995.7	1,021.4	913.5	909.3	940.2	925.5	929.5	836.0	856.9	852.4	809.9	848.8	837.7
Trachea, bronchus, and lung	145.8	181.1	268.1	267.7	227.8	255.5	213.3	212.8	207.3	196.8	211.0	185.1	188.5	166.0	168.4	166.0	157.4
Colorectal	94.1	78.8	82.4	103.5	93.8	102.9	82.5	92.2	107.2	102.5	95.8	104.5	90.0	103.3	90.2	94.5	102.0
Prostate[4]	23.7	66.7	42.0	51.1	44.5	36.3	37.6	31.9	41.5	36.2	36.8	30.8	36.7	32.6	39.0	32.6	27.7
Breast[5]	114.2	205.5	213.4	195.9	174.1	139.2	158.2	149.0	142.7	135.4	145.0	121.7	120.0	108.5	110.9	129.7	124.0

NA = Not available.

X = Not applicable.

[1]Underlying cause of death code was coded according to the 9th Revision of the *International Classification of Diseases* (*ICD*) in 1980-1998.

[2]Age-adjusted rates are calculated using the year 2000 standard population. Prior to 2001, age-adjusted rates were calculated using standard million proportions based on rounded population numbers. Starting with 2001 data, unrounded population numbers are used to calculate age-adjusted rates.

[3]Starting with 1999 data, cause of death is coded according to *ICD*-10.

[4]Rate for male population only.

[5]Rate for female population only.

[6]Starting with 2011 data, the rules for selecting Renal failure as the underlying cause of death were changed, affecting the number of deaths in the Nephritis, nephrotic syndrome and nephrosis and Diabetes categories. These changes directly affect deaths with mention of Renal failure and other associated conditions, such as Diabetes mellitus with renal complications. The result is a decrease in the number of deaths for Nephritis, nephrotic syndrome and nephrosis and an increase in the number of deaths for Diabetes mellitus. Therefore, trend data for these two causes of death should be interpreted with caution.

[7]Data for Alzheimer's disease are only presented for data years 1999 and beyond due to large differences in death rates caused by changes in the *ICD* coding of the causes of death between *ICD-9* and *ICD-10*.

[8]Figures for 2001 include September 11th-related deaths for which death certificates were filed as of October 24, 2002.

[9]The race groups White, Black, Asian or Pacific Islander, and American Indian or Alaska Native include persons of Hispanic and non-Hispanic origin. Persons of Hispanic origin may be of any race. Death rates for Hispanic, American Indian or Alaska Native, and Asian or Pacific Islander persons should be interpreted with caution because of inconsistencies in reporting Hispanic origin or race on the death certificate (death rate numerators) compared with population figures (death rate denominators). The net effect of misclassification is an underestimation of deaths and death rates for races other than White and Black.

Table 2-25. Years of Potential Life Lost Before Age 75 for Selected Causes of Death, by Sex, Race, and Hispanic Origin, Selected Years, 1980–2016—*Continued*

(Years lost before 75 per 100,000 population; data are based on death certificates.)

Sex, race, Hispanic origin, and cause of death[1]	Crude 2016[3]	Age-adjusted[2] 1980[2]	1990[2]	1995[2]	2000[3]	2005[3]	2006[3]	2007[3]	2008[3]	2009[3]	2010[3]	2011[3]	2012[3]	2013[3]	2014[3]	2015[3]	2016[3]
Chronic lower respiratory diseases	137.9	89.3	129.0	145.3	151.8	146.8	134.3	157.6	156.1	138.4	154.5	137.6	133.2	135.6	140.5	158.2	147.6
Influenza and pneumonia	93.3	307.9	206.3	199.7	124.0	102.5	89.4	94.1	141.5	174.5	99.3	100.5	80.8	109.0	129.0	75.5	100.0
Chronic liver disease and cirrhosis	541.9	1,190.3	535.1	604.8	519.4	459.3	433.2	509.7	504.0	477.1	510.8	518.8	553.3	562.2	549.9	605.3	596.1
Diabetes mellitus[6]	291.0	305.5	292.3	360.6	305.6	327.7	301.7	268.3	264.5	260.4	267.6	297.1	286.4	281.7	279.4	300.7	319.8
Alzheimer's disease[7]	9.0	X	X	X	*	*	*	9.9	5.8	6.7	8.8	7.7	6.2	5.7	6.7	5.3	10.1
Human immunodeficiency virus (HIV) disease	22.5	X	70.1	246.9	68.4	81.4	67.4	69.3	57.3	49.5	46.1	32.1	32.1	33.8	29.5	36.2	25.2
Unintentional injuries	1,614.9	3,541.0	2,183.9	1,980.9	1,700.1	1,670.0	1,637.4	1,581.6	1,482.0	1,481.4	1,377.7	1,437.1	1,505.2	1,388.2	1,509.3	1,523.6	1,629.0
Motor vehicle-related injuries	669.8	2,102.4	1,301.5	1,210.3	1,032.2	894.0	891.4	790.8	698.6	667.4	570.6	614.2	637.0	575.7	605.4	638.0	656.2
Drug overdose	591.4	92.9	119.5	161.5	180.1	302.0	317.6	359.3	433.5	479.0	449.6	479.1	514.1	487.3	537.8	543.5	614.3
Nephritis, nephrotic syndrome and nephrosis[6]	74.2	NA	88.5	70.3	102.0	94.6	112.2	85.9	94.9	92.3	81.7	68.3	67.5	73.7	80.5	74.1	81.1
Suicide[8]	564.1	515.0	495.9	445.2	403.1	446.5	427.4	403.5	411.9	415.3	437.9	423.4	437.6	463.0	437.1	497.7	546.1
Homicide[8]	286.1	628.9	434.2	432.7	278.5	298.4	284.7	237.4	264.2	253.3	256.4	234.4	244.5	227.8	239.0	256.2	279.4

ASIAN OR PACIFIC ISLANDER[8]

All causes	3,214.8	5,378.4	4,705.2	4,333.2	3,811.1	3,433.5	3,361.3	3,262.2	3,154.7	3,114.2	3,061.2	3,014.4	3,049.4	3,050.9	2,954.4	3,049.7	3,176.8
Diseases of heart	417.3	952.8	702.2	664.9	567.9	505.8	465.0	443.0	431.6	433.2	400.1	403.8	404.0	413.1	402.1	400.6	400.9
Ischemic heart disease	250.3	697.7	486.6	440.6	381.1	322.5	302.2	289.2	275.4	270.5	250.6	255.7	248.3	250.4	239.8	240.1	238.6
Cerebrovascular diseases	143.5	266.9	233.5	220.0	199.4	160.5	161.9	149.6	152.5	141.7	148.3	136.5	136.0	134.3	121.8	129.5	139.0
Malignant neoplasms	868.1	1,218.6	1,166.4	1,122.1	1,033.8	931.0	899.0	871.2	854.5	834.4	874.7	853.6	855.5	830.7	799.4	809.9	833.5
Trachea, bronchus, and lung	138.5	238.2	204.7	197.0	185.8	167.1	169.3	158.9	156.2	144.6	148.2	146.6	145.2	136.7	136.5	130.5	130.4
Colorectal	88.8	115.9	105.1	99.5	91.6	77.7	80.3	80.2	83.7	78.3	87.6	84.5	85.6	87.0	79.1	80.8	85.3
Prostate[4]	17.0	17.0	32.4	25.3	18.8	20.3	18.1	16.3	16.1	16.3	17.0	18.2	14.7	14.4	16.8	18.6	16.7
Breast[5]	166.0	222.2	216.5	237.8	200.8	175.0	169.7	151.0	155.2	149.7	156.9	156.5	161.7	146.5	160.6	155.1	154.4
Chronic lower respiratory diseases	31.1	56.4	72.8	65.8	56.5	35.4	36.6	34.8	33.8	34.3	33.2	34.2	30.6	35.0	32.7	28.0	29.4
Influenza and pneumonia	41.8	79.3	74.0	64.3	48.6	39.3	36.0	35.5	39.9	61.5	38.4	43.3	33.5	36.4	42.8	36.1	40.9
Chronic liver disease and cirrhosis	46.9	85.6	72.4	48.4	44.8	43.2	44.0	40.5	40.6	45.2	41.7	40.9	37.8	42.9	41.6	44.0	45.1
Diabetes mellitus[6]	84.2	83.1	74.0	83.5	77.0	77.1	79.7	77.5	74.9	72.8	69.5	72.3	77.0	74.0	73.8	75.4	79.9
Alzheimer's disease[7]	3.7	X	X	X	3.5	3.1	2.0	2.8	3.4	2.3	3.2	2.7	3.8	3.6	2.6	4.3	3.5
Human immunodeficiency virus (HIV) disease	10.5	X	77.0	110.4	19.9	16.6	15.4	14.6	18.0	11.6	10.7	10.0	9.9	11.2	9.8	11.0	10.2
Unintentional injuries	369.1	742.7	636.6	525.7	425.7	393.5	389.4	385.3	332.3	308.0	303.0	306.6	311.8	308.5	307.0	328.6	361.9
Motor vehicle-related injuries	155.4	472.6	445.5	351.9	263.4	228.9	229.0	210.7	184.2	154.0	147.9	138.5	135.9	136.5	141.2	140.4	153.5
Drug overdose	112.6	*	17.6	24.5	25.9	40.6	45.1	49.8	43.7	50.5	46.5	62.9	64.9	71.5	67.6	84.3	106.7
Nephritis, nephrotic syndrome and nephrosis[6]	31.5	NA	26.7	23.8	33.6	31.5	36.2	31.8	33.9	35.5	38.1	26.7	29.9	31.1	29.1	32.3	30.3
Suicide[8]	244.4	217.1	200.6	211.1	168.6	158.0	175.8	190.3	170.4	182.0	199.7	190.2	207.6	206.0	203.1	222.0	237.8
Homicide[8]	71.4	201.1	205.8	202.3	113.1	123.3	113.8	89.4	85.6	80.0	68.8	78.0	68.3	64.4	59.7	60.6	70.0

HISPANIC OR LATINO[9,10]

All causes	4,651.5	NA	7,963.3	7,426.7	6,037.6	5,701.1	5,556.2	5,377.7	5,153.6	5,055.4	4,795.1	4,681.7	4,678.4	4,668.1	4,676.8	4,750.4	4,926.0
Diseases of heart	478.0	NA	1,082.0	962.0	821.3	726.9	687.8	664.6	629.0	630.2	598.1	585.0	570.7	571.0	567.9	578.0	574.1
Ischemic heart disease	266.2	NA	756.6	665.8	564.6	483.5	447.0	417.0	396.6	381.9	366.6	351.7	341.7	340.0	334.1	339.9	330.7
Cerebrovascular diseases	123.8	NA	238.0	232.0	207.8	184.8	184.6	175.4	162.5	155.8	150.4	149.0	144.3	145.5	140.2	141.1	147.2
Malignant neoplasms	764.5	NA	1,232.2	1,172.0	1,098.2	1,016.7	988.5	986.6	971.7	955.1	951.2	925.6	947.3	927.9	909.3	900.6	900.3
Trachea, bronchus, and lung	69.7	NA	193.7	173.9	152.1	138.2	125.1	125.7	122.9	117.4	115.0	108.6	107.3	102.9	96.8	96.9	88.4
Colorectal	74.7	NA	100.2	97.9	101.4	86.5	91.7	92.6	92.8	92.3	94.0	88.7	86.7	92.8	87.4	92.4	90.5
Prostate[4]	25.3	NA	47.7	60.8	42.9	42.1	44.3	43.9	41.5	37.3	38.2	38.1	37.0	35.9	36.5	37.8	35.8
Breast[5]	153.7	NA	299.3	257.7	230.7	194.9	200.6	190.7	184.0	186.0	180.0	176.2	192.5	181.2	183.4	169.0	179.5
Chronic lower respiratory diseases	47.1	NA	78.8	82.1	68.5	62.2	56.9	56.2	59.1	58.6	59.6	54.3	53.2	56.2	52.7	54.3	56.7
Influenza and pneumonia	55.7	NA	130.1	108.5	76.0	69.1	64.8	54.7	65.8	114.1	57.5	59.3	53.1	64.3	79.1	54.3	62.7
Chronic liver disease and cirrhosis	183.7	NA	329.1	281.4	252.1	210.7	202.2	210.2	208.4	207.5	201.6	209.3	209.5	206.1	216.4	219.2	216.9
Diabetes mellitus[6]	134.8	NA	177.8	228.8	215.6	202.4	181.4	178.1	171.8	161.6	158.5	160.2	160.0	161.6	160.9	163.1	164.8
Alzheimer's disease[7]	6.9	X	X	X	6.9	7.8	8.9	7.7	8.5	7.2	8.4	8.2	7.7	8.5	8.9	10.2	10.0
Human immunodeficiency virus (HIV) disease	34.9	X	600.1	865.0	209.4	140.2	130.2	115.9	98.5	86.5	74.9	69.5	55.2	52.5	49.5	47.0	39.3
Unintentional injuries	931.5	NA	1,190.6	1,017.9	920.1	966.1	980.6	907.4	812.0	755.5	708.7	727.9	719.5	735.9	740.1	808.7	914.7
Motor vehicle-related injuries	424.4	NA	740.8	593.0	540.2	558.0	553.9	493.3	414.2	379.5	340.3	334.3	346.0	344.8	348.3	370.7	402.5
Drug overdose	332.0	NA	121.9	173.9	145.9	179.5	196.4	200.4	200.5	194.7	191.2	213.1	207.7	224.3	234.1	269.1	339.2
Nephritis, nephrotic syndrome and nephrosis[6]	50.7	NA	54.4	35.3	62.0	65.9	69.6	68.9	69.2	73.5	67.7	56.3	57.1	57.5	56.3	60.1	61.5
Suicide[8]	244.6	NA	256.2	245.1	188.5	190.9	183.2	196.5	179.9	191.9	193.6	195.0	198.1	195.6	214.3	215.4	238.7
Homicide[8]	250.8	NA	720.8	575.4	335.1	336.2	328.1	311.5	289.7	267.9	238.0	221.5	215.4	199.3	197.6	213.5	234.5

NA = Not available.
X = Not applicable.
* = Rates based on fewer than 20 deaths are considered unreliable and are not shown.
[1]Underlying cause of death code was coded according to the 9th Revision of the *International Classification of Diseases* (*ICD*) in 1980-1998.
[2]Age-adjusted rates are calculated using the year 2000 standard population. Prior to 2001, age-adjusted rates were calculated using standard million proportions based on rounded population numbers. Starting with 2001 data, unrounded population numbers are used to calculate age-adjusted rates.
[3]Starting with 1999 data, cause of death is coded according to *ICD*-10.
[4]Rate for male population only.
[5]Rate for female population only.
[6]Starting with 2011 data, the rules for selecting Renal failure as the underlying cause of death were changed, affecting the number of deaths in the Nephritis, nephrotic syndrome and nephrosis and Diabetes categories. These changes directly affect deaths with mention of Renal failure and other associated conditions, such as Diabetes mellitus with renal complications. The result is a decrease in the number of deaths for Nephritis, nephrotic syndrome and nephrosis and an increase in the number of deaths for Diabetes mellitus. Therefore, trend data for these two causes of death should be interpreted with caution.
[7]Data for Alzheimer's disease are only presented for data years 1999 and beyond due to large differences in death rates caused by changes in the *ICD* coding of the causes of death between *ICD–9* and *ICD–10*.
[8]Figures for 2001 include September 11th-related deaths for which death certificates were filed as of October 24, 2002.
[9]The race groups White, Black, Asian or Pacific Islander, and American Indian or Alaska Native include persons of Hispanic and non-Hispanic origin. Persons of Hispanic origin may be of any race. Death rates for Hispanic, American Indian or Alaska Native, and Asian or Pacific Islander persons should be interpreted with caution because of inconsistencies in reporting Hispanic origin or race on the death certificate (death rate numerators) compared with population figures (death rate denominators). The net effect of misclassification is an underestimation of deaths and death rates for races other than White and Black.
[10]Prior to 1997, excludes data from states lacking an Hispanic origin item on the death certificate.

Table 2-25. Years of Potential Life Lost Before Age 75 for Selected Causes of Death, by Sex, Race, and Hispanic Origin, Selected Years, 1980–2016—*Continued*

(Years lost before 75 per 100,000 population; data are based on death certificates.)

Sex, race, Hispanic origin, and cause of death[1]	Crude	Age-adjusted[2]															
	2016[3]	1980[2]	1990[2]	1995[2]	2000[3]	2005[3]	2006[3]	2007[3]	2008[3]	2009[3]	2010[3]	2011[3]	2012[3]	2013[3]	2014[3]	2015[3]	2016[3]
WHITE, NOT HISPANIC OR LATINO[10]																	
All causes	7,879.6	NA	8,022.5	7,607.5	6,960.5	6,903.8	6,863.2	6,791.1	6,753.3	6,643.9	6,545.3	6,614.9	6,560.4	6,593.2	6,659.4	6,799.9	7,021.0
Diseases of heart	1,202.9	NA	1,504.0	1,368.2	1,175.1	1,045.9	1,023.4	988.3	982.9	948.9	943.2	939.9	929.3	930.5	932.4	939.2	939.9
Ischemic heart disease	719.3	NA	1,127.2	988.7	824.7	692.9	671.9	641.7	633.6	598.9	590.8	582.3	574.7	560.9	553.6	546.4	539.1
Cerebrovascular diseases	177.0	NA	210.1	199.6	183.0	155.5	154.2	149.2	145.0	143.3	139.1	135.5	135.2	130.3	134.9	134.1	138.3
Malignant neoplasms	1,712.7	NA	1,974.1	1,814.2	1,668.4	1,532.2	1,503.3	1,471.1	1,447.7	1,443.8	1,421.5	1,400.2	1,383.3	1,362.2	1,349.1	1,320.0	1,292.6
Trachea, bronchus, and lung	415.0	NA	566.8	507.0	460.3	414.5	400.3	389.8	378.3	370.5	359.1	347.4	337.7	327.2	318.6	304.0	282.9
Colorectal	156.1	NA	162.1	147.8	136.2	120.6	121.6	122.6	123.2	121.7	121.2	122.2	122.4	122.1	122.3	123.0	123.2
Prostate[4]	65.7	NA	89.2	73.6	54.9	46.8	47.0	45.6	45.9	43.0	45.9	41.9	42.4	42.3	42.2	41.0	42.3
Breast[5]	285.7	NA	451.5	389.3	322.3	283.8	275.8	263.4	260.5	264.0	252.6	249.0	243.5	242.3	235.4	234.1	231.6
Chronic lower respiratory diseases	289.4	NA	188.1	190.6	193.8	192.9	182.2	185.2	195.8	193.3	189.1	193.4	190.0	195.9	195.5	197.1	198.1
Influenza and pneumonia	90.9	NA	112.3	105.8	76.4	77.1	70.7	66.9	75.7	98.0	67.8	79.8	64.5	80.5	91.1	72.3	76.5
Chronic liver disease and cirrhosis	231.6	NA	162.4	151.4	150.9	148.0	147.6	155.8	158.7	160.6	166.9	172.6	179.6	183.9	188.6	200.7	198.2
Diabetes mellitus[6]	197.4	NA	131.2	142.8	150.2	151.4	150.0	144.3	142.5	139.8	136.7	147.4	143.0	147.0	150.6	156.2	156.6
Alzheimer's disease[7]	25.1	X	X	X	11.7	12.6	12.6	13.1	13.4	12.5	12.7	12.6	12.1	12.1	12.3	13.8	15.2
Human immunodeficiency virus (HIV) disease	22.8	X	271.2	362.1	76.0	57.0	52.0	46.2	41.3	34.7	31.3	27.8	26.9	25.7	24.7	21.1	21.8
Unintentional injuries	1,459.0	NA	1,114.7	1,026.1	1,041.4	1,214.1	1,263.4	1,282.1	1,240.1	1,157.4	1,183.0	1,227.3	1,210.5	1,214.6	1,253.8	1,365.1	1,559.9
Motor vehicle-related injuries	409.1	NA	715.7	618.0	588.8	586.9	583.4	569.7	508.9	441.9	430.6	426.3	431.0	407.4	398.9	417.6	439.2
Drug overdose	802.5	NA	68.3	105.4	169.4	342.2	403.3	442.2	461.2	467.6	494.0	540.8	533.1	561.8	613.2	700.8	869.1
Nephritis, nephrotic syndrome and nephrosis[6]	71.2	NA	34.5	35.7	51.1	54.9	57.1	56.0	57.0	56.6	55.3	49.5	49.8	51.2	52.7	53.7	54.3
Suicide[8]	529.7	NA	433.0	427.7	389.2	421.2	427.9	439.5	458.3	465.2	483.8	502.5	510.2	512.9	531.3	554.1	557.8
Homicide[9]	104.1	NA	162.0	148.6	113.2	110.7	111.6	117.4	118.5	105.1	103.4	103.4	106.6	100.6	98.4	106.2	115.9
BLACK, NOT HISPANIC OR LATINO[10]																	
All causes	10,650.4	---	---	---	13,204.9	12,193.6	11,954.9	11,546.3	11,035.7	10,743.2	10,243.4	10,098.7	9,972.4	9,969.1	9,898.7	10,144.1	10,505.2
Diseases of heart	1,749.2	---	---	---	2,320.2	2,068.2	1,986.4	1,920.6	1,874.4	1,826.2	1,749.9	1,710.3	1,706.3	1,714.1	1,702.8	1,701.9	1,734.0
Ischemic heart disease	797.8	---	---	---	1,321.6	1,084.4	1,035.9	971.3	932.0	884.4	843.0	830.2	817.4	805.0	781.2	765.9	778.0
Cerebrovascular diseases	334.4	---	---	---	517.9	447.7	436.0	419.5	398.8	374.8	371.4	351.5	338.5	332.0	335.2	336.1	331.2
Malignant neoplasms	1,701.1	---	---	---	2,341.8	2,082.7	2,014.4	1,970.3	1,921.5	1,881.3	1,856.5	1,833.9	1,781.7	1,730.7	1,709.5	1,660.0	1,637.3
Trachea, bronchus, and lung	330.8	---	---	---	604.1	513.0	497.0	469.5	439.3	429.8	418.1	399.8	389.6	375.0	353.6	329.1	305.4
Colorectal	186.3	---	---	---	227.4	200.4	199.5	199.1	198.8	191.5	195.1	192.1	183.0	181.0	183.0	179.5	182.8
Prostate[4]	119.2	---	---	---	174.1	142.7	137.8	135.1	128.2	132.2	130.8	123.3	117.1	113.5	111.6	109.7	117.0
Breast[5]	396.4	---	---	---	511.4	495.1	457.7	452.8	436.4	429.9	437.1	437.0	421.8	406.5	400.9	394.2	392.9
Chronic lower respiratory diseases	218.3	---	---	---	237.9	213.3	199.4	194.6	205.0	202.3	194.1	200.5	200.6	208.4	200.2	206.0	208.0
Influenza and pneumonia	131.5	---	---	---	165.2	148.9	130.6	126.4	134.0	159.3	114.3	129.0	110.6	128.7	135.3	119.7	130.0
Chronic liver disease and cirrhosis	125.3	---	---	---	189.5	139.5	127.4	130.2	124.8	123.3	123.9	127.2	119.6	126.1	122.8	126.3	123.1
Diabetes mellitus[6]	350.8	---	---	---	391.6	384.0	378.6	360.3	333.9	328.1	327.8	336.7	328.9	336.8	335.0	342.8	347.9
Alzheimer's disease[7]	14.0	X	X	X	8.5	11.0	10.5	9.9	11.0	10.7	10.2	10.3	9.6	10.1	11.5	13.5	13.5
Human immunodeficiency virus (HIV) disease	187.5	X	---	---	779.5	608.5	582.1	536.6	451.6	413.9	344.2	299.3	269.7	249.0	233.4	213.4	196.1
Unintentional injuries	1,324.0	---	---	---	1,182.9	1,168.3	1,208.6	1,153.3	1,019.8	972.6	937.5	962.2	968.8	1,001.5	1,033.7	1,134.6	1,334.0
Motor vehicle-related injuries	526.0	---	---	---	598.3	550.2	559.5	537.7	463.1	437.9	413.0	406.7	425.1	424.9	425.4	471.7	522.4
Drug overdose	478.7	---	---	---	199.6	258.3	303.2	268.3	237.2	228.9	227.7	249.7	249.7	276.0	300.7	355.4	495.6
Nephritis, nephrotic syndrome and nephrosis[6]	185.0	---	---	---	222.0	222.0	221.9	217.3	214.5	208.7	200.3	182.3	179.8	173.0	174.0	182.3	183.0
Suicide[8]	252.1	---	---	---	213.4	200.9	193.0	193.2	203.9	196.8	204.4	212.1	219.7	216.6	216.2	223.7	248.7
Homicide[9]	1,074.0	---	---	---	970.9	1,007.9	1,044.0	1,010.2	944.4	878.5	866.5	863.8	894.5	863.4	831.7	964.9	1,045.7

NA = Not available.
X = Not applicable.
* = Rates based on fewer than 20 deaths are considered unreliable and are not shown.
[1]Underlying cause of death code was coded according to the 9th Revision of the *International Classification of Diseases (ICD)* in 1980-1998.
[2]Age-adjusted rates are calculated using the year 2000 standard population. Prior to 2001, age-adjusted rates were calculated using standard million proportions based on rounded population numbers. Starting with 2001 data, unrounded population numbers are used to calculate age-adjusted rates.
[3]Starting with 1999 data, cause of death is coded according to *ICD-10*.
[4]Rate for male population only.
[5]Rate for female population only.
[6]Starting with 2011 data, the rules for selecting Renal failure as the underlying cause of death were changed, affecting the number of deaths in the Nephritis, nephrotic syndrome and nephrosis and Diabetes categories. These changes directly affect deaths with mention of Renal failure and other associated conditions, such as Diabetes mellitus with renal complications. The result is a decrease in the number of deaths for Nephritis, nephrotic syndrome and nephrosis and an increase in the number of deaths for Diabetes mellitus. Therefore, trend data for these two causes of death should be interpreted with caution.
[7]Data for Alzheimer's disease are only presented for data years 1999 and beyond due to large differences in death rates caused by changes in the *ICD* coding of the causes of death between *ICD-9* and *ICD-10*.
[8]Figures for 2001 include September 11th-related deaths for which death certificates were filed as of October 24, 2002.
[10]Prior to 1997, excludes data from states lacking an Hispanic origin item on the death certificate.

Table 2-26. Number of Deaths, Death Rates, and Age-Adjusted Death Rates for Major Causes of Death, by State and Territory, 2017

(Number, rates per 100,000 population, age–adjusted rates per 100,000 U.S. standard population.)

State and territory	All causes			Human immunodefciency virus (HIV) disease (B20–B24)			Malignant neoplasms (C00–C97)			Diabetes mellitus (E10–E14)		
	Number	Rate	Age-adjusted rate[1]	Number	Rate	Age-adjusted rate[1]	Number	Rate	Age-adjusted rate[1]	Number	Rate	Age-adjusted rate[1]
United States[2]	2,813,503	863.8	731.9	5,698	1.7	1.6	599,108	183.9	152.5	83,564	25.7	21.5
Alabama	53,238	1,092.1	917.7	95	1.9	2.0	10,410	213.5	170.0	1,173	24.1	19.8
Alaska	4,411	596.2	708.8	3	*	*	926	125.2	139.2	130	17.6	19.3
Arizona	57,758	823.2	678.5	90	1.3	1.2	12,008	171.1	135.8	2,054	29.3	23.7
Arkansas	32,588	1,084.7	900.1	45	1.5	1.4	6,517	216.9	173.6	1,180	39.3	32.4
California	268,189	678.3	618.7	635	1.6	1.5	59,516	150.5	136.7	9,595	24.3	22.1
Colorado	38,063	678.8	663.4	55	1.0	0.9	7,829	139.6	130.9	1,017	18.1	17.2
Connecticut	31,312	872.6	651.2	52	1.4	1.1	6,608	184.2	139.5	694	19.3	14.5
Delaware	9,178	954.1	749.6	16	*	*	2,085	216.7	160.4	244	25.4	19.1
District of Columbia	4,965	715.4	725.4	68	9.8	9.3	1,031	148.6	152.8	138	19.9	20.1
Florida	203,636	970.4	672.1	754	3.6	3.2	45,131	215.1	145.9	6,172	29.4	20.2
Georgia	83,098	796.8	793.7	337	3.2	3.1	17,135	164.3	154.9	2,348	22.5	21.5
Hawaii	11,390	797.9	584.9	12	*	*	2,456	172.0	128.6	299	20.9	15.9
Idaho	14,011	816.0	741.8	8	*	*	3,020	175.9	153.2	394	22.9	20.3
Illinois	109,721	857.1	724.2	140	1.1	1.0	24,150	188.6	157.9	2,927	22.9	19.2
Indiana	65,597	983.9	848.6	75	1.1	1.0	13,462	201.9	170.0	2,096	31.4	26.6
Iowa	30,530	970.5	737.0	18	*	*	6,449	205.0	158.0	918	29.2	22.8
Kansas	27,063	929.0	771.2	24	0.8	0.8	5,494	188.6	157.2	874	30.0	25.2
Kentucky	48,212	1,082.4	929.9	51	1.1	1.1	10,145	227.8	185.7	1,474	33.1	27.7
Louisiana	45,804	977.8	881.1	164	3.5	3.4	9,513	203.1	174.9	1,272	27.2	23.9
Maine	14,676	1,098.6	771.6	8	*	*	3,391	253.8	170.8	395	29.6	19.7
Maryland	49,926	824.9	718.1	199	3.3	2.8	10,796	178.4	151.5	1,439	23.8	20.3
Massachusetts	58,803	857.2	677.1	78	1.1	0.9	12,934	188.5	149.3	1,321	19.3	15.1
Michigan	97,602	979.7	783.5	84	0.8	0.8	20,671	207.5	161.3	2,798	28.1	22.1
Minnesota	44,371	795.7	656.4	37	0.7	0.6	9,896	177.5	146.8	1,312	23.5	19.3
Mississippi	32,280	1,081.7	951.3	112	3.8	3.7	6,526	218.7	183.1	1,164	39.0	33.3
Missouri	61,876	1,012.1	820.1	71	1.2	1.1	12,971	212.2	167.2	1,605	26.3	21.0
Montana	10,200	971.0	757.5	3	*	*	2,145	204.2	152.6	292	27.8	21.6
Nebraska	16,878	879.0	726.0	10	*	*	3,502	182.4	152.6	575	29.9	25.0
Nevada	24,657	822.4	765.5	58	1.9	1.8	5,283	176.2	155.3	609	20.3	18.3
New Hampshire	12,504	931.2	717.2	6	*	*	2,760	205.5	153.5	340	25.3	19.2
New Jersey	74,846	831.1	667.5	196	2.2	1.8	16,264	180.6	144.6	1,908	21.2	16.9
New Mexico	18,673	894.3	754.7	13	*	*	3,620	173.4	138.3	673	32.2	26.5
New York	155,358	782.7	623.6	461	2.3	2.1	34,956	176.1	141.2	4,176	21.0	16.8
North Carolina	93,157	906.8	785.6	210	2.0	1.8	19,474	189.6	157.1	2,903	28.3	23.6
North Dakota	6,415	849.2	692.7	2	*	*	1,280	169.4	142.6	194	25.7	21.8
Ohio	123,648	1,060.6	849.7	128	1.1	1.0	25,643	219.9	171.2	3,740	32.1	25.2
Oklahoma	40,452	1,029.1	902.4	44	1.1	1.2	8,203	208.7	177.3	1,398	35.6	30.6
Oregon	36,624	884.0	717.2	42	1.0	0.9	8,083	195.1	154.2	1,243	30.0	23.9
Pennsylvania	135,656	1,059.4	777.3	154	1.2	1.1	28,387	221.7	161.0	3,704	28.9	21.0
Rhode Island	10,157	958.5	713.4	12	*	*	2,154	203.3	154.2	275	26.0	18.8
South Carolina	49,441	984.0	828.0	151	3.0	2.7	10,356	206.1	162.7	1,535	30.6	24.5
South Dakota	7,996	919.4	736.6	3	*	*	1,715	197.2	156.9	263	30.2	24.9
Tennessee	70,096	1,043.7	897.1	139	2.1	1.9	14,302	213.0	173.4	1,915	28.5	24.0
Texas	198,106	699.9	735.7	622	2.2	2.2	40,668	143.7	146.5	5,832	20.6	21.2
Utah	18,035	581.4	700.1	9	*	*	3,161	101.9	120.3	596	19.2	22.9
Vermont	6,007	963.2	714.9	4	*	*	1,434	229.9	164.5	163	26.1	19.2
Virginia	68,579	809.7	719.4	106	1.3	1.1	15,064	177.9	152.6	1,967	23.2	20.1
Washington	56,995	769.6	688.6	52	0.7	0.6	12,664	171.0	148.4	1,812	24.5	21.6
West Virginia	23,276	1,281.8	957.1	9	*	*	4,654	256.3	179.4	864	47.6	34.0
Wisconsin	52,681	909.0	722.0	28	0.5	0.4	11,318	195.3	153.2	1,433	24.7	19.4
Wyoming	4,768	823.0	714.5	5	*	*	948	163.6	136.1	121	20.9	18.1
Puerto Rico	30,777	922.2	658.0	181	5.4	4.9	5,210	156.1	109.1	3,238	97.0	66.6
Virgin Islands	707	659.1	625.6	1	*	*	115	107.2	92.5	38	35.4	34.1
Guam	990	591.5	870.8	–	*	*	182	108.7	146.1	29	17.3	21.8
American Samoa	304	590.2	1,087.7	–	*	*	41	79.6	153.0	33	64.1	116.8
Northern Marianas	232	443.9	805.3	–	*	*	45	86.1	135.2	18	*	*

– = Quantity zero.
* = Rate does not meet NCHS standards of reliability.
[1]Death rates are affected by the population composition of the area. Age-adjusted death rates should be used for comparisons between areas.
[2]Excludes data for Puerto Rico, Virgin Islands, Guam, American Samoa and Northern Marianas.

Table 2-26. Number of Deaths, Death Rates, and Age-Adjusted Death Rates for Major Causes of Death, by State and Territory, 2017—*Continued*

(Number, rates per 100,000 population, age–adjusted rates per 100,000 U.S. standard population.)

State and territory	Parkinson's disease (G20–G21)			Alzheimer's disease (G30)			Disease of the heart (I00–I09, I11, I13, I20–I51)			Essential hypertension and hypertensive renal disease (I10, I12, I15)		
	Number	Rate	Age-adjusted rate[1]	Number	Rate	Age-adjusted rate[1]	Number	Rate	Age-adjusted rate[1]	Number	Rate	Age-adjusted rate[1]
United States[2]	31,963	9.8	8.4	121,404	37.3	31.0	647,457	198.8	165.0	35,316	10.8	9.0
Alabama	555	11.4	9.6	2,563	52.6	45.2	13,110	268.9	223.2	531	10.9	9.1
Alaska	36	4.9	7.4	98	13.2	22.1	814	110.0	135.0	40	5.4	6.6
Arizona	754	10.7	8.7	3,058	43.6	35.1	12,398	176.7	141.9	1,019	14.5	11.7
Arkansas	295	9.8	8.0	1,436	47.8	39.4	8,270	275.3	223.8	399	13.3	11.0
California	3,370	8.5	8.1	16,238	41.1	37.1	62,797	158.8	142.9	5,596	14.2	12.8
Colorado	490	8.7	9.4	1,830	32.6	34.2	7,060	125.9	122.7	298	5.3	5.2
Connecticut	350	9.8	7.1	1,077	30.0	20.4	7,138	198.9	141.6	366	10.2	7.0
Delaware	107	11.1	8.5	377	39.2	30.5	1,990	206.9	158.4	51	5.3	4.1
District of Columbia	37	5.3	5.6	125	18.0	17.6	1,284	185.0	189.8	76	11.0	11.4
Florida	2,571	12.3	7.9	6,980	33.3	20.7	46,440	221.3	145.8	2,622	12.5	8.3
Georgia	844	8.1	8.9	4,290	41.1	46.0	18,389	176.3	175.8	1,220	11.7	11.6
Hawaii	145	10.2	7.2	465	32.6	19.7	2,575	180.4	129.8	124	8.7	6.1
Idaho	206	12.0	11.1	672	39.1	36.6	3,084	179.6	162.4	94	5.5	5.0
Illinois	1,274	10.0	8.5	4,021	31.4	25.6	25,394	198.4	163.3	1,327	10.4	8.4
Indiana	730	10.9	9.6	2,771	41.6	35.3	14,445	216.7	183.2	814	12.2	10.3
Iowa	377	12.0	9.0	1,597	50.8	35.3	7,180	228.2	167.4	399	12.7	9.1
Kansas	359	12.3	10.1	894	30.7	24.3	5,723	196.5	157.9	264	9.1	7.2
Kentucky	443	9.9	8.7	1,765	39.6	35.0	10,343	232.2	195.9	441	9.9	8.5
Louisiana	477	10.2	9.5	2,188	46.7	43.7	11,260	240.4	214.4	371	7.9	7.1
Maine	200	15.0	10.4	601	45.0	30.4	2,844	212.9	143.5	117	8.8	6.0
Maryland	573	9.5	8.6	1,191	19.7	17.1	11,653	192.5	164.5	584	9.6	8.3
Massachusetts	625	9.1	7.3	1,841	26.8	19.9	12,140	177.0	134.6	620	9.0	6.9
Michigan	1,049	10.5	8.5	4,428	44.4	34.5	25,187	252.8	196.1	938	9.4	7.3
Minnesota	675	12.1	10.2	2,474	44.4	34.9	8,230	147.6	119.1	590	10.6	8.3
Mississippi	279	9.3	8.4	1,626	54.5	49.5	7,944	266.2	231.6	551	18.5	15.8
Missouri	621	10.2	8.1	2,545	41.6	32.3	14,820	242.4	191.1	700	11.5	9.0
Montana	100	9.5	7.6	285	27.1	20.9	2,164	206.0	155.0	94	8.9	6.8
Nebraska	225	11.7	9.8	698	36.4	28.5	3,581	186.5	149.3	274	14.3	11.3
Nevada	251	8.4	8.3	779	26.0	27.3	6,417	214.0	199.3	302	10.1	9.7
New Hampshire	168	12.5	10.0	436	32.5	24.8	2,721	202.6	149.7	100	7.4	5.6
New Jersey	798	8.9	7.2	2,829	31.4	23.6	18,840	209.2	162.3	808	9.0	7.0
New Mexico	224	10.7	8.9	572	27.4	22.7	3,896	186.6	151.4	155	7.4	6.1
New York	1449	7.3	5.8	3,521	17.7	13.2	44,092	222.1	171.2	2,699	13.6	10.4
North Carolina	1007	9.8	8.7	4,289	41.7	37.3	18,808	183.1	156.5	962	9.4	8.0
North Dakota	81	10.7	8.5	387	51.2	36.5	1,326	175.5	137.8	104	13.8	10.7
Ohio	1297	11.1	8.7	5,117	43.9	33.6	28,008	240.2	186.2	1,383	11.9	9.1
Oklahoma	376	9.5	8.4	1,752	44.6	39.3	10,772	274.0	237.2	478	12.2	10.5
Oregon	465	11.2	9.3	1,850	44.7	36.0	6,942	167.6	134.0	560	13.5	10.6
Pennsylvania	1557	12.2	8.6	4,213	32.9	21.7	32,312	252.3	176.0	1,025	8.0	5.5
Rhode Island	110	10.4	7.9	435	41.1	27.3	2,339	220.7	155.7	93	8.8	6.3
South Carolina	507	10.1	8.7	2,549	50.7	44.9	10,418	207.3	172.0	575	11.4	9.5
South Dakota	89	10.2	8.1	444	51.1	36.9	1,710	196.6	150.1	102	11.7	8.7
Tennessee	716	10.7	9.3	3,522	52.4	46.7	16,019	238.5	202.2	722	10.8	9.3
Texas	2338	8.3	9.4	9,545	33.7	38.5	45,346	160.2	169.2	2,304	8.1	8.7
Utah	234	7.5	9.8	991	31.9	42.1	3,749	120.9	150.2	173	5.6	6.9
Vermont	81	13.0	9.7	370	59.3	42.9	1,332	213.6	152.5	79	12.7	9.1
Virginia	836	9.9	9.1	2,549	30.1	27.6	14,861	175.5	154.5	681	8.0	7.1
Washington	671	9.1	8.6	3,710	50.1	46.0	11,582	156.4	138.8	637	8.6	7.7
West Virginia	204	11.2	8.0	770	42.4	30.6	4,849	267.0	192.0	323	17.8	13.0
Wisconsin	690	11.9	9.5	2,428	41.9	31.6	11,860	204.6	157.6	502	8.7	6.6
Wyoming	48	8.3	7.2	212	36.6	32.7	1,001	172.8	148.9	29	5.0	4.2
Puerto Rico	188	5.6	3.7	2,339	70.1	45.4	5,557	166.5	113.6	568	17.0	11.2
Virgin Islands	10	*	*	39	36.4	43.2	153	142.6	124.6	29	27.0	26.9
Guam	2	*	*	4	*	*	336	200.8	316.5	5	*	*
American Samoa	–	*	*	1	*	*	79	153.4	260.4	6	*	*
Northern Marianas	–	*	*	1	*	*	39	74.6	117.9	5	*	*

– = Quantity zero.
* = Rate does not meet NCHS standards of reliability.
[1]Death rates are affected by the population composition of the area. Age-adjusted death rates should be used for comparisons between areas.
[2]Excludes data for Puerto Rico, Virgin Islands, Guam, American Samoa and Northern Marianas.

Table 2-26. Number of Deaths, Death Rates, and Age-Adjusted Death Rates for Major Causes of Death, by State and Territory, 2017—*Continued*

(Number, rates per 100,000 population, age–adjusted rates per 100,000 U.S. standard population.)

State and territory	Cerebrovascular disease (I60–I69)			Influenza and pneumonia (J09–J18)			Chronic lower respiratory disease (J40–J47)			Chronic liver disease and cirrhosis (K70,K73–K74)		
	Number	Rate	Age-adjusted rate[1]	Number	Rate	Age-adjusted rate[1]	Number	Rate	Age-adjusted rate[1]	Number	Rate	Age-adjusted rate[1]
United States[2]	146,383	44.9	37.6	55,672	17.1	14.3	160,201	49.2	40.9	41,743	12.8	10.9
Alabama	2,931	60.1	50.0	1,176	24.1	20.2	3,484	71.5	57.8	756	15.5	12.7
Alaska	190	25.7	35.1	66	8.9	11.7	204	27.6	35.9	121	16.4	15.1
Arizona	2,681	38.2	30.8	876	12.5	10.1	3,802	54.2	42.7	1,137	16.2	14.3
Arkansas	1,612	53.7	43.8	720	24.0	19.8	2,517	83.8	66.7	399	13.3	11.3
California	16,355	41.4	37.6	6,340	16.0	14.6	13,881	35.1	32.2	5,325	13.5	12.1
Colorado	1,988	35.5	35.8	577	10.3	10.1	2,604	46.4	45.6	865	15.4	14.0
Connecticut	1,403	39.1	27.8	675	18.8	13.1	1,471	41.0	30.4	407	11.3	9.1
Delaware	571	59.4	46.2	184	19.1	14.9	526	54.7	40.7	106	11.0	8.9
District of Columbia	246	35.4	35.9	79	11.4	11.4	137	19.7	19.6	53	7.6	7.7
Florida	12,602	60.1	38.9	3,057	14.6	9.6	12,619	60.1	39.0	3,098	14.8	11.2
Georgia	4,399	42.2	43.5	1,400	13.4	13.8	4,866	46.7	46.2	1,146	11.0	9.8
Hawaii	764	53.5	37.5	637	44.6	29.6	378	26.5	19.0	132	9.2	7.5
Idaho	726	42.3	38.5	255	14.9	13.7	925	53.9	47.2	197	11.5	10.2
Illinois	6,020	47.0	38.9	2,402	18.8	15.6	5,732	44.8	37.6	1,407	11.0	9.3
Indiana	3,150	47.2	40.2	1,078	16.2	13.8	4,375	65.6	55.2	900	13.5	11.6
Iowa	1,416	45.0	32.8	578	18.4	13.2	1,939	61.6	46.5	337	10.7	9.2
Kansas	1,355	46.5	37.7	546	18.7	15.0	1,832	62.9	51.7	317	10.9	9.7
Kentucky	2,050	46.0	39.4	932	20.9	18.1	3,480	78.1	64.5	682	15.3	12.8
Louisiana	2,460	52.5	47.4	785	16.8	15.1	2,467	52.7	46.6	543	11.6	10.0
Maine	736	55.1	37.5	301	22.5	15.2	982	73.5	48.7	196	14.7	10.4
Maryland	2,820	46.6	40.2	990	16.4	14.0	2,079	34.4	29.9	484	8.0	6.6
Massachusetts	2,367	34.5	26.5	1,433	20.9	15.9	2,842	41.4	32.4	766	11.2	9.2
Michigan	5,002	50.2	39.3	1,798	18.0	14.2	5,688	57.1	44.3	1,323	13.3	10.9
Minnesota	2,250	40.3	32.6	697	12.5	9.9	2,464	44.2	36.3	568	10.2	8.6
Mississippi	1,723	57.7	51.1	782	26.2	23.0	2,037	68.3	58.3	437	14.6	12.6
Missouri	3,159	51.7	41.0	1,281	21.0	16.7	3,940	64.4	50.7	690	11.3	9.3
Montana	487	46.4	35.6	185	17.6	13.3	752	71.6	53.5	195	18.6	16.1
Nebraska	760	39.6	31.5	393	20.5	16.1	1,224	63.7	52.6	211	11.0	9.9
Nevada	1,137	37.9	35.9	636	21.2	19.6	1,633	54.5	50.0	458	15.3	13.3
New Hampshire	514	38.3	28.9	230	17.1	13.1	755	56.2	43.0	162	12.1	9.1
New Jersey	3,474	38.6	30.2	1,337	14.8	11.7	3,227	35.8	28.6	797	8.9	7.3
New Mexico	878	42.0	34.7	338	16.2	13.6	1,143	54.7	44.2	605	29.0	26.8
New York	6,264	31.6	24.6	4,517	22.8	17.7	7,258	36.6	28.9	1,671	8.4	7.1
North Carolina	5,098	49.6	43.0	2,076	20.2	17.5	5,540	53.9	45.3	1,273	12.4	10.3
North Dakota	337	44.6	35.4	147	19.5	15.3	358	47.4	38.3	87	11.5	11.0
Ohio	6,425	55.1	42.8	2,243	19.2	14.9	7,312	62.7	48.5	1,603	13.7	11.2
Oklahoma	1,947	49.5	43.3	625	15.9	13.9	3,035	77.2	65.8	670	17.0	15.0
Oregon	2,066	49.9	39.9	573	13.8	11.1	2,088	50.4	39.7	642	15.5	12.6
Pennsylvania	6,700	52.3	36.5	2,718	21.2	14.6	6,667	52.1	37.1	1,336	10.4	8.0
Rhode Island	425	40.1	29.4	206	19.4	13.9	521	49.2	36.2	148	14.0	11.2
South Carolina	2,691	53.6	44.9	723	14.4	12.3	2,983	59.4	47.9	812	16.2	13.1
South Dakota	414	47.6	36.7	217	25.0	19.0	505	58.1	45.3	153	17.6	17.2
Tennessee	3,519	52.4	45.0	1,656	24.7	21.3	4,657	69.3	57.4	1,038	15.5	12.8
Texas	10,790	38.1	41.3	2,954	10.4	11.2	10,650	37.6	40.5	4,107	14.5	13.9
Utah	888	28.6	36.2	334	10.8	13.3	826	26.6	32.1	243	7.8	8.8
Vermont	249	39.9	28.8	86	13.8	9.7	375	60.1	43.0	71	11.4	8.8
Virginia	3,555	42.0	37.5	1,245	14.7	13.1	3,363	39.7	34.9	970	11.5	9.6
Washington	3,028	40.9	36.9	1,041	14.1	12.6	3,177	42.9	38.0	982	13.3	11.4
West Virginia	1,058	58.3	41.8	458	25.2	18.2	1,681	92.6	64.3	337	18.6	14.0
Wisconsin	2,513	43.4	33.5	974	16.8	12.9	2,834	48.9	38.3	679	11.7	9.5
Wyoming	190	32.8	28.4	115	19.9	17.5	366	63.2	53.8	101	17.4	14.2
Puerto Rico	1,216	36.4	24.8	818	24.5	16.7	1,176	35.2	23.5	294	8.8	6.2
Virgin Islands	47	43.8	39.8	6	*	*	10	*	*	7	*	*
Guam	52	31.1	44.0	17	*	*	18	*	*	27	16.1	17.7
American Samoa	18	*	*	6	*	*	8	*	*	2	*	*
Northern Marianas	23	44.0	140.9	5	*	*	7	*	*	2	*	*

* = Rate does not meet NCHS standards of reliability.
[1]Death rates are affected by the population composition of the area. Age-adjusted death rates should be used for comparisons between areas.
[2]Excludes data for Puerto Rico, Virgin Islands, Guam, American Samoa and Northern Marianas.

Table 2-26. Number of Deaths, Death Rates, and Age-Adjusted Death Rates for Major Causes of Death, by State and Territory, 2017—*Continued*

(Number, rates per 100,000 population, age–adjusted rates per 100,000 U.S. standard population.)

State and territory	Nephritis, nephrotic syndrome, and nephrosis (N00–N07, N–17–N19, N–25–N27) Number	Rate	Age-adjusted rate[1]	Accidents (V01–X59, Y85–Y86) Number	Rate	Age-adjusted rate[1]	Motor vehicle accidents[3] Number	Rate	Age-adjusted rate[1]	Intentional self–harm (suicide) (*U03, X60–X84, Y87.0) Number	Rate	Age-adjusted rate[1]
United States[2]	50,633	15.5	13.0	169,936	52.2	49.4	40,231	12.4	12.0	47,173	14.5	14.0
Alabama	980	20.1	16.5	2,703	55.4	53.8	1,034	21.2	20.9	836	17.1	16.6
Alaska	54	7.3	9.9	436	58.9	63.7	101	13.7	14.2	200	27.0	27.0
Arizona	540	7.7	6.2	4,184	59.6	56.2	1,017	14.5	14.2	1,327	18.9	18.2
Arkansas	725	24.1	19.7	1,625	54.1	51.8	579	19.3	18.9	631	21.0	20.8
California	3,887	9.8	8.9	13,840	35.0	33.1	4,194	10.6	10.3	4,312	10.9	10.5
Colorado	503	9.0	8.9	3,037	54.2	53.6	678	12.1	11.8	1,181	21.1	20.3
Connecticut	554	15.4	11.2	2,078	57.9	53.2	293	8.2	7.8	405	11.3	10.5
Delaware	205	21.3	16.1	608	63.2	61.9	127	13.2	12.9	112	11.6	11.6
District of Columbia	67	9.7	10.0	427	61.5	61.0	33	4.8	4.7	47	6.8	6.6
Florida	3,172	15.1	10.1	13,059	62.2	56.1	3,229	15.4	14.8	3,227	15.4	14.0
Georgia	1,942	18.6	18.6	4,712	45.2	45.2	1,556	14.9	14.6	1,451	13.9	13.6
Hawaii	208	14.6	10.7	585	41.0	35.7	106	7.4	7.2	227	15.9	15.2
Idaho	170	9.9	9.0	876	51.0	49.8	271	15.8	15.5	392	22.8	23.2
Illinois	2,565	20.0	16.8	6,019	47.0	44.4	1,232	9.6	9.3	1,474	11.5	11.2
Indiana	1,440	21.6	18.5	3,978	59.7	58.7	917	13.8	13.5	1,092	16.4	16.3
Iowa	367	11.7	8.8	1,536	48.8	42.7	396	12.6	12.0	479	15.2	15.0
Kansas	541	18.6	15.0	1,567	53.8	49.4	461	15.8	15.6	553	19.0	19.1
Kentucky	1,024	23.0	19.4	3,264	73.3	72.9	831	18.7	18.3	770	17.3	16.9
Louisiana	1,076	23.0	20.6	2,780	59.3	58.8	825	17.6	17.6	720	15.4	15.2
Maine	260	19.5	13.0	990	74.1	68.0	190	14.2	13.7	274	20.5	18.9
Maryland	830	13.7	11.9	2,408	39.8	36.9	574	9.5	9.2	630	10.4	9.8
Massachusetts	1,193	17.4	13.4	3,821	55.7	51.5	416	6.1	5.7	682	9.9	9.5
Michigan	1,874	18.8	14.7	5,623	56.4	53.0	1,057	10.6	10.2	1,457	14.6	14.1
Minnesota	537	9.6	7.7	2,788	50.0	44.6	452	8.1	7.8	783	14.0	13.8
Mississippi	741	24.8	21.7	1,738	58.2	56.3	771	25.8	25.7	445	14.9	15.0
Missouri	1,515	24.8	19.6	3,776	61.8	58.8	999	16.3	16.0	1,151	18.8	18.5
Montana	129	12.3	9.2	579	55.1	50.2	179	17.0	17.0	311	29.6	28.9
Nebraska	226	11.8	9.5	811	42.2	38.5	260	13.5	13.3	275	14.3	14.7
Nevada	299	10.0	9.0	1,496	49.9	47.8	353	11.8	11.2	627	20.9	20.3
New Hampshire	169	12.6	9.4	907	67.5	62.9	108	8.0	7.3	265	19.7	18.9
New Jersey	1,591	17.7	13.9	4,482	49.8	47.3	647	7.2	6.7	795	8.8	8.3
New Mexico	330	15.8	12.9	1,460	69.9	68.2	399	19.1	19.3	491	23.5	23.3
New York	2,296	11.6	9.1	7,687	38.7	35.5	1,146	5.8	5.5	1,696	8.5	8.1
North Carolina	2,040	19.9	17.0	5,985	58.3	56.3	1,520	14.8	14.4	1,521	14.8	14.3
North Dakota	122	16.2	12.9	339	44.9	41.3	118	15.6	15.4	154	20.4	20.1
Ohio	2,237	19.2	15.0	8,971	76.9	75.1	1,322	11.3	11.1	1,740	14.9	14.8
Oklahoma	461	11.7	10.2	2,563	65.2	62.5	723	18.4	18.1	756	19.2	19.1
Oregon	377	9.1	7.3	2,076	50.1	44.7	509	12.3	11.7	825	19.9	19.0
Pennsylvania	2,898	22.6	15.9	9,527	74.4	70.2	1,262	9.9	9.5	2,030	15.9	15.0
Rhode Island	176	16.6	11.6	718	67.8	60.0	105	9.9	9.4	129	12.2	11.8
South Carolina	950	18.9	15.5	3,147	62.6	60.2	1,059	21.1	20.8	838	16.7	16.3
South Dakota	75	8.6	6.8	537	61.7	56.1	165	19.0	18.9	191	22.0	22.5
Tennessee	1,140	17.0	14.4	4,435	66.0	63.0	1,088	16.2	15.7	1,166	17.4	16.8
Texas	4,256	15.0	16.0	10,763	38.0	38.8	3,892	13.8	13.8	3,778	13.3	13.4
Utah	384	12.4	15.3	1,238	39.9	44.2	293	9.4	9.9	663	21.4	22.7
Vermont	29	4.6	3.3	394	63.2	56.9	81	13.0	12.3	112	18.0	18.3
Virginia	1,618	19.1	16.9	3,922	46.3	44.0	896	10.6	10.1	1,179	13.9	13.4
Washington	439	5.9	5.2	3,455	46.7	44.0	663	9.0	8.8	1,297	17.5	16.9
West Virginia	436	24.0	17.1	1,892	104.2	100.3	337	18.6	18.2	393	21.6	21.1
Wisconsin	922	15.9	12.5	3,746	64.6	58.3	657	11.3	10.9	926	16.0	15.4
Wyoming	63	10.9	9.5	348	60.1	56.9	110	19.0	19.1	157	27.1	26.9
Puerto Rico	890	26.7	18.3	966	28.9	23.3	317	9.5	8.5	247	7.4	6.5
Virgin Islands	17	*	*	36	33.6	34.1	11	*	*	10	*	*
Guam	26	15.5	24.2	44	26.3	27.1	18	*	*	36	21.5	24.6
American Samoa	9	*	*	16	*	*	2	*	*	3	*	*
Northern Marianas	7	*	*	22	42.1	55.0	6	*	*	8	*	*

* = Rate does not meet NCHS standards of reliability.
[1]Death rates are affected by the population composition of the area. Age-adjusted death rates should be used for comparisons between areas.
[2]Excludes data for Puerto Rico, Virgin Islands, Guam, American Samoa and Northern Marianas.
[3]*ICD–10* codes for Motor vehicle accidents are V02–V04,V09.0,V09.2,V12–V14,V19.0–V19.2,V19.4–V19.6,V20–V79,V80.3–V80.5,V81.0–V81.1,V82.0–V82.1,V83–V86,V87.0–V87.8,V88.0–V88.8,V89.0, and V89.

Table 2-26. Number of Deaths, Death Rates, and Age-Adjusted Death Rates for Major Causes of Death, by State and Territory, 2017—Continued

(Number, rates per 100,000 population, age–adjusted rates per 100,000 U.S. standard population.)

State and territory	Assault (homicide) (*U01–*U02,X85–Y09, Y87.1) Number	Rate	Age-adjusted rate[1]	Alcohol–induced causes[4] Number	Rate	Age-adjusted rate[1]	Drug–induced causes[5] Number	Rate	Age-adjusted rate[1]	Injury by firearms[6] Number	Rate	Age-adjusted rate[1]
United States[2]	19,510	6.0	6.2	35,823	11.0	9.6	73,990	22.7	22.8	39,773	12.2	12.0
Alabama	602	12.3	12.9	387	7.9	6.8	960	19.7	20.3	1,124	23.1	22.9
Alaska	78	10.5	10.6	159	21.5	20.2	158	21.4	21.6	180	24.3	24.5
Arizona	441	6.3	6.6	1,228	17.5	16.2	1,628	23.2	23.6	1,134	16.2	15.8
Arkansas	278	9.3	9.8	261	8.7	7.9	481	16.0	16.7	613	20.4	20.3
California	2,022	5.1	5.1	5,096	12.9	11.6	5,302	13.4	12.7	3,184	8.1	7.9
Colorado	261	4.7	4.6	1,018	18.2	16.5	1,050	18.7	18.1	779	13.9	13.4
Connecticut	109	3.0	3.2	354	9.9	8.2	1,103	30.7	31.8	188	5.2	5.1
Delaware	63	6.5	6.9	104	10.8	9.2	342	35.6	37.5	111	11.5	11.7
District of Columbia	117	16.9	15.6	63	9.1	9.3	322	46.4	45.6	100	14.4	13.1
Florida	1,269	6.0	6.4	2,598	12.4	9.9	5,347	25.5	26.3	2,724	13.0	12.4
Georgia	810	7.8	7.9	848	8.1	7.3	1,629	15.6	15.5	1,623	15.6	15.4
Hawaii	35	2.5	2.5	95	6.7	5.8	221	15.5	15.0	39	2.7	2.5
Idaho	50	2.9	3.0	221	12.9	11.6	264	15.4	15.9	280	16.3	16.4
Illinois	1,120	8.7	9.0	1,116	8.7	7.7	2,812	22.0	21.9	1,543	12.1	12.1
Indiana	456	6.8	7.2	722	10.8	9.6	1,925	28.9	30.5	1,016	15.2	15.3
Iowa	104	3.3	3.4	404	12.8	11.5	357	11.3	12.0	293	9.3	9.0
Kansas	185	6.4	6.5	314	10.8	9.8	360	12.4	12.7	466	16.0	16.0
Kentucky	310	7.0	7.3	484	10.9	9.6	1,662	37.3	39.5	730	16.4	16.2
Louisiana	653	13.9	14.4	341	7.3	6.6	1,138	24.3	25.1	1,008	21.5	21.7
Maine	19	*	*	194	14.5	11.3	443	33.2	35.7	172	12.9	11.7
Maryland	587	9.7	10.2	393	6.5	5.5	2,296	37.9	37.0	742	12.3	12.3
Massachusetts	171	2.5	2.6	683	10.0	8.4	2,323	33.9	33.9	262	3.8	3.7
Michigan	588	5.9	6.3	1,049	10.5	9.1	3,034	30.5	31.3	1,138	11.4	11.3
Minnesota	122	2.2	2.2	641	11.5	10.0	825	14.8	14.8	465	8.3	8.2
Mississippi	360	12.1	12.7	214	7.2	6.3	387	13.0	13.3	632	21.2	21.5
Missouri	655	10.7	11.3	556	9.1	7.9	1,426	23.3	24.3	1,307	21.4	21.5
Montana	42	4.0	4.3	249	23.7	20.7	132	12.6	12.9	244	23.2	22.5
Nebraska	50	2.6	2.7	245	12.8	11.8	163	8.5	8.7	160	8.3	8.3
Nevada	221	7.4	7.6	513	17.1	14.8	698	23.3	22.2	508	16.9	16.7
New Hampshire	17	*	*	176	13.1	10.3	479	35.7	37.8	146	10.9	10.4
New Jersey	352	3.9	4.1	647	7.2	6.3	2,752	30.6	30.7	478	5.3	5.3
New Mexico	173	8.3	8.5	659	31.6	30.6	515	24.7	26.0	394	18.9	18.5
New York	577	2.9	3.0	1,584	8.0	7.0	4,117	20.7	20.4	772	3.9	3.7
North Carolina	679	6.6	6.9	1,019	9.9	8.4	2,515	24.5	25.1	1,430	13.9	13.7
North Dakota	15	*	*	111	14.7	14.0	73	9.7	9.8	103	13.6	13.2
Ohio	828	7.1	7.5	1,219	10.5	8.9	5,299	45.5	47.9	1,589	13.6	13.7
Oklahoma	318	8.1	8.5	605	15.4	14.1	805	20.5	20.8	681	17.3	17.2
Oregon	127	3.1	3.1	879	21.2	17.4	676	16.3	15.4	528	12.7	12.1
Pennsylvania	791	6.2	6.6	930	7.3	6.0	5,495	42.9	45.0	1,636	12.8	12.5
Rhode Island	19	*	*	123	11.6	9.6	322	30.4	31.2	43	4.1	3.9
South Carolina	444	8.8	9.3	631	12.6	10.5	1,052	20.9	21.3	893	17.8	17.7
South Dakota	34	3.9	4.2	181	20.8	20.2	81	9.3	9.5	101	11.6	11.9
Tennessee	557	8.3	8.8	804	12.0	10.2	1,898	28.3	28.4	1,246	18.6	18.4
Texas	1,653	5.8	5.8	2,325	8.2	7.9	3,120	11.0	11.0	3,513	12.4	12.4
Utah	79	2.5	2.6	259	8.3	9.3	691	22.3	23.7	410	13.2	14.0
Vermont	15	*	*	94	15.1	11.8	145	23.2	25.0	70	11.2	11.7
Virginia	455	5.4	5.4	696	8.2	7.1	1,558	18.4	18.4	1,041	12.3	11.9
Washington	266	3.6	3.6	1,152	15.6	13.4	1,309	17.7	16.8	849	11.5	11.1
West Virginia	112	6.2	6.5	264	14.5	11.6	1,023	56.3	60.5	348	19.2	18.6
Wisconsin	202	3.5	3.7	780	13.5	11.2	1,205	20.8	21.6	624	10.8	10.6
Wyoming	19	*	*	135	23.3	20.3	72	12.4	12.7	113	19.5	18.8
Puerto Rico	684	20.5	22.0	192	5.8	4.2	86	2.6	2.6	649	19.4	20.8
Virgin Islands	54	50.3	57.0	13	*	*	–	*	*	54	50.3	57.2
Guam	7	*	*	2	*	*	2	*	*	4	*	*
American Samoa	–	*	*	–	*	*	–	*	*	–	*	*
Northern Marianas	2	*	*	5	*	*	–	*	*	1	*	*

– = Quantity zero.
* = Rate does not meet NCHS standards of reliability.
[1]Death rates are affected by the population composition of the area. Age-adjusted death rates should be used for comparisons between areas.
[2]Excludes data for Puerto Rico, Virgin Islands, Guam, American Samoa and Northern Marianas.
[4]Causes of death attributable to alcohol-induced mortality include *ICD–10* codes E24.4, F10, G31.2, G62.1, G72.1, I42.6, K29.2, K70, K85.2, K86.0, R78.0, X45,X65, and Y15.
[5]Causes of death attributable to drug-induced mortality include *ICD–10* codes D52.1, D59.0, D59.2, D61.1, D64.2, E06.4, E16.0, E23.1, E24.2, E27.3, E66.1, F11.1–F11.5, F11.7–F11.9, F12.1–F12.5, F12.7–F12.9, F13.1–F13.5, F13.7–F13.9, F14.1–F14.5, F14.7–F14.9, F15.1–F15.5, F15.7–F15.9, F16.1–F16.5, F16.7–F16.9, F17.3–F17.5, F17.7–F17.9, F18.1–F18.5, F18.7–F18.9, F19.1–F19.5, F19.7–F19.9, G21.1, G24.0, G25.1, G25.4, G25.6, G44.4, G62.0, G72.0, I95.2, J70.2–J70.4, K85.3, L10.5, L27.0–L27.1, M10.2, M32.0, M80.4, M81.4, M83.5, M87.1, R50.2, R78.1–R78.5, X40–X44, X60–X64, X85, and Y10–Y14.
[6]*ICD–10* codes for Injury by firearms are *U01.4, W 32–W 34, X72–X74, X93–X95, Y22–Y24, and Y35.0.

Table 2-27. Death Rates for All Causes, by Sex, Race, Hispanic Origin, and Age, Selected Years 1950–2016

(Deaths per 100,000 resident population; data are based on death certificates.)

Sex, race, Hispanic origin, and age	1950[1]	1960[1]	1970	1980	1985	1990	1995	2000	2005	2006
All Persons										
All ages, age-adjusted[2]	1,446.0	1,339.2	1,222.6	1,039.1	988.1	938.7	909.8	869.0	815.0	791.8
All ages, crude	963.8	954.7	945.3	878.3	876.9	863.8	868.3	854.0	828.4	813.1
Under 1 year	3,299.2	2,696.4	2,142.4	1,288.3	1,088.1	971.9	780.3	736.7	710.2	705.8
1 to 4 years	139.4	109.1	84.5	63.9	51.8	46.8	40.4	32.4	29.9	29.1
5 to 14 years	60.1	46.6	41.3	30.6	26.5	24.0	22.2	18.0	16.3	15.2
15 to 24 years	128.1	106.3	127.7	115.4	94.9	99.2	93.4	79.9	80.7	81.4
25 to 34 years	178.7	146.4	157.4	135.5	124.4	139.2	137.3	101.4	106.8	109.0
35 to 44 years	358.7	299.4	314.5	227.9	207.7	223.2	239.4	198.9	194.9	192.0
45 to 54 years	853.9	756.0	730.0	584.0	519.3	473.4	454.3	425.6	431.9	427.5
55 to 64 years	1,901.0	1,735.1	1,658.8	1,346.3	1,294.2	1,196.9	1,104.7	992.2	898.5	881.3
65 to 74 years	4,104.3	3,822.1	3,582.7	2,994.9	2,862.8	2,648.6	2,549.0	2,399.1	2,109.7	2,031.4
75 to 84 years	9,331.1	8,745.2	8,004.4	6,692.6	6,398.7	6,007.2	5,811.3	5,666.5	5,251.8	5,096.1
85 years and over	20,196.9	19,857.5	16,344.9	15,980.3	15,712.4	15,327.4	15,248.6	15,524.4	14,982.4	14,426.7
Male										
All ages, age-adjusted[2]	1,674.2	1,609.0	1,542.1	1,348.1	1,278.1	1,202.8	1,143.9	1,053.8	971.9	943.5
All ages, crude	1,106.1	1,104.5	1,090.3	976.9	948.6	918.4	900.8	853.0	831.7	819.6
Under 1 year	3,728.0	3,059.3	2,410.0	1,428.5	1,219.9	1,082.8	856.3	806.5	782.2	773.5
1 to 4 years	151.7	119.5	93.2	72.6	58.5	52.4	44.5	35.9	34.0	31.3
5 to 14 years	70.9	55.7	50.5	36.7	31.8	28.5	26.4	20.9	18.5	17.5
15 to 24 years	167.9	152.1	188.5	172.3	138.9	147.4	137.4	114.9	117.1	118.5
25 to 34 years	216.5	187.9	215.3	196.1	179.6	204.3	198.0	138.6	148.6	152.7
35 to 44 years	428.8	372.8	402.6	299.2	278.9	310.4	331.0	255.2	246.3	242.4
45 to 54 years	1,067.1	992.2	958.5	767.3	671.6	610.3	589.9	542.8	548.2	541.4
55 to 64 years	2,395.3	2,309.5	2,282.7	1,815.1	1,711.4	1,553.4	1,400.7	1,230.7	1,119.8	1,097.5
65 to 74 years	4,931.4	4,914.4	4,873.8	4,105.2	3,856.3	3,491.5	3,263.8	2,979.6	2,566.0	2,464.5
75 to 84 years	10,426.0	10,178.4	10,010.2	8,816.7	8,501.6	7,888.6	7,399.6	6,972.6	6,300.3	6,103.8
85 years and over	21,636.0	21,186.3	17,821.5	18,801.1	18,614.1	18,056.6	17,861.0	17,501.4	16,538.9	15,910.1
Female										
All ages, age-adjusted[2]	1,236.0	1,105.3	971.4	817.9	784.5	750.9	739.4	731.4	692.3	672.2
All ages, crude	823.5	809.2	807.8	785.3	809.1	812.0	837.2	855.0	825.1	806.9
Under 1 year	2,854.6	2,321.3	1,863.7	1,141.7	950.6	855.7	700.5	663.4	634.9	635.0
1 to 4 years	126.7	98.4	75.4	54.7	44.8	41.0	36.0	28.7	25.6	26.9
5 to 14 years	48.9	37.3	31.8	24.2	21.0	19.3	17.9	15.0	13.9	12.7
15 to 24 years	89.1	61.3	68.1	57.5	49.6	49.0	47.3	43.1	42.2	42.3
25 to 34 years	142.7	106.6	101.6	75.9	69.4	74.2	76.1	63.5	64.7	65.0
35 to 44 years	290.3	229.4	231.1	159.3	138.7	137.9	149.3	143.2	144.0	142.2
45 to 54 years	641.5	526.7	517.2	412.9	375.2	342.7	324.1	312.5	319.5	317.4
55 to 64 years	1,404.8	1,196.4	1,098.9	934.3	925.6	878.8	835.2	772.2	692.4	680.0
65 to 74 years	3,333.2	2,871.8	2,579.7	2,144.7	2,096.9	1,991.2	1,975.8	1,921.2	1,721.3	1,661.0
75 to 84 years	8,399.6	7,633.1	6,677.6	5,440.1	5,162.1	4,883.1	4,818.6	4,814.7	4,532.3	4,397.2
85 years and over	19,194.7	19,008.4	15,518.0	14,746.9	14,553.9	14,274.3	14,242.3	14,719.2	14,290.8	13,753.8
White Male[3]										
All ages, age-adjusted[2]	1,642.5	1,586.0	1,513.7	1,317.6	1,249.8	1,165.9	1,107.5	1,029.4	952.9	925.8
All ages, crude	1,089.5	1,098.5	1,086.7	983.3	963.6	930.9	921.0	887.8	873.5	862.3
Under 1 year	3,400.5	2,694.1	2,113.2	1,230.3	1,056.5	896.1	720.7	667.6	664.5	653.2
1 to 4 years	135.5	104.9	83.6	66.1	52.8	45.9	39.0	32.6	31.7	28.4
5 to 14 years	67.2	52.7	48.0	35.0	30.1	26.4	24.3	19.8	17.1	16.5
15 to 24 years	152.4	143.7	170.8	167.0	134.2	131.3	120.1	105.8	110.6	112.2
25 to 34 years	185.3	163.2	176.6	171.3	158.8	176.1	171.9	124.1	136.2	141.7
35 to 44 years	380.9	332.6	343.5	257.4	243.1	268.2	286.8	233.6	232.4	228.8
45 to 54 years	984.5	932.2	882.9	698.9	611.7	548.7	528.3	496.9	512.1	508.6
55 to 64 years	2,304.4	2,225.2	2,202.6	1,728.5	1,625.8	1,467.2	1,319.3	1,163.3	1,061.3	1,043.2
65 to 74 years	4,864.9	4,848.4	4,810.1	4,035.7	3,770.7	3,397.7	3,173.3	2,905.7	2,511.6	2,409.6
75 to 84 years	10,526.3	10,299.6	10,098.8	8,829.8	8,486.1	7,844.9	7,347.3	6,933.1	6,277.9	6,089.7
85 years and over	22,116.3	21,750.0	18,551.7	19,097.3	18,980.1	18,268.3	18,050.7	17,716.4	16,693.3	16,059.2
Black or African American Male[3]										
All ages, age-adjusted[2]	1,909.1	1,811.1	1,873.9	1,697.8	1,634.5	1,644.5	1,585.7	1,403.5	1,281.3	1,239.5
All ages, crude	1,257.7	1,181.7	1,186.6	1,034.1	989.3	1,008.0	960.2	834.1	796.1	781.4
Under 1 year	NA	5,306.8	4,298.9	2,586.7	2,219.9	2,112.4	1,664.7	1,567.6	1,478.6	1,449.5
1 to 4 years[4]	1,412.6	208.5	150.5	110.5	90.1	85.8	73.1	54.5	48.7	49.3
5 to 14 years	95.1	75.1	67.1	47.4	42.3	41.2	38.5	28.2	26.4	24.2
15 to 24 years	289.7	212.0	320.6	209.1	173.6	252.2	246.6	181.4	170.8	169.5
25 to 34 years	503.5	402.5	559.5	407.3	351.9	430.8	407.4	261.0	264.8	265.0

NOTE: Starting with *Health, United States, 2003*, rates for 1991–1999 were revised using intercensal population estimates based on the 1990 and 2000 Censuses. For 2000, population estimates are bridged-race April 1 census counts. Starting with *Health, United States, 2012*, rates for 2001–2009 were revised using intercensal population estimates based on the 2000 and 2010 Censuses. For 2010, population estimates are bridged-race April 1 census counts. Rates for 2011 and beyond were computed using 2010-based postcensal estimates. Age groups were selected to minimize the presentation of unstable age-specific death rates based on small numbers of deaths and for consistency among comparison groups. Starting with 2003 data, some states began to collect information on more than one race on the death certificate, according to 1997 Office of Management and Budget (OMB) standards. The multiple-race data for these states were bridged to the single-race categories of the 1977 OMB standards, for comparability with other states. NA = Not available.

[1]Includes deaths of persons who were not residents of the 50 states and the District of Columbia (DC).
[2]Age-adjusted rates are calculated using the year 2000 standard population. Prior to 2001, age-adjusted rates were calculated using standard million proportions based on rounded population numbers. Starting with 2001 data, unrounded population numbers are used to calculate age-adjusted rates.
[3]The race groups, White, Black, Asian or Pacific Islander, and American Indian and Alaska Native, include persons of Hispanic and non-Hispanic origin. Persons of Hispanic origin may be of any race. Death rates for Hispanic, American Indian or Alaska Native, and Asian or Pacific Islander persons should be interpreted with caution because of inconsistencies in reporting Hispanic origin or race on the death certificate (death rate numerators) compared with population figures (death rate denominators). The net effect of misclassification is an underestimation of deaths and death rates for races other than White and Black.
[4]In 1950, rate is for the age group under 5 years.

Table 2-27. Death Rates for All Causes, by Sex, Race, Hispanic Origin, and Age, Selected Years 1950–2016—Continued

(Deaths per 100,000 resident population; data are based on death certificates.)

Sex, race, Hispanic origin, and age	2007	2008	2009	2010	2011	2012	2013	2014	2015	2016
All Persons										
All ages, age-adjusted[2]	775.3	774.9	749.6	747.0	741.3	732.8	731.9	724.6	733.1	728.8
All ages, crude	804.6	812.9	794.5	799.5	807.3	810.2	821.5	823.7	844.0	849.3
Under 1 year	702.5	678.9	659.7	623.4	600.1	599.3	594.7	588.0	589.6	583.4
1 to 4 years	29.4	29.3	27.4	26.5	26.3	26.3	25.5	24.0	24.9	25.3
5 to 14 years	15.2	13.9	13.8	12.9	13.2	12.6	13.0	12.7	13.2	13.4
15 to 24 years	78.8	74.2	69.8	67.7	67.7	66.4	64.8	65.5	69.5	74.9
25 to 34 years	107.2	105.1	104.4	102.9	104.7	105.4	106.1	108.4	116.7	129.0
35 to 44 years	186.0	181.0	180.0	170.5	172.0	170.7	172.0	175.2	180.1	192.2
45 to 54 years	420.3	419.6	418.1	407.1	409.8	405.4	406.1	404.8	404.0	405.5
55 to 64 years	866.7	867.1	856.7	851.9	849.4	854.2	860.0	870.3	875.3	883.8
65 to 74 years	1,976.0	1,958.4	1,888.7	1,875.1	1,846.2	1,802.5	1,802.1	1,786.3	1,796.8	1,788.6
75 to 84 years	4,987.1	4,998.1	4,820.2	4,790.2	4,753.0	4,674.5	4,648.1	4,564.2	4,579.2	4,474.8
85 years and over	14,160.9	14,332.4	13,660.1	13,934.3	13,779.3	13,678.6	13,660.4	13,407.9	13,673.9	13,392.1
Male										
All ages, age-adjusted[2]	922.9	918.8	890.9	887.1	875.3	865.1	863.6	855.1	863.2	861.0
All ages, crude	813.1	820.3	807.2	812.0	818.7	824.5	839.1	846.4	868.0	880.2
Under 1 year	768.2	742.7	725.0	680.2	652.1	651.5	650.5	638.6	639.2	633.7
1 to 4 years	32.3	32.7	30.1	29.6	29.1	29.2	28.6	26.7	28.0	27.7
5 to 14 years	17.3	15.8	15.6	14.6	15.2	14.4	14.6	14.9	15.0	15.0
15 to 24 years	114.3	108.0	100.0	97.6	97.7	95.3	92.6	93.8	99.5	107.7
25 to 34 years	149.5	146.8	142.7	141.5	143.0	144.3	145.4	148.8	160.5	178.1
35 to 44 years	235.3	227.1	225.5	212.5	213.7	212.8	213.8	216.7	226.0	244.2
45 to 54 years	529.8	526.2	520.3	505.9	507.3	500.8	500.7	496.5	495.6	497.9
55 to 64 years	1,086.5	1,089.8	1,078.4	1,075.5	1,071.1	1,080.2	1,088.4	1,098.2	1,103.9	1,112.0
65 to 74 years	2,398.6	2,372.3	2,290.5	2,275.1	2,236.2	2,186.4	2,186.0	2,175.5	2,190.0	2,186.1
75 to 84 years	5,948.6	5,939.4	5,725.8	5,693.7	5,610.8	5,500.6	5,474.2	5,369.2	5,376.3	5,258.6
85 years and over	15,620.2	15,709.6	15,142.9	15,414.3	15,069.8	14,974.4	14,911.6	14,642.2	14,795.8	14,533.8
Female										
All ages, age-adjusted[2]	658.1	659.9	636.8	634.9	632.4	624.7	623.5	616.7	624.2	617.5
All ages, crude	796.4	805.8	782.1	787.4	796.3	796.4	804.4	801.7	820.7	819.3
Under 1 year	633.6	612.5	591.5	564.0	545.8	544.6	536.1	535.0	537.7	530.7
1 to 4 years	26.5	25.8	24.6	23.3	23.3	23.2	22.4	21.3	21.6	22.9
5 to 14 years	12.9	11.9	12.0	11.1	11.1	10.8	11.2	10.5	11.2	11.8
15 to 24 years	41.3	38.6	38.1	36.4	36.2	36.0	35.6	35.8	38.1	40.4
25 to 34 years	64.6	63.1	65.6	64.0	65.9	65.8	66.0	67.2	72.1	78.6
35 to 44 years	137.2	135.3	134.9	128.9	130.7	129.0	130.5	134.1	134.5	140.7
45 to 54 years	314.4	316.4	319.1	311.4	315.2	312.7	314.1	315.6	315.0	315.6
55 to 64 years	661.8	659.6	650.1	643.5	642.9	643.8	647.4	658.2	662.3	671.2
65 to 74 years	1,612.8	1,601.0	1,540.5	1,527.5	1,505.8	1,466.1	1,464.6	1,444.2	1,450.9	1,439.3
75 to 84 years	4,313.2	4,331.8	4,172.2	4,137.7	4,124.2	4,062.5	4,029.1	3,955.1	3,971.3	3,873.8
85 years and over	13,486.3	13,684.3	12,951.6	13,219.2	13,143.4	13,030.0	13,021.6	12,765.7	13,080.8	12,780.9
White Male[3]										
All ages, age-adjusted[2]	907.1	907.1	880.5	878.5	870.2	860.0	859.2	853.4	861.9	858.9
All ages, crude	857.8	870.6	858.2	866.1	876.4	882.8	899.1	909.4	932.9	944.0
Under 1 year	653.2	635.8	611.2	584.3	560.6	558.5	566.4	551.3	541.8	537.4
1 to 4 years	29.4	30.5	28.3	27.4	27.2	27.3	26.2	23.8	24.9	25.0
5 to 14 years	16.2	14.6	14.5	13.8	14.5	13.3	13.9	14.0	14.1	14.1
15 to 24 years	108.1	102.4	94.9	91.8	92.5	89.7	87.1	88.3	92.3	99.8
25 to 34 years	140.4	139.3	135.9	135.6	138.0	139.3	139.8	145.3	157.0	175.5
35 to 44 years	222.7	218.3	216.8	206.6	208.9	207.2	208.0	212.6	221.3	239.1
45 to 54 years	501.9	504.8	502.3	491.9	495.1	489.0	491.7	488.9	487.4	489.1
55 to 64 years	1,034.7	1,044.0	1,032.2	1,033.0	1,033.3	1,043.5	1,050.7	1,063.8	1,070.9	1,077.8
65 to 74 years	2,345.4	2,324.8	2,245.3	2,232.4	2,199.7	2,150.5	2,152.0	2,143.3	2,159.9	2,149.5
75 to 84 years	5,939.7	5,938.3	5,737.1	5,703.6	5,650.4	5,529.5	5,507.2	5,419.1	5,426.8	5,305.6
85 years and over	15,776.0	15,922.9	15,362.2	15,640.3	15,335.7	15,271.5	15,220.4	15,000.3	15,202.8	14,942.0
Black or African American Male[3]										
All ages, age-adjusted[2]	1,204.8	1,168.0	1,123.1	1,104.0	1,067.1	1,058.6	1,052.8	1,034.0	1,040.3	1,049.5
All ages, crude	768.1	750.6	735.3	725.4	719.4	728.0	739.3	742.6	765.3	789.5
Under 1 year	1,406.0	1,343.0	1,357.2	1,206.5	1,149.9	1,147.3	1,120.1	1,125.4	1,150.2	1,133.8
1 to 4 years[4]	47.6	48.2	41.9	42.9	42.7	41.6	40.6	42.2	45.7	43.4
5 to 14 years	23.9	22.6	22.2	19.6	20.5	21.3	19.6	21.0	21.0	21.2
15 to 24 years	165.5	156.2	142.5	142.8	140.3	138.7	135.5	135.4	150.9	164.2
25 to 34 years	251.0	235.7	226.1	216.7	212.2	212.8	218.6	212.1	229.0	248.6

NOTE: Starting with *Health, United States, 2003*, rates for 1991–1999 were revised using intercensal population estimates based on the 1990 and 2000 Censuses. For 2000, population estimates are bridged-race April 1 census counts. Starting with *Health, United States, 2012*, rates for 2001–2009 were revised using intercensal population estimates based on the 2000 and 2010 Censuses. For 2010, population estimates are bridged-race April 1 census counts. Rates for 2011 and beyond were computed using 2010-based postcensal estimates. Age groups were selected to minimize the presentation of unstable age-specific death rates based on small numbers of deaths and for consistency among comparison groups. Starting with 2003 data, some states began to collect information on more than one race on the death certificate, according to 1997 Office of Management and Budget (OMB) standards. The multiple-race data for these states were bridged to the single-race categories of the 1977 OMB standards, for comparability with other states.
[2]Age-adjusted rates are calculated using the year 2000 standard population. Prior to 2001, age-adjusted rates were calculated using standard million proportions based on rounded population numbers. Starting with 2001 data, unrounded population numbers are used to calculate age-adjusted rates.
[3]The race groups, White, Black, Asian or Pacific Islander, and American Indian and Alaska Native, include persons of Hispanic and non-Hispanic origin. Persons of Hispanic origin may be of any race. Death rates for Hispanic, American Indian or Alaska Native, and Asian or Pacific Islander persons should be interpreted with caution because of inconsistencies in reporting Hispanic origin or race on the death certificate (death rate numerators) compared with population figures (death rate denominators). The net effect of misclassification is an underestimation of deaths and death rates for races other than White and Black.
[4]In 1950, rate is for the age group under 5 years.

Table 2-27. Death Rates for All Causes, by Sex, Race, Hispanic Origin, and Age, Selected Years 1950–2016—*Continued*

(Deaths per 100,000 resident population; data are based on death certificates.)

Sex, race, Hispanic origin, and age	1950[1]	1960[1]	1970	1980	1985	1990	1995	2000	2005	2006
35 to 44 years	878.1	762.0	956.6	689.8	630.2	699.6	716.8	453.0	394.1	389.1
45 to 54 years	1,905.0	1,624.8	1,777.5	1,479.9	1,292.9	1,261.0	1,238.9	1,017.7	923.1	891.5
55 to 64 years	3,773.2	3,316.4	3,256.9	2,873.0	2,779.8	2,618.4	2,382.0	2,080.1	1,877.9	1,805.8
65 to 74 years	5,310.3	5,798.7	5,803.2	5,131.1	5,172.4	4,946.1	4,707.8	4,253.5	3,606.8	3,511.6
75 to 84 years[5]	10,101.9	8,605.1	9,454.9	9,231.6	9,262.3	9,129.5	8,862.0	8,486.0	7,674.6	7,381.4
85 years and over	NA	14,844.8	12,222.3	16,098.8	15,774.2	16,954.9	17,016.0	16,791.0	16,769.2	16,110.0
American Indian or Alaska Native Male[3]										
All ages, age-adjusted[2]	NA	NA	NA	1,111.5	926.1	916.2	932.0	841.5	824.5	780.8
All ages, crude	NA	NA	NA	597.1	492.5	476.4	459.4	415.6	428.4	413.7
Under 1 year	NA	NA	NA	1,598.1	1,080.0	1,056.6	696.0	700.2	600.5	706.2
1 to 4 years[4]	NA	NA	NA	82.7	105.3	77.4	73.3	44.9	49.8	39.5
5 to 14 years	NA	NA	NA	43.7	39.2	33.4	27.0	20.2	19.7	14.1
15 to 24 years	NA	NA	NA	311.1	214.4	219.8	182.1	136.2	126.7	133.1
25 to 34 years	NA	NA	NA	360.6	275.0	256.1	263.6	179.1	191.6	176.3
35 to 44 years	NA	NA	NA	556.8	363.5	365.4	377.4	295.2	304.7	298.7
45 to 54 years	NA	NA	NA	871.3	687.9	619.9	601.0	520.0	541.6	534.2
55 to 64 years	NA	NA	NA	1,547.5	1,319.1	1,211.3	1,276.0	1,090.4	1,076.8	974.9
65 to 74 years	NA	NA	NA	2,968.4	2,692.3	2,461.7	2,660.8	2,478.3	2,243.8	2,127.5
75 to 84 years[5]	NA	NA	NA	5,607.0	5,572.7	5,389.2	5,787.7	5,351.2	4,877.8	4,722.6
85 years and over	NA	NA	NA	12,635.2	8,900.0	11,243.9	10,604.7	10,725.8	11,841.9	10,735.7
Asian or Pacific Islander Male[3]										
All ages, age-adjusted[2]	NA	NA	NA	786.5	755.4	716.4	693.4	624.2	560.6	544.9
All ages, crude	NA	NA	NA	375.3	344.6	334.3	341.4	332.9	326.6	323.4
Under 1 year	NA	NA	NA	816.5	750.0	605.3	468.3	529.4	439.3	457.8
1 to 4 years	NA	NA	NA	50.9	43.4	45.0	28.0	23.3	19.7	17.4
5 to 14 years	NA	NA	NA	23.4	22.5	20.7	19.6	12.9	13.5	10.7
15 to 24 years	NA	NA	NA	80.8	76.0	76.0	73.0	55.2	51.2	54.7
25 to 34 years	NA	NA	NA	83.5	77.3	79.6	75.4	55.0	54.9	53.5
35 to 44 years	NA	NA	NA	128.3	114.4	130.8	124.9	104.9	96.5	92.3
45 to 54 years	NA	NA	NA	342.3	284.8	287.1	273.0	249.7	242.4	232.9
55 to 64 years	NA	NA	NA	881.1	869.4	789.1	714.2	642.4	540.4	546.1
65 to 74 years	NA	NA	NA	2,236.1	2,102.0	2,041.4	1,894.8	1,661.0	1,388.9	1,315.0
75 to 84 years	NA	NA	NA	5,389.5	5,551.2	5,008.6	4,729.9	4,328.2	3,875.2	3,730.6
85 years and over	NA	NA	NA	13,753.6	12,750.0	12,446.3	13,252.0	12,125.3	11,343.4	11,154.9
Hispanic or Latino Male[3,6]										
All ages, age-adjusted[2]	NA	NA	NA	NA	NA	NA	NA	818.1	771.2	732.3
All ages, crude	NA	NA	NA	NA	NA	NA	NA	331.3	335.6	326.1
Under 1 year	NA	NA	NA	NA	NA	NA	NA	637.1	637.6	613.6
1 to 4 years	NA	NA	NA	NA	NA	NA	NA	31.5	33.0	28.9
5 to 14 years	NA	NA	NA	NA	NA	NA	NA	17.9	15.1	16.0
15 to 24 years	NA	NA	NA	NA	NA	NA	NA	107.7	112.3	111.8
25 to 34 years	NA	NA	NA	NA	NA	NA	NA	120.2	123.0	121.7
35 to 44 years	NA	NA	NA	NA	NA	NA	NA	211.0	188.8	184.6
45 to 54 years	NA	NA	NA	NA	NA	NA	NA	439.0	421.7	409.6
55 to 64 years	NA	NA	NA	NA	NA	NA	NA	965.7	880.2	849.4
65 to 74 years	NA	NA	NA	NA	NA	NA	NA	2,287.9	2,052.2	1,936.1
75 to 84 years	NA	NA	NA	NA	NA	NA	NA	5,395.3	5,096.5	4,739.5
85 years and over	NA	NA	NA	NA	NA	NA	NA	13,086.2	12,746.1	12,135.6
White, not Hispanic or Latino Male[6]										
All ages, age-adjusted[2]	NA	NA	NA	NA	NA	NA	NA	1,035.4	961.5	935.7
All ages, crude	NA	NA	NA	NA	NA	NA	NA	978.5	978.1	969.4
Under 1 year	NA	NA	NA	NA	NA	NA	NA	658.7	656.4	647.8
1 to 4 years	NA	NA	NA	NA	NA	NA	NA	32.4	30.6	27.4
5 to 14 years	NA	NA	NA	NA	NA	NA	NA	20.0	17.5	16.2
15 to 24 years	NA	NA	NA	NA	NA	NA	NA	103.5	107.6	109.6
25 to 34 years	NA	NA	NA	NA	NA	NA	NA	123.0	137.7	145.0
35 to 44 years	NA	NA	NA	NA	NA	NA	NA	233.9	238.4	235.3
45 to 54 years	NA	NA	NA	NA	NA	NA	NA	497.7	518.8	516.8
55 to 64 years	NA	NA	NA	NA	NA	NA	NA	1,170.9	1,070.8	1,054.0
65 to 74 years	NA	NA	NA	NA	NA	NA	NA	2,930.5	2,536.0	2,435.4
75 to 84 years	NA	NA	NA	NA	NA	NA	NA	6,977.8	6,329.5	6,154.5
85 years and over	NA	NA	NA	NA	NA	NA	NA	17,853.2	16,840.7	16,206.8

NOTE: Starting with *Health, United States, 2003*, rates for 1991–1999 were revised using intercensal population estimates based on the 1990 and 2000 Censuses. For 2000, population estimates are bridged-race April 1 census counts. Starting with *Health, United States, 2012*, rates for 2001–2009 were revised using intercensal population estimates based on the 2000 and 2010 Censuses. For 2010, population estimates are bridged-race April 1 census counts. Rates for 2011 and beyond were computed using 2010-based postcensal estimates. Age groups were selected to minimize the presentation of unstable age-specific death rates based on small numbers of deaths and for consistency among comparison groups. Starting with 2003 data, some states began to collect information on more than one race on the death certificate, according to 1997 Office of Management and Budget (OMB) standards. The multiple-race data for these states were bridged to the single-race categories of the 1977 OMB standards, for comparability with other states.
NA = Not available.
[1]Includes deaths of persons who were not residents of the 50 states and the District of Columbia (DC).
[2]Age-adjusted rates are calculated using the year 2000 standard population. Prior to 2001, age-adjusted rates were calculated using standard million proportions based on rounded population numbers. Starting with 2001 data, unrounded population numbers are used to calculate age-adjusted rates.
[3]The race groups, White, Black, Asian or Pacific Islander, and American Indian and Alaska Native, include persons of Hispanic and non-Hispanic origin. Persons of Hispanic origin may be of any race. Death rates for Hispanic, American Indian or Alaska Native, and Asian or Pacific Islander persons should be interpreted with caution because of inconsistencies in reporting Hispanic origin or race on the death certificate (death rate numerators) compared with population figures (death rate denominators). The net effect of misclassification is an underestimation of deaths and death rates for races other than White and Black.
[4]In 1950, rate is for the age group under 5 years.
[5]In 1950, rate is for the age group 75 years and over.
[6]Prior to 1997, excludes data from states lacking an Hispanic-origin item on the death certificate.

Table 2-27. Death Rates for All Causes, by Sex, Race, Hispanic Origin, and Age, Selected Years 1950–2016—Continued

(Deaths per 100,000 resident population; data are based on death certificates.)

Sex, race, Hispanic origin, and age	2007	2008	2009	2010	2011	2012	2013	2014	2015	2016
35 to 44 years	374.3	342.0	336.8	307.5	304.8	306.1	312.4	308.5	325.8	350.3
45 to 54 years	842.5	790.7	760.4	716.3	706.3	696.3	678.8	671.8	678.1	687.9
55 to 64 years	1,774.9	1,723.4	1,707.1	1,662.1	1,623.4	1,615.8	1,628.0	1,611.5	1,612.9	1,623.2
65 to 74 years	3,428.7	3,347.9	3,250.1	3,205.6	3,127.2	3,077.9	3,064.4	3,047.4	3,041.8	3,081.0
75 to 84 years[5]	7,142.9	7,084.2	6,727.9	6,721.5	6,358.9	6,416.8	6,362.4	6,172.6	6,204.5	6,134.4
85 years and over	15,879.4	15,380.0	14,562.9	14,715.3	14,159.4	13,775.7	13,657.1	13,291.7	13,066.3	13,028.7
American Indian or Alaska Native Male[3]										
All ages, age-adjusted[2]	780.3	757.2	709.0	730.2	691.7	690.5	689.2	685.4	693.6	693.2
All ages, crude	411.1	408.7	389.9	397.5	395.1	410.2	416.5	433.2	454.7	471.2
Under 1 year	646.4	600.1	548.7	542.5	486.5	528.4	493.4	509.7	486.4	524.3
1 to 4 years[4]	42.0	34.6	31.2	34.3	28.8	34.2	41.5	41.0	35.2	29.4
5 to 14 years	17.9	14.7	15.5	18.1	13.1	16.8	12.1	12.3	15.2	14.9
15 to 24 years	119.2	122.0	121.0	116.4	107.0	107.9	98.0	103.8	101.1	115.2
25 to 34 years	175.6	171.3	154.9	156.2	161.9	175.3	172.7	179.1	191.4	214.6
35 to 44 years	285.4	262.9	275.6	258.2	250.9	248.6	244.4	264.4	281.4	284.9
45 to 54 years	507.1	535.2	486.7	496.1	500.6	500.8	506.4	508.5	543.5	525.1
55 to 64 years	973.7	961.8	941.0	951.2	894.8	939.2	937.8	984.7	994.2	1,012.7
65 to 74 years	2,105.8	2,128.4	1,969.9	1,971.0	1,908.1	1,948.9	1,845.9	1,830.2	1,840.6	1,871.4
75 to 84 years[5]	4,737.9	4,729.6	4,342.4	4,451.8	4,240.5	4,190.2	4,224.5	4,097.9	4,171.0	4,015.6
85 years and over	11,274.5	9,880.9	9,174.7	10,268.1	9,169.4	8,618.1	9,034.3	8,610.4	8,277.3	8,251.1
Asian or Pacific Islander Male[3]										
All ages, age-adjusted[2]	525.9	518.5	509.2	512.1	490.7	484.1	487.8	462.0	467.6	464.6
All ages, crude	318.7	320.0	321.2	327.0	328.6	332.8	347.4	341.3	354.5	363.6
Under 1 year	462.5	443.8	412.0	434.4	410.0	430.9	408.9	384.3	437.8	449.2
1 to 4 years	24.3	16.8	19.3	19.3	15.4	16.3	19.3	14.3	15.1	16.1
5 to 14 years	11.4	11.5	11.0	8.4	9.2	9.0	11.1	9.9	10.3	9.6
15 to 24 years	52.2	41.5	41.3	43.0	42.5	41.5	42.2	44.7	48.6	52.1
25 to 34 years	47.9	50.9	50.3	52.6	53.9	54.9	54.2	54.1	55.7	58.3
35 to 44 years	92.0	89.1	93.7	83.5	84.2	92.0	88.5	83.0	84.5	98.5
45 to 54 years	227.6	219.3	226.5	213.7	216.8	216.5	220.4	212.3	205.3	210.8
55 to 64 years	514.8	516.3	509.9	519.0	502.8	505.9	517.6	519.9	507.9	521.6
65 to 74 years	1,278.2	1,273.1	1,218.8	1,226.0	1,167.1	1,109.2	1,126.4	1,107.1	1,130.7	1,133.8
75 to 84 years	3,650.5	3,595.7	3,456.9	3,438.7	3,311.2	3,218.0	3,239.9	3,047.8	3,091.6	3,019.4
85 years and over	10,580.0	10,492.8	10,477.3	10,824.5	10,143.4	10,116.5	10,142.8	9,263.1	9,405.8	9,074.8
Hispanic or Latino Male[3,6]										
All ages, age-adjusted[2]	711.4	695.3	675.5	677.7	647.3	643.9	639.8	626.8	628.9	631.8
All ages, crude	321.6	316.0	311.8	310.8	309.7	316.5	323.7	330.1	343.2	356.8
Under 1 year	616.5	605.0	569.5	556.8	487.6	509.1	501.1	508.3	500.4	511.5
1 to 4 years	28.4	29.0	25.9	25.0	25.5	23.5	23.1	20.1	22.0	21.1
5 to 14 years	15.3	12.3	14.1	11.4	12.5	12.3	11.7	12.5	12.2	12.2
15 to 24 years	104.2	91.9	87.6	79.4	78.5	76.4	72.9	75.4	82.2	87.3
25 to 34 years	117.4	112.3	107.1	100.9	98.5	100.0	99.9	103.6	111.8	127.7
35 to 44 years	173.7	165.5	158.5	146.2	142.4	142.7	143.3	149.4	152.8	164.6
45 to 54 years	404.3	377.2	376.9	351.9	357.3	342.7	348.0	341.0	340.2	342.5
55 to 64 years	836.0	837.0	818.9	815.1	791.0	816.3	797.4	787.7	788.2	804.1
65 to 74 years	1,884.2	1,854.9	1,789.2	1,775.0	1,722.4	1,679.1	1,710.4	1,655.1	1,674.3	1,668.9
75 to 84 years	4,612.2	4,563.6	4,396.7	4,461.9	4,303.5	4,250.9	4,218.1	4,103.3	4,127.1	4,054.0
85 years and over	11,719.4	11,453.4	11,225.7	11,779.8	10,707.8	10,799.6	10,596.0	10,318.0	10,145.7	10,139.3
White, not Hispanic or Latino Male[6]										
All ages, age-adjusted[2]	918.4	920.2	893.7	892.5	887.2	876.2	876.8	872.3	881.3	879.5
All ages, crude	968.3	987.5	975.7	987.5	1,004.1	1,011.2	1,032.1	1,045.4	1,072.5	1,085.6
Under 1 year	647.5	627.9	604.4	575.9	572.6	558.2	571.5	549.9	541.1	530.9
1 to 4 years	29.1	30.3	28.3	27.5	27.0	27.9	26.9	24.9	25.5	26.2
5 to 14 years	16.1	15.1	14.2	14.3	14.8	13.3	14.4	14.2	14.5	14.5
15 to 24 years	106.8	103.2	94.4	93.4	94.8	92.0	89.6	90.6	93.4	101.8
25 to 34 years	145.0	145.1	142.1	143.6	147.9	149.0	149.9	155.8	168.1	187.5
35 to 44 years	230.7	227.9	227.9	219.1	223.8	221.7	223.1	227.4	238.1	257.9
45 to 54 years	510.5	518.2	515.4	508.1	512.3	508.0	511.5	511.2	510.0	513.3
55 to 64 years	1,046.7	1,056.2	1,045.1	1,046.2	1,050.0	1,058.0	1,069.0	1,085.3	1,093.3	1,100.6
65 to 74 years	2,372.1	2,350.7	2,269.9	2,256.9	2,227.4	2,175.8	2,174.3	2,170.0	2,184.0	2,175.8
75 to 84 years	6,008.4	6,009.9	5,810.0	5,770.3	5,727.3	5,599.2	5,582.7	5,499.0	5,500.5	5,382.6
85 years and over	15,946.0	16,114.4	15,552.9	15,816.6	15,568.2	15,504.4	15,485.9	15,286.4	15,526.0	15,274.6

NOTE: Starting with *Health, United States, 2003*, rates for 1991–1999 were revised using intercensal population estimates based on the 1990 and 2000 Censuses. For 2000, population estimates are bridged-race April 1 census counts. Starting with *Health, United States, 2012*, rates for 2001–2009 were revised using intercensal population estimates based on the 2000 and 2010 Censuses. For 2010, population estimates are bridged-race April 1 census counts. Rates for 2011 and beyond were computed using 2010-based postcensal estimates. Age groups were selected to minimize the presentation of unstable age-specific death rates based on small numbers of deaths and for consistency among comparison groups. Starting with 2003 data, some states began to collect information on more than one race on the death certificate, according to 1997 Office of Management and Budget (OMB) standards. The multiple-race data for these states were bridged to the single-race categories of the 1977 OMB standards, for comparability with other states.

[2]Age-adjusted rates are calculated using the year 2000 standard population. Prior to 2001, age-adjusted rates were calculated using standard million proportions based on rounded population numbers. Starting with 2001 data, unrounded population numbers are used to calculate age-adjusted rates.

[3]The race groups, White, Black, Asian or Pacific Islander, and American Indian and Alaska Native, include persons of Hispanic and non-Hispanic origin. Persons of Hispanic origin may be of any race. Death rates for Hispanic, American Indian or Alaska Native, and Asian or Pacific Islander persons should be interpreted with caution because of inconsistencies in reporting Hispanic origin or race on the death certificate (death rate numerators) compared with population figures (death rate denominators). The net effect of misclassification is an underestimation of deaths and death rates for races other than White and Black.

[4]In 1950, rate is for the age group under 5 years.

[5]In 1950, rate is for the age group 75 years and over.

[6]Prior to 1997, excludes data from states lacking an Hispanic-origin item on the death certificate.

Table 2-27. Death Rates for All Causes, by Sex, Race, Hispanic Origin, and Age, Selected Years 1950–2016—Continued

(Deaths per 100,000 resident population; data are based on death certificates.)

Sex, race, Hispanic origin, and age	1950[1]	1960[1]	1970	1980	1985	1990	1995	2000	2005	2006
Black, not Hispanic or Latino Male[6]										
All ages, age-adjusted[2]	NA	NA	NA	NA	NA	NA	NA	1,422.0	1,306.1	1,267.0
All ages, crude	NA	NA	NA	NA	NA	NA	NA	859.5	828.4	816.5
Under 1 year	NA	NA	NA	NA	NA	NA	NA	1,623.2	1,576.8	1,562.6
1 to 4 years	NA	NA	NA	NA	NA	NA	NA	56.1	50.7	51.6
5 to 14 years	NA	NA	NA	NA	NA	NA	NA	29.1	27.4	25.4
15 to 24 years	NA	NA	NA	NA	NA	NA	NA	187.2	178.1	177.0
25 to 34 years	NA	NA	NA	NA	NA	NA	NA	270.2	277.6	280.7
35 to 44 years	NA	NA	NA	NA	NA	NA	NA	462.7	407.0	403.4
45 to 54 years	NA	NA	NA	NA	NA	NA	NA	1,036.2	945.1	914.6
55 to 64 years	NA	NA	NA	NA	NA	NA	NA	2,111.4	1,915.9	1,847.1
65 to 74 years	NA	NA	NA	NA	NA	NA	NA	4,303.9	3,669.9	3,575.2
75 to 84 years	NA	NA	NA	NA	NA	NA	NA	8,551.0	7,771.6	7,500.3
85 years and over	NA	NA	NA	NA	NA	NA	NA	16,944.8	16,993.5	16,363.7
White Female[3]										
All ages, age-adjusted[2]	1,198.0	1,074.4	944.0	796.1	764.3	728.8	718.7	715.3	680.9	662.3
All ages, crude	803.3	800.9	812.6	806.1	840.1	846.9	883.2	912.3	888.1	870.3
Under 1 year	2,566.8	2,007.7	1,614.6	962.5	799.3	690.0	574.4	550.5	535.5	533.3
1 to 4 years	112.2	85.2	66.1	49.3	40.0	36.1	31.3	25.5	23.5	24.3
5 to 14 years	45.1	34.7	29.9	22.9	19.5	17.9	16.5	14.1	12.9	12.0
15 to 24 years	71.5	54.9	61.6	55.5	48.1	45.9	43.7	41.1	41.5	41.8
25 to 34 years	112.8	85.0	84.1	65.4	59.4	61.5	62.9	55.1	59.0	60.2
35 to 44 years	235.8	191.1	193.3	138.2	121.9	117.4	125.5	125.7	131.3	130.1
45 to 54 years	546.4	458.8	462.9	372.7	341.7	309.3	291.9	281.4	291.8	292.6
55 to 64 years	1,293.8	1,078.9	1,014.9	876.2	869.1	822.7	783.4	730.9	659.7	649.9
65 to 74 years	3,242.8	2,779.3	2,470.7	2,066.6	2,027.1	1,923.5	1,913.2	1,868.3	1,687.6	1,631.5
75 to 84 years	8,481.5	7,696.6	6,698.7	5,401.7	5,111.6	4,839.1	4,775.3	4,785.3	4,526.1	4,397.1
85 years and over	19,679.5	19,477.7	15,980.2	14,979.6	14,745.4	14,400.6	14,405.8	14,890.7	14,438.0	13,905.7
Black or African American Female[3]										
All ages, age-adjusted[2]	1,545.5	1,369.7	1,228.7	1,033.3	994.4	975.1	955.9	927.6	862.7	828.4
All ages, crude	1,002.0	905.0	829.2	733.3	734.2	747.9	743.2	733.0	699.2	678.3
Under 1 year	NA	4,162.2	3,368.8	2,123.7	1,821.4	1,735.5	1,399.9	1,279.8	1,203.3	1,215.9
1 to 4 years[4]	1,139.3	173.3	129.4	84.4	71.1	67.6	59.5	45.3	38.2	41.2
5 to 14 years	72.8	53.8	43.8	30.5	28.6	27.5	25.4	20.0	19.0	17.0
15 to 24 years	213.1	107.5	111.9	70.5	59.6	68.7	68.9	58.3	50.3	50.2
25 to 34 years	393.3	273.2	231.0	150.0	137.6	159.5	162.8	121.8	110.2	107.0
35 to 44 years	758.1	568.5	533.0	323.9	276.5	298.6	324.9	271.9	248.4	243.0
45 to 54 years	1,576.4	1,177.0	1,043.9	768.2	667.6	639.4	612.1	588.3	562.0	540.9
55 to 64 years	3,089.4	2,510.9	1,986.2	1,561.0	1,532.5	1,452.6	1,354.3	1,227.2	1,083.0	1,052.9
65 to 74 years	4,000.2	4,064.2	3,860.9	3,057.4	2,967.8	2,865.7	2,837.5	2,689.6	2,300.8	2,196.1
75 to 84 years[5]	8,347.0	6,730.0	6,691.5	6,212.1	6,078.0	5,688.3	5,671.9	5,696.5	5,278.5	5,042.4
85 years and over	NA	13,052.6	10,706.6	12,367.2	12,703.0	13,309.5	13,073.3	13,941.3	14,183.6	13,535.1
American Indian or Alaska Native Female[3]										
All ages, age-adjusted[2]	NA	NA	NA	662.4	577.2	561.8	643.9	604.5	601.8	589.0
All ages, crude	NA	NA	NA	380.1	342.5	330.4	360.1	346.1	354.8	347.6
Under 1 year	NA	NA	NA	1,352.6	910.5	688.7	780.6	492.2	500.1	453.5
1 to 4 years	NA	NA	NA	87.5	54.8	37.8	54.4	39.8	31.3	34.0
5 to 14 years	NA	NA	NA	33.5	23.0	25.5	20.0	17.7	14.5	13.6
15 to 24 years	NA	NA	NA	90.3	72.8	69.0	60.4	58.9	61.5	56.3
25 to 34 years	NA	NA	NA	178.5	121.5	102.3	106.3	84.8	80.8	80.7
35 to 44 years	NA	NA	NA	286.0	185.6	156.4	171.9	171.9	171.2	176.1
45 to 54 years	NA	NA	NA	491.4	415.5	380.9	349.1	284.9	338.9	311.6
55 to 64 years	NA	NA	NA	837.1	851.9	805.9	876.2	772.1	675.6	656.8
65 to 74 years	NA	NA	NA	1,765.5	1,630.3	1,679.4	1,935.6	1,899.8	1,770.0	1,639.8
75 to 84 years	NA	NA	NA	3,612.9	3,200.0	3,073.2	4,067.6	3,850.0	3,812.8	3,967.9
85 years and over	NA	NA	NA	8,567.4	7,740.0	8,201.1	9,201.8	9,118.2	9,752.1	9,413.5

NOTE: Starting with Health, United States, 2003, rates for 1991–1999 were revised using intercensal population estimates based on the 1990 and 2000 Censuses. For 2000, population estimates are bridged-race April 1 census counts. Starting with Health, United States, 2012, rates for 2001–2009 were revised using intercensal population estimates based on the 2000 and 2010 Censuses. For 2010, population estimates are bridged-race April 1 census counts. Rates for 2011 and beyond were computed using 2010-based postcensal estimates. Age groups were selected to minimize the presentation of unstable age-specific death rates based on small numbers of deaths and for consistency among comparison groups. Starting with 2003 data, some states began to collect information on more than one race on the death certificate, according to 1997 Office of Management and Budget (OMB) standards. The multiple-race data for these states were bridged to the single-race categories of the 1977 OMB standards, for comparability with other states.
NA = Not available.
[1]Includes deaths of persons who were not residents of the 50 states and the District of Columbia (DC).
[2]Age-adjusted rates are calculated using the year 2000 standard population. Prior to 2001, age-adjusted rates were calculated using standard million proportions based on rounded population numbers. Starting with 2001 data, unrounded population numbers are used to calculate age-adjusted rates.
[3]The race groups, White, Black, Asian or Pacific Islander, and American Indian and Alaska Native, include persons of Hispanic and non-Hispanic origin. Persons of Hispanic origin may be of any race. Death rates for Hispanic, American Indian or Alaska Native, and Asian or Pacific Islander persons should be interpreted with caution because of inconsistencies in reporting Hispanic origin or race on the death certificate (death rate numerators) compared with population figures (death rate denominators). The net effect of misclassification is an underestimation of deaths and death rates for races other than White and Black.
[4]In 1950, rate is for the age group under 5 years.
[5]In 1950, rate is for the age group 75 years and over.
[6]Prior to 1997, excludes data from states lacking an Hispanic-origin item on the death certificate.

Table 2-27. Death Rates for All Causes, by Sex, Race, Hispanic Origin, and Age, Selected Years 1950–2016—Continued

(Deaths per 100,000 resident population; data are based on death certificates.)

Sex, race, Hispanic origin, and age	2007	2008	2009	2010	2011	2012	2013	2014	2015	2016
Black, not Hispanic or Latino Male[6]										
All ages, age-adjusted[2]	1,233.2	1,195.4	1,150.5	1,131.7	1,098.3	1,086.4	1,083.3	1,060.3	1,070.1	1,081.2
All ages, crude	804.9	787.8	773.2	764.5	760.4	768.5	782.5	783.3	809.4	836.2
Under 1 year	1,508.9	1,430.2	1,450.4	1,281.5	1,228.9	1,218.2	1,192.3	1,185.7	1,215.0	1,203.6
1 to 4 years	51.1	50.8	45.1	45.4	45.7	45.0	43.3	45.1	48.9	46.2
5 to 14 years	25.2	23.8	23.4	20.7	21.9	22.5	20.8	22.3	22.4	22.4
15 to 24 years	172.7	164.2	149.7	150.8	148.6	146.5	143.7	142.7	159.2	173.6
25 to 34 years	265.7	249.7	239.5	230.8	226.7	226.6	233.0	225.7	243.1	263.1
35 to 44 years	390.0	357.1	352.1	321.1	321.1	322.4	330.2	325.5	344.6	372.2
45 to 54 years	867.1	813.0	783.9	739.1	730.1	720.0	705.6	694.6	703.6	715.6
55 to 64 years	1,815.6	1,763.9	1,744.6	1,705.0	1,667.7	1,657.2	1,672.2	1,650.4	1,656.8	1,667.8
65 to 74 years	3,497.3	3,415.7	3,320.6	3,274.7	3,203.3	3,146.5	3,137.2	3,110.5	3,109.3	3,156.2
75 to 84 years	7,260.4	7,204.8	6,845.2	6,849.1	6,498.5	6,550.1	6,501.4	6,287.9	6,345.5	6,277.6
85 years and over	16,163.7	15,638.4	14,823.8	14,974.2	14,516.7	14,006.7	13,959.7	13,532.9	13,344.0	13,320.0
White Female[3]										
All ages, age-adjusted[2]	649.4	653.7	631.3	630.8	630.3	623.8	623.6	617.6	627.0	619.4
All ages, crude	860.6	874.6	849.3	857.3	868.9	869.9	879.4	876.7	899.2	895.0
Under 1 year	537.1	525.0	502.3	488.0	469.8	471.5	456.8	457.6	455.1	444.3
1 to 4 years	24.1	23.8	22.6	21.6	21.7	21.7	20.1	19.6	19.7	20.7
5 to 14 years	12.5	11.4	11.1	10.6	10.5	10.4	10.6	10.0	10.6	11.0
15 to 24 years	41.1	37.6	37.1	36.2	36.0	35.5	35.5	35.5	37.8	39.2
25 to 34 years	60.7	59.2	62.9	61.4	63.6	64.6	64.6	66.9	72.0	78.8
35 to 44 years	127.2	126.8	128.2	122.8	124.9	124.1	126.8	130.7	131.7	138.3
45 to 54 years	291.4	296.1	301.6	295.1	301.8	300.1	303.4	305.8	306.6	306.2
55 to 64 years	632.5	633.2	624.8	617.8	619.2	620.5	623.4	635.1	640.4	648.4
65 to 74 years	1,584.0	1,577.5	1,517.9	1,504.9	1,491.2	1,450.9	1,453.2	1,433.1	1,443.8	1,428.5
75 to 84 years	4,319.4	4,352.9	4,190.9	4,165.4	4,158.2	4,110.6	4,072.0	4,001.3	4,028.0	3,920.5
85 years and over	13,636.6	13,868.7	13,132.7	13,419.3	13,380.8	13,281.9	13,316.1	13,079.1	13,442.5	13,145.9
Black or African American Female[3]										
All ages, age-adjusted[2]	808.1	792.0	763.3	752.5	739.8	723.9	720.6	713.3	710.8	712.9
All ages, crude	668.2	661.8	645.6	642.7	643.4	642.3	651.1	655.5	665.7	679.5
Under 1 year	1,160.8	1,105.1	1,070.0	994.4	962.3	944.4	980.7	956.3	970.0	985.9
1 to 4 years[4]	41.0	36.3	37.7	33.2	33.8	33.0	33.4	31.9	32.0	34.0
5 to 14 years	16.6	15.8	16.6	14.5	14.6	14.0	14.8	14.3	15.0	16.3
15 to 24 years	47.5	48.8	46.6	43.3	43.5	43.6	41.2	42.5	45.8	51.6
25 to 34 years	102.1	97.2	97.5	92.9	94.9	89.5	91.0	88.6	92.9	100.4
35 to 44 years	226.4	218.2	207.7	199.3	198.5	192.9	187.9	193.9	191.8	197.9
45 to 54 years	528.3	515.1	500.5	481.0	467.6	461.5	454.4	455.8	447.0	456.0
55 to 64 years	1,021.0	1,000.1	983.7	972.2	952.3	950.4	962.2	974.8	969.6	980.8
65 to 74 years	2,159.9	2,101.7	2,041.2	2,021.2	1,969.2	1,918.7	1,909.2	1,880.2	1,864.4	1,884.8
75 to 84 years[5]	4,918.6	4,843.3	4,694.0	4,580.9	4,535.3	4,396.0	4,418.0	4,356.8	4,310.0	4,296.2
85 years and over	13,323.3	13,177.9	12,378.5	12,589.9	12,364.2	12,149.6	11,929.2	11,656.8	11,741.3	11,472.3
American Indian or Alaska Native Female[3]										
All ages, age-adjusted[2]	565.2	548.7	536.4	541.7	522.5	512.3	508.3	514.1	511.3	501.6
All ages, crude	339.0	332.9	332.4	332.4	338.1	340.9	348.2	363.5	375.8	379.8
Under 1 year	528.3	437.3	444.2	366.4	411.6	425.9	305.9	412.5	431.0	369.4
1 to 4 years	30.3	35.8	23.5	24.4	25.1	22.7	25.5	20.4	26.5	31.6
5 to 14 years	9.9	13.1	16.2	10.5	12.3	9.6	10.9	10.8	13.7	12.1
15 to 24 years	53.1	49.4	56.3	43.6	45.4	47.7	42.8	46.8	47.1	54.0
25 to 34 years	77.8	83.6	81.9	85.6	88.0	98.8	93.5	88.0	104.7	118.4
35 to 44 years	164.3	177.6	171.8	146.6	164.9	162.2	172.4	179.0	170.5	180.1
45 to 54 years	309.8	300.0	346.5	326.2	336.6	329.6	334.5	354.3	354.2	352.6
55 to 64 years	659.0	626.3	603.9	623.8	611.5	587.2	616.6	606.2	622.2	615.2
65 to 74 years	1,589.6	1,528.3	1,472.4	1,481.7	1,376.1	1,390.3	1,314.7	1,368.6	1,360.3	1,274.3
75 to 84 years	3,656.9	3,472.8	3,332.7	3,391.9	3,300.8	3,256.9	3,221.9	3,226.6	3,192.5	3,197.9
85 years and over	9,155.0	9,024.2	8,619.3	9,277.9	8,448.2	7,987.3	8,008.4	7,893.5	7,636.6	7,180.9

NOTE: Starting with *Health, United States, 2003*, rates for 1991–1999 were revised using intercensal population estimates based on the 1990 and 2000 Censuses. For 2000, population estimates are bridged-race April 1 census counts. Starting with *Health, United States, 2012*, rates for 2001–2009 were revised using intercensal population estimates based on the 2000 and 2010 Censuses. For 2010, population estimates are bridged-race April 1 census counts. Rates for 2011 and beyond were computed using 2010-based postcensal estimates. Age groups were selected to minimize the presentation of unstable age-specific death rates based on small numbers of deaths and for consistency among comparison groups. Starting with 2003 data, some states began to collect information on more than one race on the death certificate, according to 1997 Office of Management and Budget (OMB) standards. The multiple-race data for these states were bridged to the single-race categories of the 1977 OMB standards, for comparability with other states.
[2]Age-adjusted rates are calculated using the year 2000 standard population. Prior to 2001, age-adjusted rates were calculated using standard million proportions based on rounded population numbers. Starting with 2001 data, unrounded population numbers are used to calculate age-adjusted rates.
[3]The race groups, White, Black, Asian or Pacific Islander, and American Indian and Alaska Native, include persons of Hispanic and non-Hispanic origin. Persons of Hispanic origin may be of any race. Death rates for Hispanic, American Indian or Alaska Native, and Asian or Pacific Islander persons should be interpreted with caution because of inconsistencies in reporting Hispanic origin or race on the death certificate (death rate numerators) compared with population figures (death rate denominators). The net effect of misclassification is an underestimation of deaths and death rates for races other than White and Black.
[4]In 1950, rate is for the age group under 5 years.
[5]In 1950, rate is for the age group 75 years and over.
[6]Prior to 1997, excludes data from states lacking an Hispanic-origin item on the death certificate.

Table 2-27. Death Rates for All Causes, by Sex, Race, Hispanic Origin, and Age, Selected Years 1950–2016—*Continued*

(Deaths per 100,000 resident population; data are based on death certificates.)

Sex, race, Hispanic origin, and age	1950[1]	1960[1]	1970	1980	1985	1990	1995	2000	2005	2006
Asian or Pacific Islander Female[3]										
All ages, age-adjusted[2]	NA	NA	NA	425.9	456.7	469.3	446.7	416.8	385.2	381.2
All ages, crude	NA	NA	NA	222.5	224.9	234.3	250.4	262.3	271.4	273.4
Under 1 year	NA	NA	NA	755.8	622.0	518.2	396.6	434.3	373.8	348.6
1 to 4 years	NA	NA	NA	35.4	36.8	32.0	24.9	20.0	16.2	19.8
5 to 14 years	NA	NA	NA	21.5	19.1	13.0	15.4	11.7	11.4	9.8
15 to 24 years	NA	NA	NA	32.3	30.7	28.8	31.1	22.4	23.1	22.2
25 to 34 years	NA	NA	NA	45.4	36.5	37.5	35.6	27.6	27.1	26.9
35 to 44 years	NA	NA	NA	89.7	77.8	69.9	66.2	65.6	57.9	56.8
45 to 54 years	NA	NA	NA	214.1	184.9	182.7	184.1	155.5	140.1	142.1
55 to 64 years	NA	NA	NA	440.8	468.0	483.4	457.7	390.9	342.8	321.9
65 to 74 years	NA	NA	NA	1,027.7	1,130.8	1,089.2	1,037.8	996.4	896.0	887.7
75 to 84 years	NA	NA	NA	2,833.6	2,873.9	3,127.9	3,089.9	2,882.4	2,613.2	2,623.3
85 years and over	NA	NA	NA	7,923.3	9,808.3	10,254.0	9,406.1	9,052.2	8,769.0	8,664.5
Hispanic or Latina Female[3,6]										
All ages, age-adjusted[2]	NA	NA	NA	NA	546.1	537.1	546.1	546.0	513.8	500.2
All ages, crude	NA	NA	NA	NA	251.9	285.4	281.9	274.6	272.7	269.0
Under 1 year	NA	NA	NA	NA	791.4	746.6	572.0	553.6	526.3	512.0
1 to 4 years	NA	NA	NA	NA	42.3	42.1	33.1	27.5	24.3	24.0
5 to 14 years	NA	NA	NA	NA	16.0	17.3	15.0	13.4	11.8	11.6
15 to 24 years	NA	NA	NA	NA	36.2	40.6	37.5	31.7	34.5	33.0
25 to 34 years	NA	NA	NA	NA	56.3	62.9	58.6	43.4	40.5	42.6
35 to 44 years	NA	NA	NA	NA	100.0	109.3	118.9	100.5	89.1	85.7
45 to 54 years	NA	NA	NA	NA	251.3	253.3	238.8	223.8	213.7	212.5
55 to 64 years	NA	NA	NA	NA	619.7	607.5	602.3	548.4	489.0	481.0
65 to 74 years	NA	NA	NA	NA	1,449.5	1,453.8	1,457.2	1,423.2	1,285.1	1,216.0
75 to 84 years	NA	NA	NA	NA	3,551.8	3,351.3	3,506.4	3,624.5	3,464.7	3,329.0
85 years and over	NA	NA	NA	NA	10,228.6	10,098.7	10,540.5	11,202.8	10,769.7	10,682.9
White, not Hispanic or Latina Female[6]										
All ages, age-adjusted[2]	NA	NA	NA	NA	754.3	734.6	721.1	721.5	690.7	672.4
All ages, crude	NA	NA	NA	NA	861.7	903.6	951.7	1,007.3	999.7	982.8
Under 1 year	NA	NA	NA	NA	763.0	655.3	553.9	530.9	522.3	526.7
1 to 4 years	NA	NA	NA	NA	36.5	34.0	30.3	24.4	22.7	23.8
5 to 14 years	NA	NA	NA	NA	19.0	17.6	16.4	13.9	13.0	11.8
15 to 24 years	NA	NA	NA	NA	47.9	46.0	44.0	42.6	42.6	43.3
25 to 34 years	NA	NA	NA	NA	59.0	60.6	62.2	56.8	63.3	64.0
35 to 44 years	NA	NA	NA	NA	122.8	116.8	124.1	128.1	138.1	137.7
45 to 54 years	NA	NA	NA	NA	335.7	312.1	293.0	285.0	299.4	300.8
55 to 64 years	NA	NA	NA	NA	853.3	834.5	789.8	742.1	672.7	662.8
65 to 74 years	NA	NA	NA	NA	1,998.1	1,940.2	1,925.9	1,891.0	1,715.2	1,660.9
75 to 84 years	NA	NA	NA	NA	5,059.1	4,887.3	4,794.9	4,819.3	4,577.1	4,451.4
85 years and over	NA	NA	NA	NA	14,560.4	14,533.1	14,450.9	14,971.7	14,560.9	14,014.9
Black, not Hispanic or Latina Female[6]										
All ages, age-adjusted[2]	NA	NA	NA	NA	NA	NA	NA	941.2	879.4	845.6
All ages, crude	NA	NA	NA	NA	NA	NA	NA	756.7	728.1	708.1
Under 1 year	NA	NA	NA	NA	NA	NA	NA	1,327.7	1,282.3	1,295.2
1 to 4 years	NA	NA	NA	NA	NA	NA	NA	47.1	39.7	43.2
5 to 14 years	NA	NA	NA	NA	NA	NA	NA	20.7	19.7	17.6
15 to 24 years	NA	NA	NA	NA	NA	NA	NA	60.1	52.2	52.2
25 to 34 years	NA	NA	NA	NA	NA	NA	NA	126.5	115.8	113.4
35 to 44 years	NA	NA	NA	NA	NA	NA	NA	278.8	257.6	253.0
45 to 54 years	NA	NA	NA	NA	NA	NA	NA	601.2	577.2	556.2
55 to 64 years	NA	NA	NA	NA	NA	NA	NA	1,249.4	1,107.0	1,077.3
65 to 74 years	NA	NA	NA	NA	NA	NA	NA	2,728.0	2,343.2	2,238.8
75 to 84 years	NA	NA	NA	NA	NA	NA	NA	5,758.6	5,353.8	5,121.7
85 years and over	NA	NA	NA	NA	NA	NA	NA	14,054.9	14,352.9	13,703.6

NOTE: Starting with *Health, United States, 2003*, rates for 1991–1999 were revised using intercensal population estimates based on the 1990 and 2000 Censuses. For 2000, population estimates are bridged-race April 1 census counts. Starting with *Health, United States, 2012*, rates for 2001–2009 were revised using intercensal population estimates based on the 2000 and 2010 Censuses. For 2010, population estimates are bridged-race April 1 census counts. Rates for 2011 and beyond were computed using 2010-based postcensal estimates. Age groups were selected to minimize the presentation of unstable age-specific death rates based on small numbers of deaths and for consistency among comparison groups. Starting with 2003 data, some states began to collect information on more than one race on the death certificate, according to 1997 Office of Management and Budget (OMB) standards. The multiple-race data for these states were bridged to the single-race categories of the 1977 OMB standards, for comparability with other states.
NA = Not available.
[1]Includes deaths of persons who were not residents of the 50 states and the District of Columbia (DC).
[2]Age-adjusted rates are calculated using the year 2000 standard population. Prior to 2001, age-adjusted rates were calculated using standard million proportions based on rounded population numbers. Starting with 2001 data, unrounded population numbers are used to calculate age-adjusted rates.
[3]The race groups, White, Black, Asian or Pacific Islander, and American Indian and Alaska Native, include persons of Hispanic and non-Hispanic origin. Persons of Hispanic origin may be of any race. Death rates for Hispanic, American Indian or Alaska Native, and Asian or Pacific Islander persons should be interpreted with caution because of inconsistencies in reporting Hispanic origin or race on the death certificate (death rate numerators) compared with population figures (death rate denominators). The net effect of misclassification is an underestimation of deaths and death rates for races other than White and Black.
[6]Prior to 1997, excludes data from states lacking an Hispanic-origin item on the death certificate.

Table 2-27. Death Rates for All Causes, by Sex, Race, Hispanic Origin, and Age, Selected Years 1950–2016—*Continued*

(Deaths per 100,000 resident population; data are based on death certificates.)

Sex, race, Hispanic origin, and age	2007	2008	2009	2010	2011	2012	2013	2014	2015	2016
Asian or Pacific Islander Female[3]										
All ages, age-adjusted[2]	369.2	372.4	361.1	359.0	349.8	348.8	343.0	331.1	338.0	335.7
All ages, crude	269.5	277.0	273.5	277.3	283.8	292.0	297.4	295.5	310.8	318.3
Under 1 year	380.0	360.7	373.7	341.8	342.5	349.0	329.3	338.6	358.1	361.1
1 to 4 years	16.8	19.3	12.7	16.3	11.8	14.8	18.4	12.5	15.0	16.9
5 to 14 years	9.0	7.9	10.0	7.9	7.9	7.2	8.8	6.5	7.3	8.8
15 to 24 years	20.5	19.1	21.1	17.0	15.9	18.4	17.7	17.8	19.1	21.2
25 to 34 years	25.4	30.4	26.0	27.1	24.6	24.4	25.7	24.8	26.2	27.0
35 to 44 years	54.3	48.0	50.8	49.0	52.5	50.4	51.5	49.1	51.1	53.2
45 to 54 years	131.7	129.9	122.0	127.9	130.2	130.3	128.0	122.3	127.6	126.2
55 to 64 years	315.0	310.2	294.8	298.8	303.7	301.5	287.2	283.2	288.0	304.0
65 to 74 years	813.6	835.8	776.8	788.7	719.4	731.9	703.9	700.5	704.8	698.9
75 to 84 years	2,566.2	2,531.2	2,472.3	2,445.5	2,446.0	2,330.6	2,346.7	2,237.5	2,263.5	2,193.1
85 years and over	8,546.0	8,859.2	8,685.4	8,590.1	8,251.9	8,469.0	8,240.4	7,945.3	8,142.0	8,070.6
Hispanic or Latina Female[3,6]										
All ages, age-adjusted[2]	484.4	484.7	466.1	463.4	452.8	452.5	448.6	437.5	438.3	436.4
All ages, crude	264.0	265.8	261.4	260.9	264.6	272.7	279.4	281.0	290.4	297.7
Under 1 year	522.8	499.2	480.1	462.9	430.2	428.9	433.7	432.1	436.6	426.3
1 to 4 years	24.1	22.8	23.4	20.2	21.3	20.0	18.4	17.2	17.5	17.6
5 to 14 years	11.9	11.0	11.8	8.9	9.5	10.0	9.9	9.7	8.6	10.3
15 to 24 years	30.8	28.4	29.1	26.3	25.6	25.5	25.6	27.2	28.5	30.4
25 to 34 years	42.0	40.2	42.5	38.9	39.2	40.0	41.4	41.3	44.8	49.4
35 to 44 years	80.7	79.3	81.0	75.2	74.1	73.6	78.3	78.5	77.7	82.6
45 to 54 years	199.9	195.4	200.0	193.9	185.7	192.0	189.6	185.3	184.0	187.2
55 to 64 years	468.8	467.0	456.8	450.1	435.9	442.8	437.2	443.3	434.6	441.5
65 to 74 years	1,149.2	1,137.4	1,106.7	1,085.5	1,077.4	1,046.7	1,039.9	1,036.7	1,048.7	1,018.2
75 to 84 years	3,299.5	3,244.7	3,160.1	3,067.4	3,085.1	3,063.5	3,037.8	2,931.3	2,937.3	2,932.3
85 years and over	10,276.7	10,636.2	9,794.3	10,237.3	9,727.2	9,805.6	9,651.3	9,250.2	9,266.4	9,106.8
White, not Hispanic or Latina Female[6]										
All ages, age-adjusted[2]	660.6	665.4	643.1	643.3	644.6	637.6	638.4	633.8	644.1	637.2
All ages, crude	976.1	995.6	969.1	981.2	998.1	998.8	1,011.5	1,011.3	1,038.5	1,034.6
Under 1 year	525.3	516.0	494.2	480.4	468.6	469.2	448.5	451.0	445.7	438.7
1 to 4 years	23.5	23.5	21.6	21.8	21.1	21.7	20.4	20.2	20.1	21.4
5 to 14 years	12.4	11.1	10.5	10.9	10.6	10.1	10.6	9.8	11.2	10.9
15 to 24 years	43.2	39.6	38.6	38.4	38.4	37.8	38.0	37.5	40.1	41.4
25 to 34 years	65.0	63.8	67.5	66.8	69.6	70.7	70.2	73.2	78.8	86.5
35 to 44 years	135.8	136.1	137.7	133.1	136.6	136.0	138.6	143.8	145.7	152.9
45 to 54 years	301.6	308.0	313.5	307.7	317.8	315.2	320.5	325.5	327.7	327.5
55 to 64 years	645.5	646.2	638.5	631.5	635.2	635.9	640.5	653.5	661.0	670.2
65 to 74 years	1,616.4	1,609.8	1,548.1	1,535.9	1,522.8	1,480.2	1,483.9	1,462.9	1,472.8	1,460.2
75 to 84 years	4,375.2	4,416.1	4,252.4	4,232.6	4,227.0	4,178.1	4,142.2	4,078.9	4,103.1	3,992.4
85 years and over	13,761.8	13,984.1	13,264.8	13,543.5	13,544.3	13,437.0	13,502.5	13,290.4	13,682.6	13,406.5
Black, not Hispanic or Latina Female[6]										
All ages, age-adjusted[2]	826.4	809.6	781.0	770.8	759.8	742.1	740.6	731.2	731.0	734.1
All ages, crude	699.9	694.0	678.5	676.9	679.2	677.3	688.4	691.4	704.3	719.7
Under 1 year	1,247.0	1,178.5	1,135.1	1,055.7	1,028.8	1,000.0	1,039.0	1,013.7	1,027.3	1,042.8
1 to 4 years	42.7	38.8	39.7	34.8	35.8	35.2	35.4	34.0	34.0	36.6
5 to 14 years	17.4	16.7	17.5	15.5	15.4	14.8	15.7	15.1	15.9	17.5
15 to 24 years	49.7	51.1	48.9	45.6	45.9	46.1	43.5	44.2	48.2	54.5
25 to 34 years	108.6	103.3	103.8	99.1	101.7	95.2	97.0	94.1	98.7	106.2
35 to 44 years	236.2	227.7	217.4	209.1	208.4	203.2	198.6	205.2	203.3	210.1
45 to 54 years	545.2	531.2	517.7	497.4	485.2	478.6	472.6	473.9	466.5	476.5
55 to 64 years	1,045.0	1,025.5	1,009.0	996.9	979.2	975.0	990.8	1,000.8	997.9	1,011.3
65 to 74 years	2,206.7	2,146.7	2,086.7	2,068.1	2,018.0	1,963.1	1,958.7	1,922.9	1,910.9	1,934.3
75 to 84 years	5,002.8	4,925.5	4,775.8	4,675.5	4,637.5	4,489.1	4,524.5	4,441.4	4,414.5	4,404.8
85 years and over	13,508.7	13,344.2	12,544.8	12,767.7	12,591.4	12,334.1	12,132.2	11,834.9	11,954.7	11,685.1

NOTE: Starting with *Health, United States, 2003*, rates for 1991–1999 were revised using intercensal population estimates based on the 1990 and 2000 Censuses. For 2000, population estimates are bridged-race April 1 census counts. Starting with *Health, United States, 2012*, rates for 2001–2009 were revised using intercensal population estimates based on the 2000 and 2010 Censuses. For 2010, population estimates are bridged-race April 1 census counts. Rates for 2011 and beyond were computed using 2010-based postcensal estimates. Age groups were selected to minimize the presentation of unstable age-specific death rates based on small numbers of deaths and for consistency among comparison groups. Starting with 2003 data, some states began to collect information on more than one race on the death certificate, according to 1997 Office of Management and Budget (OMB) standards. The multiple-race data for these states were bridged to the single-race categories of the 1977 OMB standards, for comparability with other states.
[2]Age-adjusted rates are calculated using the year 2000 standard population. Prior to 2001, age-adjusted rates were calculated using standard million proportions based on rounded population numbers. Starting with 2001 data, unrounded population numbers are used to calculate age-adjusted rates.
[3]The race groups, White, Black, Asian or Pacific Islander, and American Indian and Alaska Native, include persons of Hispanic and non-Hispanic origin. Persons of Hispanic origin may be of any race. Death rates for Hispanic, American Indian or Alaska Native, and Asian or Pacific Islander persons should be interpreted with caution because of inconsistencies in reporting Hispanic origin or race on the death certificate (death rate numerators) compared with population figures (death rate denominators). The net effect of misclassification is an underestimation of deaths and death rates for races other than White and Black.
[6]Prior to 1997, excludes data from states lacking an Hispanic-origin item on the death certificate.

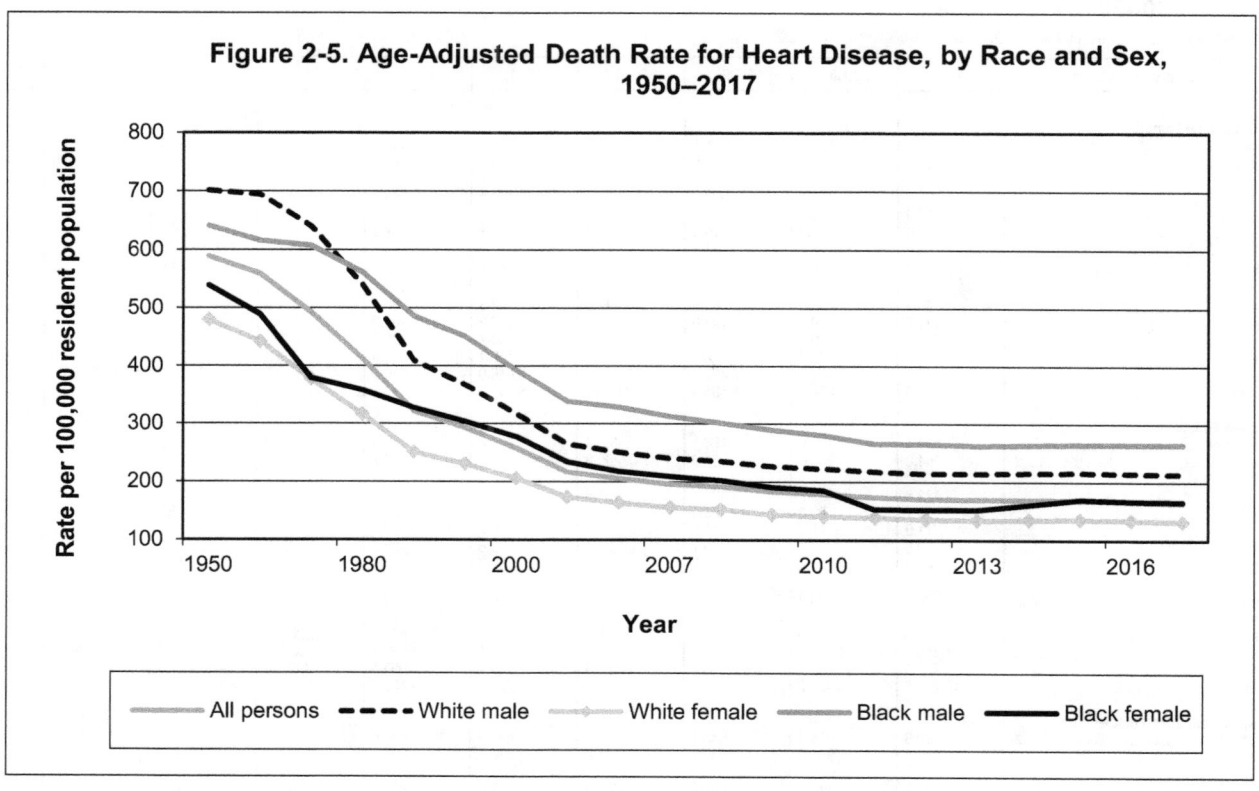

Figure 2-5. Age-Adjusted Death Rate for Heart Disease, by Race and Sex, 1950–2017

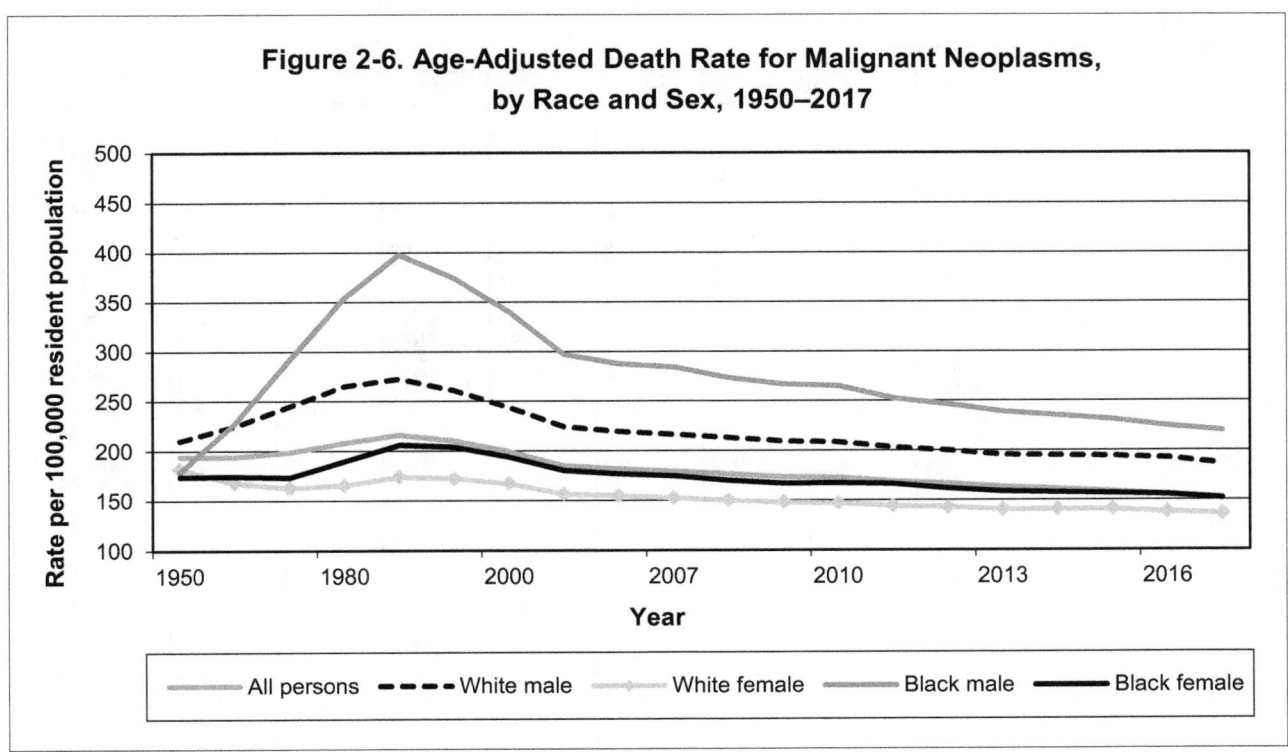

Figure 2-6. Age-Adjusted Death Rate for Malignant Neoplasms, by Race and Sex, 1950–2017

Table 2-28. Death Rates for Diseases of the Heart, by Sex, Race, Hispanic Origin, and Age, Selected Years, 1950–2016

(Deaths per 100,000 resident population; data are based on death certificates.)

Sex, race, Hispanic origin, and age	1950[1,2]	1960[1,2]	1970[2]	1980[2]	1985[2]	1990[2]	1995[2]	2000[3]	2005[3]	2006[3]
All Persons										
All ages, age-adjusted[4]	588.8	559.0	492.7	412.1	375.0	321.8	293.4	257.6	216.8	205.5
All ages, crude	356.8	369.0	362.0	336.0	324.1	289.5	277.0	252.6	220.7	211.7
Under 1 year	4.1	6.6	13.1	22.8	25.0	20.1	17.4	13.0	8.9	8.6
1 to 4 years	1.6	1.3	1.7	2.6	2.2	1.9	1.6	1.2	0.9	1.0
5 to 14 years	3.9	1.3	0.8	0.9	1.0	0.9	0.8	0.7	0.6	0.6
15 to 24 years	8.2	4.0	3.0	2.9	2.8	2.5	2.8	2.6	2.6	2.5
25 to 34 years	20.9	15.6	11.4	8.3	8.3	7.6	8.2	7.4	8.3	8.4
35 to 44 years	88.3	74.6	66.7	44.6	38.1	31.4	31.8	29.2	29.2	28.5
45 to 54 years	309.2	271.8	238.4	180.2	153.8	120.5	109.6	94.2	89.7	88.0
55 to 64 years	804.3	737.9	652.3	494.1	443.0	367.3	320.1	261.2	212.8	205.1
65 to 74 years	1,857.2	1,740.5	1,558.2	1,218.6	1,089.8	894.3	795.4	665.6	512.3	483.0
75 to 84 years	4,311.0	4,089.4	3,683.8	2,993.1	2,693.1	2,295.7	2,050.5	1,780.3	1,458.5	1,378.0
85 years and over	9,152.5	9,317.8	7,891.3	7,777.1	7,384.1	6,739.9	6,391.5	5,926.1	5,188.3	4,877.6
Male										
All ages, age-adjusted[4]	699.0	687.6	634.0	538.9	488.0	412.4	371.0	320.0	268.2	254.9
All ages, crude	424.7	439.5	422.5	368.6	344.1	297.6	278.5	249.8	222.3	215.3
Under 1 year	4.7	7.8	15.1	25.5	27.8	21.9	17.7	13.3	9.6	9.1
1 to 4 years	1.7	1.4	1.9	2.8	2.2	1.9	1.7	1.4	1.0	1.1
5 to 14 years	3.5	1.4	0.9	1.0	0.9	0.9	0.8	0.8	0.6	0.7
15 to 24 years	8.3	4.2	3.7	3.7	3.5	3.1	3.5	3.2	3.5	3.2
25 to 34 years	24.4	20.1	15.2	11.4	11.6	10.3	11.0	9.6	11.2	11.6
35 to 44 years	120.4	112.7	103.2	68.7	58.6	48.1	46.9	41.4	41.3	40.1
45 to 54 years	441.2	420.4	376.4	282.6	237.8	183.0	166.1	140.2	131.6	128.9
55 to 64 years	1,100.5	1,066.9	987.2	746.8	659.1	537.3	460.1	371.7	303.9	293.4
65 to 74 years	2,310.2	2,291.3	2,170.3	1,728.0	1,535.8	1,250.0	1,095.3	898.3	680.1	646.9
75 to 84 years	4,825.8	4,742.4	4,534.8	3,834.3	3,496.9	2,968.2	2,622.9	2,248.1	1,815.1	1,722.7
85 years and over	9,661.4	9,788.9	8,426.2	8,752.7	8,251.8	7,418.4	6,993.5	6,430.0	5,713.2	5,359.2
Female										
All ages, age-adjusted[4]	486.6	447.0	381.6	320.8	294.5	257.0	236.6	210.9	177.5	167.2
All ages, crude	289.7	300.6	304.5	305.1	305.2	281.8	275.5	255.3	219.0	208.2
Under 1 year	3.4	5.4	10.9	20.0	22.0	18.3	17.0	12.5	8.2	8.0
1 to 4 years	1.6	1.1	1.6	2.5	2.2	1.9	1.5	1.0	0.9	0.9
5 to 14 years	4.3	1.2	0.8	0.9	1.0	0.8	0.7	0.5	0.6	0.6
15 to 24 years	8.2	3.7	2.3	2.1	2.1	1.8	2.1	2.1	1.7	1.8
25 to 34 years	17.6	11.3	7.7	5.3	5.0	5.0	5.4	5.2	5.3	5.1
35 to 44 years	57.0	38.2	32.2	21.4	18.3	15.1	17.0	17.2	17.2	17.1
45 to 54 years	177.8	127.5	109.9	84.5	74.4	61.0	55.4	49.8	49.1	48.4
55 to 64 years	507.0	429.4	351.6	272.1	252.1	215.7	192.6	159.3	128.0	122.8
65 to 74 years	1,434.9	1,261.3	1,082.7	828.6	746.1	616.8	554.9	474.0	369.5	342.8
75 to 84 years	3,873.0	3,582.7	3,120.8	2,497.0	2,220.4	1,893.8	1,692.7	1,475.1	1,213.8	1,139.0
85 years and over	8,798.1	9,016.8	7,591.8	7,350.5	7,037.6	6,478.1	6,159.6	5,720.9	4,955.1	4,659.1
White Male[5]										
All ages, age-adjusted[4]	701.4	694.5	640.2	539.6	487.3	409.2	367.0	316.7	264.8	251.1
All ages, crude	434.2	454.6	438.3	384.0	360.3	312.7	294.4	265.8	237.3	229.5
45 to 54 years	424.1	413.2	365.7	269.8	225.5	170.6	153.9	130.7	122.0	120.0
55 to 64 years	1,082.6	1,056.0	979.3	730.6	640.1	516.7	439.2	351.8	286.4	276.9
65 to 74 years	2,309.4	2,297.9	2,177.2	1,729.7	1,522.7	1,230.5	1,071.8	877.8	661.1	624.6
75 to 84 years	4,908.0	4,839.9	4,617.6	3,883.2	3,527.0	2,983.4	2,625.6	2,247.0	1,812.9	1,717.2
85 years and over	9,952.3	10,135.8	8,818.0	8,958.0	8,481.7	7,558.7	7,125.1	6,560.8	5,824.6	5,450.2
Black or African American Male[5]										
All ages, age-adjusted[4]	641.5	615.2	607.3	561.4	533.9	485.4	451.3	392.5	338.8	328.3
All ages, crude	348.4	330.6	330.3	301.0	288.6	256.8	239.1	211.1	194.0	190.5
45 to 54 years	624.1	514.0	512.8	433.4	385.2	328.9	308.6	247.2	231.1	222.2
55 to 64 years	1,434.0	1,236.8	1,135.4	987.2	935.3	824.0	740.5	631.2	527.6	502.5
65 to 74 years	2,140.1	2,281.4	2,237.8	1,847.2	1,839.2	1,632.9	1,514.1	1,268.8	1,002.5	999.7
75 to 84 years[6]	4,107.9	3,533.6	3,783.4	3,578.8	3,436.6	3,107.1	2,908.7	2,597.6	2,206.2	2,126.5
85 years and over	NA	6,037.9	5,367.6	6,819.5	6,393.5	6,479.6	6,088.5	5,633.5	5,137.1	4,968.8
American Indian or Alaska Native Male[5]										
All ages, age-adjusted[4]	NA	NA	NA	320.5	280.5	264.1	256.4	222.2	191.7	186.1
All ages, crude	NA	NA	NA	130.6	117.9	108.0	101.0	90.1	82.8	83.1

NOTE: Starting with *Health, United States, 2003*, rates for 1991–1999 were revised using intercensal population estimates based on the 1990 and 2000 Censuses. For 2000, population estimates are bridged-race April 1 census counts. Starting with *Health, United States, 2012*, rates for 2001–2009 were revised using intercensal population estimates based on the 2000 and 2010 Censuses. For 2010, population estimates are bridged-race April 1 census counts. Rates for 2011 and beyond were computed using 2010-based postcensal estimates. Age groups were selected to minimize the presentation of unstable age-specific death rates based on small numbers of deaths and for consistency among comparison groups. Starting with 2003 data, some states began to collect information on more than one race on the death certificate, according to 1997 Office of Management and Budget (OMB) standards. The multiple-race data for these states were bridged to the single-race categories of the 1977 OMB standards, for comparability with other states.
NA = Not available.
[1]Includes deaths of persons who were not residents of the 50 states and the District of Columbia (DC).
[2]Underlying cause of death was coded according to the 6th revision of the *International Classification of Diseases* (ICD) in 1950, 7th revision in 1960, 8th revision in 1970, and 9th revision in 1980–1998.
[3]Starting with 1999 data, cause of death is coded according to *ICD–10*.
[4]Age-adjusted rates are calculated using the year 2000 standard population. Prior to 2001, age-adjusted rates were calculated using standard million proportions based on rounded population numbers. Starting with 2001 data, unrounded population numbers are used to calculate age-adjusted rates.
[5]The race groups, White, Black, Asian or Pacific Islander, and American Indian and Alaska Native, include persons of Hispanic and non-Hispanic origin. Persons of Hispanic origin may be of any race. Death rates for Hispanic, American Indian or Alaska Native, and Asian or Pacific Islander persons should be interpreted with caution because of inconsistencies in reporting Hispanic origin or race on the death certificate (death rate numerators) compared with population figures (death rate denominators). The net effect of misclassification is an underestimation of deaths and death rates for races other than White and Black.
[6]In 1950, rate is for the age group 75 years and over.

Table 2-28. Death Rates for Diseases of the Heart, by Sex, Race, Hispanic Origin, and Age, Selected Years, 1950–2016—*Continued*

(Deaths per 100,000 resident population; data are based on death certificates.)

Sex, race, Hispanic origin, and age	2007[3]	2008[3]	2009[3]	2010[3]	2011[3]	2012[3]	2013[3]	2014[3]	2015[3]	2016[3]
All Persons										
All ages, age-adjusted[4]	196.1	192.1	182.8	179.1	173.7	170.5	169.8	167.0	168.5	165.5
All ages, crude	204.5	202.8	195.4	193.6	191.5	191.0	193.3	192.7	197.2	196.6
Under 1 year	10.2	9.6	9.6	8.3	7.7	8.5	7.8	8.0	7.3	7.4
1 to 4 years	1.1	1.2	0.9	1.0	1.0	1.0	1.1	0.9	0.9	0.7
5 to 14 years	0.6	0.6	0.5	0.5	0.5	0.4	0.4	0.5	0.5	0.5
15 to 24 years	2.5	2.5	2.4	2.4	2.3	2.2	2.1	2.2	2.3	2.2
25 to 34 years	8.1	8.1	7.8	7.8	7.9	7.6	7.6	7.7	8.0	7.7
35 to 44 years	27.7	26.9	26.7	25.8	26.2	25.9	25.6	25.6	25.6	25.9
45 to 54 years	85.2	85.2	82.3	81.6	80.7	79.7	80.3	80.1	79.3	79.5
55 to 64 years	197.8	195.3	190.0	186.6	183.2	184.6	184.6	185.8	188.1	189.6
65 to 74 years	454.8	441.4	422.8	409.2	399.0	388.3	390.3	385.2	389.5	392.5
75 to 84 years	1,308.6	1,271.7	1,210.8	1,172.0	1,134.7	1,103.7	1,095.1	1,070.2	1,071.6	1,037.1
85 years and over	4,668.1	4,598.4	4,316.9	4,285.2	4,111.6	4,046.1	4,013.9	3,920.9	3,986.5	3,873.4
Male										
All ages, age-adjusted[4]	243.7	238.5	229.4	225.1	218.1	214.7	214.5	210.9	211.8	209.1
All ages, crude	209.2	208.2	203.7	202.5	201.2	202.3	206.5	207.1	211.7	213.3
Under 1 year	11.2	10.3	10.5	9.8	7.9	9.6	8.7	8.6	7.5	7.2
1 to 4 years	1.0	1.2	0.9	1.1	1.0	1.0	1.2	0.9	1.0	0.8
5 to 14 years	0.6	0.6	0.5	0.5	0.5	0.5	0.4	0.5	0.5	0.5
15 to 24 years	3.2	3.3	3.1	3.2	3.0	2.9	2.8	2.7	3.0	2.8
25 to 34 years	10.9	10.8	10.6	10.7	10.5	10.4	10.2	10.3	10.3	10.2
35 to 44 years	39.2	37.4	37.5	36.0	36.6	35.8	35.5	34.8	35.1	35.5
45 to 54 years	124.6	122.9	119.8	117.8	116.7	114.3	115.1	113.5	112.1	112.5
55 to 64 years	285.1	280.8	274.1	269.5	263.6	266.4	267.3	268.1	269.4	271.3
65 to 74 years	610.0	594.0	571.1	553.0	540.4	527.7	530.9	525.7	529.7	536.4
75 to 84 years	1,631.9	1,584.3	1,514.8	1,475.7	1,426.6	1,388.1	1,382.4	1,354.8	1,354.4	1,312.0
85 years and over	5,154.3	5,083.6	4,862.8	4,833.6	4,622.7	4,582.7	4,564.2	4,453.4	4,495.1	4,403.5
Female										
All ages, age-adjusted[4]	159.0	155.9	146.6	143.3	138.7	135.5	134.3	131.8	133.6	130.4
All ages, crude	199.9	197.7	187.3	184.9	182.0	180.2	180.6	178.6	183.1	180.4
Under 1 year	9.2	8.8	8.8	6.8	7.5	7.3	6.9	7.4	7.2	7.6
1 to 4 years	1.2	1.1	1.0	0.9	1.0	0.9	0.9	0.9	0.9	0.7
5 to 14 years	0.5	0.5	0.5	0.4	0.5	0.4	0.4	0.4	0.5	0.4
15 to 24 years	1.8	1.6	1.6	1.5	1.5	1.5	1.5	1.6	1.5	1.5
25 to 34 years	5.3	5.4	5.0	4.9	5.3	4.8	4.9	5.0	5.6	5.2
35 to 44 years	16.2	16.4	16.0	15.6	15.9	16.0	15.7	16.4	16.2	16.4
45 to 54 years	47.1	48.8	46.0	46.5	45.9	46.0	46.6	47.5	47.4	47.4
55 to 64 years	116.4	115.6	111.6	109.3	108.4	108.4	107.5	109.3	112.3	113.5
65 to 74 years	321.4	309.7	294.2	284.2	275.7	266.2	266.8	261.7	266.2	266.0
75 to 84 years	1,082.0	1,050.4	993.3	952.7	920.7	893.0	879.8	854.8	855.9	826.4
85 years and over	4,443.3	4,370.0	4,056.0	4,020.3	3,859.7	3,777.5	3,732.9	3,643.8	3,717.6	3,589.7
White Male[5]										
All ages, age-adjusted[4]	240.3	235.8	226.6	222.9	216.9	213.1	213.1	210.0	211.2	208.4
All ages, crude	223.6	223.3	218.4	217.8	217.1	218.0	222.6	223.9	229.1	230.4
45 to 54 years	117.0	117.1	113.1	111.2	110.8	108.3	109.8	107.7	106.6	106.2
55 to 64 years	269.3	266.9	258.9	257.0	251.7	253.2	254.0	255.9	256.5	258.8
65 to 74 years	590.1	573.9	551.1	536.3	524.9	513.5	516.0	512.7	516.8	522.0
75 to 84 years	1,629.3	1,580.9	1,516.2	1,475.1	1,434.2	1,392.6	1,389.0	1,361.5	1,362.9	1,321.7
85 years and over	5,252.0	5,192.6	4,972.4	4,943.1	4,754.6	4,712.4	4,701.6	4,603.9	4,663.2	4,574.4
Black or African American Male[5]										
All ages, age-adjusted[4]	312.4	301.2	289.0	280.6	266.1	265.3	262.8	259.5	258.6	258.1
All ages, crude	184.7	180.5	178.1	174.6	171.0	174.7	177.2	178.7	182.8	187.2
45 to 54 years	207.9	192.4	194.1	190.9	184.1	182.4	178.3	179.5	177.3	186.0
55 to 64 years	489.8	465.5	463.2	437.8	425.2	435.9	430.0	425.5	430.9	433.1
65 to 74 years	941.0	925.0	893.3	847.8	825.5	805.5	807.5	794.6	801.5	813.5
75 to 84 years[6]	1,992.0	1,958.6	1,821.7	1,807.1	1,680.2	1,677.7	1,660.0	1,651.4	1,644.6	1,590.6
85 years and over	4,751.8	4,519.0	4,260.8	4,202.7	3,846.9	3,822.1	3,754.5	3,693.0	3,583.2	3,561.3
American Indian or Alaska Native Male[5]										
All ages, age-adjusted[4]	175.5	163.5	162.2	158.7	153.4	152.5	152.3	149.7	148.0	147.7
All ages, crude	79.3	76.5	76.5	75.0	76.9	78.3	82.3	84.4	87.4	88.4

NOTE: Starting with *Health, United States, 2003*, rates for 1991–1999 were revised using intercensal population estimates based on the 1990 and 2000 Censuses. For 2000, population estimates are bridged-race April 1 census counts. Starting with *Health, United States, 2012*, rates for 2001–2009 were revised using intercensal population estimates based on the 2000 and 2010 Censuses. For 2010, population estimates are bridged-race April 1 census counts. Rates for 2011 and beyond were computed using 2010-based postcensal estimates. Age groups were selected to minimize the presentation of unstable age-specific death rates based on small numbers of deaths and for consistency among comparison groups. Starting with 2003 data, some states began to collect information on more than one race on the death certificate, according to 1997 Office of Management and Budget (OMB) standards. The multiple-race data for these states were bridged to the single-race categories of the 1977 OMB standards, for comparability with other states.
[3]Starting with 1999 data, cause of death is coded according to *ICD–10*.
[4]Age-adjusted rates are calculated using the year 2000 standard population. Prior to 2001, age-adjusted rates were calculated using standard million proportions based on rounded population numbers. Starting with 2001 data, unrounded population numbers are used to calculate age-adjusted rates.
[5]The race groups, White, Black, Asian or Pacific Islander, and American Indian and Alaska Native, include persons of Hispanic and non-Hispanic origin. Persons of Hispanic origin may be of any race. Death rates for Hispanic, American Indian or Alaska Native, and Asian or Pacific Islander persons should be interpreted with caution because of inconsistencies in reporting Hispanic origin or race on the death certificate (death rate numerators) compared with population figures (death rate denominators). The net effect of misclassification is an underestimation of deaths and death rates for races other than White and Black.
[6]In 1950, rate is for the age group 75 years and over.

Table 2-28. Death Rates for Diseases of the Heart, by Sex, Race, Hispanic Origin, and Age, Selected Years, 1950–2016—*Continued*

(Deaths per 100,000 resident population; data are based on death certificates.)

Sex, race, Hispanic origin, and age	1950[1,2]	1960[1,2]	1970[2]	1980[2]	1985[2]	1990[2]	1995[2]	2000[3]	2005[3]	2006[3]
45 to 54 years	NA	NA	NA	238.1	209.1	173.8	136.2	108.5	103.2	107.8
55 to 64 years	NA	NA	NA	496.3	438.3	411.0	375.7	285.0	263.4	242.6
65 to 74 years	NA	NA	NA	1,009.4	984.6	839.1	938.2	748.2	551.9	568.4
75 to 84 years	NA	NA	NA	2,062.2	2,118.2	1,788.8	1,858.5	1,655.7	1,253.6	1,323.6
85 years and over	NA	NA	NA	4,413.7	2,766.7	3,860.3	3,306.5	3,318.3	3,529.4	2,942.8
Asian or Pacific Islander Male[5]										
All ages, age-adjusted[4]	NA	NA	NA	286.9	258.9	220.7	214.5	185.5	149.4	145.4
All ages, crude	NA	NA	NA	119.8	103.5	88.7	93.2	90.6	81.7	80.6
45 to 54 years	NA	NA	NA	112.0	81.1	70.4	69.8	61.1	58.1	55.8
55 to 64 years	NA	NA	NA	306.7	291.2	226.1	205.4	182.6	143.9	144.1
65 to 74 years	NA	NA	NA	852.4	753.5	623.5	581.0	482.5	370.9	340.7
75 to 84 years	NA	NA	NA	2,010.9	2,025.6	1,642.2	1,533.8	1,354.7	1,014.6	996.4
85 years and over	NA	NA	NA	5,923.0	4,937.5	4,617.8	4,888.9	4,154.2	3,518.6	3,497.0
Hispanic or Latino Male[5,7]										
All ages, age-adjusted[4,7]	NA	NA	NA	NA	296.6	270.0	260.8	238.2	210.5	193.7
All ages, crude	NA	NA	NA	NA	92.1	91.0	83.1	74.7	72.3	68.2
45 to 54 years	NA	NA	NA	NA	128.1	116.4	102.0	84.3	78.7	76.7
55 to 64 years	NA	NA	NA	NA	398.8	363.0	311.2	264.8	220.4	203.7
65 to 74 years	NA	NA	NA	NA	971.1	829.9	784.6	684.8	567.9	512.3
75 to 84 years	NA	NA	NA	NA	2,150.0	1,971.3	1,854.0	1,733.2	1,541.7	1,380.2
85 years and over	NA	NA	NA	NA	4,912.5	4,711.9	5,104.0	4,897.5	4,442.3	4,190.2
White, Not Hispanic or Latino Male[7]										
All ages, age-adjusted[4]	NA	NA	NA	NA	480.4	413.6	369.1	319.9	267.9	254.6
All ages, crude	NA	NA	NA	NA	362.8	336.5	320.6	297.5	269.9	262.3
45 to 54 years	NA	NA	NA	NA	219.9	172.8	155.9	134.3	126.6	124.9
55 to 64 years	NA	NA	NA	NA	610.6	521.3	443.2	356.3	290.6	281.8
65 to 74 years	NA	NA	NA	NA	1,471.3	1,243.4	1,077.0	885.1	664.8	630.1
75 to 84 years	NA	NA	NA	NA	3,512.8	3,007.7	2,635.3	2,261.9	1,823.1	1,732.6
85 years and over	NA	NA	NA	NA	8,538.4	7,663.4	7,156.4	6,606.6	5,876.4	5,495.9
Black, Not Hispanic or Latino Male[7]										
All ages, age-adjusted[4]	NA	NA	NA	NA	NA	NA	NA	396.6	344.2	334.4
All ages, crude	NA	NA	NA	NA	NA	NA	NA	217.6	202.2	199.2
45 to 54 years	NA	NA	NA	NA	NA	NA	NA	252.5	236.7	227.7
55 to 64 years	NA	NA	NA	NA	NA	NA	NA	639.6	537.4	513.4
65 to 74 years	NA	NA	NA	NA	NA	NA	NA	1,281.7	1,019.7	1,016.8
75 to 84 years	NA	NA	NA	NA	NA	NA	NA	2,615.1	2,229.2	2,158.4
85 years and over	NA	NA	NA	NA	NA	NA	NA	5,677.2	5,199.8	5,041.8
White Female[5]										
All ages, age-adjusted[4]	479.2	441.7	376.7	315.9	289.1	250.9	230.8	205.6	173.2	163.4
All ages, crude	290.5	306.5	313.8	319.2	321.8	298.4	294.7	274.5	236.9	225.9
45 to 54 years	142.4	103.4	91.4	71.2	62.5	50.2	45.5	40.9	40.9	40.9
55 to 64 years	460.7	383.0	317.7	248.1	227.1	192.4	172.0	141.3	113.8	110.6
65 to 74 years	1,401.6	1,229.8	1,044.0	796.7	713.3	583.6	523.2	445.2	349.2	323.0
75 to 84 years	3,926.2	3,629.7	3,143.5	2,493.6	2,207.5	1,874.3	1,670.3	1,452.4	1,195.1	1,124.4
85 years and over	9,086.9	9,280.8	7,839.9	7,501.6	7,170.0	6,563.4	6,251.3	5,801.4	5,017.5	4,721.8
Black or African American Female[5]										
All ages, age-adjusted[4]	538.9	488.9	435.6	378.6	357.7	327.5	304.0	277.6	234.5	218.1
All ages, crude	289.9	268.5	261.0	249.7	250.3	237.0	226.3	212.6	184.0	172.9
45 to 54 years	526.8	360.7	290.9	202.4	176.2	155.3	141.5	125.0	114.1	109.6
55 to 64 years	1,210.7	952.3	710.5	530.1	510.7	442.0	386.0	332.8	266.9	245.8
65 to 74 years	1,659.4	1,680.5	1,553.2	1,210.3	1,149.9	1,017.5	938.2	815.2	604.2	567.1
75 to 84 years[6]	3,499.3	2,926.9	2,964.1	2,707.2	2,533.4	2,250.9	2,100.7	1,913.1	1,599.6	1,465.7
85 years and over	NA	5,650.0	5,003.8	5,796.5	5,686.5	5,766.1	5,448.5	5,298.7	4,841.3	4,493.7

NOTE: Starting with *Health, United States, 2003,* rates for 1991–1999 were revised using intercensal population estimates based on the 1990 and 2000 Censuses. For 2000, population estimates are bridged-race April 1 census counts. Starting with *Health, United States, 2012,* rates for 2001–2009 were revised using intercensal population estimates based on the 2000 and 2010 Censuses. For 2010, population estimates are bridged-race April 1 census counts. Rates for 2011 and beyond were computed using 2010-based postcensal estimates. Age groups were selected to minimize the presentation of unstable age-specific death rates based on small numbers of deaths and for consistency among comparison groups. Starting with 2003 data, some states began to collect information on more than one race on the death certificate, according to 1997 Office of Management and Budget (OMB) standards. The multiple-race data for these states were bridged to the single-race categories of the 1977 OMB standards, for comparability with other states. NA = Not available.
[1] Includes deaths of persons who were not residents of the 50 states and the District of Columbia (DC).
[2] Underlying cause of death was coded according to the 6th revision of the *International Classification of Diseases (ICD)* in 1950, 7th revision in 1960, 8th revision in 1970, and 9th revision in 1980–1998.
[3] Starting with 1999 data, cause of death is coded according to *ICD-10.*
[4] Age-adjusted rates are calculated using the year 2000 standard population. Prior to 2001, age-adjusted rates were calculated using standard million proportions based on rounded population numbers. Starting with 2001 data, unrounded population numbers are used to calculate age-adjusted rates.
[5] The race groups, White, Black, Asian or Pacific Islander, and American Indian and Alaska Native, include persons of Hispanic and non-Hispanic origin. Persons of Hispanic origin may be of any race. Death rates for Hispanic, American Indian or Alaska Native, and Asian or Pacific Islander persons should be interpreted with caution because of inconsistencies in reporting Hispanic origin or race on the death certificate (death rate numerators) compared with population figures (death rate denominators). The net effect of misclassification is an underestimation of deaths and death rates for races other than White and Black.
[6] In 1950, rate is for the age group 75 years and over.
[7] Prior to 1997, excludes data from states lacking an Hispanic-origin item on the death certificate.

Table 2-28. Death Rates for Diseases of the Heart, by Sex, Race, Hispanic Origin, and Age, Selected Years, 1950–2016—Continued

(Deaths per 100,000 resident population; data are based on death certificates.)

Sex, race, Hispanic origin, and age	2007[3]	2008[3]	2009[3]	2010[3]	2011[3]	2012[3]	2013[3]	2014[3]	2015[3]	2016[3]
45 to 54 years	99.5	106.1	86.4	98.0	91.8	87.4	101.6	95.9	102.2	92.4
55 to 64 years	221.4	219.4	230.2	217.2	210.6	198.5	206.2	217.2	231.7	192.4
65 to 74 years	515.2	520.5	518.1	425.1	470.4	451.5	465.2	444.0	408.5	442.6
75 to 84 years	1,276.2	1,058.5	1,097.2	1,042.6	1,068.8	1,138.9	1,071.8	978.2	1,042.1	1,015.1
85 years and over	2,805.9	2,684.7	2,560.7	2,833.1	2,395.7	2,278.2	2,269.1	2,415.9	2,184.3	2,330.2
Asian or Pacific Islander Male[5]										
All ages, age-adjusted[4]	134.4	133.0	130.2	127.2	115.1	116.1	118.4	109.1	109.7	106.6
All ages, crude	76.6	77.3	78.4	77.0	74.2	76.8	81.9	78.4	80.9	81.5
45 to 54 years	51.1	50.8	54.1	49.2	52.7	51.8	50.9	53.4	49.0	47.1
55 to 64 years	129.4	131.3	129.2	119.3	112.9	118.4	133.3	121.4	121.2	123.2
65 to 74 years	314.8	308.0	307.6	294.4	270.3	255.1	274.9	250.5	254.1	266.5
75 to 84 years	935.0	924.3	874.4	855.5	772.1	748.7	754.6	726.6	718.6	685.3
85 years and over	3,162.6	3,170.9	3,080.5	3,132.9	2,695.9	2,842.2	2,848.5	2,459.7	2,543.8	2,380.8
Hispanic or Latino Male[5,7]										
All ages, age-adjusted[4]	183.1	171.2	169.4	165.1	152.2	151.6	151.5	145.7	146.4	144.6
All ages, crude	66.5	63.7	65.0	64.1	62.5	64.3	66.9	67.4	70.7	72.2
45 to 54 years	74.3	68.4	71.0	66.1	66.0	61.7	63.5	64.0	64.8	64.1
55 to 64 years	203.0	196.6	195.5	185.9	172.3	177.5	178.0	169.5	176.4	176.4
65 to 74 years	482.5	459.1	452.0	424.5	412.9	406.1	416.6	391.6	395.6	397.4
75 to 84 years	1,303.4	1,219.9	1,211.9	1,160.9	1,092.7	1,069.1	1,057.5	1,019.7	1,046.6	996.7
85 years and over	3,875.4	3,569.9	3,486.6	3,577.9	3,076.1	3,147.0	3,106.2	2,987.5	2,883.7	2,918.0
White, Not Hispanic or Latino Male[7]										
All ages, age-adjusted[4]	244.0	240.0	230.4	226.9	221.6	217.7	217.9	215.2	216.3	213.9
All ages, crude	256.4	257.3	251.8	251.8	252.4	253.2	259.0	261.0	267.0	269.0
45 to 54 years	122.0	123.0	118.4	117.2	117.1	115.2	117.2	115.0	113.8	113.9
55 to 64 years	273.8	271.5	263.1	261.9	258.0	259.1	260.2	263.6	263.4	266.6
65 to 74 years	595.7	579.8	555.4	542.2	530.9	518.3	520.2	518.9	522.2	528.6
75 to 84 years	1,645.5	1,599.4	1,531.7	1,491.4	1,452.9	1,409.6	1,408.1	1,382.1	1,379.4	1,341.5
85 years and over	5,310.7	5,263.8	5,042.8	5,006.6	4,841.0	4,796.1	4,794.2	4,703.8	4,781.2	4,690.7
Black, Not Hispanic or Latino Male[7]										
All ages, age-adjusted[4]	318.5	307.6	294.9	286.3	272.8	270.9	269.1	265.2	264.9	265.0
All ages, crude	193.7	189.7	187.3	183.9	180.7	184.3	187.4	188.5	193.2	198.4
45 to 54 years	214.2	198.1	199.6	197.1	191.2	189.1	185.6	185.9	184.1	193.9
55 to 64 years	500.7	475.9	473.0	448.6	436.1	447.3	440.9	434.4	441.8	444.9
65 to 74 years	958.7	945.1	912.2	864.3	843.1	821.2	823.8	808.5	816.9	831.0
75 to 84 years	2,019.9	1,988.5	1,845.0	1,832.9	1,711.1	1,705.6	1,688.9	1,677.9	1,676.7	1,624.4
85 years and over	4,818.6	4,594.9	4,336.9	4,264.2	3,939.8	3,866.3	3,824.4	3,759.0	3,655.5	3,636.4
White Female[5]										
All ages, age-adjusted[4]	155.4	152.5	143.4	140.4	136.5	133.4	132.0	130.0	132.4	128.7
All ages, crude	216.9	215.0	203.7	201.5	198.8	196.7	196.8	195.1	200.6	196.6
45 to 54 years	40.2	41.3	39.5	40.7	40.5	40.7	41.0	42.2	42.4	42.4
55 to 64 years	104.4	103.4	99.7	98.2	98.0	97.8	95.9	98.8	101.6	102.6
65 to 74 years	301.1	292.6	276.8	268.4	261.3	251.7	252.5	247.6	253.8	252.0
75 to 84 years	1,069.4	1,038.5	982.3	941.6	912.8	888.1	871.8	849.0	855.3	817.2
85 years and over	4,496.0	4,437.7	4,119.8	4,086.7	3,938.3	3,855.8	3,821.0	3,746.8	3,835.1	3,705.8
Black or African American Female[5]										
All ages, age-adjusted[4]	209.8	202.5	191.0	185.3	176.2	172.7	172.1	167.7	165.7	166.4
All ages, crude	168.1	164.8	157.6	154.8	150.3	150.9	153.4	152.3	153.9	157.1
45 to 54 years	105.3	109.7	99.5	96.6	91.6	92.6	94.2	94.9	92.4	93.9
55 to 64 years	236.4	234.1	228.5	218.6	209.2	211.1	213.0	211.0	214.3	216.0
65 to 74 years	550.8	514.0	498.5	475.9	461.6	449.3	450.8	437.9	433.5	446.2
75 to 84 years[6]	1,388.4	1,342.1	1,272.0	1,227.2	1,158.4	1,114.8	1,122.2	1,085.7	1,050.5	1,081.3
85 years and over	4,399.9	4,153.1	3,833.3	3,783.8	3,559.7	3,513.5	3,425.3	3,269.8	3,282.5	3,165.8

NOTE: Starting with *Health, United States, 2003*, rates for 1991–1999 were revised using intercensal population estimates based on the 1990 and 2000 Censuses. For 2000, population estimates are bridged-race April 1 census counts. Starting with *Health, United States, 2012*, rates for 2001–2009 were revised using intercensal population estimates based on the 2000 and 2010 Censuses. For 2010, population estimates are bridged-race April 1 census counts. Rates for 2011 and beyond were computed using 2010-based postcensal estimates. Age groups were selected to minimize the presentation of unstable age-specific death rates based on small numbers of deaths and for consistency among comparison groups. Starting with 2003 data, some states began to collect information on more than one race on the death certificate, according to 1997 Office of Management and Budget (OMB) standards. The multiple-race data for these states were bridged to the single-race categories of the 1977 OMB standards, for comparability with other states.
[3]Starting with 1999 data, cause of death is coded according to *ICD–10*.
[4]Age-adjusted rates are calculated using the year 2000 standard population. Prior to 2001, age-adjusted rates were calculated using standard million proportions based on rounded population numbers. Starting with 2001 data, unrounded population numbers are used to calculate age-adjusted rates.
[5]The race groups, White, Black, Asian or Pacific Islander, and American Indian and Alaska Native, include persons of Hispanic and non-Hispanic origin. Persons of Hispanic origin may be of any race. Death rates for Hispanic, American Indian or Alaska Native, and Asian or Pacific Islander persons should be interpreted with caution because of inconsistencies in reporting Hispanic origin or race on the death certificate (death rate numerators) compared with population figures (death rate denominators). The net effect of misclassification is an underestimation of deaths and death rates for races other than White and Black.
[6]In 1950, rate is for the age group 75 years and over.
[7]Prior to 1997, excludes data from states lacking an Hispanic-origin item on the death certificate.

Table 2-28. Death Rates for Diseases of the Heart, by Sex, Race, Hispanic Origin, and Age, Selected Years, 1950–2016—*Continued*

(Deaths per 100,000 resident population; data are based on death certificates.)

Sex, race, Hispanic origin, and age	1950[1,2]	1960[1,2]	1970[2]	1980[2]	1985[2]	1990[2]	1995[2]	2000[3]	2005[3]	2006[3]
American Indian or Alaska Native Female[5]										
All ages, age-adjusted[4]	NA	NA	NA	175.4	170.0	153.1	164.8	143.6	129.3	126.1
All ages, crude	NA	NA	NA	80.3	84.3	77.5	80.2	71.9	66.8	65.3
45 to 54 years	NA	NA	NA	65.2	59.2	62.0	62.4	40.2	48.2	38.0
55 to 64 years	NA	NA	NA	193.5	230.8	197.0	200.7	149.4	118.0	119.8
65 to 74 years	NA	NA	NA	577.2	472.7	492.8	514.2	391.8	346.6	318.9
75 to 84 years	NA	NA	NA	1,364.3	1,258.8	1,050.3	1,184.3	1,044.1	896.3	993.4
85 years and over	NA	NA	NA	2,893.3	3,180.0	2,868.7	3,118.1	3,146.3	2,962.1	2,672.2
Asian or Pacific Islander Female[5]										
All ages, age-adjusted[4]	NA	NA	NA	132.3	149.4	149.2	137.6	115.7	97.5	93.7
All ages, crude	NA	NA	NA	57.0	60.3	62.0	66.3	65.0	63.6	62.1
45 to 54 years	NA	NA	NA	28.6	23.8	17.5	20.8	15.9	15.5	15.6
55 to 64 years	NA	NA	NA	92.9	103.0	99.0	89.5	68.8	55.2	46.8
65 to 74 years	NA	NA	NA	313.3	341.0	323.9	288.3	229.6	192.3	185.3
75 to 84 years	NA	NA	NA	1,053.2	1,056.5	1,130.9	1,001.8	866.2	705.4	664.5
85 years and over	NA	NA	NA	3,211.0	4,208.3	4,161.2	3,942.4	3,367.2	2,881.1	2,856.6
Hispanic or Latina Female[5,7]										
All ages, age-adjusted[4]	NA	NA	NA	NA	195.9	177.2	173.8	163.7	139.4	130.1
All ages, crude	NA	NA	NA	NA	75.0	79.4	76.5	71.5	64.9	61.4
45 to 54 years	NA	NA	NA	NA	46.6	43.5	32.0	28.2	25.9	26.9
55 to 64 years	NA	NA	NA	NA	184.7	153.2	141.0	111.2	91.7	85.9
65 to 74 years	NA	NA	NA	NA	534.1	460.4	419.0	366.3	304.3	271.5
75 to 84 years	NA	NA	NA	NA	1,457.3	1,259.7	1,231.3	1,169.4	1,002.0	924.0
85 years and over	NA	NA	NA	NA	4,528.6	4,440.3	4,653.1	4,605.8	3,968.1	3,735.5
White, not Hispanic or Latina Female[7]										
All ages, age-adjusted[4]	NA	NA	NA	NA	287.2	252.6	231.5	206.8	174.8	165.2
All ages, crude	NA	NA	NA	NA	334.2	320.0	319.7	304.9	268.3	256.8
45 to 54 years	NA	NA	NA	NA	61.3	50.2	46.1	41.9	42.5	42.4
55 to 64 years	NA	NA	NA	NA	219.6	193.6	172.0	142.9	115.3	112.3
65 to 74 years	NA	NA	NA	NA	700.5	584.7	525.2	448.5	351.7	325.9
75 to 84 years	NA	NA	NA	NA	2,201.7	1,890.2	1,674.9	1,458.9	1,202.9	1,133.4
85 years and over	NA	NA	NA	NA	7,164.2	6,615.2	6,265.8	5,822.7	5,049.4	4,753.9
Black, not Hispanic or Latina Female[7]										
All ages, age-adjusted[4]	NA	NA	NA	NA	NA	NA	NA	281.0	238.3	221.9
All ages, crude	NA	NA	NA	NA	NA	NA	NA	219.5	191.7	180.6
45 to 54 years	NA	NA	NA	NA	NA	NA	NA	127.8	117.1	113.2
55 to 64 years	NA	NA	NA	NA	NA	NA	NA	339.3	273.0	252.3
65 to 74 years	NA	NA	NA	NA	NA	NA	NA	827.1	614.1	577.6
75 to 84 years	NA	NA	NA	NA	NA	NA	NA	1,931.9	1,620.0	1,487.4
85 years and over	NA	NA	NA	NA	NA	NA	NA	5,330.8	4,893.6	4,541.9

NOTE: Starting with *Health, United States, 2003,* rates for 1991–1999 were revised using intercensal population estimates based on the 1990 and 2000 Censuses. For 2000, population estimates are bridged-race April 1 census counts. Starting with *Health, United States, 2012,* rates for 2001–2009 were revised using intercensal population estimates based on the 2000 and 2010 Censuses. For 2010, population estimates are bridged-race April 1 census counts. Rates for 2011 and beyond were computed using 2010-based postcensal estimates. Age groups were selected to minimize the presentation of unstable age-specific death rates based on small numbers of deaths and for consistency among comparison groups. Starting with 2003 data, some states began to collect information on more than one race on the death certificate, according to 1997 Office of Management and Budget (OMB) standards. The multiple-race data for these states were bridged to the single-race categories of the 1977 OMB standards, for comparability with other states. NA = Not available.

[1]Includes deaths of persons who were not residents of the 50 states and the District of Columbia (DC).
[2]Underlying cause of death was coded according to the 6th revision of the *International Classification of Diseases* (*ICD*) in 1950, 7th revision in 1960, 8th revision in 1970, and 9th revision in 1980–1998.
[3]Starting with 1999 data, cause of death is coded according to *ICD–10.*
[4]Age-adjusted rates are calculated using the year 2000 standard population. Prior to 2001, age-adjusted rates were calculated using standard million proportions based on rounded population numbers. Starting with 2001 data, unrounded population numbers are used to calculate age-adjusted rates.
[5]The race groups, White, Black, Asian or Pacific Islander, and American Indian and Alaska Native, include persons of Hispanic and non-Hispanic origin. Persons of Hispanic origin may be of any race. Death rates for Hispanic, American Indian or Alaska Native, and Asian or Pacific Islander persons should be interpreted with caution because of inconsistencies in reporting Hispanic origin or race on the death certificate (death rate numerators) compared with population figures (death rate denominators). The net effect of misclassification is an underestimation of deaths and death rates for races other than White and Black.
[7]Prior to 1997, excludes data from states lacking an Hispanic-origin item on the death certificate.

Table 2-28. Death Rates for Diseases of the Heart, by Sex, Race, Hispanic Origin, and Age, Selected Years, 1950–2016—Continued

(Deaths per 100,000 resident population; data are based on death certificates.)

Sex, race, Hispanic origin, and age	2007[3]	2008[3]	2009[3]	2010[3]	2011[3]	2012[3]	2013[3]	2014[3]	2015[3]	2016[3]
American Indian or Alaska Native Female[5]										
All ages, age-adjusted[4]	112.2	106.8	104.6	103.5	99.4	92.9	93.9	94.0	94.0	89.1
All ages, crude	59.0	56.9	56.9	55.9	57.3	55.7	58.4	61.0	63.8	63.0
45 to 54 years	32.8	35.1	42.0	37.7	40.9	39.4	37.3	40.8	44.0	40.3
55 to 64 years	103.3	99.9	102.1	89.0	99.3	83.9	100.5	90.4	93.9	102.1
65 to 74 years	284.5	260.0	262.7	248.1	225.8	245.0	220.1	269.0	247.5	229.6
75 to 84 years	829.1	764.1	734.4	684.7	715.5	698.2	664.6	657.3	690.7	662.9
85 years and over	2,487.8	2,469.0	2,352.1	2,614.1	2,259.3	1,874.7	2,089.2	1,931.7	1,813.0	1,660.8
Asian or Pacific Islander Female[5]										
All ages, age-adjusted[4]	88.5	88.5	83.6	81.2	76.2	74.0	73.3	68.2	68.5	68.4
All ages, crude	60.0	61.7	59.4	59.0	59.1	59.6	61.8	59.2	61.9	63.8
45 to 54 years	11.7	12.7	11.4	10.6	12.0	10.5	12.5	11.9	12.3	10.2
55 to 64 years	44.8	48.5	38.6	40.6	42.1	40.9	41.7	34.9	40.6	38.6
65 to 74 years	164.6	158.0	150.2	141.6	125.4	126.8	124.7	124.8	122.1	121.4
75 to 84 years	635.0	637.8	594.4	574.3	551.7	505.2	521.0	485.4	469.3	475.7
85 years and over	2,733.3	2,730.3	2,644.6	2,581.8	2,364.5	2,381.5	2,272.4	2,097.2	2,131.6	2,127.5
Hispanic or Latina Female[5,7]										
All ages, age-adjusted[4]	123.2	117.6	109.6	107.8	101.2	98.6	97.0	92.4	93.0	92.6
All ages, crude	59.0	57.3	54.9	54.6	54.1	54.7	55.9	55.3	57.8	59.2
45 to 54 years	22.9	23.7	23.8	24.5	22.3	21.9	22.2	21.3	21.8	21.7
55 to 64 years	80.0	77.9	74.0	72.3	71.3	71.9	63.1	70.2	64.7	66.1
65 to 74 years	246.9	242.4	224.5	212.2	202.2	192.3	195.8	190.0	196.6	190.5
75 to 84 years	884.3	799.9	793.7	756.0	720.3	711.9	702.3	657.5	654.8	671.8
85 years and over	3,568.0	3,486.5	3,080.0	3,140.3	2,868.0	2,781.3	2,738.8	2,558.9	2,599.1	2,542.8
White, not Hispanic or Latina Female[7]										
All ages, age-adjusted[4]	157.3	154.6	145.4	142.5	138.8	135.8	134.6	133.0	135.6	131.7
All ages, crude	247.7	246.5	234.3	232.2	230.0	227.5	228.0	226.9	233.6	228.9
45 to 54 years	42.2	43.5	41.5	42.9	43.1	43.5	44.0	45.8	46.3	46.4
55 to 64 years	106.2	105.3	101.7	100.3	100.2	99.9	99.0	101.4	105.5	106.6
65 to 74 years	304.6	295.6	279.9	271.9	265.3	255.5	256.3	251.3	257.3	255.9
75 to 84 years	1,078.5	1,052.0	992.3	951.5	923.8	898.1	881.3	862.1	867.6	825.7
85 years and over	4,528.6	4,470.5	4,161.5	4,122.8	3,985.5	3,903.8	3,876.5	3,813.8	3,907.6	3,780.8
Black, not Hispanic or Latina Female[7]										
All ages, age-adjusted[4]	213.8	206.2	194.7	189.1	180.3	176.5	176.4	171.5	169.9	170.8
All ages, crude	176.1	172.8	165.6	163.0	158.7	159.2	162.2	160.7	162.8	166.5
45 to 54 years	108.8	113.4	102.8	99.8	95.2	96.2	97.7	98.9	96.3	98.5
55 to 64 years	241.8	239.7	234.1	224.2	215.4	216.4	219.6	216.7	220.3	222.7
65 to 74 years	563.3	523.2	510.4	486.5	473.7	459.2	461.1	447.9	444.0	458.5
75 to 84 years	1,409.4	1,361.7	1,292.3	1,250.4	1,182.1	1,136.6	1,148.8	1,104.5	1,074.4	1,106.3
85 years and over	4,454.4	4,203.6	3,874.6	3,828.1	3,616.3	3,561.1	3,478.7	3,313.2	3,335.4	3,213.4

NOTE: Starting with *Health, United States, 2003*, rates for 1991–1999 were revised using intercensal population estimates based on the 1990 and 2000 Censuses. For 2000, population estimates are bridged-race April 1 census counts. Starting with *Health, United States, 2012*, rates for 2001–2009 were revised using intercensal population estimates based on the 2000 and 2010 Censuses. For 2010, population estimates are bridged-race April 1 census counts. Rates for 2011 and beyond were computed using 2010-based postcensal estimates. Age groups were selected to minimize the presentation of unstable age-specific death rates based on small numbers of deaths and for consistency among comparison groups. Starting with 2003 data, some states began to collect information on more than one race on the death certificate, according to 1997 Office of Management and Budget (OMB) standards. The multiple-race data for these states were bridged to the single-race categories of the 1977 OMB standards, for comparability with other states.
[3]Starting with 1999 data, cause of death is coded according to *ICD–10*.
[4]Age-adjusted rates are calculated using the year 2000 standard population. Prior to 2001, age-adjusted rates were calculated using standard million proportions based on rounded population numbers. Starting with 2001 data, unrounded population numbers are used to calculate age-adjusted rates.
[5]The race groups, White, Black, Asian or Pacific Islander, and American Indian and Alaska Native, include persons of Hispanic and non-Hispanic origin. Persons of Hispanic origin may be of any race. Death rates for Hispanic, American Indian or Alaska Native, and Asian or Pacific Islander persons should be interpreted with caution because of inconsistencies in reporting Hispanic origin or race on the death certificate (death rate numerators) compared with population figures (death rate denominators). The net effect of misclassification is an underestimation of deaths and death rates for races other than White and Black.
[7]Prior to 1997, excludes data from states lacking an Hispanic-origin item on the death certificate.

Table 2-29. Death Rates for Cerebrovascular Diseases, by Sex, Race, Hispanic Origin, and Age, Selected Years, 1950–2016

(Deaths per 100,000 resident population; data are based on death certificates.)

Sex, race, Hispanic origin, and age	1950[1,2]	1960[1,2]	1970[2]	1980[2]	1985[2]	1990[2]	1995[2]	2000[3]	2005[3]	2006[3]
All Persons										
All ages, age-adjusted[4]	180.7	177.9	147.7	96.2	76.4	65.3	63.1	60.9	48.0	44.8
All ages, crude	104.0	108.0	101.9	75.0	64.2	57.8	59.2	59.6	48.6	46.0
Under 1 year	5.1	4.1	5.0	4.4	3.6	3.8	5.9	3.3	3.1	3.5
1 to 4 years	0.9	0.8	1.0	0.5	0.3	0.3	0.4	0.3	0.4	0.3
5 to 14 years	0.5	0.7	0.7	0.3	0.2	0.2	0.2	0.2	0.2	0.2
15 to 24 years	1.6	1.8	1.6	1.0	0.8	0.6	0.5	0.5	0.5	0.5
25 to 34 years	4.2	4.7	4.5	2.6	2.2	2.2	1.7	1.5	1.4	1.3
35 to 44 years	18.7	14.7	15.6	8.5	7.2	6.4	6.5	5.8	5.2	5.1
45 to 54 years	70.4	49.2	41.6	25.2	21.2	18.7	17.4	16.0	15.0	14.6
55 to 64 years	194.2	147.3	115.8	65.1	54.7	47.9	45.6	41.0	32.7	32.9
65 to 74 years	554.7	469.2	384.1	219.0	172.4	144.2	136.2	128.6	99.8	94.9
75 to 84 years	1,499.6	1,491.3	1,254.2	786.9	600.1	498.0	477.1	461.3	358.4	333.9
85 years and over	2,990.1	3,680.5	3,014.3	2,283.7	1,858.5	1,628.9	1,607.2	1,589.2	1,239.7	1,131.7
Male										
All ages, age-adjusted[4]	186.4	186.1	157.4	102.2	79.9	68.5	65.9	62.4	48.4	45.2
All ages, crude	102.5	104.5	94.5	63.4	52.4	46.7	47.2	46.9	39.0	37.2
Under 1 year	6.4	5.0	5.8	5.0	4.6	4.4	6.4	3.8	3.6	4.0
1 to 4 years	1.1	0.9	1.2	0.4	0.4	0.3	0.4	*	0.5	0.3
5 to 14 years	0.5	0.7	0.8	0.3	0.2	0.2	0.2	0.2	0.3	0.3
15 to 24 years	1.8	1.9	1.8	1.1	0.7	0.7	0.5	0.5	0.4	0.5
25 to 34 years	4.2	4.5	4.4	2.6	2.2	2.1	1.8	1.5	1.5	1.5
35 to 44 years	17.5	14.6	15.7	8.7	7.4	6.8	7.0	5.8	5.3	5.4
45 to 54 years	67.9	52.2	44.4	27.2	23.1	20.5	19.5	17.5	16.5	16.4
55 to 64 years	205.2	163.8	138.7	74.6	63.4	54.3	52.7	47.2	38.2	38.3
65 to 74 years	589.6	530.7	449.5	258.6	201.0	166.6	154.7	145.0	111.6	105.8
75 to 84 years	1,543.6	1,555.9	1,361.6	866.3	659.4	551.1	517.7	490.8	370.0	341.4
85 years and over	3,048.6	3,643.1	2,895.2	2,193.6	1,723.8	1,528.5	1,522.1	1,484.3	1,136.7	1,036.8
Female										
All ages, age-adjusted[4]	175.8	170.7	140.0	91.7	73.3	62.6	60.5	59.1	47.0	43.9
All ages, crude	105.6	111.4	109.0	85.9	75.3	68.4	70.7	71.8	57.9	54.4
Under 1 year	3.7	3.2	4.0	3.8	2.7	3.1	5.3	2.7	2.7	3.0
1 to 4 years	0.7	0.7	0.7	0.5	0.3	0.3	0.3	0.4	0.3	0.4
5 to 14 years	0.4	0.6	0.6	0.3	0.3	0.2	0.1	0.2	0.2	0.2
15 to 24 years	1.5	1.6	1.4	0.8	0.8	0.6	0.4	0.5	0.5	0.5
25 to 34 years	4.3	4.9	4.7	2.6	2.1	2.2	1.6	1.5	1.3	1.2
35 to 44 years	19.9	14.8	15.6	8.4	6.9	6.1	6.0	5.7	5.1	4.9
45 to 54 years	72.9	46.3	39.0	23.3	19.4	17.0	15.3	14.5	13.6	13.0
55 to 64 years	183.1	131.8	95.3	56.8	47.1	42.2	39.1	35.3	27.7	28.0
65 to 74 years	522.1	415.7	333.3	188.7	150.4	126.7	121.4	115.1	89.7	85.6
75 to 84 years	1,462.2	1,441.1	1,183.1	740.1	565.1	466.2	451.8	442.1	350.4	328.6
85 years and over	2,949.4	3,704.4	3,081.0	2,323.1	1,912.3	1,667.6	1,640.0	1,632.0	1,285.5	1,174.8
White Male[5]										
All ages, age-adjusted[4]	182.1	181.6	153.7	98.7	77.1	65.5	62.9	59.8	46.0	42.8
All ages, crude	100.5	102.7	93.5	63.1	52.5	46.9	48.0	48.4	40.1	38.1
45 to 54 years	53.7	40.9	35.6	21.7	18.0	15.4	14.7	13.6	12.9	12.9
55 to 64 years	182.2	139.0	119.9	64.0	54.5	45.7	44.2	39.7	31.5	31.3
65 to 74 years	569.7	501.0	420.0	239.8	185.9	152.9	142.1	133.8	101.3	95.3
75 to 84 years	1,556.3	1,564.8	1,361.6	852.7	648.1	539.2	503.8	480.0	361.0	333.4
85 years and over	3,127.1	3,734.8	3,018.1	2,230.8	1,758.7	1,545.4	1,536.0	1,490.7	1,138.5	1,037.0
Black or African American Male[5]										
All ages, age-adjusted[4]	228.8	238.5	206.4	142.0	112.5	102.2	97.0	89.6	72.7	68.8
All ages, crude	122.0	122.9	108.8	73.0	59.2	53.0	49.8	46.1	40.1	39.0
45 to 54 years	211.9	166.1	136.1	82.1	71.1	68.4	62.3	49.5	43.6	42.1
55 to 64 years	522.8	439.9	343.4	189.7	160.5	141.7	130.8	115.4	99.6	101.1
65 to 74 years	783.6	899.2	780.1	472.3	379.4	326.9	297.0	268.5	215.9	209.3
75 to 84 years[6]	1,504.9	1,475.2	1,445.7	1,066.3	813.2	721.5	705.9	659.2	504.2	470.4
85 years and over	NA	2,700.0	1,963.1	1,873.2	1,427.4	1,421.5	1,410.1	1,458.8	1,194.3	1,076.0

NOTE: Starting with *Health, United States*, 2003, rates for 1991–1999 were revised using intercensal population estimates based on the 1990 and 2000 Censuses. For 2000, population estimates are bridged-race April 1 census counts. Starting with *Health, United States*, 2012, rates for 2001–2009 were revised using intercensal population estimates based on the 2000 and 2010 Censuses. For 2010, population estimates are bridged-race April 1 census counts. Rates for 2011 and beyond were computed using 2010-based postcensal estimates. Age groups were selected to minimize the presentation of unstable age-specific death rates based on small numbers of deaths and for consistency among comparison groups. Starting with 2003 data, some states began to collect information on more than one race on the death certificate, according to 1997 Office of Management and Budget (OMB) standards. The multiple-race data for these states were bridged to the single-race categories of the 1977 OMB standards, for comparability with other states. NA = Not available.

* = Rates based on fewer than 20 deaths are considered unreliable and are not shown.

[1] Includes deaths of persons who were not residents of the 50 states and the District of Columbia (DC).

[2] Underlying cause of death was coded according to the 6th revision of the *International Classification of Diseases* (*ICD*) in 1950, 7th revision in 1960, 8th revision in 1970, and 9th revision in 1980–1998.

[3] Starting with 1999 data, cause of death is coded according to *ICD–10*.

[4] Age-adjusted rates are calculated using the year 2000 standard population. Prior to 2001, age-adjusted rates were calculated using standard million proportions based on rounded population numbers. Starting with 2001 data, unrounded population numbers are used to calculate age-adjusted rates.

[5] The race groups, White, Black, Asian or Pacific Islander, and American Indian and Alaska Native, include persons of Hispanic and non-Hispanic origin. Persons of Hispanic origin may be of any race. Death rates for Hispanic, American Indian or Alaska Native, and Asian or Pacific Islander persons should be interpreted with caution because of inconsistencies in reporting Hispanic origin or race on the death certificate (death rate numerators) compared with population figures (death rate denominators). The net effect of misclassification is an underestimation of deaths and death rates for races other than White and Black.

[6] In 1950, rate is for the age group 75 years and over.

Table 2-29. Death Rates for Cerebrovascular Diseases, by Sex, Race, Hispanic Origin, and Age, Selected Years, 1950–2016—Continued

(Deaths per 100,000 resident population; data are based on death certificates.)

Sex, race, Hispanic origin, and age	2007³	2008³	2009³	2010³	2011³	2012³	2013³	2014³	2015³	2016³
All Persons										
All ages, age-adjusted⁴	43.5	42.1	39.6	39.1	37.9	36.9	36.2	36.5	37.6	37.3
All ages, crude	45.1	44.1	42.0	41.9	41.4	40.9	40.8	41.7	43.7	44.0
Under 1 year	3.2	3.4	3.7	3.3	3.4	2.6	2.7	2.4	2.2	3.1
1 to 4 years	0.3	0.4	0.3	0.3	0.3	0.3	0.2	0.2	0.3	0.3
5 to 14 years	0.2	0.2	0.2	0.2	0.2	0.2	0.2	0.2	0.2	0.2
15 to 24 years	0.5	0.4	0.4	0.4	0.4	0.4	0.3	0.4	0.4	0.3
25 to 34 years	1.3	1.3	1.3	1.3	1.3	1.3	1.2	1.3	1.3	1.3
35 to 44 years	5.0	4.8	4.6	4.6	4.2	4.3	4.2	4.3	4.4	4.6
45 to 54 years	14.5	13.7	13.7	13.1	12.8	12.8	12.4	12.3	12.3	12.5
55 to 64 years	31.7	30.6	29.7	29.3	29.4	28.7	28.9	29.3	29.6	29.7
65 to 74 years	91.4	87.3	82.8	81.7	78.2	75.7	74.2	74.5	75.5	76.0
75 to 84 years	320.8	313.3	294.9	288.3	285.4	272.2	268.9	265.7	273.0	265.5
85 years and over	1,110.7	1,071.0	992.2	993.8	943.7	931.2	906.0	929.7	975.8	972.9
Male										
All ages, age-adjusted⁴	43.7	42.2	39.9	39.3	37.9	37.1	36.7	36.9	37.8	37.5
All ages, crude	36.5	35.8	34.5	34.5	34.1	34.1	34.5	35.3	36.8	37.3
Under 1 year	3.6	3.3	4.4	3.2	3.6	2.6	3.0	2.6	2.6	3.7
1 to 4 years	0.2	0.4	0.3	0.3	0.4	0.4	0.3	*	0.3	0.3
5 to 14 years	0.2	0.2	0.2	0.3	0.2	0.2	0.2	0.2	0.2	0.3
15 to 24 years	0.5	0.5	0.5	0.5	0.5	0.5	0.4	0.5	0.4	0.4
25 to 34 years	1.3	1.5	1.5	1.3	1.3	1.4	1.3	1.5	1.4	1.5
35 to 44 years	5.4	5.2	5.1	5.0	4.5	4.8	4.7	5.0	4.9	5.3
45 to 54 years	16.2	15.3	15.3	14.9	14.5	14.2	14.2	14.0	13.6	14.1
55 to 64 years	37.5	35.5	35.0	34.7	34.9	34.5	35.1	35.2	35.4	35.8
65 to 74 years	102.7	97.6	94.2	92.0	88.1	85.7	85.0	85.1	86.3	86.5
75 to 84 years	328.2	320.4	300.9	295.2	289.7	277.7	277.9	272.8	282.2	277.0
85 years and over	998.9	965.2	891.6	892.0	840.0	832.1	808.4	832.0	863.3	848.4
Female										
All ages, age-adjusted⁴	42.7	41.4	38.8	38.3	37.2	36.1	35.2	35.6	36.9	36.5
All ages, crude	53.4	52.1	49.2	49.1	48.4	47.6	46.9	47.9	50.3	50.5
Under 1 year	2.7	3.6	3.0	3.4	3.1	2.6	2.5	2.1	1.9	2.5
1 to 4 years	0.4	0.4	0.3	0.3	*	0.3	*	*	*	0.3
5 to 14 years	0.2	0.2	0.1	0.2	0.2	0.2	0.2	0.2	0.2	0.2
15 to 24 years	0.4	0.4	0.4	0.4	0.4	0.3	0.3	0.3	0.4	0.3
25 to 34 years	1.3	1.2	1.2	1.2	1.2	1.1	1.1	1.2	1.1	1.1
35 to 44 years	4.6	4.5	4.2	4.2	4.0	3.8	3.7	3.7	3.9	3.9
45 to 54 years	12.9	12.2	12.2	11.4	11.0	11.4	10.6	10.7	11.0	11.0
55 to 64 years	26.3	26.1	24.8	24.3	24.4	23.3	23.1	23.8	24.3	24.0
65 to 74 years	81.7	78.4	72.9	72.8	69.6	67.0	64.8	65.2	66.0	66.8
75 to 84 years	315.5	308.2	290.6	283.4	282.1	268.2	262.1	260.3	266.0	256.7
85 years and over	1,162.4	1,120.8	1,040.2	1,043.0	994.9	980.9	955.8	980.6	1,035.3	1,039.5
White Male⁵										
All ages, age-adjusted⁴	41.3	40.2	38.0	37.6	36.2	35.4	35.0	35.2	36.1	35.9
All ages, crude	37.5	37.0	35.7	35.8	35.4	35.3	35.8	36.7	38.2	38.8
45 to 54 years	13.1	12.0	12.7	12.2	11.8	11.4	11.7	11.9	11.2	11.9
55 to 64 years	31.2	29.9	29.3	29.0	29.3	29.4	29.9	29.6	29.8	31.0
65 to 74 years	92.3	88.2	86.2	83.3	80.3	78.1	77.6	77.3	78.2	78.6
75 to 84 years	317.3	313.3	292.9	288.3	283.4	270.9	271.1	265.3	273.5	268.9
85 years and over	999.3	968.9	896.0	903.2	846.2	838.2	815.2	841.4	878.9	856.5
Black or African American Male⁵										
All ages, age-adjusted⁴	68.7	63.5	58.8	56.6	55.3	53.8	54.1	55.1	55.5	55.2
All ages, crude	39.1	36.8	35.0	34.5	34.5	34.1	35.1	36.5	37.5	37.8
45 to 54 years	39.4	39.4	34.5	33.6	33.9	33.4	30.7	29.6	30.4	29.6
55 to 64 years	94.7	85.1	84.5	83.2	81.4	76.0	78.1	79.4	78.4	74.1
65 to 74 years	212.4	195.0	182.8	182.6	172.0	164.9	165.0	169.8	169.9	169.4
75 to 84 years⁶	490.1	443.5	412.7	398.0	384.7	385.0	387.4	393.2	410.8	403.6
85 years and over	1,061.7	1,002.8	887.4	804.5	826.7	796.8	814.1	827.6	804.3	848.6

NOTE: Starting with *Health, United States, 2003,* rates for 1991–1999 were revised using intercensal population estimates based on the 1990 and 2000 Censuses. For 2000, population estimates are bridged-race April 1 census counts. Starting with *Health, United States, 2012,* rates for 2001–2009 were revised using intercensal population estimates based on the 2000 and 2010 Censuses. For 2010, population estimates are bridged-race April 1 census counts. Rates for 2011 and beyond were computed using 2010-based postcensal estimates. Age groups were selected to minimize the presentation of unstable age-specific death rates based on small numbers of deaths and for consistency among comparison groups. Starting with 2003 data, some states began to collect information on more than one race on the death certificate, according to 1997 Office of Management and Budget (OMB) standards. The multiple-race data for these states were bridged to the single-race categories of the 1977 OMB standards, for comparability with other states.
* = Rates based on fewer than 20 deaths are considered unreliable and are not shown.
³Starting with 1999 data, cause of death is coded according to *ICD–10.*
⁴Age-adjusted rates are calculated using the year 2000 standard population. Prior to 2001, age-adjusted rates were calculated using standard million proportions based on rounded population numbers. Starting with 2001 data, unrounded population numbers are used to calculate age-adjusted rates.
⁵The race groups, White, Black, Asian or Pacific Islander, and American Indian and Alaska Native, include persons of Hispanic and non-Hispanic origin. Persons of Hispanic origin may be of any race. Death rates for Hispanic, American Indian or Alaska Native, and Asian or Pacific Islander persons should be interpreted with caution because of inconsistencies in reporting Hispanic origin or race on the death certificate (death rate numerators) compared with population figures (death rate denominators). The net effect of misclassification is an underestimation of deaths and death rates for races other than White and Black.
⁶In 1950, rate is for the age group 75 years and over.

Table 2-29. Death Rates for Cerebrovascular Diseases, by Sex, Race, Hispanic Origin, and Age, Selected Years, 1950–2016—Continued

(Deaths per 100,000 resident population; data are based on death certificates.)

Sex, race, Hispanic origin, and age	1950[1,2]	1960[1,2]	1970[2]	1980[2]	1985[2]	1990[2]	1995[2]	2000[3]	2005[3]	2006[3]
American Indian or Alaska Native Male[5]										
All ages, age-adjusted[4]	NA	NA	NA	66.4	48.4	44.3	51.7	46.1	35.0	28.4
All ages, crude	NA	NA	NA	23.1	18.4	16.0	18.4	16.8	14.0	12.5
45 to 54 years	NA	NA	NA	*	*	*	25.5	13.3	12.6	14.7
55 to 64 years	NA	NA	NA	72.0	38.4	39.8	42.6	48.6	34.5	33.2
65 to 74 years	NA	NA	NA	170.5	196.2	120.3	156.4	144.7	112.5	82.1
75 to 84 years	NA	NA	NA	523.9	372.7	325.9	351.2	373.3	255.8	196.1
85 years and over	NA	NA	NA	1,384.7	733.3	949.8	1,072.4	834.9	655.7	490.5
Asian or Pacific Islander Male[5]										
All ages, age-adjusted[4]	NA	NA	NA	71.4	65.2	59.1	64.0	58.0	43.9	42.5
All ages, crude	NA	NA	NA	28.7	24.0	23.3	27.5	27.2	23.3	23.1
45 to 54 years	NA	NA	NA	17.0	13.9	15.6	16.5	15.0	14.4	13.5
55 to 64 years	NA	NA	NA	59.9	48.8	51.8	59.6	49.3	33.1	36.0
65 to 74 years	NA	NA	NA	197.9	155.6	167.9	155.6	135.6	103.9	107.7
75 to 84 years	NA	NA	NA	619.5	583.7	483.9	521.9	438.7	347.8	305.1
85 years and over	NA	NA	NA	1,399.0	1,387.5	1,196.6	1,382.1	1,415.6	1,007.2	1,014.1
Hispanic or Latino Male[5,7]										
All ages, age-adjusted[4]	NA	NA	NA	NA	57.5	46.5	51.2	50.5	41.6	39.4
All ages, crude	NA	NA	NA	NA	17.2	15.6	16.2	15.8	14.5	14.4
45 to 54 years	NA	NA	NA	NA	23.6	20.0	20.3	18.1	18.0	17.3
55 to 64 years	NA	NA	NA	NA	64.0	49.2	46.9	48.8	40.5	41.4
65 to 74 years	NA	NA	NA	NA	163.3	126.4	138.1	136.1	107.4	101.4
75 to 84 years	NA	NA	NA	NA	394.7	356.6	373.3	392.9	308.5	308.9
85 years and over	NA	NA	NA	NA	1,181.2	866.3	1,079.5	1,029.9	870.3	748.4
White, Not Hispanic or Latino Male[7]										
All ages, age-adjusted[4]	NA	NA	NA	NA	74.8	66.3	62.8	59.9	46.0	42.7
All ages, crude	NA	NA	NA	NA	52.1	50.6	51.9	53.9	45.1	42.9
45 to 54 years	NA	NA	NA	NA	15.9	14.9	13.9	13.0	12.1	12.2
55 to 64 years	NA	NA	NA	NA	50.4	45.1	43.3	38.7	30.5	30.0
65 to 74 years	NA	NA	NA	NA	178.2	154.5	141.4	133.1	100.5	94.3
75 to 84 years	NA	NA	NA	NA	635.2	547.3	506.2	482.3	363.0	333.7
85 years and over	NA	NA	NA	NA	1,729.1	1,578.7	1,544.8	1,505.9	1,148.7	1,048.5
Black, Not Hispanic or Latino Male[7]										
All ages, age-adjusted[4]	NA	NA	NA	NA	NA	NA	NA	90.8	74.1	70.2
All ages, crude	NA	NA	NA	NA	NA	NA	NA	47.7	42.0	40.9
45 to 54 years	NA	NA	NA	NA	NA	NA	NA	50.4	44.7	43.2
55 to 64 years	NA	NA	NA	NA	NA	NA	NA	116.9	102.4	103.6
65 to 74 years	NA	NA	NA	NA	NA	NA	NA	272.1	219.9	213.1
75 to 84 years	NA	NA	NA	NA	NA	NA	NA	664.9	510.5	478.1
85 years and over	NA	NA	NA	NA	NA	NA	NA	1,479.5	1,213.5	1,091.8
White Female[5]										
All ages, age-adjusted[4]	169.7	165.0	135.5	89.0	70.7	60.3	58.6	57.3	45.3	42.3
All ages, crude	103.3	110.1	109.8	88.6	78.2	71.6	75.1	76.9	62.0	58.3
45 to 54 years	55.0	33.8	30.5	18.6	15.5	13.5	12.6	11.2	10.5	10.4
55 to 64 years	156.9	103.0	78.1	48.6	39.9	35.8	33.3	30.2	23.7	23.9
65 to 74 years	498.1	383.3	303.2	172.5	137.6	116.1	111.7	107.3	82.6	78.6
75 to 84 years	1,471.3	1,444.7	1,176.8	728.8	551.7	456.5	443.4	434.2	343.4	321.6
85 years and over	3,017.9	3,795.7	3,167.6	2,362.7	1,938.0	1,685.9	1,656.7	1,646.7	1,292.6	1,182.1
Black or African American Female[5]										
All ages, age-adjusted[4]	238.4	232.5	189.3	119.6	99.2	84.0	79.4	76.2	62.4	58.4
All ages, crude	128.3	127.7	112.2	77.8	68.5	60.7	59.1	58.3	48.8	46.2
45 to 54 years	248.9	166.2	119.4	61.8	50.8	44.1	36.0	38.1	34.6	30.9
55 to 64 years	567.7	452.0	272.4	138.4	113.5	96.9	85.6	76.4	58.7	59.8
65 to 74 years	754.4	830.5	673.5	361.7	285.1	236.7	222.3	190.9	151.0	146.0
75 to 84 years[6]	1,496.7	1,413.1	1,338.3	917.5	752.4	595.0	565.1	549.2	451.5	416.8
85 years and over	NA	2,578.9	2,210.5	1,891.6	1,653.4	1,495.2	1,518.4	1,556.5	1,282.5	1,176.9
American Indian or Alaska Native Female[5]										
All ages, age-adjusted[4]	NA	NA	NA	51.2	44.3	38.4	46.3	43.7	41.1	35.4
All ages, crude	NA	NA	NA	22.0	21.5	19.3	22.0	21.5	21.3	17.2

NOTE: Starting with *Health, United States, 2003*, rates for 1991–1999 were revised using intercensal population estimates based on the 1990 and 2000 Censuses. For 2000, population estimates are bridged-race April 1 census counts. Starting with *Health, United States, 2012*, rates for 2001–2009 were revised using intercensal population estimates based on the 2000 and 2010 Censuses. For 2010, population estimates are bridged-race April 1 census counts. Rates for 2011 and beyond were computed using 2010-based postcensal estimates. Age groups were selected to minimize the presentation of unstable age-specific death rates based on small numbers of deaths and for consistency among comparison groups. Starting with 2003 data, some states began to collect information on more than one race on the death certificate, according to 1997 Office of Management and Budget (OMB) standards. The multiple-race data for these states were bridged to the single-race categories of the 1977 OMB standards, for comparability with other states. NA = Not available.

* = Rates based on fewer than 20 deaths are considered unreliable and are not shown.
[1]Includes deaths of persons who were not residents of the 50 states and the District of Columbia (DC).
[2]Underlying cause of death was coded according to the 6th revision of the *International Classification of Diseases* (*ICD*) in 1950, 7th revision in 1960, 8th revision in 1970, and 9th revision in 1980–1998.
[3]Starting with 1999 data, cause of death is coded according to *ICD–10*.
[4]Age-adjusted rates are calculated using the year 2000 standard population. Prior to 2001, age-adjusted rates were calculated using standard million proportions based on rounded population numbers. Starting with 2001 data, unrounded population numbers are used to calculate age-adjusted rates.
[5]The race groups, White, Black, Asian or Pacific Islander, and American Indian and Alaska Native, include persons of Hispanic and non-Hispanic origin. Persons of Hispanic origin may be of any race. Death rates for Hispanic, American Indian or Alaska Native, and Asian or Pacific Islander persons should be interpreted with caution because of inconsistencies in reporting Hispanic origin or race on the death certificate (death rate numerators) compared with population figures (death rate denominators). The net effect of misclassification is an underestimation of deaths and death rates for races other than White and Black.
[6]In 1950, rate is for the age group 75 years and over.
[7]Prior to 1997, excludes data from states lacking an Hispanic-origin item on the death certificate.

Table 2-29. Death Rates for Cerebrovascular Diseases, by Sex, Race, Hispanic Origin, and Age, Selected Years, 1950–2016—*Continued*

(Deaths per 100,000 resident population; data are based on death certificates.)

Sex, race, Hispanic origin, and age	2007[3]	2008[3]	2009[3]	2010[3]	2011[3]	2012[3]	2013[3]	2014[3]	2015[3]	2016[3]
American Indian or Alaska Native Male[5]										
All ages, age-adjusted[4]	35.6	27.5	32.0	29.8	25.8	25.5	22.7	25.3	24.5	23.9
All ages, crude	13.9	11.7	12.7	12.0	11.8	12.0	11.3	13.0	13.4	13.0
45 to 54 years	12.3	13.0	14.4	11.7	10.4	10.7	9.2	8.4	10.9	8.7
55 to 64 years	34.8	28.1	25.2	22.1	29.0	26.9	23.8	29.8	23.8	24.0
65 to 74 years	82.2	94.5	68.4	68.0	66.8	84.4	72.5	74.7	76.5	58.4
75 to 84 years	300.5	193.8	288.5	267.5	226.3	172.2	191.0	193.0	183.3	193.1
85 years and over	709.9	492.5	629.2	580.4	425.6	506.3	348.3	463.9	424.5	464.4
Asian or Pacific Islander Male[5]										
All ages, age-adjusted[4]	37.9	36.2	35.4	35.2	33.5	33.2	31.2	29.4	31.3	31.4
All ages, crude	21.2	20.9	20.8	21.5	21.2	21.7	21.3	20.7	22.8	23.5
45 to 54 years	14.6	13.1	12.9	14.7	12.9	13.2	15.7	11.0	11.9	12.1
55 to 64 years	31.0	31.3	31.1	31.7	31.4	30.0	27.7	30.0	32.2	29.9
65 to 74 years	88.9	88.2	76.2	84.9	75.6	78.1	73.0	66.4	73.0	73.0
75 to 84 years	282.8	265.1	278.0	260.0	258.2	239.3	230.5	217.2	239.8	221.8
85 years and over	888.2	835.2	800.0	778.7	746.2	776.0	686.7	666.1	669.1	726.9
Hispanic or Latino Male[5,7]										
All ages, age-adjusted[4]	38.1	37.3	34.0	33.9	32.6	32.0	31.8	32.1	34.2	34.0
All ages, crude	14.1	13.9	13.1	13.2	13.3	13.5	14.0	14.6	15.9	16.5
45 to 54 years	16.7	15.4	14.7	14.3	13.9	13.5	13.8	13.3	11.5	13.3
55 to 64 years	43.2	35.3	33.7	31.9	35.2	33.3	33.9	33.2	32.7	34.2
65 to 74 years	95.6	90.6	92.6	84.4	80.4	75.5	82.1	77.0	86.4	86.7
75 to 84 years	278.6	292.2	253.0	266.5	245.4	248.1	242.1	245.8	265.9	257.0
85 years and over	778.3	758.4	678.8	679.1	665.4	644.9	620.6	656.6	706.9	700.6
White, Not Hispanic or Latino Male[7]										
All ages, age-adjusted[4]	41.1	40.0	37.9	37.5	36.1	35.3	34.9	35.1	35.8	35.7
All ages, crude	42.3	41.9	40.6	40.7	40.3	40.3	40.8	41.8	43.5	44.0
45 to 54 years	12.4	11.3	12.1	11.6	11.2	10.8	11.0	11.3	10.9	11.3
55 to 64 years	29.7	29.1	28.6	28.4	28.3	28.5	29.0	28.7	28.9	30.0
65 to 74 years	91.5	87.4	85.1	82.6	79.8	77.7	76.6	76.7	76.5	76.9
75 to 84 years	318.6	313.6	294.7	288.6	284.9	271.2	272.0	265.8	272.0	268.3
85 years and over	1,008.2	976.7	906.2	913.2	854.8	848.0	825.6	851.2	887.3	866.0
Black, Not Hispanic or Latino Male[7]										
All ages, age-adjusted[4]	70.1	64.8	60.2	58.1	57.0	55.1	55.6	56.5	57.0	56.7
All ages, crude	41.0	38.7	37.0	36.6	36.6	36.1	37.2	38.7	39.8	40.2
45 to 54 years	40.5	40.4	35.8	34.9	35.1	34.5	31.9	30.8	31.4	31.0
55 to 64 years	97.0	87.1	86.4	85.9	83.8	78.2	80.4	81.8	80.9	76.5
65 to 74 years	216.1	198.7	187.1	187.5	176.5	169.1	169.4	173.8	174.5	174.1
75 to 84 years	499.0	451.2	421.0	406.8	395.0	395.1	397.4	401.7	419.9	412.8
85 years and over	1,082.2	1,020.7	903.6	819.8	849.5	806.2	833.9	847.2	823.6	866.1
White Female[5]										
All ages, age-adjusted[4]	41.2	39.9	37.6	37.2	36.2	35.2	34.2	34.7	35.9	35.5
All ages, crude	57.3	56.0	53.1	53.0	52.3	51.5	50.6	51.8	54.4	54.3
45 to 54 years	10.0	9.5	9.6	9.1	9.0	9.3	9.0	8.8	9.5	9.1
55 to 64 years	22.3	21.9	21.1	20.6	21.1	19.8	19.8	20.4	21.1	20.8
65 to 74 years	75.0	72.8	67.5	66.8	64.6	62.3	60.0	60.2	61.4	61.8
75 to 84 years	310.6	302.0	286.4	280.2	278.0	265.4	257.7	257.1	260.1	251.4
85 years and over	1,168.7	1,129.7	1,052.0	1,052.8	1,008.1	994.7	970.4	995.7	1,055.0	1,055.5
Black or African American Female[5]										
All ages, age-adjusted[4]	56.4	54.8	50.0	49.6	47.0	45.4	44.7	45.2	46.7	46.4
All ages, crude	45.1	44.2	41.0	41.1	39.6	39.2	39.2	40.5	42.5	43.1
45 to 54 years	32.4	30.1	28.8	26.7	23.6	25.0	21.1	22.4	21.3	22.2
55 to 64 years	57.0	57.5	53.5	51.3	48.2	48.8	47.7	48.4	48.1	47.4
65 to 74 years	140.5	127.4	122.5	126.2	116.7	111.2	109.1	112.6	110.1	113.6
75 to 84 years	389.1	399.3	360.1	347.2	342.0	321.6	333.0	322.6	345.3	326.8
85 years and over	1,166.7	1,106.4	989.6	1,001.5	948.1	927.2	894.1	934.0	977.5	997.4
American Indian or Alaska Native Female[5]										
All ages, age-adjusted[4]	32.8	27.2	27.0	26.5	27.9	24.8	25.5	25.0	24.4	23.5
All ages, crude	16.7	14.2	14.4	14.2	15.9	14.4	15.4	15.7	16.1	15.7

NOTE: Starting with *Health, United States, 2003*, rates for 1991–1999 were revised using intercensal population estimates based on the 1990 and 2000 Censuses. For 2000, population estimates are bridged-race April 1 census counts. Starting with *Health, United States, 2012*, rates for 2001–2009 were revised using intercensal population estimates based on the 2000 and 2010 Censuses. For 2010, population estimates are bridged-race April 1 census counts. Rates for 2011 and beyond were computed using 2010-based postcensal estimates. Age groups were selected to minimize the presentation of unstable age-specific death rates based on small numbers of deaths and for consistency among comparison groups. Starting with 2003 data, some states began to collect information on more than one race on the death certificate, according to 1997 Office of Management and Budget (OMB) standards. The multiple-race data for these states were bridged to the single-race categories of the 1977 OMB standards, for comparability with other states.
[3]Starting with 1999 data, cause of death is coded according to *ICD–10*.
[4]Age-adjusted rates are calculated using the year 2000 standard population. Prior to 2001, age-adjusted rates were calculated using standard million proportions based on rounded population numbers. Starting with 2001 data, unrounded population numbers are used to calculate age-adjusted rates.
[5]The race groups, White, Black, Asian or Pacific Islander, and American Indian and Alaska Native, include persons of Hispanic and non-Hispanic origin. Persons of Hispanic origin may be of any race. Death rates for Hispanic, American Indian or Alaska Native, and Asian or Pacific Islander persons should be interpreted with caution because of inconsistencies in reporting Hispanic origin or race on the death certificate (death rate numerators) compared with population figures (death rate denominators). The net effect of misclassification is an underestimation of deaths and death rates for races other than White and Black.
[6]In 1950, rate is for the age group 75 years and over.
[7]Prior to 1997, excludes data from states lacking an Hispanic-origin item on the death certificate.

Table 2-29. Death Rates for Cerebrovascular Diseases, by Sex, Race, Hispanic Origin, and Age, Selected Years, 1950–2016—*Continued*

(Deaths per 100,000 resident population; data are based on death certificates.)

Sex, race, Hispanic origin, and age	1950[1,2]	1960[1,2]	1970[2]	1980[2]	1985[2]	1990[2]	1995[2]	2000[3]	2005[3]	2006[3]
45 to 54 years	NA	NA	NA	*	*	*	*	14.4	16.3	*
55 to 64 years	NA	NA	NA	*	40.4	40.7	41.5	37.9	34.6	15.5
65 to 74 years	NA	NA	NA	128.3	118.2	100.5	114.8	79.5	114.5	78.0
75 to 84 years	NA	NA	NA	404.2	317.6	282.0	364.4	391.1	304.7	283.4
85 years and over	NA	NA	NA	1,095.5	980.0	776.2	983.9	931.5	865.8	919.7
Asian or Pacific Islander Female[5]										
All ages, age-adjusted[4]	NA	NA	NA	60.8	54.8	54.9	48.3	49.1	38.3	37.0
All ages, crude	NA	NA	NA	26.4	23.3	24.3	24.2	28.7	25.6	25.5
45 to 54 years	NA	NA	NA	20.3	15.1	19.7	15.6	13.3	9.7	10.2
55 to 64 years	NA	NA	NA	43.7	49.0	42.1	37.6	33.3	26.4	27.8
65 to 74 years	NA	NA	NA	136.1	129.9	124.0	101.0	102.8	80.1	79.9
75 to 84 years	NA	NA	NA	446.6	387.0	396.6	381.8	386.0	278.1	295.2
85 years and over	NA	NA	NA	1,545.2	1,383.3	1,395.0	1,197.0	1,246.6	1,044.6	890.5
Hispanic or Latina Female[5,7]										
All ages, age-adjusted[4]	NA	NA	NA	NA	47.5	43.7	42.7	43.0	36.0	35.0
All ages, crude	NA	NA	NA	NA	18.2	20.1	19.4	19.4	17.3	17.1
45 to 54 years	NA	NA	NA	NA	15.8	15.2	15.1	12.4	11.9	11.6
55 to 64 years	NA	NA	NA	NA	35.3	38.5	36.5	31.9	26.9	27.5
65 to 74 years	NA	NA	NA	NA	108.6	102.6	102.3	95.2	75.4	76.5
75 to 84 years	NA	NA	NA	NA	340.0	308.5	307.3	311.3	270.3	248.5
85 years and over	NA	NA	NA	NA	1,185.7	1,055.3	1,021.0	1,108.9	905.5	901.5
White, not Hispanic or Latina Female[7]										
All ages, age-adjusted[4]	NA	NA	NA	NA	69.7	61.0	58.7	57.6	45.6	42.5
All ages, crude	NA	NA	NA	NA	80.8	77.2	81.5	85.5	70.1	66.0
45 to 54 years	NA	NA	NA	NA	14.3	13.2	12.3	10.9	10.2	10.1
55 to 64 years	NA	NA	NA	NA	37.8	35.7	32.6	29.9	23.2	23.4
65 to 74 years	NA	NA	NA	NA	133.2	116.9	111.4	107.6	82.9	78.3
75 to 84 years	NA	NA	NA	NA	550.8	461.9	445.9	438.3	347.0	325.2
85 years and over	NA	NA	NA	NA	1,920.7	1,714.7	1,666.8	1,661.6	1,306.0	1,192.2
Black, not Hispanic or Latina Female[7]										
All ages, age-adjusted[4]	NA	NA	NA	NA	NA	NA	NA	77.2	63.4	59.5
All ages, crude	NA	NA	NA	NA	NA	NA	NA	60.3	50.9	48.3
45 to 54 years	NA	NA	NA	NA	NA	NA	NA	39.2	35.6	31.8
55 to 64 years	NA	NA	NA	NA	NA	NA	NA	77.8	60.2	61.2
65 to 74 years	NA	NA	NA	NA	NA	NA	NA	194.1	153.0	149.0
75 to 84 years	NA	NA	NA	NA	NA	NA	NA	553.8	457.4	423.1
85 years and over	NA	NA	NA	NA	NA	NA	NA	1,570.4	1,300.2	1,193.3

NOTE: Starting with *Health, United States, 2003*, rates for 1991–1999 were revised using intercensal population estimates based on the 1990 and 2000 Censuses. For 2000, population estimates are bridged-race April 1 census counts. Starting with *Health, United States, 2012*, rates for 2001–2009 were revised using intercensal population estimates based on the 2000 and 2010 Censuses. For 2010, population estimates are bridged-race April 1 census counts. Rates for 2011 and beyond were computed using 2010-based postcensal estimates. Age groups were selected to minimize the presentation of unstable age-specific death rates based on small numbers of deaths and for consistency among comparison groups. Starting with 2003 data, some states began to collect information on more than one race on the death certificate, according to 1997 Office of Management and Budget (OMB) standards. The multiple-race data for these states were bridged to the single-race categories of the 1977 OMB standards, for comparability with other states. NA = Not available.

* = Rates based on fewer than 20 deaths are considered unreliable and are not shown.
[1]Includes deaths of persons who were not residents of the 50 states and the District of Columbia (DC).
[2]Underlying cause of death was coded according to the 6th revision of the *International Classification of Diseases* (*ICD*) in 1950, 7th revision in 1960, 8th revision in 1970, and 9th revision in 1980–1998.
[3]Starting with 1999 data, cause of death is coded according to *ICD–10.*
[4]Age-adjusted rates are calculated using the year 2000 standard population. Prior to 2001, age-adjusted rates were calculated using standard million proportions based on rounded population numbers. Starting with 2001 data, unrounded population numbers are used to calculate age-adjusted rates.
[5]The race groups, White, Black, Asian or Pacific Islander, and American Indian and Alaska Native, include persons of Hispanic and non-Hispanic origin. Persons of Hispanic origin may be of any race. Death rates for Hispanic, American Indian or Alaska Native, and Asian or Pacific Islander persons should be interpreted with caution because of inconsistencies in reporting Hispanic origin or race on the death certificate (death rate numerators) compared with population figures (death rate denominators). The net effect of misclassification is an underestimation of deaths and death rates for races other than White and Black.
[7]Prior to 1997, excludes data from states lacking an Hispanic-origin item on the death certificate.

Table 2-29. Death Rates for Cerebrovascular Diseases, by Sex, Race, Hispanic Origin, and Age, Selected Years, 1950–2016—*Continued*

(Deaths per 100,000 resident population; data are based on death certificates.)

Sex, race, Hispanic origin, and age	2007[3]	2008[3]	2009[3]	2010[3]	2011[3]	2012[3]	2013[3]	2014[3]	2015[3]	2016[3]
45 to 54 years	8.9	9.3	11.6	10.6	11.2	7.2	9.0	11.2	11.2	9.4
55 to 64 years	22.5	24.4	24.6	22.4	19.2	20.0	19.1	21.6	19.8	17.0
65 to 74 years	82.2	54.5	69.3	59.4	64.2	58.8	60.6	52.4	58.2	44.7
75 to 84 years	211.4	221.3	169.7	173.6	237.7	205.5	187.2	183.2	176.0	190.4
85 years and over	879.0	615.3	692.2	700.0	550.3	531.3	593.6	618.8	559.4	528.4
Asian or Pacific Islander Female[5]										
All ages, age-adjusted[4]	35.5	34.2	31.2	31.4	30.0	28.9	27.9	27.2	28.3	29.9
All ages, crude	24.8	24.7	22.9	23.5	23.7	23.7	23.8	23.8	25.5	28.0
45 to 54 years	9.6	10.2	9.4	7.9	9.1	9.2	8.6	8.6	7.6	9.5
55 to 64 years	24.1	24.6	20.6	22.1	22.5	20.0	18.2	18.4	18.3	19.2
65 to 74 years	70.9	74.9	61.4	65.6	55.8	56.3	54.0	52.3	51.3	54.9
75 to 84 years	269.8	247.2	237.1	218.4	237.2	213.4	203.0	197.9	219.2	215.0
85 years and over	935.0	898.2	814.3	872.8	758.7	770.1	754.6	747.4	757.6	835.9
Hispanic or Latina Female[5,7]										
All ages, age-adjusted[4]	33.5	32.0	30.4	30.2	29.0	28.2	27.6	28.3	30.4	30.1
All ages, crude	16.6	16.0	15.6	15.7	15.7	15.8	16.1	16.9	18.8	19.3
45 to 54 years	10.8	10.0	9.1	9.2	9.5	8.8	9.1	7.7	8.8	8.4
55 to 64 years	25.0	20.7	22.9	22.1	21.0	19.9	19.7	17.2	19.3	19.9
65 to 74 years	70.8	65.9	58.4	60.6	59.2	59.3	53.6	54.7	54.0	57.9
75 to 84 years	252.1	248.9	234.0	221.6	233.9	217.6	211.4	219.7	230.0	221.7
85 years and over	845.7	804.0	774.8	799.3	692.5	705.9	698.4	744.6	831.1	822.9
White, not Hispanic or Latina Female[7]										
All ages, age-adjusted[4]	41.5	40.2	37.8	37.4	36.5	35.5	34.5	35.0	36.2	35.8
All ages, crude	65.3	64.0	60.8	60.8	60.2	59.2	58.3	59.7	62.4	62.5
45 to 54 years	9.8	9.3	9.6	9.0	8.8	9.2	8.8	8.9	9.4	9.1
55 to 64 years	21.9	21.8	20.7	20.3	20.9	19.6	19.6	20.6	21.0	20.6
65 to 74 years	75.0	73.1	68.0	66.9	64.8	62.1	60.2	60.3	61.5	61.7
75 to 84 years	313.7	304.6	289.1	283.4	280.6	268.1	260.3	259.0	260.9	252.5
85 years and over	1,181.4	1,142.1	1,062.9	1,063.0	1,022.8	1,008.1	984.3	1,009.2	1,066.0	1,068.7
Black, not Hispanic or Latina Female[7]										
All ages, age-adjusted[4]	57.6	55.9	51.1	50.7	48.2	46.4	45.9	46.3	47.9	47.8
All ages, crude	47.4	46.4	43.1	43.4	41.9	41.4	41.5	42.8	45.0	45.9
45 to 54 years	33.4	31.0	29.8	27.6	24.6	26.0	22.0	23.4	22.3	23.3
55 to 64 years	58.6	58.9	54.8	52.7	49.8	50.1	49.3	49.8	49.7	49.2
65 to 74 years	143.8	129.6	125.2	129.0	119.3	113.9	112.0	115.9	112.5	117.0
75 to 84 years	396.0	407.8	366.6	355.5	348.9	328.6	341.3	328.9	353.5	336.1
85 years and over	1,184.0	1,118.7	1,004.9	1,016.4	969.4	941.5	908.5	950.2	994.7	1,018.8

NOTE: Starting with *Health, United States, 2003*, rates for 1991–1999 were revised using intercensal population estimates based on the 1990 and 2000 Censuses. For 2000, population estimates are bridged-race April 1 census counts. Starting with *Health, United States, 2012*, rates for 2001–2009 were revised using intercensal population estimates based on the 2000 and 2010 Censuses. For 2010, population estimates are bridged-race April 1 census counts. Rates for 2011 and beyond were computed using 2010-based postcensal estimates. Age groups were selected to minimize the presentation of unstable age-specific death rates based on small numbers of deaths and for consistency among comparison groups. Starting with 2003 data, some states began to collect information on more than one race on the death certificate, according to 1997 Office of Management and Budget (OMB) standards. The multiple-race data for these states were bridged to the single-race categories of the 1977 OMB standards, for comparability with other states.
[3]Starting with 1999 data, cause of death is coded according to *ICD–10*.
[4]Age-adjusted rates are calculated using the year 2000 standard population. Prior to 2001, age-adjusted rates were calculated using standard million proportions based on rounded population numbers. Starting with 2001 data, unrounded population numbers are used to calculate age-adjusted rates.
[5]The race groups, White, Black, Asian or Pacific Islander, and American Indian and Alaska Native, include persons of Hispanic and non-Hispanic origin. Persons of Hispanic origin may be of any race. Death rates for Hispanic, American Indian or Alaska Native, and Asian or Pacific Islander persons should be interpreted with caution because of inconsistencies in reporting Hispanic origin or race on the death certificate (death rate numerators) compared with population figures (death rate denominators). The net effect of misclassification is an underestimation of deaths and death rates for races other than White and Black.
[7]Prior to 1997, excludes data from states lacking an Hispanic-origin item on the death certificate.

Table 2-30. Death Rates for Malignant Neoplasms, by Sex, Race, Hispanic Origin, and Age, Selected Years, 1950–2016

(Deaths per 100,000 resident population; data are based on death certificates.)

Sex, race, Hispanic origin, and age	1950[1,2]	1960[1,2]	1970[2]	1980[2]	1985[2]	1990[2]	1995[2]	2000[3]	2005[3]	2006[3]
All Persons										
All ages, age-adjusted[4]	193.9	193.9	198.6	207.9	211.3	216.0	209.9	199.6	185.1	181.8
All ages, crude	139.8	149.2	162.8	183.9	194.0	203.2	202.2	196.5	189.3	187.6
Under 1 year	8.7	7.2	4.7	3.2	3.1	2.3	1.8	2.4	1.9	1.9
1 to 4 years	11.7	10.9	7.5	4.5	3.8	3.5	3.1	2.7	2.4	2.4
5 to 14 years	6.7	6.8	6.0	4.3	3.5	3.1	2.7	2.5	2.5	2.2
15 to 24 years	8.6	8.3	8.3	6.3	5.4	4.9	4.5	4.4	4.0	3.8
25 to 34 years	20.0	19.5	16.5	13.7	13.2	12.6	11.6	9.8	9.2	9.3
35 to 44 years	62.7	59.7	59.5	48.6	45.9	43.3	40.1	36.6	33.5	32.2
45 to 54 years	175.1	177.0	182.5	180.0	170.1	158.9	140.4	127.5	118.6	116.3
55 to 64 years	390.7	396.8	423.0	436.1	454.6	449.6	412.3	366.7	323.9	317.7
65 to 74 years	698.8	713.9	754.2	817.9	845.5	872.3	863.3	816.3	733.2	716.3
75 to 84 years	1,153.3	1,127.4	1,169.2	1,232.3	1,271.8	1,348.5	1,355.4	1,335.6	1,272.8	1,259.2
85 years and over	1,451.0	1,450.0	1,320.7	1,594.6	1,615.4	1,752.9	1,797.7	1,819.4	1,778.2	1,748.3
Male										
All ages, age-adjusted[4]	208.1	225.1	247.6	271.2	274.4	280.4	267.5	248.9	227.2	221.7
All ages, crude	142.9	162.5	182.1	205.3	213.4	221.3	216.3	207.2	200.0	197.8
Under 1 year	9.7	7.7	4.4	3.7	3.0	2.4	1.9	2.6	2.2	1.9
1 to 4 years	12.5	12.4	8.3	5.2	4.3	3.7	3.6	3.0	2.7	2.5
5 to 14 years	7.4	7.6	6.7	4.9	3.9	3.5	3.0	2.7	2.7	2.4
15 to 24 years	9.7	10.2	10.4	7.8	6.4	5.7	5.4	5.1	4.8	4.6
25 to 34 years	17.7	18.8	16.3	13.4	13.2	12.6	11.3	9.2	9.2	9.0
35 to 44 years	45.6	48.9	53.0	44.0	42.4	38.5	36.3	32.7	29.3	27.8
45 to 54 years	156.2	170.8	183.5	188.7	175.2	162.5	141.5	130.9	121.7	119.1
55 to 64 years	413.1	459.9	511.8	520.8	536.9	532.9	475.1	415.8	365.8	359.4
65 to 74 years	791.5	890.5	1,006.8	1,093.2	1,105.2	1,122.2	1,083.0	1,001.9	883.1	852.5
75 to 84 years	1,332.6	1,389.4	1,588.3	1,790.5	1,839.7	1,914.4	1,847.9	1,760.6	1,636.8	1,611.8
85 years and over	1,668.3	1,741.2	1,720.8	2,369.5	2,451.8	2,739.9	2,818.7	2,710.7	2,576.2	2,500.3
Female										
All ages, age-adjusted[4]	182.3	168.7	163.2	166.7	171.2	175.7	173.6	167.6	156.7	154.7
All ages, crude	136.8	136.4	144.4	163.6	175.7	186.0	188.8	186.2	178.9	177.8
Under 1 year	7.6	6.8	5.0	2.7	3.2	2.2	1.8	2.3	1.5	1.9
1 to 4 years	10.8	9.3	6.7	3.7	3.4	3.2	2.6	2.5	2.1	2.2
5 to 14 years	6.0	6.0	5.2	3.6	3.1	2.8	2.3	2.2	2.2	2.0
15 to 24 years	7.6	6.5	6.2	4.8	4.3	4.1	3.5	3.6	3.3	3.1
25 to 34 years	22.2	20.1	16.7	14.0	13.2	12.6	11.9	10.4	9.2	9.6
35 to 44 years	79.3	70.0	65.6	53.1	49.2	48.1	43.8	40.4	37.6	36.5
45 to 54 years	194.0	183.0	181.5	171.8	165.3	155.5	139.3	124.2	115.7	113.5
55 to 64 years	368.2	337.7	343.2	361.7	381.8	375.2	355.1	321.3	284.8	278.9
65 to 74 years	612.3	560.2	557.9	607.1	645.3	677.4	687.1	663.6	605.6	599.8
75 to 84 years	1,000.7	924.1	891.9	903.1	937.8	1,010.3	1,047.5	1,058.5	1,023.0	1,014.6
85 years and over	1,299.7	1,263.9	1,096.7	1,255.7	1,281.4	1,372.1	1,404.4	1,456.4	1,423.6	1,407.2
White Male[5]										
All ages, age-adjusted[4]	210.0	224.7	244.8	265.1	267.1	272.2	260.6	243.9	224.3	219.3
All ages, crude	147.2	166.1	185.1	208.7	218.1	227.7	225.3	218.1	212.8	211.1
25 to 34 years	17.7	18.8	16.2	13.6	13.1	12.3	11.0	9.2	8.8	9.0
35 to 44 years	44.5	46.3	50.1	41.1	39.8	35.8	34.1	30.9	28.9	27.2
45 to 54 years	150.8	164.1	172.0	175.4	162.0	149.9	132.7	123.5	116.3	114.3
55 to 64 years	409.4	450.9	498.1	497.4	512.0	508.2	456.0	401.9	354.2	350.4
65 to 74 years	798.7	887.3	997.0	1,070.7	1,076.5	1,090.7	1,056.1	984.3	875.6	845.8
75 to 84 years	1,367.6	1,413.7	1,592.7	1,779.7	1,817.1	1,883.2	1,817.4	1,736.0	1,629.2	1,606.9
85 years and over	1,732.7	1,791.4	1,772.2	2,375.6	2,449.1	2,715.1	2,789.4	2,693.7	2,558.2	2,487.9
Black or African American Male[5]										
All ages, age-adjusted[4]	178.9	227.6	291.9	353.4	373.9	397.9	374.3	340.3	297.2	287.2
All ages, crude	106.6	136.7	171.6	205.5	214.9	221.9	204.8	188.5	174.7	171.2
25 to 34 years	18.0	18.4	18.8	14.1	14.9	15.7	14.8	10.1	12.4	10.4
35 to 44 years	55.7	72.9	81.3	73.8	69.9	64.3	57.2	48.4	36.1	36.2
45 to 54 years	211.7	244.7	311.2	333.0	315.9	302.6	243.9	214.2	181.1	176.1
55 to 64 years	490.8	579.7	689.2	812.5	851.3	859.2	738.1	626.4	546.0	518.2
65 to 74 years	636.5	938.5	1,168.9	1,417.2	1,532.8	1,613.9	1,541.4	1,363.8	1,139.4	1,106.8
75 to 84 years[6]	853.5	1,053.3	1,624.8	2,029.6	2,229.6	2,478.3	2,449.8	2,351.8	2,019.5	1,976.0
85 years and over	NA	1,155.2	1,387.0	2,393.9	2,629.0	3,238.3	3,395.5	3,264.8	3,258.8	3,102.5

NOTE: Starting with *Health, United States, 2003*, rates for 1991–1999 were revised using intercensal population estimates based on the 1990 and 2000 Censuses. For 2000, population estimates are bridged-race April 1 census counts. Starting with *Health, United States, 2012*, rates for 2001–2009 were revised using intercensal population estimates based on the 2000 and 2010 Censuses. For 2010, population estimates are bridged-race April 1 census counts. Rates for 2011 and beyond were computed using 2010-based postcensal estimates. Age groups were selected to minimize the presentation of unstable age-specific death rates based on small numbers of deaths and for consistency among comparison groups. Starting with 2003 data, some states began to collect information on more than one race on the death certificate, according to 1997 Office of Management and Budget (OMB) standards. The multiple-race data for these states were bridged to the single-race categories of the 1977 OMB standards, for comparability with other states.

NA = Not available.

[1] Includes deaths of persons who were not residents of the 50 states and the District of Columbia (DC).

[2] Underlying cause of death was coded according to the 6th revision of the *International Classification of Diseases (ICD)* in 1950, 7th revision in 1960, 8th revision in 1970, and 9th revision in 1980–1998.

[3] Starting with 1999 data, cause of death is coded according to *ICD–10*.

[4] Age-adjusted rates are calculated using the year 2000 standard population. Prior to 2001, age-adjusted rates were calculated using standard million proportions based on rounded population numbers. Starting with 2001 data, unrounded population numbers are used to calculate age-adjusted rates.

[5] The race groups, White, Black, Asian or Pacific Islander, and American Indian and Alaska Native, include persons of Hispanic and non-Hispanic origin. Persons of Hispanic origin may be of any race. Death rates for Hispanic, American Indian or Alaska Native, and Asian or Pacific Islander persons should be interpreted with caution because of inconsistencies in reporting Hispanic origin or race on the death certificate (death rate numerators) compared with population figures (death rate denominators). The net effect of misclassification is an underestimate of deaths and death rates for races other than White and Black.

[6] In 1950, rate is for the age group 75 years and over.

Table 2-30. Death Rates for Malignant Neoplasms, by Sex, Race, Hispanic Origin, and Age, Selected Years, 1950–2016—*Continued*

(Deaths per 100,000 resident population; data are based on death certificates.)

Sex, race, Hispanic origin, and age	2007³	2008³	2009³	2010³	2011³	2012³	2013³	2014³	2015³	2016³
All Persons										
All ages, age-adjusted⁴	179.3	176.4	173.5	172.8	169.0	166.5	163.2	161.2	158.5	155.8
All ages, crude	186.9	186.0	185.0	186.2	185.1	185.6	185.0	185.6	185.4	185.1
Under 1 year	1.7	1.7	1.8	1.6	1.8	1.6	1.6	1.3	1.3	1.7
1 to 4 years	2.3	2.4	2.2	2.1	2.2	2.4	2.1	2.0	2.2	2.4
5 to 14 years	2.4	2.2	2.2	2.2	2.1	2.2	2.2	2.1	2.1	2.1
15 to 24 years	3.8	3.8	3.8	3.7	3.7	3.6	3.4	3.6	3.4	3.3
25 to 34 years	8.7	8.8	9.0	8.8	8.4	8.7	8.6	8.3	8.4	8.5
35 to 44 years	31.0	30.1	30.2	28.8	28.8	28.0	28.1	27.8	26.9	26.9
45 to 54 years	114.2	113.4	112.8	111.6	109.3	108.5	105.5	103.2	99.7	96.5
55 to 64 years	311.4	304.7	301.7	300.1	295.8	293.2	288.2	287.6	284.1	280.6
65 to 74 years	702.9	688.4	668.2	666.1	647.6	632.2	616.9	603.1	594.3	578.3
75 to 84 years	1,250.1	1,230.9	1,213.0	1,202.2	1,179.1	1,161.7	1,139.4	1,125.9	1,100.8	1,081.7
85 years and over	1,739.4	1,724.6	1,699.3	1,729.5	1,676.2	1,658.9	1,635.4	1,632.9	1,628.6	1,620.3
Male										
All ages, age-adjusted⁴	218.8	214.9	210.9	209.9	204.0	200.3	196.0	192.9	189.2	185.4
All ages, crude	197.8	197.5	196.8	198.3	197.2	197.9	197.6	198.4	198.3	197.7
Under 1 year	1.8	2.3	2.2	1.5	1.9	1.7	1.5	1.1	1.5	1.8
1 to 4 years	2.3	2.6	2.2	2.4	2.2	2.7	2.2	2.2	2.4	2.5
5 to 14 years	2.4	2.2	2.3	2.3	2.3	2.4	2.2	2.3	2.2	2.3
15 to 24 years	4.5	4.6	4.5	4.5	4.3	4.1	3.8	4.2	3.9	4.0
25 to 34 years	8.5	8.8	8.8	8.6	8.1	8.4	8.6	8.2	8.2	8.1
35 to 44 years	26.8	26.2	26.1	25.2	24.9	24.0	24.0	24.0	23.0	22.9
45 to 54 years	117.4	117.7	115.3	113.8	110.7	110.1	106.5	102.9	99.4	94.4
55 to 64 years	353.9	349.3	345.9	344.9	340.4	336.9	331.3	330.3	325.5	318.8
65 to 74 years	834.1	817.0	790.4	789.2	765.8	746.7	726.2	711.9	701.7	684.1
75 to 84 years	1,593.3	1,563.1	1,538.3	1,514.2	1,478.5	1,447.6	1,414.5	1,387.5	1,355.8	1,324.6
85 years and over	2,508.4	2,444.4	2,412.2	2,452.6	2,339.8	2,303.1	2,272.6	2,250.4	2,220.2	2,218.4
Female										
All ages, age-adjusted⁴	152.3	149.6	147.4	146.7	144.0	142.1	139.5	138.1	135.9	134.0
All ages, crude	176.3	174.8	173.7	174.4	173.4	173.7	172.8	173.2	172.9	172.8
Under 1 year	1.6	1.1	1.5	1.6	1.6	1.5	1.8	1.6	1.1	1.6
1 to 4 years	2.2	2.2	2.1	1.9	2.1	2.2	1.9	1.8	2.0	2.2
5 to 14 years	2.3	2.2	2.0	2.2	1.9	2.0	2.1	1.8	2.0	1.9
15 to 24 years	3.2	3.0	3.0	2.8	3.0	3.0	3.0	2.9	2.8	2.5
25 to 34 years	8.9	8.7	9.1	9.0	8.6	8.9	8.6	8.5	8.6	8.9
35 to 44 years	35.3	34.0	34.2	32.3	32.8	31.9	32.1	31.6	30.7	30.9
45 to 54 years	111.0	109.2	110.4	109.4	108.0	107.0	104.6	103.4	100.0	98.5
55 to 64 years	271.8	263.3	260.6	258.5	254.1	252.5	248.1	247.9	245.4	245.1
65 to 74 years	590.3	577.3	562.2	559.1	544.5	531.9	520.8	507.5	499.8	485.4
75 to 84 years	1,009.6	995.9	980.1	977.0	959.6	950.0	933.3	928.0	906.4	895.4
85 years and over	1,383.9	1,385.9	1,358.6	1,380.1	1,349.1	1,336.4	1,310.1	1,311.7	1,315.8	1,300.1
White Male⁵										
All ages, age-adjusted⁴	216.3	212.9	209.2	208.2	203.1	199.7	195.5	193.0	189.7	185.9
All ages, crude	211.2	211.5	211.0	212.7	212.0	213.1	213.0	214.4	214.7	214.0
25 to 34 years	8.5	8.8	8.9	8.8	8.1	8.5	8.5	8.4	8.4	8.3
35 to 44 years	26.4	25.6	25.9	25.2	25.2	24.2	23.9	24.0	23.1	22.9
45 to 54 years	112.8	113.9	112.5	111.6	108.6	108.2	105.7	102.3	98.8	94.4
55 to 64 years	344.1	340.4	335.8	334.9	332.4	329.4	323.1	323.5	320.5	312.0
65 to 74 years	827.3	811.1	784.2	782.8	759.5	742.8	723.3	707.6	698.7	680.7
75 to 84 years	1,588.2	1,560.4	1,538.3	1,511.6	1,485.2	1,453.0	1,421.7	1,400.4	1,369.4	1,338.8
85 years and over	2,488.1	2,437.8	2,412.5	2,453.5	2,347.1	2,318.7	2,290.7	2,279.7	2,251.6	2,256.5
Black or African American Male⁵										
All ages, age-adjusted⁴	284.2	273.1	266.7	264.8	252.6	246.1	238.7	231.9	224.8	220.3
All ages, crude	171.3	168.4	168.2	169.0	166.4	166.4	165.6	165.1	163.8	164.2
25 to 34 years	9.9	9.9	10.4	9.2	9.2	9.1	10.2	8.3	8.7	8.3
35 to 44 years	33.6	33.7	31.3	30.1	28.9	26.6	27.3	28.8	26.3	26.6
45 to 54 years	171.1	165.4	157.4	150.9	145.6	145.0	132.4	128.8	123.8	114.4
55 to 64 years	516.3	501.3	502.0	496.7	478.4	468.8	464.0	450.5	437.4	433.0
65 to 74 years	1,083.8	1,047.3	1,038.6	1,027.8	1,004.1	970.2	941.5	925.8	895.8	880.7
75 to 84 years⁶	1,929.9	1,875.6	1,835.3	1,826.8	1,705.6	1,685.7	1,633.2	1,569.4	1,526.9	1,489.5
85 years and over	3,230.0	2,956.8	2,791.3	2,854.6	2,675.3	2,540.2	2,465.6	2,378.6	2,316.0	2,298.6

NOTE: Starting with *Health, United States, 2003*, rates for 1991–1999 were revised using intercensal population estimates based on the 1990 and 2000 Censuses. For 2000, population estimates are bridged-race April 1 census counts. Starting with *Health, United States, 2012*, rates for 2001–2009 were revised using intercensal population estimates based on the 2000 and 2010 Censuses. For 2010, population estimates are bridged-race April 1 census counts. Rates for 2011 and beyond were computed using 2010-based postcensal estimates. Age groups were selected to minimize the presentation of unstable age-specific death rates based on small numbers of deaths and for consistency among comparison groups. Starting with 2003 data, some states began to collect information on more than one race on the death certificate, according to 1997 Office of Management and Budget (OMB) standards. The multiple-race data for these states were bridged to the single-race categories of the 1977 OMB standards, for comparability with other states.
³Starting with 1999 data, cause of death is coded according to *ICD–10*.
⁴Age-adjusted rates are calculated using the year 2000 standard population. Prior to 2001, age-adjusted rates were calculated using standard million proportions based on rounded population numbers. Starting with 2001 data, unrounded population numbers are used to calculate age-adjusted rates.
⁵The race groups, White, Black, Asian or Pacific Islander, and American Indian and Alaska Native, include persons of Hispanic and non-Hispanic origin. Persons of Hispanic origin may be of any race. Death rates for Hispanic, American Indian or Alaska Native, and Asian or Pacific Islander persons should be interpreted with caution because of inconsistencies in reporting Hispanic origin or race on the death certificate (death rate numerators) compared with population figures (death rate denominators). The net effect of misclassification is an underestimation of deaths and death rates for races other than White and Black.
⁶In 1950, rate is for the age group 75 years and over.

Table 2-30. Death Rates for Malignant Neoplasms, by Sex, Race, Hispanic Origin, and Age, Selected Years, 1950–2016—*Continued*

(Deaths per 100,000 resident population; data are based on death certificates.)

Sex, race, Hispanic origin, and age	1950[1,2]	1960[1,2]	1970[2]	1980[2]	1985[2]	1990[2]	1995[2]	2000[3]	2005[3]	2006[3]
American Indian or Alaska Native Male[5]										
All ages, age-adjusted[4]	NA	NA	NA	140.5	142.1	145.8	169.0	155.8	158.5	146.0
All ages, crude	NA	NA	NA	58.1	62.8	61.4	67.8	67.0	73.0	66.0
25 to 34 years	NA	NA	NA	*	*	*	*	*	*	*
35 to 44 years	NA	NA	NA	*	28.8	22.8	14.3	21.4	24.3	13.3
45 to 54 years	NA	NA	NA	86.9	89.4	86.9	79.2	70.3	75.2	67.3
55 to 64 years	NA	NA	NA	213.4	276.6	246.2	279.8	255.6	257.7	211.0
65 to 74 years	NA	NA	NA	613.0	584.6	530.6	684.7	648.0	619.3	578.3
75 to 84 years	NA	NA	NA	936.4	963.6	1,038.4	1,346.3	1,152.5	1,138.4	1,143.9
85 years and over	NA	NA	NA	1,471.2	1,133.3	1,654.4	1,549.0	1,584.2	1,832.2	1,653.0
Asian or Pacific Islander Male[5]										
All ages, age-adjusted[4]	NA	NA	NA	165.2	173.4	172.5	164.3	150.8	137.4	131.6
All ages, crude	NA	NA	NA	81.9	82.6	82.7	83.7	85.2	84.8	82.6
25 to 34 years	NA	NA	NA	6.3	10.0	9.2	8.2	7.4	7.1	6.9
35 to 44 years	NA	NA	NA	29.4	25.7	27.7	26.1	26.1	20.6	20.4
45 to 54 years	NA	NA	NA	108.2	98.0	92.6	82.4	78.5	75.9	70.3
55 to 64 years	NA	NA	NA	298.5	315.0	274.6	244.8	229.2	197.5	195.6
65 to 74 years	NA	NA	NA	581.2	631.3	687.2	614.3	559.4	487.0	455.0
75 to 84 years	NA	NA	NA	1,147.6	1,251.2	1,229.9	1,167.2	1,086.1	1,022.0	974.7
85 years and over	NA	NA	NA	1,798.7	1,800.0	1,837.0	2,081.3	1,823.2	1,716.2	1,685.3
Hispanic or Latino Male[5,7]										
All ages, age-adjusted[4]	NA	NA	NA	NA	161.3	174.7	180.9	171.7	162.4	153.5
All ages, crude	NA	NA	NA	NA	56.1	65.5	65.4	61.3	63.2	60.9
25 to 34 years	NA	NA	NA	NA	9.7	8.0	8.4	6.9	6.9	6.5
35 to 44 years	NA	NA	NA	NA	22.9	22.5	24.7	20.1	18.5	16.8
45 to 54 years	NA	NA	NA	NA	83.5	96.6	85.0	79.4	76.7	72.4
55 to 64 years	NA	NA	NA	NA	259.0	294.0	281.6	253.1	238.1	226.4
65 to 74 years	NA	NA	NA	NA	598.2	655.5	697.9	651.2	610.3	582.5
75 to 84 years	NA	NA	NA	NA	1,210.5	1,233.4	1,359.8	1,306.4	1,219.2	1,158.8
85 years and over	NA	NA	NA	NA	1,743.8	2,019.4	2,018.6	2,049.7	2,013.0	1,852.2
White, Not Hispanic or Latino Male[7]										
All ages, age-adjusted[4]	NA	NA	NA	NA	259.0	276.7	263.5	247.7	228.4	223.7
All ages, crude	NA	NA	NA	NA	217.4	246.2	246.0	244.4	242.5	241.7
25 to 34 years	NA	NA	NA	NA	13.5	12.8	11.2	9.7	9.3	9.5
35 to 44 years	NA	NA	NA	NA	39.1	36.8	34.8	32.3	30.8	29.2
45 to 54 years	NA	NA	NA	NA	159.9	153.9	135.6	127.2	120.7	119.1
55 to 64 years	NA	NA	NA	NA	496.4	520.6	464.9	412.0	363.1	360.0
65 to 74 years	NA	NA	NA	NA	1,044.2	1,109.0	1,069.9	1,002.1	893.3	863.5
75 to 84 years	NA	NA	NA	NA	1,765.5	1,906.6	1,825.4	1,750.2	1,650.0	1,630.1
85 years and over	NA	NA	NA	NA	2,327.3	2,744.4	2,810.8	2,714.1	2,578.7	2,511.9
Black, Not Hispanic or Latino Male[7]										
All ages, age-adjusted[4]	NA	NA	NA	NA	NA	NA	NA	344.8	302.6	293.1
All ages, crude	NA	NA	NA	NA	NA	NA	NA	194.9	182.4	179.5
25 to 34 years	NA	NA	NA	NA	NA	NA	NA	10.5	13.0	11.1
35 to 44 years	NA	NA	NA	NA	NA	NA	NA	49.6	37.4	37.9
45 to 54 years	NA	NA	NA	NA	NA	NA	NA	219.0	185.6	181.1
55 to 64 years	NA	NA	NA	NA	NA	NA	NA	637.4	558.5	531.8
65 to 74 years	NA	NA	NA	NA	NA	NA	NA	1,382.7	1,160.0	1,127.9
75 to 84 years	NA	NA	NA	NA	NA	NA	NA	2,372.3	2,047.5	2,010.3
85 years and over	NA	NA	NA	NA	NA	NA	NA	3,290.1	3,307.3	3,146.8
White Female[5]										
All ages, age-adjusted[4]	182.0	167.7	162.5	165.2	169.9	174.0	172.1	166.9	156.4	154.7
All ages, crude	139.9	139.8	149.4	170.3	184.4	196.1	200.6	199.4	192.3	191.5
25 to 34 years	20.9	18.8	16.3	13.5	12.7	11.9	11.2	10.1	8.8	9.3
35 to 44 years	74.5	66.6	62.4	50.9	47.3	46.2	41.9	38.2	36.2	35.2
45 to 54 years	185.8	175.7	177.3	166.4	161.6	150.9	135.0	120.1	110.9	109.9
55 to 64 years	362.5	329.0	338.6	355.5	376.3	368.5	350.3	319.7	282.2	277.1
65 to 74 years	616.5	562.1	554.7	605.2	644.9	675.1	685.6	665.6	611.5	606.1
75 to 84 years	1,026.6	939.3	903.5	905.4	938.2	1,011.8	1,047.9	1,063.4	1,032.0	1,023.5
85 years and over	1,348.3	1,304.9	1,126.6	1,266.8	1,285.4	1,372.3	1,405.4	1,459.1	1,426.4	1,413.0

NOTE: Starting with *Health, United States, 2003*, rates for 1991–1999 were revised using intercensal population estimates based on the 1990 and 2000 Censuses. For 2000, population estimates are bridged-race April 1 census counts. Starting with *Health, United States, 2012*, rates for 2001–2009 were revised using intercensal population estimates based on the 2000 and 2010 Censuses. For 2010, population estimates are bridged-race April 1 census counts. Rates for 2011 and beyond were computed using 2010-based postcensal estimates. Age groups were selected to minimize the presentation of unstable age-specific death rates based on small numbers of deaths and for consistency among comparison groups. Starting with 2003 data, some states began to collect information on more than one race on the death certificate, according to 1997 Office of Management and Budget (OMB) standards. The multiple-race data for these states were bridged to the single-race categories of the 1977 OMB standards, for comparability with other states.
NA = Not available.
* = Rates based on fewer than 20 deaths are considered unreliable and are not shown.
[1] Includes deaths of persons who were not residents of the 50 states and the District of Columbia (DC).
[2] Underlying cause of death was coded according to the 6th revision of the *International Classification of Diseases* (*ICD*) in 1950, 7th revision in 1960, 8th revision in 1970, and 9th revision in 1980–1998.
[3] Starting with 1999 data, cause of death is coded according to *ICD–10*.
[4] Age-adjusted rates are calculated using the year 2000 standard population. Prior to 2001, age-adjusted rates were calculated using standard million proportions based on rounded population numbers. Starting with 2001 data, unrounded population numbers are used to calculate age-adjusted rates.
[5] The race groups, White, Black, Asian or Pacific Islander, and American Indian and Alaska Native, include persons of Hispanic and non-Hispanic origin. Persons of Hispanic origin may be of any race. Death rates for Hispanic, American Indian or Alaska Native, and Asian or Pacific Islander persons should be interpreted with caution because of inconsistencies in reporting Hispanic origin or race on the death certificate (death rate numerators) compared with population figures (death rate denominators). The net effect of misclassification is an underestimation of deaths and death rates for races other than White and Black.
[7] Prior to 1997, excludes data from states lacking an Hispanic-origin item on the death certificate.

Table 2-30. Death Rates for Malignant Neoplasms, by Sex, Race, Hispanic Origin, and Age, Selected Years, 1950–2016—Continued

(Deaths per 100,000 resident population; data are based on death certificates.)

Sex, race, Hispanic origin, and age	2007[3]	2008[3]	2009[3]	2010[3]	2011[3]	2012[3]	2013[3]	2014[3]	2015[3]	2016[3]
American Indian or Alaska Native Male[5]										
All ages, age-adjusted[4]	150.7	151.8	132.8	151.0	132.7	127.9	132.3	130.4	127.1	122.4
All ages, crude	70.1	72.7	66.4	74.1	68.0	70.5	73.6	76.1	77.5	78.6
25 to 34 years	*	*	6.5	7.4	*	*	6.2	*	5.4	*
35 to 44 years	13.7	17.7	12.3	13.4	11.3	14.2	13.1	15.2	14.7	14.5
45 to 54 years	69.3	82.5	73.2	70.0	70.6	65.9	61.9	58.7	70.0	57.4
55 to 64 years	248.4	225.4	229.6	249.5	197.2	216.2	233.5	221.2	202.7	232.1
65 to 74 years	558.7	620.8	541.3	597.7	523.8	558.4	477.8	520.7	505.3	493.1
75 to 84 years	1,112.3	1,144.2	936.9	1,104.4	1,018.5	885.2	1,009.1	1,015.8	971.8	902.0
85 years and over	1,876.3	1,588.6	1,390.1	1,741.3	1,459.3	1,288.7	1,488.1	1,256.3	1,229.2	1,161.0
Asian or Pacific Islander Male[5]										
All ages, age-adjusted[4]	134.8	132.8	131.0	131.0	125.7	123.1	120.9	116.4	116.7	114.4
All ages, crude	85.5	86.3	86.7	88.6	89.0	89.0	90.5	90.2	92.5	93.2
25 to 34 years	6.2	6.8	5.7	6.5	6.8	7.4	6.5	6.0	5.3	5.9
35 to 44 years	19.5	18.9	21.2	18.2	16.1	19.4	20.3	15.9	18.0	18.8
45 to 54 years	72.9	69.5	67.5	67.4	67.6	65.9	67.6	64.6	61.6	61.4
55 to 64 years	187.0	189.4	193.4	195.2	193.7	186.7	186.4	190.7	179.8	187.7
65 to 74 years	461.2	464.1	425.8	446.2	436.6	396.5	387.5	399.6	410.2	390.1
75 to 84 years	1,046.7	1,004.1	988.2	980.4	917.6	936.3	899.5	839.8	843.2	828.8
85 years and over	1,693.4	1,689.0	1,762.0	1,707.2	1,626.3	1,577.7	1,575.3	1,468.0	1,492.8	1,419.4
Hispanic or Latino Male[5,7]										
All ages, age-adjusted[4]	151.7	151.4	148.6	149.4	144.9	141.9	138.8	135.9	133.8	132.7
All ages, crude	61.6	62.8	62.9	64.2	65.0	66.3	66.9	68.0	69.4	70.7
25 to 34 years	6.7	8.0	7.7	7.2	6.7	7.6	7.8	7.1	7.7	7.2
35 to 44 years	18.2	18.2	18.0	16.5	16.4	17.3	16.4	17.2	17.0	17.0
45 to 54 years	75.2	71.7	70.7	69.7	69.2	67.6	66.4	65.1	63.3	60.8
55 to 64 years	223.1	228.8	222.9	225.4	224.3	224.8	217.4	207.8	208.8	206.6
65 to 74 years	566.8	565.5	545.9	552.0	528.2	524.3	515.6	497.9	487.9	478.7
75 to 84 years	1,133.4	1,137.6	1,128.7	1,118.7	1,104.5	1,068.1	1,051.3	1,026.5	1,016.4	1,016.3
85 years and over	1,855.9	1,820.3	1,794.7	1,861.2	1,728.5	1,652.6	1,606.6	1,624.9	1,573.7	1,568.0
White, Not Hispanic or Latino Male[7]										
All ages, age-adjusted[4]	220.8	217.2	213.6	212.6	207.6	204.0	200.0	197.7	194.3	190.5
All ages, crude	242.6	243.3	243.5	245.8	245.6	247.0	247.3	249.3	249.7	249.1
25 to 34 years	8.9	8.9	9.1	9.1	8.4	8.5	8.5	8.6	8.4	8.4
35 to 44 years	28.0	27.1	27.6	27.0	27.2	25.7	25.6	25.6	24.5	24.3
45 to 54 years	117.2	119.3	117.9	117.2	114.4	114.2	111.9	108.5	105.0	100.6
55 to 64 years	354.0	349.4	345.4	344.2	341.8	338.6	332.9	335.0	331.7	323.1
65 to 74 years	845.7	827.6	800.4	798.5	775.7	757.4	737.2	722.1	713.1	695.0
75 to 84 years	1,614.0	1,583.8	1,561.8	1,534.4	1,508.2	1,475.9	1,444.8	1,424.1	1,391.1	1,359.3
85 years and over	2,514.5	2,464.5	2,440.5	2,480.8	2,377.1	2,353.6	2,330.5	2,319.1	2,294.1	2,304.1
Black, Not Hispanic or Latino Male[7]										
All ages, age-adjusted[4]	290.5	278.9	272.8	271.1	259.4	252.3	245.4	237.5	231.0	226.4
All ages, crude	180.1	177.2	177.3	178.6	176.3	176.2	175.9	174.7	174.0	174.5
25 to 34 years	10.6	10.4	11.0	9.7	9.8	9.7	11.0	8.9	9.0	8.9
35 to 44 years	35.0	35.1	32.7	31.6	30.5	28.1	28.8	30.5	27.9	28.3
45 to 54 years	176.8	170.2	162.4	155.7	150.5	149.9	137.7	133.3	129.0	119.1
55 to 64 years	529.4	514.6	514.0	510.2	492.3	480.8	477.7	463.2	450.9	445.9
65 to 74 years	1,105.0	1,068.5	1,061.6	1,050.8	1,028.4	994.0	965.7	946.3	916.4	903.8
75 to 84 years	1,964.9	1,908.3	1,871.2	1,865.7	1,746.5	1,725.1	1,673.1	1,602.2	1,564.7	1,526.0
85 years and over	3,299.0	3,007.2	2,846.7	2,907.2	2,738.7	2,590.6	2,528.0	2,420.1	2,374.6	2,352.4
White Female[5]										
All ages, age-adjusted[4]	152.3	149.8	147.9	146.9	144.0	142.5	140.2	138.8	136.8	134.8
All ages, crude	190.0	188.7	187.8	188.2	186.8	187.5	186.8	187.2	187.1	186.7
25 to 34 years	8.8	8.6	9.1	8.8	8.3	8.7	8.5	8.3	8.6	8.9
35 to 44 years	34.2	32.8	33.6	31.3	31.4	31.0	31.8	31.2	29.9	30.1
45 to 54 years	107.4	106.0	108.4	106.5	105.0	104.5	103.0	101.8	98.7	96.5
55 to 64 years	269.5	261.7	258.9	255.3	250.6	249.7	245.4	244.9	242.1	241.6
65 to 74 years	595.9	581.9	567.1	563.7	549.2	535.5	526.4	512.4	505.9	490.3
75 to 84 years	1,018.1	1,008.3	991.2	988.6	970.1	962.1	945.4	943.2	922.7	912.1
85 years and over	1,392.7	1,393.2	1,370.0	1,389.8	1,359.9	1,351.4	1,326.5	1,329.0	1,338.3	1,326.3

NOTE: Starting with *Health, United States, 2003,* rates for 1991–1999 were revised using intercensal population estimates based on the 1990 and 2000 Censuses. For 2000, population estimates are bridged-race April 1 census counts. Starting with *Health, United States, 2012,* rates for 2001–2009 were revised using intercensal population estimates based on the 2000 and 2010 Censuses. For 2010, population estimates are bridged-race April 1 census counts. Rates for 2011 and beyond were computed using 2010-based postcensal estimates. Age groups were selected to minimize the presentation of unstable age-specific death rates based on small numbers of deaths and for consistency among comparison groups. Starting with 2003 data, some states began to collect information on more than one race on the death certificate, according to 1997 Office of Management and Budget (OMB) standards. The multiple-race data for these states were bridged to the single-race categories of the 1977 OMB standards, for comparability with other states.
* = Rates based on fewer than 20 deaths are considered unreliable and are not shown.
[3]Starting with 1999 data, cause of death is coded according to *ICD–10.*
[4]Age-adjusted rates are calculated using the year 2000 standard population. Prior to 2001, age-adjusted rates were calculated using standard million proportions based on rounded population numbers. Starting with 2001 data, unrounded population numbers are used to calculate age-adjusted rates.
[5]The race groups, White, Black, Asian or Pacific Islander, and American Indian and Alaska Native, include persons of Hispanic and non-Hispanic origin. Persons of Hispanic origin may be of any race. Death rates for Hispanic, American Indian or Alaska Native, and Asian or Pacific Islander persons should be interpreted with caution because of inconsistencies in reporting Hispanic origin or race on the death certificate (death rate numerators) compared with population figures (death rate denominators). The net effect of misclassification is an underestimation of deaths and death rates for races other than White and Black.
[7]Prior to 1997, excludes data from states lacking an Hispanic-origin item on the death certificate.

Table 2-30. Death Rates for Malignant Neoplasms, by Sex, Race, Hispanic Origin, and Age, Selected Years, 1950–2016—*Continued*

(Deaths per 100,000 resident population; data are based on death certificates.)

Sex, race, Hispanic origin, and age	1950[1,2]	1960[1,2]	1970[2]	1980[2]	1985[2]	1990[2]	1995[2]	2000[3]	2005[3]	2006[3]
Black or African American Female[5]										
All ages, age-adjusted[4]	174.1	174.3	173.4	189.5	195.5	205.9	203.8	193.8	180.3	176.6
All ages, crude	111.8	113.8	117.3	136.5	145.2	156.1	155.8	151.8	148.1	146.5
25 to 34 years	34.3	31.0	20.9	18.3	17.2	18.7	16.5	13.5	12.7	12.6
35 to 44 years	119.8	102.4	94.6	73.5	69.0	67.4	61.7	58.9	52.1	50.3
45 to 54 years	277.0	254.8	228.6	230.2	212.4	209.9	190.6	173.9	164.5	156.6
55 to 64 years	484.6	442.7	404.8	450.4	474.9	482.4	444.9	391.0	358.6	349.1
65 to 74 years	477.3	541.6	615.8	662.4	704.2	773.2	803.5	753.1	667.7	659.8
75 to 84 years[6]	605.3	696.3	763.3	923.9	986.3	1,059.9	1,120.8	1,124.0	1,074.9	1,068.2
85 years and over	NA	728.9	791.5	1,159.9	1,284.2	1,431.3	1,446.2	1,527.7	1,514.6	1,469.8
American Indian or Alaska Native Female[5]										
All ages, age-adjusted[4]	NA	NA	NA	94.0	93.0	106.9	117.7	108.3	108.9	111.9
All ages, crude	NA	NA	NA	50.4	52.5	62.1	64.5	61.3	65.7	66.7
25 to 34 years	NA	NA	NA	*	*	*	10.2	*	*	*
35 to 44 years	NA	NA	NA	36.9	23.4	31.0	29.7	23.7	20.7	21.8
45 to 54 years	NA	NA	NA	96.9	90.1	104.5	76.9	59.7	79.1	66.3
55 to 64 years	NA	NA	NA	198.4	192.3	213.3	213.2	200.9	194.6	185.3
65 to 74 years	NA	NA	NA	350.8	378.8	438.9	437.0	458.3	473.0	464.9
75 to 84 years	NA	NA	NA	446.4	505.9	554.3	819.9	714.0	742.4	801.6
85 years and over	NA	NA	NA	786.5	700.0	843.7	1,039.4	983.2	802.0	971.7
Asian or Pacific Islander Female[5]										
All ages, age-adjusted[4]	NA	NA	NA	93.0	99.6	103.0	107.4	100.7	96.2	94.2
All ages, crude	NA	NA	NA	54.1	57.5	60.5	69.5	72.1	75.0	74.5
25 to 34 years	NA	NA	NA	9.5	9.9	7.3	9.9	8.1	7.3	6.9
35 to 44 years	NA	NA	NA	38.7	33.1	29.8	27.6	28.9	25.0	24.7
45 to 54 years	NA	NA	NA	99.8	91.3	93.9	94.4	78.2	73.9	72.0
55 to 64 years	NA	NA	NA	174.7	195.5	196.2	203.5	176.5	166.2	155.0
65 to 74 years	NA	NA	NA	301.9	330.8	346.2	343.3	357.4	324.7	327.1
75 to 84 years	NA	NA	NA	522.1	589.1	641.4	681.0	650.1	626.8	625.7
85 years and over	NA	NA	NA	800.0	908.3	971.7	1,092.7	988.5	1,060.1	1,006.7
Hispanic or Latina Female[5,7]										
All ages, age-adjusted[4]	NA	NA	NA	NA	101.5	111.9	110.8	110.8	104.9	103.8
All ages, crude	NA	NA	NA	NA	49.8	60.7	58.7	58.5	58.3	58.5
25 to 34 years	NA	NA	NA	NA	9.7	9.7	8.5	7.8	7.0	8.4
35 to 44 years	NA	NA	NA	NA	30.9	34.8	30.7	30.7	26.6	27.5
45 to 54 years	NA	NA	NA	NA	90.1	100.5	89.7	84.7	78.9	77.1
55 to 64 years	NA	NA	NA	NA	199.2	205.4	203.0	192.5	170.8	172.5
65 to 74 years	NA	NA	NA	NA	356.4	404.8	398.0	410.0	380.6	368.2
75 to 84 years	NA	NA	NA	NA	600.0	663.0	706.2	716.5	708.7	687.8
85 years and over	NA	NA	NA	NA	907.1	1,022.7	1,028.6	1,056.5	1,045.6	1,073.8
White, not Hispanic or Latina Female[7]										
All ages, age-adjusted[4]	NA	NA	NA	NA	167.1	177.5	174.7	170.0	160.1	158.4
All ages, crude	NA	NA	NA	NA	187.1	210.6	217.3	220.6	216.6	216.5
25 to 34 years	NA	NA	NA	NA	12.2	11.9	11.5	10.5	9.1	9.4
35 to 44 years	NA	NA	NA	NA	47.2	47.0	42.7	38.9	37.8	36.3
45 to 54 years	NA	NA	NA	NA	158.8	154.9	137.8	123.0	114.2	113.4
55 to 64 years	NA	NA	NA	NA	372.7	379.5	359.3	328.9	291.7	286.3
65 to 74 years	NA	NA	NA	NA	638.4	688.5	697.9	681.0	629.1	625.1
75 to 84 years	NA	NA	NA	NA	917.8	1,027.2	1,056.1	1,075.3	1,048.9	1,042.3
85 years and over	NA	NA	NA	NA	1,241.5	1,385.7	1,411.6	1,468.7	1,440.0	1,424.6
Black, not Hispanic or Latina Female[7]										
All ages, age-adjusted[4]	NA	NA	NA	NA	NA	NA	NA	196.9	183.9	180.2
All ages, crude	NA	NA	NA	NA	NA	NA	NA	156.9	154.4	153.0
25 to 34 years	NA	NA	NA	NA	NA	NA	NA	14.0	13.3	13.4
35 to 44 years	NA	NA	NA	NA	NA	NA	NA	60.4	53.8	52.5
45 to 54 years	NA	NA	NA	NA	NA	NA	NA	177.5	169.0	161.1
55 to 64 years	NA	NA	NA	NA	NA	NA	NA	398.8	366.6	356.3
65 to 74 years	NA	NA	NA	NA	NA	NA	NA	763.6	680.5	671.9
75 to 84 years	NA	NA	NA	NA	NA	NA	NA	1,138.4	1,091.9	1,085.5
85 years and over	NA	NA	NA	NA	NA	NA	NA	1,541.6	1,530.0	1,489.8

NOTE: Starting with *Health, United States, 2003*, rates for 1991–1999 were revised using intercensal population estimates based on the 1990 and 2000 Censuses. For 2000, population estimates are bridged-race April 1 census counts. Starting with *Health, United States, 2012*, rates for 2001–2009 were revised using intercensal population estimates based on the 2000 and 2010 Censuses. For 2010, population estimates are bridged-race April 1 census counts. Rates for 2011 and beyond were computed using 2010-based postcensal estimates. Age groups were selected to minimize the presentation of unstable age-specific death rates based on small numbers of deaths and for consistency among comparison groups. Starting with 2003 data, some states began to collect information on more than one race on the death certificate, according to 1997 Office of Management and Budget (OMB) standards. The multiple-race data for these states were bridged to the single-race categories of the 1977 OMB standards, for comparability with other states. NA = Not available.

* =. Rates based on fewer than 20 deaths are considered unreliable and are not shown.
[1]Includes deaths of persons who were not residents of the 50 states and the District of Columbia (DC).
[2]Underlying cause of death was coded according to the 6th revision of the *International Classification of Diseases* (*ICD*) in 1950, 7th revision in 1960, 8th revision in 1970, and 9th revision in 1980–1998.
[3]Starting with 1999 data, cause of death is coded according to *ICD–10*.
[4]Age-adjusted rates are calculated using the year 2000 standard population. Prior to 2001, age-adjusted rates were calculated using standard million proportions based on rounded population numbers. Starting with 2001 data, unrounded population numbers are used to calculate age-adjusted rates.
[5]The race groups, White, Black, Asian or Pacific Islander, and American Indian and Alaska Native, include persons of Hispanic and non-Hispanic origin. Persons of Hispanic origin may be of any race. Death rates for Hispanic, American Indian or Alaska Native, and Asian or Pacific Islander persons should be interpreted with caution because of inconsistencies in reporting Hispanic origin or race on the death certificate (death rate numerators) compared with population figures (death rate denominators). The net effect of misclassification is an underestimation of deaths and death rates for races other than White and Black.
[6]In 1950, rate is for the age group 75 years and over.
[7]Prior to 1997, excludes data from states lacking an Hispanic-origin item on the death certificate.

Table 2-30. Death Rates for Malignant Neoplasms, by Sex, Race, Hispanic Origin, and Age, Selected Years, 1950–2016—Continued

(Deaths per 100,000 resident population; data are based on death certificates.)

Sex, race, Hispanic origin, and age	2007³	2008³	2009³	2010³	2011³	2012³	2013³	2014³	2015³	2016³
Black or African American Female⁵										
All ages, age-adjusted⁴	174.9	170.1	167.0	167.1	166.1	161.7	158.5	156.8	152.2	151.4
All ages, crude	146.5	144.2	143.5	145.5	147.5	146.3	146.2	147.5	146.2	148.2
25 to 34 years	12.0	10.4	11.4	10.8	12.2	12.1	10.4	11.2	10.9	10.8
35 to 44 years	47.9	47.7	44.6	44.5	46.4	42.5	40.7	40.5	40.9	39.1
45 to 54 years	153.5	149.0	145.7	146.4	144.9	140.2	134.8	133.4	126.2	128.2
55 to 64 years	343.6	330.7	327.2	331.1	327.6	320.9	320.0	321.9	317.2	314.8
65 to 74 years	665.7	652.1	638.2	631.0	623.1	617.8	593.4	583.7	566.7	562.3
75 to 84 years⁶	1,075.1	1,021.3	1,026.7	1,008.2	1,010.4	985.6	984.3	960.8	925.2	926.0
85 years and over	1,405.0	1,427.8	1,345.7	1,418.6	1,390.9	1,318.4	1,306.5	1,297.5	1,267.9	1,246.9
American Indian or Alaska Native Female⁵										
All ages, age-adjusted⁴	105.8	105.6	102.2	102.0	92.6	99.1	94.3	88.5	93.0	88.8
All ages, crude	63.6	64.2	64.4	64.8	61.3	66.7	65.8	63.4	69.2	68.7
25 to 34 years	*	*	6.6	6.3	*	*	6.4	*	6.5	6.4
35 to 44 years	17.0	22.5	20.4	14.2	16.2	16.1	18.8	17.5	18.0	20.9
45 to 54 years	67.6	64.3	70.5	68.7	68.4	62.5	69.1	67.1	62.7	68.8
55 to 64 years	180.8	169.8	183.1	185.9	160.7	176.2	155.1	139.5	161.3	160.0
65 to 74 years	438.2	443.9	414.4	432.2	375.6	394.4	373.0	359.8	350.7	318.2
75 to 84 years	757.7	732.5	696.4	682.3	621.8	753.5	656.2	611.5	654.8	632.4
85 years and over	937.1	986.0	863.4	885.7	828.6	763.3	844.8	817.9	884.0	740.7
Asian or Pacific Islander Female⁵										
All ages, age-adjusted⁴	91.7	91.8	89.6	93.5	91.5	90.9	86.0	86.2	86.2	84.6
All ages, crude	73.4	74.4	73.7	78.5	79.8	80.9	78.6	80.6	82.7	83.3
25 to 34 years	5.4	7.8	5.8	7.1	5.1	5.6	6.4	6.2	5.3	6.0
35 to 44 years	23.7	20.5	21.3	21.7	23.3	23.2	22.1	21.7	21.7	25.0
45 to 54 years	67.7	67.1	60.2	69.5	69.9	71.2	63.6	64.1	67.1	66.3
55 to 64 years	155.2	145.6	144.9	152.6	155.9	149.9	139.7	143.8	146.6	153.1
65 to 74 years	301.7	316.1	300.8	314.4	299.6	290.3	280.7	278.8	279.5	268.5
75 to 84 years	624.4	633.4	618.7	654.5	640.9	626.5	601.5	597.1	589.1	557.4
85 years and over	1,019.8	1,027.2	1,053.5	994.4	957.6	1,012.6	925.7	963.7	941.5	896.6
Hispanic or Latina Female⁵,⁷										
All ages, age-adjusted⁴	101.7	100.1	99.8	99.4	97.5	99.3	97.3	95.7	93.6	94.0
All ages, crude	58.1	57.8	58.4	59.0	59.4	62.4	63.0	63.6	64.2	65.9
25 to 34 years	8.6	7.7	7.4	8.4	7.2	8.1	8.8	7.2	8.3	8.4
35 to 44 years	25.9	25.0	24.4	23.5	24.0	24.4	25.4	25.4	25.2	26.7
45 to 54 years	74.0	69.8	70.8	74.0	66.2	73.2	69.1	68.6	67.9	67.4
55 to 64 years	172.7	175.2	170.0	165.9	161.6	165.1	164.7	163.2	161.4	162.5
65 to 74 years	360.4	346.3	351.7	355.2	348.2	342.8	342.0	335.9	330.6	319.5
75 to 84 years	687.2	684.5	665.4	657.6	672.0	662.9	656.7	636.6	621.7	640.6
85 years and over	1,005.8	1,020.6	1,061.0	1,043.4	1,006.5	1,073.7	996.6	1,004.3	946.7	943.4
White, not Hispanic or Latina Female⁷										
All ages, age-adjusted⁴	156.1	153.6	151.8	150.6	147.9	146.0	143.9	142.7	140.6	138.5
All ages, crude	215.6	214.7	214.2	215.0	213.9	214.4	214.0	215.1	215.1	214.8
25 to 34 years	8.6	8.7	9.3	8.8	8.4	8.6	8.1	8.4	8.4	8.8
35 to 44 years	35.6	34.1	35.4	32.8	32.8	32.3	32.9	32.3	30.6	30.3
45 to 54 years	111.3	110.3	113.1	110.5	110.4	108.8	108.0	107.1	103.7	101.3
55 to 64 years	278.1	269.2	266.9	263.4	259.0	257.9	253.3	253.3	250.6	250.1
65 to 74 years	615.2	600.9	584.6	580.4	566.0	551.1	541.4	527.0	520.4	504.8
75 to 84 years	1,037.7	1,028.1	1,012.4	1,010.4	990.3	983.0	966.6	967.1	945.6	933.1
85 years and over	1,407.8	1,407.4	1,382.3	1,403.8	1,375.6	1,362.4	1,343.5	1,345.8	1,360.0	1,350.9
Black, not Hispanic or Latina Female⁷										
All ages, age-adjusted⁴	178.7	173.8	171.0	171.4	170.6	165.7	163.0	160.8	156.6	155.9
All ages, crude	153.5	151.4	151.1	153.5	155.9	154.4	154.8	155.8	154.9	157.1
25 to 34 years	12.8	11.1	12.3	11.4	13.1	12.9	11.1	12.0	11.6	11.4
35 to 44 years	49.8	49.7	46.6	46.7	48.7	44.6	43.0	42.7	43.2	41.6
45 to 54 years	158.5	153.9	150.9	151.5	150.4	145.2	140.3	138.2	131.7	133.9
55 to 64 years	351.0	338.9	335.9	339.5	336.8	329.1	329.2	330.8	326.5	324.7
65 to 74 years	679.2	666.3	651.1	646.6	637.4	632.1	608.6	596.5	581.1	576.9
75 to 84 years	1,093.0	1,037.9	1,046.1	1,029.2	1,033.5	1,007.0	1,007.9	980.3	947.1	948.8
85 years and over	1,425.7	1,444.1	1,364.3	1,442.0	1,417.1	1,336.0	1,327.2	1,318.2	1,289.9	1,269.7

NOTE: Starting with *Health, United States, 2003*, rates for 1991–1999 were revised using intercensal population estimates based on the 1990 and 2000 Censuses. For 2000, population estimates are bridged-race April 1 census counts. Starting with *Health, United States, 2012*, rates for 2001–2009 were revised using intercensal population estimates based on the 2000 and 2010 Censuses. For 2010, population estimates are bridged-race April 1 census counts. Rates for 2011 and beyond were computed using 2010-based postcensal estimates. Age groups were selected to minimize the presentation of unstable age-specific death rates based on small numbers of deaths and for consistency among comparison groups. Starting with 2003 data, some states began to collect information on more than one race on the death certificate, according to 1997 Office of Management and Budget (OMB) standards. The multiple-race data for these states were bridged to the single-race categories of the 1977 OMB standards, for comparability with other states.
* = . Rates based on fewer than 20 deaths are considered unreliable and are not shown.
³Starting with 1999 data, cause of death is coded according to *ICD–10*.
⁴Age-adjusted rates are calculated using the year 2000 standard population. Prior to 2001, age-adjusted rates were calculated using standard million proportions based on rounded population numbers. Starting with 2001 data, unrounded population numbers are used to calculate age-adjusted rates.
⁵The race groups, White, Black, Asian or Pacific Islander, and American Indian and Alaska Native, include persons of Hispanic and non-Hispanic origin. Persons of Hispanic origin may be of any race. Death rates for Hispanic, American Indian or Alaska Native, and Asian or Pacific Islander persons should be interpreted with caution because of inconsistencies in reporting Hispanic origin or race on the death certificate (death rate numerators) compared with population figures (death rate denominators). The net effect of misclassification is an underestimation of deaths and death rates for races other than White and Black.
⁶In 1950, rate is for the age group 75 years and over.
⁷Prior to 1997, excludes data from states lacking an Hispanic-origin item on the death certificate.

Table 2-31. Death Rates for Malignant Neoplasms of the Trachea, Bronchus, and Lung, by Sex, Race, Hispanic Origin, and Age, Selected Years, 1950–2016

(Deaths per 100,000 resident population; data are based on death certificates.)

Sex, race, Hispanic origin, and age	1950[1,2]	1960[1,2]	1970[2]	1980[2]	1985[2]	1990[2]	1995[2]	2000[3]	2005[3]	2006[3]
All Persons										
All ages, age-adjusted[4]	15.0	24.1	37.1	49.9	54.6	59.3	58.4	56.1	52.7	51.5
All ages, crude	12.2	20.3	32.1	45.8	51.5	56.8	56.8	55.3	53.9	53.2
Under 25 years	0.1	0.0	0.1	0.0	0.0	0.0	0.0	0.0	0.0	0.0
25 to 34 years	0.8	1.0	0.9	0.6	0.6	0.7	0.6	0.5	0.3	0.4
35 to 44 years	4.5	6.8	11.0	9.2	7.8	6.8	6.0	6.1	5.3	4.7
45 to 54 years	20.4	29.6	43.4	54.1	50.9	46.8	37.5	31.6	29.7	29.1
55 to 64 years	48.7	75.3	109.1	138.2	153.8	160.6	141.6	122.4	102.4	98.1
65 to 74 years	59.7	108.1	164.5	233.3	261.2	288.4	295.4	284.2	256.3	249.3
75 to 84 years	55.8	91.5	163.2	240.5	282.0	333.3	358.9	370.8	375.0	372.1
85 years and over	42.3	65.6	101.7	176.0	195.2	242.5	279.9	302.1	328.2	327.1
Male										
All ages, age-adjusted[4]	24.6	43.6	67.5	85.2	88.6	91.1	84.2	76.7	69.1	67.0
All ages, crude	19.9	35.4	53.4	68.6	72.5	75.1	70.5	65.5	62.1	60.9
Under 25 years	0.0	0.0	0.1	0.1	*	0.0	0.1	*	*	*
25 to 34 years	1.1	1.4	1.3	0.8	0.7	0.9	0.7	0.5	0.4	0.4
35 to 44 years	7.1	10.5	16.1	11.9	10.0	8.5	7.0	6.9	5.5	4.8
45 to 54 years	35.0	50.6	67.5	76.0	67.5	59.7	46.3	38.5	35.1	33.8
55 to 64 years	83.8	139.3	189.7	213.6	223.5	222.9	185.3	154.0	126.3	120.2
65 to 74 years	98.7	204.3	320.8	403.9	416.2	430.4	414.3	377.9	324.8	312.9
75 to 84 years	82.6	167.1	330.8	488.8	537.6	572.9	553.8	532.2	511.1	503.8
85 years and over	62.5	107.7	194.0	368.1	433.2	513.2	540.3	521.2	519.9	508.9
Female										
All ages, age-adjusted[4]	5.8	7.5	13.1	24.4	30.6	37.1	40.4	41.3	40.6	40.1
All ages, crude	4.5	6.4	11.9	24.3	31.7	39.4	43.6	45.4	46.0	45.7
Under 25 years	0.1	0.0	0.0	*	*	*	*	*	*	*
25 to 34 years	0.5	0.5	0.5	0.5	0.6	0.5	0.6	0.5	0.3	0.4
35 to 44 years	1.9	3.2	6.1	6.5	5.6	5.2	5.0	5.3	5.1	4.6
45 to 54 years	5.8	9.2	21.0	33.7	35.2	34.5	29.1	25.0	24.5	24.6
55 to 64 years	13.6	15.4	36.8	72.0	92.1	105.0	101.9	93.3	80.0	77.4
65 to 74 years	23.3	24.4	43.1	102.7	141.8	177.6	200.0	206.9	197.9	195.0
75 to 84 years	32.9	32.8	52.4	94.1	131.7	190.1	237.2	265.6	281.6	280.8
85 years and over	28.2	38.8	50.0	91.9	100.2	138.1	179.6	212.8	243.1	244.6
White Male[5]										
All ages, age-adjusted[4]	25.1	43.6	67.1	83.8	86.8	89.0	82.6	75.7	68.8	66.7
All ages, crude	20.8	36.4	54.6	70.2	74.5	77.8	74.0	69.4	66.6	65.4
45 to 54 years	35.1	49.2	63.3	70.9	62.7	55.2	43.2	35.7	33.5	31.9
55 to 64 years	85.4	139.2	186.8	205.6	214.2	213.7	178.9	150.8	122.6	117.4
65 to 74 years	101.5	207.5	325.0	401.0	409.5	422.1	408.0	374.9	326.5	313.8
75 to 84 years	85.5	170.4	336.7	493.5	540.3	572.2	550.8	529.9	514.5	506.9
85 years and over	67.4	109.4	199.6	374.1	440.0	516.3	539.3	522.4	517.6	511.1
Black or African American Male[5]										
All ages, age-adjusted[4]	17.8	42.6	75.4	107.6	117.2	125.4	115.1	101.1	86.1	83.0
All ages, crude	12.1	28.1	47.7	66.6	71.2	73.7	65.6	58.3	52.8	51.7
45 to 54 years	34.4	68.4	115.4	133.8	122.5	114.9	85.2	70.7	55.4	55.0
55 to 64 years	68.3	146.8	234.3	321.1	351.5	358.6	288.5	223.5	191.3	175.9
65 to 74 years	53.8	168.3	300.5	472.3	539.6	585.4	559.5	488.8	393.5	385.4
75 to 84 years[6]	36.2	107.3	271.6	472.9	556.4	645.4	667.1	642.5	565.7	563.0
85 years and over	NA	82.8	137.0	311.3	382.3	499.5	583.0	562.8	601.6	539.6
American Indian or Alaska Native Male[5]										
All ages, age-adjusted[4]	NA	NA	NA	31.7	41.2	47.5	53.6	42.9	42.6	39.6
All ages, crude	NA	NA	NA	14.2	18.4	20.0	21.8	18.1	20.1	18.4
45 to 54 years	NA	NA	NA	*	*	26.6	23.8	14.5	18.2	16.5
55 to 64 years	NA	NA	NA	72.0	85.1	97.8	98.9	86.0	79.5	61.0
65 to 74 years	NA	NA	NA	202.8	223.1	194.3	261.5	184.8	190.3	200.4
75 to 84 years	NA	NA	NA	*	263.6	356.2	409.7	367.9	341.1	330.9
85 years and over	NA	NA	NA	*	*	*	*	*	*	*
Asian or Pacific Islander Male[5]										
All ages, age-adjusted[4]	NA	NA	NA	43.3	42.7	44.2	41.0	40.9	37.1	36.6
All ages, crude	NA	NA	NA	22.1	20.4	20.7	20.7	22.7	22.4	22.7

NOTE: Starting with *Health, United States, 2003*, rates for 1991–1999 were revised using intercensal population estimates based on the 1990 and 2000 Censuses. For 2000, population estimates are bridged-race April 1 census counts. Starting with *Health, United States, 2012*, rates for 2001–2009 were revised using intercensal population estimates based on the 2000 and 2010 Censuses. For 2010, population estimates are bridged-race April 1 census counts. Rates for 2011 and beyond were computed using 2010-based postcensal estimates. Age groups were selected to minimize the presentation of unstable age-specific death rates based on small numbers of deaths and for consistency among comparison groups. Starting with 2003 data, some states began to collect information on more than one race on the death certificate, according to 1997 Office of Management and Budget (OMB) standards. The multiple-race data for these states were bridged to the single-race categories of the 1977 OMB standards, for comparability with other states.
NA = Not available.
* = Rates based on fewer than 20 deaths are considered unreliable and are not shown.
0.0 = Quantity more than zero but less than 0.05.
[1]Includes deaths of persons who were not residents of the 50 states and the District of Columbia (DC).
[2]Underlying cause of death was coded according to the 6th revision of the *International Classification of Diseases (ICD)* in 1950, 7th revision in 1960, 8th revision in 1970, and 9th revision in 1980–1998.
[3]Starting with 1999 data, cause of death is coded according to *ICD–10.*
[4]Age-adjusted rates are calculated using the year 2000 standard population. Prior to 2001, age-adjusted rates were calculated using standard million proportions based on rounded population numbers. Starting with 2001 data, unrounded population numbers are used to calculate age-adjusted rates.
[5]The race groups, White, Black, Asian or Pacific Islander, and American Indian and Alaska Native, include persons of Hispanic and non-Hispanic origin. Persons of Hispanic origin may be of any race. Death rates for Hispanic, American Indian or Alaska Native, and Asian or Pacific Islander persons should be interpreted with caution because of inconsistencies in reporting Hispanic origin or race on the death certificate (death rate numerators) compared with population figures (death rate denominators). The net effect of misclassification is an underestimation of deaths and death rates for races other than White and Black.
[6]In 1950, rate is for the age group 75 years and over.

Table 2-31. Death Rates for Malignant Neoplasms of the Trachea, Bronchus, and Lung, by Sex, Race, Hispanic Origin, and Age, Selected Years, 1950–2016—*Continued*

(Deaths per 100,000 resident population; data are based on death certificates.)

Sex, race, Hispanic origin, and age	2007[3]	2008[3]	2009[3]	2010[3]	2011[3]	2012[3]	2013[3]	2014[3]	2015[3]	2016[3]
All Persons										
All ages, age-adjusted[4]	50.6	49.5	48.4	47.6	46.0	44.9	43.4	42.1	40.5	38.4
All ages, crude	52.7	52.2	51.6	51.3	50.4	50.2	49.4	48.8	47.9	46.1
Under 25 years	0.0	0.0	0.0	0.0	0.0	0.0	0.0	0.0	0.0	0.0
25 to 34 years	0.3	0.4	0.4	0.4	0.3	0.4	0.3	0.3	0.3	0.3
35 to 44 years	4.3	3.8	3.7	3.3	3.1	2.9	2.8	2.7	2.5	2.2
45 to 54 years	28.4	28.2	27.8	26.9	25.7	25.1	23.9	22.4	20.5	18.6
55 to 64 years	94.2	90.2	87.5	85.4	83.5	81.5	79.9	78.5	76.8	73.2
65 to 74 years	244.5	235.5	228.6	223.9	214.3	206.1	196.6	189.4	181.0	167.9
75 to 84 years	369.5	366.7	359.8	357.2	345.9	339.6	328.5	321.2	306.4	295.4
85 years and over	328.0	332.9	328.0	332.4	323.7	323.7	320.0	311.7	316.1	305.2
Male										
All ages, age-adjusted[4]	64.9	63.5	61.4	60.3	57.7	56.1	53.7	51.7	49.5	46.7
All ages, crude	59.7	59.3	58.2	57.8	56.6	56.1	55.1	54.1	52.9	50.8
Under 25 years	0.0	0.1	0.0	*	0.0	0.0	*	*	*	*
25 to 34 years	0.4	0.4	0.4	0.4	0.3	0.5	0.3	0.3	0.3	0.3
35 to 44 years	4.3	4.0	3.7	3.2	3.1	2.9	2.8	2.9	2.6	2.4
45 to 54 years	32.1	32.3	31.0	30.0	28.1	27.7	25.9	23.8	22.1	19.8
55 to 64 years	114.7	111.1	107.9	104.9	102.5	98.3	96.9	93.8	92.1	86.2
65 to 74 years	302.8	291.2	279.4	274.9	262.8	250.0	236.0	229.5	217.1	203.6
75 to 84 years	490.9	482.0	470.5	461.9	442.4	432.0	413.4	395.7	378.3	360.3
85 years and over	505.2	511.0	489.1	492.3	467.3	473.4	463.0	442.8	434.4	417.9
Female										
All ages, age-adjusted[4]	40.1	39.1	38.6	38.1	37.1	36.4	35.5	34.7	33.5	31.9
All ages, crude	46.0	45.3	45.1	45.0	44.4	44.4	44.0	43.7	43.0	41.5
Under 25 years	*	*	*	0.0	*	*	*	*	0.0	*
25 to 34 years	0.3	0.3	0.3	0.4	0.3	0.3	0.3	0.3	0.3	0.2
35 to 44 years	4.4	3.6	3.6	3.3	3.1	2.9	2.9	2.6	2.4	2.0
45 to 54 years	24.8	24.3	24.7	23.8	23.3	22.6	21.9	21.0	18.8	17.3
55 to 64 years	75.2	70.7	68.4	67.2	65.7	65.9	64.2	64.2	62.7	61.2
65 to 74 years	194.3	187.4	184.5	179.5	171.9	167.5	161.9	154.2	149.1	136.6
75 to 84 years	284.4	285.1	280.6	281.7	275.3	271.1	264.9	264.8	251.5	245.6
85 years and over	246.0	249.1	251.0	255.2	252.9	248.7	246.9	243.5	253.6	244.9
White Male[5]										
All ages, age-adjusted[4]	64.6	63.4	61.3	60.1	57.7	56.0	53.7	51.8	49.7	46.9
All ages, crude	64.1	63.9	62.8	62.3	61.2	60.6	59.5	58.7	57.4	55.1
45 to 54 years	30.4	31.0	30.3	28.8	27.4	26.9	25.6	23.7	22.0	20.0
55 to 64 years	112.2	108.9	105.2	101.8	100.7	96.4	94.6	92.1	91.1	84.8
65 to 74 years	303.8	293.3	280.7	275.7	262.9	250.8	236.5	230.2	216.9	202.8
75 to 84 years	493.6	484.0	474.3	465.5	446.7	434.4	416.8	400.4	383.5	366.1
85 years and over	500.5	509.4	489.5	495.0	471.0	475.7	466.8	446.6	439.6	424.1
Black or African American Male[5]										
All ages, age-adjusted[4]	81.5	77.8	75.0	73.7	69.6	68.6	65.7	61.9	58.6	54.9
All ages, crude	51.0	49.2	48.7	48.7	47.2	47.3	46.8	45.0	43.7	42.0
45 to 54 years	52.0	48.7	45.1	45.2	40.4	40.6	35.2	31.0	28.8	24.3
55 to 64 years	168.6	159.0	158.1	155.4	145.4	138.4	141.0	131.4	124.4	117.1
65 to 74 years	376.3	345.5	348.8	341.3	333.1	312.8	302.6	287.7	275.3	262.3
75 to 84 years[6]	544.2	544.3	516.0	509.1	479.7	494.6	465.7	435.1	407.5	382.8
85 years and over	618.3	591.2	526.6	521.8	473.9	485.0	458.5	456.0	433.4	405.3
American Indian or Alaska Native Male[5]										
All ages, age-adjusted[4]	43.7	44.3	35.4	41.6	38.1	35.9	34.4	34.1	32.1	30.0
All ages, crude	20.0	20.8	17.7	20.8	18.9	19.4	18.2	19.8	19.0	19.2
45 to 54 years	12.8	16.7	14.4	19.7	16.4	13.0	10.7	8.8	13.1	8.7
55 to 64 years	77.4	66.2	65.4	67.6	52.9	59.7	55.8	53.2	42.0	58.1
65 to 74 years	200.2	221.0	183.2	213.2	164.1	185.8	131.3	177.8	160.5	142.0
75 to 84 years	339.5	361.5	249.4	325.8	333.2	259.8	299.3	292.1	276.2	242.6
85 years and over	422.6	333.6	*	276.4	328.3	310.7	369.4	193.3	229.9	207.3
Asian or Pacific Islander Male[5]										
All ages, age-adjusted[4]	35.9	36.1	34.8	33.8	32.9	32.7	30.6	29.6	29.5	28.4
All ages, crude	22.0	22.9	22.3	22.5	22.7	22.9	22.3	22.4	23.0	22.8

NOTE: Starting with *Health, United States, 2003,* rates for 1991–1999 were revised using intercensal population estimates based on the 1990 and 2000 Censuses. For 2000, population estimates are bridged-race April 1 census counts. Starting with *Health, United States, 2012,* rates for 2001–2009 were revised using intercensal population estimates based on the 2000 and 2010 Censuses. For 2010, population estimates are bridged-race April 1 census counts. Rates for 2011 and beyond were computed using 2010-based postcensal estimates. Age groups were selected to minimize the presentation of unstable age-specific death rates based on small numbers of deaths and for consistency among comparison groups. Starting with 2003 data, some states began to collect information on more than one race on the death certificate, according to 1997 Office of Management and Budget (OMB) standards. The multiple-race data for these states were bridged to the single-race categories of the 1977 OMB standards, for comparability with other states.
* = Rates based on fewer than 20 deaths are considered unreliable and are not shown.
0.0 = Quantity more than zero but less than 0.05.
[3]Starting with 1999 data, cause of death is coded according to *ICD–10.*
[4]Age-adjusted rates are calculated using the year 2000 standard population. Prior to 2001, age-adjusted rates were calculated using standard million proportions based on rounded population numbers. Starting with 2001 data, unrounded population numbers are used to calculate age-adjusted rates.
[5]The race groups, White, Black, Asian or Pacific Islander, and American Indian and Alaska Native, include persons of Hispanic and non-Hispanic origin. Persons of Hispanic origin may be of any race. Death rates for Hispanic, American Indian or Alaska Native, and Asian or Pacific Islander persons should be interpreted with caution because of inconsistencies in reporting Hispanic origin or race on the death certificate (death rate numerators) compared with population figures (death rate denominators). The net effect of misclassification is an underestimation of deaths and death rates for races other than White and Black.
[6]In 1950, rate is for the age group 75 years and over.

Table 2-31. Death Rates for Malignant Neoplasms of the Trachea, Bronchus, and Lung, by Sex, Race, Hispanic Origin, and Age, Selected Years, 1950–2016—*Continued*

(Deaths per 100,000 resident population; data are based on death certificates.)

Sex, race, Hispanic origin, and age	1950[1,2]	1960[1,2]	1970[2]	1980[2]	1985[2]	1990[2]	1995[2]	2000[3]	2005[3]	2006[3]
45 to 54 years	NA	NA	NA	33.3	21.7	18.8	18.6	17.2	15.6	18.1
55 to 64 years	NA	NA	NA	94.4	98.1	74.4	64.4	61.4	56.7	55.7
65 to 74 years	NA	NA	NA	174.3	180.8	215.8	184.0	183.2	142.6	139.7
75 to 84 years	NA	NA	NA	301.3	295.3	307.5	296.6	323.2	295.0	295.5
85 years and over	NA	NA	NA	*	350.0	421.3	439.0	378.0	439.5	401.3
Hispanic or Latino Male[5,7]										
All ages, age-adjusted[4]	NA	NA	NA	NA	39.2	44.1	42.2	39.0	35.2	32.3
All ages, crude	NA	NA	NA	NA	12.9	16.2	14.8	13.3	13.1	12.1
45 to 54 years	NA	NA	NA	NA	16.7	21.5	17.5	14.8	12.1	10.6
55 to 64 years	NA	NA	NA	NA	68.6	80.7	69.9	58.6	52.5	45.1
65 to 74 years	NA	NA	NA	NA	169.9	195.5	192.0	167.3	153.1	142.0
75 to 84 years	NA	NA	NA	NA	292.1	313.4	324.4	327.5	295.5	268.2
85 years and over	NA	NA	NA	NA	393.8	420.7	382.8	368.8	338.1	339.4
White, Not Hispanic or Latino Male[7]										
All ages, age-adjusted[4]	NA	NA	NA	NA	84.2	91.1	84.1	77.9	71.3	69.3
All ages, crude	NA	NA	NA	NA	74.5	84.7	81.5	78.9	77.4	76.4
45 to 54 years	NA	NA	NA	NA	62.6	57.8	44.9	37.7	36.2	34.6
55 to 64 years	NA	NA	NA	NA	209.8	221.0	184.8	157.7	128.6	123.7
65 to 74 years	NA	NA	NA	NA	398.4	431.4	416.0	387.3	339.1	326.6
75 to 84 years	NA	NA	NA	NA	518.2	580.4	554.8	537.7	526.6	520.7
85 years and over	NA	NA	NA	NA	413.8	520.9	542.7	527.3	525.1	517.8
Black, Not Hispanic or Latino Male[7]										
All ages, age-adjusted[4]	NA	NA	NA	NA	NA	NA	NA	102.6	87.9	84.7
All ages, crude	NA	NA	NA	NA	NA	NA	NA	60.3	55.2	54.2
45 to 54 years	NA	NA	NA	NA	NA	NA	NA	72.4	56.7	56.6
55 to 64 years	NA	NA	NA	NA	NA	NA	NA	227.1	195.5	180.9
65 to 74 years	NA	NA	NA	NA	NA	NA	NA	495.4	401.5	392.6
75 to 84 years	NA	NA	NA	NA	NA	NA	NA	649.5	575.5	573.0
85 years and over	NA	NA	NA	NA	NA	NA	NA	567.1	611.9	547.0
White Female[5]										
All ages, age-adjusted[4]	5.9	6.8	13.1	24.5	31.0	37.6	41.1	42.3	41.7	41.2
All ages, crude	4.7	5.9	12.3	25.6	33.9	42.4	47.5	49.9	50.7	50.6
45 to 54 years	5.7	9.0	20.9	33.0	35.4	34.6	29.3	24.8	24.1	24.1
55 to 64 years	13.7	15.1	37.2	71.9	92.4	105.7	104.0	96.1	82.2	79.9
65 to 74 years	23.7	24.8	42.9	104.6	145.5	181.3	203.8	213.2	205.6	203.3
75 to 84 years	34.0	32.7	52.6	95.2	134.8	194.6	243.3	272.7	288.9	288.9
85 years and over	29.3	39.1	50.6	92.4	99.3	138.3	181.0	215.9	245.9	248.8
Black or African American Female[5]										
All ages, age-adjusted[4]	4.5	6.8	13.7	24.8	29.7	36.8	38.8	39.8	39.9	38.8
All ages, crude	2.8	4.3	9.4	18.3	22.5	28.1	29.5	30.8	32.5	32.0
45 to 54 years	7.5	11.3	23.9	43.4	39.1	41.3	34.5	32.9	33.2	34.2
55 to 64 years	12.9	17.9	33.5	79.9	103.5	117.9	106.9	95.3	86.3	80.8
65 to 74 years	14.0	18.1	46.1	88.0	117.2	164.3	196.2	194.1	181.3	175.6
75 to 84 years[6]	*	31.3	49.1	79.4	101.2	148.1	183.2	224.3	254.2	252.0
85 years and over	NA	34.2	44.8	85.8	114.3	134.9	158.9	185.9	228.4	213.0
American Indian or Alaska Native Female[5]										
All ages, age-adjusted[4]	NA	NA	NA	11.7	14.2	19.3	25.9	24.8	30.0	26.9
All ages, crude	NA	NA	NA	6.0	8.2	11.2	13.8	14.0	17.8	16.1
45 to 54 years	NA	NA	NA	*	*	22.9	*	12.1	17.2	11.0
55 to 64 years	NA	NA	NA	*	38.5	53.7	45.7	52.6	54.9	57.1
65 to 74 years	NA	NA	NA	*	93.9	78.5	134.6	151.5	165.1	143.1
75 to 84 years	NA	NA	NA	*	*	111.8	209.5	136.3	204.1	183.2
85 years and over	NA	NA	NA	*	*	*	*	*	*	*
Asian or Pacific Islander Female[5]										
All ages, age-adjusted[4]	NA	NA	NA	15.4	14.4	18.9	21.4	18.4	18.5	18.1
All ages, crude	NA	NA	NA	8.4	7.9	10.5	13.0	12.6	13.9	13.9
45 to 54 years	NA	NA	NA	13.5	12.5	11.3	11.6	9.9	10.6	10.0
55 to 64 years	NA	NA	NA	24.6	26.0	38.3	37.6	30.4	27.3	26.6

NOTE: Starting with *Health, United States, 2003*, rates for 1991–1999 were revised using intercensal population estimates based on the 1990 and 2000 Censuses. For 2000, population estimates are bridged-race April 1 census counts. Starting with *Health, United States, 2012*, rates for 2001–2009 were revised using intercensal population estimates based on the 2000 and 2010 Censuses. For 2010, population estimates are bridged-race April 1 census counts. Rates for 2011 and beyond were computed using 2010-based postcensal estimates. Age groups were selected to minimize the presentation of unstable age-specific death rates based on small numbers of deaths and for consistency among comparison groups. Starting with 2003 data, some states began to collect information on more than one race on the death certificate, according to 1997 Office of Management and Budget (OMB) standards. The multiple-race data for these states were bridged to the single-race categories of the 1977 OMB standards, for comparability with other states.
NA = Not available.
* = Rates based on fewer than 20 deaths are considered unreliable and are not shown.
[1] Includes deaths of persons who were not residents of the 50 states and the District of Columbia (DC).
[2] Underlying cause of death was coded according to the 6th revision of the *International Classification of Diseases* (*ICD*) in 1950, 7th revision in 1960, 8th revision in 1970, and 9th revision in 1980–1998.
[3] Starting with 1999 data, cause of death is coded according to *ICD–10*.
[4] Age-adjusted rates are calculated using the year 2000 standard population. Prior to 2001, age-adjusted rates were calculated using standard million proportions based on rounded population numbers. Starting with 2001 data, unrounded population numbers are used to calculate age-adjusted rates.
[5] The race groups, White, Black, Asian or Pacific Islander, and American Indian and Alaska Native, include persons of Hispanic and non-Hispanic origin. Persons of Hispanic origin may be of any race. Death rates for Hispanic, American Indian or Alaska Native, and Asian or Pacific Islander persons should be interpreted with caution because of inconsistencies in reporting Hispanic origin or race on the death certificate (death rate numerators) compared with population figures (death rate denominators). The net effect of misclassification is an underestimation of deaths and death rates for races other than White and Black.
[6] In 1950, rate is for the age group 75 years and over.
[7] Prior to 1997, excludes data from states lacking an Hispanic-origin item on the death certificate.

Table 2-31. Death Rates for Malignant Neoplasms of the Trachea, Bronchus, and Lung, by Sex, Race, Hispanic Origin, and Age, Selected Years, 1950–2016—*Continued*

(Deaths per 100,000 resident population; data are based on death certificates.)

Sex, race, Hispanic origin, and age	2007[3]	2008[3]	2009[3]	2010[3]	2011[3]	2012[3]	2013[3]	2014[3]	2015[3]	2016[3]
45 to 54 years	17.0	16.3	13.1	13.8	12.2	13.0	12.7	13.1	11.2	11.1
55 to 64 years	43.4	49.5	49.6	51.1	45.0	45.3	42.5	44.7	44.5	43.4
65 to 74 years	132.5	136.5	117.7	127.0	131.3	114.8	110.3	108.9	116.5	111.4
75 to 84 years	311.1	303.2	304.9	286.4	276.1	279.4	257.5	239.8	239.4	229.3
85 years and over	423.9	416.6	429.9	382.0	370.7	411.4	387.3	363.2	347.3	332.3
Hispanic or Latino Male[5,7]										
All ages, age-adjusted[4,7]	31.6	32.2	29.8	29.6	28.7	26.8	26.2	25.0	24.3	22.7
All ages, crude	12.0	12.4	11.8	11.9	12.0	11.7	11.8	11.6	11.7	11.2
45 to 54 years	10.4	9.8	10.3	9.0	8.3	8.5	8.0	7.2	6.0	5.7
55 to 64 years	42.3	43.5	38.5	40.1	39.4	35.6	35.6	31.4	32.8	30.3
65 to 74 years	142.4	137.2	128.6	126.2	120.2	116.4	110.8	107.0	103.4	91.9
75 to 84 years	260.0	278.1	263.3	256.3	240.6	237.3	225.4	216.1	211.0	206.5
85 years and over	335.3	337.7	290.7	307.9	330.3	258.0	282.7	276.0	267.7	241.4
White, Not Hispanic or Latino Male[7]										
All ages, age-adjusted[4]	67.2	65.9	63.9	62.7	60.3	58.5	56.3	54.4	52.2	49.4
All ages, crude	75.2	75.1	74.2	73.8	72.7	72.2	71.0	70.2	68.6	66.2
45 to 54 years	33.1	34.0	33.2	31.8	30.6	29.9	28.7	26.9	25.2	23.0
55 to 64 years	118.6	114.9	111.6	107.8	106.9	102.8	101.0	99.0	98.0	91.6
65 to 74 years	316.1	305.0	292.3	287.3	274.4	261.3	246.6	240.3	226.1	212.5
75 to 84 years	508.2	496.7	487.7	479.3	461.0	448.1	430.8	414.3	396.2	378.2
85 years and over	508.0	517.1	499.5	504.4	478.2	488.3	478.0	457.5	451.0	437.9
Black, Not Hispanic or Latino Male[7]										
All ages, age-adjusted[4]	83.3	79.4	76.7	75.6	71.6	70.5	67.5	63.6	60.3	56.5
All ages, crude	53.5	51.8	51.4	51.6	50.2	50.2	49.7	47.9	46.5	44.7
45 to 54 years	53.5	50.2	46.5	46.9	41.9	41.9	36.6	32.2	29.9	25.3
55 to 64 years	173.2	163.5	162.1	159.8	149.7	142.1	145.1	135.9	128.5	120.8
65 to 74 years	384.0	352.3	356.2	350.0	342.0	320.9	310.2	295.8	282.3	269.5
75 to 84 years	552.1	554.3	525.5	519.4	493.2	508.5	478.5	445.4	418.4	394.0
85 years and over	630.9	600.6	540.1	534.4	484.3	496.2	470.5	465.0	444.9	411.6
White Female[5]										
All ages, age-adjusted[4]	41.3	40.4	40.0	39.3	38.3	37.6	36.7	36.0	34.9	33.1
All ages, crude	51.0	50.5	50.4	50.0	49.3	49.4	48.9	48.7	48.1	46.4
45 to 54 years	24.8	24.7	25.2	24.3	23.9	23.0	22.6	21.7	19.7	18.1
55 to 64 years	77.6	73.1	70.1	68.9	67.2	68.0	66.0	66.3	64.8	62.9
65 to 74 years	202.5	195.6	193.6	187.4	179.6	174.3	169.0	161.4	156.2	143.4
75 to 84 years	293.1	294.1	289.8	290.5	284.9	280.7	274.1	275.3	263.0	256.0
85 years and over	250.5	253.1	257.3	258.3	256.3	254.5	250.9	247.7	260.2	250.2
Black or African American Female[5]										
All ages, age-adjusted[4]	37.9	36.8	35.8	36.5	35.4	34.7	34.1	32.7	30.7	29.8
All ages, crude	31.5	30.8	30.5	31.4	31.2	31.1	31.3	30.7	29.5	29.2
45 to 54 years	31.9	28.3	29.0	27.7	26.8	25.9	24.0	23.2	18.8	17.7
55 to 64 years	76.6	74.1	76.3	74.0	73.3	71.0	71.9	69.8	67.4	67.6
65 to 74 years	176.3	168.3	161.4	163.1	156.9	158.2	151.0	142.3	136.2	123.9
75 to 84 years[6]	250.1	249.0	243.2	249.2	240.5	239.8	235.8	227.5	209.6	212.8
85 years and over	212.0	226.3	197.6	249.3	236.8	211.2	224.9	220.8	218.6	224.9
American Indian or Alaska Native Female[5]										
All ages, age-adjusted[4]	27.4	27.4	25.1	26.3	23.9	25.6	22.9	22.7	22.5	21.2
All ages, crude	16.3	15.9	15.5	16.0	15.3	16.9	15.6	15.8	16.9	16.1
45 to 54 years	9.7	10.9	12.7	13.2	13.8	13.0	12.3	14.4	12.3	10.8
55 to 64 years	49.7	41.2	50.5	40.3	39.5	44.9	31.1	28.0	44.5	37.0
65 to 74 years	157.7	126.8	119.4	141.8	110.2	116.5	124.9	114.4	103.2	97.8
75 to 84 years	192.2	218.7	197.5	185.9	189.7	203.3	174.6	179.3	159.0	176.1
85 years and over	*	236.6	*	200.0	168.3	183.2	137.0	161.4	179.8	127.4
Asian or Pacific Islander Female[5]										
All ages, age-adjusted[4]	18.9	18.1	18.3	18.3	18.6	17.8	18.0	17.6	16.8	16.3
All ages, crude	14.8	14.2	14.5	14.9	15.8	15.5	16.0	16.0	15.8	15.8
45 to 54 years	10.3	9.5	8.7	8.8	8.5	10.9	9.3	9.0	9.7	8.6
55 to 64 years	31.8	25.8	25.1	28.0	29.0	25.1	24.3	25.2	24.2	25.5

NOTE: Starting with *Health, United States, 2003*, rates for 1991–1999 were revised using intercensal population estimates based on the 1990 and 2000 Censuses. For 2000, population estimates are bridged-race April 1 census counts. Starting with *Health, United States, 2012*, rates for 2001–2009 were revised using intercensal population estimates based on the 2000 and 2010 Censuses. For 2010, population estimates are bridged-race April 1 census counts. Rates for 2011 and beyond were computed using 2010-based postcensal estimates. Age groups were selected to minimize the presentation of unstable age-specific death rates based on small numbers of deaths and for consistency among comparison groups. Starting with 2003 data, some states began to collect information on more than one race on the death certificate, according to 1997 Office of Management and Budget (OMB) standards. The multiple-race data for these states were bridged to the single-race categories of the 1977 OMB standards, for comparability with other states.
* = Rates based on fewer than 20 deaths are considered unreliable and are not shown.
[3]Starting with 1999 data, cause of death is coded according to *ICD–10*.
[4]Age-adjusted rates are calculated using the year 2000 standard population. Prior to 2001, age-adjusted rates were calculated using standard million proportions based on rounded population numbers. Starting with 2001 data, unrounded population numbers are used to calculate age-adjusted rates.
[5]The race groups, White, Black, Asian or Pacific Islander, and American Indian and Alaska Native, include persons of Hispanic and non-Hispanic origin. Persons of Hispanic origin may be of any race. Death rates for Hispanic, American Indian or Alaska Native, and Asian or Pacific Islander persons should be interpreted with caution because of inconsistencies in reporting Hispanic origin or race on the death certificate (death rate numerators) compared with population figures (death rate denominators). The net effect of misclassification is an underestimation of deaths and death rates for races other than White and Black.
[6]In 1950, rate is for the age group 75 years and over.
[7]Prior to 1997, excludes data from states lacking an Hispanic-origin item on the death certificate.

Table 2-31. Death Rates for Malignant Neoplasms of the Trachea, Bronchus, and Lung, by Sex, Race, Hispanic Origin, and Age, Selected Years, 1950–2016—*Continued*

(Deaths per 100,000 resident population; data are based on death certificates.)

Sex, race, Hispanic origin, and age	1950[1,2]	1960[1,2]	1970[2]	1980[2]	1985[2]	1990[2]	1995[2]	2000[3]	2005[3]	2006[3]
65 to 74 years	NA	NA	NA	62.4	60.7	71.6	84.2	77.0	73.9	74.2
75 to 84 years	NA	NA	NA	117.7	97.8	137.9	153.5	135.0	144.6	135.0
85 years and over	NA	NA	NA	*	*	172.9	235.5	175.3	184.4	190.7
Hispanic or Latina Female[5,7]										
All ages, age-adjusted[4]	NA	NA	NA	NA	10.9	14.1	14.3	14.7	14.8	14.0
All ages, crude	NA	NA	NA	NA	4.9	7.2	7.1	7.2	7.7	7.4
45 to 54 years	NA	NA	NA	NA	6.8	8.7	7.1	7.1	7.0	6.2
55 to 64 years	NA	NA	NA	NA	17.4	25.1	25.5	22.2	20.2	18.8
65 to 74 years	NA	NA	NA	NA	49.1	66.8	59.2	66.0	62.8	64.9
75 to 84 years	NA	NA	NA	NA	73.6	94.3	111.0	112.3	118.3	111.1
85 years and over	NA	NA	NA	NA	110.7	118.2	128.3	137.5	153.2	128.7
White, not Hispanic or Latina Female[7]										
All ages, age-adjusted[4]	NA	NA	NA	NA	31.7	39.0	42.5	44.1	43.8	43.5
All ages, crude	NA	NA	NA	NA	35.6	46.2	52.3	56.4	58.7	58.9
45 to 54 years	NA	NA	NA	NA	36.6	36.6	31.0	26.4	26.1	26.4
55 to 64 years	NA	NA	NA	NA	93.4	111.3	109.4	102.2	87.9	85.7
65 to 74 years	NA	NA	NA	NA	149.4	186.4	210.4	222.9	217.5	215.2
75 to 84 years	NA	NA	NA	NA	138.1	199.1	247.2	279.2	298.6	299.8
85 years and over	NA	NA	NA	NA	100.9	139.0	181.6	218.0	249.1	253.4
Black, not Hispanic or Latina Female[7]										
All ages, age-adjusted[4]	NA	NA	NA	NA	NA	NA	NA	40.4	40.9	39.7
All ages, crude	NA	NA	NA	NA	NA	NA	NA	31.9	34.0	33.5
45 to 54 years	NA	NA	NA	NA	NA	NA	NA	33.6	34.3	35.4
55 to 64 years	NA	NA	NA	NA	NA	NA	NA	97.0	88.5	82.7
65 to 74 years	NA	NA	NA	NA	NA	NA	NA	196.9	184.8	179.7
75 to 84 years	NA	NA	NA	NA	NA	NA	NA	227.3	259.6	256.0
85 years and over	NA	NA	NA	NA	NA	NA	NA	188.4	232.8	216.4

NOTE: Starting with *Health, United States, 2003*, rates for 1991–1999 were revised using intercensal population estimates based on the 1990 and 2000 Censuses. For 2000, population estimates are bridged-race April 1 census counts. Starting with *Health, United States, 2012*, rates for 2001–2009 were revised using intercensal population estimates based on the 2000 and 2010 Censuses. For 2010, population estimates are bridged-race April 1 census counts. Rates for 2011 and beyond were computed using 2010-based postcensal estimates. Age groups were selected to minimize the presentation of unstable age-specific death rates based on small numbers of deaths and for consistency among comparison groups. Starting with 2003 data, some states began to collect information on more than one race on the death certificate, according to 1997 Office of Management and Budget (OMB) standards. The multiple-race data for these states were bridged to the single-race categories of the 1977 OMB standards, for comparability with other states. NA = Not available.

* = Rates based on fewer than 20 deaths are considered unreliable and are not shown.

[1]Includes deaths of persons who were not residents of the 50 states and the District of Columbia (DC).

[2]Underlying cause of death was coded according to the 6th revision of the *International Classification of Diseases* (*ICD*) in 1950, 7th revision in 1960, 8th revision in 1970, and 9th revision in 1980–1998.

[3]Starting with 1999 data, cause of death is coded according to *ICD–10*.

[4]Age-adjusted rates are calculated using the year 2000 standard population. Prior to 2001, age-adjusted rates were calculated using standard million proportions based on rounded population numbers. Starting with 2001 data, unrounded population numbers are used to calculate age-adjusted rates.

[5]The race groups, White, Black, Asian or Pacific Islander, and American Indian and Alaska Native, include persons of Hispanic and non-Hispanic origin. Persons of Hispanic origin may be of any race. Death rates for Hispanic, American Indian or Alaska Native, and Asian or Pacific Islander persons should be interpreted with caution because of inconsistencies in reporting Hispanic origin or race on the death certificate (death rate numerators) compared with population figures (death rate denominators). The net effect of misclassification is an underestimation of deaths and death rates for races other than White and Black.

[7]Prior to 1997, excludes data from states lacking an Hispanic-origin item on the death certificate.

Table 2-31. Death Rates for Malignant Neoplasms of the Trachea, Bronchus, and Lung, by Sex, Race, Hispanic Origin, and Age, Selected Years, 1950–2016—*Continued*

(Deaths per 100,000 resident population; data are based on death certificates.)

Sex, race, Hispanic origin, and age	2007[3]	2008[3]	2009[3]	2010[3]	2011[3]	2012[3]	2013[3]	2014[3]	2015[3]	2016[3]
65 to 74 years	73.0	73.8	68.0	67.0	70.6	68.6	63.9	59.3	64.4	57.4
75 to 84 years	145.2	148.6	153.9	160.3	149.1	142.8	150.2	149.3	134.7	131.6
85 years and over	193.6	168.3	203.9	171.1	200.8	181.7	207.4	199.6	183.2	183.5
Hispanic or Latina Female[5,7]										
All ages, age-adjusted[4]	14.9	14.2	13.6	13.8	13.3	13.6	13.2	13.3	12.9	12.1
All ages, crude	7.9	7.7	7.5	7.7	7.6	8.0	8.0	8.3	8.4	8.0
45 to 54 years	6.5	7.1	5.9	7.1	5.7	6.0	5.4	5.1	5.3	5.2
55 to 64 years	21.8	20.8	20.5	19.3	18.5	20.5	18.9	19.3	19.5	18.5
65 to 74 years	65.9	62.0	58.5	51.7	54.2	51.7	52.9	53.0	51.1	42.7
75 to 84 years	115.3	111.2	104.0	117.3	108.6	110.8	107.2	109.7	104.7	106.0
85 years and over	152.0	137.7	144.9	143.4	144.8	152.4	146.7	151.9	139.5	133.5
White, not Hispanic or Latina Female[7]										
All ages, age-adjusted[4]	43.5	42.7	42.3	41.7	40.7	39.9	39.0	38.4	37.3	35.4
All ages, crude	59.5	59.2	59.3	59.0	58.5	58.6	58.2	58.1	57.6	55.7
45 to 54 years	27.2	27.1	28.0	26.9	26.8	25.8	25.6	24.8	22.5	20.7
55 to 64 years	83.0	78.3	75.1	74.0	72.4	73.3	71.4	72.1	70.4	68.7
65 to 74 years	214.3	207.3	205.6	199.5	191.3	185.5	179.5	171.6	166.2	153.2
75 to 84 years	304.5	306.5	303.1	303.0	298.7	294.2	288.1	289.7	277.0	269.5
85 years and over	254.5	258.2	262.3	263.8	261.9	259.6	256.8	253.1	267.8	258.4
Black, not Hispanic or Latina Female[7]										
All ages, age-adjusted[4]	38.9	37.7	36.7	37.3	36.3	35.6	35.1	33.6	31.5	30.7
All ages, crude	33.1	32.4	32.2	33.1	33.0	33.0	33.3	32.6	31.3	31.1
45 to 54 years	33.0	29.3	30.1	28.6	27.9	26.9	25.0	24.3	19.7	18.5
55 to 64 years	78.6	76.2	78.4	75.9	75.6	73.1	74.3	72.0	69.3	69.8
65 to 74 years	180.8	172.0	164.9	167.1	160.2	162.3	155.4	146.1	139.8	127.6
75 to 84 years	255.2	254.2	249.6	253.7	246.1	246.0	242.5	232.7	214.2	219.0
85 years and over	215.2	227.7	201.6	252.2	241.4	215.0	229.7	225.1	222.9	230.6

NOTE: Starting with *Health, United States, 2003,* rates for 1991–1999 were revised using intercensal population estimates based on the 1990 and 2000 Censuses. For 2000, population estimates are bridged-race April 1 census counts. Starting with *Health, United States, 2012,* rates for 2001–2009 were revised using intercensal population estimates based on the 2000 and 2010 Censuses. For 2010, population estimates are bridged-race April 1 census counts. Rates for 2011 and beyond were computed using 2010-based postcensal estimates. Age groups were selected to minimize the presentation of unstable age-specific death rates based on small numbers of deaths and for consistency among comparison groups. Starting with 2003 data, some states began to collect information on more than one race on the death certificate, according to 1997 Office of Management and Budget (OMB) standards. The multiple-race data for these states were bridged to the single-race categories of the 1977 OMB standards, for comparability with other states.
[3]Starting with 1999 data, cause of death is coded according to *ICD–10.*
[4]Age-adjusted rates are calculated using the year 2000 standard population. Prior to 2001, age-adjusted rates were calculated using standard million proportions based on rounded population numbers. Starting with 2001 data, unrounded population numbers are used to calculate age-adjusted rates.
[5]The race groups, White, Black, Asian or Pacific Islander, and American Indian and Alaska Native, include persons of Hispanic and non-Hispanic origin. Persons of Hispanic origin may be of any race. Death rates for Hispanic, American Indian or Alaska Native, and Asian or Pacific Islander persons should be interpreted with caution because of inconsistencies in reporting Hispanic origin or race on the death certificate (death rate numerators) compared with population figures (death rate denominators). The net effect of misclassification is an underestimation of deaths and death rates for races other than White and Black.
[7]Prior to 1997, excludes data from states lacking an Hispanic-origin item on the death certificate.

Table 2-32. Death Rates for Malignant Neoplasms of the Breast Among Females, by Race, Hispanic Origin, and Age, Selected Years, 1950–2016

(Deaths per 100,000 resident population; data are based on death certificates.)

Sex, race, Hispanic origin, and age	1950[1,2]	1960[1,2]	1970[2]	1980[2]	1985[2]	1990[2]	1995[2]	2000[3]	2005[3]	2006[3]
All Females										
All ages, age-adjusted[4]	31.9	31.7	32.1	31.9	33.0	33.3	30.5	26.8	24.2	23.6
All ages, crude	24.7	26.1	28.4	30.6	32.8	34.0	32.2	29.2	27.4	26.9
Under 25 years	*	*	*	*	*	*	*	*	*	*
25 to 34 years	3.8	3.8	3.9	3.3	3.0	2.9	2.6	2.3	1.8	1.9
35 to 44 years	20.8	20.2	20.4	17.9	17.5	17.8	14.9	12.4	11.4	10.8
45 to 54 years	46.9	51.4	52.6	48.1	47.1	45.4	41.0	33.0	28.7	27.6
55 to 64 years	69.9	70.8	77.6	80.5	84.2	78.6	69.4	59.3	54.0	53.1
65 to 74 years	95.0	90.0	93.8	101.1	107.8	111.7	102.8	88.3	78.5	76.1
75 to 84 years	139.8	129.9	127.4	126.4	136.2	146.3	140.1	128.9	119.6	119.4
85 years and over	195.5	191.9	157.1	169.3	178.5	196.8	200.2	205.7	191.2	183.1
White Female[5]										
All ages, age-adjusted[4]	32.4	32.0	32.5	32.1	33.1	33.2	30.1	26.3	23.6	23.1
All ages, crude	25.7	27.2	29.9	32.3	34.7	35.9	33.8	30.7	28.5	28.2
25 to 34 years	20.8	19.7	20.2	17.3	16.8	17.1	14.0	11.3	10.3	9.9
45 to 54 years	47.1	51.2	53.0	48.1	46.8	44.3	38.9	31.2	26.3	25.7
55 to 64 years	70.9	71.8	79.3	81.3	84.7	78.5	68.3	57.9	52.1	51.6
65 to 74 years	96.3	91.6	95.9	103.7	109.9	113.3	103.3	89.3	78.7	76.4
75 to 84 years	143.6	132.8	129.6	128.4	138.8	148.2	141.4	130.2	120.9	120.4
85 years and over	204.2	199.7	161.9	171.7	180.9	198.0	202.6	205.5	191.6	182.7
Black or African American Female[5]										
All ages, age-adjusted[4]	25.3	27.9	28.9	31.7	34.6	38.1	38.0	34.5	32.8	31.6
All ages, crude	16.4	18.7	19.7	22.9	25.9	29.0	29.6	27.9	28.2	27.3
25 to 34 years	21.0	24.8	24.4	24.1	26.1	25.8	22.9	20.9	20.1	18.8
45 to 54 years	46.5	54.4	52.0	52.7	55.5	60.5	61.9	51.5	49.5	44.0
55 to 64 years	64.3	63.2	64.7	79.9	90.4	93.1	89.1	80.9	79.6	74.6
65 to 74 years	67.0	72.3	77.3	84.3	100.7	112.2	117.9	98.6	94.5	89.5
75 to 84 years[6]	81.0	87.5	101.8	114.1	117.6	140.5	147.2	139.8	126.9	138.6
85 years and over	NA	92.1	112.1	149.9	159.4	201.5	192.7	238.7	223.8	221.1
American Indian or Alaska Native Female[5]										
All ages, age-adjusted[4]	NA	NA	NA	10.8	12.1	13.7	15.0	13.6	15.5	13.0
All ages, crude	NA	NA	NA	6.1	6.9	8.6	9.0	8.7	9.3	8.7
25 to 34 years	NA	NA	NA	*	*	*	*	*	*	*
45 to 54 years	NA	NA	NA	*	*	23.9	21.6	14.4	11.9	14.4
55 to 64 years	NA	NA	NA	*	*	*	37.4	40.0	20.3	29.6
65 to 74 years	NA	NA	NA	*	*	*	46.3	42.5	65.4	42.5
75 to 84 years	NA	NA	NA	*	*	*	*	71.8	124.2	57.3
85 years and over	NA	NA	NA	*	*	*	*	*	*	*
Asian or Pacific Islander Female[5]										
All ages, age-adjusted[4]	NA	NA	NA	11.9	13.2	13.7	13.9	12.3	12.2	12.1
All ages, crude	NA	NA	NA	8.2	8.6	9.3	10.8	10.2	10.6	10.6
25 to 34 years	NA	NA	NA	10.4	7.2	8.4	8.0	8.1	6.7	5.2
45 to 54 years	NA	NA	NA	23.4	21.9	26.4	29.1	22.3	18.2	19.2
55 to 64 years	NA	NA	NA	35.7	39.5	33.8	37.9	31.3	34.0	32.0
65 to 74 years	NA	NA	NA	*	32.5	38.5	36.6	34.7	31.7	38.7
75 to 84 years	NA	NA	NA	*	50.0	48.0	42.3	37.5	53.9	44.1
85 years and over	NA	NA	NA	*	*	*	*	68.2	69.7	78.9
Hispanic or Latina Female[5,7]										
All ages, age-adjusted[4]	NA	NA	NA	NA	16.3	19.5	18.7	16.9	15.3	15.2
All ages, crude	NA	NA	NA	NA	8.8	11.5	10.6	9.7	9.2	9.4
25 to 34 years	NA	NA	NA	NA	10.4	11.7	9.5	8.7	7.9	7.8
45 to 54 years	NA	NA	NA	NA	26.4	32.8	27.7	23.9	19.7	19.4
55 to 64 years	NA	NA	NA	NA	43.5	45.8	45.0	39.1	34.4	36.0
65 to 74 years	NA	NA	NA	NA	40.9	64.8	58.0	54.9	46.7	47.0
75 to 84 years	NA	NA	NA	NA	64.5	67.2	80.9	74.9	75.4	71.1
85 years and over	NA	NA	NA	NA	85.7	102.8	115.6	105.8	113.0	109.1
White, not Hispanic or Latina Female[7]										
All ages, age-adjusted[4]	NA	NA	NA	NA	33.0	33.9	30.6	26.8	24.2	23.6
All ages, crude	NA	NA	NA	NA	35.6	38.5	36.6	33.8	32.0	31.7

NOTE: Starting with *Health, United States, 2003*, rates for 1991–1999 were revised using intercensal population estimates based on the 1990 and 2000 Censuses. For 2000, population estimates are bridged-race April 1 census counts. Starting with *Health, United States, 2012*, rates for 2001–2009 were revised using intercensal population estimates based on the 2000 and 2010 Censuses. For 2010, population estimates are bridged-race April 1 census counts. Rates for 2011 and beyond were computed using 2010-based postcensal estimates. Age groups were selected to minimize the presentation of unstable age-specific death rates based on small numbers of deaths and for consistency among comparison groups. Starting with 2003 data, some states began to collect information on more than one race on the death certificate, according to 1997 Office of Management and Budget (OMB) standards. The multiple-race data for these states were bridged to the single-race categories of the 1977 OMB standards, for comparability with other states.
NA = Not available.
* = Rates based on fewer than 20 deaths are considered unreliable and are not shown.
[1] Includes deaths of persons who were not residents of the 50 states and the District of Columbia (DC).
[2] Underlying cause of death was coded according to the 6th revision of the *International Classification of Diseases (ICD)* in 1950, 7th revision in 1960, 8th revision in 1970, and 9th revision in 1980–1998.
[3] Starting with 1999 data, cause of death is coded according to *ICD–10*.
[4] Age-adjusted rates are calculated using the year 2000 standard population. Prior to 2001, age-adjusted rates were calculated using standard million proportions based on rounded population numbers. Starting with 2001 data, unrounded population numbers are used to calculate age-adjusted rates.
[5] The race groups, White, Black, Asian or Pacific Islander, and American Indian and Alaska Native, include persons of Hispanic and non-Hispanic origin. Persons of Hispanic origin may be of any race. Death rates for Hispanic, American Indian or Alaska Native, and Asian or Pacific Islander populations should be interpreted with caution because of inconsistencies in reporting Hispanic origin or race on the death certificate (death rate numerators) compared with population figures (death rate denominators). The net effect of misclassification is an underestimation of deaths and death rates for races other than White and Black.
[6] In 1950, rate is for the age group 75 years and over.
[7] Prior to 1997, excludes data from states lacking an Hispanic-origin item on the death certificate.

Table 2-32. Death Rates for Malignant Neoplasms of the Breast Among Females, by Race, Hispanic Origin, and Age, Selected Years, 1950–2016—Continued

(Deaths per 100,000 resident population; data are based on death certificates.)

Sex, race, Hispanic origin, and age	2007[3]	2008[3]	2009[3]	2010[3]	2011[3]	2012[3]	2013[3]	2014[3]	2015[3]	2016[3]
All Females										
All ages, age-adjusted[4]	23.0	22.6	22.3	22.1	21.6	21.3	20.8	20.6	20.3	20.1
All ages, crude	26.5	26.3	26.1	26.1	25.9	25.8	25.5	25.5	25.4	25.3
Under 25 years	*	*	*	*	*	*	*	*	*	*
25 to 34 years	1.7	1.6	1.7	1.6	1.7	1.7	1.6	1.6	1.8	2.0
35 to 44 years	10.1	10.1	10.5	9.8	9.9	9.7	9.6	9.7	9.0	9.4
45 to 54 years	26.7	26.2	26.2	25.7	25.2	25.2	24.6	23.8	23.7	23.5
55 to 64 years	50.7	49.2	47.9	47.7	46.2	45.4	44.1	43.3	43.3	41.3
65 to 74 years	76.3	75.6	73.4	73.9	72.5	70.0	68.4	67.5	66.7	64.9
75 to 84 years	116.6	113.8	112.6	109.1	108.2	106.9	104.4	104.2	101.7	102.6
85 years and over	184.7	182.7	178.0	185.8	176.5	177.3	173.0	174.0	173.3	169.6
White Female[5]										
All ages, age-adjusted[4]	22.5	22.1	21.9	21.5	21.0	20.8	20.4	20.1	19.8	19.6
All ages, crude	27.7	27.4	27.4	27.3	26.9	26.9	26.7	26.6	26.6	26.5
25 to 34 years	9.2	9.1	9.8	8.8	8.9	8.8	8.8	8.9	8.2	8.6
45 to 54 years	24.8	24.5	24.8	23.9	23.4	23.5	23.0	22.0	22.0	21.5
55 to 64 years	49.0	47.8	46.4	45.9	44.1	43.5	42.5	41.4	41.4	39.8
65 to 74 years	76.5	74.9	73.2	73.3	71.9	69.6	68.4	67.4	66.4	64.6
75 to 84 years	117.4	114.4	113.1	110.2	108.8	107.8	105.0	105.2	102.5	103.7
85 years and over	185.5	182.9	179.2	186.8	178.3	178.8	174.9	175.9	175.4	172.7
Black or African American Female[5]										
All ages, age-adjusted[4]	31.3	30.9	30.2	30.3	30.2	29.4	28.3	28.1	27.7	27.3
All ages, crude	27.4	27.3	26.9	27.5	27.8	27.5	26.7	27.0	27.0	26.9
25 to 34 years	18.0	17.7	17.6	18.3	17.6	16.8	16.3	16.0	15.1	15.2
45 to 54 years	43.6	42.2	40.6	40.9	41.0	40.1	39.2	39.1	38.2	39.8
55 to 64 years	73.8	69.2	68.5	70.5	69.7	67.6	63.7	64.4	63.8	57.7
65 to 74 years	93.8	97.8	92.4	97.4	95.8	89.7	86.6	85.9	86.6	85.1
75 to 84 years[6]	135.6	133.4	136.4	123.2	130.4	129.7	126.1	122.6	117.8	122.8
85 years and over	213.2	224.0	201.9	214.6	199.2	204.4	193.1	196.4	196.4	188.2
American Indian or Alaska Native Female[5]										
All ages, age-adjusted[4]	13.0	12.5	12.2	11.5	10.8	10.8	10.1	10.8	12.8	12.1
All ages, crude	8.8	8.6	8.4	8.0	7.6	7.9	7.5	8.0	9.7	9.4
25 to 34 years	*	*	*	*	*	*	*	*	*	*
45 to 54 years	16.2	12.1	12.0	13.2	11.2	10.8	11.2	9.4	11.5	13.7
55 to 64 years	33.1	33.1	29.9	25.2	21.8	22.5	20.6	19.3	22.5	21.3
65 to 74 years	37.8	50.7	51.3	34.3	38.5	46.8	38.2	40.2	42.6	38.5
75 to 84 years	54.9	55.3	53.2	61.1	59.4	64.1	50.5	61.7	71.9	77.3
85 years and over	*	*	*	*	*	*	*	*	144.8	108.5
Asian or Pacific Islander Female[5]										
All ages, age-adjusted[4]	11.0	11.5	11.1	11.9	11.3	11.3	11.1	11.6	11.7	10.7
All ages, crude	9.7	10.3	10.1	10.8	10.7	10.9	10.8	11.5	11.7	11.1
25 to 34 years	5.7	6.2	5.4	5.4	6.4	6.4	5.7	6.4	5.9	6.7
45 to 54 years	14.9	15.2	15.5	17.0	15.7	16.7	15.6	16.8	15.7	13.8
55 to 64 years	27.6	29.2	28.8	28.4	29.3	27.8	27.2	27.6	29.1	29.6
65 to 74 years	34.9	39.5	34.6	37.9	34.6	37.1	32.7	35.1	34.3	31.4
75 to 84 years	50.7	52.3	46.4	53.2	46.7	40.3	48.6	47.7	55.9	42.9
85 years and over	61.0	56.5	72.9	77.5	71.4	77.4	82.8	81.3	74.0	66.4
Hispanic or Latina Female[5,7]										
All ages, age-adjusted[4]	14.8	14.6	14.8	14.4	14.1	14.7	14.6	14.5	13.5	13.9
All ages, crude	9.2	9.1	9.4	9.2	9.3	10.0	10.0	10.3	9.8	10.4
25 to 34 years	7.2	7.2	7.0	6.2	7.0	7.2	7.2	7.7	7.1	7.5
45 to 54 years	19.0	17.0	19.0	18.6	17.3	20.3	18.0	17.4	15.7	16.8
55 to 64 years	33.4	34.6	32.6	32.7	29.6	31.8	31.2	31.5	30.9	31.0
65 to 74 years	47.7	45.9	46.3	49.0	46.3	45.7	46.3	47.0	40.0	43.7
75 to 84 years	68.6	69.7	72.4	61.8	68.5	63.9	73.3	69.3	67.1	64.3
85 years and over	109.0	111.5	111.4	117.8	108.7	121.8	112.0	116.3	108.5	111.7
White, not Hispanic or Latina Female[7]										
All ages, age-adjusted[4]	23.1	22.6	22.5	22.1	21.6	21.3	20.9	20.6	20.4	20.1
All ages, crude	31.3	31.1	31.0	31.0	30.7	30.6	30.3	30.2	30.4	30.2

NOTE: Starting with *Health, United States, 2003*, rates for 1991–1999 were revised using intercensal population estimates based on the 1990 and 2000 Censuses. For 2000, population estimates are bridged-race April 1 census counts. Starting with *Health, United States, 2012*, rates for 2001–2009 were revised using intercensal population estimates based on the 2000 and 2010 Censuses. For 2010, population estimates are bridged-race April 1 census counts. Rates for 2011 and beyond were computed using 2010-based postcensal estimates. Age groups were selected to minimize the presentation of unstable age-specific death rates based on small numbers of deaths and for consistency among comparison groups. Starting with 2003 data, some states began to collect information on more than one race on the death certificate, according to 1997 Office of Management and Budget (OMB) standards. The multiple-race data for these states were bridged to the single-race categories of the 1977 OMB standards, for comparability with other states.

* = Rates based on fewer than 20 deaths are considered unreliable and are not shown.

[3]Starting with 1999 data, cause of death is coded according to *ICD–10*.

[4]Age-adjusted rates are calculated using the year 2000 standard population. Prior to 2001, age-adjusted rates were calculated using standard million proportions based on rounded population numbers. Starting with 2001 data, unrounded population numbers are used to calculate age-adjusted rates.

[5]The race groups, White, Black, Asian or Pacific Islander, and American Indian and Alaska Native, include persons of Hispanic and non-Hispanic origin. Persons of Hispanic origin may be of any race. Death rates for Hispanic, American Indian or Alaska Native, and Asian or Pacific Islander persons should be interpreted with caution because of inconsistencies in reporting Hispanic origin or race on the death certificate (death rate numerators) compared with population figures (death rate denominators). The net effect of misclassification is an underestimation of deaths and death rates for races other than White and Black.

[6]In 1950, rate is for the age group 75 years and over.

[7]Prior to 1997, excludes data from states lacking an Hispanic-origin item on the death certificate.

Table 2-32. Death Rates for Malignant Neoplasms of the Breast Among Females, by Race, Hispanic Origin, and Age, Selected Years, 1950–2016—*Continued*

(Deaths per 100,000 resident population; data are based on death certificates.)

Sex, race, Hispanic origin, and age	1950[1,2]	1960[1,2]	1970[2]	1980[2]	1985[2]	1990[2]	1995[2]	2000[3]	2005[3]	2006[3]
25 to 34 years	NA	NA	NA	NA	16.9	17.5	14.4	11.6	10.7	10.1
45 to 54 years	NA	NA	NA	NA	46.8	45.2	39.5	31.7	26.9	26.4
55 to 64 years	NA	NA	NA	NA	85.1	80.6	69.5	59.2	53.5	53.0
65 to 74 years	NA	NA	NA	NA	108.6	115.7	105.4	91.4	81.2	78.8
75 to 84 years	NA	NA	NA	NA	139.4	151.4	143.2	132.2	123.3	123.3
85 years and over	NA	NA	NA	NA	175.6	201.5	204.4	208.3	194.7	185.5
Black, not Hispanic or Latina Female[7]										
All ages, age-adjusted[4]	NA	NA	NA	NA	NA	NA	NA	35.1	33.5	32.3
All ages, crude	NA	NA	NA	NA	NA	NA	NA	28.9	29.4	28.5
25 to 34 years	NA	NA	NA	NA	NA	NA	NA	21.5	20.9	19.7
45 to 54 years	NA	NA	NA	NA	NA	NA	NA	52.5	50.9	45.2
55 to 64 years	NA	NA	NA	NA	NA	NA	NA	82.5	81.3	75.7
65 to 74 years	NA	NA	NA	NA	NA	NA	NA	100.1	95.9	90.6
75 to 84 years	NA	NA	NA	NA	NA	NA	NA	141.5	128.6	141.1
85 years and over	NA	NA	NA	NA	NA	NA	NA	241.6	226.4	224.7

NOTE: Starting with *Health, United States, 2003*, rates for 1991–1999 were revised using intercensal population estimates based on the 1990 and 2000 Censuses. For 2000, population estimates are bridged-race April 1 census counts. Starting with *Health, United States, 2012*, rates for 2001–2009 were revised using intercensal population estimates based on the 2000 and 2010 Censuses. For 2010, population estimates are bridged-race April 1 census counts. Rates for 2011 and beyond were computed using 2010-based postcensal estimates. Age groups were selected to minimize the presentation of unstable age-specific death rates based on small numbers of deaths and for consistency among comparison groups. Starting with 2003 data, some states began to collect information on more than one race on the death certificate, according to 1997 Office of Management and Budget (OMB) standards. The multiple-race data for these states were bridged to the single-race categories of the 1977 OMB standards, for comparability with other states.
NA = Not available.
[1] Includes deaths of persons who were not residents of the 50 states and the District of Columbia (DC).
[2] Underlying cause of death was coded according to the 6th revision of the *International Classification of Diseases* (*ICD*) in 1950, 7th revision in 1960, 8th revision in 1970, and 9th revision in 1980–1998.
[3] Starting with 1999 data, cause of death is coded according to *ICD–10*.
[4] Age-adjusted rates are calculated using the year 2000 standard population. Prior to 2001, age-adjusted rates were calculated using standard million proportions based on rounded population numbers. Starting with 2001 data, unrounded population numbers are used to calculate age-adjusted rates.
[7] Prior to 1997, excludes data from states lacking an Hispanic-origin item on the death certificate.

Table 2-32. Death Rates for Malignant Neoplasms of the Breast Among Females, by Race, Hispanic Origin, and Age, Selected Years, 1950–2016—*Continued*

(Deaths per 100,000 resident population; data are based on death certificates.)

Sex, race, Hispanic origin, and age	2007[3]	2008[3]	2009[3]	2010[3]	2011[3]	2012[3]	2013[3]	2014[3]	2015[3]	2016[3]
25 to 34 years	9.4	9.4	10.3	9.3	9.3	9.0	9.1	9.1	8.3	8.7
45 to 54 years	25.4	25.3	25.4	24.5	24.2	23.8	23.6	22.6	23.0	22.3
55 to 64 years	50.4	48.9	47.6	47.1	45.4	44.6	43.5	42.2	42.3	40.6
65 to 74 years	78.9	77.2	75.3	75.1	74.1	71.6	70.1	69.1	68.7	66.3
75 to 84 years	120.4	117.2	115.9	113.6	111.6	111.1	107.3	108.1	105.2	107.0
85 years and over	188.8	185.8	182.3	189.9	181.7	181.8	178.5	179.4	179.5	176.7
Black, not Hispanic or Latina Female[7]										
All ages, age-adjusted[4]	32.1	31.8	31.0	31.3	31.2	30.2	29.2	28.8	28.5	28.2
All ages, crude	28.8	28.7	28.3	29.0	29.4	28.9	28.3	28.4	28.6	28.5
25 to 34 years	18.7	18.5	18.3	19.3	18.5	17.7	17.3	16.8	15.9	16.3
45 to 54 years	45.0	43.7	42.1	42.4	42.7	41.5	40.7	40.4	39.7	41.5
55 to 64 years	75.6	71.1	70.2	72.3	71.7	69.1	65.3	66.2	65.4	59.4
65 to 74 years	95.7	99.9	94.8	100.1	98.2	91.5	89.0	87.4	89.1	87.3
75 to 84 years	137.8	136.3	139.0	126.3	132.9	132.0	129.1	125.1	121.2	125.6
85 years and over	216.0	228.5	204.2	218.4	203.4	205.6	195.7	197.8	198.6	191.3

NOTE: Starting with *Health, United States, 2003,* rates for 1991–1999 were revised using intercensal population estimates based on the 1990 and 2000 Censuses. For 2000, population estimates are bridged-race April 1 census counts. Starting with *Health, United States, 2012,* rates for 2001–2009 were revised using intercensal population estimates based on the 2000 and 2010 Censuses. For 2010, population estimates are bridged-race April 1 census counts. Rates for 2011 and beyond were computed using 2010-based postcensal estimates. Age groups were selected to minimize the presentation of unstable age-specific death rates based on small numbers of deaths and for consistency among comparison groups. Starting with 2003 data, some states began to collect information on more than one race on the death certificate, according to 1997 Office of Management and Budget (OMB) standards. The multiple-race data for these states were bridged to the single-race categories of the 1977 OMB standards, for comparability with other states.
[3]Starting with 1999 data, cause of death is coded according to *ICD–10.*
[4]Age-adjusted rates are calculated using the year 2000 standard population. Prior to 2001, age-adjusted rates were calculated using standard million proportions based on rounded population numbers. Starting with 2001 data, unrounded population numbers are used to calculate age-adjusted rates.
[7]Prior to 1997, excludes data from states lacking an Hispanic-origin item on the death certificate.

Table 2-33. Death Rates for Motor Vehicle–Related Injuries, by Sex, Race, Hispanic Origin, and Age, Selected Years, 1950–2016

(Deaths per 100,000 resident population; data are based on death certificates.)

Sex, race, Hispanic origin, and age	1950[1,2]	1960[1,2]	1970[2]	1980[2]	1985	1990[2]	1995	2000[3]	2005[3]	2006[3]
All Persons										
All ages, age-adjusted[4]	24.6	23.1	27.6	22.3	18.6	18.5	16.3	15.4	15.2	15.0
All ages, crude	23.1	21.3	26.9	23.5	19.3	18.8	16.3	15.4	15.3	15.2
Under 1 year	8.4	8.1	9.8	7.0	4.9	4.9	4.7	4.4	3.6	3.5
1 to 14 years	9.8	8.6	10.5	8.2	7.0	6.0	5.3	4.3	3.7	3.4
1 to 4 years	11.5	10.0	11.5	9.2	7.2	6.3	5.2	4.2	3.9	3.7
5 to 14 years	8.8	7.9	10.2	7.9	6.9	5.9	5.3	4.3	3.6	3.3
15 to 24 years	34.4	38.0	47.2	44.8	35.7	34.1	28.9	26.9	25.7	25.7
15 to 19 years	29.6	33.9	43.6	43.0	33.5	33.1	28.1	26.0	23.1	22.6
20 to 24 years	38.8	42.9	51.3	46.6	37.6	35.0	29.7	28.0	28.3	28.9
25 to 34 years	24.6	24.3	30.9	29.1	23.0	23.6	19.2	17.3	18.4	18.7
35 to 44 years	20.3	19.3	24.9	20.9	17.2	16.9	15.3	15.3	15.5	15.4
45 to 64 years	25.2	23.0	26.5	18.0	15.4	15.7	14.1	14.3	14.8	14.8
45 to 54 years	22.2	21.4	25.5	18.6	15.2	15.6	13.8	14.2	15.1	15.3
55 to 64 years	29.0	25.1	27.9	17.4	15.6	15.9	14.5	14.4	14.5	14.1
65 years and over	43.1	34.7	36.2	22.5	21.7	23.1	22.6	21.4	20.1	19.0
65 to 74 years	39.1	31.4	32.8	19.2	17.9	18.6	17.5	16.5	16.5	15.2
75 to 84 years	52.7	41.8	43.5	28.1	27.4	29.1	28.4	25.7	22.9	22.2
85 years and over	45.1	37.9	34.2	27.6	26.5	31.2	31.0	30.4	27.3	25.5
Male										
All ages, age-adjusted[4]	38.5	35.4	41.5	33.6	27.2	26.5	22.8	21.7	21.9	21.5
All ages, crude	35.4	31.8	39.7	35.3	28.0	26.7	22.4	21.3	21.8	21.6
Under 1 year	9.1	8.6	9.3	7.3	5.0	5.0	4.9	4.6	3.6	3.4
1 to 14 years	12.3	10.7	13.0	10.0	8.5	7.0	6.1	4.9	4.1	3.7
1 to 4 years	13.0	11.5	12.9	10.2	8.3	6.9	5.6	4.7	4.3	3.9
5 to 14 years	11.9	10.4	13.1	9.9	8.6	7.0	6.3	5.0	4.1	3.7
15 to 24 years	56.7	61.2	73.2	68.4	52.7	49.5	40.5	37.4	36.3	36.3
15 to 19 years	46.3	51.7	64.1	62.6	46.5	45.5	36.1	33.9	29.9	29.5
20 to 24 years	66.7	73.2	84.4	74.3	58.2	53.3	45.0	41.2	42.8	43.4
25 to 34 years	40.8	40.1	49.4	46.3	35.9	35.7	28.1	25.5	27.9	28.5
35 to 44 years	32.5	29.9	37.7	31.7	25.2	24.7	21.7	22.0	22.5	22.1
45 to 64 years	37.7	33.3	38.9	26.5	22.0	21.9	19.5	20.2	21.6	21.6
45 to 54 years	33.6	31.6	37.2	27.6	21.9	22.0	19.3	20.4	22.2	22.6
55 to 64 years	43.1	35.6	40.9	25.4	22.1	21.7	19.6	19.8	20.7	20.3
65 years and over	66.6	52.1	54.4	33.9	30.4	32.1	30.7	29.5	28.4	26.4
65 to 74 years	59.1	45.8	47.3	27.3	23.0	24.2	22.2	21.7	22.8	20.7
75 to 84 years	85.0	66.0	68.2	44.3	41.3	41.2	39.9	35.6	32.1	30.4
85 years and over	78.1	62.7	63.1	56.1	55.3	64.5	61.5	57.5	49.0	45.6
Female										
All ages, age-adjusted[4]	11.5	11.7	14.9	11.8	10.7	11.0	10.3	9.5	8.9	8.8
All ages, crude	10.9	11.0	14.7	12.3	11.0	11.3	10.4	9.7	9.1	9.0
Under 1 year	7.6	7.5	10.4	6.7	4.7	4.9	4.5	4.2	3.7	3.5
1 to 14 years	7.2	6.3	7.9	6.3	5.4	4.9	4.4	3.7	3.1	3.1
1 to 4 years	10.0	8.4	10.0	8.1	6.0	5.6	4.8	3.8	3.4	3.5
5 to 14 years	5.7	5.4	7.2	5.7	5.1	4.7	4.2	3.6	3.0	2.9
15 to 24 years	12.6	15.1	21.6	20.8	18.2	17.9	16.8	15.9	14.5	14.5
15 to 19 years	12.9	16.0	22.7	22.8	20.1	20.0	19.7	17.5	15.9	15.4
20 to 24 years	12.2	14.0	20.4	18.9	16.7	16.0	13.8	14.2	13.2	13.6
25 to 34 years	9.3	9.2	13.0	12.2	10.1	11.5	10.2	8.8	8.9	8.8
35 to 44 years	8.5	9.1	12.9	10.4	9.4	9.2	9.0	8.8	8.6	8.8
45 to 64 years	12.6	13.1	15.3	10.3	9.5	10.1	9.0	8.7	8.4	8.3
45 to 54 years	10.9	11.6	14.5	10.2	9.0	9.6	8.4	8.2	8.2	8.2
55 to 64 years	14.9	15.2	16.2	10.5	9.9	10.8	9.9	9.5	8.8	8.5
65 years and over	21.9	20.3	23.1	15.0	15.8	17.2	17.0	15.8	14.1	13.6
65 to 74 years	20.6	19.0	21.6	13.0	14.0	14.1	13.7	12.3	11.1	10.5
75 to 84 years	25.2	23.0	27.2	18.5	19.2	21.9	21.2	19.2	16.5	16.5
85 years and over	22.1	22.0	18.0	15.2	15.0	18.3	19.3	19.3	17.6	16.4
White Male[5]										
All ages, age-adjusted[4]	37.9	34.8	40.4	33.8	27.2	26.3	22.6	21.8	22.4	22.1
All ages, crude	35.1	31.5	39.1	35.9	28.3	26.7	22.4	21.6	22.5	22.2
Under 1 year	9.1	8.8	9.1	7.0	4.6	4.8	4.3	4.2	3.4	3.3
1 to 14 years	12.4	10.6	12.5	9.8	8.3	6.6	5.9	4.8	4.1	3.6

NOTE: Starting with *Health, United States, 2003*, rates for 1991–1999 were revised using intercensal population estimates based on the 1990 and 2000 Censuses. For 2000, population estimates are bridged-race April 1 census counts. Starting with *Health, United States, 2012*, rates for 2001–2009 were revised using intercensal population estimates based on the 2000 and 2010 Censuses. For 2010, population estimates are bridged-race April 1 census counts. Rates for 2011 and beyond were computed using 2010-based postcensal estimates. Age groups were selected to minimize the presentation of unstable age-specific death rates based on small numbers of deaths and for consistency among comparison groups. Starting with 2003 data, some states began to collect information on more than one race on the death certificate, according to 1997 Office of Management and Budget (OMB) standards. The multiple-race data for these states were bridged to the single-race categories of the 1977 OMB standards, for comparability with other states.
[1]Includes deaths of persons who were not residents of the 50 states and the District of Columbia (DC).
[2]Underlying cause of death was coded according to the 6th revision of the *International Classification of Diseases (ICD)* in 1950, 7th revision in 1960, 8th revision in 1970, and 9th revision in 1980–1998.
[3]Starting with 1999 data, cause of death is coded according to *ICD–10*.
[4]Age-adjusted rates are calculated using the year 2000 standard population. Prior to 2001, age-adjusted rates were calculated using standard million proportions based on rounded population numbers. Starting with 2001 data, unrounded population numbers are used to calculate age-adjusted rates.
[5]The race groups, White, Black, Asian or Pacific Islander, and American Indian and Alaska Native, include persons of Hispanic and non-Hispanic origin. Persons of Hispanic origin may be of any race. Death rates for Hispanic, American Indian or Alaska Native, and Asian or Pacific Islander persons should be interpreted with caution because of inconsistencies in reporting Hispanic origin or race on the death certificate (death rate numerators) compared with population figures (death rate denominators). The net effect of misclassification is an underestimation of deaths and death rates for races other than White and Black.

Table 2-33. Death Rates for Motor Vehicle–Related Injuries, by Sex, Race, Hispanic Origin, and Age, Selected Years, 1950–2016—*Continued*

(Deaths per 100,000 resident population; data are based on death certificates.)

Sex, race, Hispanic origin, and age	2007³	2008³	2009³	2010³	2011³	2012³	2013³	2014³	2015³	2016³
All Persons										
All ages, age-adjusted⁴	14.4	12.9	11.6	11.3	11.1	11.4	10.9	10.8	11.4	12.1
All ages, crude	14.6	13.1	11.8	11.4	11.3	11.6	11.2	11.1	11.7	12.5
Under 1 year	3.0	2.5	2.4	2.0	2.4	1.8	1.7	1.7	1.8	2.3
1 to 14 years	3.2	2.6	2.5	2.3	2.3	2.2	2.2	2.2	2.2	2.4
1 to 4 years	3.4	2.9	2.9	2.8	2.6	2.9	2.7	2.5	2.6	2.6
5 to 14 years	3.2	2.5	2.4	2.2	2.1	2.0	2.1	2.0	2.1	2.3
15 to 24 years	24.5	20.6	17.6	16.6	16.2	16.1	15.2	15.3	15.9	16.6
15 to 19 years	21.4	17.4	15.2	13.6	13.2	12.6	11.4	11.9	12.4	12.7
20 to 24 years	27.7	24.0	20.2	19.7	19.1	19.3	18.8	18.3	19.2	20.2
25 to 34 years	17.8	16.3	14.5	14.0	13.7	14.5	13.9	13.9	14.7	16.1
35 to 44 years	14.9	13.4	12.2	11.6	11.3	11.8	11.4	11.1	11.9	12.9
45 to 64 years	14.1	13.3	12.2	11.9	11.9	12.4	12.1	12.0	12.8	13.5
45 to 54 years	14.9	13.7	12.7	12.0	12.3	12.6	12.2	12.1	12.8	13.4
55 to 64 years	13.2	12.8	11.5	11.9	11.5	12.2	11.9	11.9	12.7	13.6
65 years and over	18.7	16.9	15.8	16.0	15.9	15.7	15.1	14.8	15.3	16.0
65 to 74 years	14.9	13.8	12.7	12.3	13.0	13.0	12.2	11.9	12.8	13.3
75 to 84 years	21.7	19.2	18.6	18.8	18.3	17.9	17.8	17.5	17.5	18.9
85 years and over	25.3	23.2	20.9	23.8	21.8	22.1	21.0	20.9	21.7	21.8
Male										
All ages, age-adjusted⁴	21.0	18.9	16.8	16.2	16.1	16.5	15.9	15.8	16.7	17.6
All ages, crude	21.0	18.9	16.9	16.3	16.3	16.6	16.1	16.0	17.0	18.0
Under 1 year	2.7	2.9	2.6	2.2	2.8	1.9	1.7	1.9	2.2	2.1
1 to 14 years	3.7	3.1	2.9	2.7	2.5	2.5	2.5	2.5	2.5	2.6
1 to 4 years	3.8	3.2	3.4	3.0	2.7	3.1	3.0	2.8	2.9	2.7
5 to 14 years	3.7	3.0	2.7	2.5	2.5	2.3	2.4	2.4	2.4	2.6
15 to 24 years	34.6	29.3	24.5	23.1	22.8	22.5	21.2	21.5	22.2	22.9
15 to 19 years	27.7	22.6	19.2	17.8	17.2	16.2	14.7	16.1	16.3	16.5
20 to 24 years	41.9	36.3	30.0	28.5	28.2	28.4	27.3	26.5	27.7	29.0
25 to 34 years	27.2	25.2	21.7	21.0	20.4	21.5	20.8	20.8	21.8	23.5
35 to 44 years	22.1	19.9	18.2	16.9	16.7	17.6	16.9	16.4	17.9	19.4
45 to 64 years	20.9	19.7	18.2	17.9	18.2	18.6	18.2	18.1	19.4	20.4
45 to 54 years	22.2	20.2	19.0	17.9	18.6	18.8	18.3	18.2	19.1	19.8
55 to 64 years	19.2	19.0	17.2	17.8	17.7	18.5	18.1	18.1	19.8	21.1
65 years and over	26.9	24.1	22.0	22.2	22.3	22.1	21.5	21.0	22.1	23.4
65 to 74 years	21.1	19.4	17.5	17.1	18.2	18.5	17.5	17.0	18.5	19.4
75 to 84 years	31.4	27.3	25.8	25.9	25.7	24.8	24.9	24.8	24.9	27.1
85 years and over	44.4	40.2	35.3	40.2	35.4	35.3	35.3	34.0	35.6	36.7
Female										
All ages, age-adjusted⁴	8.2	7.2	6.7	6.5	6.3	6.5	6.2	6.1	6.4	6.9
All ages, crude	8.4	7.4	6.9	6.8	6.5	6.7	6.4	6.3	6.7	7.1
Under 1 year	3.3	2.0	2.1	1.8	1.9	1.8	1.8	1.5	1.3	2.5
1 to 14 years	2.8	2.2	2.2	2.0	2.0	1.9	1.9	1.8	1.9	2.1
1 to 4 years	3.1	2.5	2.5	2.5	2.6	2.6	2.3	2.3	2.3	2.5
5 to 14 years	2.6	2.0	2.0	1.8	1.8	1.7	1.8	1.6	1.8	2.0
15 to 24 years	13.8	11.5	10.5	9.9	9.4	9.3	8.9	8.7	9.3	9.9
15 to 19 years	14.8	11.8	10.9	9.2	9.0	8.9	7.9	7.6	8.4	8.8
20 to 24 years	12.8	11.2	10.0	10.5	9.7	9.8	9.9	9.7	10.2	10.8
25 to 34 years	8.5	7.4	7.2	6.9	7.0	7.4	6.9	6.8	7.5	8.5
35 to 44 years	7.8	7.0	6.2	6.2	6.0	6.2	5.9	5.8	6.1	6.5
45 to 64 years	7.7	7.2	6.5	6.3	5.9	6.4	6.3	6.2	6.4	6.9
45 to 54 years	7.8	7.4	6.6	6.3	6.1	6.5	6.3	6.2	6.7	7.1
55 to 64 years	7.5	6.9	6.3	6.3	5.7	6.4	6.2	6.1	6.1	6.6
65 years and over	12.6	11.5	11.1	11.3	10.9	10.8	10.0	9.9	10.0	10.2
65 to 74 years	9.6	8.9	8.5	8.2	8.4	8.2	7.5	7.5	7.8	8.0
75 to 84 years	15.0	13.5	13.5	13.7	12.8	12.9	12.5	12.0	11.9	12.6
85 years and over	16.5	15.3	14.0	15.9	15.1	15.5	13.7	14.1	14.4	13.8
White Male⁵										
All ages, age-adjusted⁴	21.6	19.6	17.3	16.7	16.6	17.0	16.3	16.1	17.0	17.8
All ages, crude	21.7	19.7	17.5	17.0	16.9	17.3	16.7	16.5	17.4	18.4
Under 1 year	2.9	2.9	2.5	2.0	2.5	1.9	1.7	1.8	1.9	1.6
1 to 14 years	3.8	3.1	2.8	2.7	2.6	2.4	2.4	2.4	2.5	2.5

NOTE: Starting with *Health, United States, 2003*, rates for 1991–1999 were revised using intercensal population estimates based on the 1990 and 2000 Censuses. For 2000, population estimates are bridged-race April 1 census counts. Starting with *Health, United States, 2012*, rates for 2001–2009 were revised using intercensal population estimates based on the 2000 and 2010 Censuses. For 2010, population estimates are bridged-race April 1 census counts. Rates for 2011 and beyond were computed using 2010-based postcensal estimates. Age groups were selected to minimize the presentation of unstable age-specific death rates based on small numbers of deaths and for consistency among comparison groups. Starting with 2003 data, some states began to collect information on more than one race on the death certificate, according to 1997 Office of Management and Budget (OMB) standards. The multiple-race data for these states were bridged to the single-race categories of the 1977 OMB standards, for comparability with other states.
³Starting with 1999 data, cause of death is coded according to *ICD–10*.
⁴Age-adjusted rates are calculated using the year 2000 standard population. Prior to 2001, age-adjusted rates were calculated using standard million proportions based on rounded population numbers. Starting with 2001 data, unrounded population numbers are used to calculate age-adjusted rates.
⁵The race groups, White, Black, Asian or Pacific Islander, and American Indian and Alaska Native, include persons of Hispanic and non-Hispanic origin. Persons of Hispanic origin may be of any race. Death rates for Hispanic, American Indian or Alaska Native, and Asian or Pacific Islander persons should be interpreted with caution because of inconsistencies in reporting Hispanic origin or race on the death certificate (death rate numerators) compared with population figures (death rate denominators). The net effect of misclassification is an underestimation of deaths and death rates for races other than White and Black.
⁶In 1950, rate is for the age group 75 years and over.
⁷Prior to 1997, excludes data from states lacking an Hispanic-origin item on the death certificate.

Table 2-33. Death Rates for Motor Vehicle–Related Injuries, by Sex, Race, Hispanic Origin, and Age, Selected Years, 1950–2016—*Continued*

(Deaths per 100,000 resident population; data are based on death certificates.)

Sex, race, Hispanic origin, and age	1950[1,2]	1960[1,2]	1970[2]	1980[2]	1985	1990[2]	1995	2000[3]	2005[3]	2006[3]
15 to 24 years	58.3	62.7	75.2	73.8	56.5	52.5	42.4	39.6	39.2	39.3
25 to 34 years	39.1	38.6	47.0	46.6	35.8	35.4	27.9	25.1	28.4	28.8
35 to 44 years	30.9	28.4	35.2	30.7	24.3	23.7	21.1	21.8	22.8	22.6
45 to 64 years	36.2	31.7	36.5	25.2	20.8	20.6	18.7	19.7	21.7	21.6
65 years and over	67.1	52.1	54.2	32.7	29.9	31.4	30.1	29.4	28.7	26.6
Black or African American Male[5]										
All ages, age-adjusted[4]	34.8	39.6	51.0	34.2	29.0	29.9	26.1	24.4	22.5	22.6
All ages, crude	37.2	33.1	44.3	31.1	27.1	28.1	24.1	22.5	21.1	21.4
Under 1 year	NA	*	10.6	7.8	*	*	8.7	6.7	*	*
1 to 14 years[6]	10.4	11.2	16.3	11.4	9.7	8.9	7.5	5.5	4.4	4.8
15 to 24 years	42.5	46.4	58.1	34.9	32.0	36.1	33.9	30.2	27.8	26.9
25 to 34 years	54.4	51.0	70.4	44.9	37.7	39.5	32.2	32.6	32.1	34.4
35 to 44 years	46.7	43.6	59.5	41.2	34.7	33.5	28.7	27.2	25.8	25.1
45 to 64 years	54.6	47.8	61.7	39.5	32.9	33.3	26.2	27.1	24.1	25.2
65 years and over	52.6	48.2	53.4	42.4	35.2	36.3	36.9	32.1	29.1	26.1
American Indian or Alaska Native Male[5]										
All ages, age-adjusted[4]	NA	NA	NA	78.9	50.9	48.3	40.7	35.8	31.5	33.5
All ages, crude	NA	NA	NA	74.6	51.7	47.6	40.1	33.6	31.3	32.2
1 to 14 years	NA	NA	NA	15.1	16.2	11.6	7.6	7.8	9.6	4.6
15 to 24 years	NA	NA	NA	126.1	77.3	75.2	69.0	56.8	44.1	47.9
25 to 34 years	NA	NA	NA	107.0	84.0	78.2	67.8	49.8	49.0	45.2
35 to 44 years	NA	NA	NA	82.8	55.8	57.0	45.2	36.3	36.9	34.3
45 to 64 years	NA	NA	NA	77.4	52.2	45.9	38.8	32.0	31.9	41.4
65 years and over	NA	NA	NA	97.0	*	43.0	*	48.5	27.8	37.4
Asian or Pacific Islander Male[5]										
All ages, age-adjusted[4]	NA	NA	NA	19.0	17.3	17.9	14.5	10.6	9.5	9.3
All ages, crude	NA	NA	NA	17.1	16.0	15.8	12.6	9.8	8.7	8.6
1 to 14 years	NA	NA	NA	8.2	5.2	6.3	4.5	2.5	1.7	2.6
15 to 24 years	NA	NA	NA	27.2	28.1	25.7	18.5	17.0	14.5	14.9
25 to 34 years	NA	NA	NA	18.8	18.4	17.0	12.4	10.4	8.9	8.4
35 to 44 years	NA	NA	NA	13.1	12.0	12.2	9.9	6.9	6.6	6.0
45 to 64 years	NA	NA	NA	13.7	13.4	15.1	14.3	10.1	9.0	8.6
65 years and over	NA	NA	NA	37.3	37.3	33.6	32.1	21.1	20.8	19.7
Hispanic or Latino Male[5,7]										
All ages, age-adjusted[4]	NA	NA	NA	NA	25.4	29.5	24.4	21.3	21.4	21.4
All ages, crude	NA	NA	NA	NA	25.6	29.2	22.4	20.1	20.8	20.9
1 to 14 years	NA	NA	NA	NA	7.7	7.2	5.7	4.4	4.6	4.4
15 to 24 years	NA	NA	NA	NA	44.9	48.2	37.1	34.7	37.6	38.1
25 to 34 years	NA	NA	NA	NA	31.2	41.0	28.8	24.9	28.0	27.6
35 to 44 years	NA	NA	NA	NA	26.3	28.0	23.2	21.6	20.9	21.6
45 to 64 years	NA	NA	NA	NA	25.9	28.9	23.0	21.7	20.2	21.6
65 years and over	NA	NA	NA	NA	22.9	35.3	37.0	28.9	27.6	24.8
White, Not Hispanic or Latino Male[7]										
All ages, age-adjusted[4]	NA	NA	NA	NA	24.9	25.7	22.1	21.7	22.2	21.8
All ages, crude	NA	NA	NA	NA	25.9	26.0	21.9	21.5	22.5	22.1
1 to 14 years	NA	NA	NA	NA	7.8	6.4	5.8	4.9	3.9	3.2
15 to 24 years	NA	NA	NA	NA	53.3	52.3	42.7	40.3	38.8	38.8
25 to 34 years	NA	NA	NA	NA	33.2	34.0	27.1	24.7	27.8	28.5
35 to 44 years	NA	NA	NA	NA	21.6	23.1	20.3	21.6	22.9	22.4
45 to 64 years	NA	NA	NA	NA	18.0	19.8	18.1	19.3	21.7	21.4
65 years and over	NA	NA	NA	NA	27.6	31.1	29.4	29.3	28.6	26.6
Black, Not Hispanic or Latino Male[7]										
All ages, age-adjusted[4]	NA	NA	NA	NA	NA	NA	NA	24.9	23.2	23.3
All ages, crude	NA	NA	NA	NA	NA	NA	NA	23.1	21.9	22.2
1 to 14 years	NA	NA	NA	NA	NA	NA	NA	5.6	4.7	5.0
15 to 24 years	NA	NA	NA	NA	NA	NA	NA	31.1	28.8	27.7
25 to 34 years	NA	NA	NA	NA	NA	NA	NA	33.6	33.7	36.4
35 to 44 years	NA	NA	NA	NA	NA	NA	NA	27.9	26.6	26.1
45 to 64 years	NA	NA	NA	NA	NA	NA	NA	27.5	24.5	25.9
65 years and over	NA	NA	NA	NA	NA	NA	NA	32.4	29.5	26.5
White Female[5]										
All ages, age-adjusted[4]	11.4	11.7	14.9	12.2	10.9	11.2	10.4	9.8	9.3	9.2
All ages, crude	10.9	11.2	14.8	12.8	11.4	11.6	10.7	10.0	9.6	9.4

NOTE: Starting with *Health, United States, 2003*, rates for 1991–1999 were revised using intercensal population estimates based on the 1990 and 2000 Censuses. For 2000, population estimates are bridged-race April 1 census counts. Starting with *Health, United States, 2012*, rates for 2001–2009 were revised using intercensal population estimates based on the 2000 and 2010 Censuses. For 2010, population estimates are bridged-race April 1 census counts. Rates for 2011 and beyond were computed using 2010-based postcensal estimates. Age groups were selected to minimize the presentation of unstable age-specific death rates based on small numbers of deaths and for consistency among comparison groups. Starting with 2003 data, some states began to collect information on more than one race on the death certificate, according to 1997 Office of Management and Budget (OMB) standards. The multiple-race data for these states were bridged to the single-race categories of the 1977 OMB standards, for comparability with other states. NA = Not available.
* = Rates based on fewer than 20 deaths are considered unreliable and are not shown.
[1]Includes deaths of persons who were not residents of the 50 states and the District of Columbia (DC).
[2]Underlying cause of death was coded according to the 6th revision of the *International Classification of Diseases (ICD)* in 1950, 7th revision in 1960, 8th revision in 1970, and 9th revision in 1980–1998.
[3]Starting with 1999 data, cause of death is coded according to *ICD–10*.
[4]Age-adjusted rates are calculated using the year 2000 standard population. Prior to 2001, age-adjusted rates were calculated using standard million proportions based on rounded population numbers. Starting with 2001 data, unrounded population numbers are used to calculate age-adjusted rates.
[5]The race groups, White, Black, Asian or Pacific Islander, and American Indian and Alaska Native, include persons of Hispanic and non-Hispanic origin. Persons of Hispanic origin may be of any race. Death rates for Hispanic, American Indian or Alaska Native, and Asian or Pacific Islander persons should be interpreted with caution because of inconsistencies in reporting Hispanic origin or race on the death certificate (death rate numerators) compared with population figures (death rate denominators). The net effect of misclassification is an underestimation of deaths and death rates for races other than White and Black.
[6]In 1950, rate is for the age group 75 years and over.
[7]Prior to 1997, excludes data from states lacking an Hispanic-origin item on the death certificate.

Table 2-33. Death Rates for Motor Vehicle–Related Injuries, by Sex, Race, Hispanic Origin, and Age, Selected Years, 1950–2016—*Continued*

(Deaths per 100,000 resident population; data are based on death certificates.)

Sex, race, Hispanic origin, and age	2007[3]	2008[3]	2009[3]	2010[3]	2011[3]	2012[3]	2013[3]	2014[3]	2015[3]	2016[3]
15 to 24 years	37.4	31.7	26.6	24.6	24.6	24.5	22.9	23.0	23.3	23.9
25 to 34 years	27.8	26.2	21.8	21.4	20.9	22.0	21.1	20.8	22.1	23.7
35 to 44 years	22.2	20.3	18.5	17.4	17.0	18.0	17.3	16.6	18.0	19.2
45 to 64 years	21.1	20.1	18.7	18.3	18.5	19.0	18.5	18.3	19.5	20.7
65 years and over	27.0	24.5	22.3	22.7	22.8	22.6	22.1	21.5	22.7	23.7
Black or African American Male[5]										
All ages, age-adjusted[4]	22.3	18.9	17.8	16.7	16.7	17.4	17.0	17.4	19.1	20.9
All ages, crude	21.0	18.0	16.7	15.9	15.8	16.6	16.4	16.8	18.7	20.3
Under 1 year	*	*	*	*	*	*	*	*	*	*
1 to 14 years[6]	4.0	3.1	3.5	3.0	2.7	3.2	3.3	2.9	3.2	3.3
15 to 24 years	26.9	22.4	18.5	19.4	17.7	17.5	17.6	18.7	21.8	23.0
25 to 34 years	32.0	27.0	26.9	24.9	22.4	25.6	25.1	25.7	26.7	30.2
35 to 44 years	27.2	23.0	21.9	19.4	20.8	20.8	20.5	21.2	23.7	27.2
45 to 64 years	24.0	21.5	19.3	19.1	20.2	20.8	20.8	21.1	24.5	23.8
65 years and over	27.4	22.9	22.8	20.0	21.3	21.8	18.5	19.8	19.6	24.7
American Indian or Alaska Native Male[5]										
All ages, age-adjusted[4]	28.6	24.1	22.7	21.1	22.5	22.2	20.0	23.4	22.8	24.5
All ages, crude	27.3	23.5	22.0	19.8	21.8	22.2	19.0	22.2	22.1	23.5
1 to 14 years	4.4	4.6	4.8	*	*	6.8	3.9	4.2	4.4	5.7
15 to 24 years	40.0	37.5	35.2	31.9	30.9	27.3	26.8	27.3	24.9	29.2
25 to 34 years	42.7	30.5	29.3	23.8	34.8	32.0	30.3	31.8	32.4	31.5
35 to 44 years	32.0	29.3	28.5	24.5	21.9	30.4	19.8	24.2	30.3	29.7
45 to 64 years	27.9	25.8	22.8	23.2	27.4	27.0	20.4	30.5	26.6	29.6
65 years and over	38.5	24.5	22.2	26.6	23.7	*	25.8	26.8	26.3	26.0
Asian or Pacific Islander Male[5]										
All ages, age-adjusted[4]	9.1	7.9	6.2	6.5	6.6	5.9	6.4	6.2	6.3	6.9
All ages, crude	8.3	7.5	5.8	6.2	6.2	5.6	5.9	6.0	6.1	6.6
1 to 14 years	1.8	1.6	1.5	*	*	*	1.5	1.2	*	1.4
15 to 24 years	15.7	11.6	8.8	9.6	9.3	8.9	8.1	8.6	9.7	9.1
25 to 34 years	7.0	8.5	7.3	7.8	6.6	5.8	5.9	8.0	6.7	6.3
35 to 44 years	6.1	6.4	4.5	4.1	4.8	3.5	5.3	4.1	3.8	5.9
45 to 64 years	7.7	7.4	5.6	6.0	6.5	6.3	5.9	5.7	6.4	7.0
65 years and over	20.9	16.1	11.9	14.6	14.9	12.5	14.3	13.1	13.5	14.5
Hispanic or Latino Male[5,7]										
All ages, age-adjusted[4]	19.4	16.7	14.7	14.0	13.7	13.9	14.2	14.3	15.2	16.1
All ages, crude	18.6	16.1	14.2	12.8	12.9	13.1	13.3	13.5	14.4	15.3
1 to 14 years	4.1	2.9	3.0	2.5	2.3	2.5	2.5	2.5	2.6	2.3
15 to 24 years	32.8	26.9	24.1	20.2	20.7	20.3	20.5	22.0	22.8	23.7
25 to 34 years	25.9	24.7	20.1	18.0	17.4	19.9	18.2	19.6	21.2	23.9
35 to 44 years	18.6	16.4	15.5	13.9	13.9	13.9	14.5	13.4	14.8	15.4
45 to 64 years	18.8	16.9	14.4	14.3	15.2	14.7	15.9	14.9	15.9	17.5
65 years and over	25.6	19.7	16.9	20.7	18.0	17.5	18.8	19.5	20.1	20.5
White, Not Hispanic or Latino Male[7]										
All ages, age-adjusted[4]	21.6	19.8	17.4	17.1	17.0	17.3	16.5	16.2	17.0	17.9
All ages, crude	22.0	20.2	17.9	17.6	17.6	18.0	17.2	16.9	17.9	18.9
1 to 14 years	3.5	3.1	2.6	2.7	2.7	2.2	2.3	2.3	2.4	2.6
15 to 24 years	37.9	32.5	26.6	25.4	25.3	25.3	23.0	22.6	22.8	23.3
25 to 34 years	27.6	26.1	21.8	21.9	21.5	22.0	21.4	20.7	21.7	23.1
35 to 44 years	22.7	20.9	18.9	18.0	17.5	18.9	17.8	17.2	18.6	20.0
45 to 64 years	21.1	20.2	19.0	18.6	18.7	19.3	18.6	18.6	19.8	21.0
65 years and over	27.0	24.7	22.6	22.7	23.0	22.9	22.3	21.5	22.8	23.8
Black, Not Hispanic or Latino Male[7]										
All ages, age-adjusted[4]	23.1	19.6	18.4	17.4	17.5	18.2	17.8	18.2	19.9	21.8
All ages, crude	21.8	18.8	17.4	16.7	16.7	17.4	17.3	17.7	19.7	21.2
1 to 14 years	4.3	3.3	3.8	3.2	2.9	3.4	3.5	3.2	3.4	3.5
15 to 24 years	27.7	23.3	19.3	20.6	18.5	18.2	18.6	19.6	22.7	24.0
25 to 34 years	33.6	28.4	28.1	26.4	24.0	27.2	26.8	27.1	28.4	31.4
35 to 44 years	28.3	24.1	22.7	20.3	22.0	21.9	21.6	22.3	25.0	28.8
45 to 64 years	24.5	22.2	19.8	19.6	20.7	21.6	22.0	21.9	25.3	24.6
65 years and over	27.8	23.4	22.8	20.2	21.9	22.2	18.8	20.3	19.9	25.2
White Female[5]										
All ages, age-adjusted[4]	8.6	7.5	6.9	6.8	6.6	6.8	6.4	6.3	6.6	7.0
All ages, crude	8.8	7.8	7.2	7.1	7.1	7.1	6.7	6.6	6.9	7.3

NOTE: Starting with *Health, United States, 2003*, rates for 1991–1999 were revised using intercensal population estimates based on the 1990 and 2000 Censuses. For 2000, population estimates are bridged-race April 1 census counts. Starting with *Health, United States, 2012*, rates for 2001–2009 were revised using intercensal population estimates based on the 2000 and 2010 Censuses. For 2010, population estimates are bridged-race April 1 census counts. Rates for 2011 and beyond were computed using 2010-based postcensal estimates. Age groups were selected to minimize the presentation of unstable age-specific death rates based on small numbers of deaths and for consistency among comparison groups. Starting with 2003 data, some states began to collect information on more than one race on the death certificate, according to 1997 Office of Management and Budget (OMB) standards. The multiple-race data for these states were bridged to the single-race categories of the 1977 OMB standards, for comparability with other states.
* = Rates based on fewer than 20 deaths are considered unreliable and are not shown.
[3] Starting with 1999 data, cause of death is coded according to *ICD–10*.
[4] Age-adjusted rates are calculated using the year 2000 standard population. Prior to 2001, age-adjusted rates were calculated using standard million proportions based on rounded population numbers. Starting with 2001 data, unrounded population numbers are used to calculate age-adjusted rates.
[5] The race groups, White, Black, Asian or Pacific Islander, and American Indian and Alaska Native, include persons of Hispanic and non-Hispanic origin. Persons of Hispanic origin may be of any race. Death rates for Hispanic, American Indian or Alaska Native, and Asian or Pacific Islander persons should be interpreted with caution because of inconsistencies in reporting Hispanic origin or race on the death certificate (death rate numerators) compared with population figures (death rate denominators). The net effect of misclassification is an underestimation of deaths and death rates for races other than White and Black.
[6] In 1950, rate is for the age group 75 years and over.
[7] Prior to 1997, excludes data from states lacking an Hispanic-origin item on the death certificate.

Table 2-33. Death Rates for Motor Vehicle–Related Injuries, by Sex, Race, Hispanic Origin, and Age, Selected Years, 1950–2016—*Continued*

(Deaths per 100,000 resident population; data are based on death certificates.)

Sex, race, Hispanic origin, and age	1950[1,2]	1960[1,2]	1970[2]	1980[2]	1985	1990[2]	1995	2000[3]	2005[3]	2006[3]
Under 1 year	7.8	7.5	10.2	7.1	3.9	4.7	4.5	3.5	3.0	3.1
1 to 14 years	7.2	6.2	7.5	6.2	5.4	4.8	4.3	3.7	3.2	3.1
15 to 24 years	12.6	15.6	22.7	23.0	20.0	19.5	18.1	17.1	15.7	15.9
25 to 34 years	9.0	9.0	12.7	12.2	10.1	11.6	10.2	8.9	9.4	9.1
35 to 44 years	8.1	8.9	12.3	10.6	9.4	9.2	8.9	8.9	9.0	9.2
45 to 64 years	12.7	13.1	15.1	10.4	9.5	9.9	8.9	8.7	8.6	8.3
65 years and over	22.2	20.8	23.7	15.3	16.2	17.4	17.5	16.2	14.5	14.0
Black or African American Female[5]										
All ages, age-adjusted[4]	9.3	10.4	14.1	8.5	8.5	9.6	9.0	8.4	7.6	7.7
All ages, crude	10.2	9.7	13.4	8.3	8.3	9.4	8.8	8.2	7.5	7.6
Under 1 year	NA	8.1	11.9	*	8.1	7.0	*	*	6.9	*
1 to 14 years[6]	7.2	6.9	10.2	6.3	5.1	5.3	4.9	3.9	3.4	3.4
15 to 24 years	11.6	9.9	13.4	8.0	9.1	9.9	10.5	11.7	10.5	9.8
25 to 34 years	10.8	9.8	13.3	10.6	9.3	11.1	10.3	9.4	7.6	8.7
35 to 44 years	11.1	11.0	16.1	8.3	9.1	9.4	9.7	8.2	7.7	8.0
45 to 64 years	11.8	12.7	16.7	9.2	9.0	10.7	9.3	9.0	8.2	8.8
65 years and over	14.3	13.2	15.7	9.5	11.2	13.5	11.4	10.4	9.9	9.5
American Indian or Alaska Native Female[5]										
All ages, age-adjusted[4]	NA	NA	NA	32.0	19.8	17.5	18.2	19.5	14.0	15.1
All ages, crude	NA	NA	NA	32.0	20.6	17.3	18.8	18.6	13.8	14.9
1 to 14 years	NA	NA	NA	15.0	9.2	8.1	8.1	6.5	*	*
15 to 24 years	NA	NA	NA	42.3	29.5	31.4	30.4	30.3	22.0	24.5
25 to 34 years	NA	NA	NA	52.5	30.2	18.8	33.7	22.3	22.1	19.1
35 to 44 years	NA	NA	NA	38.1	27.0	18.2	17.2	22.0	15.7	17.7
45 to 64 years	NA	NA	NA	32.6	19.5	17.6	15.7	17.8	10.6	13.5
65 years and over	NA	NA	NA	*	*	*	*	24.0	*	17.1
Asian or Pacific Islander Female[5]										
All ages, age-adjusted[4]	NA	NA	NA	9.3	8.8	10.4	8.6	6.7	5.7	5.4
All ages, crude	NA	NA	NA	8.2	7.9	9.0	7.7	5.9	5.3	5.1
1 to 14 years	NA	NA	NA	7.4	5.0	3.6	3.2	2.3	1.5	1.7
15 to 24 years	NA	NA	NA	7.4	7.4	11.4	11.5	6.0	7.0	6.3
25 to 34 years	NA	NA	NA	7.3	8.4	7.3	4.8	4.5	3.4	3.2
35 to 44 years	NA	NA	NA	8.6	7.0	7.5	5.9	4.9	4.3	4.1
45 to 64 years	NA	NA	NA	8.5	8.6	11.8	10.4	6.4	6.4	6.0
65 years and over	NA	NA	NA	18.6	20.5	24.3	18.9	18.5	13.9	13.6
Hispanic or Latina Female[5,7]										
All ages, age-adjusted[4]	NA	NA	NA	NA	8.8	9.6	8.8	7.9	7.8	7.6
All ages, crude	NA	NA	NA	NA	7.9	8.9	8.0	7.2	7.3	7.0
1 to 14 years	NA	NA	NA	NA	4.8	4.8	4.3	3.9	3.3	3.1
15 to 24 years	NA	NA	NA	NA	10.1	11.6	11.8	10.6	12.7	10.9
25 to 34 years	NA	NA	NA	NA	7.5	9.4	7.2	6.5	7.1	6.8
35 to 44 years	NA	NA	NA	NA	8.8	8.0	7.9	7.3	7.3	7.1
45 to 64 years	NA	NA	NA	NA	9.4	11.4	9.3	8.3	7.4	8.0
65 years and over	NA	NA	NA	NA	14.8	14.9	14.6	13.4	11.4	12.0
White, not Hispanic or Latina Female[7]										
All ages, age-adjusted[4]	NA	NA	NA	NA	10.4	11.3	10.5	10.0	9.5	9.4
All ages, crude	NA	NA	NA	NA	10.9	11.7	10.9	10.3	9.9	9.8
1 to 14 years	NA	NA	NA	NA	4.9	4.7	4.2	3.5	3.0	3.0
15 to 24 years	NA	NA	NA	NA	20.2	20.4	19.0	18.4	16.3	16.9
25 to 34 years	NA	NA	NA	NA	9.8	11.7	10.5	9.3	9.9	9.6
35 to 44 years	NA	NA	NA	NA	8.6	9.3	8.9	9.0	9.2	9.4
45 to 64 years	NA	NA	NA	NA	8.6	9.7	8.6	8.7	8.6	8.3
65 years and over	NA	NA	NA	NA	15.3	17.5	17.5	16.3	14.7	14.1
Black, not Hispanic or Latina Female[7]										
All ages, age-adjusted[4]	NA	NA	NA	NA	NA	NA	NA	8.7	7.8	8.0
All ages, crude	NA	NA	NA	NA	NA	NA	NA	8.5	7.7	7.9
1 to 14 years	NA	NA	NA	NA	NA	NA	NA	4.0	3.6	3.5
15 to 24 years	NA	NA	NA	NA	NA	NA	NA	12.3	10.8	10.2
25 to 34 years	NA	NA	NA	NA	NA	NA	NA	9.8	8.0	9.3
35 to 44 years	NA	NA	NA	NA	NA	NA	NA	8.5	7.9	8.3
45 to 64 years	NA	NA	NA	NA	NA	NA	NA	9.2	8.4	8.9
65 years and over	NA	NA	NA	NA	NA	NA	NA	10.4	10.2	9.5

NOTE: Starting with *Health, United States, 2003,* rates for 1991–1999 were revised using intercensal population estimates based on the 1990 and 2000 Censuses. For 2000, population estimates are bridged-race April 1 census counts. Starting with *Health, United States, 2012,* rates for 2001–2009 were revised using intercensal population estimates based on the 2000 and 2010 Censuses. For 2010, population estimates are bridged-race April 1 census counts. Rates for 2011 and beyond were computed using 2010-based postcensal estimates. Age groups were selected to minimize the presentation of unstable age-specific death rates based on small numbers of deaths and for consistency among comparison groups. Starting with 2003 data, some states began to collect information on more than one race on the death certificate, according to 1997 Office of Management and Budget (OMB) standards. The multiple-race data for these states were bridged to the single-race categories of the 1977 OMB standards, for comparability with other states.
NA = Not available.
* = Rates based on fewer than 20 deaths are considered unreliable and are not shown.
[1] Includes deaths of persons who were not residents of the 50 states and the District of Columbia (DC).
[2] Underlying cause of death was coded according to the 6th revision of the *International Classification of Diseases (ICD)* in 1950, 7th revision in 1960, 8th revision in 1970, and 9th revision in 1980–1998.
[3] Starting with 1999 data, cause of death is coded according to *ICD–10.*
[4] Age-adjusted rates are calculated using the year 2000 standard population. Prior to 2001, age-adjusted rates were calculated using standard million proportions based on rounded population numbers. Starting with 2001 data, unrounded population numbers are used to calculate age-adjusted rates.
[5] The race groups, White, Black, Asian or Pacific Islander, and American Indian and Alaska Native, include persons of Hispanic and non-Hispanic origin. Persons of Hispanic origin may be of any race. Death rates for Hispanic, American Indian or Alaska Native, and Asian or Pacific Islander persons should be interpreted with caution because of inconsistencies in reporting Hispanic origin or race on the death certificate (death rate numerators) compared with population figures (death rate denominators). The net effect of misclassification is an underestimation of deaths and death rates for races other than White and Black.
[6] In 1950, rate is for the age group 75 years and over.
[7] Prior to 1997, excludes data from states lacking an Hispanic-origin item on the death certificate.

Table 2-33. Death Rates for Motor Vehicle–Related Injuries, by Sex, Race, Hispanic Origin, and Age, Selected Years, 1950–2016—Continued

(Deaths per 100,000 resident population; data are based on death certificates.)

Sex, race, Hispanic origin, and age	2007³	2008³	2009³	2010³	2011³	2012³	2013³	2014³	2015³	2016³
Under 1 year	2.9	1.8	1.5	1.9	1.4	1.6	1.7	1.5	*	2.4
1 to 14 years	2.7	2.1	2.1	2.1	2.0	1.9	1.8	1.8	1.8	2.0
15 to 24 years	15.1	12.6	11.3	10.8	10.1	10.0	9.5	9.2	9.8	10.2
25 to 34 years	9.0	7.6	7.4	7.1	7.3	7.6	7.1	7.1	7.7	8.8
35 to 44 years	8.1	7.4	6.5	6.5	6.4	6.6	6.1	6.1	6.4	6.7
45 to 64 years	7.8	7.3	6.6	6.4	6.1	6.5	6.4	6.3	6.6	7.0
65 years and over	13.0	11.8	11.4	11.5	11.3	11.3	10.4	10.3	10.3	10.4
Black or African American Female⁵										
All ages, age-adjusted⁴	7.0	6.4	6.2	5.9	5.7	5.9	5.7	5.6	6.1	7.1
All ages, crude	6.9	6.3	6.1	5.8	5.7	5.9	5.7	5.6	6.1	7.1
Under 1 year	*	*	*	*	*	*	*	*	*	*
1 to 14 years⁶	3.3	2.5	2.6	2.0	2.3	2.4	2.3	2.3	2.6	3.1
15 to 24 years	9.5	8.4	8.1	7.8	7.6	7.7	7.7	7.7	8.9	10.3
25 to 34 years	7.5	7.1	7.6	6.8	7.1	7.4	7.2	6.9	7.8	9.0
35 to 44 years	7.0	6.7	6.0	5.8	5.4	5.7	6.4	5.7	6.1	7.3
45 to 64 years	7.4	7.0	6.5	6.3	5.9	6.5	6.2	6.2	6.3	7.1
65 years and over	8.7	8.4	7.9	8.6	7.6	7.7	5.9	6.4	6.8	7.6
American Indian or Alaska Native Female⁵										
All ages, age-adjusted⁴	13.5	12.8	11.8	10.6	10.8	10.2	11.0	10.1	11.2	11.3
All ages, crude	13.5	12.4	11.7	10.0	10.5	10.1	10.7	10.0	11.2	11.0
1 to 14 years	*	*	*	*	*	*	4.9	*	*	*
15 to 24 years	21.4	17.4	19.8	13.4	14.7	16.2	13.6	16.5	13.8	15.5
25 to 34 years	19.4	19.2	13.8	17.7	18.0	15.1	17.0	13.4	21.2	18.5
35 to 44 years	18.8	15.3	16.9	13.1	11.3	11.6	14.2	12.0	12.6	14.5
45 to 64 years	10.8	10.3	11.7	8.4	8.7	10.5	8.7	9.7	11.9	9.8
65 years and over	*	17.8	*	14.8	14.4	*	*	*	*	11.6
Asian or Pacific Islander Female⁵										
All ages, age-adjusted⁴	5.0	4.2	3.8	3.9	3.3	3.3	3.4	3.2	3.6	3.7
All ages, crude	4.6	3.9	3.5	3.6	3.1	3.3	3.4	3.2	3.6	3.7
1 to 14 years	*	1.4	1.5	*	*	*	*	*	*	1.2
15 to 24 years	6.7	4.5	4.3	3.3	3.7	3.0	3.0	3.0	3.4	3.4
25 to 34 years	2.9	3.1	2.9	3.1	1.9	2.8	2.5	2.5	2.6	2.7
35 to 44 years	2.7	2.2	2.1	2.0	2.3	1.7	*	2.0	1.7	1.6
45 to 64 years	5.4	4.4	3.0	4.3	3.0	4.2	4.1	3.3	4.0	4.0
65 years and over	13.4	12.1	11.4	12.2	10.2	8.7	10.8	9.4	11.2	11.6
Hispanic or Latina Female⁵,⁷										
All ages, age-adjusted⁴	6.8	5.5	5.5	5.3	4.8	5.3	5.2	5.0	5.2	6.1
All ages, crude	6.3	5.0	5.1	4.9	4.5	4.9	4.8	4.7	5.0	5.8
1 to 14 years	2.7	2.1	2.3	2.0	1.7	1.9	1.7	1.9	1.8	2.0
15 to 24 years	10.1	7.8	7.8	7.7	6.3	7.2	7.4	7.5	7.7	9.4
25 to 34 years	6.6	5.4	5.5	5.0	5.1	5.4	5.1	5.3	6.1	7.5
35 to 44 years	6.7	4.8	4.6	4.5	4.6	4.5	4.7	4.1	4.6	4.8
45 to 64 years	6.7	5.1	5.5	5.6	4.8	5.6	5.3	5.3	5.2	6.3
65 years and over	10.5	10.7	9.5	9.4	8.6	9.2	9.0	8.1	8.3	9.0
White, not Hispanic or Latina Female⁷										
All ages, age-adjusted⁴	8.8	7.9	7.1	7.0	6.9	7.0	6.6	6.5	6.8	7.1
All ages, crude	9.2	8.3	7.5	7.5	7.3	7.5	7.1	7.0	7.3	7.6
1 to 14 years	2.6	2.1	1.9	2.0	2.1	1.8	1.8	1.7	1.8	1.9
15 to 24 years	16.2	13.7	12.0	11.4	11.0	10.7	10.0	9.6	10.3	10.2
25 to 34 years	9.5	8.1	7.7	7.6	7.7	8.2	7.5	7.5	8.0	9.0
35 to 44 years	8.3	7.9	6.8	6.9	6.7	7.0	6.4	6.6	6.8	7.2
45 to 64 years	7.9	7.6	6.7	6.4	6.2	6.6	6.5	6.4	6.7	7.0
65 years and over	13.1	11.8	11.5	11.6	11.5	11.4	10.5	10.4	10.5	10.5
Black, not Hispanic or Latina Female⁷										
All ages, age-adjusted⁴	7.2	6.6	6.4	6.1	5.9	6.2	6.0	5.8	6.3	7.4
All ages, crude	7.2	6.6	6.4	6.1	5.9	6.3	6.0	5.9	6.4	7.4
1 to 14 years	3.4	2.6	2.8	2.1	2.4	2.6	2.5	2.4	2.7	3.4
15 to 24 years	10.0	8.8	8.4	8.2	8.0	8.2	8.0	8.0	9.1	10.8
25 to 34 years	8.0	7.6	7.9	7.3	7.6	7.9	7.7	7.4	8.2	9.5
35 to 44 years	7.3	6.9	6.2	6.2	5.7	6.1	6.9	6.1	6.4	7.6
45 to 64 years	7.6	7.3	6.7	6.4	6.0	6.7	6.4	6.3	6.5	7.2
65 years and over	8.9	8.5	8.0	8.7	7.8	7.8	5.9	6.4	7.0	7.7

NOTE: Starting with *Health, United States, 2003*, rates for 1991–1999 were revised using intercensal population estimates based on the 1990 and 2000 Censuses. For 2000, population estimates are bridged-race April 1 census counts. Starting with *Health, United States, 2012*, rates for 2001–2009 were revised using intercensal population estimates based on the 2000 and 2010 Censuses. For 2010, population estimates are bridged-race April 1 census counts. Rates for 2011 and beyond were computed using 2010-based postcensal estimates. Age groups were selected to minimize the presentation of unstable age-specific death rates based on small numbers of deaths and for consistency among comparison groups. Starting with 2003 data, some states began to collect information on more than one race on the death certificate, according to 1997 Office of Management and Budget (OMB) standards. The multiple-race data for these states were bridged to the single-race categories of the 1977 OMB standards, for comparability with other states.
* = Rates based on fewer than 20 deaths are considered unreliable and are not shown.
³Starting with 1999 data, cause of death is coded according to *ICD-10*.
⁴Age-adjusted rates are calculated using the year 2000 standard population. Prior to 2001, age-adjusted rates were calculated using standard million proportions based on rounded population numbers. Starting with 2001 data, unrounded population numbers are used to calculate age-adjusted rates.
⁵The race groups, White, Black, Asian or Pacific Islander, and American Indian and Alaska Native, include persons of Hispanic and non-Hispanic origin. Persons of Hispanic origin may be of any race. Death rates for Hispanic, American Indian or Alaska Native, and Asian or Pacific Islander persons should be interpreted with caution because of inconsistencies in reporting Hispanic origin or race on the death certificate (death rate numerators) compared with population figures (death rate denominators). The net effect of misclassification is an underestimate of deaths and death rates for races other than White and Black.
⁶In 1950, rate is for the age group 75 years and over.
⁷Prior to 1997, excludes data from states lacking an Hispanic-origin item on the death certificate.

Table 2-34. Occupant and Alcohol-Impaired Driving Deaths, by State, 2005–2014

(Number.)

State	Alcohol-impaired driving deaths	Occupant deaths
United States	113,001	255,297
Alabama	2,997	7,754
Alaska	205	439
Arizona	1,636	4,526
Arkansas	2,656	5,712
California	9,791	20,733
Colorado	1,599	3,521
Connecticut	1,049	1,806
Delaware	430	767
District of Columbia	96	130
Florida	8,053	16,041
Georgia	3,513	10,406
Hawaii	453	587
Idaho	661	1,725
Illinois	3,554	7,348
Indiana	2,171	5,966
Iowa	967	2,970
Kansas	1,142	3,248
Kentucky	1,900	6,133
Louisiana	2,875	6,073
Maine	454	1,231
Maryland	1,586	3,454
Massachusetts	1,309	2,465
Michigan	2,710	6,699
Minnesota	1,274	3,248
Mississippi	2,367	6,100
Missouri	3,004	7,219
Montana	897	1,778
Nebraska	631	1,919
Nevada	968	1,962
New Hampshire	386	853
New Jersey	1,747	3,832
New Mexico	1,166	2,766
New York	3,605	7,013
North Carolina	3,996	10,093
North Dakota	539	1,078
Ohio	3,457	8,223
Oklahoma	2,095	5,711
Oregon	1,129	2,735
Pennsylvania	4,355	9,656
Rhode Island	265	429
South Carolina	3,723	6,648
South Dakota	469	1,107
Tennessee	3,154	8,357
Texas	13,171	24,013
Utah	456	1,882
Vermont	199	535
Virginia	2,518	6,335
Washington	1,799	3,542
West Virginia	1,040	2,762
Wisconsin	2,300	4,572
Wyoming	484	1,195

Note: Alcohol-Impaired Driving Fatalities 2003-2012; All persons killed in crashes involving a driver with BAC >= .08 g/dL. Occupant Fatalities 2003-2012; All occupants killed where body type = 1-79.Source: Fatality Analysis Reporting System (FARS) 2003-2011 and 2012 ARF.

Table 2-35. Death Rates for Drug Overdoses, by Sex, Race, Hispanic Origin, and Age, Selected Years, 1999–2016

(Deaths per 100,000 resident population.)

Sex, race, Hispanic origin, and age	1999	2000	2001	2002	2003	2004	2005	2006	2007	2008	2009	2010	2011	2012	2013	2014	2015	2016
									Drug poisoning deaths per 100,000 resident population[1]									
All Persons																		
All ages, age-adjusted[2]	6.1	6.2	6.8	8.2	8.9	9.4	10.1	11.5	11.9	11.9	11.9	12.3	13.2	13.1	13.8	14.7	16.3	19.8
All ages, crude	6.0	6.2	6.8	8.2	8.9	9.4	10.1	11.5	12.0	12.0	12.1	12.4	13.3	13.2	13.9	14.8	16.3	19.7
Under 15 years	0.1	0.1	0.2	0.2	0.2	0.2	0.2	0.2	0.2	0.2	0.2	0.2	0.2	0.2	0.2	0.2	0.2	0.2
15 to 24 years	3.2	3.7	4.2	5.1	6.0	6.6	6.9	8.1	8.2	8.0	7.7	8.2	8.6	8.0	8.3	8.6	9.7	12.4
25 to 34 years	8.1	7.9	8.6	10.5	11.4	11.9	13.6	16.1	16.8	16.8	17.2	18.4	20.2	20.1	20.9	23.1	26.9	34.6
35 to 44 years	14.0	14.3	15.5	18.1	18.9	19.3	19.6	21.7	21.4	21.1	20.5	20.8	22.5	22.1	23.0	25.0	28.3	35.0
45 to 54 years	11.1	11.6	13.0	16.2	17.9	19.3	21.1	24.1	25.1	25.2	25.4	25.1	26.7	26.9	27.5	28.2	30.0	34.5
55 to 64 years	4.2	4.2	4.7	6.0	6.9	7.8	9.0	10.5	12.2	12.9	13.7	15.0	15.9	16.6	19.2	20.3	21.8	25.6
65 to 74 years	2.4	2.0	2.4	2.8	2.9	2.9	3.2	3.5	4.0	4.6	4.7	4.7	5.4	5.8	6.4	6.9	7.2	8.2
75 to 84 years	2.8	2.4	2.5	2.8	2.7	2.9	3.1	3.3	3.2	3.3	3.8	3.4	3.4	3.4	3.6	3.6	3.6	3.4
85 years and over	3.8	4.4	3.7	4.4	4.1	4.0	4.1	4.4	4.5	4.1	4.4	4.7	4.2	4.3	4.3	4.1	4.4	4.0
Male																		
All ages, age-adjusted[2]	8.2	8.3	9.0	10.6	11.5	11.8	12.8	14.8	14.9	14.9	14.8	15.0	16.1	16.1	17.0	18.3	20.8	26.2
All ages, crude	8.2	8.4	9.0	10.6	11.5	11.9	12.9	14.9	15.1	15.0	15.0	15.2	16.3	16.3	17.2	18.4	20.8	26.1
Under 15 years	0.1	0.2	0.2	0.2	0.2	0.2	0.2	0.2	0.3	0.2	0.2	0.3	0.2	0.2	0.2	0.2	0.2	0.2
15 to 24 years	4.5	5.3	6.1	7.3	8.8	9.6	10.0	12.0	12.0	11.9	11.3	11.6	12.4	11.4	11.7	12.1	13.3	17.5
25 to 34 years	11.5	11.3	12.0	14.7	15.7	16.6	18.7	22.7	23.4	23.6	24.0	25.0	27.5	27.0	28.6	31.9	37.9	48.9
35 to 44 years	19.2	19.5	20.6	23.4	24.3	23.8	24.4	27.5	26.7	25.6	25.2	24.9	26.8	27.1	28.1	30.8	36.3	46.9
45 to 54 years	15.2	15.7	17.0	20.3	22.6	23.8	25.8	29.7	29.2	29.6	29.1	28.5	30.4	30.4	31.5	32.9	35.3	42.5
55 to 64 years	4.9	4.4	5.3	6.8	7.8	8.6	10.6	12.3	14.0	14.8	16.0	17.3	18.5	19.4	22.7	23.5	26.2	32.2
65 to 74 years	2.7	2.1	2.7	2.8	2.9	2.9	3.3	3.5	4.4	4.8	4.8	4.5	5.4	6.2	6.9	7.3	8.5	10.0
75 to 84 years	2.5	2.5	2.6	3.1	2.9	2.8	3.4	3.2	3.2	3.2	3.5	3.6	3.4	3.2	3.7	3.8	3.9	3.7
85 years and over	4.4	5.9	3.6	5.7	4.8	4.8	5.2	4.7	4.9	4.4	5.2	5.1	4.3	5.3	5.9	4.3	5.0	4.6
Female																		
All ages, age-adjusted[2]	3.9	4.1	4.6	5.8	6.4	6.9	7.3	8.2	8.8	8.9	9.1	9.6	10.2	10.2	10.6	11.1	11.8	13.4
All ages, crude	3.9	4.1	4.6	5.8	6.4	6.9	7.4	8.3	9.0	9.0	9.2	9.8	10.3	10.3	10.7	11.3	11.9	13.5
Under 15 years	0.1	0.1	0.1	0.2	0.1	0.2	0.2	0.2	0.2	0.2	0.2	0.2	0.2	0.2	0.2	0.2	0.3	0.2
15 to 24 years	1.8	1.9	2.2	2.8	3.1	3.3	3.5	3.9	4.2	4.0	4.1	4.6	4.6	4.4	4.8	5.0	5.9	7.0
25 to 34 years	4.6	4.6	5.2	6.2	7.1	7.2	8.5	9.5	10.1	9.9	10.4	11.9	12.8	13.1	13.0	14.1	15.7	19.9
35 to 44 years	8.7	9.2	10.4	12.8	13.7	14.8	14.8	15.9	16.1	16.5	16.0	16.8	18.2	17.1	18.0	19.2	20.5	23.3
45 to 54 years	7.2	7.7	9.1	12.2	13.5	15.0	16.5	18.6	21.0	21.0	21.8	21.8	23.1	23.4	23.6	23.7	24.9	26.7
55 to 64 years	3.5	3.9	4.2	5.2	6.1	7.0	7.5	8.8	10.5	11.1	11.6	12.9	13.5	14.0	15.9	17.2	17.6	19.5
65 to 74 years	2.1	2.0	2.2	2.8	2.9	3.0	3.1	3.6	3.7	4.4	4.6	4.8	5.3	5.5	5.9	6.5	6.1	6.5
75 to 84 years	3.0	2.3	2.4	2.6	2.6	2.9	2.9	3.3	3.2	3.3	3.9	3.3	3.4	3.5	3.4	3.5	3.3	3.2
85 years and over	3.5	3.9	3.7	3.9	3.8	3.7	3.7	4.2	4.3	4.0	3.9	4.5	4.2	3.8	3.5	4.0	4.1	3.6
All Ages, Age-Adjusted[2,3]																		
White male	8.1	8.4	9.2	11.1	12.2	12.6	13.6	15.7	16.3	16.5	16.4	16.8	18.1	18.1	19.0	20.4	23.2	28.8
Black or African American male	11.5	10.8	11.0	11.5	11.3	11.1	12.8	15.2	13.0	11.3	10.8	10.1	11.0	11.3	12.9	13.8	16.8	24.0
American Indian or Alaska Native male	5.7	6.1	5.9	8.2	9.4	11.2	10.8	13.0	10.5	13.5	14.2	11.8	12.9	12.8	12.9	15.9	16.0	17.7
Asian or Pacific Islander male	1.5	1.4	1.6	1.9	1.7	2.1	2.2	2.3	2.2	2.1	2.8	2.5	3.2	3.1	3.2	3.3	4.1	4.7
Hispanic or Latino male	8.6	7.1	6.7	8.0	8.3	7.5	8.4	9.1	8.7	8.4	8.2	7.6	8.1	8.5	9.2	9.3	10.9	13.9
White, not Hispanic or Latino male	8.0	8.6	9.6	11.6	12.9	13.7	14.7	17.2	18.0	18.3	18.3	19.0	20.5	20.4	21.4	23.2	26.2	32.7
Black, not Hispanic or Latino male	11.5	10.9	11.2	11.7	11.6	11.4	13.0	15.7	13.3	11.6	11.1	10.5	11.3	11.6	13.3	14.2	17.3	24.7
White female	4.0	4.3	4.9	6.2	6.9	7.5	8.0	9.0	9.8	10.1	10.3	10.9	11.7	11.6	12.1	12.7	13.6	15.2
Black or African American female	3.9	4.1	4.4	5.0	5.2	5.5	6.0	6.3	6.3	5.4	5.6	5.7	5.9	6.0	6.3	7.0	7.5	10.0
American Indian or Alaska Native female	4.6	3.7	5.2	5.6	7.3	7.9	8.6	7.9	9.9	8.8	9.6	9.7	10.7	12.2	11.6	11.2	11.3	13.1
Asian or Pacific Islander female	1.0	0.8	0.8	1.1	1.2	1.1	1.3	1.4	1.6	1.3	1.3	1.5	1.6	1.4	1.5	1.7	1.5	1.8
Hispanic or Latina female	2.2	2.0	2.2	2.7	2.9	2.9	3.0	3.4	3.1	3.2	3.5	3.6	4.0	4.0	4.1	4.1	4.4	5.0
White, not Hispanic or Latina female	4.3	4.5	5.3	6.8	7.5	8.3	8.8	10.0	11.0	11.4	11.6	12.5	13.3	13.2	13.8	14.6	15.8	17.7
Black, not Hispanic or Latina female	4.0	4.2	4.4	5.1	5.4	5.6	6.2	6.5	6.5	5.6	5.6	5.8	5.9	6.2	6.2	6.5	7.3	10.4

NOTE: Rates for 1999 were computed using intercensal population estimates based on the 1990 and 2000 Censuses. Rates for 2000 were computed based on 2000 bridged-race April 1 census counts. Starting with *Health, United States, 2012*, rates for 2001–2009 were revised using intercensal population estimates based on the 2000 and 2010 Censuses. Rates for 2010 were based on 2010 bridged-race April 1 census counts. Rates for 2011 and beyond were computed using 2010-based postcensal estimates. Age groups were selected to minimize the presentation of unstable age-specific death rates based on small numbers of deaths and for consistency among comparison groups. For additional injury-related statistics, see the Web-based Injury Statistics Query and Reporting System (WISQARS), available from: https://www.cdc.gov/injury/wisqars/index.html. Starting with 2003 data, some states allowed the reporting of more than one race on the death certificate. The multiple-race data for these states were bridged to the single-race categories of the 1977 Office of Management and Budget standards, for comparability with other states.

[1] Drug overdose was coded using underlying cause of death according to the 10th revision of the *International Classification of Diseases* (*ICD–10*). Drug overdose deaths include those resulting from accidental or intentional overdose of a drug, being given the wrong drug, taking the wrong drug in error, taking a drug inadvertently, or other misuses of drugs. These deaths are from all manners and intents, including unintentional, suicide, homicide, legal intervention, operations of war, and undetermined intent.

[2] Age-adjusted rates are calculated using the year 2000 standard population with unrounded population numbers.

[3] The race groups White, Black, Asian or Pacific Islander, and American Indian or Alaska Native include persons of Hispanic and non-Hispanic origin. Persons of Hispanic origin may be of any race. Death rates for Hispanic, American Indian or Alaska Native, and Asian or Pacific Islander persons should be interpreted with caution because of inconsistencies in reporting Hispanic origin or race on the death certificate (death rate numerators) compared with population figures (death rate denominators). The net effect of misclassification is an underestimation of deaths and death rates for races other than White and Black.

Table 2-35. Death Rates for Drug Overdoses, by Sex, Race, Hispanic Origin, and Age, Selected Years, 1999–2016—*Continued*

(Deaths per 100,000 resident population.)

Sex, race, Hispanic origin, and age	1999	2000	2001	2002	2003	2004	2005	2006	2007	2008	2009	2010	2011	2012	2013	2014	2015	2016
	Drug overdose deaths involving any opioid per 100,000 resident population (T40.0–T40.4, 40.6)[4]																	
All Persons																		
All ages, age-adjusted[2]	2.9	3.0	3.3	4.1	4.5	4.7	5.1	5.9	6.1	6.4	6.6	6.8	7.3	7.4	7.9	9.0	10.4	13.3
All ages, crude	2.9	3.0	3.3	4.1	4.5	4.7	5.0	5.9	6.1	6.4	6.7	6.8	7.3	7.4	7.9	9.0	10.3	13.1
Under 15 years	*	0.1	0.1	0.1	0.1	0.1	0.1	0.1	0.1	0.1	0.1	0.1	0.1	0.1	0.1	0.1	0.1	0.1
15 to 24 years	1.6	1.9	2.3	2.9	3.4	3.8	4.0	4.9	5.0	5.3	5.1	5.5	5.8	5.3	5.7	6.2	7.0	9.3
25 to 34 years	4.1	4.1	4.4	5.6	6.2	6.6	7.4	9.0	9.6	10.0	10.7	11.4	12.6	12.8	13.8	16.2	19.4	25.9
35 to 44 years	7.2	7.3	7.8	9.5	9.6	9.7	9.6	10.8	11.0	11.2	11.3	11.6	12.4	12.6	13.3	15.6	18.4	24.1
45 to 54 years	5.4	5.8	6.6	8.4	9.2	9.6	10.7	12.2	12.5	13.2	13.4	13.2	14.0	14.2	14.8	16.1	17.6	21.2
55 to 64 years	1.5	1.6	2.0	2.4	2.9	3.4	3.9	4.8	5.6	6.2	7.0	7.4	7.8	8.3	9.9	11.1	12.4	15.2
65 to 74 years	0.5	0.5	0.5	0.8	0.9	1.0	1.2	1.2	1.4	1.7	1.9	1.7	2.1	2.3	2.7	3.3	3.5	4.2
75 to 84 years	0.4	0.3	0.4	0.5	0.5	0.6	0.7	0.8	0.7	0.7	0.9	0.8	0.8	1.0	0.9	1.0	1.2	1.2
85 years and over	*	*	0.5	0.8	0.7	0.8	1.0	0.8	1.1	0.8	0.8	1.3	0.9	0.9	1.0	1.1	0.9	0.9
Male																		
All ages, age-adjusted[2]	4.3	4.4	4.8	5.7	6.1	6.3	6.6	7.8	8.0	8.4	8.7	8.7	9.4	9.5	10.2	11.7	13.7	18.1
All ages, crude	4.4	4.4	4.8	5.8	6.2	6.3	6.7	7.9	8.1	8.5	8.7	8.8	9.4	9.5	10.3	11.7	13.7	17.9
Under 15 years	*	0.1	0.1	0.1	0.1	0.1	0.1	0.1	0.1	0.1	0.1	0.2	0.1	0.1	0.1	0.1	0.1	0.1
15 to 24 years	2.4	2.9	3.6	4.3	5.2	5.9	6.0	7.5	7.6	8.1	7.7	8.0	8.6	7.9	8.2	8.9	9.8	13.4
25 to 34 years	6.3	6.2	6.6	8.2	8.9	9.4	10.5	13.1	13.9	14.7	15.6	16.2	17.9	17.8	19.7	23.4	28.2	37.3
35 to 44 years	10.9	10.7	11.0	12.9	13.0	12.5	12.3	14.2	14.1	14.4	14.8	14.7	15.6	16.3	16.9	20.1	24.5	33.3
45 to 54 years	8.2	8.6	9.4	11.4	12.3	12.3	13.6	15.3	14.8	16.0	15.8	15.4	16.3	16.6	17.4	19.2	21.2	26.8
55 to 64 years	2.0	1.9	2.4	3.1	3.6	4.1	4.7	5.6	6.5	7.3	8.3	8.7	9.2	10.1	11.9	13.4	15.3	19.3
65 to 74 years	0.7	0.5	0.6	0.8	1.0	1.0	1.0	1.3	1.4	1.8	1.9	1.6	2.0	2.4	2.8	3.4	4.4	5.3
75 to 84 years	0.5	*	0.5	0.5	0.4	0.5	0.6	0.7	0.6	0.6	0.8	0.8	0.8	0.9	1.0	1.0	1.2	1.4
85 years and over	*	*	*	*	*	*	*	*	1.4	*	1.3	1.4	*	1.0	1.5	0.9	0.9	1.0
Female																		
All ages, age-adjusted[2]	1.4	1.6	1.9	2.6	2.8	3.1	3.4	3.9	4.3	4.4	4.6	4.9	5.2	5.3	5.6	6.3	7.1	8.5
All ages, crude	1.4	1.6	1.9	2.6	2.8	3.1	3.4	3.9	4.3	4.4	4.7	4.9	5.3	5.3	5.6	6.3	7.0	8.4
Under 15 years	*	*	*	*	*	0.1	*	0.1	0.1	0.1	0.1	0.1	0.1	0.1	0.1	0.1	0.1	0.1
15 to 24 years	0.7	0.7	1.0	1.4	1.5	1.6	1.8	2.1	2.3	2.3	2.5	2.8	2.9	2.7	3.0	3.3	4.1	4.9
25 to 34 years	2.0	2.0	2.3	3.0	3.3	3.6	4.3	4.8	5.3	5.2	5.8	6.6	7.3	7.7	7.7	8.8	10.5	14.1
35 to 44 years	3.5	3.8	4.6	6.1	6.2	6.8	6.9	7.4	7.8	8.0	8.0	8.5	9.3	8.9	9.8	11.2	12.5	15.0
45 to 54 years	2.7	3.1	3.8	5.5	6.2	7.0	7.8	9.3	10.2	10.5	11.1	11.1	11.7	12.0	12.2	13.1	14.0	15.8
55 to 64 years	1.1	1.4	1.5	1.8	2.3	2.8	3.2	4.0	4.7	5.1	5.8	6.2	6.4	6.7	7.9	9.0	9.8	11.5
65 to 74 years	0.4	0.5	0.5	0.9	0.8	1.0	1.4	1.2	1.4	1.6	1.9	1.8	2.1	2.2	2.6	3.1	2.8	3.3
75 to 84 years	0.4	*	0.4	0.4	0.6	0.7	0.7	0.8	0.8	0.9	1.0	0.8	0.7	1.0	0.8	1.1	1.1	1.1
85 years and over	*	*	*	0.6	0.8	*	0.9	0.9	0.9	0.9	0.6	1.2	0.9	0.9	0.8	1.2	0.9	0.8
All Ages, Age-Adjusted[2,3]																		
White male	4.4	4.5	5.0	6.1	6.7	7.0	7.4	8.7	9.1	9.7	9.9	10.1	10.8	11.0	11.7	13.4	15.8	20.4
Black or African American male	5.7	5.6	5.3	5.3	5.0	4.4	4.8	6.0	4.6	4.5	4.7	4.1	4.7	5.1	6.3	7.4	9.1	14.7
American Indian or Alaska Native male	3.2	3.4	3.0	4.4	5.1	6.2	5.7	6.9	5.8	8.0	10.0	6.3	7.2	7.9	7.2	9.7	9.3	10.2
Asian or Pacific Islander male	*	0.5	0.4	0.5	0.5	0.7	0.9	0.8	0.7	0.7	0.9	0.9	1.3	1.1	1.3	1.4	1.7	2.3
Hispanic or Latino male	5.8	4.5	4.2	4.8	5.1	4.3	4.5	4.9	4.9	5.1	4.8	4.1	4.6	5.0	5.6	5.7	6.7	9.2
White, not Hispanic or Latino male	4.1	4.4	5.1	6.4	7.0	7.6	8.0	9.6	10.1	10.8	11.1	11.6	12.4	12.5	13.3	15.5	18.1	23.4
Black, not Hispanic or Latino male	5.7	5.7	5.4	5.4	5.1	4.5	4.8	6.2	4.7	4.5	4.9	4.3	4.9	5.3	6.5	7.6	9.3	15.1
White female	1.5	1.7	2.1	2.8	3.1	3.5	3.8	4.4	4.9	5.0	5.3	5.6	6.1	6.1	6.6	7.4	8.2	9.7
Black or African American female	1.5	1.5	1.6	2.0	2.0	2.0	2.1	2.4	2.4	2.3	2.4	2.5	2.6	2.8	3.0	3.6	4.0	5.9
American Indian or Alaska Native female	1.9	1.4	2.5	2.6	3.3	3.3	4.6	3.6	5.2	5.2	5.3	5.7	5.9	6.8	6.5	5.8	6.5	7.6
Asian or Pacific Islander female	*	*	*	*	*	0.3	0.4	0.4	0.4	0.5	0.4	0.5	0.5	0.5	0.4	0.6	0.5	0.8
Hispanic or Latina female	1.0	0.8	1.0	1.5	1.3	1.4	1.4	1.6	1.5	1.6	1.6	1.6	1.9	1.9	2.1	2.3	2.4	3.0
White, not Hispanic or Latino female	1.6	1.8	2.2	3.1	3.4	3.9	4.3	4.9	5.5	5.7	6.1	6.5	7.0	7.0	7.6	8.5	9.6	11.4
Black, not Hispanic or Latina female	1.6	1.6	1.6	2.0	2.1	2.1	2.2	2.5	2.5	2.4	2.5	2.6	2.7	2.9	3.1	3.7	4.1	6.1

NOTE: Rates for 1999 were computed using intercensal population estimates based on the 1990 and 2000 Censuses. Rates for 2000 were computed based on 2000 bridged-race April 1 census counts. Starting with *Health, United States, 2012*, rates for 2001–2009 were revised using intercensal population estimates based on the 2000 and 2010 Censuses. Rates for 2010 were based on 2010 bridged-race April 1 census counts. Rates for 2011 and beyond were computed using 2010-based postcensal estimates. Age groups were selected to minimize the presentation of unstable age-specific death rates based on small numbers of deaths and for consistency among comparison groups. For additional injury-related statistics, see the Web-based Injury Statistics Query and Reporting System (WISQARS), available from: https://www.cdc.gov/injury/wisqars/index.html. Starting with 2003 data, some states allowed the reporting of more than one race on the death certificate. The multiple-race data for these states are bridged to the single-race categories of the 1977 Office of Management and Budget standards, for comparability with other states.

* = Rates based on fewer than 20 deaths are considered unreliable and are not shown.

[2] Age-adjusted rates are calculated using the year 2000 standard population with unrounded population numbers.

[3] The race groups White, Black, Asian or Pacific Islander, and American Indian or Alaska Native include persons of Hispanic and non-Hispanic origin. Persons of Hispanic origin may be of any race. Death rates for Hispanic, American Indian or Alaska Native, and Asian or Pacific Islander persons should be interpreted with caution because of inconsistencies in reporting Hispanic origin or race on the death certificate (death rate numerators) compared with population figures (death rate denominators). The net effect of misclassification is an underestimation of deaths and death rates for races other than White and Black.

[4] Drug overdose deaths involving opioids include those with an underlying cause of drug overdose and with an opioid mentioned in the *ICD–10* multiple causes of death. The Any opioid category is defined by multiple cause-of-death codes T40.0–T40.4 and T40.6. The Natural and semisynthetic opioids category, which includes codeine, oxycodone, and morphine, among other drugs, is defined by multiple cause-of-death code T40.2. The Other synthetic opioids (other than methadone) category, which includes fentanyl, tramadol, and propoxyphene (removed from the market in 2010), is defined by multiple cause-of-death code T40.4. A sharp increase in deaths involving synthetic opioids, other than methadone, in 2014 coincided with law enforcement reports of increased availability of illicitly manufactured, or nonpharmaceutical, fentanyl. Illicitly manufactured fentanyl cannot be distinguished from pharmaceutical fentanyl in death certificate data. For more information, see the Centers for Disease Control and Prevention's health advisory: Increases in fentanyl drug confiscations and fentanyl-related overdose fatalities. 2015. Available from: https://emergency.cdc.gov/han/han00384.asp, and Rudd RA, Aleshire N, Zibbell JE, Gladden M. Increases in drug and opioid overdose deaths—United States, 2000–2014. MMWR Morb Mortal Wkly Rep 64(50–51):1378–82. 2016 . Available from: https://www.cdc.gov/mmwr/preview/mmwrhtml/mm6450a3.htm?s_cid=mm6450a3_w. Drug overdose deaths involving heroin include those with an underlying cause of drug overdose and with heroin mentioned in the *ICD–10* multiple causes of death. Metabolic breakdown of heroin into morphine in the body can make it difficult to distinguish between deaths from heroin and deaths from morphine based on the information on the death certificate. Some deaths reported to involve morphine could be deaths from heroin. This may result in an undercount of heroin-related deaths. For more information, see Hedegaard H, Chen LH, Warner M. Drug-poisoning deaths involving heroin: United States, 2000–2013. NCHS Data Brief, no 190. Hyattsville, MD: National Center for Health Statistics. 2015. Available from: https://www.cdc.gov/nchs/data/databriefs/db190.htm. See Appendix I, National Vital Statistics System (NVSS), Mortality Multiple Cause-of-Death File, See Appendix II, Cause of death; Table IV. Drug overdose deaths may involve multiple drugs. Deaths involving multiple drugs, for example heroin and oxycodone, are included in the death rate for natural and semisynthetic opioids and the death rate for heroin. For more information on the type of drugs commonly involved in drug-overdose deaths, see: Warner M, Trinidad JP, Bastian BA, Minin o AM, Hedegaard H. Drugs most frequently involved in drug overdose deaths: United States, 2010–2014. National Vital Statistics Reports; vol 65 no 10. Hyattsville, MD: National Center for Health Statistics. 2016. Available from: https://www.cdc.gov/nchs/data/nvsr/nvsr65/nvsr65_10.pdf. In 1999–2016, 15%–25% of drug-overdose deaths did not include specific information on the death certificate on the type of drug that was involved. Some of these deaths could have potentially involved heroin or opioids. For more information, see Warner M, Hedegaard H, Chen LH. Trends in drug-poisoning deaths involving opioid analgesics and heroin: United States, 1999–2012. NCHS Health E-Stats. 2014. Available from: https://www.cdc.gov/nchs/data/hestat/drug_poisoning/drug_poisoning.htm. For more information on the enhancement of mortality statistics using information from the death certificate, see: Trinidad JP, Warner M, Bastian BA, Minin o AM, Hedegaard H. Using literal text from the death certificate to enhance mortality statistics: Characterizing drug involvement in deaths. National Vital Statistics Reports; vol 65 no 9. Hyattsville, MD: National Center for Health Statistics. 2016. Available from: https://www.cdc.gov/nchs/data/nvsr/nvsr65/nvsr65_09.pdf.

Table 2-35. Death Rates for Drug Overdoses, by Sex, Race, Hispanic Origin, and Age, Selected Years, 1999–2016—*Continued*

(Deaths per 100,000 resident population.)

Sex, race, Hispanic origin, and age	1999	2000	2001	2002	2003	2004	2005	2006	2007	2008	2009	2010	2011	2012	2013	2014	2015	2016
	Drug overdose deaths involving natural and semisynthetic opioids per 100,000 resident population (T40.2)[4]																	
All Persons																		
All ages, age-adjusted[2]	1.0	1.0	1.2	1.5	1.7	1.8	1.9	2.3	2.7	3.0	3.1	3.5	3.7	3.5	3.5	3.8	3.9	4.4
All ages, crude	1.0	1.0	1.2	1.5	1.7	1.8	2.0	2.4	2.7	3.0	3.2	3.5	3.8	3.5	3.6	3.8	4.0	4.5
Under 15 years	*	*	0.0	0.0	0.0	0.1	0.0	0.0	0.1	0.1	0.1	0.1	0.1	0.1	0.1	0.1	0.1	0.1
15 to 24 years	0.5	0.5	0.9	0.9	1.1	1.2	1.2	1.6	1.8	2.0	2.0	2.4	2.4	1.9	1.7	1.7	1.6	2.3
25 to 34 years	1.3	1.3	1.4	1.9	2.1	2.1	2.5	3.2	3.8	4.1	4.5	5.3	5.6	4.9	4.9	4.9	5.3	6.3
35 to 44 years	2.3	2.4	2.8	3.4	3.5	3.6	3.7	4.2	4.8	5.2	5.5	6.1	6.5	6.2	5.9	6.5	6.9	7.7
45 to 54 years	2.0	2.2	2.5	3.3	3.6	3.9	4.4	5.1	5.8	6.5	6.8	7.3	7.9	7.6	7.8	8.0	8.1	8.7
55 to 64 years	0.7	0.7	0.9	1.1	1.4	1.7	1.9	2.4	3.0	3.4	3.7	4.2	4.5	4.7	5.4	6.1	6.4	7.2
65 to 74 years	0.3	0.3	0.3	0.4	0.5	0.5	0.7	0.7	0.8	1.0	1.2	1.1	1.4	1.6	1.7	2.1	2.1	2.3
75 to 84 years	0.2	*	0.2	0.3	0.3	0.4	0.4	0.4	0.4	0.4	0.5	0.6	0.6	0.6	0.6	0.8	0.9	0.9
85 years and over	*	*	*	*	0.5	*	0.6	0.5	0.7	0.5	0.5	0.9	0.7	0.7	0.8	0.7	0.7	0.6
Male																		
All ages, age-adjusted[2]	1.4	1.4	1.6	2.0	2.2	2.2	2.4	2.9	3.3	3.7	3.8	4.3	4.4	4.0	4.1	4.2	4.4	5.2
All ages, crude	1.4	1.5	1.7	2.0	2.2	2.3	2.4	2.9	3.3	3.7	3.9	4.4	4.5	4.1	4.1	4.3	4.5	5.3
Under 15 years	*	*	*	*	*	*	*	*	*	0.1	0.1	0.1	0.1	0.1	0.1	0.1	0.1	0.1
15 to 24 years	0.7	0.8	1.3	1.3	1.7	1.8	1.9	2.3	2.6	3.0	2.8	3.5	3.3	2.7	2.6	2.3	2.2	3.3
25 to 34 years	2.0	1.9	2.0	2.7	2.9	2.9	3.4	4.4	5.2	5.9	6.3	7.1	7.5	6.3	6.4	6.5	7.0	8.4
35 to 44 years	3.6	3.4	3.7	4.4	4.5	4.5	4.4	5.3	5.8	6.3	6.6	7.5	7.7	7.1	6.6	7.2	7.8	9.1
45 to 54 years	2.8	3.1	3.3	4.2	4.5	4.7	5.3	5.8	6.4	7.4	7.6	8.3	8.6	8.0	8.2	8.4	8.2	9.3
55 to 64 years	0.8	0.7	0.9	1.3	1.6	1.8	2.0	2.6	3.3	3.7	4.1	4.7	5.0	5.0	5.7	6.3	6.8	7.8
65 to 74 years	0.4	0.3	0.3	0.4	0.5	0.5	0.5	0.7	0.8	1.1	1.2	1.0	1.2	1.6	1.6	1.9	2.3	2.4
75 to 84 years	*	*	*	*	*	*	0.4	*	*	*	0.5	0.5	0.6	0.5	0.7	0.7	0.9	0.9
85 years and over	*	*	*	*	*	*	*	*	*	*	*	*	*	*	*	1.1	*	*
Female																		
All ages, age-adjusted[2]	0.5	0.6	0.8	1.1	1.2	1.3	1.5	1.8	2.1	2.3	2.4	2.7	3.0	3.0	3.0	3.3	3.4	3.6
All ages, crude	0.5	0.6	0.8	1.1	1.2	1.3	1.5	1.8	2.1	2.3	2.5	2.8	3.0	3.0	3.1	3.4	3.4	3.7
Under 15 years	*	*	*	*	*	*	*	*	0.1	0.1	*	*	*	*	*	0.1	0.1	0.1
15 to 24 years	0.3	0.3	0.3	0.5	0.5	0.5	0.6	0.8	0.9	0.9	1.0	1.3	1.4	1.1	0.9	0.9	1.0	1.2
25 to 34 years	0.7	0.8	0.8	1.1	1.3	1.3	1.6	2.0	2.4	2.4	2.7	3.4	3.6	3.5	3.3	3.2	3.5	4.2
35 to 44 years	1.1	1.4	1.9	2.4	2.5	2.8	2.9	3.2	3.9	4.2	4.4	4.8	5.3	5.3	5.2	5.9	6.1	6.3
45 to 54 years	1.1	1.3	1.8	2.4	2.8	3.2	3.5	4.5	5.2	5.6	6.0	6.4	7.1	7.2	7.3	7.7	7.9	8.1
55 to 64 years	0.6	0.7	0.8	1.0	1.3	1.5	1.7	2.3	2.6	3.1	3.4	3.6	4.0	4.5	5.0	5.9	5.9	6.5
65 to 74 years	0.2	0.3	0.3	0.5	0.5	0.6	0.8	0.8	0.8	1.0	1.1	1.3	1.5	1.5	1.8	2.3	1.9	2.3
75 to 84 years	*	*	*	0.3	0.4	0.4	0.5	0.4	0.4	0.6	0.6	0.5	0.5	0.7	0.6	0.8	0.9	0.8
85 years and over	*	*	*	*	*	*	*	0.6	*	0.7	*	0.8	0.7	0.6	0.7	0.8	0.7	0.5
All Ages, Age-Adjusted[2,3]																		
White male	1.6	1.6	1.8	2.2	2.5	2.6	2.7	3.3	3.8	4.3	4.5	5.1	5.3	4.7	4.7	4.9	5.1	6.0
Black or African American male	1.0	0.9	0.9	1.0	0.9	1.1	1.1	1.2	1.2	1.4	1.5	1.5	1.5	1.5	1.8	2.2	2.3	3.1
American Indian or Alaska Native male	*	*	*	2.0	1.6	2.2	2.2	3.2	2.2	3.3	4.2	3.6	3.1	4.2	3.6	4.4	4.3	3.6
Asian or Pacific Islander male	*	*	*	0.4	*	*	0.3	0.4	0.3	0.3	0.5	0.5	0.7	0.5	0.6	0.6	0.6	0.7
Hispanic or Latino male	2.3	1.5	1.4	1.7	1.7	1.4	1.5	1.7	2.0	2.0	1.9	1.6	1.9	1.7	2.0	1.7	1.8	2.1
White, not Hispanic or Latino male	1.4	1.6	1.9	2.4	2.6	2.8	3.0	3.6	4.2	4.8	5.0	5.9	6.0	5.4	5.4	5.6	6.0	7.0
Black, not Hispanic or Latino male	1.0	0.9	0.9	1.0	0.9	1.1	1.2	1.3	1.2	1.4	1.5	1.5	1.6	1.6	1.8	2.2	2.4	3.3
White female	0.6	0.7	0.9	1.2	1.4	1.5	1.7	2.1	2.4	2.6	2.8	3.2	3.5	3.5	3.5	3.8	3.9	4.2
Black or African American female	0.3	0.3	0.4	0.6	0.6	0.7	0.8	0.8	0.9	1.0	1.2	1.3	1.3	1.5	1.5	1.7	1.8	2.2
American Indian or Alaska Native female	*	*	*	*	1.6	1.5	1.9	1.2	2.7	2.1	3.0	2.8	3.0	3.6	3.7	3.8	3.3	3.5
Asian or Pacific Islander female	*	*	*	*	*	*	*	*	*	*	0.4	0.3	0.4	0.3	0.4	0.2	0.3	0.4
Hispanic or Latina female	0.3	0.3	0.3	0.6	0.5	0.6	0.6	0.8	0.7	0.8	0.8	0.8	0.9	1.1	1.0	1.1	1.1	1.2
White, not Hispanic or Latino female	0.6	0.8	1.0	1.3	1.5	1.7	1.9	2.3	2.7	3.0	3.2	3.6	4.1	3.9	4.0	4.4	4.6	4.9
Black, not Hispanic or Latina female	0.3	0.3	0.4	0.6	0.6	0.7	0.8	0.9	0.9	1.1	1.2	1.3	1.4	1.5	1.5	1.8	1.9	2.3

NOTE: Rates for 1999 were computed using intercensal population estimates based on the 1990 and 2000 Censuses. Rates for 2000 were computed based on 2000 bridged-race April 1 census counts. Starting with *Health, United States, 2012*, rates for 2001–2009 were revised using intercensal population estimates based on the 2000 and 2010 Censuses. Rates for 2010 were based on 2010 bridged-race April 1 census counts. Rates for 2011 and beyond were computed using 2010-based postcensal estimates. Age groups were selected to minimize the presentation of unstable age-specific death rates based on small numbers of deaths and for consistency among comparison groups. For additional injury-related statistics, see the Web-based Injury Statistics Query and Reporting System (WISQARS), available from: https://www.cdc.gov/injury/wisqars/index.html. Starting with 2003 data, some states allowed the reporting of more than one race on the death certificate. The multiple-race data for these states were bridged to the single-race categories of the 1977 Office of Management and Budget standards, for comparability with other states.

0.0 = Rate more than zero but less than 0.05.

* = Rates based on fewer than 20 deaths are considered unreliable and are not shown.

[2]Age-adjusted rates are calculated using the year 2000 standard population with unrounded population numbers.

[3]The race groups White, Black, Asian or Pacific Islander, and American Indian or Alaska Native include persons of Hispanic and non-Hispanic origin. Persons of Hispanic origin may be of any race. Death rates for Hispanic, American Indian or Alaska Native, and Asian or Pacific Islander persons should be interpreted with caution because of inconsistencies in reporting Hispanic origin or race on the death certificate (death rate numerators) compared with population figures (death rate denominators). The net effect of misclassification is an underestimation of deaths and death rates for races other than White and Black.

[4]Drug overdose deaths involving opioids include those with an underlying cause of drug overdose and with an opioid mentioned in the *ICD–10* multiple causes of death. The Any opioid category is defined by multiple cause-of-death codes T40.0–T40.4 and T40.6. The Natural and semisynthetic opioids category, which includes codeine, oxycodone, and morphine, among other drugs, is defined by multiple cause-of-death code T40.2. The Other synthetic opioids (other than methadone) category, which includes fentanyl, tramadol, and propoxyphene (removed from the market in 2010), is defined by multiple cause-of-death code T40.4. A sharp increase in deaths involving synthetic opioids, other than methadone, in 2014 coincided with law enforcement reports of increased availability of illicitly manufactured, or nonpharmaceutical, fentanyl. Illicitly manufactured fentanyl cannot be distinguished from pharmaceutical fentanyl in death certificate data. For more information, see the Centers for Disease Control and Prevention's health advisory: Increases in fentanyl drug confiscations and fentanyl-related overdose fatalities. 2015. Available from: https://emergency.cdc.gov/han/han00384.asp, and Rudd RA, Aleshire N, Zibbell JE, Gladden M. Increases in drug and opioid overdose deaths—United States, 2000–2014. MMWR Morb Mortal Wkly Rep 64(50–51):1378–82. 2016 . Available from: https://www.cdc.gov/mmwr/preview/mmwrhtml/mm6450a3.htm?s_cid=mm6450a3_w. Drug overdose deaths involving heroin include those with an underlying cause of drug overdose and with heroin mentioned in the *ICD–10* multiple causes of death. Metabolic breakdown of heroin into morphine in the body can make it difficult to distinguish between deaths from heroin and deaths from morphine based on the information on the death certificate. Some deaths reported to involve morphine could be deaths from heroin. This may result in an undercount of heroin-related deaths. For more information, see Hedegaard H, Chen LH, Warner M. Drug-poisoning deaths involving heroin: United States, 2000–2013. NCHS Data Brief, no 190. Hyattsville, MD: National Center for Health Statistics. 2015. Available from: https://www.cdc.gov/nchs/data/databriefs/db190.htm. See Appendix I, National Vital Statistics System (NVSS), Mortality Multiple Cause-of-Death File, See Appendix II, Cause of death; Table IV. Drug overdose deaths may involve multiple drugs. Deaths involving multiple drugs, for example heroin and oxycodone, are included in the death rate for natural and semisynthetic opioids and the death rate for heroin. For more information on the type of drugs commonly involved in drug-overdose deaths, see: Warner M, Trinidad JP, Bastian BA, Minin o AM, Hedegaard H. Drugs most frequently involved in drug overdose deaths: United States, 2010–2014. National Vital Statistics Reports; vol 65 no 10. Hyattsville, MD: National Center for Health Statistics. 2016. Available from: https://www.cdc.gov/nchs/data/nvsr/nvsr65/nvsr65_10.pdf. In 1999–2016, 15%–25% of drug-overdose deaths did not include specific information on the death certificate on the type of drug that was involved. Some of these deaths could have potentially involved heroin or opioids. For more information, see: Warner M, Hedegaard H, Chen LH. Trends in drug-poisoning deaths involving opioid analgesics and heroin: United States, 1999–2012. NCHS Health E-Stats. 2014. Available from: https://www.cdc.gov/nchs/data/hestat/drug_poisoning/drug_poisoning.htm. For more information on the enhancement of mortality statistics using information from the death certificate, see: Trinidad JP, Warner M, Bastian BA, Minin o AM, Hedegaard H. Using literal text from the death certificate to enhance mortality statistics: Characterizing drug involvement in deaths. National Vital Statistics Reports; vol 65 no 9. Hyattsville, MD: National Center for Health Statistics. 2016. Available from: https://www.cdc.gov/nchs/data/nvsr/nvsr65/nvsr65_09.pdf.

Table 2-35. Death Rates for Drug Overdoses, by Sex, Race, Hispanic Origin, and Age, Selected Years, 1999–2016—Continued

(Deaths per 100,000 resident population.)

Sex, race, Hispanic origin, and age	1999	2000	2001	2002	2003	2004	2005	2006	2007	2008	2009	2010	2011	2012	2013	2014	2015	2016
	Drug overdose deaths involving methadone per 100,000 resident population (T40.3)[4]																	
All Persons																		
All ages, age-adjusted[2]	0.3	0.4	0.5	0.8	1.0	1.3	1.5	1.8	1.8	1.6	1.5	1.5	1.4	1.2	1.1	1.1	1.0	1.0
All ages, crude	0.3	0.4	0.5	0.8	1.0	1.3	1.5	1.8	1.8	1.6	1.5	1.5	1.4	1.3	1.1	1.1	1.0	1.0
Under 15 years	*	*	*	*	*	0.0	0.0	0.0	0.0	0.1	*	0.0	*	*	*	*	*	*
15 to 24 years	0.1	0.2	0.4	0.7	1.1	1.4	1.4	1.9	2.0	1.6	1.4	1.3	1.1	0.8	0.6	0.5	0.5	0.4
25 to 34 years	0.4	0.5	0.7	1.2	1.4	2.1	2.5	3.1	3.3	2.8	2.7	2.8	2.6	2.3	2.0	1.8	1.7	1.7
35 to 44 years	0.8	0.9	1.2	1.8	2.2	2.6	2.8	3.2	3.0	2.6	2.5	2.4	2.5	2.2	2.1	1.9	1.8	2.0
45 to 54 years	0.5	0.7	1.0	1.7	2.1	2.5	3.0	3.5	3.5	3.3	3.0	2.8	2.7	2.3	2.1	2.0	2.0	1.8
55 to 64 years	0.1	0.2	0.3	0.4	0.5	0.7	1.0	1.1	1.4	1.2	1.5	1.5	1.5	1.5	1.5	1.6	1.6	1.7
65 to 74 years	*	*	*	0.1	*	0.2	0.2	0.3	0.2	0.2	0.3	0.2	0.3	0.3	0.4	0.3	0.4	0.4
75 to 84 years	*	*	*	*	*	*	*	*	*	*	*	*	*	*	*	*	*	*
85 years and over	*	*	*	*	*	*	*	*	*	*	*	*	*	*	*	*	*	*
Male																		
All ages, age-adjusted[2]	0.4	0.4	0.7	1.0	1.3	1.7	2.0	2.4	2.4	2.1	2.0	1.9	1.8	1.6	1.4	1.3	1.2	1.3
All ages, crude	0.4	0.5	0.7	1.1	1.4	1.7	2.0	2.5	2.4	2.1	2.0	1.9	1.8	1.6	1.4	1.3	1.2	1.3
Under 15 years	*	*	*	*	*	*	*	*	0.1	*	*	*	*	*	*	*	*	*
15 to 24 years	0.2	0.3	0.6	1.1	1.7	2.3	2.2	3.0	3.0	2.5	2.2	1.9	1.7	1.2	0.9	0.8	0.7	0.6
25 to 34 years	0.5	0.6	0.9	1.6	1.8	2.9	3.4	4.5	4.8	4.1	3.8	4.0	3.5	3.2	2.6	2.4	2.2	2.2
35 to 44 years	1.0	1.1	1.5	2.1	2.6	3.1	3.5	4.0	3.7	3.2	3.2	2.9	3.0	2.7	2.3	2.2	2.1	2.4
45 to 54 years	0.7	0.9	1.4	2.1	2.6	3.0	3.7	4.3	4.1	3.9	3.3	3.2	3.0	2.5	2.3	2.1	2.0	2.0
55 to 64 years	*	0.2	0.4	0.5	0.7	0.8	1.3	1.4	1.7	1.5	1.9	1.9	1.7	1.9	1.8	1.9	1.8	2.1
65 to 74 years	*	*	*	*	*	*	*	0.3	*	0.3	0.4	0.2	0.3	0.3	0.4	0.4	0.6	0.5
75 to 84 years	*	*	*	*	*	*	*	*	*	*	*	*	*	*	*	*	*	*
85 years and over	*	*	*	*	*	*	*	*	*	*	*	*	*	*	*	*	*	*
Female																		
All ages, age-adjusted[2]	0.2	0.2	0.3	0.6	0.7	0.9	1.0	1.2	1.3	1.1	1.1	1.1	1.1	0.9	0.9	0.9	0.8	0.8
All ages, crude	0.2	0.2	0.3	0.6	0.7	0.9	1.0	1.2	1.3	1.1	1.1	1.0	1.1	0.9	0.9	0.9	0.8	0.8
Under 15 years	*	*	*	*	*	*	*	*	*	*	*	*	*	*	*	*	*	*
15 to 24 years	*	*	0.2	0.3	0.4	0.5	0.6	0.7	0.9	0.7	0.6	0.6	0.4	0.4	0.3	0.3	0.2	0.2
25 to 34 years	0.3	0.3	0.4	0.7	0.9	1.3	1.5	1.7	1.8	1.6	1.6	1.6	1.7	1.5	1.3	1.2	1.1	1.2
35 to 44 years	0.6	0.7	0.9	1.4	1.8	2.1	2.1	2.4	2.4	2.0	1.8	1.9	2.0	1.7	1.9	1.6	1.5	1.6
45 to 54 years	0.4	0.5	0.7	1.2	1.5	1.9	2.4	2.7	2.9	2.7	2.6	2.4	2.4	2.1	1.8	1.9	1.9	1.7
55 to 64 years	*	*	0.2	0.3	0.4	0.6	0.7	0.8	1.0	0.9	1.0	1.2	1.2	1.1	1.3	1.3	1.4	1.4
65 to 74 years	*	*	*	*	*	*	0.2	0.2	*	0.2	0.2	0.2	0.2	0.2	0.4	0.3	0.3	0.2
75 to 84 years	*	*	*	*	*	*	*	*	*	*	*	*	*	*	*	*	*	*
85 years and over	*	*	*	*	*	*	*	*	*	*	*	*	*	*	*	*	*	*
All Ages, Age-Adjusted[2,3]																		
White male	0.4	0.5	0.7	1.2	1.6	2.0	2.3	2.8	2.8	2.5	2.3	2.3	2.1	1.8	1.6	1.5	1.4	1.4
Black or African American male	0.2	0.3	0.4	0.5	0.5	0.6	0.9	1.0	1.0	0.8	0.8	0.7	0.7	0.7	0.7	0.6	0.7	0.8
American Indian or Alaska Native male	*	*	*	*	*	2.0	1.8	2.1	1.6	2.3	2.6	1.6	1.9	1.4	1.0	1.2	1.1	1.0
Asian or Pacific Islander male	*	*	*	*	*	*	*	*	*	*	*	*	0.2	0.2	*	*	*	*
Hispanic or Latino male	0.4	0.2	0.4	0.4	0.6	0.6	0.7	0.8	0.9	0.8	0.7	0.8	0.6	0.7	0.6	0.6	0.6	0.7
White, not Hispanic or Latino male	0.4	0.5	0.8	1.4	1.7	2.3	2.6	3.3	3.3	2.9	2.7	2.6	2.4	2.1	1.8	1.7	1.6	1.6
Black, not Hispanic or Latino male	0.2	0.2	0.4	0.5	0.5	0.7	0.9	1.0	1.0	0.7	0.8	0.7	0.8	0.7	0.7	0.6	0.7	0.8
White female	0.2	0.3	0.4	0.7	0.8	1.0	1.2	1.3	1.4	1.3	1.2	1.2	1.2	1.1	1.1	1.0	1.0	0.9
Black or African American female	0.2	0.2	0.2	0.3	0.3	0.5	0.5	0.7	0.7	0.5	0.5	0.5	0.6	0.4	0.5	0.6	0.5	0.6
American Indian or Alaska Native female	*	*	*	*	*	*	1.4	1.4	1.5	1.7	1.2	1.9	1.3	1.5	1.3	*	*	*
Asian or Pacific Islander female	*	*	*	*	*	*	*	*	*	*	*	*	*	*	*	*	*	*
Hispanic or Latina female	*	0.1	0.2	0.2	0.3	0.3	0.4	0.4	0.3	0.4	0.4	0.4	0.4	0.3	0.3	0.3	0.3	0.3
White, not Hispanic or Latina female	0.2	0.3	0.4	0.7	0.9	1.2	1.3	1.5	1.7	1.5	1.4	1.4	1.4	1.3	1.2	1.2	1.1	1.1
Black, not Hispanic or Latina female	0.2	0.2	0.2	0.3	0.3	0.5	0.5	0.6	0.7	0.5	0.5	0.5	0.6	0.4	0.5	0.6	0.5	0.6

NOTE: Rates for 1999 were computed using intercensal population estimates based on the 1990 and 2000 Censuses. Rates for 2000 were computed based on 2000 bridged-race April 1 census counts. Starting with *Health, United States, 2012*, rates for 2001–2009 were revised using intercensal population estimates based on the 2000 and 2010 Censuses. Rates for 2010 were based on 2010 bridged-race April 1 census counts. Rates for 2011 and beyond were computed using 2010-based postcensal estimates. Age groups were selected to minimize the presentation of unstable age-specific death rates based on small numbers of deaths and for consistency among comparison groups. For additional injury-related statistics, see the Web-based Injury Statistics Query and Reporting System (WISQARS), available from: https://www.cdc.gov/injury/wisqars/index.html. Starting with 2003 data, some states allowed the reporting of more than one race on the death certificate. The multiple-race data for these states were bridged to the single-race categories of the 1977 Office of Management and Budget standards, for comparability with other states.

0.0 = Rate more than zero but less than 0.05.

* = Rates based on fewer than 20 deaths are considered unreliable and are not shown.

[2]Age-adjusted rates are calculated using the year 2000 standard population with unrounded population numbers.

[3]The race groups White, Black, Asian or Pacific Islander, and American Indian or Alaska Native include persons of Hispanic and non-Hispanic origin. Persons of Hispanic origin may be of any race. Death rates for Hispanic, American Indian or Alaska Native, and Asian or Pacific Islander persons should be interpreted with caution because of inconsistencies in reporting Hispanic origin or race on the death certificate (death rate numerators) compared with population figures (death rate denominators). The net effect of misclassification is an underestimation of deaths and death rates for races other than White and Black.

[4]Drug overdose deaths involving opioids include those with an underlying cause of drug overdose and with an opioid mentioned in the *ICD–10* multiple causes of death. The Any opioid category is defined by multiple cause-of-death codes T40.0–T40.4 and T40.6. The Natural and semisynthetic opioids category, which includes codeine, oxycodone, and morphine, among other drugs, is defined by multiple cause-of-death code T40.2. The Other synthetic opioids (other than methadone) category, which includes fentanyl, tramadol, and propoxyphene (removed from the market in 2010), is defined by multiple cause-of-death code T40.4. A sharp increase in deaths involving synthetic opioids, other than methadone, in 2014 coincided with law enforcement reports of increased availability of illicitly manufactured, or nonpharmaceutical, fentanyl. Illicitly manufactured fentanyl cannot be distinguished from pharmaceutical fentanyl in death certificate data. For more information, see the Centers for Disease Control and Prevention's health advisory: Increases in fentanyl drug confiscations and fentanyl-related overdose fatalities. 2015. Available from: https://emergency.cdc.gov/han/han00384.asp, and Rudd RA, Aleshire N, Zibbell JE, Gladden M. Increases in drug and opioid overdose deaths—United States, 2000–2014. MMWR Morb Mortal Wkly Rep 64(50–51):1378–82. 2016 . Available from: https://www.cdc.gov/mmwr/preview/mmwrhtml/mm6450a3.htm?s_cid=mm6450a3_w. Drug overdose deaths involving heroin include those with an underlying cause of drug overdose and with heroin mentioned in the *ICD–10* multiple causes of death. Metabolic breakdown of heroin into morphine in the body can make it difficult to distinguish between deaths from heroin and deaths from morphine based on the information on the death certificate. Some deaths reported to involve morphine could be deaths from heroin. For more information, see Hedegaard H, Chen LH, Warner M. Drug-poisoning deaths involving heroin: United States, 2000–2013. NCHS Data Brief, no 190. Hyattsville, MD: National Center for Health Statistics. 2015. Available from: https://www.cdc.gov/nchs/data/databriefs/db190.htm. See Appendix I, National Vital Statistics System (NVSS), Mortality Multiple Cause-of-Death File, See Appendix II, Cause of death; Table IV. Drug overdose deaths may involve multiple drugs. Deaths involving multiple drugs, for example heroin and oxycodone, are included in the death rate for natural and semisynthetic opioids and the death rate for heroin. For more information on the type of drugs commonly involved in drug-overdose deaths, see: Warner M, Trinidad JP, Bastian BA, Minin o AM, Hedegaard H. Drugs most frequently involved in drug overdose deaths: United States, 2010–2014. National Vital Statistics Reports; vol 65 no 10. Hyattsville, MD: National Center for Health Statistics. 2016. Available from: https://www.cdc.gov/nchs/data/nvsr/nvsr65/nvsr65_10.pdf. In 1999–2016, 15%–25% of drug-overdose deaths did not include specific information on the death certificate on the type of drug that was involved. Some of these deaths could have potentially involved heroin or opioids. For more information, see: Warner M, Hedegaard H, Chen LH. Trends in drug-poisoning deaths involving opioid analgesics and heroin: United States, 1999–2012. NCHS Health E-Stats. 2014. Available from: https://www.cdc.gov/nchs/data/hestat/drug_poisoning/drug_poisoning.htm. For more information on the enhancement of mortality statistics using information from the death certificate, see: Trinidad JP, Warner M, Bastian BA, Minin o AM, Hedegaard H. Using literal text from the death certificate to enhance mortality statistics: Characterizing drug involvement in deaths. National Vital Statistics Reports; vol 65 no 9. Hyattsville, MD: National Center for Health Statistics. 2016. Available from: https://www. cdc.gov/nchs/data/nvsr/nvsr65/nvsr65_09.pdf.

Table 2-35. Death Rates for Drug Overdoses, by Sex, Race, Hispanic Origin, and Age, Selected Years, 1999–2016—Continued

(Deaths per 100,000 resident population.)

Sex, race, Hispanic origin, and age	1999	2000	2001	2002	2003	2004	2005	2006	2007	2008	2009	2010	2011	2012	2013	2014	2015	2016
	Drug overdose deaths involving other synthetic opioids (other than methadone) per 100,000 resident population (T40.4)[4]																	
All Persons																		
All ages, age-adjusted[2]	0.3	0.3	0.3	0.4	0.5	0.6	0.6	0.9	0.7	0.8	1.0	1.0	0.8	0.8	1.0	1.8	3.1	6.2
All ages, crude	0.3	0.3	0.3	0.5	0.5	0.6	0.6	0.9	0.7	0.8	1.0	1.0	0.9	0.8	1.0	1.7	3.0	6.0
Under 15 years	*	*	*	*	*	*	*	*	*	*	*	*	*	*	*	*	*	*
15 to 24 years	0.1	0.1	0.1	0.2	0.3	0.3	0.3	0.6	0.4	0.4	0.5	0.5	0.5	0.4	0.5	1.2	2.3	4.5
25 to 34 years	0.3	0.2	0.4	0.5	0.6	0.7	0.7	1.3	1.0	1.0	1.2	1.4	1.2	1.3	1.5	3.4	6.6	13.6
35 to 44 years	0.6	0.7	0.8	1.0	1.1	1.2	1.2	1.7	1.3	1.4	1.7	1.7	1.4	1.4	1.6	3.1	5.6	11.9
45 to 54 years	0.5	0.6	0.7	0.9	1.0	1.3	1.3	1.9	1.6	1.7	2.2	2.1	1.9	1.8	2.0	3.1	4.6	9.0
55 to 64 years	0.2	0.3	0.3	0.4	0.4	0.4	0.5	0.8	0.8	0.9	1.2	1.2	1.1	1.1	1.4	1.9	2.9	5.4
65 to 74 years	0.1	*	*	0.2	0.2	0.2	0.2	0.2	0.3	0.3	0.5	0.3	0.3	0.4	0.4	0.5	0.7	1.3
75 to 84 years	*	*	*	*	*	*	0.2	0.2	0.2	*	0.2	0.2	0.2	0.2	*	0.2	0.2	0.2
85 years and over	*	*	*	*	*	*	*	*	*	*	*	*	*	*	*	*	0.2	*
Male																		
All ages, age-adjusted[2]	0.3	0.3	0.4	0.5	0.5	0.6	0.6	1.1	0.8	0.8	1.0	1.0	0.9	0.9	1.1	2.2	4.2	8.9
All ages, crude	0.3	0.3	0.4	0.5	0.5	0.6	0.6	1.1	0.8	0.8	1.0	1.0	0.9	0.9	1.1	2.2	4.1	8.7
Under 15 years	*	*	*	*	*	*	*	*	*	*	*	*	*	*	*	*	*	*
15 to 24 years	0.1	0.1	0.2	0.3	0.3	0.4	0.5	1.0	0.6	0.6	0.7	0.7	0.7	0.6	0.8	1.7	3.2	6.4
25 to 34 years	0.4	0.3	0.4	0.7	0.8	0.9	0.9	1.8	1.4	1.2	1.5	1.8	1.5	1.5	2.0	4.8	9.8	20.0
35 to 44 years	0.7	0.7	0.9	1.1	1.3	1.4	1.3	2.2	1.5	1.5	1.8	1.8	1.4	1.6	1.7	3.9	7.9	17.4
45 to 54 years	0.6	0.7	0.7	0.9	1.0	1.2	1.3	2.2	1.4	1.7	2.1	1.9	1.8	1.7	1.9	3.6	5.8	12.4
55 to 64 years	0.2	0.2	0.3	0.3	0.3	0.3	0.4	0.8	0.6	0.7	1.0	1.1	1.0	1.1	1.4	2.0	3.6	7.5
65 to 74 years	*	*	*	*	*	*	*	*	0.2	0.3	0.3	*	0.3	0.3	0.3	0.4	0.8	1.7
75 to 84 years	*	*	*	*	*	*	*	*	*	*	*	*	*	*	*	*	*	*
85 years and over	*	*	*	*	*	*	*	*	*	*	*	*	*	*	*	*	*	*
Female																		
All ages, age-adjusted[2]	0.2	0.3	0.3	0.4	0.4	0.5	0.5	0.7	0.7	0.7	0.9	0.9	0.8	0.7	0.9	1.3	1.9	3.5
All ages, crude	0.2	0.3	0.3	0.4	0.4	0.5	0.5	0.7	0.7	0.7	0.9	0.9	0.8	0.7	0.9	1.3	1.9	3.4
Under 15 years	*	*	*	*	*	*	*	*	*	*	*	*	*	*	*	*	*	*
15 to 24 years	*	*	*	0.1	0.2	0.1	0.1	0.3	0.2	0.2	0.2	0.4	0.3	0.2	0.3	0.6	1.3	2.5
25 to 34 years	0.2	0.2	0.3	0.4	0.4	0.5	0.6	0.7	0.7	0.7	0.9	1.0	0.9	1.0	1.0	1.9	3.3	7.1
35 to 44 years	0.5	0.6	0.7	0.9	1.0	1.1	1.1	1.3	1.2	1.3	1.5	1.5	1.4	1.1	1.4	2.3	3.4	6.5
45 to 54 years	0.5	0.6	0.7	0.9	1.0	1.4	1.3	1.7	1.8	1.7	2.3	2.2	1.9	1.9	2.2	2.6	3.4	5.8
55 to 64 years	0.3	0.4	0.4	0.5	0.4	0.6	0.6	0.8	0.9	1.0	1.4	1.3	1.1	1.1	1.5	1.7	2.1	3.5
65 to 74 years	*	*	*	0.3	0.2	0.3	0.3	0.2	0.4	0.4	0.7	0.5	0.3	0.4	0.5	0.6	0.6	0.9
75 to 84 years	*	*	*	*	*	*	*	*	*	*	0.3	*	*	0.3	*	*	*	*
85 years and over	*	*	*	*	*	*	*	*	*	*	*	*	*	*	*	*	*	*
All Ages, Age-Adjusted[2,3]																		
White male	0.3	0.3	0.4	0.5	0.6	0.7	0.7	1.2	0.9	1.0	1.2	1.2	1.1	1.1	1.2	2.5	4.8	9.9
Black or African American male	*	0.1	0.2	0.1	0.2	0.2	0.2	1.5	0.2	0.2	0.3	0.3	0.3	0.3	0.5	1.5	3.1	8.4
American Indian or Alaska Native male	*	*	*	*	*	*	*	*	*	1.3	1.8	*	*	*	*	1.5	1.5	3.1
Asian or Pacific Islander male	*	*	*	*	*	*	*	*	*	*	*	*	*	*	*	0.2	0.4	1.0
Hispanic or Latino male	0.2	*	*	0.1	0.2	0.2	0.2	0.5	0.2	0.2	0.3	0.2	0.3	0.3	0.4	0.7	1.4	4.2
White, not Hispanic or Latino male	0.3	0.4	0.5	0.6	0.7	0.8	0.8	1.3	1.1	1.1	1.3	1.5	1.3	1.3	1.5	3.0	5.8	11.5
Black, not Hispanic or Latino male	*	0.1	0.2	0.1	0.2	0.2	0.2	1.6	0.3	0.2	0.3	0.3	0.3	0.3	0.5	1.5	3.2	8.6
White female	0.3	0.3	0.3	0.5	0.5	0.6	0.6	0.8	0.8	0.8	1.0	1.1	0.9	0.9	1.0	1.5	2.3	4.0
Black or African American female	*	*	0.1	0.2	0.1	0.2	0.2	0.4	0.2	0.2	0.3	0.4	0.3	0.3	0.4	0.7	1.1	2.9
American Indian or Alaska Native female	*	*	*	*	*	*	*	*	*	1.1	1.3	1.0	*	1.1	*	0.9	1.1	1.9
Asian or Pacific Islander female	*	*	*	*	*	*	*	*	*	*	*	*	*	*	*	*	*	0.3
Hispanic or Latina female	*	*	*	0.2	0.1	0.2	0.1	0.2	0.2	0.2	0.3	0.3	0.2	0.2	0.3	0.4	0.4	1.1
White, not Hispanic or Latina female	0.3	0.3	0.4	0.5	0.6	0.7	0.7	0.9	0.9	0.9	1.2	1.2	1.0	1.0	1.2	1.8	2.7	4.8
Black, not Hispanic or Latina female	*	*	0.1	0.2	0.1	0.2	0.3	0.5	0.3	0.3	0.4	0.4	0.4	0.3	0.5	0.7	1.1	3.0

NOTE: Rates for 1999 were computed using intercensal population estimates based on the 1990 and 2000 Censuses. Rates for 2000 were computed based on 2000 bridged-race April 1 census counts. Starting with *Health, United States, 2012*, rates for 2001–2009 were revised using intercensal population estimates based on the 2000 and 2010 Censuses. Rates for 2010 were based on 2010 bridged-race April 1 census counts. Rates for 2011 and beyond were computed using 2010-based postcensal estimates. Age groups were selected to minimize the presentation of unstable age-specific death rates based on small numbers of deaths and for consistency among comparison groups. For additional injury-related statistics, see the Web-based Injury Statistics Query and Reporting System (WISQARS), available from: https://www.cdc.gov/injury/wisqars/index.html. Starting with 2003 data, some states allowed the reporting of more than one race on the death certificate. The multiple-race data for these states were bridged to the single-race categories of the 1977 Office of Management and Budget standards, for comparability with other states.

* = Rates based on fewer than 20 deaths are considered unreliable and are not shown.

[2]Age-adjusted rates are calculated using the year 2000 standard population with unrounded population numbers.

[3]The race groups White, Black, Asian or Pacific Islander, and American Indian or Alaska Native include persons of Hispanic and non-Hispanic origin. Persons of Hispanic origin may be of any race. Death rates for Hispanic, American Indian or Alaska Native, and Asian or Pacific Islander persons should be interpreted with caution because of inconsistencies in reporting Hispanic origin or race on the death certificate (death rate numerators) compared with population figures (death rate denominators). The net effect of misclassification is an underestimation of deaths and death rates for races other than White and Black.

[4]Drug overdose deaths involving opioids include those with an underlying cause of drug overdose and with an opioid mentioned in the *ICD-10* multiple causes of death. The Any opioid category is defined by multiple cause-of-death codes T40.0–T40.4 and T40.6. The Natural and semisynthetic opioids category, which includes codeine, oxycodone, and morphine, among other drugs, is defined by multiple cause-of-death code T40.2. The Other synthetic opioids (other than methadone) category, which includes fentanyl, tramadol, and propoxyphene (removed from the market in 2010), is defined by multiple cause-of-death code T40.4. A sharp increase in deaths involving synthetic opioids, other than methadone, in 2014 coincided with law enforcement reports of increased availability of illicitly manufactured, or nonpharmaceutical, fentanyl. Illicitly manufactured fentanyl cannot be distinguished from pharmaceutical fentanyl in death certificate data. For more information, see the Centers for Disease Control and Prevention's health advisory: Increases in fentanyl drug confiscations and fentanyl-related overdose fatalities. 2015. Available from: https://emergency.cdc.gov/han/han00384.asp, and Rudd RA, Aleshire N, Zibbell JE, Gladden M. Increases in drug and opioid overdose deaths—United States, 2000–2014. MMWR Morb Mortal Wkly Rep 64(50–51):1378–82. 2016 . Available from: https://www.cdc.gov/mmwr/preview/mmwrhtml/mm6450a3.htm?s_cid=mm6450a3_w. Drug overdose deaths involving heroin include those with an underlying cause of drug overdose and with heroin mentioned in the *ICD-10* multiple causes of death. Metabolic breakdown of heroin into morphine in the body can make it difficult to distinguish between deaths from heroin and deaths from morphine based on the information on the death certificate. Some deaths reported to involve morphine could be deaths from heroin. This may result in an undercount of heroin-related deaths. For more information, see Hedegaard H, Chen LH, Warner M. Drug-poisoning deaths involving heroin: United States, 2000–2013. NCHS Data Brief, no 190. Hyattsville, MD: National Center for Health Statistics. 2015. Available from: https://www.cdc.gov/nchs/data/databriefs/db190.htm. See Appendix I, National Vital Statistics System (NVSS), Mortality Multiple Cause-of-Death File, See Appendix II, Cause of death; Table IV. Drug overdose deaths may involve multiple drugs. Deaths involving multiple drugs, for example heroin and oxycodone, are included in the death rate for natural and semisynthetic opioids and the death rate for heroin. For more information on the type of drugs commonly involved in drug-overdose deaths, see: Warner M, Trinidad JP, Bastian BA, Minin o AM, Hedegaard H. Drugs most frequently involved in drug overdose deaths: United States, 2010–2014. National Vital Statistics Reports; vol 65 no 10. Hyattsville, MD: National Center for Health Statistics. 2016. Available from: https://www.cdc.gov/nchs/data/nvsr/nvsr65/nvsr65_10.pdf. In 1999–2016, 15%–25% of drug-overdose deaths did not include specific information on the death certificate on the type of drug that was involved. Some of these deaths could have potentially involved heroin or opioids. For more information, see: Warner M, Hedegaard H, Chen LH. Trends in drug-poisoning deaths involving opioid analgesics and heroin: United States, 1999–2012. NCHS Health E-Stats. 2014. Available from: https://www.cdc.gov/nchs/data/hestat/drug_poisoning/drug_poisoning.htm. For more information on the enhancement of mortality statistics using information from the death certificate, see: Trinidad JP, Warner M, Bastian BA, Minin o AM, Hedegaard H. Using literal text from the death certificate to enhance mortality statistics: Characterizing drug involvement in deaths. National Vital Statistics Reports; vol 65 no 9. Hyattsville, MD: National Center for Health Statistics. 2016. Available from: https://www.cdc.gov/nchs/data/nvsr/nvsr65/nvsr65_09.pdf.

Table 2-35. Death Rates for Drug Overdoses, by Sex, Race, Hispanic Origin, and Age, Selected Years, 1999–2016—*Continued*

(Deaths per 100,000 resident population.)

Sex, race, Hispanic origin, and age	1999	2000	2001	2002	2003	2004	2005	2006	2007	2008	2009	2010	2011	2012	2013	2014	2015	2016
	Drug overdose deaths involving heroin per 100,000 resident population (T40.1)[4]																	
All Persons																		
All ages, age-adjusted[2]	0.7	0.7	0.6	0.7	0.7	0.6	0.7	0.7	0.8	1.0	1.1	1.0	1.4	1.9	2.7	3.4	4.1	4.9
All ages, crude	0.7	0.7	0.6	0.7	0.7	0.6	0.7	0.7	0.8	1.0	1.1	1.0	1.4	1.9	2.6	3.3	4.0	4.8
Under 15 years	*	*	*	*	*	*	*	*	*	*	*	*	*	*	*	*	*	*
15 to 24 years	0.5	0.6	0.5	0.6	0.6	0.6	0.7	0.7	0.8	1.1	1.2	1.2	1.8	2.2	2.9	3.3	3.8	4.0
25 to 34 years	1.0	1.0	1.0	1.1	1.1	1.1	1.2	1.2	1.5	2.0	2.3	2.2	3.4	4.6	6.3	8.0	9.7	11.3
35 to 44 years	1.8	1.5	1.5	1.7	1.5	1.2	1.2	1.3	1.4	1.7	1.8	1.6	2.2	3.1	4.4	5.9	7.4	9.0
45 to 54 years	1.3	1.2	1.2	1.4	1.5	1.2	1.4	1.4	1.5	1.7	1.8	1.4	2.0	2.8	3.7	4.7	5.6	7.0
55 to 64 years	0.3	0.3	0.3	0.3	0.3	0.4	0.4	0.4	0.4	0.7	0.7	0.7	1.0	1.3	2.1	2.7	3.4	4.3
65 to 74 years	*	*	*	*	*	*	*	*	*	0.1	0.1	*	0.2	0.1	0.3	0.5	0.6	0.9
75 to 84 years	*	*	*	*	*	*	*	*	*	*	*	*	*	*	*	*	*	*
85 years and over	*	*	*	*	*	*	*	*	*	*	*	*	*	*	*	*	*	*
Male																		
All ages, age-adjusted[2]	1.2	1.1	1.0	1.2	1.2	1.1	1.1	1.2	1.3	1.6	1.8	1.6	2.3	3.1	4.2	5.2	6.3	7.5
All ages, crude	1.2	1.1	1.0	1.2	1.2	1.1	1.1	1.2	1.4	1.7	1.8	1.6	2.3	3.0	4.2	5.2	6.2	7.4
Under 15 years	*	*	*	*	*	*	*	*	*	*	*	*	*	*	*	*	*	*
15 to 24 years	0.8	0.9	0.8	0.9	1.0	1.0	1.0	1.2	1.3	1.8	1.8	1.9	2.8	3.2	4.2	4.8	5.2	5.7
25 to 34 years	1.6	1.7	1.6	1.7	1.9	1.9	2.0	2.1	2.4	3.3	3.9	3.5	5.4	7.1	9.9	12.3	14.8	17.1
35 to 44 years	3.0	2.6	2.3	2.8	2.4	2.0	1.9	2.1	2.4	2.8	3.0	2.8	3.6	5.1	6.9	9.2	11.4	13.8
45 to 54 years	2.3	2.2	2.0	2.5	2.6	2.0	2.3	2.3	2.6	2.7	3.0	2.4	3.2	4.5	6.0	7.2	8.7	10.6
55 to 64 years	0.5	0.4	0.5	0.6	0.6	0.6	0.7	0.8	0.8	1.2	1.3	1.1	1.7	2.3	3.6	4.4	5.6	6.8
65 to 74 years	*	*	*	*	*	*	*	*	*	*	*	*	0.3	0.3	0.5	0.9	1.1	1.7
75 to 84 years	*	*	*	*	*	*	*	*	*	*	*	*	*	*	*	*	*	*
85 years and over	*	*	*	*	*	*	*	*	*	*	*	*	*	*	*	*	*	*
Female																		
All ages, age-adjusted[2]	0.2	0.2	0.2	0.2	0.2	0.2	0.3	0.2	0.3	0.4	0.4	0.4	0.6	0.8	1.2	1.6	2.0	2.4
All ages, crude	0.2	0.2	0.2	0.2	0.2	0.2	0.3	0.2	0.3	0.4	0.4	0.4	0.6	0.8	1.1	1.5	1.9	2.3
Under 15 years	*	*	*	*	*	*	*	*	*	*	*	*	*	*	*	*	*	*
15 to 24 years	0.2	0.2	0.2	0.3	0.3	0.3	0.3	0.3	0.3	0.5	0.5	0.6	0.9	1.1	1.5	1.7	2.2	2.1
25 to 34 years	0.3	0.4	0.3	0.4	0.3	0.4	0.5	0.4	0.5	0.6	0.7	0.9	1.4	2.0	2.6	3.7	4.6	5.4
35 to 44 years	0.6	0.5	0.6	0.6	0.5	0.5	0.5	0.4	0.4	0.7	0.6	0.6	0.8	1.1	1.9	2.6	3.5	4.1
45 to 54 years	0.3	0.3	0.3	0.4	0.5	0.4	0.5	0.5	0.5	0.7	0.7	0.5	0.8	1.1	1.6	2.2	2.7	3.6
55 to 64 years	*	*	*	*	0.1	*	*	*	0.2	0.2	0.2	0.3	0.3	0.4	0.7	1.0	1.5	1.9
65 to 74 years	*	*	*	*	*	*	*	*	*	*	*	*	*	*	*	*	0.2	0.3
75 to 84 years	*	*	*	*	*	*	*	*	*	*	*	*	*	*	*	*	*	*
85 years and over	*	*	*	*	*	*	*	*	*	*	*	*	*	*	*	*	*	*
All Ages, Age-Adjusted[2,3]																		
White male	1.2	1.1	1.1	1.2	1.3	1.1	1.1	1.2	1.5	1.9	2.0	1.8	2.6	3.5	4.7	6.0	7.2	8.3
Black or African American male	1.4	1.6	1.3	1.6	1.3	1.1	1.3	1.2	1.3	1.3	1.5	1.2	1.6	2.1	3.4	4.1	5.0	7.1
American Indian or Alaska Native male	*	*	*	*	*	*	*	*	*	1.1	1.7	*	1.3	1.7	2.6	3.5	4.0	4.3
Asian or Pacific Islander male	*	*	*	*	*	*	*	*	*	*	*	*	0.3	0.3	0.5	0.6	0.8	0.8
Hispanic or Latino male	2.0	1.6	1.4	1.8	1.8	1.3	1.4	1.4	1.4	1.7	1.7	1.5	1.7	2.2	2.6	3.2	3.8	4.4
White, not Hispanic or Latino male	1.1	1.0	1.0	1.2	1.2	1.1	1.1	1.3	1.5	1.9	2.1	1.9	2.9	3.9	5.3	6.7	8.1	9.4
Black, not Hispanic or Latino male	1.4	1.7	1.3	1.6	1.3	1.1	1.3	1.3	1.3	1.3	1.6	1.3	1.6	2.2	3.5	4.2	5.1	7.3
White female	0.2	0.2	0.2	0.2	0.2	0.2	0.3	0.2	0.3	0.4	0.4	0.4	0.6	0.9	1.3	1.8	2.3	2.7
Black or African American female	0.3	0.3	0.3	0.3	0.3	0.3	0.3	0.3	0.3	0.3	0.3	0.3	0.4	0.6	0.7	1.1	1.3	2.0
American Indian or Alaska Native female	*	*	*	*	*	*	*	*	*	*	*	*	1.0	*	1.0	1.2	1.8	2.2
Asian or Pacific Islander female	*	*	*	*	*	*	*	*	*	*	*	*	*	*	*	*	0.2	0.2
Hispanic or Latina female	0.2	0.1	0.2	0.3	0.2	0.2	0.2	0.2	0.2	0.3	0.2	0.2	0.3	0.4	0.5	0.7	0.8	1.1
White, not Hispanic or Latina female	0.2	0.2	0.2	0.3	0.3	0.3	0.3	0.2	0.3	0.4	0.5	0.5	0.7	1.1	1.5	2.1	2.7	3.1
Black, not Hispanic or Latina female	0.3	0.3	0.3	0.3	0.3	0.3	0.3	0.3	0.3	0.3	0.3	0.3	0.4	0.5	0.7	1.1	1.1	2.0

NOTE: Rates for 1999 were computed using intercensal population estimates based on the 1990 and 2000 Censuses. Rates for 2000 were computed based on 2000 bridged-race April 1 census counts. Starting with *Health, United States, 2012,* rates for 2001–2009 were revised using intercensal population estimates based on the 2000 and 2010 Censuses. Rates for 2010 were based on 2010 bridged-race April 1 census counts. Rates for 2011 and beyond were computed using 2010-based postcensal estimates. Age groups were selected to minimize the presentation of unstable age-specific death rates based on small numbers of deaths and for consistency among comparison groups. For additional injury-related statistics, see the Web-based Injury Statistics Query and Reporting System (WISQARS), available from: https://www.cdc.gov/injury/wisqars/index.html. Starting with 2003 data, some states allowed the reporting of more than one race on the death certificate. The multiple-race data for these states were bridged to the single-race categories of the 1977 Office of Management and Budget standards, for comparability with other states.

* = Rates based on fewer than 20 deaths are considered unreliable and are not shown.

[2] Age-adjusted rates are calculated using the year 2000 standard population with unrounded population numbers.

[3] The race groups White, Black, Asian or Pacific Islander, and American Indian or Alaska Native include persons of Hispanic and non-Hispanic origin. Persons of Hispanic origin may be of any race. Death rates for Hispanic, American Indian or Alaska Native, and Asian or Pacific Islander persons should be interpreted with caution because of inconsistencies in reporting Hispanic origin or race on the death certificate (death rate numerators) compared with population figures (death rate denominators). The net effect of misclassification is an underestimation of deaths and death rates for races other than White and Black.

[4] Drug overdose deaths involving opioids include those with an underlying cause of drug overdose and with an opioid mentioned in the *ICD–10* multiple causes of death. The Any opioid category is defined by multiple cause-of-death codes T40.0–T40.4 and T40.6. The Natural and semisynthetic opioids category, which includes codeine, oxycodone, and morphine, among other drugs, is defined by multiple cause-of-death code T40.2. The Other synthetic opioids (other than methadone) category, which includes fentanyl, tramadol, and propoxyphene (removed from the market in 2010), is defined by multiple cause-of-death code T40.4. A sharp increase in deaths involving synthetic opioids, other than methadone, in 2014 coincided with law enforcement reports of increased availability of illicitly manufactured, or nonpharmaceutical, fentanyl. Illicitly manufactured fentanyl cannot be distinguished from pharmaceutical fentanyl in death certificate data. For more information, see the Centers for Disease Control and Prevention's health advisory: Increases in fentanyl drug confiscations and fentanyl-related overdose fatalities. 2015. Available from: https://emergency.cdc.gov/han/han00384.asp, and Rudd RA, Aleshire N, Zibbell JE, Gladden M. Increases in drug and opioid overdose deaths—United States, 2000–2014. MMWR Morb Mortal Wkly Rep 64(50–51):1378–82. 2016 . Available from: https://www.cdc.gov/mmwr/preview/mmwrhtml/mm6450a3.htm?s_cid=mm6450a3_w. Drug overdose deaths involving heroin include those with an underlying cause of drug overdose and with heroin mentioned in the *ICD–10* multiple causes of death. Metabolic breakdown of heroin into morphine in the body can make it difficult to distinguish between deaths from heroin and deaths from morphine based on the information on the death certificate. Some deaths reported to involve morphine could be deaths from heroin. This may result in an undercount of heroin-related deaths. For more information, see Hedegaard H, Chen LH, Warner M. Drug-poisoning deaths involving heroin: United States, 2000–2013. NCHS Data Brief, no 190. Hyattsville, MD: National Center for Health Statistics. 2015. Available from: https://www.cdc.gov/nchs/data/databriefs/db190.htm. See Appendix I, National Vital Statistics System (NVSS), Mortality Multiple Cause-of-Death File, See Appendix II, Cause of death; Table IV. Drug overdose deaths may involve multiple drugs. Deaths involving multiple drugs, for example heroin and oxycodone, are included in the death rate for natural and semisynthetic opioids and the death rate for heroin. For more information on the type of drugs commonly involved in drug-overdose deaths, see: Warner M, Trinidad JP, Bastian BA, Minin o AM, Hedegaard H. Drugs most frequently involved in drug overdose deaths: United States, 2010–2014. National Vital Statistics Reports; vol 65 no 10. Hyattsville, MD: National Center for Health Statistics. 2016. Available from: https://www.cdc.gov/nchs/data/nvsr/nvsr65/nvsr65_10.pdf. In 1999–2016, 15%–25% of drug-overdose deaths did not include specific information on the death certificate on the type of drug that was involved. Some of these deaths could have potentially involved heroin or opioids. For more information, see: Warner M, Hedegaard H, Chen LH. Trends in drug-poisoning deaths involving opioid analgesics and heroin: United States, 1999–2012. NCHS Health E-Stats. 2014. Available from: https://www.cdc.gov/nchs/data/hestat/drug_poisoning/drug_poisoning.htm. For more information on the enhancement of mortality statistics using information from the death certificate, see: Trinidad JP, Warner M, Bastian BA, Minin o AM, Hedegaard H. Using literal text from the death certificate to enhance mortality statistics: Characterizing drug involvement in deaths. National Vital Statistics Reports; vol 65 no 9. Hyattsville, MD: National Center for Health Statistics. 2016. Available from: https://www.cdc.gov/nchs/data/nvsr/nvsr65/nvsr65_09.pdf.

This page is intentionally left blank

Table 2-36. Death Rates for Homicide, by Sex, Race, Hispanic Origin, and Age, Selected Years, 1950–2016

(Deaths per 100,000 resident population; data are based on death certificates.)

Sex, race, Hispanic origin, and age	1950[1,2]	1960[1,2]	1970[2]	1980[2]	1985[2]	1990[2]	1995	2000[3]	2005[3]	2006[3]
All Persons										
All ages, age-adjusted[4]	5.1	5.0	8.8	10.4	7.9	9.4	8.3	5.9	6.1	6.2
All ages, crude	5.0	4.6	8.1	10.6	8.2	9.9	8.5	6.0	6.1	6.2
Under 1 year	4.4	4.8	4.3	5.9	5.4	8.4	8.2	9.2	7.6	8.3
1 to 14 years	0.6	0.6	1.1	1.5	1.6	1.8	1.9	1.3	1.3	1.3
1 to 4 years	0.6	0.7	1.9	2.5	2.5	2.5	2.9	2.3	2.4	2.3
5 to 14 years	0.5	0.5	0.9	1.2	1.2	1.5	1.5	0.9	0.8	1.0
15 to 24 years	5.8	5.6	11.3	15.4	11.7	19.7	19.6	12.6	12.9	13.3
15 to 19 years	3.9	3.9	7.7	10.5	8.4	16.9	17.8	9.5	9.7	10.5
20 to 24 years	8.5	7.7	15.6	20.2	14.6	22.2	21.5	16.0	16.2	16.3
25 to 44 years	8.9	8.5	14.9	17.5	13.1	14.7	11.9	8.7	9.5	9.4
25 to 34 years	9.3	9.2	16.2	19.3	14.6	17.4	14.4	10.4	12.1	12.0
35 to 44 years	8.4	7.8	13.5	14.9	11.1	11.6	9.4	7.1	7.1	7.0
45 to 64 years	5.0	5.3	8.7	9.0	6.9	6.3	5.4	4.0	4.0	4.3
45 to 54 years	5.9	6.1	10.0	11.0	8.1	7.5	6.0	4.7	4.8	5.1
55 to 64 years	3.9	4.1	7.1	7.0	5.7	5.0	4.4	3.0	2.8	3.2
65 years and over	3.0	2.7	4.6	5.5	4.3	4.0	3.1	2.4	2.3	2.1
65 to 74 years	3.2	2.8	4.9	5.7	4.3	3.8	3.2	2.4	2.3	2.1
75 to 84 years	2.5	2.3	4.0	5.2	4.3	4.3	3.0	2.4	2.2	2.1
85 years and over	2.3	2.4	4.2	5.3	4.1	4.6	3.2	2.4	2.3	2.1
Male										
All ages, age-adjusted[4]	7.9	7.5	14.3	16.6	12.2	14.8	12.8	9.0	9.7	9.8
All ages, crude	7.7	6.8	13.1	17.1	12.8	15.9	13.4	9.3	9.9	10.0
Under 1 year	4.5	4.7	4.5	6.3	5.6	8.8	9.0	10.4	8.4	9.6
1 to 14 years	0.6	0.6	1.2	1.6	1.8	2.0	2.2	1.5	1.4	1.6
1 to 4 years	0.5	0.7	1.9	2.7	2.5	2.7	3.1	2.5	2.6	2.6
5 to 14 years	0.6	0.5	1.0	1.2	1.4	1.7	1.9	1.1	1.0	1.2
15 to 24 years	8.6	8.4	18.2	24.0	18.2	32.5	32.8	20.9	21.9	22.7
15 to 19 years	5.5	5.7	12.1	15.9	12.8	27.8	29.1	15.5	16.4	17.8
20 to 24 years	13.5	11.8	25.6	32.2	23.0	36.9	36.5	26.7	27.5	27.8
25 to 44 years	13.8	12.8	24.4	28.9	20.6	23.5	18.2	13.3	15.3	15.1
25 to 34 years	14.4	13.9	26.8	31.9	22.8	27.7	22.5	16.7	20.3	20.1
35 to 44 years	13.2	11.7	21.7	24.5	17.6	18.6	14.0	10.3	10.7	10.5
45 to 64 years	8.1	8.1	14.8	15.2	11.0	10.2	8.3	6.0	6.2	6.5
45 to 54 years	9.5	9.4	16.8	18.4	12.7	11.9	9.2	6.9	7.6	7.7
55 to 64 years	6.3	6.4	12.1	11.8	9.1	8.0	7.0	4.6	4.3	4.8
65 years and over	4.8	4.3	7.7	8.8	6.2	5.8	4.2	3.3	3.0	2.8
65 to 74 years	5.2	4.6	8.5	9.2	6.5	5.8	4.5	3.4	3.2	2.9
75 to 84 years	3.9	3.7	5.9	8.1	5.7	5.7	3.7	3.2	2.6	2.6
85 years and over	2.5	3.6	7.4	7.5	5.0	6.7	4.1	3.3	3.0	2.5
Female										
All ages, age-adjusted[4]	2.4	2.6	3.7	4.4	3.8	4.0	3.7	2.8	2.5	2.6
All ages, crude	2.4	2.4	3.4	4.5	3.9	4.2	3.8	2.8	2.5	2.5
Under 1 year	4.2	4.9	4.1	5.6	5.2	8.0	7.4	7.9	6.8	6.9
1 to 14 years	0.6	0.5	1.0	1.4	1.4	1.6	1.5	1.1	1.1	1.1
1 to 4 years	0.7	0.7	1.9	2.2	2.4	2.3	2.6	2.1	2.1	2.0
5 to 14 years	0.5	0.4	0.7	1.1	1.0	1.2	1.0	0.7	0.7	0.7
15 to 24 years	3.0	2.8	4.6	6.6	5.1	6.2	5.9	3.9	3.4	3.5
15 to 19 years	2.4	1.9	3.2	4.9	3.9	5.4	5.8	3.1	2.5	2.8
20 to 24 years	3.7	3.8	6.2	8.2	6.1	7.0	6.0	4.7	4.3	4.2
25 to 44 years	4.2	4.3	5.8	6.4	5.7	6.0	5.6	4.0	3.7	3.6
25 to 34 years	4.5	4.6	6.0	6.9	6.4	7.1	6.3	4.1	3.8	3.8
35 to 44 years	3.8	4.0	5.7	5.7	4.9	4.8	4.9	4.0	3.6	3.5
45 to 64 years	1.9	2.5	3.1	3.4	3.2	2.8	2.6	2.1	1.9	2.2
45 to 54 years	2.3	2.9	3.7	4.1	3.7	3.2	2.9	2.5	2.2	2.6
55 to 64 years	1.4	2.0	2.5	2.8	2.7	2.3	2.1	1.6	1.4	1.7
65 years and over	1.4	1.3	2.3	3.3	3.0	2.8	2.4	1.8	1.7	1.6
65 to 74 years	1.3	1.3	2.2	3.0	2.6	2.2	2.1	1.6	1.5	1.3
75 to 84 years	1.4	1.3	2.7	3.5	3.4	3.4	2.6	2.0	1.9	1.8
85 years and over	2.1	1.6	2.5	4.3	3.8	3.8	2.9	2.0	2.0	1.9
White Male[5]										
All ages, age-adjusted[4]	3.8	3.9	7.2	10.4	7.7	8.3	7.3	5.2	5.4	5.5
All ages, crude	3.6	3.6	6.6	10.7	8.1	8.8	7.5	5.2	5.5	5.5

[1]Includes deaths of persons who were not residents of the 50 states and the District of Columbia.
[2]Underlying cause of death was coded according to the 6th Revision of the *International Classification of Diseases* (*ICD*) in 1950, 7th Revision in 1960, 8th Revision in 1970, and 9th Revision in 1980-1998.
[3]Starting with 1999 data, cause of death is coded according to *ICD*-10.
[4]Age-adjusted rates are calculated using the year 2000 standard population. Prior to 2001, age-adjusted rates were calculated using standard million proportions based on rounded population numbers. Starting with 2001 data, unrounded population numbers are used to calculate age-adjusted rates.
[5]The race groups, White, Black, Asian or Pacific Islander, and American Indian or Alaska Native, include persons of Hispanic and non-Hispanic origin. Persons of Hispanic origin may be of any race. Death rates for the American Indian or Alaska Native, Asian or Pacific Islander, and Hispanic populations are known to be underestimated.

Table 2-36. Death Rates for Homicide, by Sex, Race, Hispanic Origin, and Age, Selected Years, 1950–2016—Continued

(Deaths per 100,000 resident population; data are based on death certificates.)

Sex, race, Hispanic origin, and age	2007[3]	2008[3]	2009[3]	2010[3]	2011[3]	2012[3]	2013[3]	2014[3]	2015[3]	2016[3]
All Persons										
All ages, age-adjusted[4]	6.1	5.9	5.5	5.3	5.3	5.4	5.2	5.1	5.7	6.2
All ages, crude	6.1	5.9	5.5	5.3	5.2	5.3	5.1	5.0	5.5	6.0
Under 1 year	8.5	8.2	7.9	7.9	7.3	7.3	7.2	6.3	6.6	7.0
1 to 14 years	1.3	1.3	1.2	1.1	1.2	1.1	1.1	1.1	1.2	1.1
1 to 4 years	2.5	2.6	2.3	2.4	2.5	2.1	2.1	2.3	2.3	2.1
5 to 14 years	0.9	0.8	0.7	0.6	0.7	0.8	0.7	0.7	0.7	0.7
15 to 24 years	12.9	12.2	11.2	10.7	10.4	10.5	9.8	9.5	10.8	11.9
15 to 19 years	10.1	9.4	8.6	8.3	7.8	7.6	6.6	6.7	7.5	8.6
20 to 24 years	15.8	15.0	13.8	13.2	13.0	13.3	12.8	12.1	13.8	15.0
25 to 44 years	9.5	9.1	8.5	8.2	8.1	8.5	8.2	8.1	9.2	10.3
25 to 34 years	12.0	11.5	10.4	10.4	10.0	10.3	9.9	9.6	11.0	12.0
35 to 44 years	7.1	6.9	6.7	6.0	6.2	6.7	6.4	6.4	7.1	8.3
45 to 64 years	4.0	4.0	3.8	3.8	3.8	3.9	3.8	3.7	4.1	4.2
45 to 54 years	4.9	4.8	4.6	4.4	4.6	4.6	4.5	4.5	4.9	5.0
55 to 64 years	3.0	2.9	2.9	2.9	2.9	3.0	3.0	2.9	3.2	3.4
65 years and over	2.0	2.1	2.2	2.0	2.0	2.0	2.0	2.0	2.0	2.0
65 to 74 years	2.1	2.3	2.2	2.1	2.0	2.1	2.0	2.1	2.0	2.0
75 to 84 years	2.0	1.8	2.0	1.9	2.0	2.0	2.1	2.0	2.1	2.0
85 years and over	1.6	2.3	2.3	2.0	2.2	1.9	1.9	1.9	1.7	1.9
Male										
All ages, age-adjusted[4]	9.7	9.3	8.6	8.4	8.3	8.5	8.2	8.0	9.1	9.9
All ages, crude	9.8	9.5	8.7	8.4	8.3	8.5	8.2	8.0	9.0	9.7
Under 1 year	9.7	9.3	9.0	8.8	8.2	8.1	8.7	7.1	7.1	7.1
1 to 14 years	1.5	1.5	1.3	1.4	1.4	1.3	1.2	1.2	1.5	1.2
1 to 4 years	2.6	2.8	2.3	2.8	2.9	2.4	2.3	2.4	2.8	2.2
5 to 14 years	1.0	0.9	0.9	0.8	0.8	0.9	0.8	0.8	0.9	0.8
15 to 24 years	21.8	20.6	18.8	18.2	17.6	17.7	16.7	16.1	18.4	20.1
15 to 19 years	17.0	15.9	14.5	14.0	13.0	12.8	11.4	11.2	12.7	14.3
20 to 24 years	26.8	25.5	23.4	22.6	22.1	22.4	21.6	20.6	23.7	25.6
25 to 44 years	15.3	14.9	13.6	13.3	13.2	13.9	13.4	13.2	15.1	17.0
25 to 34 years	20.2	19.3	17.0	17.3	16.6	17.1	16.4	15.9	18.4	20.1
35 to 44 years	10.7	10.7	10.3	9.2	9.6	10.6	10.1	10.3	11.5	13.4
45 to 64 years	6.1	6.1	5.7	5.6	5.7	5.8	5.7	5.7	6.3	6.5
45 to 54 years	7.3	7.3	6.8	6.7	6.8	7.0	6.9	6.9	7.6	7.7
55 to 64 years	4.5	4.4	4.2	4.3	4.4	4.4	4.3	4.3	4.8	5.2
65 years and over	2.8	2.8	3.0	2.6	2.7	2.8	2.8	2.7	2.7	2.7
65 to 74 years	3.1	3.1	3.2	2.9	2.7	3.0	2.9	2.9	2.9	2.9
75 to 84 years	2.8	2.4	2.6	2.1	2.7	2.5	2.5	2.2	2.3	2.6
85 years and over	1.6	2.5	3.1	2.2	2.5	2.2	2.9	2.2	1.9	1.8
Female										
All ages, age-adjusted[4]	2.5	2.4	2.4	2.3	2.2	2.2	2.1	2.1	2.2	2.5
All ages, crude	2.5	2.4	2.4	2.2	2.2	2.2	2.1	2.1	2.2	2.4
Under 1 year	7.2	7.1	6.8	6.9	6.2	6.5	5.5	5.4	6.1	6.8
1 to 14 years	1.2	1.1	1.1	0.9	1.0	1.0	0.9	1.0	0.9	1.0
1 to 4 years	2.4	2.4	2.4	1.9	2.2	1.8	2.0	2.2	1.8	2.1
5 to 14 years	0.7	0.6	0.5	0.5	0.5	0.6	0.5	0.6	0.5	0.6
15 to 24 years	3.4	3.3	3.1	2.9	2.9	2.9	2.6	2.5	2.8	3.3
15 to 19 years	2.7	2.6	2.5	2.3	2.2	2.0	1.6	1.9	2.1	2.6
20 to 24 years	4.2	4.0	3.7	3.4	3.5	3.7	3.6	3.1	3.5	3.9
25 to 44 years	3.6	3.3	3.4	3.1	3.1	3.0	3.0	2.9	3.1	3.5
25 to 34 years	3.7	3.6	3.7	3.3	3.3	3.3	3.2	3.2	3.5	3.8
35 to 44 years	3.5	3.1	3.1	2.9	2.8	2.8	2.7	2.6	2.8	3.3
45 to 64 years	2.1	2.0	2.1	2.0	2.0	2.0	2.0	1.8	1.9	2.1
45 to 54 years	2.5	2.4	2.4	2.3	2.4	2.3	2.3	2.2	2.2	2.4
55 to 64 years	1.5	1.5	1.6	1.7	1.5	1.6	1.7	1.5	1.7	1.8
65 years and over	1.4	1.6	1.6	1.6	1.6	1.5	1.4	1.5	1.5	1.4
65 to 74 years	1.2	1.6	1.5	1.4	1.4	1.3	1.3	1.3	1.2	1.3
75 to 84 years	1.5	1.3	1.5	1.8	1.5	1.7	1.7	1.8	1.9	1.5
85 years and over	1.6	2.3	2.0	2.0	2.1	1.7	1.4	1.8	1.7	1.9
White Male[5]										
All ages, age-adjusted[4]	5.5	5.5	4.9	4.7	4.6	4.6	4.4	4.3	4.7	5.2
All ages, crude	5.5	5.5	4.9	4.7	4.6	4.6	4.4	4.3	4.6	5.1

[3]Starting with 1999 data, cause of death is coded according to *ICD*-10.
[4]Age-adjusted rates are calculated using the year 2000 standard population. Prior to 2001, age-adjusted rates were calculated using standard million proportions based on rounded population numbers. Starting with 2001 data, unrounded population numbers are used to calculate age-adjusted rates.
[5]The race groups, White, Black, Asian or Pacific Islander, and American Indian or Alaska Native, include persons of Hispanic and non-Hispanic origin. Persons of Hispanic origin may be of any race. Death rates for the American Indian or Alaska Native, Asian or Pacific Islander, and Hispanic populations are known to be underestimated.

Table 2-36. Death Rates for Homicide, by Sex, Race, Hispanic Origin, and Age, Selected Years, 1950–2016—*Continued*

(Deaths per 100,000 resident population; data are based on death certificates.)

Sex, race, Hispanic origin, and age	1950[1,2]	1960[1,2]	1970[2]	1980[2]	1985[2]	1990[2]	1995	2000[3]	2005[3]	2006[3]
Under 1 year	4.3	3.8	2.9	4.3	3.8	6.4	7.1	8.2	6.9	7.6
1 to 14 years	0.4	0.5	0.7	1.2	1.3	1.3	1.5	1.2	1.0	1.1
15 to 24 years	3.2	5.0	7.6	15.1	10.7	15.2	15.9	9.9	10.6	10.7
25 to 44 years	5.4	5.5	11.6	17.2	12.7	13.0	10.4	7.4	8.2	8.0
25 to 34 years	4.9	5.7	12.5	18.5	13.7	14.7	12.1	8.4	10.2	9.8
35 to 44 years	6.1	5.2	10.8	15.2	11.3	11.1	8.7	6.5	6.5	6.5
45 to 64 years	4.8	4.6	8.3	9.8	7.4	6.9	5.5	4.1	4.3	4.4
65 years and over	3.8	3.1	5.4	6.7	4.4	4.1	2.9	2.5	2.2	2.1
Black or African American Male[5]										
All ages, age-adjusted[4]	47.0	42.3	78.2	69.4	48.4	63.1	51.1	35.4	37.6	38.0
All ages, crude	44.7	35.0	66.0	65.7	48.3	68.5	54.5	37.2	39.6	40.4
Under 1 year	NA	10.3	14.3	18.6	16.7	21.4	20.3	23.3	16.4	21.4
1 to 14 years[6]	1.8	1.5	4.4	4.1	4.2	5.8	5.8	3.1	3.9	4.0
15 to 24 years	53.8	43.2	98.3	82.6	64.8	137.1	129.4	85.3	83.5	87.3
25 to 44 years	92.8	80.5	140.2	130.0	86.1	105.4	75.8	55.8	64.6	64.2
25 to 34 years	104.3	86.4	154.5	142.9	94.0	123.7	95.1	73.9	89.8	89.9
35 to 44 years	80.0	74.4	124.0	109.3	74.0	81.2	54.9	38.5	40.5	39.5
45 to 64 years	46.0	44.6	82.3	70.6	46.0	41.4	33.4	21.9	21.6	22.5
65 years and over	16.5	17.3	33.3	30.9	26.1	25.7	20.3	12.8	11.8	9.9
American Indian or Alaska Native Male[5]										
All ages, age-adjusted[4]	NA	NA	NA	23.3	19.1	16.7	14.4	10.7	10.1	10.5
All ages, crude	NA	NA	NA	23.1	18.4	16.6	15.7	10.7	10.9	11.2
15 to 24 years	NA	NA	NA	35.4	27.1	25.1	28.0	17.0	19.3	19.2
25 to 44 years	NA	NA	NA	39.2	28.2	25.7	24.6	17.0	14.7	16.1
45 to 64 years	NA	NA	NA	22.1	21.2	14.8	12.0	*	10.0	8.4
Asian or Pacific Islander Male[5]										
All ages, age-adjusted[4]	NA	NA	NA	9.1	5.5	7.3	7.2	4.3	4.3	4.2
All ages, crude	NA	NA	NA	8.3	5.7	7.9	7.5	4.4	4.5	4.4
15 to 24 years	NA	NA	NA	9.3	8.0	14.9	17.2	7.8	9.7	10.2
25 to 44 years	NA	NA	NA	11.3	8.6	9.6	7.4	4.6	4.9	4.1
45 to 64 years	NA	NA	NA	10.4	5.2	7.0	7.7	6.1	4.1	4.7
Hispanic or Latino Male[5,7]										
All ages, age-adjusted[4]	NA	NA	NA	NA	24.9	27.4	20.4	11.8	12.1	11.7
All ages, crude	NA	NA	NA	NA	27.2	31.0	23.5	13.4	13.7	13.2
Under 1 year	NA	NA	NA	NA	*	8.7	5.9	6.6	6.0	9.7
1 to 14 years	NA	NA	NA	NA	1.5	3.1	3.2	1.7	1.5	1.6
15 to 24 years	NA	NA	NA	NA	42.1	55.4	54.7	28.5	29.0	28.7
25 to 44 years	NA	NA	NA	NA	46.7	46.4	28.8	17.2	19.0	17.6
25 to 34 years	NA	NA	NA	NA	50.6	50.9	33.0	19.9	23.7	21.3
35 to 44 years	NA	NA	NA	NA	39.8	39.3	22.8	13.5	13.2	13.1
45 to 64 years	NA	NA	NA	NA	19.6	20.5	14.7	9.1	8.3	8.4
65 years and over	NA	NA	NA	NA	8.9	9.4	5.8	4.4	4.6	3.3
White, not Hispanic or Latino Male[7]										
All ages, age-adjusted[4]	NA	NA	NA	NA	6.1	5.6	4.8	3.6	3.6	3.6
All ages, crude	NA	NA	NA	NA	6.2	5.8	4.9	3.6	3.6	3.7
Under 1 year	NA	NA	NA	NA	4.6	5.4	6.8	8.3	7.3	6.8
1 to 14 years	NA	NA	NA	NA	1.2	0.9	1.1	1.0	0.8	0.9
15 to 24 years	NA	NA	NA	NA	7.6	7.5	7.2	4.7	4.8	4.8
25 to 44 years	NA	NA	NA	NA	9.2	8.7	7.2	5.2	5.2	5.2
25 to 34 years	NA	NA	NA	NA	9.3	9.3	7.7	5.2	5.6	5.6
35 to 44 years	NA	NA	NA	NA	9.1	8.0	6.7	5.2	4.9	4.9
45 to 64 years	NA	NA	NA	NA	6.3	5.7	4.6	3.6	3.8	3.9
65 years and over	NA	NA	NA	NA	4.4	3.7	2.6	2.3	2.1	2.1
Black, not Hispanic or Latino Male[7]										
All ages, age-adjusted[4]	NA	NA	NA	NA	NA	NA	NA	36.4	39.1	39.7
All ages, crude	NA	NA	NA	NA	NA	NA	NA	38.3	41.1	42.1
Under 1 year	NA	NA	NA	NA	NA	NA	NA	24.9	17.2	21.9
1 to 14 years	NA	NA	NA	NA	NA	NA	NA	3.2	4.1	4.2
15 to 24 years	NA	NA	NA	NA	NA	NA	NA	88.1	87.2	91.6
25 to 44 years	NA	NA	NA	NA	NA	NA	NA	57.4	67.1	67.3
25 to 34 years	NA	NA	NA	NA	NA	NA	NA	76.5	94.0	95.2
35 to 44 years	NA	NA	NA	NA	NA	NA	NA	39.4	41.9	41.0
45 to 64 years	NA	NA	NA	NA	NA	NA	NA	22.2	22.1	22.9
65 years and over	NA	NA	NA	NA	NA	NA	NA	12.9	12.1	10.0

NA = Not available

* = Rates based on fewer than 20 deaths are considered unreliable and are not shown.

[1]Includes deaths of persons who were not residents of the 50 states and the District of Columbia.

[2]Underlying cause of death was coded according to the 6th Revision of the *International Classification of Diseases* (*ICD*) in 1950, 7th Revision in 1960, 8th Revision in 1970, and 9th Revision in 1980-1998.

[3]Starting with 1999 data, cause of death is coded according to *ICD*-10.

[4]Age-adjusted rates are calculated using the year 2000 standard population. Prior to 2001, age-adjusted rates were calculated using standard million proportions based on rounded population numbers. Starting with 2001 data, unrounded population numbers are used to calculate age-adjusted rates.

[5]The race groups, White, Black, Asian or Pacific Islander, and American Indian or Alaska Native, include persons of Hispanic and non-Hispanic origin. Persons of Hispanic origin may be of any race. Death rates for the American Indian or Alaska Native, Asian or Pacific Islander, and Hispanic populations are known to be underestimated.

[6]In 1950, rate is for the age group under 15 years.

[7]Prior to 1997, excludes data from states lacking an Hispanic-origin item on the death certificate.

Table 2-36. Death Rates for Homicide, by Sex, Race, Hispanic Origin, and Age, Selected Years, 1950–2016—Continued

(Deaths per 100,000 resident population; data are based on death certificates.)

Sex, race, Hispanic origin, and age	2007[3]	2008[3]	2009[3]	2010[3]	2011[3]	2012[3]	2013[3]	2014[3]	2015[3]	2016[3]
Under 1 year	8.1	7.7	7.1	8.5	6.5	6.4	6.8	5.8	5.9	5.7
1 to 14 years	1.0	1.1	1.0	1.0	1.1	1.0	0.9	0.9	1.0	0.8
15 to 24 years	10.5	10.2	9.1	8.2	7.6	7.5	7.1	6.5	7.3	8.2
25 to 44 years	8.4	8.3	7.3	6.9	6.8	7.1	6.5	6.8	7.2	8.4
25 to 34 years	10.4	9.9	8.3	8.3	7.9	8.1	7.4	7.5	8.0	9.3
35 to 44 years	6.5	6.9	6.3	5.5	5.6	6.0	5.6	6.0	6.3	7.5
45 to 64 years	4.2	4.4	4.1	4.1	4.1	4.1	4.0	4.0	4.4	4.5
65 years and over	2.2	2.3	2.5	2.1	2.3	2.4	2.4	2.2	2.3	2.2
Black or African American Male[5]										
All ages, age-adjusted[4]	37.1	34.4	32.0	31.5	31.2	32.8	31.6	30.6	35.4	38.0
All ages, crude	39.3	36.5	33.8	33.4	33.0	34.5	33.1	32.1	37.3	39.8
Under 1 year	19.8	17.5	18.7	12.3	17.0	17.6	17.9	13.9	13.4	14.7
1 to 14 years	3.9	3.7	3.2	3.4	3.1	3.2	2.6	3.1	3.7	3.1
15 to 24 years	83.9	76.7	70.7	71.0	69.4	70.8	66.6	65.0	74.9	81.4
25 to 44 years	63.3	60.1	56.4	55.9	55.4	59.2	57.9	54.8	65.5	70.4
25 to 34 years	86.2	82.2	74.1	76.1	72.5	73.9	73.2	67.7	81.4	83.8
35 to 44 years	40.7	38.0	38.0	34.5	36.5	42.6	40.4	39.7	46.4	53.9
45 to 64 years	21.5	19.9	18.0	17.6	18.4	18.8	18.4	18.2	20.4	21.1
65 years and over	10.6	8.4	8.8	8.0	6.8	7.5	7.3	8.4	7.2	8.0
American Indian or Alaska Native Male[5]										
All ages, age-adjusted[4]	7.9	9.2	8.9	8.8	8.9	9.0	8.2	9.1	9.8	9.9
All ages, crude	8.5	9.6	9.3	9.5	9.0	9.4	8.3	9.2	9.9	10.0
15 to 24 years	12.2	13.2	15.8	17.6	11.2	12.4	7.1	12.1	15.2	12.3
25 to 44 years	15.0	16.1	15.0	14.8	13.8	15.3	15.4	13.6	15.1	17.4
45 to 64 years	5.8	7.8	7.5	6.5	10.9	9.7	8.0	9.7	10.1	10.1
Asian or Pacific Islander Male[5]										
All ages, age-adjusted[4]	3.1	2.9	2.8	2.6	2.9	2.5	2.3	2.2	2.3	2.5
All ages, crude	3.3	3.1	3.0	2.7	2.9	2.7	2.3	2.3	2.4	2.6
15 to 24 years	6.3	5.9	4.4	4.0	4.2	3.8	3.5	3.4	2.9	3.8
25 to 44 years	3.9	3.5	3.2	3.3	4.1	3.7	2.7	3.0	3.1	3.3
45 to 64 years	3.3	2.8	3.7	3.1	2.0	2.9	2.5	2.5	2.8	3.2
Hispanic or Latino Male[5,7]										
All ages, age-adjusted[4]	11.1	10.3	9.7	8.7	7.9	7.9	7.3	7.2	7.9	8.6
All ages, crude	12.4	11.4	10.5	9.5	8.6	8.5	7.8	7.6	8.4	9.2
Under 1 year	8.1	7.4	5.7	7.0	5.8	5.0	6.8	4.5	*	5.0
1 to 14 years	1.2	1.2	1.2	1.1	1.3	0.9	0.9	0.7	1.2	0.9
15 to 24 years	27.1	24.5	22.9	19.7	17.6	17.1	15.3	14.2	16.5	17.6
25 to 44 years	16.9	15.8	14.2	13.2	12.0	12.3	11.0	11.6	12.2	14.6
25 to 34 years	21.3	18.8	16.5	16.8	14.6	14.7	13.3	13.1	14.3	17.5
35 to 44 years	11.7	12.3	11.5	8.9	9.0	9.5	8.4	9.9	9.9	11.4
45 to 64 years	7.7	7.5	6.9	6.9	5.9	5.9	6.1	5.6	6.3	6.1
65 years and over	3.9	3.1	4.9	3.2	3.5	3.3	2.9	3.3	2.9	2.8
White, not Hispanic or Latino Male[7]										
All ages, age-adjusted[4]	3.8	3.9	3.4	3.3	3.4	3.5	3.4	3.3	3.6	3.9
All ages, crude	3.7	3.9	3.4	3.3	3.4	3.5	3.3	3.3	3.5	3.8
Under 1 year	7.6	7.4	7.3	8.7	6.9	6.8	6.5	6.5	7.0	6.1
1 to 14 years	0.9	1.0	0.8	0.9	1.0	1.0	0.9	0.9	1.0	0.8
15 to 24 years	5.0	5.2	4.1	4.1	3.9	3.9	3.9	3.5	3.8	4.4
25 to 44 years	5.7	5.9	4.9	4.7	4.9	5.1	4.9	4.9	5.3	6.1
25 to 34 years	6.4	6.6	5.2	5.0	5.4	5.5	5.2	5.3	5.5	6.3
35 to 44 years	5.1	5.3	4.7	4.4	4.5	4.8	4.6	4.6	5.0	5.9
45 to 64 years	3.7	3.9	3.7	3.6	3.7	3.7	3.6	3.6	3.9	4.1
65 years and over	2.0	2.2	2.3	2.0	2.2	2.3	2.3	2.0	2.2	2.1
Black, not Hispanic or Latino Male[7]										
All ages, age-adjusted[4]	39.0	36.2	33.7	33.1	33.0	34.8	33.5	32.4	37.6	40.4
All ages, crude	41.1	38.2	35.4	35.0	34.9	36.5	35.1	34.0	39.6	42.3
Under 1 year	21.1	18.6	19.9	13.0	17.7	19.0	18.7	13.9	14.0	15.1
1 to 14 years	4.2	4.0	3.5	3.6	3.3	3.4	2.8	3.3	4.0	3.3
15 to 24 years	88.0	80.9	74.6	74.9	73.9	75.4	71.0	69.0	79.6	86.8
25 to 44 years	66.5	63.3	59.5	58.9	58.9	63.1	61.6	58.5	70.0	75.3
25 to 34 years	91.4	87.5	78.9	81.1	77.6	79.3	78.1	72.9	87.2	89.7
35 to 44 years	42.6	39.5	39.7	35.8	38.6	45.2	43.0	41.8	49.5	57.7
45 to 64 years	22.2	20.4	18.4	18.0	19.0	19.4	19.1	18.7	21.2	21.9
65 years and over	10.9	8.6	8.9	8.2	6.8	7.4	7.5	8.6	7.3	8.1

* = Rates based on fewer than 20 deaths are considered unreliable and are not shown.
[3]Starting with 1999 data, cause of death is coded according to *ICD*-10.
[4]Age-adjusted rates are calculated using the year 2000 standard population. Prior to 2001, age-adjusted rates were calculated using standard million proportions based on rounded population numbers. Starting with 2001 data, unrounded population numbers are used to calculate age-adjusted rates.
[5]The race groups, White, Black, Asian or Pacific Islander, and American Indian or Alaska Native, include persons of Hispanic and non-Hispanic origin. Persons of Hispanic origin may be of any race. Death rates for the American Indian or Alaska Native, Asian or Pacific Islander, and Hispanic populations are known to be underestimated.
[7]Prior to 1997, excludes data from states lacking an Hispanic-origin item on the death certificate.

Table 2-36. Death Rates for Homicide, by Sex, Race, Hispanic Origin, and Age, Selected Years, 1950–2016—*Continued*

(Deaths per 100,000 resident population; data are based on death certificates.)

Sex, race, Hispanic origin, and age	1950[1,2]	1960[1,2]	1970[2]	1980[2]	1985[2]	1990[2]	1995	2000[3]	2005[3]	2006[3]
White Female[4]										
All ages, age-adjusted[4]	1.4	1.5	2.3	3.2	2.9	2.7	2.7	2.1	1.9	2.0
All ages, crude	1.4	1.4	2.1	3.2	2.9	2.8	2.7	2.1	1.9	1.9
Under 1 year	3.9	3.5	2.9	4.3	4.3	5.1	5.1	5.0	5.7	6.6
1 to 14 years	0.4	0.4	0.7	1.1	1.1	1.0	1.1	0.8	0.8	0.8
15 to 24 years	1.3	1.5	2.7	4.7	3.6	4.0	4.0	2.7	2.3	2.4
25 to 44 years	2.0	2.1	3.3	4.2	4.1	3.8	3.7	2.9	2.8	2.5
45 to 64 years	1.5	1.7	2.1	2.6	2.6	2.3	2.2	1.8	1.5	1.8
65 years and over	1.2	1.2	1.9	2.9	2.6	2.2	2.0	1.6	1.6	1.5
Black or African American Female[4]										
All ages, age-adjusted[4]	11.1	11.4	14.7	13.2	10.6	12.5	10.4	7.1	6.0	6.4
All ages, crude	11.5	10.4	13.2	13.5	11.0	13.4	10.9	7.2	6.1	6.5
Under 1 year	NA	13.8	10.7	12.8	10.7	22.8	20.1	22.2	12.9	11.3
1 to 14 years[6]	1.8	1.2	3.1	3.3	3.3	4.7	3.4	2.7	2.3	2.5
15 to 24 years	16.5	11.9	17.7	18.4	14.2	18.9	16.4	10.7	8.7	9.3
25 to 44 years	22.5	22.7	25.3	22.6	17.8	21.0	17.1	11.0	9.3	10.1
45 to 64 years	6.8	10.3	13.4	10.8	7.9	6.5	5.9	4.5	4.8	5.1
65 years and over	3.6	3.0	7.4	8.0	7.8	9.4	6.8	3.5	3.0	2.5
American Indian or Alaska Native Female[4]										
All ages, age-adjusted[4]	NA	NA	NA	8.1	4.8	4.6	5.3	3.0	3.5	2.6
All ages, crude	NA	NA	NA	7.7	4.5	4.8	5.1	2.9	3.6	2.6
15 to 24 years	NA	NA	NA	*	*	*	*	*	*	*
25 to 44 years	NA	NA	NA	13.7	*	6.9	8.3	5.9	5.4	5.2
45 to 64 years	NA	NA	NA	*	*	*	*	*	*	*
Asian or Pacific Islander Female[5]										
All ages, age-adjusted[4]	NA	NA	NA	3.1	2.6	2.8	2.4	1.7	1.5	1.3
All ages, crude	NA	NA	NA	3.1	2.8	2.8	2.6	1.7	1.5	1.4
15 to 24 years	NA	NA	NA	*	*	*	*	*	2.5	*
25 to 44 years	NA	NA	NA	4.6	2.9	3.8	3.6	2.2	1.6	1.6
45 to 64 years	NA	NA	NA	*	*	*	2.2	2.0	1.2	1.9
Hispanic or Latina Female[5,7]										
All ages, age-adjusted[4]	NA	NA	NA	NA	4.1	4.3	4.0	2.8	2.3	2.3
All ages, crude	NA	NA	NA	NA	4.3	4.7	4.2	2.8	2.4	2.4
Under 1 year	NA	NA	NA	NA	*	*	*	7.4	6.2	6.2
1 to 14 years	NA	NA	NA	NA	1.5	1.9	1.8	1.0	1.0	1.0
15 to 24 years	NA	NA	NA	NA	5.7	8.1	6.4	3.7	3.4	3.6
25 to 44 years	NA	NA	NA	NA	6.8	6.1	5.6	3.7	3.3	3.1
45 to 64 years	NA	NA	NA	NA	3.2	3.3	3.4	2.9	1.9	1.8
65 years and over	NA	NA	NA	NA	*	*	2.4	2.4	*	*
White, not Hispanic or Latina Female[7]										
All ages, age-adjusted[4]	NA	NA	NA	NA	2.9	2.5	2.3	1.9	1.8	1.8
All ages, crude	NA	NA	NA	NA	2.9	2.5	2.3	1.9	1.8	1.8
Under 1 year	NA	NA	NA	NA	4.1	4.4	4.4	4.1	5.3	6.5
1 to 14 years	NA	NA	NA	NA	1.0	0.8	0.9	0.8	0.7	0.8
15 to 24 years	NA	NA	NA	NA	3.5	3.3	3.4	2.3	2.0	2.1
25 to 44 years	NA	NA	NA	NA	3.9	3.5	3.3	2.7	2.7	2.3
45 to 64 years	NA	NA	NA	NA	3.6	2.2	1.9	1.6	1.4	1.8
65 years and over	NA	NA	NA	NA	2.6	2.2	1.9	1.6	1.6	1.5
Black, not Hispanic or Latina Female[7]										
All ages, age-adjusted[4]	NA	NA	NA	NA	NA	NA	NA	7.2	6.3	6.7
All ages, crude	NA	NA	NA	NA	NA	NA	NA	7.4	6.3	6.8
Under 1 year	NA	NA	NA	NA	NA	NA	NA	23.3	14.0	12.0
1 to 14 years	NA	NA	NA	NA	NA	NA	NA	2.8	2.4	2.6
15 to 24 years	NA	NA	NA	NA	NA	NA	NA	11.0	9.0	9.7
25 to 44 years	NA	NA	NA	NA	NA	NA	NA	11.3	9.7	10.6
45 to 64 years	NA	NA	NA	NA	NA	NA	NA	4.5	4.9	5.3
65 years and over	NA	NA	NA	NA	NA	NA	NA	3.5	3.0	2.5

NA = Not available

* = Rates based on fewer than 20 deaths are considered unreliable and are not shown.

[1]Includes deaths of persons who were not residents of the 50 states and the District of Columbia.

[2]Underlying cause of death was coded according to the 6th Revision of the *International Classification of Diseases* (*ICD*) in 1950, 7th Revision in 1960, 8th Revision in 1970, and 9th Revision in 1980-1998.

[3]Starting with 1999 data, cause of death is coded according to *ICD*-10.

[4]Age-adjusted rates are calculated using the year 2000 standard population. Prior to 2001, age-adjusted rates were calculated using standard million proportions based on rounded population numbers. Starting with 2001 data, unrounded population numbers are used to calculate age-adjusted rates.

[5]The race groups, White, Black, Asian or Pacific Islander, and American Indian or Alaska Native, include persons of Hispanic and non-Hispanic origin. Persons of Hispanic origin may be of any race. Death rates for the American Indian or Alaska Native, Asian or Pacific Islander, and Hispanic populations are known to be underestimated.

[6]In 1950, rate is for the age group under 15 years.

[7]Prior to 1997, excludes data from states lacking an Hispanic-origin item on the death certificate.

Table 2-36. Death Rates for Homicide, by Sex, Race, Hispanic Origin, and Age, Selected Years, 1950–2016—*Continued*

(Deaths per 100,000 resident population; data are based on death certificates.)

Sex, race, Hispanic origin, and age	2007[3]	2008[3]	2009[3]	2010[3]	2011[3]	2012[3]	2013[3]	2014[3]	2015[3]	2016[3]
White Female[4]										
All ages, age-adjusted[4]	2.0	1.9	1.9	1.8	1.8	1.8	1.7	1.7	1.8	1.9
All ages, crude	1.9	1.9	1.9	1.8	1.8	1.8	1.7	1.7	1.7	1.8
Under 1 year	6.4	5.6	5.1	5.8	4.9	5.9	4.3	4.5	4.2	5.5
1 to 14 years	0.9	0.8	0.9	0.7	0.8	0.8	0.7	0.8	0.7	0.7
15 to 24 years	2.5	2.2	2.1	2.0	1.9	1.9	1.8	1.7	1.9	2.1
25 to 44 years	2.8	2.7	2.7	2.4	2.5	2.4	2.3	2.3	2.5	2.8
45 to 64 years	1.7	1.8	1.8	1.7	1.7	1.7	1.7	1.5	1.7	1.8
65 years and over	1.3	1.5	1.5	1.6	1.4	1.4	1.4	1.5	1.4	1.3
Black or African American Female[4]										
All ages, age-adjusted[4]	6.0	5.4	5.2	5.0	4.9	4.9	4.9	4.7	4.9	5.7
All ages, crude	6.1	5.5	5.3	5.1	5.0	4.9	4.9	4.7	4.9	5.7
Under 1 year	11.7	15.4	15.4	13.9	11.9	11.5	12.4	10.8	15.8	13.2
1 to 14 years[6]	2.7	2.5	2.2	2.0	2.2	2.0	2.1	2.2	1.9	2.5
15 to 24 years	8.6	9.3	8.0	7.5	8.1	8.0	6.9	7.0	7.5	9.2
25 to 44 years	9.1	7.6	7.8	7.4	7.0	7.1	7.2	6.7	7.4	8.4
45 to 64 years	4.8	3.7	4.0	4.2	3.9	3.9	4.3	3.7	3.7	4.3
65 years and over	2.6	2.3	2.2	1.8	2.3	2.2	2.0	2.4	2.0	2.3
American Indian or Alaska Native Female[4]										
All ages, age-adjusted[4]	3.1	3.1	2.9	2.5	2.8	2.4	2.4	2.5	2.5	3.5
All ages, crude	3.0	3.2	3.0	2.5	2.7	2.6	2.4	2.4	2.5	3.5
15 to 24 years	*	*	*	*	*	*	*	*	*	*
25 to 44 years	4.4	3.9	*	4.7	*	3.6	3.7	4.2	4.1	5.6
45 to 64 years	*	*	*	*	*	*	*	*	*	*
Asian or Pacific Islander Female[5]										
All ages, age-adjusted[4]	1.3	1.2	1.3	1.2	1.3	1.2	0.9	1.0	1.0	1.2
All ages, crude	1.3	1.2	1.3	1.2	1.3	1.2	0.9	1.0	1.0	1.2
15 to 24 years	*	*	*	*	*	*	*	*	*	*
25 to 44 years	1.8	1.3	1.5	1.3	1.5	1.2	1.3	0.8	1.0	1.1
45 to 64 years	1.5	1.1	1.6	1.4	1.3	1.6	1.1	1.5	1.0	1.3
Hispanic or Latina Female[5,7]										
All ages, age-adjusted[4]	2.2	2.3	2.2	1.8	1.8	1.8	1.6	1.7	1.8	1.8
All ages, crude	2.4	2.4	2.2	1.8	1.9	1.8	1.6	1.8	1.8	1.9
Under 1 year	7.1	5.4	6.1	6.6	3.9	4.6	4.0	4.6	4.2	4.4
1 to 14 years	1.2	1.1	1.1	0.5	0.9	0.8	0.7	1.0	0.5	0.7
15 to 24 years	3.2	3.3	3.0	2.6	2.3	2.2	2.5	2.7	2.4	2.5
25 to 44 years	3.2	3.1	2.9	2.5	2.8	2.4	2.4	2.3	2.5	2.7
45 to 64 years	1.7	2.0	2.0	1.6	1.5	1.8	1.2	1.4	1.7	1.5
65 years and over	*	1.6	1.3	1.3	*	*	*	*	1.2	1.2
White, not Hispanic or Latina Female[7]										
All ages, age-adjusted[4]	1.9	1.8	1.8	1.8	1.7	1.7	1.7	1.6	1.7	1.8
All ages, crude	1.8	1.8	1.8	1.7	1.7	1.7	1.7	1.6	1.7	1.8
Under 1 year	5.9	5.7	4.2	5.3	5.0	6.1	4.4	4.4	4.4	5.9
1 to 14 years	0.8	0.7	0.8	0.7	0.7	0.8	0.7	0.7	0.7	0.7
15 to 24 years	2.2	1.8	1.7	1.8	1.7	1.7	1.6	1.3	1.7	1.8
25 to 44 years	2.6	2.5	2.5	2.4	2.3	2.4	2.2	2.3	2.4	2.7
45 to 64 years	1.7	1.7	1.7	1.7	1.7	1.7	1.8	1.5	1.7	1.8
65 years and over	1.3	1.5	1.5	1.6	1.5	1.4	1.5	1.5	1.4	1.3
Black, not Hispanic or Latina Female[7]										
All ages, age-adjusted[4]	6.3	5.6	5.4	5.2	5.2	5.1	5.1	4.8	5.1	6.0
All ages, crude	6.3	5.7	5.5	5.3	5.3	5.1	5.2	4.9	5.2	6.0
Under 1 year	12.7	16.2	16.5	15.1	12.6	11.4	12.8	10.4	15.9	14.1
1 to 14 years	2.7	2.6	2.3	2.2	2.3	2.0	2.2	2.3	2.1	2.7
15 to 24 years	9.0	9.8	8.4	7.9	8.6	8.4	7.2	7.2	8.0	9.9
25 to 44 years	9.6	8.0	8.1	7.9	7.4	7.5	7.7	7.1	7.8	8.9
45 to 64 years	4.9	3.8	4.1	4.3	4.1	3.9	4.5	3.8	3.9	4.5
65 years and over	2.7	2.4	2.2	1.9	2.4	2.2	2.1	2.4	2.1	2.4

* = Rates based on fewer than 20 deaths are considered unreliable and are not shown.
[3]Starting with 1999 data, cause of death is coded according to *ICD*-10.
[4]Age-adjusted rates are calculated using the year 2000 standard population. Prior to 2001, age-adjusted rates were calculated using standard million proportions based on rounded population numbers. Starting with 2001 data, unrounded population numbers are used to calculate age-adjusted rates.
[5]The race groups, White, Black, Asian or Pacific Islander, and American Indian or Alaska Native, include persons of Hispanic and non-Hispanic origin. Persons of Hispanic origin may be of any race. Death rates for the American Indian or Alaska Native, Asian or Pacific Islander, and Hispanic populations are known to be underestimated.
[6]In 1950, rate is for the age group under 15 years.
[7]Prior to 1997, excludes data from states lacking an Hispanic-origin item on the death certificate.

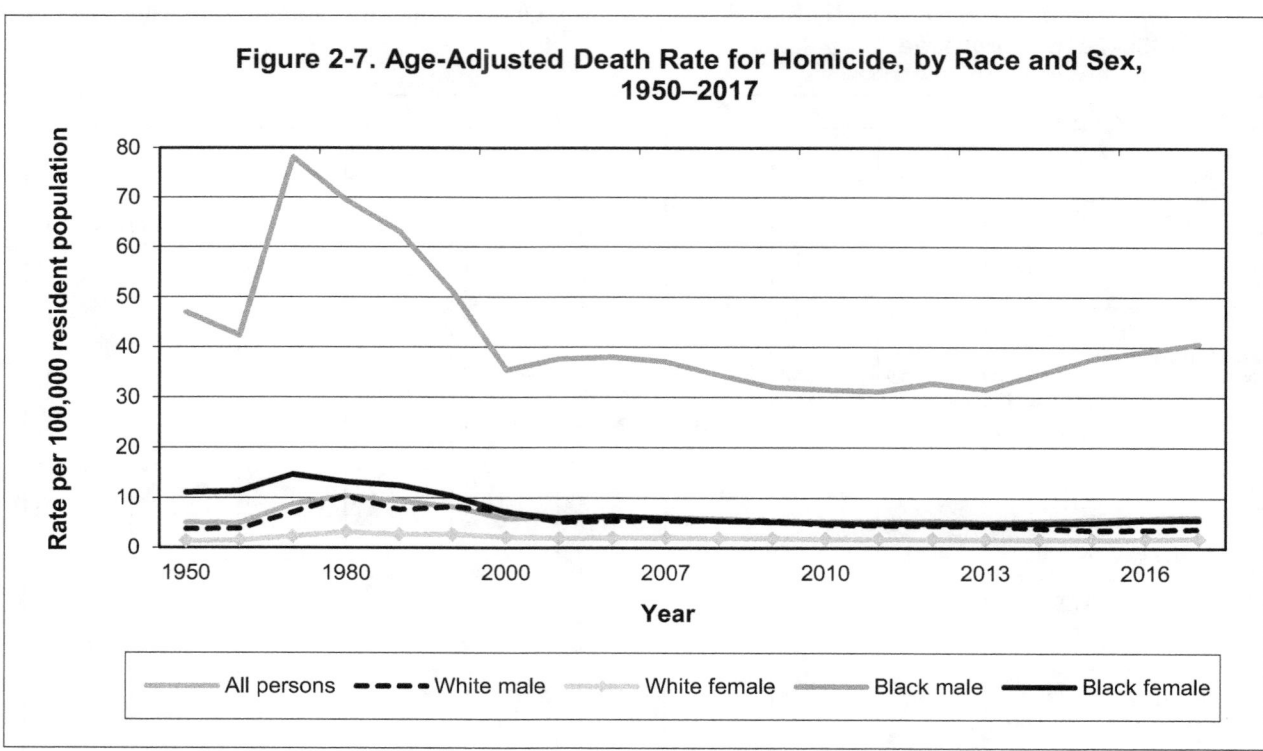

Figure 2-7. Age-Adjusted Death Rate for Homicide, by Race and Sex, 1950–2017

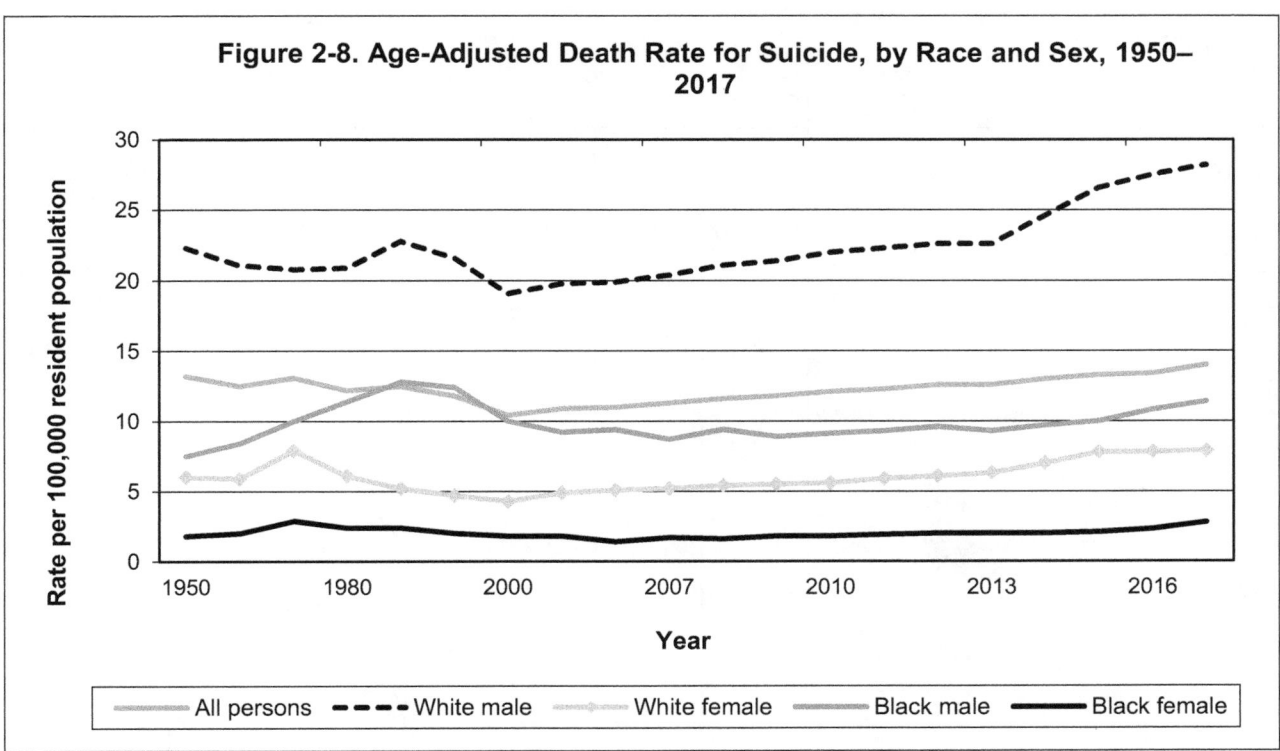

Figure 2-8. Age-Adjusted Death Rate for Suicide, by Race and Sex, 1950–2017

Table 2-37. Death Rates for Suicide, by Sex, Race, Hispanic Origin, and Age, Selected Years, 1950–2016

(Deaths per 100,000 resident population; data are based on death certificates.)

Sex, race, Hispanic origin, and age	1950[1,2]	1960[1,2]	1970[2]	1980[2]	1985	1990[2]	1995	2000[3]	2005[3]	2006[3]
All Persons										
All ages, age-adjusted[4]	13.2	12.5	13.1	12.2	12.5	12.5	11.8	10.4	10.9	11.0
All ages, crude	11.4	10.6	11.6	11.9	12.4	12.4	11.7	10.4	11.0	11.2
Under 1 year	X	X	X	X	X	X	X	X	X	X
1 to 4 years	X	X	X	X	X	X	X	X	X	X
5 to 14 years	0.2	0.3	0.3	0.4	0.8	0.8	0.9	0.7	0.7	0.5
15 to 24 years	4.5	5.2	8.8	12.3	12.8	13.2	13.0	10.2	9.9	9.8
15 to 19 years	2.7	3.6	5.9	8.5	9.9	11.1	10.3	8.0	7.5	7.1
20 to 24 years	6.2	7.1	12.2	16.1	15.4	15.1	15.8	12.5	12.4	12.5
25 to 44 years	11.6	12.2	15.4	15.6	15.0	15.2	15.1	13.4	13.9	14.0
25 to 34 years	9.1	10.0	14.1	16.0	15.3	15.2	15.0	12.0	12.7	12.7
35 to 44 years	14.3	14.2	16.9	15.4	14.6	15.3	15.1	14.5	15.1	15.2
45 to 64 years	23.5	22.0	20.6	15.9	16.3	15.3	13.9	13.5	15.3	16.0
45 to 54 years	20.9	20.7	20.0	15.9	15.7	14.8	14.4	14.4	16.5	17.2
55 to 64 years	26.8	23.7	21.4	15.9	16.8	16.0	13.2	12.1	13.7	14.4
65 years and over	30.0	24.5	20.8	17.6	20.4	20.5	17.9	15.2	14.7	14.3
65 to 74 years	29.6	23.0	20.8	16.9	18.7	17.9	15.7	12.5	12.4	12.4
75 to 84 years	31.1	27.9	21.2	19.1	23.9	24.9	20.6	17.6	16.8	15.8
85 years and over	28.8	26.0	19.0	19.2	19.4	22.2	21.3	19.6	18.3	17.3
Male										
All ages, age-adjusted[4]	21.2	20.0	19.8	19.9	21.1	21.5	20.3	17.7	18.1	18.1
All ages, crude	17.8	16.5	16.8	18.6	20.0	20.4	19.5	17.1	17.8	17.9
Under 1 year	X	X	X	X	X	X	X	X	X	X
1 to 4 years	X	X	X	X	X	X	X	X	X	X
5 to 14 years	0.3	0.4	0.5	0.6	1.2	1.1	1.3	1.2	1.0	0.7
15 to 24 years	6.5	8.2	13.5	20.2	21.0	22.0	22.0	17.1	16.1	16.0
15 to 19 years	3.5	5.6	8.8	13.8	15.8	18.1	17.1	13.0	11.8	11.3
20 to 24 years	9.3	11.5	19.3	26.8	25.7	25.7	27.0	21.4	20.4	21.0
25 to 44 years	17.2	17.9	20.9	24.0	23.7	24.4	24.4	21.3	22.1	22.1
25 to 34 years	13.4	14.7	19.8	25.0	24.7	24.8	24.8	19.6	20.6	20.5
35 to 44 years	21.3	21.0	22.1	22.5	22.3	23.9	24.0	22.8	23.4	23.5
45 to 64 years	37.1	34.4	30.0	23.7	25.3	24.3	22.2	21.3	23.9	24.6
45 to 54 years	32.0	31.6	27.9	22.9	23.6	23.2	22.5	22.4	25.2	26.2
55 to 64 years	43.6	38.1	32.7	24.5	27.1	25.7	21.8	19.4	22.0	22.5
65 years and over	52.8	44.0	38.4	35.0	40.9	41.6	36.2	31.1	29.5	28.4
65 to 74 years	50.5	39.6	36.0	30.4	33.9	32.2	28.5	22.7	22.3	22.2
75 to 84 years	58.3	52.5	42.8	42.3	53.1	56.1	44.9	38.6	35.5	32.9
85 years and over	58.3	57.4	42.4	50.6	56.2	65.9	62.7	57.5	49.9	48.0
Female										
All ages, age-adjusted[4]	5.6	5.6	7.4	5.7	5.2	4.8	4.3	4.0	4.4	4.5
All ages, crude	5.1	4.9	6.6	5.5	5.2	4.8	4.3	4.0	4.5	4.6
Under 1 year	X	X	X	X	X	X	X	X	X	X
1 to 4 years	X	X	X	X	X	X	X	X	X	X
5 to 14 years	0.1	0.1	0.2	0.2	0.4	0.4	0.4	0.3	0.3	0.3
15 to 24 years	2.6	2.2	4.2	4.3	4.3	3.9	3.6	3.0	3.5	3.2
15 to 19 years	1.8	1.6	2.9	3.0	3.7	3.7	3.1	2.7	3.0	2.8
20 to 24 years	3.3	2.9	5.7	5.5	4.9	4.1	4.2	3.2	4.0	3.6
25 to 44 years	6.2	6.6	10.2	7.7	6.5	6.2	5.8	5.4	5.8	5.9
25 to 34 years	4.9	5.5	8.6	7.1	5.9	5.6	5.1	4.3	4.7	4.7
35 to 44 years	7.5	7.7	11.9	8.5	7.1	6.8	6.4	6.4	6.8	7.0
45 to 64 years	9.9	10.2	12.0	8.9	8.0	7.1	6.1	6.2	7.2	7.7
45 to 54 years	9.9	10.2	12.6	9.4	8.3	6.9	6.6	6.7	8.0	8.4
55 to 64 years	9.9	10.2	11.4	8.4	7.8	7.3	5.3	5.4	6.0	6.8
65 years and over	9.4	8.4	8.1	6.1	6.6	6.4	5.4	4.0	4.0	3.9
65 to 74 years	10.1	8.4	9.0	6.5	6.9	6.7	5.4	4.0	4.0	4.0
75 to 84 years	8.1	8.9	7.0	5.5	6.7	6.3	5.4	4.0	4.0	4.0
85 years and over	8.2	6.0	5.9	5.5	4.7	5.4	5.4	4.2	4.3	3.3
White Male[5]										
All ages, age-adjusted[4]	22.3	21.1	20.8	20.9	22.4	22.8	21.6	19.1	19.8	19.9
All ages, crude	19.0	17.6	18.0	19.9	21.6	22.0	21.1	18.8	19.9	20.0

NOTE: Starting with *Health, United States, 2003*, rates for 1991–1999 were revised using intercensal population estimates based on the 1990 and 2000 Censuses. For 2000, population estimates are bridged-race April 1 census counts. Starting with *Health, United States, 2012*, rates for 2001–2009 were revised using intercensal population estimates based on the 2000 and 2010 Censuses. For 2010, population estimates are bridged-race April 1 census counts. Rates for 2011 and beyond were computed using 2010-based postcensal estimates. Age groups were selected to minimize the presentation of unstable age-specific death rates based on small numbers of deaths and for consistency among comparison groups. Starting with 2003 data, some states began to collect information on more than one race on the death certificate, according to 1997 Office of Management and Budget (OMB) standards. The multiple-race data for these states were bridged to the single-race categories of the 1977 OMB standards, for comparability with other states. X = Not applicable.

[1] Includes deaths of persons who were not residents of the 50 states and the District of Columbia (DC).
[2] Underlying cause of death was coded according to the 6th revision of the *International Classification of Diseases* (*ICD*) in 1950, 7th revision in 1960, 8th revision in 1970, and 9th revision in 1980–1998.
[3] Starting with 1999 data, cause of death is coded according to *ICD–10*.
[4] Age-adjusted rates are calculated using the year 2000 standard population. Prior to 2001, age-adjusted rates were calculated using standard million proportions based on rounded population numbers. Starting with 2001 data, unrounded population numbers are used to calculate age-adjusted rates.
[5] The race groups, White, Black, Asian or Pacific Islander, and American Indian and Alaska Native, include persons of Hispanic and non-Hispanic origin. Persons of Hispanic origin may be of any race. Death rates for Hispanic, American Indian or Alaska Native, and Asian or Pacific Islander persons should be interpreted with caution because of inconsistencies in reporting Hispanic origin or race on the death certificate (death rate numerators) compared with population figures (death rate denominators). The net effect of misclassification is an underestimation of deaths and death rates for races other than White and Black.

Table 2-37. Death Rates for Suicide, by Sex, Race, Hispanic Origin, and Age, Selected Years, 1950–2016—Continued

(Deaths per 100,000 resident population; data are based on death certificates.)

Sex, race, Hispanic origin, and age	2007[3]	2008[3]	2009[3]	2010[3]	2011[3]	2012[3]	2013[3]	2014[3]	2015[3]	2016[3]
All Persons										
All ages, age-adjusted[4]	11.3	11.6	11.8	12.1	12.3	12.6	12.6	13.0	13.3	13.5
All ages, crude	11.5	11.8	12.0	12.4	12.7	12.9	13.0	13.4	13.7	13.9
Under 1 year	X	X	X	X	X	X	X	X	X	X
1 to 4 years	X	X	X	X	X	X	X	X	X	X
5 to 14 years	0.5	0.5	0.6	0.7	0.7	0.8	1.0	1.0	1.0	1.1
15 to 24 years	9.6	9.9	10.0	10.5	11.0	11.1	11.1	11.6	12.5	13.2
15 to 19 years	6.7	7.2	7.5	7.5	8.3	8.3	8.3	8.7	9.8	10.0
20 to 24 years	12.6	12.7	12.6	13.6	13.6	13.7	13.7	14.2	15.1	16.1
25 to 44 years	14.5	14.6	14.6	15.0	15.4	15.7	15.5	15.8	16.4	16.9
25 to 34 years	13.3	13.2	13.1	14.0	14.6	14.7	14.8	15.1	15.7	16.5
35 to 44 years	15.7	15.9	16.1	16.0	16.2	16.7	16.2	16.6	17.1	17.4
45 to 64 years	16.7	17.5	17.9	18.6	18.6	19.1	19.0	19.5	19.6	19.2
45 to 54 years	17.7	18.6	19.2	19.6	19.8	20.0	19.7	20.2	20.3	19.7
55 to 64 years	15.3	16.0	16.4	17.5	17.1	18.0	18.1	18.8	18.9	18.7
65 years and over	14.3	14.8	14.8	14.9	15.3	15.4	16.1	16.7	16.6	16.7
65 to 74 years	12.4	13.6	13.7	13.7	14.1	14.0	15.0	15.6	15.2	15.4
75 to 84 years	16.2	16.1	15.8	15.7	16.5	16.8	17.1	17.5	17.9	18.2
85 years and over	17.0	16.4	16.4	17.6	16.9	17.8	18.6	19.3	19.4	19.0
Male										
All ages, age-adjusted[4]	18.5	19.0	19.2	19.8	20.0	20.4	20.3	20.7	21.1	21.4
All ages, crude	18.4	19.0	19.3	19.9	20.2	20.6	20.6	21.1	21.5	21.8
Under 1 year	X	X	X	X	X	X	X	X	X	X
1 to 4 years	X	X	X	X	X	X	X	X	X	X
5 to 14 years	0.6	0.7	0.8	0.9	1.0	1.1	1.2	1.3	1.2	1.3
15 to 24 years	15.7	16.0	16.1	16.9	17.6	17.4	17.3	18.2	19.4	20.5
15 to 19 years	10.8	11.3	11.6	11.7	12.9	12.5	12.4	13.0	14.2	14.8
20 to 24 years	20.9	21.0	20.8	22.2	22.3	22.0	21.9	22.9	24.2	25.9
25 to 44 years	22.9	22.8	23.0	23.6	24.0	24.5	24.1	24.4	25.2	26.2
25 to 34 years	21.5	21.2	21.0	22.5	23.1	23.4	23.4	23.8	24.7	26.0
35 to 44 years	24.2	24.4	24.9	24.6	24.9	25.7	24.8	25.0	25.9	26.3
45 to 64 years	25.7	27.4	27.9	29.2	28.9	29.5	29.0	29.7	29.5	29.1
45 to 54 years	27.0	28.6	29.3	30.4	30.1	30.2	29.6	30.0	30.1	29.4
55 to 64 years	23.9	25.8	26.1	27.7	27.3	28.7	28.3	29.4	28.9	28.7
65 years and over	28.4	29.2	29.1	29.0	29.4	29.5	30.9	31.4	31.0	31.0
65 to 74 years	22.0	24.3	24.3	23.9	24.4	24.1	26.0	26.6	26.2	25.9
75 to 84 years	33.8	33.5	32.9	32.3	33.8	34.2	34.7	34.9	35.2	36.0
85 years and over	46.6	43.0	44.0	47.3	44.1	46.9	48.5	49.9	48.2	48.0
Female										
All ages, age-adjusted[4]	4.6	4.8	4.9	5.0	5.2	5.4	5.5	5.8	6.0	6.0
All ages, crude	4.8	4.9	5.0	5.2	5.4	5.5	5.7	6.0	6.2	6.2
Under 1 year	X	X	X	X	X	X	X	X	X	X
1 to 4 years	X	X	X	X	X	X	X	X	X	X
5 to 14 years	0.3	0.3	0.5	0.4	0.4	0.4	0.7	0.7	0.8	0.9
15 to 24 years	3.1	3.5	3.6	3.9	4.0	4.5	4.5	4.6	5.3	5.4
15 to 19 years	2.4	3.0	3.2	3.1	3.5	3.9	3.9	4.2	5.1	5.0
20 to 24 years	3.9	4.0	4.1	4.7	4.5	4.9	5.2	5.0	5.5	5.8
25 to 44 years	6.2	6.3	6.2	6.4	6.8	6.8	6.8	7.2	7.5	7.6
25 to 34 years	5.0	5.1	5.1	5.3	6.0	5.9	6.1	6.3	6.6	6.7
35 to 44 years	7.3	7.4	7.4	7.5	7.6	7.7	7.6	8.2	8.4	8.5
45 to 64 years	8.1	8.1	8.5	8.6	8.8	9.1	9.4	9.8	10.2	9.9
45 to 54 years	8.7	9.0	9.3	9.0	9.8	10.2	10.0	10.7	10.7	10.3
55 to 64 years	7.2	6.9	7.4	8.0	7.6	8.0	8.7	8.9	9.7	9.4
65 years and over	3.9	4.1	4.0	4.2	4.5	4.5	4.6	5.0	5.1	5.3
65 to 74 years	4.2	4.4	4.6	4.8	5.2	5.2	5.4	5.9	5.7	6.2
75 to 84 years	3.8	3.8	3.6	3.7	3.8	3.9	3.9	4.3	4.6	4.5
85 years and over	3.4	3.8	3.2	3.3	3.5	3.2	3.3	3.4	4.2	3.5
White Male[5]										
All ages, age-adjusted[4]	20.4	21.1	21.4	22.0	22.3	22.6	22.6	23.3	23.6	23.9
All ages, crude	20.7	21.5	21.9	22.6	23.0	23.3	23.4	24.2	24.6	24.8

NOTE: Starting with *Health, United States, 2003*, rates for 1991–1999 were revised using intercensal population estimates based on the 1990 and 2000 Censuses. For 2000, population estimates are bridged-race April 1 census counts. Starting with *Health, United States, 2012*, rates for 2001–2009 were revised using intercensal population estimates based on the 2000 and 2010 Censuses. For 2010, population estimates are bridged-race April 1 census counts. Rates for 2011 and beyond were computed using 2010-based postcensal estimates. Age groups were selected to minimize the presentation of unstable age-specific death rates based on small numbers of deaths and for consistency among comparison groups. Starting with 2003 data, some states began to collect information on more than one race on the death certificate, according to 1997 Office of Management and Budget (OMB) standards. The multiple-race data for these states were bridged to the single-race categories of the 1977 OMB standards, for comparability with other states.

X = Not applicable.

[3]Starting with 1999 data, cause of death is coded according to *ICD–10*.

[4]Age-adjusted rates are calculated using the year 2000 standard population. Prior to 2001, age-adjusted rates were calculated using standard million proportions based on rounded population numbers. Starting with 2001 data, unrounded population numbers are used to calculate age-adjusted rates.

[5]The race groups, White, Black, Asian or Pacific Islander, and American Indian and Alaska Native, include persons of Hispanic and non-Hispanic origin. Persons of Hispanic origin may be of any race. Death rates for Hispanic, American Indian or Alaska Native, and Asian or Pacific Islander persons should be interpreted with caution because of inconsistencies in reporting Hispanic origin or race on the death certificate (death rate numerators) compared with population figures (death rate denominators). The net effect of misclassification is an underestimation of deaths and death rates for races other than White and Black.

Table 2-37. Death Rates for Suicide, by Sex, Race, Hispanic Origin, and Age, Selected Years, 1950–2016—*Continued*

(Deaths per 100,000 resident population; data are based on death certificates.)

Sex, race, Hispanic origin, and age	1950[1,2]	1960[1,2]	1970[2]	1980[2]	1985	1990[2]	1995	2000[3]	2005[3]	2006[3]
15 to 24 years	6.6	8.6	13.9	21.4	22.3	23.2	23.1	17.9	17.3	17.2
25 to 44 years	17.9	18.5	21.5	24.6	24.8	25.4	25.8	22.9	24.2	24.2
45 to 64 years	39.3	36.5	31.9	25.0	27.0	26.0	23.9	23.2	26.6	27.5
65 years and over	55.8	46.7	41.1	37.2	43.7	44.2	38.5	33.3	32.0	30.8
65 to 74 years	53.2	42.0	38.7	32.5	35.8	34.2	30.1	24.3	24.5	24.3
75 to 84 years	61.9	55.7	45.5	45.5	57.0	60.2	47.7	41.1	38.0	35.4
85 years and over	61.9	61.3	45.8	52.8	60.9	70.3	67.9	61.6	53.1	50.8
Black or African American Male[5]										
All ages, age-adjusted[4]	7.5	8.4	10.0	11.4	11.8	12.8	12.4	10.0	9.2	9.4
All ages, crude	6.3	6.4	8.0	10.3	11.0	12.0	11.7	9.4	8.7	8.8
15 to 24 years	4.9	4.1	10.5	12.3	13.3	15.1	17.8	14.2	11.4	10.5
25 to 44 years	9.8	12.6	16.1	19.2	17.8	19.6	18.3	14.3	14.0	14.5
45 to 64 years	12.7	13.0	12.4	11.8	12.9	13.1	11.5	9.9	9.1	9.5
65 years and over	9.0	9.9	8.7	11.4	15.8	14.9	14.6	11.5	10.2	10.3
65 to 74 years	10.0	11.3	8.7	11.1	16.7	14.7	13.8	11.1	8.1	8.4
75 to 84 years[6]	*	*	*	10.5	15.6	14.4	16.7	12.1	12.9	11.6
85 years and over	NA	*	*	*	*	*	*	*	*	*
American Indian or Alaska Native Male[5]										
All ages, age-adjusted[4]	NA	NA	NA	19.3	17.9	20.1	17.4	16.0	17.3	16.5
All ages, crude	NA	NA	NA	20.9	20.3	20.9	18.0	15.9	17.6	16.8
15 to 24 years	NA	NA	NA	45.3	42.0	49.1	30.8	26.2	28.6	30.6
25 to 44 years	NA	NA	NA	31.2	30.2	27.8	29.1	24.5	27.0	23.3
45 to 64 years	NA	NA	NA	*	*	*	13.6	15.4	15.6	16.5
65 years and over	NA	NA	NA	*	*	*	*	*	*	*
Asian or Pacific Islander Male[5]										
All ages, age-adjusted[4]	NA	NA	NA	10.7	9.3	9.6	9.6	8.6	7.3	7.8
All ages, crude	NA	NA	NA	8.8	8.4	8.7	9.0	7.9	7.1	7.8
15 to 24 years	NA	NA	NA	10.8	14.2	13.5	14.4	9.1	6.5	10.6
25 to 44 years	NA	NA	NA	11.0	9.3	10.6	10.8	9.9	9.6	9.3
45 to 64 years	NA	NA	NA	13.0	10.4	9.7	8.7	9.7	8.9	9.7
65 years and over	NA	NA	NA	18.6	16.7	16.8	18.9	15.4	11.2	10.8
Hispanic or Latino Male[5,7]										
All ages, age-adjusted[4]	NA	NA	NA	NA	11.0	13.7	12.7	10.3	9.6	9.0
All ages, crude	NA	NA	NA	NA	9.8	11.4	10.9	8.4	8.4	8.0
15 to 24 years	NA	NA	NA	NA	13.8	14.7	16.0	10.9	11.3	10.7
25 to 44 years	NA	NA	NA	NA	14.8	16.2	14.5	11.2	11.8	11.5
45 to 64 years	NA	NA	NA	NA	12.3	16.1	14.2	12.0	10.8	10.4
65 years and over	NA	NA	NA	NA	14.7	23.4	21.0	19.5	14.7	12.7
White, not Hispanic or Latino Male[7]										
All ages, age-adjusted[4]	NA	NA	NA	NA	22.9	23.5	22.3	20.2	21.4	21.6
All ages, crude	NA	NA	NA	NA	22.3	23.1	22.2	20.4	22.1	22.4
15 to 24 years	NA	NA	NA	NA	22.6	24.4	24.0	19.5	18.8	18.8
25 to 44 years	NA	NA	NA	NA	25.1	26.4	27.1	25.1	27.1	27.4
45 to 64 years	NA	NA	NA	NA	27.3	26.8	24.5	24.0	28.2	29.3
65 years and over	NA	NA	NA	NA	46.4	45.4	39.0	33.9	33.0	31.9
Black, not Hispanic or Latino Male[7]										
All ages, age-adjusted[4]	NA	NA	NA	NA	NA	NA	NA	10.2	9.5	9.6
All ages, crude	NA	NA	NA	NA	NA	NA	NA	9.6	9.0	9.1
15 to 24 years	NA	NA	NA	NA	NA	NA	NA	14.6	11.9	10.9
25 to 44 years	NA	NA	NA	NA	NA	NA	NA	14.7	14.6	15.1
45 to 64 years	NA	NA	NA	NA	NA	NA	NA	9.8	9.3	9.6
65 years and over	NA	NA	NA	NA	NA	NA	NA	11.8	10.0	10.3
White Female[5]										
All ages, age-adjusted[4]	6.0	5.9	7.9	6.1	5.7	5.2	4.7	4.3	4.9	5.1
All ages, crude	5.5	5.3	7.1	5.9	5.6	5.3	4.8	4.4	5.0	5.3
15 to 24 years	2.7	2.3	4.2	4.6	4.7	4.2	3.8	3.1	3.7	3.4
25 to 44 years	6.6	7.0	11.0	8.1	7.4	6.6	6.3	6.0	6.6	6.9

NOTE: Starting with *Health, United States, 2003*, rates for 1991–1999 were revised using intercensal population estimates based on the 1990 and 2000 Censuses. For 2000, population estimates are bridged-race April 1 census counts. Starting with *Health, United States, 2012*, rates for 2001–2009 were revised using intercensal population estimates based on the 2000 and 2010 Censuses. For 2010, population estimates are bridged-race April 1 census counts. Rates for 2011 and beyond were computed using 2010-based postcensal estimates. Age groups were selected to minimize the presentation of unstable age-specific death rates based on small numbers of deaths and for consistency among comparison groups. Starting with 2003 data, some states began to collect information on more than one race on the death certificate, according to 1997 Office of Management and Budget (OMB) standards. The multiple-race data for these states were bridged to the single-race categories of the 1977 OMB standards, for comparability with other states.
NA = Not available.
* = Rates based on fewer than 20 deaths are considered unreliable and are not shown.
[1]Includes deaths of persons who were not residents of the 50 states and the District of Columbia (DC).
[2]Underlying cause of death was coded according to the 6th revision of the *International Classification of Diseases* (ICD) in 1950, 7th revision in 1960, 8th revision in 1970, and 9th revision in 1980–1998.
[3]Starting with 1999 data, cause of death is coded according to *ICD–10*.
[4]Age-adjusted rates are calculated using the year 2000 standard population. Prior to 2001, age-adjusted rates were calculated using standard million proportions based on rounded population numbers. Starting with 2001 data, unrounded population numbers are used to calculate age-adjusted rates.
[5]The race groups, White, Black, Asian or Pacific Islander, and American Indian and Alaska Native, include persons of Hispanic and non-Hispanic origin. Persons of Hispanic origin may be of any race. Death rates for Hispanic, American Indian or Alaska Native, and Asian or Pacific Islander persons should be interpreted with caution because of inconsistencies in reporting Hispanic origin or race on the death certificate (death rate numerators) compared with population figures (death rate denominators). The net effect of misclassification is an underestimation of deaths and death rates for races other than White and Black.
[6]In 1950, rate is for the age group 75 years and over.
[7]Prior to 1997, excludes data from states lacking an Hispanic-origin item on the death certificate.

Table 2-37. Death Rates for Suicide, by Sex, Race, Hispanic Origin, and Age, Selected Years, 1950–2016—Continued

(Deaths per 100,000 resident population; data are based on death certificates.)

Sex, race, Hispanic origin, and age	2007[3]	2008[3]	2009[3]	2010[3]	2011[3]	2012[3]	2013[3]	2014[3]	2015[3]	2016[3]
15 to 24 years	16.9	17.2	17.6	18.3	19.3	19.0	18.7	19.9	20.9	21.9
25 to 44 years	25.3	25.4	25.7	26.2	26.8	27.2	26.8	27.5	28.6	29.2
45 to 64 years	28.8	30.8	31.4	33.0	32.8	33.5	33.0	34.0	33.8	33.2
65 years and over	30.9	31.6	31.5	31.7	32.1	32.2	34.1	34.7	34.3	34.4
65 to 74 years	24.1	26.3	26.6	26.3	26.7	26.4	28.9	29.5	29.1	28.8
75 to 84 years	36.2	36.1	35.3	34.9	36.8	37.0	38.1	38.3	38.6	39.7
85 years and over	50.1	45.8	46.9	50.8	47.0	50.7	52.6	54.4	52.5	52.5
Black or African American Male[5]										
All ages, age-adjusted[4]	8.7	9.4	8.9	9.1	9.3	9.6	9.3	9.5	9.6	10.2
All ages, crude	8.3	9.0	8.5	8.7	9.0	9.2	9.0	9.2	9.4	10.1
15 to 24 years	10.1	12.0	10.4	11.1	11.5	11.4	11.5	12.0	12.9	14.7
25 to 44 years	13.9	13.9	13.2	14.5	14.4	15.3	14.4	14.4	14.8	16.4
45 to 64 years	9.0	9.8	9.6	9.5	9.5	9.6	10.0	9.9	9.7	9.6
65 years and over	8.5	10.8	9.6	8.3	9.4	9.6	8.4	8.9	8.6	8.7
65 to 74 years	7.9	10.4	8.0	7.6	9.1	8.4	7.8	7.7	7.3	8.0
75 to 84 years[6]	11.2	11.8	11.9	9.9	8.4	12.5	9.1	11.0	11.2	10.6
85 years and over	*	*	*	*	*	*	*	*	*	*
American Indian or Alaska Native Male[5]										
All ages, age-adjusted[4]	15.9	15.4	14.6	15.5	16.4	17.4	18.1	16.4	18.8	20.7
All ages, crude	16.2	15.4	15.1	16.1	16.1	17.5	17.9	16.0	18.5	20.7
15 to 24 years	26.8	29.0	28.9	30.6	27.6	29.3	29.1	23.5	29.5	32.6
25 to 44 years	24.9	22.7	20.4	20.9	24.2	24.3	26.6	26.2	27.3	33.6
45 to 64 years	14.4	11.1	15.4	17.8	14.9	19.1	18.3	15.1	20.8	19.8
65 years and over	*	*	*	*	*	*	*	13.4	13.2	11.8
Asian or Pacific Islander Male[5]										
All ages, age-adjusted[4]	8.8	7.9	8.7	9.5	8.7	9.4	9.1	8.9	9.1	10.1
All ages, crude	8.4	7.5	8.4	9.3	8.6	9.3	9.2	9.0	9.2	10.3
15 to 24 years	11.4	7.1	8.0	10.9	9.6	9.7	11.9	12.9	15.6	16.3
25 to 44 years	9.7	8.5	9.7	10.6	10.6	11.8	11.9	9.7	9.6	11.9
45 to 64 years	10.6	10.9	12.1	12.8	11.1	12.3	10.9	12.1	10.9	11.8
65 years and over	13.1	14.8	15.3	14.9	13.3	12.9	10.9	11.6	12.6	12.1
Hispanic or Latino Male[5,7]										
All ages, age-adjusted[4]	10.3	9.5	9.9	9.9	9.4	9.5	9.3	10.3	9.9	10.9
All ages, crude	8.8	8.0	8.5	8.5	8.4	8.5	8.3	9.2	9.0	10.1
15 to 24 years	10.4	9.5	10.7	10.7	10.7	11.5	10.1	11.6	12.8	13.5
25 to 44 years	12.5	11.2	11.4	11.2	11.7	11.4	11.5	12.6	12.2	14.6
45 to 64 years	13.1	11.6	12.6	12.9	11.6	12.0	11.4	12.4	11.4	12.7
65 years and over	16.6	16.7	16.0	15.7	13.7	13.5	14.2	15.9	14.5	13.7
White, not Hispanic or Latino Male[7]										
All ages, age-adjusted[4]	22.1	23.1	23.4	24.2	24.8	25.2	25.3	25.9	26.6	26.6
All ages, crude	23.1	24.3	24.7	25.7	26.2	26.7	26.9	27.7	28.3	28.3
15 to 24 years	18.6	19.2	19.4	20.4	21.9	21.2	21.4	22.4	23.4	24.5
25 to 44 years	28.6	29.1	29.5	30.3	31.0	31.7	31.2	31.8	33.5	33.5
45 to 64 years	30.5	33.0	33.6	35.4	35.5	36.3	36.1	37.2	37.2	36.5
65 years and over	31.8	32.5	32.5	32.7	33.4	33.6	35.6	36.1	35.9	36.1
Black, not Hispanic or Latino Male[7]										
All ages, age-adjusted[4]	9.0	9.7	9.3	9.4	9.7	10.0	9.7	9.7	10.0	10.6
All ages, crude	8.6	9.3	8.8	9.1	9.4	9.6	9.5	9.5	9.8	10.6
15 to 24 years	10.5	12.6	10.8	11.5	12.0	12.0	12.2	12.4	13.1	15.4
25 to 44 years	14.5	14.6	13.9	15.1	15.3	15.9	15.3	15.1	15.5	17.1
45 to 64 years	9.1	9.9	9.8	9.8	9.8	9.9	10.1	9.8	10.0	10.0
65 years and over	8.6	10.9	9.8	8.4	9.3	10.0	8.6	8.9	8.8	8.9
White Female[5]										
All ages, age-adjusted[4]	5.2	5.4	5.5	5.6	5.9	6.1	6.3	6.6	6.9	6.9
All ages, crude	5.4	5.6	5.7	5.9	6.1	6.3	6.5	6.9	7.2	7.2
15 to 24 years	3.4	3.6	3.8	4.2	4.4	4.6	5.0	5.0	5.6	5.5
25 to 44 years	7.0	7.2	7.2	7.1	7.3	7.7	7.7	7.8	8.4	8.8

NOTE: Starting with *Health, United States, 2003*, rates for 1991–1999 were revised using intercensal population estimates based on the 1990 and 2000 Censuses. For 2000, population estimates are bridged-race April 1 census counts. Starting with *Health, United States, 2012*, rates for 2001–2009 were revised using intercensal population estimates based on the 2000 and 2010 Censuses. For 2010, population estimates are bridged-race April 1 census counts. Rates for 2011 and beyond were computed using 2010-based postcensal estimates. Age groups were selected to minimize the presentation of unstable age-specific death rates based on small numbers of deaths and for consistency among comparison groups. Starting with 2003 data, some states began to collect information on more than one race on the death certificate, according to 1997 Office of Management and Budget (OMB) standards. The multiple-race data for these states were bridged to the single-race categories of the 1977 OMB standards, for comparability with other states.
* = Rates based on fewer than 20 deaths are considered unreliable and are not shown.
[3]Starting with 1999 data, cause of death is coded according to *ICD–10*.
[4]Age-adjusted rates are calculated using the year 2000 standard population. Prior to 2001, age-adjusted rates were calculated using standard million proportions based on rounded population numbers. Starting with 2001 data, unrounded population numbers are used to calculate age-adjusted rates.
[5]The race groups, White, Black, Asian or Pacific Islander, and American Indian and Alaska Native, include persons of Hispanic and non-Hispanic origin. Persons of Hispanic origin may be of any race. Death rates for Hispanic, American Indian or Alaska Native, and Asian or Pacific Islander persons should be interpreted with caution because of inconsistencies in reporting Hispanic origin or race on the death certificate (death rate numerators) compared with population figures (death rate denominators). The net effect of misclassification is an underestimation of deaths and death rates for races other than White and Black.
[6]In 1950, rate is for the age group 75 years and over.
[7]Prior to 1997, excludes data from states lacking an Hispanic-origin item on the death certificate.

Table 2-37. Death Rates for Suicide, by Sex, Race, Hispanic Origin, and Age, Selected Years, 1950–2016—*Continued*

(Deaths per 100,000 resident population; data are based on death certificates.)

Sex, race, Hispanic origin, and age	1950[1,2]	1960[1,2]	1970[2]	1980[2]	1985	1990[2]	1995	2000[3]	2005[3]	2006[3]
45 to 64 years	10.6	10.9	13.0	9.6	8.7	7.7	6.7	6.9	8.1	8.8
65 years and over	9.9	8.8	8.5	6.4	6.9	6.8	5.7	4.3	4.2	4.1
Black or African American Female[5]										
All ages, age-adjusted[4]	1.8	2.0	2.9	2.4	2.3	2.4	2.0	1.8	1.8	1.4
All ages, crude	1.5	1.6	2.6	2.2	2.1	2.3	2.0	1.7	1.8	1.4
15 to 24 years	1.8	*	3.8	2.3	2.0	2.3	2.2	2.2	1.7	1.7
25 to 44 years	2.3	3.0	4.8	4.3	3.2	3.8	3.3	2.6	2.8	2.0
45 to 64 years	2.7	3.1	2.9	2.5	2.8	2.9	2.0	2.1	2.4	1.9
65 years and over	*	*	2.6	*	2.7	1.9	2.1	1.3	1.5	*
American Indian or Alaska Native Female[5]										
All ages, age-adjusted[4]	NA	NA	NA	4.7	4.1	3.6	3.9	3.8	4.2	4.5
All ages, crude	NA	NA	NA	4.7	4.4	3.7	3.8	4.0	4.4	4.7
15 to 24 years	NA	NA	NA	*	*	*	*	*	9.1	7.9
25 to 44 years	NA	NA	NA	10.7	*	*	6.4	7.2	6.6	6.9
45 to 64 years	NA	NA	NA	*	*	*	*	*	*	*
65 years and over	NA	NA	NA	*	*	*	*	*	*	*
Asian or Pacific Islander Female[5]										
All ages, age-adjusted[4]	NA	NA	NA	5.5	5.0	4.1	4.1	2.8	3.2	3.3
All ages, crude	NA	NA	NA	4.7	4.3	3.4	3.7	2.7	3.1	3.2
15 to 24 years	NA	NA	NA	*	5.8	3.9	4.8	2.7	3.2	3.5
25 to 44 years	NA	NA	NA	5.4	4.2	3.8	3.6	3.3	3.3	3.2
45 to 64 years	NA	NA	NA	7.9	5.4	5.0	4.7	3.2	3.7	4.1
65 years and over	NA	NA	NA	*	13.6	8.5	8.6	5.2	6.9	7.0
Hispanic or Latina Female[5,7]										
All ages, age-adjusted[4]	NA	NA	NA	NA	1.9	2.3	2.0	1.7	1.8	1.8
All ages, crude	NA	NA	NA	NA	1.6	2.2	1.8	1.5	1.6	1.7
15 to 24 years	NA	NA	NA	NA	2.1	3.1	2.4	2.0	2.5	2.5
25 to 44 years	NA	NA	NA	NA	2.1	3.1	2.5	2.1	2.2	2.3
45 to 64 years	NA	NA	NA	NA	3.2	2.5	2.8	2.5	2.1	2.4
65 years and over	NA	NA	NA	NA	*	*	*	*	2.0	1.7
White, not Hispanic or Latina Female[7]										
All ages, age-adjusted[4]	NA	NA	NA	NA	6.1	5.4	4.9	4.7	5.3	5.6
All ages, crude	NA	NA	NA	NA	6.2	5.6	5.1	4.9	5.6	5.9
15 to 24 years	NA	NA	NA	NA	4.7	4.3	4.0	3.3	4.0	3.5
25 to 44 years	NA	NA	NA	NA	7.7	7.0	6.6	6.7	7.5	7.9
45 to 64 years	NA	NA	NA	NA	9.2	8.0	6.9	7.3	8.7	9.5
65 years and over	NA	NA	NA	NA	7.5	7.0	5.8	4.4	4.4	4.3
Black, not Hispanic or Latina Female[7]										
All ages, age-adjusted[4]	NA	NA	NA	NA	NA	NA	NA	1.8	1.9	1.4
All ages, crude	NA	NA	NA	NA	NA	NA	NA	1.7	1.8	1.4
15 to 24 years	NA	NA	NA	NA	NA	NA	NA	2.3	1.7	1.8
25 to 44 years	NA	NA	NA	NA	NA	NA	NA	2.7	2.9	2.1
45 to 64 years	NA	NA	NA	NA	NA	NA	NA	2.2	2.4	1.9
65 years and over	NA	NA	NA	NA	NA	NA	NA	1.3	1.4	*

NOTE: Starting with *Health, United States, 2003*, rates for 1991–1999 were revised using intercensal population estimates based on the 1990 and 2000 Censuses. For 2000, population estimates are bridged-race April 1 census counts. Starting with *Health, United States, 2012*, rates for 2001–2009 were revised using intercensal population estimates based on the 2000 and 2010 Censuses. For 2010, population estimates are bridged-race April 1 census counts. Rates for 2011 and beyond were computed using 2010-based postcensal estimates. Age groups were selected to minimize the presentation of unstable age-specific death rates based on small numbers of deaths and for consistency among comparison groups. Starting with 2003 data, some states began to collect information on more than one race on the death certificate, according to 1997 Office of Management and Budget (OMB) standards. The multiple-race data for these states were bridged to the single-race categories of the 1977 OMB standards, for comparability with other states. NA = Not available.

* = Rates based on fewer than 20 deaths are considered unreliable and are not shown.
[1]Includes deaths of persons who were not residents of the 50 states and the District of Columbia (DC).
[2]Underlying cause of death was coded according to the 6th revision of the *International Classification of Diseases (ICD)* in 1950, 7th revision in 1960, 8th revision in 1970, and 9th revision in 1980–1998.
[3]Starting with 1999 data, cause of death is coded according to *ICD–10*.
[4]Age-adjusted rates are calculated using the year 2000 standard population. Prior to 2001, age-adjusted rates were calculated using standard million proportions based on rounded population numbers. Starting with 2001 data, unrounded population numbers are used to calculate age-adjusted rates.
[5]The race groups, White, Black, Asian or Pacific Islander, and American Indian and Alaska Native, include persons of Hispanic and non-Hispanic origin. Persons of Hispanic origin may be of any race. Death rates for Hispanic, American Indian or Alaska Native, and Asian or Pacific Islander persons should be interpreted with caution because of inconsistencies in reporting Hispanic origin or race on the death certificate (death rate numerators) compared with population figures (death rate denominators). The net effect of misclassification is an underestimation of deaths and death rates for races other than White and Black.
[7]Prior to 1997, excludes data from states lacking an Hispanic-origin item on the death certificate.

Table 2-37. Death Rates for Suicide, by Sex, Race, Hispanic Origin, and Age, Selected Years, 1950–2016—*Continued*

(Deaths per 100,000 resident population; data are based on death certificates.)

Sex, race, Hispanic origin, and age	2007[3]	2008[3]	2009[3]	2010[3]	2011[3]	2012[3]	2013[3]	2014[3]	2015[3]	2016[3]
45 to 64 years	9.3	9.4	9.6	9.9	10.2	10.6	10.9	11.5	11.9	11.6
65 years and over	4.2	4.4	4.4	4.5	4.8	4.9	5.1	5.5	5.6	5.8
Black or African American Female[5]										
All ages, age-adjusted[4]	1.7	1.6	1.8	1.8	1.9	2.0	2.0	2.1	2.0	2.4
All ages, crude	1.7	1.6	1.8	1.8	1.9	2.0	2.0	2.1	2.1	2.4
15 to 24 years	1.6	2.4	2.1	2.0	2.3	2.8	2.6	2.6	3.6	4.0
25 to 44 years	2.7	2.5	2.7	2.8	3.1	3.1	2.9	2.9	2.7	3.6
45 to 64 years	2.2	1.6	2.5	2.1	2.0	2.4	2.7	2.7	2.6	2.3
65 years and over	*	1.2	1.0	*	1.2	*	*	1.3	0.9	1.4
American Indian or Alaska Native Female[5]										
All ages, age-adjusted[4]	4.3	4.9	5.4	6.1	5.0	4.3	5.3	5.5	6.5	6.4
All ages, crude	4.3	5.1	5.6	5.9	5.0	4.5	5.4	5.6	6.6	6.4
15 to 24 years	6.7	8.6	11.1	10.4	7.1	9.7	9.4	9.6	11.7	11.8
25 to 44 years	5.8	6.2	7.5	7.4	7.8	6.6	7.5	9.7	8.8	10.7
45 to 64 years	*	6.5	5.9	6.2	5.8	*	6.6	*	6.9	4.1
65 years and over	*	*	*	*	*	*	*	*	*	*
Asian or Pacific Islander Female[5]										
All ages, age-adjusted[4]	3.4	3.5	3.5	3.4	3.4	3.6	3.0	3.4	4.0	3.6
All ages, crude	3.4	3.5	3.5	3.4	3.5	3.7	3.1	3.5	4.1	3.7
15 to 24 years	3.2	3.9	4.4	3.5	3.1	5.5	3.6	4.1	4.9	6.3
25 to 44 years	4.3	4.5	3.9	4.1	4.3	3.9	3.7	4.0	4.5	3.7
45 to 64 years	3.9	3.7	4.7	4.7	4.6	4.3	3.9	4.2	5.2	4.5
65 years and over	5.3	5.8	4.8	4.3	5.1	5.3	3.3	5.2	5.2	4.7
Hispanic or Latina Female[5,7]										
All ages, age-adjusted[4]	1.8	1.8	2.0	2.1	2.0	2.2	2.3	2.5	2.6	2.6
All ages, crude	1.7	1.7	1.8	2.0	1.9	2.1	2.2	2.4	2.6	2.5
15 to 24 years	2.0	2.2	2.3	3.1	2.9	2.9	3.3	3.4	3.9	3.8
25 to 44 years	2.6	2.2	2.5	2.4	2.6	2.7	2.8	3.0	3.2	3.5
45 to 64 years	2.7	2.7	2.5	2.8	2.7	3.2	3.2	3.5	3.8	3.3
65 years and over	*	1.6	2.3	2.2	1.6	2.1	1.2	2.1	1.9	1.8
White, not Hispanic or Latina Female[7]										
All ages, age-adjusted[4]	5.8	6.0	6.1	6.2	6.7	6.9	7.1	7.5	7.8	7.9
All ages, crude	6.1	6.3	6.5	6.7	7.0	7.2	7.5	7.9	8.3	8.2
15 to 24 years	3.7	3.9	4.1	4.4	4.8	5.1	5.4	5.4	6.1	6.1
25 to 44 years	8.1	8.4	8.3	8.6	9.1	9.2	9.3	9.8	10.3	10.3
45 to 64 years	10.0	10.1	10.5	10.7	11.1	11.6	12.0	12.6	13.1	13.0
65 years and over	4.4	4.6	4.5	4.7	5.1	5.1	5.4	5.8	6.0	6.2
Black, not Hispanic or Latina Female[7]										
All ages, age-adjusted[4]	1.7	1.7	1.9	1.9	1.9	2.1	2.0	2.1	2.1	2.4
All ages, crude	1.7	1.7	1.9	1.8	1.9	2.1	2.1	2.1	2.1	2.5
15 to 24 years	1.6	2.6	2.2	2.1	2.4	2.9	2.7	2.7	3.7	4.0
25 to 44 years	2.8	2.6	2.8	2.9	3.2	3.3	3.0	3.0	2.9	3.8
45 to 64 years	2.3	1.7	2.5	2.2	2.0	2.4	2.7	2.7	2.6	2.3
65 years and over	*	1.2	1.0	*	1.2	*	*	1.3	0.9	1.4

NOTE: Starting with *Health, United States, 2003*, rates for 1991–1999 were revised using intercensal population estimates based on the 1990 and 2000 Censuses. For 2000, population estimates are bridged-race April 1 census counts. Starting with *Health, United States, 2012*, rates for 2001–2009 were revised using intercensal population estimates based on the 2000 and 2010 Censuses. For 2010, population estimates are bridged-race April 1 census counts. Rates for 2011 and beyond were computed using 2010-based postcensal estimates. Age groups were selected to minimize the presentation of unstable age-specific death rates based on small numbers of deaths and for consistency among comparison groups. Starting with 2003 data, some states began to collect information on more than one race on the death certificate, according to 1997 Office of Management and Budget (OMB) standards. The multiple-race data for these states were bridged to the single-race categories of the 1977 OMB standards, for comparability with other states.
* = Rates based on fewer than 20 deaths are considered unreliable and are not shown.
[3]Starting with 1999 data, cause of death is coded according to *ICD–10*.
[4]Age-adjusted rates are calculated using the year 2000 standard population. Prior to 2001, age-adjusted rates were calculated using standard million proportions based on rounded population numbers. Starting with 2001 data, unrounded population numbers are used to calculate age-adjusted rates.
[5]The race groups, White, Black, Asian or Pacific Islander, and American Indian and Alaska Native, include persons of Hispanic and non-Hispanic origin. Persons of Hispanic origin may be of any race. Death rates for Hispanic, American Indian or Alaska Native, and Asian or Pacific Islander persons should be interpreted with caution because of inconsistencies in reporting Hispanic origin or race on the death certificate (death rate numerators) compared with population figures (death rate denominators). The net effect of misclassification is an underestimation of deaths and death rates for races other than White and Black.
[7]Prior to 1997, excludes data from states lacking an Hispanic-origin item on the death certificate.

Table 2-38. Death Rates for Firearm-Related Injuries, by Sex, Race, Hispanic Origin, and Age, Selected Years, 1970–2016

(Deaths per 100,000 resident population; data are based on death certificates.)

Sex, race, Hispanic origin, and age	1970[1]	1980[1]	1985	1990[1]	1995[1]	2000[2]	2005[2]	2006[2]
All Persons								
All ages, age-adjusted[3]	14.3	14.8	13.1	14.6	13.4	10.2	10.3	10.3
All ages, crude	13.1	14.9	13.3	14.9	13.5	10.2	10.4	10.4
Under 1 year	*	*	*	*	*	*	*	*
1 to 14 years	1.6	1.4	1.4	1.5	1.6	0.7	0.7	0.7
1 to 4 years	1.0	0.7	0.7	0.6	0.6	0.3	0.4	0.4
5 to 14 years	1.7	1.6	1.8	1.9	1.9	0.9	0.8	0.9
15 to 24 years	15.5	20.6	17.2	25.8	26.7	16.8	16.1	16.7
15 to 19 years	11.4	14.7	13.3	23.3	24.1	12.9	12.2	12.9
20 to 24 years	20.3	26.4	20.6	28.1	29.2	20.9	20.0	20.7
25 to 44 years	20.9	22.5	17.9	19.3	16.9	13.1	13.8	13.6
25 to 34 years	22.2	24.3	19.3	21.8	19.6	14.5	16.1	15.7
35 to 44 years	19.6	20.0	16.0	16.3	14.3	11.9	11.7	11.6
45 to 64 years	17.6	15.2	14.3	13.6	11.7	10.0	10.6	10.6
45 to 54 years	18.1	16.4	14.7	13.9	12.0	10.5	11.2	11.2
55 to 64 years	17.0	13.9	13.9	13.3	11.3	9.4	9.7	9.7
65 years and over	13.8	13.5	15.6	16.0	14.1	12.2	11.8	11.3
65 to 74 years	14.5	13.8	15.1	14.4	12.8	10.6	10.2	9.9
75 to 84 years	13.4	13.4	17.7	19.4	16.3	13.9	13.6	12.9
85 years and over	10.2	11.6	12.2	14.7	14.4	14.2	13.0	12.5
Male								
All ages, age-adjusted[3]	24.8	25.9	23.1	26.1	23.8	18.1	18.5	18.2
All ages, crude	22.2	25.7	22.8	26.2	23.6	17.8	18.4	18.2
Under 1 year	*	*	*	*	*	*	*	*
1 to 14 years	2.3	2.0	2.1	2.2	2.3	1.1	1.0	1.0
1 to 4 years	1.2	0.9	0.8	0.7	0.8	0.4	0.5	0.5
5 to 14 years	2.7	2.5	2.7	2.9	2.9	1.4	1.2	1.2
15 to 24 years	26.4	34.8	29.1	44.7	46.5	29.4	28.5	29.5
15 to 19 years	19.2	24.5	22.4	40.1	41.6	22.4	21.5	22.7
20 to 24 years	35.1	45.2	35.0	49.1	51.5	37.0	35.7	36.6
25 to 44 years	34.1	38.1	29.7	32.6	28.4	22.0	23.7	23.2
25 to 34 years	36.5	41.4	32.1	37.0	33.2	24.9	28.2	27.6
35 to 44 years	31.6	33.2	26.6	27.4	23.6	19.4	19.5	19.2
45 to 64 years	31.0	25.9	24.5	23.4	20.0	17.1	18.2	17.8
45 to 54 years	30.7	27.3	24.4	23.2	20.1	17.6	18.9	18.6
55 to 64 years	31.3	24.5	24.6	23.7	19.8	16.3	17.2	16.8
65 years and over	29.7	29.7	34.2	35.3	30.7	26.4	25.1	24.0
65 to 74 years	29.5	27.8	30.0	28.2	25.1	20.3	19.3	18.8
75 to 84 years	31.0	33.0	42.7	46.9	37.8	32.2	30.5	28.8
85 years and over	26.2	34.9	38.2	49.3	47.1	44.7	39.3	37.3
Female								
All ages, age-adjusted[3]	4.8	4.7	4.2	4.2	3.8	2.8	2.7	2.7
All ages, crude	4.4	4.7	4.2	4.3	3.8	2.8	2.7	2.8
Under 1 year	*	*	*	*	*	*	*	*
1 to 14 years	0.8	0.7	0.7	0.8	0.8	0.3	0.4	0.4
1 to 4 years	0.9	0.5	0.5	0.5	0.5	*	0.3	*
5 to 14 years	0.8	0.7	0.8	1.0	0.9	0.4	0.4	0.4
15 to 24 years	4.8	6.1	5.0	6.0	5.9	3.5	3.0	3.1
15 to 19 years	3.5	4.6	3.9	5.7	5.6	2.9	2.4	2.5
20 to 24 years	6.4	7.7	5.9	6.3	6.1	4.2	3.6	3.8
25 to 44 years	8.3	7.4	6.2	6.1	5.5	4.2	3.9	3.9
25 to 34 years	8.4	7.5	6.6	6.7	5.8	4.0	3.8	3.7
35 to 44 years	8.2	7.2	5.8	5.4	5.2	4.4	4.0	4.1
45 to 64 years	5.4	5.4	5.0	4.5	3.9	3.4	3.3	3.6
45 to 54 years	6.4	6.2	5.6	4.9	4.2	3.6	3.7	4.0
55 to 64 years	4.2	4.6	4.5	4.0	3.5	3.0	2.8	3.1
65 years and over	2.4	2.5	3.2	3.1	2.8	2.2	2.1	1.9
65 to 74 years	2.8	3.1	3.6	3.6	3.0	2.5	2.5	2.2
75 to 84 years	1.7	1.7	3.0	2.9	2.8	2.0	2.1	1.8
85 years and over	*	1.3	1.8	1.3	1.8	1.7	1.4	1.2
White Male[4]								
All ages, age-adjusted[3]	19.7	22.1	21.0	22.0	20.1	15.9	15.9	15.5
All ages, crude	17.6	21.8	20.7	21.8	19.9	15.6	16.0	15.6

NOTE: Starting with *Health, United States, 2003,* rates for 1991–1999 were revised using intercensal population estimates based on the 1990 and 2000 Censuses. For 2000, population estimates are bridged-race April 1 census counts. Starting with *Health, United States, 2012,* rates for 2001–2009 were revised using intercensal population estimates based on the 2000 and 2010 Censuses. For 2010, population estimates are bridged-race April 1 census counts. Rates for 2011 and beyond were computed using 2010-based postcensal estimates. Age groups were selected to minimize the presentation of unstable age-specific death rates based on small numbers of deaths and for consistency among comparison groups. Starting with 2003 data, some states began to collect information on more than one race on the death certificate, according to 1997 Office of Management and Budget (OMB) standards. The multiple-race data for these states were bridged to the single-race categories of the 1977 OMB standards, for comparability with other states.
[1]Underlying cause of death was coded according to the 6th revision of the *International Classification of Diseases (ICD)* in 1950, 7th revision in 1960, 8th revision in 1970, and 9th revision in 1980–1998.
[2]Starting with 1999 data, cause of death is coded according to *ICD–10.*
[3]Age-adjusted rates are calculated using the year 2000 standard population. Prior to 2001, age-adjusted rates were calculated using standard million proportions based on rounded population numbers. Starting with 2001 data, unrounded population numbers are used to calculate age-adjusted rates.
[4]The race groups, White, Black, Asian or Pacific Islander, and American Indian and Alaska Native, include persons of Hispanic and non-Hispanic origin. Persons of Hispanic origin may be of any race. Death rates for Hispanic, American Indian or Alaska Native, and Asian or Pacific Islander persons should be interpreted with caution because of inconsistencies in reporting Hispanic origin or race on the death certificate (death rate numerators) compared with population figures (death rate denominators). The net effect of misclassification is an underestimation of deaths and death rates for races other than White and Black.

Table 2-38. Death Rates for Firearm-Related Injuries, by Sex, Race, Hispanic Origin, and Age, Selected Years, 1970–2016—Continued

(Deaths per 100,000 resident population; data are based on death certificates.)

Sex, race, Hispanic origin, and age	2007[2]	2008[2]	2009[2]	2010[2]	2011[2]	2012[2]	2013[2]	2014[2]	2015[2]	2016[2]
All Persons										
All ages, age-adjusted[3]	10.3	10.3	10.1	10.1	10.2	10.5	10.4	10.3	11.1	11.8
All ages, crude	10.4	10.4	10.2	10.3	10.4	10.7	10.6	10.5	11.3	12.0
Under 1 year	*	*	*	*	*	*	*	*	*	*
1 to 14 years	0.7	0.6	0.6	0.6	0.7	0.7	0.7	0.8	0.8	0.8
1 to 4 years	0.4	0.5	0.4	0.4	0.5	0.4	0.4	0.4	0.5	0.6
5 to 14 years	0.8	0.7	0.7	0.7	0.8	0.8	0.8	0.9	0.9	0.9
15 to 24 years	16.0	15.4	14.4	14.2	14.4	14.7	14.1	14.0	15.7	17.2
15 to 19 years	12.1	11.7	11.1	10.6	10.7	10.7	9.7	9.9	11.3	12.6
20 to 24 years	20.1	19.3	18.0	17.9	18.0	18.5	18.1	17.7	19.8	21.6
25 to 44 years	13.8	13.5	13.2	13.3	13.4	13.8	13.9	13.4	15.0	16.4
25 to 34 years	15.9	15.4	14.5	15.0	15.0	15.3	15.3	14.7	16.8	18.2
35 to 44 years	12.0	11.8	11.9	11.7	11.7	12.4	12.3	12.1	13.1	14.5
45 to 64 years	10.6	11.2	11.4	11.6	11.7	12.0	11.9	11.8	12.0	12.3
45 to 54 years	11.1	11.5	11.8	12.0	12.2	12.4	12.3	12.2	12.4	12.8
55 to 64 years	10.1	10.8	10.8	11.1	11.0	11.6	11.5	11.4	11.7	11.9
65 years and over	11.3	11.8	11.9	11.7	12.1	12.2	12.5	12.7	12.7	12.7
65 to 74 years	9.8	10.7	10.9	10.7	10.9	10.8	11.3	11.5	11.3	11.4
75 to 84 years	13.1	13.2	13.3	12.7	13.7	14.1	14.1	13.9	14.5	14.7
85 years and over	12.7	12.5	12.5	13.2	13.1	13.6	13.9	15.0	14.5	14.3
Male										
All ages, age-adjusted[3]	18.3	18.3	17.8	17.9	18.0	18.5	18.3	18.0	19.4	20.5
All ages, crude	18.3	18.3	17.9	18.0	18.1	18.7	18.5	18.3	19.6	20.7
Under 1 year	*	*	*	*	*	*	*	*	*	*
1 to 14 years	1.0	0.9	0.9	1.0	1.0	1.0	1.0	1.1	1.1	1.1
1 to 4 years	0.5	0.6	0.5	0.6	0.6	0.5	0.6	0.5	0.6	0.7
5 to 14 years	1.1	1.0	1.0	1.1	1.1	1.1	1.2	1.3	1.2	1.3
15 to 24 years	28.2	27.0	25.3	25.0	25.0	25.6	24.4	24.3	27.4	29.7
15 to 19 years	21.2	20.4	19.3	18.4	18.4	18.5	17.0	17.2	19.5	21.4
20 to 24 years	35.5	34.0	31.6	31.8	31.5	32.4	31.2	30.8	34.7	37.6
25 to 44 years	23.8	23.3	22.4	22.9	22.7	23.6	23.7	22.8	25.6	27.9
25 to 34 years	28.0	27.1	25.0	26.4	25.9	26.4	26.3	25.2	28.8	31.3
35 to 44 years	19.8	19.6	19.9	19.3	19.4	20.7	20.8	20.1	22.1	24.1
45 to 64 years	18.2	19.2	19.3	19.9	19.8	20.5	20.1	19.8	20.2	20.7
45 to 54 years	18.6	19.4	19.6	20.3	20.1	20.4	20.4	19.9	20.5	21.1
55 to 64 years	17.7	19.0	19.1	19.3	19.5	20.5	19.8	19.8	19.9	20.4
65 years and over	24.0	24.7	24.8	24.1	24.8	25.0	25.3	25.7	25.5	25.5
65 to 74 years	18.7	20.3	20.6	20.0	20.3	20.2	20.9	21.5	21.1	20.9
75 to 84 years	29.0	29.0	28.8	27.5	29.5	30.1	29.8	29.2	30.2	30.9
85 years and over	37.4	35.5	35.7	37.4	36.1	37.5	38.3	40.7	38.9	38.4
Female										
All ages, age-adjusted[3]	2.7	2.7	2.8	2.7	2.9	3.0	3.0	3.0	3.2	3.4
All ages, crude	2.7	2.8	2.8	2.7	2.9	3.0	3.0	3.0	3.2	3.5
Under 1 year	*	*	*	*	*	*	*	*	*	*
1 to 14 years	0.4	0.4	0.3	0.3	0.4	0.4	0.4	0.5	0.5	0.5
1 to 4 years	0.4	0.4	0.4	0.3	0.3	0.3	0.3	0.4	0.4	0.5
5 to 14 years	0.4	0.4	0.3	0.3	0.4	0.5	0.4	0.5	0.5	0.5
15 to 24 years	3.2	3.2	3.1	2.9	3.2	3.2	3.2	3.1	3.4	4.1
15 to 19 years	2.5	2.4	2.4	2.3	2.5	2.4	2.0	2.3	2.7	3.4
20 to 24 years	3.9	4.0	3.7	3.5	3.8	3.9	4.3	3.9	4.1	4.8
25 to 44 years	3.9	3.8	3.9	3.8	4.0	4.0	4.0	4.0	4.4	4.9
25 to 34 years	3.6	3.6	3.9	3.5	3.9	4.0	4.1	3.9	4.5	4.8
35 to 44 years	4.2	4.0	3.9	4.1	4.0	4.1	4.0	4.1	4.3	4.9
45 to 64 years	3.4	3.6	3.8	3.7	3.9	4.0	4.1	4.1	4.3	4.4
45 to 54 years	3.7	3.9	4.3	3.8	4.5	4.6	4.5	4.7	4.5	4.6
55 to 64 years	3.0	3.1	3.2	3.4	3.1	3.3	3.8	3.6	4.0	4.1
65 years and over	2.0	2.1	2.2	2.2	2.3	2.3	2.4	2.5	2.5	2.6
65 to 74 years	2.2	2.4	2.6	2.6	2.7	2.6	2.8	2.7	2.7	3.0
75 to 84 years	2.0	2.0	2.2	2.1	2.1	2.3	2.3	2.4	2.6	2.3
85 years and over	1.2	1.6	1.3	1.5	1.7	1.6	1.5	1.6	1.7	1.5
White Male[4]										
All ages, age-adjusted[3]	15.8	16.1	15.9	16.1	16.2	16.5	16.5	16.3	17.0	17.8
All ages, crude	15.9	16.4	16.2	16.5	16.6	17.0	17.1	17.0	17.7	18.5

NOTE: Starting with *Health, United States, 2003*, rates for 1991–1999 were revised using intercensal population estimates based on the 1990 and 2000 Censuses. For 2000, population estimates are bridged-race April 1 census counts. Starting with *Health, United States, 2012*, rates for 2001–2009 were revised using intercensal population estimates based on the 2000 and 2010 Censuses. For 2010, population estimates are bridged-race April 1 census counts. Rates for 2011 and beyond were computed using 2010-based postcensal estimates. Age groups were selected to minimize the presentation of unstable age-specific death rates based on small numbers of deaths and for consistency among comparison groups. Starting with 2003 data, some states began to collect information on more than one race on the death certificate, according to 1997 Office of Management and Budget (OMB) standards. The multiple-race data for these states were bridged to the single-race categories of the 1977 OMB standards, for comparability with other states.
[2]Starting with 1999 data, cause of death is coded according to *ICD-10*.
[3]Age-adjusted rates are calculated using the year 2000 standard population. Prior to 2001, age-adjusted rates were calculated using standard million proportions based on rounded population numbers. Starting with 2001 data, unrounded population numbers are used to calculate age-adjusted rates.
[4]The race groups, White, Black, Asian or Pacific Islander, and American Indian and Alaska Native, include persons of Hispanic and non-Hispanic origin. Persons of Hispanic origin may be of any race. Death rates for Hispanic, American Indian or Alaska Native, and Asian or Pacific Islander persons should be interpreted with caution because of inconsistencies in reporting Hispanic origin or race on the death certificate (death rate numerators) compared with population figures (death rate denominators). The net effect of misclassification is an underestimation of deaths and death rates for races other than White and Black.

Table 2-38. Death Rates for Firearm-Related Injuries, by Sex, Race, Hispanic Origin, and Age, Selected Years, 1970–2016—Continued

(Deaths per 100,000 resident population; data are based on death certificates.)

Sex, race, Hispanic origin, and age	1970[1]	1980[1]	1985	1990[1]	1995[1]	2000[2]	2005[2]	2006[2]
1 to 14 years	1.8	1.9	2.1	1.9	1.9	1.0	0.8	0.8
15 to 24 years	16.9	28.4	24.1	29.5	30.8	19.6	18.3	18.4
25 to 44 years	24.2	29.5	25.0	25.7	23.2	18.0	18.4	17.9
25 to 34 years	24.3	31.1	26.3	27.8	25.2	18.1	19.4	18.5
35 to 44 years	24.1	27.1	23.3	23.3	21.2	17.9	17.5	17.3
45 to 64 years	27.4	23.3	23.6	22.8	19.5	17.4	19.0	18.4
65 years and over	29.9	30.1	35.4	36.8	32.2	28.2	27.0	25.8
Black or African American Male[4]								
All ages, age-adjusted[3]	70.8	60.1	40.9	56.3	49.2	34.2	36.7	37.6
All ages, crude	60.8	57.7	41.3	61.9	52.9	36.1	38.6	39.8
1 to 14 years	5.3	3.0	2.7	4.4	4.4	1.8	2.1	2.2
15 to 24 years	97.3	77.9	61.3	138.0	138.7	89.3	86.2	90.9
25 to 44 years	126.2	114.1	71.8	90.3	70.2	54.1	64.8	64.8
25 to 34 years	145.6	128.4	79.8	108.6	92.3	74.8	92.1	92.8
35 to 44 years	104.2	92.3	59.2	66.1	46.3	34.3	38.6	37.8
45 to 64 years	71.1	55.6	36.9	34.5	28.3	18.4	17.2	18.5
65 years and over	30.6	29.7	26.3	23.9	21.8	13.8	13.5	13.2
American Indian or Alaska Native Male[4]								
All ages, age-adjusted[3]	NA	24.0	23.6	19.4	19.4	13.1	14.4	13.3
All ages, crude	NA	27.5	24.4	20.5	20.9	13.2	14.9	13.7
15 to 24 years	NA	55.3	39.8	49.1	40.9	26.9	28.6	27.8
25 to 44 years	NA	43.9	40.3	25.4	31.2	16.6	21.3	19.0
45 to 64 years	NA	*	21.2	*	14.2	12.2	12.1	10.1
65 years and over	NA	*	*	*	*	*	*	*
Asian or Pacific Islander Male[4]								
All ages, age-adjusted[3]	NA	7.8	7.3	8.8	9.2	6.0	5.1	5.2
All ages, crude	NA	8.2	7.3	9.4	10.0	6.2	5.4	5.5
15 to 24 years	NA	10.8	12.6	21.0	24.3	9.3	10.9	12.9
25 to 44 years	NA	12.8	9.8	10.9	10.6	8.1	6.4	5.7
45 to 64 years	NA	10.4	6.7	8.1	8.2	7.4	5.7	5.6
65 years and over	NA	*	*	*	*	*	*	*
Hispanic or Latino Male[4,5]								
All ages, age-adjusted[3]	NA	NA	24.2	27.6	23.8	13.6	13.4	12.8
All ages, crude	NA	NA	26.0	29.9	26.2	14.2	14.3	13.8
1 to 14 years	NA	NA	1.4	2.6	2.8	1.0	0.7	1.1
15 to 24 years	NA	NA	42.0	55.5	61.7	30.8	30.8	31.1
25 to 44 years	NA	NA	43.2	42.7	31.4	17.3	19.7	18.5
25 to 34 years	NA	NA	47.3	47.3	36.4	20.3	24.4	22.5
35 to 44 years	NA	NA	35.9	35.4	24.2	13.2	13.9	13.5
45 to 64 years	NA	NA	19.2	21.4	17.2	12.0	9.2	8.6
65 years and over	NA	NA	12.4	19.1	16.5	12.2	10.2	8.0
White, not Hispanic or Latino Male[5]								
All ages, age-adjusted[3]	NA	NA	20.2	20.6	18.6	15.5	15.5	15.1
All ages, crude	NA	NA	19.9	20.4	18.5	15.7	16.1	15.8
1 to 14 years	NA	NA	2.0	1.6	1.6	1.0	0.9	0.7
15 to 24 years	NA	NA	22.0	24.1	23.5	16.2	14.1	14.1
25 to 44 years	NA	NA	23.0	23.3	21.4	17.9	17.7	17.4
25 to 34 years	NA	NA	23.7	24.7	22.5	17.2	17.4	16.7
35 to 44 years	NA	NA	22.0	21.6	20.4	18.4	17.9	18.0
45 to 64 years	NA	NA	23.0	22.7	19.5	17.8	20.0	19.5
65 years and over	NA	NA	37.3	37.4	32.5	29.0	28.1	27.0
Black, not Hispanic or Latino Male[5]								
All ages, age-adjusted[3]	NA	NA	NA	NA	NA	35.2	38.2	39.4
All ages, crude	NA	NA	NA	NA	NA	37.1	40.1	41.5
1 to 14 years	NA	NA	NA	NA	NA	1.8	2.2	2.3
15 to 24 years	NA	NA	NA	NA	NA	92.2	90.3	95.3
25 to 44 years	NA	NA	NA	NA	NA	55.8	67.5	68.0
25 to 34 years	NA	NA	NA	NA	NA	77.6	96.7	98.5
35 to 44 years	NA	NA	NA	NA	NA	35.3	40.0	39.2
45 to 64 years	NA	NA	NA	NA	NA	18.5	17.6	18.9
65 years and over	NA	NA	NA	NA	NA	14.1	13.6	13.3

NOTE: Starting with *Health, United States, 2003*, rates for 1991–1999 were revised using intercensal population estimates based on the 1990 and 2000 Censuses. For 2000, population estimates are bridged-race April 1 census counts. Starting with *Health, United States, 2012*, rates for 2001–2009 were revised using intercensal population estimates based on the 2000 and 2010 Censuses. For 2010, population estimates are bridged-race April 1 census counts. Rates for 2011 and beyond were computed using 2010-based postcensal estimates. Age groups were selected to minimize the presentation of unstable age-specific death rates based on small numbers of deaths and for consistency among comparison groups. Starting with 2003 data, some states began to collect information on more than one race on the death certificate, according to 1997 Office of Management and Budget (OMB) standards. The multiple-race data for these states were bridged to the single-race categories of the 1977 OMB standards, for comparability with other states. NA = Not available.

[1] Underlying cause of death was coded according to the 6th revision of the *International Classification of Diseases* (*ICD*) in 1950, 7th revision in 1960, 8th revision in 1970, and 9th revision in 1980–1998.

[2] Starting with 1999 data, cause of death is coded according to *ICD–10.*

[3] Age-adjusted rates are calculated using the year 2000 standard population. Prior to 2001, age-adjusted rates were calculated using standard million proportions based on rounded population numbers. Starting with 2001 data, unrounded population numbers are used to calculate age-adjusted rates.

[4] The race groups, White, Black, Asian or Pacific Islander, and American Indian and Alaska Native, include persons of Hispanic and non-Hispanic origin. Persons of Hispanic origin may be of any race. Death rates for Hispanic, American Indian or Alaska Native, and Asian or Pacific Islander persons should be interpreted with caution because of inconsistencies in reporting Hispanic origin or race on the death certificate (death rate numerators) compared with population figures (death rate denominators). The net effect of misclassification is an underestimation of deaths and death rates for races other than White and Black.

[5] Prior to 1997, excludes data from states lacking an Hispanic-origin item on the death certificate.

Table 2-38. Death Rates for Firearm-Related Injuries, by Sex, Race, Hispanic Origin, and Age, Selected Years, 1970–2016—Continued

(Deaths per 100,000 resident population; data are based on death certificates.)

Sex, race, Hispanic origin, and age	2007[2]	2008[2]	2009[2]	2010[2]	2011[2]	2012[2]	2013[2]	2014[2]	2015[2]	2016[2]
1 to 14 years	0.7	0.7	0.8	0.8	0.9	0.9	1.0	1.0	0.9	1.0
15 to 24 years	17.5	17.7	16.9	16.2	16.5	16.7	16.0	16.1	17.5	19.1
25 to 44 years	18.9	18.6	18.1	18.6	18.4	18.8	18.9	18.4	20.0	21.6
25 to 34 years	19.8	19.1	17.9	19.1	19.1	19.2	19.1	18.7	20.5	22.3
35 to 44 years	18.0	18.2	18.2	18.0	17.7	18.4	18.8	18.2	19.4	20.8
45 to 64 years	19.0	20.5	20.5	21.3	21.3	22.0	21.6	21.4	21.6	21.8
65 years and over	26.0	26.6	26.9	26.5	27.1	27.4	28.0	28.3	28.3	28.3
Black or African American Male[4]										
All ages, age-adjusted[3]	36.2	34.3	32.3	31.8	31.7	33.4	32.1	31.5	36.4	39.6
All ages, crude	38.5	36.2	33.7	33.4	33.2	34.8	33.5	32.9	38.1	41.5
1 to 14 years	2.2	2.0	1.6	1.9	1.4	1.5	1.4	1.9	2.1	2.2
15 to 24 years	87.7	79.7	72.8	73.2	72.4	74.2	69.9	68.9	79.7	87.4
25 to 44 years	63.3	60.8	57.2	57.3	57.4	61.1	60.2	57.4	68.1	74.0
25 to 34 years	88.5	85.3	76.0	78.2	75.5	77.1	76.6	71.3	84.9	90.2
35 to 44 years	38.4	36.2	37.7	35.2	37.5	43.1	41.5	41.0	47.9	53.9
45 to 64 years	18.1	16.9	17.1	16.5	16.3	17.0	16.7	16.9	18.7	20.6
65 years and over	10.9	13.2	12.1	9.4	10.7	11.1	8.8	10.9	10.0	10.5
American Indian or Alaska Native Male[4]										
All ages, age-adjusted[3]	11.0	11.7	11.4	11.7	11.9	13.5	12.9	12.9	14.4	16.2
All ages, crude	11.1	11.7	11.6	12.5	11.7	13.4	12.5	12.4	14.2	15.9
15 to 24 years	20.8	22.2	22.2	26.0	19.0	21.2	18.4	17.7	26.4	21.3
25 to 44 years	14.2	17.3	16.3	16.9	17.1	20.1	18.8	19.3	18.7	25.1
45 to 64 years	10.6	7.1	11.1	11.1	11.6	14.3	13.5	12.6	14.0	17.8
65 years and over	*	*	*	*	*	*	*	*	*	12.4
Asian or Pacific Islander Male[4]										
All ages, age-adjusted[3]	5.0	4.2	4.4	4.2	4.0	4.4	4.1	3.7	4.4	5.0
All ages, crude	5.1	4.4	4.5	4.4	4.1	4.6	4.3	3.8	4.7	5.1
15 to 24 years	9.7	7.5	5.4	6.8	5.7	6.3	5.9	6.3	8.0	8.4
25 to 44 years	5.9	5.2	6.2	6.0	5.7	6.4	6.4	4.8	6.0	6.5
45 to 64 years	5.6	4.7	5.2	4.4	4.4	5.0	4.6	4.1	5.0	5.8
65 years and over	4.5	4.4	4.7	3.9	4.0	4.0	*	3.4	3.7	4.0
Hispanic or Latino Male[4,5]										
All ages, age-adjusted[3]	12.9	11.7	11.4	10.5	9.8	10.1	9.4	9.4	10.1	11.2
All ages, crude	13.4	12.0	11.4	10.5	9.9	10.1	9.4	9.4	10.2	11.4
1 to 14 years	0.8	0.5	0.7	0.6	0.7	0.6	0.5	0.5	0.5	0.5
15 to 24 years	28.4	24.9	23.3	20.9	19.2	19.6	17.4	17.2	19.6	21.7
25 to 44 years	18.2	16.6	15.5	14.4	13.9	14.4	13.8	14.1	15.0	17.8
25 to 34 years	22.5	19.4	18.0	18.0	17.0	17.3	16.2	15.7	17.7	21.2
35 to 44 years	12.9	13.2	12.4	10.2	10.2	11.0	11.1	12.3	11.9	13.9
45 to 64 years	9.7	9.0	9.5	9.1	8.0	8.2	8.2	7.9	8.0	8.5
65 years and over	11.2	10.3	10.8	9.9	9.6	9.7	8.1	7.8	9.1	8.4
White, not Hispanic or Latino Male[5]										
All ages, age-adjusted[3]	15.5	16.2	16.1	16.6	16.9	17.2	17.5	17.3	18.0	18.7
All ages, crude	16.3	17.1	17.0	17.6	18.0	18.5	18.8	18.7	19.4	20.0
1 to 14 years	0.7	0.7	0.7	0.9	1.0	1.0	1.2	1.2	1.0	1.2
15 to 24 years	13.7	14.9	14.2	14.2	15.1	15.2	15.1	15.4	16.4	17.7
25 to 44 years	18.7	18.9	18.4	19.4	19.4	19.8	20.2	19.4	21.2	22.4
25 to 34 years	18.5	18.5	17.4	18.9	19.3	19.3	19.7	19.2	20.9	22.1
35 to 44 years	18.8	19.2	19.4	19.9	19.6	20.3	20.8	19.7	21.5	22.7
45 to 64 years	20.0	21.8	21.8	22.8	23.0	23.8	23.5	23.4	23.7	24.0
65 years and over	27.0	27.7	27.9	27.6	28.4	28.7	29.6	29.9	29.8	30.0
Black, not Hispanic or Latino Male[5]										
All ages, age-adjusted[3]	38.0	36.2	34.0	33.4	33.5	35.3	34.0	33.3	38.6	42.2
All ages, crude	40.3	38.0	35.4	35.1	35.1	36.8	35.5	34.8	40.3	44.1
1 to 14 years	2.3	2.2	1.7	2.0	1.5	1.5	1.5	2.0	2.3	2.4
15 to 24 years	92.0	84.1	76.9	77.3	76.9	79.0	74.5	73.0	84.5	93.3
25 to 44 years	66.5	64.2	60.4	60.5	61.1	65.0	64.1	61.2	72.7	79.1
25 to 34 years	93.8	91.0	81.0	83.5	80.9	82.5	81.7	76.6	90.9	96.5
35 to 44 years	40.3	37.8	39.5	36.6	39.6	45.6	44.2	43.3	50.9	57.6
45 to 64 years	18.6	17.3	17.5	17.0	16.8	17.6	17.3	17.3	19.3	21.5
65 years and over	11.2	13.3	12.5	9.5	10.8	11.4	9.2	11.1	10.3	10.9

NOTE: Starting with *Health, United States, 2003*, rates for 1991–1999 were revised using intercensal population estimates based on the 1990 and 2000 Censuses. For 2000, population estimates are bridged-race April 1 census counts. Starting with *Health, United States, 2012*, rates for 2001–2009 were revised using intercensal population estimates based on the 2000 and 2010 Censuses. For 2010, population estimates are bridged-race April 1 census counts. Rates for 2011 and beyond were computed using 2010-based postcensal estimates. Age groups were selected to minimize the presentation of unstable age-specific death rates based on small numbers of deaths and for consistency among comparison groups. Starting with 2003 data, some states began to collect information on more than one race on the death certificate, according to 1997 Office of Management and Budget (OMB) standards. The multiple-race data for these states were bridged to the single-race categories of the 1977 OMB standards, for comparability with other states.
[2]Starting with 1999 data, cause of death is coded according to *ICD-10*.
[3]Age-adjusted rates are calculated using the year 2000 standard population. Prior to 2001, age-adjusted rates were calculated using standard million proportions based on rounded population numbers. Starting with 2001 data, unrounded population numbers are used to calculate age-adjusted rates.
[4]The race groups, White, Black, Asian or Pacific Islander, and American Indian and Alaska Native, include persons of Hispanic and non-Hispanic origin. Persons of Hispanic origin may be of any race. Death rates for Hispanic, American Indian or Alaska Native, and Asian or Pacific Islander persons should be interpreted with caution because of inconsistencies in reporting Hispanic origin or race on the death certificate (death rate numerators) compared with population figures (death rate denominators). The net effect of misclassification is an underestimation of deaths and death rates for races other than White and Black.
[5]Prior to 1997, excludes data from states lacking an Hispanic-origin item on the death certificate.

Table 2-38. Death Rates for Firearm-Related Injuries, by Sex, Race, Hispanic Origin, and Age, Selected Years, 1970–2016—*Continued*

(Deaths per 100,000 resident population; data are based on death certificates.)

Sex, race, Hispanic origin, and age	1970[1]	1980[1]	1985	1990[1]	1995[1]	2000[2]	2005[2]	2006[2]
White Female[4]								
All ages, age-adjusted[3]	4.0	4.2	3.9	3.8	3.5	2.7	2.6	2.6
All ages, crude	3.7	4.1	4.0	3.8	3.5	2.7	2.6	2.7
15 to 24 years	3.4	5.1	4.4	4.8	4.5	2.8	2.3	2.3
25 to 44 years	6.9	6.2	5.6	5.3	4.9	3.9	3.8	3.6
45 to 64 years	5.0	5.1	5.0	4.5	4.0	3.5	3.5	3.9
65 years and over	2.2	2.5	3.2	3.1	2.8	2.4	2.3	2.1
Black or African American Female[4]								
All ages, age-adjusted[3]	11.1	8.7	6.4	7.3	6.2	3.9	3.6	3.9
All ages, crude	10.0	8.8	6.5	7.8	6.5	4.0	3.7	4.1
15 to 24 years	15.2	12.3	8.3	13.3	13.2	7.6	6.6	7.5
25 to 44 years	19.4	16.1	11.4	12.4	9.8	6.5	6.0	6.9
45 to 64 years	10.2	8.2	5.8	4.8	4.1	3.1	2.7	2.6
65 years and over	4.3	3.1	3.7	3.1	2.6	1.3	1.3	1.0
American Indian or Alaska Native Female[4]								
All ages, age-adjusted[3]	NA	5.8	3.9	3.3	3.8	2.9	2.2	2.1
All ages, crude	NA	5.8	4.1	3.4	4.1	2.9	2.3	2.1
15 to 24 years	NA	*	*	*	*	*	*	*
25 to 44 years	NA	10.2	*	*	7.0	5.5	*	*
45 to 64 years	NA	*	*	*	*	*	*	*
65 years and over	NA	*	*	*	*	*	*	*
Asian or Pacific Islander Female[4]								
All ages, age-adjusted[3]	NA	2.0	1.5	1.9	2.0	1.1	0.9	0.9
All ages, crude	NA	2.1	1.7	2.1	2.1	1.2	0.9	1.0
15 to 24 years	NA	*	*	*	3.9	*	2.0	*
25 to 44 years	NA	3.2	2.2	2.7	2.7	1.5	0.9	1.2
45 to 64 years	NA	*	*	*	*	*	*	1.2
65 years and over	NA	*	*	*	*	*	*	*
Hispanic or Latina Female[4,5]								
All ages, age-adjusted[3]	NA	NA	2.9	3.3	3.1	1.8	1.5	1.4
All ages, crude	NA	NA	3.2	3.6	3.3	1.8	1.5	1.5
15 to 24 years	NA	NA	5.1	6.9	6.1	2.9	2.4	2.5
25 to 44 years	NA	NA	5.5	5.1	4.7	2.5	2.6	2.2
45 to 64 years	NA	NA	2.2	2.4	2.4	2.2	1.2	1.3
65 years and over	NA	NA	*	*	*	*	*	*
White, not Hispanic or Latina Female[5]								
All ages, age-adjusted[3]	NA	NA	4.0	3.7	3.4	2.8	2.7	2.7
All ages, crude	NA	NA	4.1	3.7	3.5	2.9	2.8	2.9
15 to 24 years	NA	NA	4.5	4.3	4.1	2.7	2.2	2.2
25 to 44 years	NA	NA	5.6	5.1	4.8	4.2	4.0	3.8
45 to 64 years	NA	NA	5.1	4.6	4.1	3.6	3.8	4.2
65 years and over	NA	NA	3.4	3.2	2.8	2.4	2.4	2.2
Black, not Hispanic or Latina Female[5]								
All ages, age-adjusted[3]	NA	NA	NA	NA	NA	4.1	3.7	4.1
All ages, crude	NA	NA	NA	NA	NA	4.2	3.8	4.2
15 to 24 years	NA	NA	NA	NA	NA	7.9	6.8	7.8
25 to 44 years	NA	NA	NA	NA	NA	6.8	6.3	7.3
45 to 64 years	NA	NA	NA	NA	NA	3.1	2.7	2.6
65 years and over	NA	NA	NA	NA	NA	1.4	1.4	1.0

NOTE: Starting with *Health, United States, 2003,* rates for 1991–1999 were revised using intercensal population estimates based on the 1990 and 2000 Censuses. For 2000, population estimates are bridged-race April 1 census counts. Starting with *Health, United States, 2012,* rates for 2001–2009 were revised using intercensal population estimates based on the 2000 and 2010 Censuses. For 2010, population estimates are bridged-race April 1 census counts. Rates for 2011 and beyond were computed using 2010-based postcensal estimates. Age groups were selected to minimize the presentation of unstable age-specific death rates based on small numbers of deaths and for consistency among comparison groups. Starting with 2003 data, some states began to collect information on more than one race on the death certificate, according to 1997 Office of Management and Budget (OMB) standards. The multiple-race data for these states were bridged to the single-race categories of the 1977 OMB standards, for comparability with other states. NA = Not available.

[1]Underlying cause of death was coded according to the 6th revision of the *International Classification of Diseases (ICD)* in 1950, 7th revision in 1960, 8th revision in 1970, and 9th revision in 1980–1998.

[2]Starting with 1999 data, cause of death is coded according to *ICD–10.*

[3]Age-adjusted rates are calculated using the year 2000 standard population. Prior to 2001, age-adjusted rates were calculated using standard million proportions based on rounded population numbers. Starting with 2001 data, unrounded population numbers are used to calculate age-adjusted rates.

[4]The race groups, White, Black, Asian or Pacific Islander, and American Indian and Alaska Native, include persons of Hispanic and non-Hispanic origin. Persons of Hispanic origin may be of any race. Death rates for Hispanic, American Indian or Alaska Native, and Asian or Pacific Islander persons should be interpreted with caution because of inconsistencies in reporting Hispanic origin or race on the death certificate (death rate numerators) compared with population figures (death rate denominators). The net effect of misclassification is an underestimation of deaths and death rates for races other than White and Black.

[5]Prior to 1997, excludes data from states lacking an Hispanic-origin item on the death certificate.

Table 2-38. Death Rates for Firearm-Related Injuries, by Sex, Race, Hispanic Origin, and Age, Selected Years, 1970–2016—Continued

(Deaths per 100,000 resident population; data are based on death certificates.)

Sex, race, Hispanic origin, and age	2007[2]	2008[2]	2009[2]	2010[2]	2011[2]	2012[2]	2013[2]	2014[2]	2015[2]	2016[2]
White Female[4]										
All ages, age-adjusted[3]	2.6	2.7	2.8	2.7	2.9	2.9	3.0	3.1	3.2	3.4
All ages, crude	2.7	2.8	2.9	2.8	3.0	3.0	3.1	3.2	3.3	3.5
15 to 24 years	2.6	2.3	2.4	2.3	2.6	2.4	2.7	2.6	2.8	3.2
25 to 44 years	3.8	3.8	3.8	3.7	3.9	4.0	3.9	4.0	4.4	4.6
45 to 64 years	3.7	4.0	4.2	4.1	4.3	4.4	4.7	4.7	4.9	4.9
65 years and over	2.1	2.3	2.5	2.5	2.6	2.5	2.7	2.7	2.8	2.8
Black or African American Female[4]										
All ages, age-adjusted[3]	3.8	3.4	3.4	3.3	3.3	3.6	3.4	3.2	3.6	4.5
All ages, crude	3.8	3.5	3.5	3.3	3.4	3.7	3.4	3.2	3.7	4.6
15 to 24 years	6.9	7.9	6.7	6.4	6.7	7.2	6.1	6.2	6.8	9.2
25 to 44 years	6.3	5.3	5.7	5.6	5.6	5.8	6.0	5.3	6.2	7.8
45 to 64 years	2.7	2.0	2.4	2.2	2.2	2.7	2.5	2.1	2.3	2.7
65 years and over	1.2	1.3	*	*	1.0	1.3	0.9	1.4	1.1	1.5
American Indian or Alaska Native Female[4]										
All ages, age-adjusted[3]	1.8	2.3	2.5	2.6	2.4	1.8	2.0	2.4	2.6	3.2
All ages, crude	1.7	2.3	2.4	2.4	2.3	1.8	2.0	2.4	2.5	3.2
15 to 24 years	*	*	*	*	*	*	*	*	*	*
25 to 44 years	*	3.5	3.6	3.7	3.3	*	*	5.6	4.3	6.1
45 to 64 years	*	*	*	*	*	*	*	*	*	*
65 years and over	*	*	*	*	*	*	*	*	*	*
Asian or Pacific Islander Female[4]										
All ages, age-adjusted[3]	0.7	0.7	0.9	0.6	0.8	0.9	0.9	0.7	0.8	1.0
All ages, crude	0.7	0.8	0.9	0.6	0.9	0.9	0.9	0.8	0.8	1.0
15 to 24 years	*	*	*	*	*	*	*	*	*	2.0
25 to 44 years	0.9	1.1	1.1	1.1	1.4	1.1	1.5	0.8	1.0	1.2
45 to 64 years	*	*	1.2	*	1.0	0.9	0.8	1.3	0.8	1.0
65 years and over	*	*	*	*	*	*	*	*	*	*
Hispanic or Latina Female[4,5]										
All ages, age-adjusted[3]	1.5	1.5	1.4	1.3	1.3	1.3	1.3	1.4	1.5	1.6
All ages, crude	1.5	1.5	1.4	1.3	1.3	1.3	1.3	1.4	1.5	1.6
15 to 24 years	2.6	2.6	2.6	2.1	2.1	1.9	2.3	2.6	2.5	2.8
25 to 44 years	2.2	1.9	1.9	1.8	2.0	2.0	2.0	1.9	2.2	2.5
45 to 64 years	1.4	1.6	1.4	1.5	1.3	1.4	1.2	1.2	1.6	1.3
65 years and over	*	*	*	*	*	*	*	*	*	*
White, not Hispanic or Latina Female[5]										
All ages, age-adjusted[3]	2.8	2.9	3.0	3.0	3.2	3.3	3.3	3.4	3.6	3.8
All ages, crude	2.9	3.0	3.1	3.1	3.3	3.4	3.5	3.6	3.7	3.9
15 to 24 years	2.5	2.2	2.2	2.3	2.6	2.5	2.8	2.6	2.9	3.2
25 to 44 years	4.1	4.2	4.3	4.2	4.4	4.5	4.4	4.6	5.0	5.2
45 to 64 years	3.9	4.2	4.5	4.4	4.7	4.9	5.2	5.2	5.4	5.5
65 years and over	2.2	2.4	2.6	2.6	2.7	2.7	2.9	2.9	3.0	3.0
Black, not Hispanic or Latina Female[5]										
All ages, age-adjusted[3]	4.0	3.6	3.5	3.4	3.5	3.8	3.6	3.4	3.8	4.8
All ages, crude	4.0	3.7	3.6	3.5	3.5	3.9	3.6	3.4	3.8	4.9
15 to 24 years	7.2	8.3	7.0	6.7	7.1	7.6	6.3	6.4	7.2	9.8
25 to 44 years	6.7	5.6	6.0	5.9	5.9	6.1	6.4	5.6	6.6	8.3
45 to 64 years	2.8	2.1	2.4	2.3	2.3	2.8	2.6	2.2	2.4	2.9
65 years and over	1.3	1.3	*	*	1.0	1.3	0.9	1.4	1.2	1.5

NOTE: Starting with *Health, United States, 2003*, rates for 1991–1999 were revised using intercensal population estimates based on the 1990 and 2000 Censuses. For 2000, population estimates are bridged-race April 1 census counts. Starting with *Health, United States, 2012*, rates for 2001–2009 were revised using intercensal population estimates based on the 2000 and 2010 Censuses. For 2010, population estimates are bridged-race April 1 census counts. Rates for 2011 and beyond were computed using 2010-based postcensal estimates. Age groups were selected to minimize the presentation of unstable age-specific death rates based on small numbers of deaths and for consistency among comparison groups. Starting with 2003 data, some states began to collect information on more than one race on the death certificate, according to 1997 Office of Management and Budget (OMB) standards. The multiple-race data for these states were bridged to the single-race categories of the 1977 OMB standards, for comparability with other states.
[2]Starting with 1999 data, cause of death is coded according to *ICD-10*.
[3]Age-adjusted rates are calculated using the year 2000 standard population. Prior to 2001, age-adjusted rates were calculated using standard million proportions based on rounded population numbers. Starting with 2001 data, unrounded population numbers are used to calculate age-adjusted rates.
[4]The race groups, White, Black, Asian or Pacific Islander, and American Indian and Alaska Native, include persons of Hispanic and non-Hispanic origin. Persons of Hispanic origin may be of any race. Death rates for Hispanic, American Indian or Alaska Native, and Asian or Pacific Islander persons should be interpreted with caution because of inconsistencies in reporting Hispanic origin or race on the death certificate (death rate numerators) compared with population figures (death rate denominators). The net effect of misclassification is an underestimation of deaths and death rates for races other than White and Black.
[5]Prior to 1997, excludes data from states lacking an Hispanic-origin item on the death certificate.

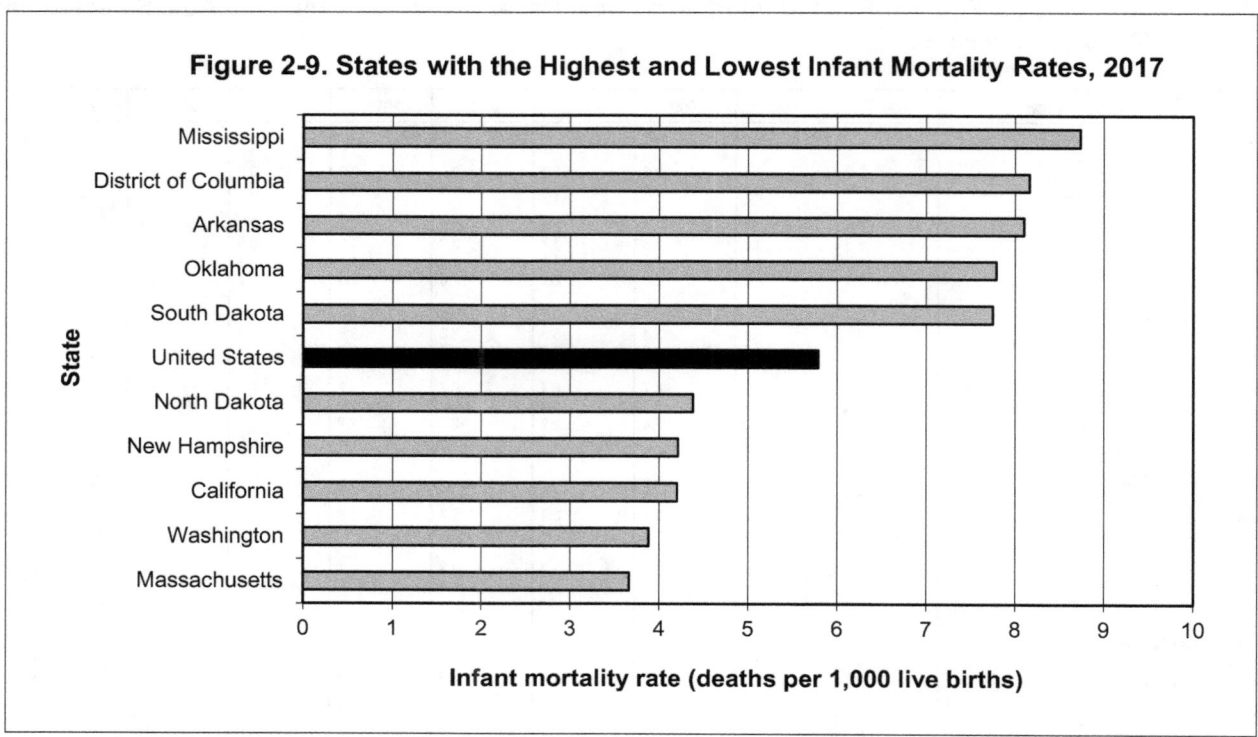

Figure 2-9. States with the Highest and Lowest Infant Mortality Rates, 2017

Table 2-39. Number of Infant Deaths and Infant Mortality Rates, by Selected Cause and Race and Hispanic Origin, 2017

(Number; rate. Infant deaths [under 1 year] per 100,000 live births in specified group. Infant deaths are based on race or Hispanic origin of decedent; live births are based on race or Hispanic origin of mother. Race and Hispanic-origin categories are consistent with 1977 Office of Management and Budget (OMB) standards.)

Cause of death (based on *International Classification of Diseases, 10th Revision*)	Number (includes races and origins not shown separately)				Rate			
	Total[1]	Non-Hispanic White[2]	Non-Hispanic Black[2]	Hispanic	Total[1]	Non-Hispanic White[2]	Non-Hispanic Black[2]	Hispanic
All causes	22,335	9,359	6,730	4,808	579.3	460.9	1,145.8	535.0
Certain intestinal infectious diseases (A00–A08)	8	–	1	4	*	*	*	*
Diarrhea and gastroenteritis of infectious origin (A09)	180	60	66	38	4.7	3.0	11.2	4.2
Tuberculosis (A16–A19)	1	–	–	1	*	*	*	*
Tetanus (A33,A35)	–	–	–	–	*	*	*	*
Diphtheria (A36)	–	–	–	–	*	*	*	*
Whooping cough (A37)	5	3	1	1	*	*	*	*
Meningococcal infection (A39)	4	2	1	1	*	*	*	*
Septicemia (A40–A41)	147	53	51	31	3.8	2.6	8.7	3.4
Congenital syphilis (A50)	7	1	3	3	*	*	*	*
Gonococcal infection (A54)	–	–	–	–	*	*	*	*
Acute poliomyelitis (A80)	–	–	–	–	*	*	*	*
Varicella (chickenpox) (B01)	–	–	–	–	*	*	*	*
Measles (B05)	–	–	–	–	*	*	*	*
Human immunodeficiency virus (HIV) disease (B20–B24)	–	–	–	–	*	*	*	*
Mumps (B26)	–	–	–	–	*	*	*	*
Candidiasis (B37)	1	–	–	1	*	*	*	*
Malaria (B50–B54)	–	–	–	–	*	*	*	*
Pneumocystosis (B59)	2	–	1	1	*	*	*	*
Malignant neoplasms (C00–C97)	57	28	9	16	1.5	1.4	*	*
In situ neoplasms, benign neoplasms and neoplasms of uncertain or unknown behavior (D00–D48)	41	18	8	10	1.1	*	*	*
Diseases of the blood and blood-forming organs and certain disorders involving the immune mechanism (D50–D89)	84	38	21	18	2.2	1.9	3.6	*
Short stature, not elsewhere classified (E34.3)	4	3	1	–	*	*	*	*
Nutritional deficiencies (E40–E64)	6	2	3	–	*	*	*	*
Cystic fibrosis (E84)	5	3	1	1	*	*	*	*
Volume depletion, disorders of fluid, electrolyte and acid- base balance (E86–E87)	55	23	16	11	1.4	1.1	*	*
Meningitis (G00,G03)	47	20	10	14	1.2	1.0	*	*
Infantile spinal muscular atrophy, type I (Werdnig-Hoffman) (G12.0)	3	3	–	–	*	*	*	*
Infantile cerebral palsy (G80)	1	–	–	1	*	*	*	*
Anoxic brain damage, not elsewhere classified (G93.1)	30	14	10	4	0.8	*	*	*
Diseases of the ear and mastoid process (H60–H93)	4	1	–	3	*	*	*	*
Diseases of the circulatory system (I00–I99)	449	190	140	75	11.6	9.4	23.8	8.3
Acute upper respiratory infections (J00–J06)	12	6	2	2	*	*	*	*
Influenza and pneumonia (J09–J18)	157	59	54	35	4.1	2.9	9.2	3.9
Acute bronchitis and acute bronchiolitis (J20–J21)	42	12	18	7	1.1	*	*	*
Bronchitis, chronic and unspecified (J40–J42)	11	4	4	3	*	*	*	*
Asthma (J45–J46)	1	–	1	–	*	*	*	*
Pneumonitis due to solids and liquids (J69)	6	4	–	–	*	*	*	*
Gastritis, duodenitis, and noninfective enteritis and colitis (K29,K50–K55)	23	9	5	6	0.6	*	*	*
Hernia of abdominal cavity and intestinal obstruction without hernia (K40–K46,K56)	34	17	6	5	0.9	*	*	*
Renal failure and other disorders of kidney (N17–N19,N25,N27)	73	29	25	15	1.9	1.4	4.3	*
Newborn affected by maternal hypertensive disorders (P00.0)	56	20	19	12	1.5	1.0	*	*
Newborn affected by other maternal conditions which may be unrelated to present pregnancy (P00.1–P00.9)	87	37	24	19	2.3	1.8	4.1	*
Newborn affected by maternal complications of pregnancy (P01)	1,432	480	492	349	37.1	23.6	83.8	38.8
Newborn affected by complications of placenta, cord and membranes (P02)	843	371	246	174	21.9	18.3	41.9	19.4
Newborn affected by other complications of labor and delivery (P03)	80	34	20	20	2.1	1.7	3.4	2.2
Newborn affected by noxious influences transmitted via placenta or breast milk (P04)	58	29	19	6	1.5	1.4	*	*
Slow fetal growth and fetal malnutrition (P05)	103	41	39	18	2.7	2.0	6.6	*
Disorders related to short gestation and low birth weight, not elsewhere classified (P07)	3,749	1,290	1,404	790	97.2	63.5	239.0	87.9
Disorders related to long gestation and high birth weight (P08)	–	–	–	–	*	*	*	*
Birth trauma (P10–P15)	12	5	3	4	*	*	*	*
Intrauterine hypoxia and birth asphyxia (P20–P21)	328	150	90	63	8.5	7.4	15.3	7.0
Respiratory distress of newborn (P22)	440	173	142	99	11.4	8.5	24.2	11.0
Other respiratory conditions originating in the perinatal period (P23–P28)	734	312	234	141	19.0	15.4	39.8	15.7
Congenital pneumonia (P23)	37	18	10	7	1.0	*	*	*
Neonatal aspiration syndromes (P24)	48	20	18	6	1.2	1.0	*	*
Interstitial emphysema and related conditions originating in the perinatal period (P25)	65	28	17	17	1.7	1.4	*	*
Pulmonary hemorrhage originating in the perinatal period (P26)	133	47	47	33	3.4	2.3	8.0	3.7

– = Quantity zero.
* = Rate does not meet NCHS standards of reliability.
[1]Only selected causes of deaths are shown; therefore, subcategories do not add to totals.
[2]Includes races and origins not shown separately.

Table 2-39. Number of Infant Deaths and Infant Mortality Rates, by Selected Cause and Race and Hispanic Origin, 2017—*Continued*

(Number; rate. Infant deaths [under 1 year] per 100,000 live births in specified group. Infant deaths are based on race or Hispanic origin of decedent; live births are based on race or Hispanic origin of mother. Race and Hispanic-origin categories are consistent with 1977 Office of Management and Budget (OMB) standards.)

Cause of death (based on *International Classification of Diseases, 10th Revision*)	Number (includes races and origins not shown separately)				Rate			
	Total[1]	Non-Hispanic White[2]	Non-Hispanic Black[2]	Hispanic	Total[1]	Non-Hispanic White[2]	Non-Hispanic Black[2]	Hispanic
Chronic respiratory disease originating in the perinatal period (P27)	121	48	50	17	3.1	2.4	8.5	*
Atelectasis (P28.0–P28.1)	257	111	75	51	6.7	5.5	12.8	5.7
Bacterial sepsis of newborn (P36)	592	219	184	135	15.4	10.8	31.3	15.0
Omphalitis of newborn with or without mild hemorrhage (P38)	–	–	–	–	*	*	*	*
Neonatal hemorrhage (P50–P52,P54)	379	176	82	99	9.8	8.7	14.0	11.0
Hemorrhagic disease of newborn (P53)	–	–	–	–	*	*	*	*
Hemolytic disease of newborn due to isoimmunization and other perinatal jaundice (P55–P59)	11	8	–	3	*	*	*	*
Hematological disorders (P60–P61)	108	49	31	21	2.8	2.4	5.3	2.3
Syndrome of infant of a diabetic mother and neonatal diabetes mellitus (P70.0–P70.2)	14	7	3	3	*	*	*	*
Necrotizing enterocolitis of newborn (P77)	338	117	119	83	8.8	5.8	20.3	9.2
Hydrops fetalis not due to hemolytic disease (P83.2)	165	84	31	43	4.3	4.1	5.3	4.8
Congenital malformations, deformations and chromosomal abnormalities (Q00–Q99)	4,580	2,200	891	1,218	118.8	108.3	151.7	135.5
Symptoms, signs and abnormal clinical and laboratory findings, not elsewhere classified (R00–R99)	2,692	1,211	943	432	69.8	59.6	160.5	48.1
Sudden infant death syndrome (R95)	1,363	651	472	186	35.4	32.1	80.4	20.7
Accidents (unintentional injuries) (V01–X59)	1,317	596	455	207	34.2	29.4	77.5	23.0
Assault (homicide) (*U01,X85-Y09)[3]	302	119	119	56	7.8	5.9	20.3	6.2
Complications of medical and surgical care (Y40–Y84)	14	8	2	4	*	*	*	*

– = Quantity zero.
* = Rate does not meet NCHS standards of reliability.
[1]Only selected causes of deaths are shown; therefore, subcategories do not add to totals.
[2]Includes races and origins not shown separately.
[3]Asterisks (*) preceding cause-of-death codes indicate they are not part of the *International Classification of Diseases, Tenth Revision.*

Table 2-40. Infant, Neonatal, and Postneonatal Mortality Rates, by Race and Sex, Selected Years, 1940–2017

(Rates are infant (under 1 year), neonatal (under 28 days), and postneonatal (28 days–11 months) deaths per 1,000 live births in specified group. Race and Hispanic-origin categories are consistent with 1977 Office of Management and Budget (OMB) standards.)

Year	Total[1] Both sexes	Male	Female	Non-Hispanic White[2] Both sexes	Male	Female	Non-Hispanic Black[2] Both sexes	Male	Female	Hispanic[3] Both sexes	Male	Female
INFANT MORTALITY RATE												
1940	47.02	52.45	41.29	NA	NA	NA	NA	NA	NA	NA	NA	NA
1950	29.21	32.75	25.48	NA	NA	NA	NA	NA	NA	NA	NA	NA
1960	26.04	29.33	22.59	NA	NA	NA	NA	NA	NA	NA	NA	NA
1970	20.01	22.37	17.52	NA	NA	NA	NA	NA	NA	NA	NA	NA
1980	12.60	13.93	11.21	NA	NA	NA	NA	NA	NA	NA	NA	NA
1990	9.22	10.26	8.13	NA	NA	NA	NA	NA	NA	NA	NA	NA
2000	6.91	7.57	6.21	5.72	6.32	5.08	14.11	15.50	12.66	5.64	6.04	5.22
2001	6.85	7.52	6.14	5.72	6.30	5.12	14.03	15.53	12.49	5.49	5.99	4.97
2002	6.97	7.64	6.27	5.86	6.54	5.14	14.32	15.39	13.23	5.64	6.14	5.11
2003	6.85	7.60	6.07	5.69	6.37	4.98	14.16	15.70	12.57	5.79	6.32	5.24
2004	6.79	7.47	6.09	5.68	6.28	5.05	14.20	15.65	12.70	5.62	6.10	5.12
2005	6.87	7.56	6.15	5.71	6.69	4.79	14.28	15.75	12.76	5.81	6.34	5.25
2006	6.69	7.32	6.03	5.59	6.15	5.00	13.78	14.98	12.53	5.52	5.99	5.03
2007	6.75	7.38	6.09	5.63	6.20	5.03	13.76	15.04	12.43	5.71	6.17	5.23
2008	6.61	7.21	5.97	5.52	6.04	4.97	13.14	14.37	11.88	5.66	6.16	5.13
2009	6.39	7.01	5.75	5.25	5.76	4.71	13.07	14.60	11.49	5.43	5.86	4.98
2010	6.15	6.69	5.57	5.10	5.54	4.64	11.99	13.08	10.85	5.47	5.96	4.96
2011	6.07	6.58	5.52	5.05	5.52	4.56	11.98	13.13	10.80	5.25	5.59	4.90
2012	5.98	6.50	5.43	4.97	5.38	4.54	11.59	12.80	10.35	5.30	5.76	4.83
2013	5.96	6.52	5.38	4.96	5.53	4.36	11.61	12.48	10.73	5.27	5.65	4.88
2014	5.82	6.31	5.30	4.81	5.26	4.34	11.37	12.33	10.39	5.22	5.63	4.79
2015	5.90	6.39	5.38	4.82	5.27	4.36	11.73	12.75	10.67	5.20	5.56	4.83
2016	5.87	6.38	5.34	4.80	5.24	4.34	11.76	12.67	10.82	5.24	5.72	4.75
2017	5.79	6.32	5.24	4.61	5.07	4.12	11.46	12.59	10.29	5.35	5.76	4.93
NEONATAL MORTALITY RATE												
1940	28.75	32.56	24.74	NA	NA	NA	NA	NA	NA	NA	NA	NA
1950	20.50	23.34	17.50	NA	NA	NA	NA	NA	NA	NA	NA	NA
1960	18.73	21.24	16.09	NA	NA	NA	NA	NA	NA	NA	NA	NA
1970	15.08	16.96	13.10	NA	NA	NA	NA	NA	NA	NA	NA	NA
1980	8.48	9.31	7.60	NA	NA	NA	NA	NA	NA	NA	NA	NA
1990	5.85	6.50	5.16	NA	NA	NA	NA	NA	NA	NA	NA	NA
2000	4.63	5.06	4.17	3.84	4.21	3.45	9.36	10.35	8.34	3.74	4.01	3.45
2001	4.54	4.97	4.08	3.82	4.17	3.45	9.20	10.16	8.20	3.65	4.08	3.21
2002	4.66	5.06	4.25	3.92	4.32	3.51	9.46	10.07	8.83	3.80	4.13	3.45
2003	4.62	5.08	4.14	3.84	4.26	3.39	9.46	10.47	8.42	3.95	4.24	3.65
2004	4.52	4.94	4.09	3.76	4.13	3.37	9.36	10.21	8.48	3.84	4.17	3.49
2005	4.54	4.93	4.12	3.74	4.26	3.24	9.40	10.33	8.44	3.92	4.29	3.52
2006	4.45	4.84	4.05	3.69	4.04	3.32	9.10	9.85	8.32	3.79	4.07	3.49
2007	4.42	4.79	4.02	3.64	3.96	3.31	8.97	9.82	8.09	3.82	4.12	3.51
2008	4.29	4.67	3.89	3.53	3.84	3.21	8.46	9.24	7.64	3.81	4.16	3.45
2009	4.18	4.53	3.81	3.42	3.68	3.14	8.42	9.34	7.46	3.63	3.89	3.36
2010	4.05	4.37	3.71	3.34	3.58	3.07	7.71	8.32	7.09	3.73	4.07	3.37
2011	4.06	4.36	3.73	3.34	3.62	3.06	7.85	8.53	7.14	3.67	3.87	3.46
2012	4.01	4.34	3.67	3.31	3.54	3.06	7.58	8.30	6.83	3.71	4.05	3.35
2013	4.04	4.37	3.68	3.33	3.67	2.97	7.66	8.16	7.14	3.73	3.99	3.45
2014	3.94	4.25	3.62	3.23	3.48	2.97	7.51	8.13	6.87	3.67	3.98	3.34
2015	3.93	4.22	3.64	3.16	3.37	2.92	7.60	8.16	7.02	3.73	4.02	3.42
2016	3.87	4.19	3.54	3.10	3.33	2.86	7.64	8.32	6.95	3.63	3.94	3.30
2017	3.84	4.19	3.49	3.05	3.34	2.74	7.28	8.04	6.51	3.73	4.00	3.46
POSTNEONATAL MORTALITY RATE												
1940	18.27	19.89	16.55	NA	NA	NA	NA	NA	NA	NA	NA	NA
1950	8.71	9.41	7.98	NA	NA	NA	NA	NA	NA	NA	NA	NA
1960	7.31	8.1	6.49	NA	NA	NA	NA	NA	NA	NA	NA	NA
1970	4.93	5.41	4.42	NA	NA	NA	NA	NA	NA	NA	NA	NA
1980	4.13	4.62	3.61	NA	NA	NA	NA	NA	NA	NA	NA	NA
1990	3.38	3.76	2.97	NA	NA	NA	NA	NA	NA	NA	NA	NA
2000	2.28	2.51	2.04	1.88	2.11	1.63	4.74	5.15	4.32	1.9	2.02	1.77
2001	2.31	2.55	2.06	1.9	2.13	1.66	4.83	5.36	4.28	1.84	1.92	1.76
2002	2.31	2.58	2.03	1.94	2.22	1.64	4.87	5.32	4.4	1.84	2.01	1.66
2003	2.23	2.52	1.94	1.86	2.11	1.59	4.7	5.23	4.15	1.84	2.08	1.59
2004	2.27	2.53	2	1.92	2.15	1.68	4.84	5.45	4.22	1.78	1.93	1.63
2005	2.34	2.63	2.03	1.98	2.43	1.55	4.88	5.41	4.32	1.89	2.05	1.73
2006	2.24	2.48	1.98	1.91	2.11	1.68	4.68	5.13	4.21	1.73	1.92	1.53
2007	2.34	2.58	2.07	1.98	2.23	1.72	4.79	5.22	4.34	1.89	2.05	1.72

NA = Not available.
[1] Includes races and origins not shown separately.
[2] Multiple-race data reported according to 1997 OMB standards were bridged to the single-race categories of 1977 OMB standards.
[3] Infant deaths are based on race or Hispanic origin of child as stated on the death certificate; live births are based on race or Hispanic origin of mother as stated on the birth certificate.

Table 2-40. Infant, Neonatal, and Postneonatal Mortality Rates, by Race and Sex, Selected Years, 1940–2017—Continued

(Rates are infant (under 1 year), neonatal (under 28 days), and postneonatal (28 days–11 months) deaths per 1,000 live births in specified group. Race and Hispanic-origin categories are consistent with 1977 Office of Management and Budget (OMB) standards.)

Year	Total[1]			Non-Hispanic White[2]			Non-Hispanic Black[2]			Hispanic[3]		
	Both sexes	Male	Female	Both sexes	Male	Female	Both sexes	Male	Female	Both sexes	Male	Female
2008	2.32	2.54	2.08	1.99	2.2	1.76	4.69	5.12	4.23	1.84	2	1.68
2009	2.22	2.48	1.94	1.83	2.07	1.57	4.65	5.26	4.03	1.8	1.96	1.62
2010	2.10	2.32	1.87	1.76	1.96	1.56	4.28	4.77	3.77	1.74	1.89	1.59
2011	2.01	2.22	1.79	1.71	1.9	1.5	4.14	4.6	3.67	1.58	1.72	1.44
2012	1.97	2.16	1.76	1.66	1.84	1.47	4.02	4.49	3.52	1.6	1.71	1.47
2013	1.93	2.15	1.7	1.63	1.86	1.38	3.96	4.31	3.59	1.54	1.66	1.43
2014	1.88	2.07	1.68	1.58	1.78	1.37	3.86	4.21	3.51	1.55	1.66	1.45
2015	1.96	2.17	1.74	1.67	1.89	1.43	4.13	4.59	3.65	1.47	1.54	1.41
2016	2.00	2.19	1.8	1.7	1.9	1.48	4.11	4.35	3.87	1.62	1.78	1.45
2017	1.95	2.13	1.76	1.56	1.73	1.38	4.17	4.55	3.78	1.62	1.76	1.47

NA = Not available.

[1]Includes races and origins not shown separately.

[2]Multiple-race data reported according to 1997 OMB standards were bridged to the single-race categories of 1977 OMB standards.

[3]Infant deaths are based on race or Hispanic origin of child as stated on the death certificate; live births are based on race or Hispanic origin of mother as stated on the birth certificate.

Table 2-41. Number of Infant Deaths and Mortality Rates, by Race, Hispanic Origin, Sex, State, and Territory, 2017

(Number; rate. Rates are infant (under 1 year), neonatal (under 28 days), and postneonatal (28 days–11 months) deaths per 1,000 live births in specified group. Race and Hispanic-origin categories are consistent with 1977 Office of Management and Budget (OMB) standards.)

Sex, state, and territory	Total[1]		Non-Hispanic White[2]		Non-Hispanic Black[2]		Hispanic	
	Number	Rate	Number	Rate	Number	Rate	Number	Rate
United States[3]	22,335	5.79	9,359	4.61	6,730	11.46	4,808	5.35
Male	12,468	6.32	5,281	5.07	3,760	12.59	2,635	5.76
Female	9,867	5.24	4,078	4.12	2,970	10.29	2,173	4.93
Alabama	434	7.36	196	5.63	205	11.17	22	4.84
Alaska	59	5.65	25	4.35	4	*	2	*
Arizona	469	5.73	145	4.21	54	11.31	205	5.96
Arkansas	307	8.18	176	7.20	94	12.89	24	5.93
California	1,973	4.18	436	3.27	222	8.40	1,089	4.95
Colorado	291	4.52	149	3.90	31	8.71	96	5.30
Connecticut	160	4.54	63	3.28	47	10.29	41	4.64
Delaware	72	6.63	19	*	38	12.82	12	*
District of Columbia	77	8.05	13	*	57	12.19	7	*
Florida	1,358	6.07	453	4.64	515	10.22	353	5.26
Georgia	932	7.21	286	4.94	525	11.52	92	5.12
Hawaii	92	5.25	16	*	12	*	21	7.86
Idaho	102	4.60	77	4.42	1	*	19	*
Illinois	912	6.10	347	4.35	352	13.28	168	5.35
Indiana	600	7.30	361	5.91	163	15.34	58	7.56
Iowa	203	5.28	145	4.79	31	10.62	22	6.24
Kansas	221	6.05	130	5.00	34	11.79	43	7.21
Kentucky	355	6.48	275	6.15	54	10.07	20	6.33
Louisiana	431	7.06	146	4.59	252	11.05	28	5.86
Maine	70	5.69	64	5.75	4	*	2	*
Maryland	460	6.42	121	3.97	257	11.14	57	4.66
Massachusetts	262	3.71	121	2.91	50	6.82	71	5.22
Michigan	755	6.78	354	4.61	306	14.04	57	7.77
Minnesota	328	4.78	171	3.58	81	9.35	25	4.98
Mississippi	322	8.62	118	6.30	188	11.60	6	*
Missouri	456	6.24	284	5.18	146	12.95	18	*
Montana	64	5.42	42	4.39	–	*	4	*
Nebraska	144	5.58	94	5.18	20	10.36	20	4.56
Nevada	208	5.82	68	4.94	52	10.44	71	5.39
New Hampshire	51	4.21	41	3.87	3	*	4	*
New Jersey	453	4.47	139	3.00	155	10.98	124	4.53
New Mexico	140	5.89	33	4.96	4	*	81	6.06
New York	1,047	4.56	381	3.37	304	8.64	230	4.33
North Carolina	847	7.05	329	5.02	360	12.38	106	5.74
North Dakota	46	4.28	27	3.33	8	*	1	*
Ohio	983	7.18	527	5.26	383	15.89	54	7.23
Oklahoma	387	7.71	183	5.92	69	14.29	63	8.47
Oregon	236	5.41	138	4.57	18	*	58	7.01
Pennsylvania	841	6.11	435	4.63	268	13.53	100	6.31
Rhode Island	66	6.20	35	5.59	15	*	13	*
South Carolina	371	6.51	164	4.99	176	10.12	26	4.98
South Dakota	94	7.75	64	7.24	8	*	3	*
Tennessee	597	7.37	325	5.98	211	12.66	50	6.51
Texas	2,237	5.86	634	4.89	529	10.70	989	5.49
Utah	285	5.87	206	5.55	8	*	52	6.64
Vermont	27	4.77	22	4.25	4	*	–	*
Virginia	592	5.90	254	4.52	219	10.11	71	5.07
Washington	341	3.89	182	3.48	50	10.23	75	4.70
West Virginia	131	7.01	114	6.64	15	*	2	*
Wisconsin	414	6.37	205	4.37	128	17.28	49	7.69
Wyoming	32	4.64	26	4.72	–	*	4	*
Puerto Rico	163	6.71	–	*	–	*	163	6.91
Virgin Islands	10	*	–	*	4	*	2	*
Guam	24	7.28	–	*	–	*	2	*
American Samoa	12	*	–	*	–	*	–	*
Northern Marianas	8	*	1	*	–	*	–	*

– = Quantity zero.
* = Rate does not meet NCHS standards of reliability.
[1]Includes races and origins not shown separately.
[2]Multiple-race data reported according to 1997 OMB standards were bridged to the single-race categories of 1977 OMB standards.
[3]Excludes data for Puerto Rico, Virgin Islands, Guam, American Samoa, and Northern Marianas.

NOTES AND DEFINITIONS

Sources of Data

A significant amount of notes and information are derived from Kochanek KD, Murphy SL, Xu JQ, Arias E. *Deaths: Final Data for 2017*. National Vital Statistics Reports; vol 68 no 9. Hyattsville, MD: National Center for Health Statistics. 2019. Life expectancy calculations are derived from information provided in Arias E, Xu JQ. *United States Life tables, 2017*. National Vital Statistics Reports; vol 68 no 7. Hyattsville, MD: National Center for Health Statistics. 2019. Infant mortality information was additionally sourced from Ely DM, Driscoll AK. *Infant Mortality in the United States, 2017: Data from the Period Linked Birth/Infant Death File*. National Vital Statistics Reports, vol 68 no 10. Hyattsville, MD: National Center for Health Statistics. 2019.

In these tables, the asterisks (*) preceding the cause-of-death codes indicate that they are not part of the *International Classification of Diseases, Tenth Revision (ICD–10), Second Edition*. Updated tables were accessed via https://www.cdc.gov/nchs/data/nvsr/nvsr66/nvsr66_06.pdf.

Tables 2-21 through 2-24 come from the Census of Fatal Occupational Injuries, which can be found on the Web site of the U.S. Department of Commerce's Bureau of Labor Statistics.

Table 2-34 can be found at https://data.cdc.gov/Motor-Vehicle/Occupant-and-Alcohol-Impaired-Driving-Deaths-in-St/haed-k2ka.

Notes on the Data

Final data in Part B are based on information from all resident death certificates filed in the 50 states and the District of Columbia. It is believed that more than 99 percent of all deaths that occur in the United States are registered.

Data shown for geographic areas are by place of residence. Beginning with 1970, mortality statistics for the United States exclude deaths of nonresidents of the United States. All data exclude fetal deaths. Mortality statistics for Puerto Rico, Virgin Islands, American Samoa, and Northern Marianas exclude deaths of nonresidents for each area. For Guam, however, mortality statistics exclude deaths that occurred to a resident of any place other than Guam or the United States.

Data in this report are based on information from all resident death certificates filed in the 50 states and the District of Columbia. More than 99 percent of deaths occurring in this country are believed to be registered. Tables showing data by state also

provide information for Puerto Rico, Guam, U.S. Virgin Islands, American Samoa, and the Commonwealth of the Northern Mariana Islands (Northern Marianas). Cause-of-death statistics presented in this report are classified in accordance with the *International Classification of Diseases, 10th Revision (ICD–10)* (5–7). Selected causes are presented primarily based on their impact on public health and future planning. Mortality data on specific demographic and medical characteristics cover all 50 states and the District of Columbia.

Measures of mortality in this report include the number of deaths; crude, age-specific, and age-adjusted death rates; infant, neonatal, and postneonatal mortality rates; life expectancy; and rate ratios. Changes in death rates in 2017 compared with 2016 and differences in death rates across demographic groups in 2017 were tested for statistical significance. Unless otherwise specified, reported differences are statistically significant.

The populations used to calculate death rates shown in this report for 1991–2017 were produced under a collaborative arrangement with the U.S. Census Bureau. Populations for 2010–2017 and the intercensal period 2001–2009 are consistent with the 2010 census. Reflecting the latest guidelines issued in 1997 by the Office of Management and Budget (OMB), the 2000 and 2010 censuses included an option for persons to report more than one race as appropriate for themselves and household members (17). Beginning with deaths occurring in 2003, some states allowed for multiple-race reporting on the death certificate. Multiple-race data for these states are bridged to single-race categories; see Technical Notes. Use of the bridged-race process will be discontinued once all states collect data on race according to 1997 OMB guidelines for the full data year. This report presents mortality statistics for Hispanic, non-Hispanic white, non-Hispanic black, non-Hispanic American Indian or Alaska Native (AIAN), and non-Hispanic Asian or Pacific Islander (API) persons.

The population data used to compute death rates by race and Hispanic origin in this report are based on special estimation procedures and are not true counts. This is the case even for the 2000 and 2010 populations. The estimation procedures used to develop these populations contain some error. Smaller population groups are affected much more than larger population groups (18). Data presented in this report and other mortality tabulations are available from the National Center for Health Statistics (NCHS), National Vital Statistics System website: https://www.cdc.gov/nchs/deaths.htm.

Cause of death statistics are in accordance with the *International Classification of Diseases, Tenth Revision (ICD-10)*.

Concepts and Definitions

Age-adjusted death rate—the death rate used to make comparisons of relative mortality risks across groups and over time. This rate should be viewed as a construct or an index rather than as a direct or actual measure of mortality risk. Statistically, it is a weighted average of the age-specific death rates, where the weights represent the fixed population proportions by age.

Age-specific death rate—deaths per 100,000 population in a specified age group, such as 1–4 years or 5–9 years for a specified period.

Cause of death—for the purpose of national mortality statistics, every death is attributed to one underlying condition, based on information reported on the death certificate and using the international rules for selecting the underlying cause of death from the conditions stated on the death certificate. The underlying cause is defined by the World Health Organization as the disease or injury that initiated the train of events leading directly to death, or the circumstances of the accident or violence that produced the fatal injury. Generally more medical information is reported on death certificates than is directly reflected in the underlying cause of death. The conditions that are not selected as underlying cause of death constitute the nonunderlying causes of death, also known as multiple cause of death.

Cause-of-death ranking—selected causes of death of public health and medical importance comprise tabulation lists and are ranked according to the number of deaths assigned to these causes. The top-ranking causes determine the leading causes of death. Certain causes on the tabulation lists are not ranked if, for example, the category title represents a group title (such as major cardiovascular diseases and symptoms, signs, and abnormal clinical and laboratory findings, not elsewhere classified); or the category title begins with the words "other" and "all other". In addition, when one of the titles that represents a subtotal (such as malignant neoplasms) is ranked, its component parts are not ranked.

Crude death rate—total deaths per 100,000 population for a specified period. The crude death rate represents the average chance of dying during a specified period for persons in the entire population.

Fetal death rate—the number of fetal deaths with stated or presumed gestation of 20 weeks or more, divided by the sum of live births plus fetal deaths, per 1,000 live births plus fetal deaths.

Infant deaths—deaths of infants under 1 year of age.

International Classification of Diseases (ICD)—used to code and classify cause-of-death data. It is developed collaboratively by the World Health Organization and 10 international centers, one of which is housed at NCHS. The purpose of it is to promote international comparability in the collection, classification, processing, and presentation of health statistics. Since 1900, it has been modified about once every 10 years, except for the 20-year interval between the ninth and tenth editions. The purpose of the revisions is to stay abreast with advances in medical science. New revisions usually introduce major disruptions in time series of mortality statistics.

Hispanic origin—includes persons of Mexican, Puerto Rican, Cuban, Central and South American, and other or unknown Latin American or Spanish origins. Persons of Hispanic origin may be of any race.

Late fetal death rate—the number of fetal deaths with stated or presumed gestation of 28 weeks or more, divided by the sum of live births plus late fetal deaths per 1,000 live births plus late fetal deaths.

Life expectancy—the average number of years of life remaining to a person at a particular age and is based on a given set of age-specific death rates, generally the mortality conditions existing in the period mentioned.

Maternal mortality rate—the number of maternal deaths per 100,000 live births. The maternal mortality rate is the measure of the likelihood that a pregnant woman will die from maternal causes.

Neonatal deaths—deaths of infants aged 0–27 days.

Perinatal mortality rate—the sum of late fetal deaths plus infant deaths within 7 days of birth divided by the sum of live births plus late fetal deaths, per 1,000 live births plus late fetal deaths.

Perinatal mortality ratio—the sum of late fetal deaths plus infant deaths within 7 days of birth divided by the number of live births, per 1,000 live births.

Postneonatal deaths—deaths of infants aged 28 days–1 year old.

Years of potential life lost (YPLL)—a measure of premature mortality. YPLL is presented for persons under 75 years of age because the average life expectancy in the United States is over 75 years. YPLL-75 is calculated using the following eight age groups: under 1 year, 1–14 years, 15–24 years, 25–34 years, 35–44 years, 45–54 years, 55–64 years, and 65–74 years. The number of deaths for each age group is multiplied by years of life lost, calculated as the difference between age 75 years and the midpoint of the age group. For the eight age groups, the midpoints are 0.5, 7.5, 19.5, 29.5, 39.5, 49.5, 59.5, and 69.5. For example, the death of a person 15–24 years of age counts as 55.5 years of life lost. Years of potential life lost is derived by summing years of life lost over all age groups.

Explanation of Life Expectancy Table

Column 1. Age (between x and $x + 1$)—Shows the age interval between the two exact ages indicated. For instance, "20–21" means the 1-year interval between the 20th and 21st birthdays.

Column 2. Probability of dying (q_x)—Shows the probability of dying between ages x and $x + 1$. For example, for males in the age interval 20–21 years, the probability of dying is 0.001147. This column forms the basis of the life table; all subsequent columns are derived from it.

Column 3. Number surviving (l_x)—Shows the number of persons from the original hypothetical cohort of 100,000 live births who survive to the beginning of each age interval. The l_x values are computed from the q_x values, which are successively applied to the remainder of the original 100,000 persons still alive at the beginning of each age interval. Thus, out of 100,000 female babies born alive, 99,477 will complete the first year of life and enter the second; 99,341 will reach age 10; 99,134 will reach age 20; and 49,264 will live to age 85.

Column 4. Number dying (d_x)—Shows the number dying in each successive age interval out of the original 100,000 live births. For example, out of 100,000 males born alive, 630 will die in the first year of life; 113 between ages 20 and 21; and 971 after reaching age 100. Each figure in column 4 is the difference between the two successive figures in column 3.

Column 5. Person-years lived (L_x)—Shows the number of person-years lived by the hypothetical life table cohort within an age interval x to $x + 1$. Each figure in column 5 represents the total time (in years) lived between two indicated birthdays by all those reaching the earlier birthday. Thus, the figure 98,692 for males in the age interval 20–21 is the total number of years lived between the 20th and 21st birthdays by the 98,749 males (column 3) who reached their 20th birthday out of 100,000 males born alive.

Column 6. Total number of person-years lived (T_x)—Shows the total number of person-years that would be lived after the beginning of the age interval x to $x + 1$ by the hypothetical life table cohort. For example, 5,626,672 is the total number of years lived after reaching age 20 by the 98,749 males reaching that age.

Column 7. Expectation of life (e_x)—The expectation of life at any given age is the average number of years remaining to be lived by those surviving to that age, based on a given set of age-specific rates of dying. It is derived by dividing the total person-years that would be lived beyond age x by the number of persons who survived to that age interval (T_x / l_x). Thus, the average remaining lifetime for males who reach age 20 is 57.0 years (5,626,672 divided by 98,749).

PART III:
HEALTH

PART III: HEALTH

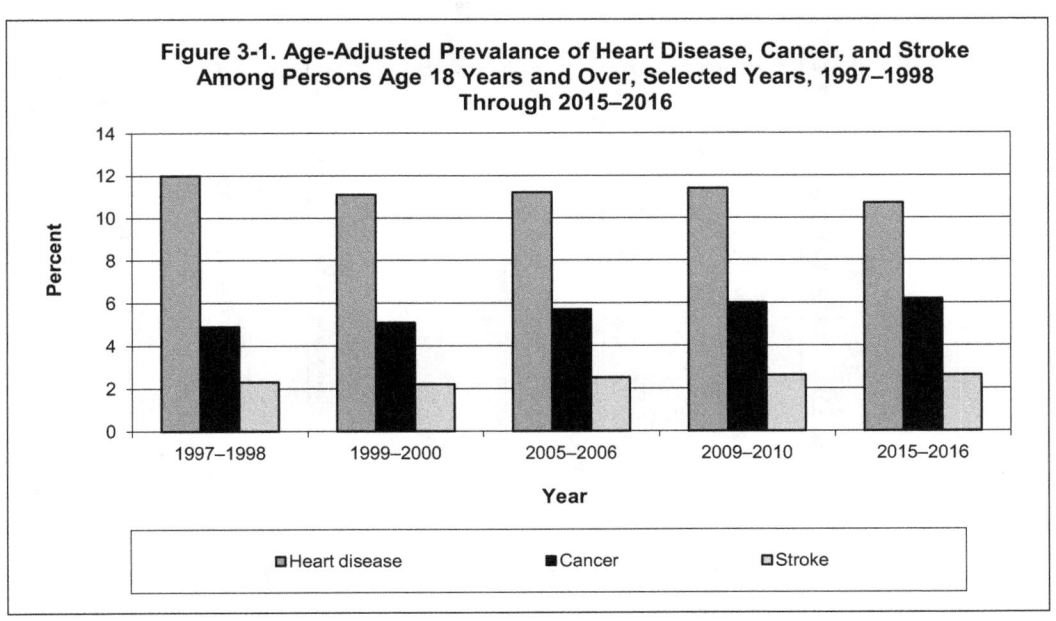

Figure 3-1. Age-Adjusted Prevalance of Heart Disease, Cancer, and Stroke Among Persons Age 18 Years and Over, Selected Years, 1997–1998 Through 2015–2016

HIGHLIGHTS

- In 2015–2016, according to age-adjusted data, 10.7 percent of people suffered from heart disease, a decline from 12.0 percent in 1997–1998. Although the percentage of people with heart disease declined, the percentage of people suffering from cancer increased from 4.9 percent to 6.2 percent, while the percentage of people suffering from a stroke increased from 2.3 percent to 2.6 percent in the same time period.

- In 2016, 16.0 percent of adults age 25 years and over were smokers of cigarettes. This percentage was down from 36.9 percent in 1974.

- Approximately 24.3 percent of Native Hawaiian and Other Pacific Islanders had no usual source of health care in 2013, compared to 16.4 percent of Whites.

- The median annual wage for healthcare practitioners and technical occupations in May 2018 was $66,440. Anesthesiologists earned the most at $267,020, while home health aides earned the least at $25,330.

DETERMINANTS AND MEASURES OF HEALTH

Table 3-1. Selected Notifiable Disease Rates and Number of New Cases, Selected Years, 1950–2016

(Cases per 100,000 population; number; data are based on reporting by state health departments.)

Disease	1950	1960	1970	1980	1985	1988	1989	1990	1991	1992	1993
Rate											
Acute hepatitis A viral infection	NA	NA	27.87	12.84	10.03	11.60	14.43	12.64	9.67	9.06	9.40
Acute hepatitis B viral infection	NA	NA	4.08	8.39	11.50	9.43	9.43	8.48	7.14	6.32	5.18
Acute hepatitis C viral infection[1]	NA	NA	NA	NA	NA	NA	NA	1.03	1.42	2.36	1.86
Diphtheria	3.83	0.51	0.21	0.00	0.00	0.00	0.00	0.00	0.00	0.00	–
Haemophilus influenzae, invasive	NA	NA	NA	NA	NA	NA	NA	NA	1.10	0.55	0.55
Lyme disease[2]	NA	NA	NA	NA	NA	NA	NA	NA	NA	NA	NA
Measles (Rubeola)	211.01	245.42	23.23	5.96	1.18	1.38	7.33	11.17	3.82	0.88	0.12
Meningococcal disease	NA	NA	1.23	1.25	1.04	1.21	1.10	0.99	0.84	0.84	1.02
Mumps	NA	NA	55.55	3.86	1.30	2.05	2.34	2.17	1.72	1.03	0.66
Pertussis (whooping cough)	79.82	8.23	2.08	0.76	1.50	1.40	1.67	1.84	1.08	1.60	2.55
Poliomyelitis, paralytic[3]	NA	1.40	0.02	0.00	0.00	0.00	0.00	0.00	0.00	0.00	0.00
Rubella (German measles)	NA	NA	27.75	1.72	0.26	0.09	0.16	0.45	0.56	0.06	0.07
Salmonellosis, excluding typhoid fever	NA	3.85	10.84	14.88	27.37	19.91	19.26	19.54	19.10	16.04	16.15
Shigellosis	15.45	6.94	6.79	8.41	7.14	12.46	10.07	10.89	9.34	9.38	12.48
Spotted fever rickettsiosis[4]	NA	NA	0.19	0.52	0.30	0.25	0.25	0.26	0.25	0.20	0.18
Tuberculosis[5]	NA	30.83	18.28	12.25	9.30	9.13	9.46	10.33	10.42	10.46	9.82
Sexually transmitted diseases[6]											
Syphilis[7]	146.02	68.78	44.80	30.30	28.39	42.75	46.63	54.32	50.88	44.73	39.48
Primary and secondary	16.73	9.06	10.80	12.00	11.40	16.55	18.57	20.26	16.98	13.26	10.21
Early latent	39.71	10.11	8.00	8.90	9.11	14.71	18.39	22.19	21.29	19.46	16.13
Late and late latent[8]	70.22	45.91	24.70	9.20	7.74	11.19	8.93	10.32	10.87	10.42	11.83
Congenital[9]	368.30	103.70	52.30	7.70	8.75	18.95	45.46	92.95	107.62	100.05	85.49
Chlamydia[10]	NA	NA	NA	NA	17.42	87.13	102.45	160.19	179.66	182.35	178.05
Gonorrhea[11]	192.50	145.40	294.20	442.10	382.98	301.86	297.09	276.43	245.84	196.04	171.07
Chancroid	3.34	0.94	0.70	0.30	0.87	2.00	1.90	1.69	1.37	0.74	0.50
Number											
Acute hepatitis A viral infection	NA	NA	56,797	29,087	23,210	28,507	35,821	31,441	24,378	23,112	24,238
Acute hepatitis B viral infection	NA	NA	8,310	19,015	26,611	23,177	23,419	21,102	18,003	16,126	13,361
Acute hepatitis C viral infection[1]	NA	NA	NA	NA	NA	NA	NA	2,553	3,582	6,010	4,786
Diphtheria	5,796	918	435	3	3	2	3	4	5	4	–
Haemophilus influenzae, invasive	NA	NA	NA	NA	NA	NA	NA	NA	2,764	1,412	1,419
Lyme disease[2]	NA	NA	NA	NA	NA	NA	NA	NA	NA	NA	NA
Measles (Rubeola)	319,124	441,703	47,351	13,506	2,822	3,396	18,193	27,786	9,643	2,237	312
Meningococcal disease	NA	NA	2,505	2,840	2,479	2,964	2,727	2,451	2,130	2,134	2,637
Mumps	NA	NA	104,953	8,576	2,982	4,866	5,712	5,292	4,264	2,572	1,692
Pertussis (whooping cough)	120,718	14,809	4,249	1,730	3,589	3,450	4,157	4,570	2,719	4,083	6,586
Poliomyelitis, paralytic[3]	NA	2,525	31	4	8	9	11	6	10	6	4
Rubella (German measles)	NA	NA	56,552	3,904	630	225	396	1,125	1,401	160	192
Salmonellosis, excluding typhoid fever	NA	6,929	22,096	33,715	65,347	48,948	47,812	48,603	48,154	40,912	41,641
Shigellosis	23,367	12,487	13,845	19,041	17,057	30,617	25,010	27,077	23,548	23,931	32,198
Spotted fever rickettsiosis[4]	464	NA	380	1,163	714	609	623	651	628	502	456
Tuberculosis[5]	NA	55,494	37,137	27,749	22,201	22,436	23,495	25,701	26,283	26,673	25,313
Sexually transmitted diseases[6]											
Syphilis[7]	217,558	122,538	91,382	68,832	67,563	104,546	115,089	135,590	128,719	114,730	102,612
Primary and secondary	23,939	16,145	21,982	27,204	27,131	40,474	45,826	50,578	42,950	34,009	26,527
Early latent	59,256	18,017	16,311	20,297	21,689	35,968	45,394	55,397	53,855	49,929	41,919
Late and late latent[8]	113,569	81,798	50,348	20,979	18,414	27,363	22,032	25,750	27,490	26,725	30,746
Congenital[9]	13,377	4,416	1,953	277	329	741	1,837	3,865	4,424	4,067	3,420
Chlamydia[10]	NA	NA	NA	NA	25,848	157,854	200,904	323,663	381,228	409,694	405,332
Gonorrhea[11]	286,746	258,933	600,072	1,004,029	911,419	738,160	733,294	690,042	621,918	502,858	444,649
Chancroid	4,977	1,680	1,416	788	2,067	4,891	4,697	4,212	3,476	1,906	1,292

– = Quantity zero.
0.0 = Quantity more than zero but less than 0.05.
NA = Not available.
[1]Anti-HCV antibody test became available May 1990. Total number of cases in 2015 and 2016 reported from 42 states.
[2]Not nationally notifiable prior to 1991. National surveillance case definition revised in 2008; probable cases not reported previously.
[3]Cases of vaccine-associated paralytic poliomyelitis caused by polio vaccine virus.
[4]Prior to 2010 data, cases of spotted fever rickettsiosis were reported as Rocky Mountain spotted fever (RMSF). Because serologic tests commonly used to diagnose RMSF exhibit cross-reactivity between spotted fever rickettsial pathogens, some cases reported as RMSF might actually be disease caused by other spotted fever rickettsial infections, and therefore are more correctly referred to as spotted fever rickettsiosis starting with 2010 data. Includes confirmed and probable cases.
[5]Case reporting for tuberculosis began in 1953. Data prior to 1975 are not comparable with subsequent years because of changes in reporting criteria effective in 1975.
[6]For 1950, data for Alaska and Hawaii were not included. Starting with 1991, data include both civilian and military cases. Cases and rates shown do not include U.S. outlying areas of Guam, Puerto Rico, and the Virgin Islands.
[7]Includes stage of syphilis not stated.
[8]Includes cases of unknown duration.
[9]Rates include all cases of congenitally acquired syphilis per 100,000 live births. Cases of congenitally acquired syphilis were reported through 1994. Starting with 1995 data, only congenital syphilis for cases under 1 year of age were reported.
[10]Prior to 1994, chlamydia was not notifiable. In 1994–1999, cases for New York were exclusively reported by New York City. Starting with 2000 data, cases for New York include the entire state.
[11]Data for 1994 do not include cases from Georgia.

Table 3-1. Selected Notifiable Disease Rates and Number of New Cases, Selected Years, 1950–2016—*Continued*

(Cases per 100,000 population; number; data are based on reporting by state health departments.)

Disease	1994	1995	1996	1997	1998	1999	2000	2001	2002	2003	2004
Rate											
Acute hepatitis A viral infection	10.29	12.13	11.70	11.22	8.59	6.25	4.91	3.77	3.13	2.66	1.95
Acute hepatitis B viral infection	4.81	4.19	4.01	3.90	3.80	2.82	2.95	2.79	2.84	2.61	2.14
Acute hepatitis C viral infection[1]	1.78	1.78	1.41	1.43	1.30	1.14	1.17	1.41	0.65	0.38	0.31
Diphtheria	0.00	–	0.01	0.01	0.00	0.00	0.00	0.00	0.00	0.00	–
Haemophilus influenzae, invasive	0.45	0.45	0.45	0.44	0.44	0.48	0.51	0.57	0.62	0.70	0.72
Lyme disease[2]	NA	NA	NA	NA	NA	NA	NA	NA	NA	NA	NA
Measles (Rubeola)	0.37	0.12	0.20	0.06	0.04	0.04	0.03	0.04	0.02	0.02	0.01
Meningococcal disease	1.11	1.25	1.30	1.24	1.01	0.92	0.83	0.83	0.64	0.61	0.47
Mumps	0.60	0.35	0.29	0.27	0.25	0.14	0.13	0.10	0.10	0.08	0.09
Pertussis (whooping cough)	1.77	1.97	2.94	2.46	2.74	2.67	2.88	2.69	3.47	4.04	8.88
Poliomyelitis, paralytic[3]	0.00	0.00	0.03	0.02	0.01	0.00	–	–	–	–	–
Rubella (German measles)	0.09	0.05	0.10	0.07	0.13	0.10	0.06	0.01	0.01	0.00	0.00
Salmonellosis, excluding typhoid fever	16.64	17.66	17.15	15.66	16.17	14.89	14.51	14.39	15.73	15.16	14.47
Shigellosis	11.44	12.32	9.80	8.64	8.74	6.43	8.41	7.19	8.37	8.19	4.99
Spotted fever rickettsiosis[4]	0.18	0.23	0.32	0.16	0.14	0.21	0.18	0.25	0.39	0.38	0.60
Tuberculosis[5]	9.36	8.70	8.04	7.42	6.79	6.43	6.01	5.68	5.36	5.17	5.09
Sexually transmitted diseases[6]											
Syphilis[7]	31.43	26.05	19.76	17.13	13.88	12.68	11.20	11.32	11.42	11.79	11.38
Primary and secondary	7.84	6.21	4.23	3.14	2.54	2.37	2.12	2.14	2.38	2.47	2.72
Early latent	12.17	10.01	7.49	6.10	4.60	4.13	3.35	3.05	2.92	2.88	2.65
Late and late latent[8]	10.49	9.12	7.56	7.50	6.43	5.97	5.53	5.95	5.95	6.30	5.89
Congenital[9]	62.03	47.77	32.94	27.88	21.39	14.65	14.29	12.57	11.44	10.56	9.12
Chlamydia[10]	192.49	187.84	190.57	205.49	231.83	247.16	251.38	274.52	289.41	301.74	316.51
Gonorrhea[11]	163.93	147.46	121.82	120.18	129.23	129.31	128.67	126.77	122.01	115.23	112.42
Chancroid	0.30	0.23	0.14	0.09	0.07	0.04	0.03	0.01	0.02	0.02	0.01
Number											
Acute hepatitis A viral infection	26,796	31,582	31,032	30,021	23,229	17,047	13,397	10,609	8,795	7,653	5,683
Acute hepatitis B viral infection	12,517	10,805	10,637	10,416	10,258	7,694	8,036	7,843	7,996	7,526	6,212
Acute hepatitis C viral infection[1]	4,470	4,576	3,716	3,816	3,518	3,111	3,197	3,976	1,835	1,102	720
Diphtheria	2	–	2	4	1	1	1	2	1	1	–
Haemophilus influenzae, invasive	1,174	1,180	1,170	1,162	1,194	1,309	1,398	1,597	1,743	2,013	2,085
Lyme disease[2]	NA	NA	NA	NA	NA	NA	NA	NA	NA	NA	NA
Measles (Rubeola)	963	309	508	138	100	100	86	116	44	56	37
Meningococcal disease	2,886	3,243	3,437	3,308	2,725	2,501	2,256	2,333	1,814	1,756	1,361
Mumps	1,537	906	751	683	666	387	338	266	270	231	258
Pertussis (whooping cough)	4,617	5,137	7,796	6,564	7,405	7,288	7,867	7,580	9,771	11,647	25,827
Poliomyelitis, paralytic[3]	8	7	7	6	3	2	–	–	–	–	–
Rubella (German measles)	227	128	238	181	364	267	176	23	18	7	10
Salmonellosis, excluding typhoid fever	43,323	45,970	45,471	41,901	43,694	40,596	39,574	40,495	44,264	43,657	42,197
Shigellosis	29,769	32,080	25,978	23,117	23,626	17,521	22,922	20,221	23,541	23,581	14,627
Spotted fever rickettsiosis[4]	465	590	831	409	365	579	495	695	1,104	1,091	1,713
Tuberculosis[5]	24,361	22,860	21,337	19,851	18,361	17,531	16,377	15,989	15,075	14,874	14,517
Sexually transmitted diseases[6]											
Syphilis[7]	82,713	69,359	53,240	46,716	38,289	35,386	31,618	32,286	32,919	34,289	33,423
Primary and secondary	20,641	16,543	11,405	8,556	7,007	6,617	5,979	6,103	6,862	7,177	7,980
Early latent	32,017	26,657	20,187	16,631	12,696	11,534	9,465	8,701	8,429	8,361	7,768
Late and late latent[8]	27,603	24,296	20,366	20,447	17,743	16,655	15,594	16,976	17,168	18,319	17,300
Congenital[9]	2,452	1,863	1,282	1,082	843	580	580	506	460	432	375
Chlamydia[10]	451,785	478,577	492,631	537,904	614,250	662,647	709,452	783,242	834,555	877,478	929,462
Gonorrhea[11]	419,602	392,651	328,169	327,665	356,492	360,813	363,136	361,705	351,852	335,104	330,132
Chancroid	782	607	386	246	189	110	78	38	48	54	30

– = Quantity zero.

0.0 = Quantity more than zero but less than 0.05.

NA = Not available.

[1]Anti-HCV antibody test became available May 1990. Total number of cases in 2015 and 2016 reported from 42 states.

[2]Not nationally notifiable prior to 1991. National surveillance case definition revised in 2008; probable cases not reported previously.

[3]Cases of vaccine-associated paralytic poliomyelitis caused by polio vaccine virus.

[4]Prior to 2010 data, cases of spotted fever rickettsiosis were reported as Rocky Mountain spotted fever (RMSF). Because serologic tests commonly used to diagnose RMSF exhibit cross-reactivity between spotted fever rickettsial pathogens, some cases reported as RMSF might actually be disease caused by other spotted fever rickettsial infections, and therefore are more correctly referred to as spotted fever rickettsiosis starting with 2010 data. Includes confirmed and probable cases.

[5]Case reporting for tuberculosis began in 1953. Data prior to 1975 are not comparable with subsequent years because of changes in reporting criteria effective in 1975.

[6]For 1950, data for Alaska and Hawaii were not included. Starting with 1991, data include both civilian and military cases. Cases and rates shown do not include U.S. outlying areas of Guam, Puerto Rico, and the Virgin Islands.

[7]Includes stage of syphilis not stated.

[8]Includes cases of unknown duration.

[9]Rates include all cases of congenitally acquired syphilis per 100,000 live births. Cases of congenitally acquired syphilis were reported through 1994. Starting with 1995 data, only congenital syphilis for cases under 1 year of age were reported.

[10]Prior to 1994, chlamydia was not notifiable. In 1994–1999, cases for New York were exclusively reported by New York City. Starting with 2000 data, cases for New York include the entire state.

[11]Data for 1994 do not include cases from Georgia.

Table 3-1. Selected Notifiable Disease Rates and Number of New Cases, Selected Years, 1950–2016—*Continued*

(Cases per 100,000 population; number; data are based on reporting by state health departments.)

Disease	2005	2006	2007	2008	2009	2010	2011	2012	2013	2014	2015	2016
Rate												
Acute hepatitis A viral infection	1.53	1.21	1.00	0.86	0.65	0.54	0.45	0.50	0.57	0.39	0.43	0.62
Acute hepatitis B viral infection	1.78	1.62	1.51	1.34	1.12	1.10	0.94	0.93	0.97	0.88	1.06	1.00
Acute hepatitis C viral infection[1]	0.23	0.26	0.28	0.29	0.27	0.29	0.42	0.59	0.71	0.73	0.81	0.97
Diphtheria	–	–	–	–	–	–	–	0.00	–	0.00	–	–
Haemophilus influenzae, invasive	0.78	0.82	0.85	0.96	0.99	1.03	1.15	1.10	1.21	1.11	1.29	1.51
Lyme disease[2]	NA	NA	NA	11.67	12.71	9.86	10.78	9.96	11.62	10.54	11.90	11.32
Measles (Rubeola)	0.02	0.02	0.01	0.05	0.02	0.02	0.06	0.02	0.06	0.21	0.06	0.03
Meningococcal disease	0.42	0.40	0.36	0.39	0.32	0.27	0.25	0.18	0.18	0.14	0.12	0.12
Mumps	0.11	2.22	0.27	0.15	0.65	0.85	0.13	0.07	0.19	0.38	0.41	1.97
Pertussis (whooping cough)	8.72	5.27	3.49	4.40	5.54	8.97	6.06	15.49	9.12	10.34	6.46	5.56
Poliomyelitis, paralytic[3]	–	–	–	–	0.00	–	–	–	0.00	–	–	–
Rubella (German measles)	0.00	0.00	0.00	0.01	0.00	0.00	0.00	0.00	0.00	0.00	0.00	0.00
Salmonellosis, excluding typhoid fever	15.43	15.45	16.03	16.92	16.18	17.73	16.79	17.27	16.13	16.14	17.15	16.67
Shigellosis	5.51	5.23	6.60	7.50	5.24	4.82	4.32	4.90	4.06	6.51	7.34	6.53
Spotted fever rickettsiosis[4]	0.66	0.80	0.77	0.85	0.60	0.65	0.91	1.44	1.08	1.18	1.31	1.33
Tuberculosis[5]	4.80	4.65	4.44	4.28	3.80	3.64	3.41	3.19	3.05	2.95	2.97	2.87
Sexually transmitted diseases[6]												
Syphilis[7]	11.23	12.34	13.57	15.22	14.60	14.85	14.78	15.90	17.87	19.90	23.24	27.25
Primary and secondary	2.94	3.26	3.80	4.44	4.56	4.46	4.48	4.99	5.50	6.27	7.43	8.61
Early latent	2.76	3.07	3.57	4.08	4.26	4.41	4.22	4.62	5.36	6.10	7.52	9.00
Late and late latent[8]	5.41	5.89	6.05	6.56	5.65	5.86	5.96	6.18	6.90	7.38	8.14	9.54
Congenital[9]	8.19	8.72	10.08	10.50	10.43	9.68	9.06	8.45	9.18	11.56	12.34	15.82
Chlamydia[10]	329.42	344.33	367.47	398.12	405.26	423.62	453.41	453.30	443.46	452.17	474.97	494.65
Gonorrhea[11]	114.57	119.70	118.03	110.75	98.10	100.19	103.29	106.66	105.34	109.79	122.96	144.99
Chancroid	0.01	0.01	0.01	0.01	0.01	0.01	0.00	0.00	0.00	0.00	0.00	0.00
Number												
Acute hepatitis A viral infection	4,488	3,579	2,979	2,585	1,987	1,670	1,398	1,562	1,781	1,239	1,390	2,007
Acute hepatitis B viral infection	5,119	4,713	4,519	4,033	3,405	3,374	2,903	2,895	3,050	2,791	3,370	3,218
Acute hepatitis C viral infection[1]	662	766	845	877	782	849	1,229	1,782	2,138	2,204	2,447	2,942
Diphtheria	–	–	–	–	–	–	–	1	–	1	–	–
Haemophilus influenzae, invasive	2,304	2,496	2,541	2,886	3,022	3,151	3,539	3,418	3,792	3,541	4,138	4,895
Lyme disease[2]	NA	NA	NA	35,198	38,468	30,158	33,097	30,831	36,307	33,461	38,069	36,429
Measles (Rubeola)	66	55	43	140	71	63	55	220	187	667	188	85
Meningococcal disease	1,245	1,194	1,077	1,172	980	833	759	551	556	433	372	375
Mumps	314	6,584	800	454	1,991	2,612	404	229	584	1,223	1,329	6,369
Pertussis (whooping cough)	25,616	15,632	10,454	13,278	16,858	27,550	18,719	48,277	28,639	32,971	20,762	17,972
Poliomyelitis, paralytic[3]	–	–	–	–	1	–	–	–	1	–	–	–
Rubella (German measles)	11	11	12	16	3	5	4	9	9	6	5	1
Salmonellosis, excluding typhoid fever	45,322	45,808	47,995	51,040	49,192	54,424	51,887	53,800	50,634	51,455	55,108	53,850
Shigellosis	16,168	15,503	19,758	22,625	15,931	14,786	13,352	15,283	12,729	20,745	23,590	21,097
Spotted fever rickettsiosis[4]	1,936	2,288	2,221	2,563	1,815	1,985	4,470	2,802	3,359	3,757	4,198	4,269
Tuberculosis[5]	14,097	13,779	13,299	12,904	11,545	11,182	10,528	9,945	9,582	9,421	9,557	9,272
Sexually transmitted diseases[6]												
Syphilis[7]	33,288	36,958	40,925	46,292	44,832	45,844	46,040	49,915	56,484	63,453	74,707	88,042
Primary and secondary	8,724	9,756	11,466	13,500	13,997	13,774	13,970	15,667	17,375	19,999	23,872	27,814
Early latent	8,176	9,186	10,768	12,401	13,066	13,604	13,136	14,503	16,929	19,452	24,173	28,924
Late and late latent[8]	16,049	17,644	18,256	19,945	17,338	18,079	18,576	19,411	21,819	23,541	26,170	30,676
Congenital[9]	339	372	435	446	431	387	358	334	361	461	492	628
Chlamydia[10]	976,445	1,030,911	1,108,374	1,210,523	1,244,180	1,307,893	1,412,791	1,422,976	1,401,906	1,441,789	1,526,658	1,598,354
Gonorrhea[11]	339,593	358,366	355,991	336,742	301,174	309,341	321,849	334,826	333,004	350,062	395,216	468,514
Chancroid	17	19	23	25	28	24	8	15	10	6	11	7

– = Quantity zero.
0.0 = Quantity more than zero but less than 0.05.
NA = Not available.
[1]Anti-HCV antibody test became available May 1990. Total number of cases in 2015 and 2016 reported from 42 states.
[2]Not nationally notifiable prior to 1991. National surveillance case definition revised in 2008; probable cases not reported previously.
[3]Cases of vaccine-associated paralytic poliomyelitis caused by polio vaccine virus.
[4]Prior to 2010 data, cases of spotted fever rickettsiosis were reported as Rocky Mountain spotted fever (RMSF). Because serologic tests commonly used to diagnose RMSF exhibit cross-reactivity between spotted fever rickettsial pathogens, some cases reported as RMSF might actually be disease caused by other spotted fever rickettsial infections, and therefore are more correctly referred to as spotted fever rickettsiosis starting with 2010 data. Includes confirmed and probable cases.
[5]Case reporting for tuberculosis began in 1953. Data prior to 1975 are not comparable with subsequent years because of changes in reporting criteria effective in 1975.
[6]For 1950, data for Alaska and Hawaii were not included. Starting with 1991, data include both civilian and military cases. Cases and rates shown do not include U.S. outlying areas of Guam, Puerto Rico, and the Virgin Islands.
[7]Includes stage of syphilis not stated.
[8]Includes cases of unknown duration.
[9]Rates include all cases of congenitally acquired syphilis per 100,000 live births. Cases of congenitally acquired syphilis were reported through 1994. Starting with 1995 data, only congenital syphilis for cases under 1 year of age were reported.
[10]Prior to 1994, chlamydia was not notifiable. In 1994–1999, cases for New York were exclusively reported by New York City. Starting with 2000 data, cases for New York include the entire state.
[11]Data for 1994 do not include cases from Georgia.

Table 3-2. Human Immunodeficiency Virus (HIV) Diagnoses, by Year of Diagnosis and Selected Characteristics, 2008–2016

(Number, percent distribution; data are based on reporting by 50 states and the District of Columbia.)

Characteristic	Year of diagnosis[1]					
	2011	2012	2013	2014	2015[2]	2016[2]
Estimated number of HIV diagnoses[3]						
All persons[4]	41,984	41,168	39,652	40,276	39,876	39,782
Sex and Age						
Male, 13 years and over	32,964	32,671	31,772	32,476	32,306	32,131
Female, 13 years and over	8,822	8,257	7,694	7,620	7,435	7,529
Age at Diagnosis						
Under 13 years	198	240	186	180	135	122
13-14 years	42	47	41	35	26	23
15-19 years	1,999	1,882	1,692	1,731	1,721	1,652
20-24 years	7,072	7,141	7,058	7,349	7,228	6,776
25-29 years	6,364	6,469	6,661	7,188	7,600	7,964
30-34 years	5,251	5,468	5,214	5,460	5,461	5,701
35-39 years	4,463	4,158	3,985	4,266	4,253	4,242
40-44 years	4,791	4,449	3,945	3,789	3,416	3,334
45-49 years	4,573	4,302	3,934	3,627	3,319	3,156
50-54 years	3,350	3,199	2,982	2,907	2,987	2,959
55-59 years	1,990	1,928	2,022	1,938	1,886	1,923
60-64 years	1,068	1,059	1,074	975	997	1,089
65 years and over	823	826	858	831	847	841
Hispanic Origin and Race[5]						
Not Hispanic or Latino						
White	11,146	11,039	10,636	10,618	10,465	10,345
Black or African American	18,992	18,258	17,470	17,530	17,432	17,528
American Indian or Alaska Native	143	176	154	187	197	243
Asian	744	784	810	938	947	977
Native Hawaiian or Other Pacific Islander	55	54	49	44	80	48
Multiple race	1,612	1,566	1,436	1,249	1,060	875
Hispanic or Latino[6]	9,292	9,291	9,097	9,710	9,695	9,766
Region of Residence						
Northeast	7,755	7,551	7,013	6,994	6,502	6,309
Midwest	5,391	5,484	5,327	5,106	5,224	5,068
South	21,291	20,493	20,020	20,345	20,442	20,588
West	7,547	7,640	7,292	7,831	7,708	7,817
Estimated Number of HIV Diagnoses per 100,000 Resident Population[3]						
All persons	13.5	13.1	12.5	12.6	12.4	12.3
Sex and Age						
Male, 13 years and over	26.1	25.6	24.7	25.0	24.7	24.3
Female, 13 years and over	6.7	6.2	5.7	5.6	5.4	5.4
Age at Diagnosis						
Under 13 years	0.4	0.5	0.4	0.3	0.3	0.2
13-14 years	0.5	0.6	0.5	0.4	0.3	0.3
15-19 years	9.2	8.8	8.0	8.2	8.2	7.8
20-24 years	31.9	31.6	30.9	32.1	31.9	30.3
25-29 years	29.9	30.2	30.9	32.7	33.9	34.8
30-34 years	25.6	26.1	24.5	25.4	25.3	26.2
35-39 years	22.8	21.3	20.3	21.5	20.9	20.4
40-44 years	22.8	21.1	18.9	18.4	16.9	16.9
45-49 years	20.6	19.8	18.5	17.4	16.0	15.1
50-54 years	14.8	14.2	13.2	12.9	13.4	13.5
55-59 years	9.8	9.3	9.5	9.0	8.7	8.7
60-64 years	6.0	5.9	5.9	5.3	5.2	5.6
65 years and over	2.0	1.9	1.9	1.8	1.8	1.7
Hispanic Origin and Race[5]						
Not Hispanic or Latino						
White	5.6	5.6	5.4	5.4	5.3	5.2
Black or African American	49.5	47.1	44.6	44.4	43.7	43.6
American Indian or Alaska Native	6.2	7.6	6.6	8.0	8.3	10.2
Asian	4.9	5.0	5.0	5.6	5.5	5.5
Native Hawaiian or Other Pacific Islander	10.8	10.4	9.2	8.1	14.4	8.5
Multiple race	27.7	26.1	23.2	19.6	16.1	12.9
Hispanic or Latino[6]	17.9	17.5	16.8	17.6	17.2	17.0
Region of Residence[7]						
Northeast	13.9	13.5	12.5	12.5	11.6	11.2
Midwest	8.0	8.1	7.9	7.5	7.7	7.5
South	18.3	17.5	16.9	17.0	16.9	16.8
West	10.4	10.4	9.8	10.4	10.2	10.2

NOTE: Data shown are for the 50 states and the District of Columbia, and include newly diagnosed and reported cases. This table does not present HIV incidence or prevalence data. Rates were calculated using vintage 2016 resident population estimates from the U.S. Census Bureau. Variations in trends among subpopulations may be due to differences in testing behaviors, targeted HIV testing initiatives, or the numbers of new HIV infections in some subpopulations. Caution should be used when interpreting data on diagnoses of HIV infection. HIV surveillance reports may not be representative of all persons with HIV for several reasons: not all infected persons have been tested and diagnosed; results of anonymous tests are not reported to the name-based HIV registries of state and local health departments; testing patterns are influenced by the extent to which testing is routinely offered to specific groups; and surveillance and reporting practices among jurisdictions differ. The data presented here are estimates of the minimum number of persons for whom HIV infection has been diagnosed and reported to the surveillance system. Data have been revised and differ from previous editions.

[1]Based on diagnoses during 2011–2016 that were reported to the Centers for Disease Control and Prevention (CDC) through June 30, 2017. infection regardless of the stage of disease (stage 0, 1, 2, 3 [AIDS], or unknown). In 2014, the criteria used to define HIV diagnoses changed. according to the 2008 HIV case definition. Starting with 2014 data, cases were classified according to the new definition. Because of the change in case definition, HIV diagnoses prior to 2014 are not strictly comparable with HIV diagnoses for 2014. The vertical line in the table represents the discontinuity in the HIV diagnosis trend.
[2]Data for 2016 are preliminary; CDC cautions against using the 2016 data in this report for assessments of trends.
[3]Numbers and rates are point estimates that result from statistical adjustments for missing risk factor information.
[4]Includes unknown sex not shown separately.
[5]Hispanic origin and race categories are mutually exclusive.
[6]Persons of Hispanic origin may be of any race.
[7]Data are based on residence at the time of diagnosis of HIV infection.

Table 3-3. Age-Adjusted Cancer Incidence Rates for Selected Cancer Sites, by Sex, Race, and Hispanic Origin, Selected Geographic Areas, Selected Years, 1990–2014

(Number of new cases per 100,000 population;[1] data are based on the Surveillance, Epidemiology, and End Results (SEER) Program's 13 population-based cancer registries.)

Site, sex, race, and Hispanic origin	1990	1995	2000	2003	2005	2010	2011	2012	2013	2014	1990–2014 APC[2]
All Sites											
All persons	475.8	471.5	475.3	463.6	461.1	451.4	444.1	430.9	423.8	417.2	†–0.5
White	483.3	477.6	485.9	474.3	473.4	463.3	456.2	441.7	434.7	430.0	†–0.5
Black or African American	515.3	539.5	526.3	514.9	506.0	484.8	478.6	467.8	452.4	423.9	†–0.8
American Indian or Alaska Native[3]	349.0	371.7	365.6	381.9	405.5	409.4	380.6	359.8	377.4	346.1	0.0
Asian or Pacific Islander	335.5	340.6	341.7	334.9	332.2	324.9	323.1	312.7	309.7	297.7	†–0.5
Hispanic or Latino[4]	356.3	360.3	362.5	359.6	365.8	350.3	353.7	340.2	332.6	327.5	†–0.4
White, not Hispanic or Latino[4]	495.2	491.3	503.8	492.4	491.5	483.9	475.8	461.4	455.7	451.9	†–0.4
Male	584.1	564.8	565.8	546.2	535.2	513.8	499.7	470.8	460.6	447.7	†–1.1
White	591.1	563.6	570.0	551.1	544.0	521.8	508.4	478.0	467.1	457.1	†–1.0
Black or African American	688.4	743.1	708.1	670.6	638.8	597.3	574.1	554.0	537.0	481.6	†–1.6
American Indian or Alaska Native[3]	397.1	424.0	372.7	447.8	427.5	460.6	409.0	351.6	391.3	348.6	–0.4
Asian or Pacific Islander	386.2	398.9	400.6	388.0	372.2	348.3	345.7	320.4	316.0	300.7	†–1.2
Hispanic or Latino[4]	417.5	440.9	436.9	425.6	427.7	400.5	394.4	369.4	350.3	343.4	†–0.9
White, not Hispanic or Latino[4]	606.7	577.5	589.2	569.4	562.1	542.7	528.7	498.1	489.8	480.1	†–0.9
Female	411.5	410.7	414.2	407.2	410.0	407.1	405.4	404.9	400.6	399.0	†–0.1
White	421.3	423.3	430.1	422.4	425.0	421.9	420.1	418.7	415.3	415.2	0.0
Black or African American	406.7	403.2	404.1	410.4	416.5	406.7	412.9	408.8	393.9	385.9	–0.1
American Indian or Alaska Native[3]	316.5	338.6	367.3	338.4	390.8	379.8	365.4	374.2	372.0	348.3	†0.5
Asian or Pacific Islander	295.7	297.9	301.2	300.1	307.3	312.6	311.1	312.0	310.6	300.0	0.1
Hispanic or Latina[4]	323.1	311.0	318.5	319.1	327.3	319.7	330.1	325.2	327.2	323.5	†0.1
White, not Hispanic or Latina[4]	430.6	436.7	446.1	439.9	442.5	441.3	438.5	437.6	434.4	435.8	0.1
Lung and Bronchus											
Male	95.0	86.9	77.8	75.5	71.5	63.1	60.9	59.0	56.7	55.0	†–2.1
White	94.1	85.0	76.3	74.3	70.8	62.9	60.3	58.1	55.7	55.1	†–2.1
Black or African American	134.2	137.0	111.7	112.1	98.1	82.2	82.8	82.0	75.7	68.1	†–2.7
American Indian or Alaska Native[3]	77.3	82.8	62.6	74.2	67.4	67.1	55.6	46.5	55.7	44.6	†–1.4
Asian or Pacific Islander	64.4	60.1	63.9	58.7	58.2	51.1	50.0	49.1	49.6	44.6	†–1.4
Hispanic or Latino[4]	59.4	52.4	45.2	46.6	44.0	34.7	35.6	34.2	34.5	32.6	†–2.1
White, not Hispanic or Latino[4]	97.4	88.4	80.2	77.9	74.6	67.2	64.3	62.1	59.4	59.0	†–2.0
Female	47.2	49.3	48.6	49.8	50.0	46.1	45.0	44.5	43.7	43.0	†–0.4
White	48.5	51.7	50.7	52.4	51.9	48.1	46.7	46.2	45.6	45.1	†–0.4
Black or African American	52.9	50.0	55.1	55.5	58.4	52.9	50.1	52.0	48.7	48.1	–0.2
American Indian or Alaska Native[3]	30.4	46.1	38.5	41.4	45.1	37.2	42.5	35.1	28.8	26.3	0.1
Asian or Pacific Islander	28.4	27.6	27.3	29.1	30.8	29.3	31.5	29.3	29.4	27.0	0.2
Hispanic or Latina[4]	26.2	25.2	24.3	24.5	23.0	24.7	24.0	23.2	24.8	21.6	†–0.5
White, not Hispanic or Latina[4]	50.8	54.8	54.4	56.6	56.4	52.0	50.8	50.5	49.6	49.8	–0.2
Colon and Rectum											
Male	72.3	63.2	62.6	58.4	54.7	47.0	45.5	43.7	42.7	42.5	†–2.2
White	73.0	62.5	62.1	57.0	54.1	45.5	43.6	42.3	40.6	41.4	†–2.3
Black or African American	73.1	75.2	73.5	76.5	67.1	57.9	57.1	56.0	56.5	46.9	†–1.6
American Indian or Alaska Native[3]	61.9	66.2	48.7	70.4	65.6	65.2	65.5	57.7	55.9	59.9	–0.2
Asian or Pacific Islander	60.9	58.8	58.0	53.4	47.8	45.6	45.7	42.4	43.2	41.1	†–1.7
Hispanic or Latino[4]	47.7	46.0	50.5	47.7	47.5	42.1	43.7	40.4	38.5	37.7	†–1.0
White, not Hispanic or Latino[4]	75.0	63.9	63.4	58.1	54.8	46.0	43.6	42.5	41.0	42.2	†–2.4
Female	50.2	45.9	46.1	43.6	41.4	36.0	34.7	33.7	32.3	33.2	†–1.7
White	49.7	45.4	45.5	42.9	40.3	34.5	33.9	32.9	31.8	33.0	†–1.7
Black or African American	61.3	54.9	58.2	55.4	54.3	46.6	42.5	41.8	38.7	38.2	†–1.5
American Indian or Alaska Native[3]	45.8	47.9	39.1	45.1	49.1	43.8	45.9	46.2	49.5	48.3	–0.1
Asian or Pacific Islander	37.8	38.9	37.5	36.4	36.8	34.6	31.7	29.0	27.9	27.8	†–1.5
Hispanic or Latina[4]	34.5	32.0	34.2	33.8	33.8	30.9	29.5	28.4	27.1	29.2	†–0.7
White, not Hispanic or Latina[4]	50.9	46.7	46.7	44.0	41.3	34.9	34.6	33.7	32.6	33.8	†–1.7
Prostate											
Male	166.9	166.6	179.1	165.6	154.2	144.0	137.6	112.3	106.4	96.1	†–2.2
White	168.5	161.3	175.0	161.8	150.2	140.2	133.6	106.6	101.6	91.9	†–2.3
Black or African American	219.6	279.8	292.3	254.4	244.7	220.7	209.7	184.3	176.7	145.4	†–2.2
American Indian or Alaska Native[3]	98.3	93.5	70.4	113.8	94.4	85.0	71.0	62.0	60.3	53.6	†–2.3
Asian or Pacific Islander	88.6	104.9	108.2	105.4	96.0	79.5	80.2	64.8	57.9	52.1	†–2.4
Hispanic or Latino[4]	119.2	141.5	150.6	139.9	133.5	119.5	111.2	95.4	85.3	78.8	†–2.1
White, not Hispanic or Latino[4]	172.2	163.6	178.8	165.3	152.8	144.2	138.0	109.3	105.4	95.4	†–2.2
Breast											
Female	129.4	130.9	134.3	124.3	124.5	123.6	127.0	126.5	126.7	125.3	†–0.3
White	134.3	136.3	140.7	129.1	129.6	127.4	130.7	129.7	129.7	128.5	†–0.3
Black or African American	117.4	123.0	122.8	123.4	119.4	123.6	129.7	131.4	127.3	124.9	†0.3
American Indian or Alaska Native[3]	69.6	96.7	100.2	95.9	107.0	91.7	105.8	99.0	91.2	102.2	0.4
Asian or Pacific Islander	87.9	88.4	95.1	92.3	95.9	100.9	103.1	104.6	108.3	104.0	†0.7
Hispanic or Latina[4]	91.2	89.4	97.2	88.4	93.4	87.8	97.0	92.6	94.6	93.8	0.1
White, not Hispanic or Latina[4]	138.6	141.8	147.0	135.7	136.2	135.5	137.5	137.3	137.4	136.8	–0.2

NOTE: Estimates are based on 13 SEER areas, November 2015 submission and differ from published estimates based on 9 SEER areas or other submission dates. The site variable distinguishes Kaposi Sarcoma and Mesothelioma as individual cancer sites. As a result, Kaposi Sarcoma and Mesothelioma cases do not contribute to other cancer sites. Estimates for 2001–2009 were computed using intercensal population estimates based on the 2000 and 2010 Censuses. Data have been revised and differ from previous editions.
† =Annual percent change (APC) is significantly different from 0 (p<0.05).
0.0 = APC is greater than –0.05 but less than 0.05.
[1]Age adjusted by 5-year age groups to the year 2000 U.S. standard population. Age-adjusted rates are based on at least 16 cases.
[2]APC has been calculated by fitting a linear regression model to the natural logarithm of the yearly rates from 1990–2014.
[3]Estimates for the American Indian or Alaska Native populations are based on the Contract Health Service Delivery Area (CHSDA) counties within SEER areas.
[4]Hispanic data exclude cases from Alaska. The race groups white, black, Asian or Pacific Islander, and American Indian or Alaska Native include persons of Hispanic and non-Hispanic origin. Persons of Hispanic origin may be of any race. The North American Association of Central Cancer Registries (NAACCR) Hispanic Identification Algorithm was used on a combination of variables to classify cases as Hispanic for analytic purposes. See the report, "NAACCR Guideline for Enhancing Hispanic-Latino Identification," for more information (available from: https://seer.cancer.gov/seerstat/variables/seer/race_ethnicity/).

Table 3-3. Age-Adjusted Cancer Incidence Rates for Selected Cancer Sites, by Sex, Race, and Hispanic Origin, Selected Geographic Areas, Selected Years, 1990–2014—Continued

(Number of new cases per 100,000 population;[1] data are based on the Surveillance, Epidemiology, and End Results (SEER) Program's 13 population-based cancer registries.)

Site, sex, race, and Hispanic origin	1990	1995	2000	2003	2005	2010	2011	2012	2013	2014	1990–2014 APC[2]
Cervix Uteri											
Female	11.9	9.9	8.9	8.2	7.9	7.2	7.0	6.9	6.6	6.8	†–2.4
White	11.2	9.2	8.9	7.9	7.8	7.2	7.2	6.8	6.5	6.9	†–2.0
Black or African American	16.7	14.9	10.7	10.8	9.4	8.5	7.8	7.7	8.2	6.5	†–3.5
American Indian or Alaska Native[3]	14.7	*	*	*	10.7	8.3	9.5	*	9.8	8.3	†–1.8
Asian or Pacific Islander	12.2	11.2	8.0	8.1	7.8	6.5	5.5	6.7	5.9	6.1	†–3.6
Hispanic or Latina[4]	21.3	17.5	17.1	14.1	13.7	10.5	9.3	9.4	8.2	8.6	†–3.9
White, not Hispanic or Latina[4]	9.7	7.8	7.1	6.5	6.4	6.2	6.5	6.0	6.0	6.4	†–1.8
Corpus and Uterus, Not Otherwise Specified											
Female	24.7	24.9	23.8	23.6	24.1	26.7	26.6	27.0	26.5	27.0	†0.4
White	26.4	26.4	25.6	25.0	25.4	27.6	27.2	28.1	26.9	27.8	†0.2
Black or African American	17.0	17.9	17.4	20.3	21.5	24.6	27.7	25.2	27.2	26.7	†2.2
American Indian or Alaska Native[3]	19.3	*	18.5	19.5	14.4	26.9	20.5	19.3	27.5	19.6	*
Asian or Pacific Islander	13.5	17.8	16.6	16.7	18.9	22.6	21.8	22.3	22.6	21.8	†1.7
Hispanic or Latina[4]	17.8	16.6	15.9	17.8	19.4	20.6	22.2	24.1	23.6	24.0	†1.7
White, not Hispanic or Latina[4]	27.1	27.5	26.8	26.0	26.2	28.6	27.7	28.4	27.1	28.2	0.1
Ovary											
Female	15.5	14.6	14.2	13.6	13.2	12.6	12.2	12.4	11.5	11.3	†–1.1
White	16.4	15.4	15.1	14.3	13.9	13.5	13.0	13.1	12.1	11.9	†–1.1
Black or African American	11.3	10.8	10.9	11.6	10.8	9.6	10.2	10.6	9.0	9.3	†–0.5
American Indian or Alaska Native[3]	21.9	*	18.9	13.4	12.2	11.9	11.6	15.7	10.9	10.7	*
Asian or Pacific Islander	11.1	10.4	10.4	10.2	11.0	9.8	9.6	9.7	9.9	9.4	†–0.5
Hispanic or Latina[4]	12.2	11.7	10.6	11.6	11.9	11.9	11.3	12.3	10.3	10.1	†–0.5
White, not Hispanic or Latina[4]	16.7	15.9	15.7	14.7	14.1	13.4	13.1	13.1	12.2	12.1	†–1.2
Oral Cavity and Pharynx											
Male	18.5	16.5	15.8	15.2	15.1	15.6	16.0	15.7	16.4	16.3	†–0.5
White	18.0	16.4	15.6	15.3	15.5	16.1	16.9	16.5	17.1	17.1	–0.1
Black or African American	25.4	22.3	19.5	17.6	15.9	13.7	13.9	14.0	14.4	14.3	†–2.6
American Indian or Alaska Native[3]	*	*	*	16.3	10.4	21.3	16.0	15.4	12.8	10.4	*
Asian or Pacific Islander	14.9	11.8	13.7	11.9	11.5	11.8	10.9	10.9	12.7	11.2	†–0.8
Hispanic or Latino[4]	10.7	12.3	9.1	8.9	9.7	8.9	10.8	10.1	9.1	9.9	–0.5
White, not Hispanic or Latino[4]	18.8	16.9	16.6	16.3	16.4	17.6	18.1	17.8	18.8	18.7	0.1
Female	7.3	7.0	6.2	6.0	6.1	6.1	6.1	6.3	6.2	5.8	†–0.8
White	7.4	7.1	6.2	5.9	6.0	6.3	6.4	6.5	6.3	6.1	†–0.7
Black or African American	6.4	6.7	5.4	6.7	7.0	5.5	5.2	4.5	5.3	4.5	†–1.6
American Indian or Alaska Native[3]	*	*	*	*	*	*	8.7	7.4	8.8	*	*
Asian or Pacific Islander	6.1	5.2	6.3	5.2	6.0	5.2	4.8	5.9	5.3	4.8	†–0.8
Hispanic or Latina[4]	4.0	3.7	3.7	3.9	3.5	4.2	3.9	3.9	4.0	4.2	–0.2
White, not Hispanic or Latina[4]	7.8	7.5	6.6	6.2	6.4	6.7	7.0	7.0	6.8	6.4	†–0.5
Stomach											
Male	14.6	13.5	12.6	11.8	11.4	10.5	10.6	10.2	10.1	10.0	†–1.7
White	12.8	11.9	10.6	10.1	9.6	9.3	9.5	8.9	8.8	8.8	†–1.6
Black or African American	21.5	18.6	18.6	18.7	17.4	13.3	14.1	14.9	14.4	12.4	†–2.2
American Indian or Alaska Native[3]	*	24.1	20.2	*	20.8	20.7	21.2	16.1	22.6	16.3	–0.5
Asian or Pacific Islander	26.9	24.3	23.0	19.2	20.2	15.3	14.3	14.9	14.8	14.6	†–2.9
Hispanic or Latino[4]	20.2	19.3	16.1	16.2	15.6	14.9	14.2	13.1	12.0	13.2	†–1.9
White, not Hispanic or Latino[4]	12.1	11.1	10.0	9.2	8.6	8.3	8.5	7.9	7.9	7.8	†–1.9
Female	6.7	6.2	6.1	6.0	5.7	5.7	5.6	5.9	5.4	5.0	†–0.9
White	5.7	5.1	5.0	5.0	4.7	4.7	4.8	5.1	4.5	4.3	†–0.9
Black or African American	10.0	9.8	8.7	9.5	8.1	8.5	9.5	8.1	7.0	7.0	†–1.3
American Indian or Alaska Native[3]	*	*	*	*	*	13.0	*	12.1	12.3	11.3	*
Asian or Pacific Islander	15.4	13.0	12.9	11.1	10.3	8.9	7.8	8.8	8.9	6.9	†–2.8
Hispanic or Latina[4]	10.8	11.2	10.6	10.3	10.2	9.4	8.8	9.7	8.8	8.7	†–1.0
White, not Hispanic or Latina[4]	5.1	4.5	4.2	4.1	3.8	3.6	3.9	4.0	3.5	3.2	†–1.6
Pancreas											
Male	13.0	12.8	12.8	12.5	13.7	13.7	14.2	14.1	14.3	14.0	†0.6
White	12.7	12.4	12.6	12.3	13.5	13.5	14.2	14.5	14.2	14.0	†0.7
Black or African American	19.3	19.2	18.2	17.4	18.3	18.6	17.0	16.1	17.9	18.3	–0.2
American Indian or Alaska Native[3]	*	*	*	*	21.2	17.4	17.7	*	14.3	*	*
Asian or Pacific Islander	11.0	10.3	10.7	10.2	11.7	11.4	12.2	10.4	12.3	10.9	0.2
Hispanic or Latino[4]	10.7	12.0	12.2	10.1	12.3	11.5	13.4	10.8	12.0	11.5	†0.7
White, not Hispanic or Latino[4]	12.8	12.4	12.7	12.7	13.6	13.8	14.3	15.0	14.5	14.4	†0.7
Female	10.0	9.9	9.9	10.4	10.8	11.3	10.6	11.4	11.2	10.8	†0.6
White	9.7	9.6	9.6	10.2	10.6	10.9	10.4	11.1	11.2	10.8	†0.7
Black or African American	12.9	15.5	12.8	14.4	16.4	15.2	15.1	15.1	13.6	13.2	–0.2
American Indian or Alaska Native[3]	*	*	20.4	*	12.4	12.9	*	12.1	*	*	*
Asian or Pacific Islander	9.9	8.1	9.2	8.1	8.0	10.4	9.2	10.0	9.6	8.8	†0.8

NOTE: Estimates are based on 13 SEER areas, November 2015 submission and differ from published estimates based on 9 SEER areas or other submission dates. The site variable distinguishes Kaposi Sarcoma and Mesothelioma as individual cancer sites. As a result, Kaposi Sarcoma and Mesothelioma cases do not contribute to other cancer sites. Estimates for 2001–2009 were computed using intercensal population estimates based on the 2000 and 2010 Censuses. Data have been revised and differ from previous editions.
† =Annual percent change (APC) is significantly different from 0 (p<0.05).
* = Estimates are considered unreliable. Data not shown if the rate is based on fewer than 16 cases for the time interval.
[1]Age adjusted by 5-year age groups to the year 2000 U.S. standard population. Age-adjusted rates are based on at least 16 cases.
[2]APC has been calculated by fitting a linear regression model to the natural logarithm of the yearly rates from 1990–2014.
[3]Estimates for the American Indian or Alaska Native populations are based on the Contract Health Service Delivery Area (CHSDA) counties within SEER areas.
[4]Hispanic data exclude cases from Alaska. The race groups white, black, Asian or Pacific Islander, and American Indian or Alaska Native include persons of Hispanic and non-Hispanic origin. Persons of Hispanic origin may be of any race. The North American Association of Central Cancer Registries (NAACCR) Hispanic Identification Algorithm was used on a combination of variables to classify cases as Hispanic for analytic purposes. See the report, "NAACCR Guideline for Enhancing Hispanic-Latino Identification," for more information (available from: https://seer.cancer.gov/seerstat/variables/seer/race_ethnicity/).

Table 3-3. Age-Adjusted Cancer Incidence Rates for Selected Cancer Sites, by Sex, Race, and Hispanic Origin, Selected Geographic Areas, Selected Years, 1990–2014—*Continued*

(Number of new cases per 100,000 population;[1] data are based on the Surveillance, Epidemiology, and End Results (SEER) Program's 13 population-based cancer registries.)

Site, sex, race, and Hispanic origin	1990	1995	2000	2003	2005	2010	2011	2012	2013	2014	1990–2014 APC[2]
Hispanic or Latina[4]	9.9	9.0	9.1	8.6	11.1	9.9	10.2	10.5	11.4	9.7	0.3
White, not Hispanic or Latina[4]	9.7	9.7	9.6	10.5	10.6	11.1	10.4	11.1	11.1	10.9	†0.7
Urinary Bladder											
Male	37.2	35.4	36.8	37.0	37.1	36.0	34.0	34.4	33.1	32.5	†–0.4
White	40.7	38.8	40.9	40.8	40.9	40.1	38.2	38.2	36.6	36.1	†–0.3
Black or African American	19.7	19.7	20.2	23.2	23.2	22.3	20.7	23.4	23.2	21.0	†0.4
American Indian or Alaska Native[3]	*	*	*	*	16.8	17.4	17.6	*	13.7	14.0	*
Asian or Pacific Islander	15.4	17.2	16.9	18.1	17.5	17.3	15.0	16.5	15.7	15.3	0.1
Hispanic or Latino[4]	22.4	17.8	20.4	20.3	20.2	18.6	20.1	19.1	18.6	19.0	–0.3
White, not Hispanic or Latino[4]	42.4	40.9	43.3	43.4	43.7	43.4	41.1	41.1	39.7	39.0	–0.1
Female	9.5	9.3	9.1	9.2	9.0	8.6	8.3	8.3	7.9	8.1	†–0.6
White	10.0	10.1	10.0	10.0	9.7	9.4	9.2	9.3	8.6	8.8	†–0.5
Black or African American	8.7	7.3	7.8	7.8	7.9	7.0	7.0	6.0	7.8	7.2	–0.5
American Indian or Alaska Native[3]	*	*	*	*	*	*	*	*	*	*	*
Asian or Pacific Islander	5.2	4.5	4.3	5.0	5.2	4.7	4.4	4.1	3.8	4.3	–0.3
Hispanic or Latina[4]	5.8	5.3	5.8	4.8	5.9	4.7	5.5	4.8	4.4	4.8	†–0.6
White, not Hispanic or Latina[4]	10.3	10.6	10.5	10.8	10.3	10.2	9.8	10.1	9.4	9.6	†–0.3
Non-Hodgkin Lymphoma											
Male	22.6	25.1	23.6	24.3	24.7	25.5	23.8	23.6	23.7	24.1	0.1
White	23.6	26.2	25.0	25.7	26.0	26.7	25.1	25.0	24.9	25.4	†0.2
Black or African American	17.7	21.7	17.6	19.4	19.7	21.5	17.4	17.4	17.8	18.8	–0.1
American Indian or Alaska Native[3]	*	*	15.3	*	24.3	19.6	10.8	13.8	10.4	9.9	*
Asian or Pacific Islander	16.7	16.5	16.4	16.3	17.9	17.6	18.1	17.7	18.4	17.6	†0.4
Hispanic or Latino[4]	17.3	21.0	20.5	19.6	19.8	23.0	20.1	19.6	19.8	19.9	0.3
White, not Hispanic or Latino[4]	24.3	26.7	25.6	26.5	27.0	27.4	25.8	26.0	25.8	26.4	†0.3
Female	14.5	15.2	16.0	17.2	16.5	17.0	15.9	16.1	15.7	15.9	†0.5
White	15.4	15.9	17.0	18.0	17.8	18.1	16.6	17.1	16.6	17.0	†0.5
Black or African American	10.4	10.3	11.9	13.5	13.3	12.8	13.0	13.6	13.1	11.8	†1.1
American Indian or Alaska Native[3]	*	*	13.5	11.7	12.2	13.0	16.5	11.1	12.9	13.1	*
Asian or Pacific Islander	9.6	12.3	11.5	12.8	9.8	12.0	12.0	11.5	10.8	11.7	0.3
Hispanic or Latina[4]	13.6	13.2	13.8	15.3	15.0	15.4	14.7	15.3	14.7	16.8	†0.8
White, not Hispanic or Latina[4]	15.6	16.2	17.3	18.4	18.1	18.5	17.0	17.3	17.0	17.0	†0.5
Leukemia											
Male	17.2	17.7	17.2	17.4	17.6	18.2	17.9	17.5	17.2	17.2	†0.1
White	18.1	19.0	18.3	18.5	19.2	19.8	19.2	18.5	18.6	18.5	†0.2
Black or African American	16.1	13.4	14.4	15.1	12.8	13.7	14.6	15.1	14.5	13.6	0.1
American Indian or Alaska Native[3]	*	*	*	*	12.3	*	9.8	14.6	11.4	13.1	*
Asian or Pacific Islander	8.4	10.2	10.6	10.5	9.4	10.2	10.4	10.6	9.1	10.2	0.0
Hispanic or Latino[4]	12.2	14.6	13.4	12.4	13.2	13.2	13.9	11.8	13.0	11.6	0.2
White, not Hispanic or Latino[4]	18.3	19.3	18.7	19.1	19.6	20.4	19.9	19.3	19.1	19.4	†0.3
Female	9.9	10.3	10.5	10.1	10.2	10.8	10.7	10.7	10.6	10.3	†0.3
White	10.3	11.0	11.1	10.7	10.7	11.6	11.5	11.5	11.5	11.1	†0.4
Black or African American	8.5	8.4	10.0	9.1	9.6	9.1	9.6	9.2	8.5	8.6	0.1
American Indian or Alaska Native[3]	*	*	*	*	*	8.7	*	7.0	8.2	*	*
Asian or Pacific Islander	5.7	6.4	6.4	6.6	6.5	6.1	6.4	6.7	6.3	6.5	0.1
Hispanic or Latina[4]	8.5	8.2	7.8	7.4	8.3	8.7	8.8	9.0	9.7	9.0	†0.6
White, not Hispanic or Latina[4]	10.3	11.1	11.1	11.2	10.8	12.0	11.8	11.6	11.5	11.2	†0.5

NOTE: Estimates are based on 13 SEER areas, November 2015 submission and differ from published estimates based on 9 SEER areas or other submission dates. The site variable distinguishes Kaposi Sarcoma and Mesothelioma as individual cancer sites. As a result, Kaposi Sarcoma and Mesothelioma cases do not contribute to other cancer sites. Estimates for 2001 –2009 were computed using intercensal population estimates based on the 2000 and 2010 Censuses. Data have been revised and differ from previous editions.
† =Annual percent change (APC) is significantly different from 0 (p<0.05).
0.0 = APC is greater than -0.05 but less than 0.05.
* = Estimates are considered unreliable. Data not shown if the rate is based on fewer than 16 cases for the time interval.
[1]Age adjusted by 5-year age groups to the year 2000 U.S. standard population. Age-adjusted rates are based on at least 16 cases.
[2]APC has been calculated by fitting a linear regression model to the natural logarithm of the yearly rates from 1990–2014.
[3]Estimates for the American Indian or Alaska Native populations are based on the Contract Health Service Delivery Area (CHSDA) counties within SEER areas.
[4]Hispanic data exclude cases from Alaska. The race groups white, black, Asian or Pacific Islander, and American Indian or Alaska Native include persons of Hispanic and non-Hispanic origin. Persons of Hispanic origin may be of any race. The North American Association of Central Cancer Registries (NAACCR) Hispanic Identification Algorithm was used on a combination of variables to classify cases as Hispanic for analytic purposes. See the report, "NAACCR Guideline for Enhancing Hispanic-Latino Identification," for more information (available from: https://seer.cancer.gov/seerstat/variables/seer/race_ethnicity/).

Table 3-4. Five-Year Relative Cancer Survival Rates for Selected Cancer Sites, by Sex and Selected Race, Selected Geographic Areas, Selected Years 1975–1977 Through 2007–2013

(Percent of patients; data are based on the Surveillance, Epidemiology, and End Results (SEER) Program's nine population-based cancer registries.)

Sex and site	White										
	1975–1977	1978–1980	1981–1983	1984–1986	1987–1989	1990–1992	1993–1995	1996–1998	1999–2001	2002–2006	2007–2013
Both Sexes											
All sites	49.8	50.0	51.3	53.6	56.7	61.4	62.4	64.4	67.2	68.8	70.1
Oral cavity and pharynx	54.0	55.4	54.0	56.3	55.9	57.9	60.1	59.9	62.2	66.1	69.2
Esophagus	5.5	5.3	7.3	10.2	10.5	12.9	13.4	14.1	18.9	19.9	22.3
Stomach	14.1	15.4	16.2	16.8	18.3	18.8	20.0	20.3	22.3	26.9	29.9
Colon	50.9	52.4	55.4	59.0	60.7	62.8	60.5	62.9	66.6	66.2	66.5
Rectum	48.3	49.7	52.0	57.0	58.7	59.9	60.6	63.5	66.5	68.9	68.5
Pancreas	2.5	2.5	2.5	2.6	3.2	4.4	3.9	4.1	5.0	6.2	8.9
Lung and bronchus	12.3	12.9	13.3	13.0	13.3	14.0	14.5	14.8	15.5	17.1	19.6
Urinary bladder	73.3	74.7	77.4	77.2	79.8	80.2	81.0	79.8	81.0	80.9	78.6
Non-Hodgkin's lymphoma	46.8	47.9	50.8	52.0	51.3	51.5	53.2	59.4	64.9	71.6	74.2
Leukemia	34.5	36.7	38.1	41.6	43.9	46.4	48.6	49.6	52.0	60.4	64.8
Male											
All sites	42.7	44.3	46.6	48.6	52.8	60.8	62.0	64.1	67.5	69.4	70.1
Oral cavity and pharynx	53.8	54.4	52.9	54.8	54.1	56.4	59.4	59.1	62.0	66.0	68.7
Esophagus	4.8	5.3	6.5	9.0	11.0	12.2	13.6	13.9	18.6	20.0	22.0
Stomach	13.1	13.6	15.4	14.3	15.5	16.1	18.9	18.6	21.0	25.5	28.1
Colon	50.5	51.3	56.2	59.6	61.4	63.1	60.7	62.9	67.9	66.6	66.4
Rectum	47.3	49.3	51.0	56.4	58.9	59.0	59.5	62.8	66.5	69.2	68.1
Pancreas	2.7	2.6	2.1	2.1	3.1	4.2	3.6	4.7	5.5	5.9	9.3
Lung and bronchus	11.1	11.5	11.7	11.2	12.0	12.5	12.6	13.1	13.3	14.8	16.9
Prostate gland	68.5	71.2	73.1	76.4	84.4	94.1	95.9	97.9	99.7	99.8	99.6
Urinary bladder	74.3	75.4	78.6	78.4	81.9	82.6	82.5	81.1	81.5	82.6	79.6
Non-Hodgkin's lymphoma	46.3	46.2	50.5	50.6	48.1	47.6	49.7	57.6	62.8	70.7	73.5
Leukemia	33.6	35.8	37.8	41.3	45.5	46.2	49.4	49.6	52.9	60.8	66.0
Female											
All sites	56.5	55.6	56.0	58.6	60.6	62.1	62.8	64.7	66.8	68.2	70.1
Colon	51.3	53.4	54.8	58.5	59.9	62.4	60.2	62.8	65.5	66.0	66.7
Rectum	49.4	50.1	53.2	57.7	58.4	61.0	61.9	64.4	66.4	68.4	69.0
Pancreas	2.3	2.5	3.0	3.1	3.3	4.5	4.2	3.6	4.4	6.6	8.3
Lung and bronchus	15.4	16.2	16.6	16.3	15.3	16.2	17.1	17.0	18.0	19.7	22.6
Melanoma of skin	86.2	87.9	87.2	91.0	91.3	91.8	92.6	92.7	94.6	95.4	95.7
Breast	75.6	75.1	77.1	80.0	85.1	86.5	87.6	89.4	90.8	91.7	92.2
Cervix uteri	69.7	68.1	67.8	68.8	72.5	70.9	74.2	73.6	73.4	70.8	70.8
Corpus uteri, not otherwise specified	88.0	83.7	82.2	84.0	83.9	85.7	84.9	85.1	85.9	85.5	85.3
Ovary	35.3	36.9	38.5	37.5	38.2	40.4	40.6	43.3	43.6	43.9	46.2
Non-Hodgkin's lymphoma	47.3	49.5	51.1	53.6	55.2	56.4	57.7	61.5	67.5	72.8	75.1

NOTE: Rates are based on follow-up of patients through 2014. The rate is the ratio of the observed survival rate for the patient group to the expected survival rate for persons in the general population similar to the patient group with respect to age, sex, race, and calendar year of observation. It estimates the chance of surviving the effects of cancer. The site variable distinguishes Kaposi sarcoma and mesothelioma as individual cancer sites. As a result, Kaposi sarcoma and mesothelioma cases are excluded from each of the sites except all sites combined. The race groups, White and Back, include persons of Hispanic and non-Hispanic origin. Due to death certificate race-ethnicity classification and other methodological issues related to developing life tables, relative survival rates for race-ethnicity groups other than White and Black are not calculated. Data have been revised and differ from previous editions.

Table 3-4. Five-Year Relative Cancer Survival Rates for Selected Cancer Sites, by Sex and Selected Race, Selected Geographic Areas, Selected Years 1975–1977 Through 2007–2013—Continued

(Percent of patients; data are based on the Surveillance, Epidemiology, and End Results (SEER) Program's nine population-based cancer registries.)

Sex and site	Black or African American										
	1975–1977	1978–1980	1981–1983	1984–1986	1987–1989	1990–1992	1993–1995	1996–1998	1999–2001	2002–2006	2007–2013
Both Sexes											
All sites	39.0	39.0	38.8	40.2	43.0	47.9	52.8	55.2	58.0	59.9	63.3
Oral cavity and pharynx	36.0	34.9	30.9	35.0	34.0	33.0	37.9	36.1	44.6	45.1	49.3
Esophagus	3.5	4.3	4.3	8.7	6.6	9.4	7.6	10.2	12.5	13.2	11.7
Stomach	16.1	16.4	16.4	19.1	18.8	22.7	19.3	22.6	23.2	28.6	31.4
Colon	44.7	48.9	48.5	49.1	52.4	53.4	51.1	53.6	52.5	55.6	56.2
Rectum	44.4	34.6	40.3	45.9	52.3	51.2	53.8	55.0	59.2	61.1	65.5
Pancreas	2.3	5.7	3.6	4.7	5.5	3.6	3.7	3.4	5.6	5.0	7.5
Lung and bronchus	11.2	11.7	11.3	11.1	10.9	10.5	12.8	12.3	12.6	13.4	17.3
Urinary bladder	50.3	54.5	59.5	59.4	62.6	63.1	60.6	62.7	67.5	63.8	65.4
Non-Hodgkin's lymphoma	48.6	51.3	49.5	46.8	45.7	42.2	42.1	54.6	55.7	62.4	67.1
Leukemia	33.4	28.2	33.9	32.7	35.0	35.7	41.3	38.6	43.3	53.3	57.8
Male											
All sites	32.7	33.3	34.2	35.5	38.9	47.6	54.5	57.9	61.1	63.6	65.9
Oral cavity and pharynx	29.7	29.8	25.4	29.5	30.0	28.2	33.0	31.2	39.4	40.7	47.0
Esophagus	2.0	3.4	3.7	8.2	5.3	9.7	7.8	8.5	10.6	11.3	10.3
Stomach	16.1	15.6	16.2	16.9	16.6	22.0	17.5	20.4	25.0	23.6	25.7
Colon	44.0	47.5	44.7	48.9	50.7	54.6	51.2	55.8	53.7	53.4	56.7
Rectum	41.4	33.5	38.1	43.4	47.7	53.7	51.4	53.6	60.1	57.6	59.1
Pancreas	2.5	4.5	3.7	3.9	5.1	3.2	3.6	3.1	3.7	4.3	7.4
Lung and bronchus	10.5	9.7	10.1	10.3	10.8	9.3	11.2	10.7	10.8	12.7	14.2
Prostate gland	60.7	62.1	62.8	65.7	71.1	84.4	91.7	94.9	97.3	97.8	97.4
Urinary bladder	56.5	62.6	64.9	62.3	67.5	65.7	67.8	65.6	71.8	68.3	70.0
Non-Hodgkin's lymphoma	42.6	47.3	49.2	44.5	41.3	38.2	35.7	53.0	49.0	58.1	63.5
Leukemia	30.4	27.3	33.4	31.5	32.7	30.5	41.6	39.0	44.5	55.3	59.0
Female											
All sites	46.2	45.6	44.4	45.5	47.7	48.2	50.6	52.1	54.3	55.8	60.3
Colon	45.3	49.8	51.5	49.3	53.8	52.3	51.0	51.8	51.5	57.4	55.7
Rectum	46.8	35.5	42.5	48.2	56.9	48.5	56.4	56.2	58.2	64.4	72.6
Pancreas	1.9	7.0	3.2	5.3	5.8	4.0	3.7	3.5	7.4	5.5	7.7
Lung and bronchus	13.8	17.8	14.9	12.8	11.1	12.7	15.7	15.0	15.2	14.4	20.7
Melanoma of skin	*	*	*	*	89.5	*	*	78.6	76.1	74.5	74.9
Breast	62.2	63.4	63.4	65.1	71.1	71.5	72.7	76.2	78.9	77.9	82.7
Cervix uteri	64.6	61.0	59.2	57.9	57.0	58.1	62.8	64.8	66.0	62.6	58.3
Corpus uteri, not otherwise specified	60.0	54.9	50.7	56.2	56.7	54.0	58.5	61.4	61.4	61.3	64.7
Ovary	41.3	38.8	37.5	39.4	33.9	35.5	41.5	39.2	35.6	37.3	38.5
Non-Hodgkin's lymphoma	55.3	56.7	49.8	49.9	51.0	47.7	54.0	57.0	63.7	67.6	71.0

NOTE: Rates are based on follow-up of patients through 2014. The rate is the ratio of the observed survival rate for the patient group to the expected survival rate for persons in the general population similar to the patient group with respect to age, sex, race, and calendar year of observation. It estimates the chance of surviving the effects of cancer. The site variable distinguishes Kaposi sarcoma and mesothelioma as individual cancer sites. As a result, Kaposi sarcoma and mesothelioma cases are excluded from each of the sites shown except all sites combined. The race groups, White and Back, include persons of Hispanic and non-Hispanic origin. Due to death certificate race-ethnicity classification and other methodological issues related to developing life tables, relative survival rates for race-ethnicity groups other than White and Black are not calculated. Data have been revised and differ from previous editions.

* = Data for population groups with fewer than 25 cases are not shown because estimates are considered unreliable.

Table 3-5. Respondent-Reported Prevalence of Heart Disease, Cancer, and Stroke Among Adults 18 Years of Age and Over, by Selected Characteristics, Selected Years, 1997–1998 Through 2015–2016

(Percent; data are based on household interviews of a sample of the civilian noninstitutionalized population.)

Characteristic	Heart disease[1]				Cancer[2]				Stroke[3]			
	1997–1998	1999–2000	2010–2011	2015–2016	1997–1998	1999–2000	2010–2011	2015–2016	1997–1998	1999–2000	2010–2011	2015–2016
18 years and over, age adjusted[4,5]	12.0	11.1	11.1	10.7	4.9	5.1	6.0	6.2	2.3	2.2	2.6	2.6
18 years and over, crude[5]	11.6	10.9	11.6	11.6	4.8	4.9	6.3	6.9	2.2	2.1	2.7	2.9
Age												
18 to 44 years	4.6	4.3	4.0	4.1	1.7	1.7	1.7	1.6	0.4	0.4	0.6	0.6
18 to 24 years	3.2	3.3	3.0	3.0	0.8	1.0	0.7	0.5	*	*	*	0.1
25 to 44 years	5.0	4.6	4.4	4.5	2.0	1.9	2.0	2.0	0.4	0.5	0.7	0.7
45 to 64 years	13.5	12.6	13.0	12.0	5.4	5.2	6.9	7.1	2.3	2.0	2.9	3.0
45 to 54 years	10.9	10.0	9.6	9.5	4.0	4.0	4.9	4.8	1.4	1.3	2.1	2.4
55 to 64 years	17.4	16.6	17.1	14.8	7.4	7.2	9.3	9.4	3.8	3.1	3.9	3.6
65 years and over	31.8	29.6	30.5	28.9	14.1	15.2	18.5	19.2	8.1	8.1	8.2	8.2
65 to 74 years	27.8	25.8	25.6	24.2	12.4	13.1	15.9	15.9	6.7	6.2	6.3	6.1
75 years and over	37.0	34.3	36.5	35.6	16.2	17.7	21.7	23.9	9.8	10.3	10.6	11.1
Sex[4]												
Male	12.3	11.9	12.4	11.8	4.1	4.4	5.5	5.5	2.6	2.4	2.6	2.7
Female	11.8	10.5	10.2	9.8	5.8	5.8	6.6	6.9	2.1	2.1	2.6	2.5
Sex and Age												
Male												
18 to 44 years	3.7	3.6	3.7	3.8	0.8	0.8	0.9	0.9	0.3	0.3	0.5	0.7
45 to 54 years	11.0	10.0	9.5	9.5	2.0	2.0	3.1	2.9	1.2	1.3	1.9	2.2
55 to 64 years	18.7	19.7	19.1	16.7	5.8	5.9	7.5	7.2	4.6	3.7	4.0	3.9
65 to 74 years	32.0	30.4	31.3	29.8	12.8	13.9	16.9	15.6	8.1	6.7	6.6	6.7
75 years and over	40.8	39.2	44.7	42.1	18.3	20.3	26.1	27.1	11.2	11.3	10.6	10.9
Female												
18 to 44 years	5.5	4.9	4.3	4.4	2.6	2.5	2.5	2.2	0.4	0.4	0.6	0.5
45 to 54 years	10.8	9.9	9.6	9.4	6.0	5.9	6.6	6.7	1.5	1.4	2.2	2.5
55 to 64 years	16.2	13.8	15.3	13.0	8.8	8.4	10.9	11.5	3.2	2.6	3.9	3.4
65 to 74 years	24.5	22.0	20.6	19.3	12.1	12.5	15.0	16.2	5.5	5.8	6.1	5.5
75 years and over	34.6	31.2	30.9	30.9	14.9	16.1	18.7	21.6	9.0	9.6	10.6	11.3
Race[4,6]												
White only	12.2	11.3	11.2	11.0	5.2	5.4	6.3	6.5	2.2	2.1	2.3	2.5
Black or African American only	11.4	10.6	10.7	9.7	3.5	3.5	5.1	4.8	3.3	3.5	4.1	3.8
American Indian or Alaska Native only	18.6	14.7	12.5	14.8	*6.5	*5.7	6.5	4.9	*5.0	*5.4	*4.7	3.1
Asian only	6.9	6.3	7.2	6.3	2.4	*2.3	3.0	3.2	*1.2	*1.2	2.4	1.3
Native Hawaiian or Other Pacific Islander only	- - -	*	*	10.5	- - -	*	*	*	- - -	*	*	0.2
Two or more races	- - -	17.0	16.7	14.4	- - -	*4.7	7.9	6.7	- - -	*4.0	*3.9	4.9
Hispanic Origin and Race[4,6]												
Hispanic or Latino	8.7	8.0	8.4	8.1	2.9	3.0	3.4	3.9	2.1	1.9	2.7	2.7
Mexican	7.5	7.4	8.4	8.3	3.0	2.8	3.2	4.2	2.5	2.0	2.6	3.0
Not Hispanic or Latino	12.2	11.4	11.4	11.1	5.1	5.2	6.3	6.5	2.3	2.2	2.6	2.6
White only	12.5	11.6	11.7	11.5	5.4	5.5	6.7	7.0	2.2	2.1	2.3	2.5
Black or African American only	11.4	10.5	10.8	9.9	3.6	3.6	5.1	4.8	3.3	3.5	4.2	3.9
Education[7,8]												
No high school diploma or GED	15.1	13.8	14.6	13.6	5.3	5.5	5.8	6.1	3.9	3.8	4.4	4.8
High school diploma or GED	12.8	11.9	12.4	11.9	5.5	5.8	6.8	6.8	2.5	2.5	3.4	3.3
Some college or more	12.7	12.0	11.9	11.5	6.0	5.9	7.4	7.5	2.1	1.9	2.3	2.4
Percent of Poverty Level[4,9]												
Below 100 percent	15.3	13.6	13.9	14.2	4.9	4.9	5.3	6.0	4.3	3.7	4.6	5.1
100 percent to 199 percent	13.2	12.0	12.3	12.1	4.8	5.3	5.9	5.5	3.1	3.2	3.7	3.5
200 percent to 399 percent	11.5	11.0	11.3	10.4	4.9	5.1	6.2	6.4	2.1	2.1	2.5	2.6
400 percent or more	11.0	10.2	9.8	9.4	5.2	5.1	6.2	6.5	1.6	1.5	1.5	1.7
Hispanic Origin and Race and Percent of Poverty Level[4,6,9]												
Hispanic or Latino												
Below 100 percent	9.7	9.7	9.4	11.1	2.2	2.3	2.9	4.1	3.0	2.0	3.4	4.2
100 percent to 199 percent	8.7	8.4	8.3	8.5	2.8	3.2	2.6	2.9	2.2	2.2	3.2	2.7

NA = Not available.

* = Estimates are considered unreliable. Starting with 2015–2016 data, the reliability of survey percentage estimates was assessed using new multistep National Center for Health Statistics data presentation standards for proportions. Prior to 2015–2016 data, the reliability of estimates for earlier years was evaluated based on relative standard errors (RSE). Data preceded by an asterisk have an RSE of 20%–30%. Data not shown have an RSE greater than 30%.

[1]Heart disease is based on self-reported responses to questions about whether respondents had ever been told by a doctor or other health professional that they had coronary heart disease, angina (angina pectoris), a heart attack (myocardial infarction), or any other kind or heart disease or heart condition.

[2]Cancer is based on self-reported responses to a question about whether respondents had ever been told by a doctor or other health professional that they had cancer or a malignancy of any kind. Excludes squamous cell and basal cell carcinomas.

[3]Stroke is based on self-reported responses to a question about whether respondents had ever been told by a doctor or other health professional that they had a stroke.

[4]Estimates are age-adjusted to the year 2000 standard population using five age groups: 18 to 44 years, 45 to 54 years, 55 to 64 years, 65 to 74 years, and 75 years and over. Age-adjusted estimates in this table may differ from other age-adjusted estimates based on the same data and presented elsewhere if different age groups are used in the adjustment procedure.

[5]Includes all other races not shown separately and unknown education level.

[6]The race groups White, Black, American Indian or Alaska Native, Asian, Native Hawaiian or Other Pacific Islander, and two or more races, include persons of Hispanic and non-Hispanic origin. Persons of Hispanic origin may be of any race. Starting with 1999 data, race-specific estimates are tabulated according to the 1997 Revisions to the Standards for the Classification of Federal Data on Race and Ethnicity and are not strictly comparable with estimates for earlier years. The five single-race categories and multiple-race categories shown in the table conform to the 1997 Standards. Starting with 1999 data, race-specific estimates are for persons who reported only one racial group; the category 2 or more races includes persons who reported more than one racial group. Prior to 1999, data were tabulated according to the 1977 Standards with four racial groups, and the Asian only category included Native Hawaiian or Other Pacific Islander. Estimates for single-race categories prior to 1999 included persons who reported one race, or if they reported more than one race, identified one race as best representing their race. Starting with 2003 data, race responses of other race and unspecified multiple race were treated as missing, and then race was imputed if these were the only race responses. Almost all persons with a race response of other race were of Hispanic origin.

[7]Estimates are for persons 25 years of age and over and are age-adjusted to the year 2000 standard population using five age groups: 25 to 44 years, 45 to 54 years, 55 to 64 years, 65 to 74 years, and 75 years and over.

[8]GED is General Educational Development high school equivalency diploma.

[9]Percent of poverty level is based on family income and family size and composition using U.S. Census Bureau poverty thresholds. Missing family income data were imputed for 1997–1998 and beyond.

Table 3-5. Respondent-Reported Prevalence of Heart Disease, Cancer, and Stroke Among Adults 18 Years of Age and Over, by Selected Characteristics, Selected Years, 1997–1998 Through 2015–2016—Continued

(Percent; data are based on household interviews of a sample of the civilian noninstitutionalized population.)

Characteristic	Heart disease[1]				Cancer[2]				Stroke[3]			
	1997–1998	1999–2000	2010–2011	2015–2016	1997–1998	1999–2000	2010–2011	2015–2016	1997–1998	1999–2000	2010–2011	2015–2016
200 percent to 399 percent	8.4	8.2	8.5	7.1	2.7	2.7	4.7	5.4	*1.8	*2.3	2.2	2.7
400 percent or more	8.4	5.6	7.5	6.5	*5.5	*4.5	3.3	3.5	*	*	*2.1	1.3
Not Hispanic or Latino												
White only												
Below 100 percent	17.8	15.2	15.8	16.9	6.3	6.2	6.8	7.9	4.4	3.8	4.4	5.2
100 percent to 199 percent	14.1	12.8	13.8	13.7	5.6	6.2	7.3	6.9	3.2	3.0	3.6	3.7
200 percent to 399 percent	12.2	11.6	11.8	11.6	5.2	5.5	6.8	7.0	2.1	2.1	2.3	2.6
400 percent or more	11.3	10.6	10.2	10.0	5.4	5.3	6.6	6.9	1.6	1.5	1.4	1.7
Black or African American only												
Below 100 percent	14.6	13.0	14.7	13.7	4.4	4.0	4.5	4.0	5.0	4.5	6.2	6.4
100 percent to 199 percent	12.9	11.2	11.2	11.7	3.3	3.2	5.2	4.3	4.2	5.1	4.6	5.0
200 percent to 399 percent	9.2	10.2	10.5	8.2	3.2	3.7	5.3	5.2	2.5	2.7	3.9	2.6
400 percent or more	9.5	8.9	7.3	7.2	4.0	4.3	5.6	5.7	*	*	*2.1	2.4
Geographic Region[4]												
Northeast	11.6	10.6	10.1	10.2	4.5	5.0	5.6	5.7	1.8	1.8	2.0	2.1
Midwest	12.1	11.4	11.5	12.4	5.1	5.2	6.7	6.6	2.3	2.2	2.6	2.7
South	12.5	11.5	12.1	10.7	5.0	5.0	6.2	6.2	2.6	2.5	2.9	2.9
West	11.1	10.4	9.9	9.3	5.1	5.0	5.5	6.1	2.1	2.0	2.4	2.6
Location of Residence[4,10]												
Within MSA	11.7	10.7	10.8	10.2	4.9	5.0	5.9	6.1	2.2	2.1	2.4	2.5
Outside MSA	12.8	12.5	13.0	13.2	5.1	5.5	6.7	6.5	2.7	2.5	3.4	3.1

NA = Not available.

* = Estimates are considered unreliable. Starting with 2015–2016 data, the reliability of survey percentage estimates was assessed using new multistep National Center for Health Statistics data presentation standards for proportions. Prior to 2015–2016 data, the reliability of estimates for earlier years was evaluated based on relative standard errors (RSE). Data preceded by an asterisk have an RSE of 20%–30%. Data not shown have an RSE greater than 30%.

[1]Heart disease is based on self-reported responses to questions about whether respondents had ever been told by a doctor or other health professional that they had coronary heart disease, angina (angina pectoris), a heart attack (myocardial infarction), or any other kind or heart disease or heart condition.

[2]Cancer is based on self-reported responses to a question about whether respondents had ever been told by a doctor or other health professional that they had cancer or a malignancy of any kind. Excludes squamous cell and basal cell carcinomas.

[3]Stroke is based on self-reported responses to a question about whether respondents had ever been told by a doctor or other health professional that they had a stroke.

[4]Estimates are age-adjusted to the year 2000 standard population using five age groups: 18 to 44 years, 45 to 54 years, 55 to 64 years, 65 to 74 years, and 75 years and over. Age-adjusted estimates in this table may differ from other age-adjusted estimates based on the same data and presented elsewhere if different age groups are used in the adjustment procedure.

[10]MSA is metropolitan statistical area. Starting with 2016 data, MSA status is determined using 2010 Census data and the 2010 standards for defining MSAs.

Table 3-6. Diabetes Prevalence and Glycemic Control Among Adults 20 Years of Age and Over, by Sex, Age, Race and Hispanic Origin, Selected Years 1988–1994 Through 2011–2014

(Percent.)

Age, race, sex, and Hispanic origin[1]	Physician-diagnosed and undiagnosed diabetes[2,3]								Physician-diagnosed diabetes[2]			
	1988–1994	1999–2002	2001–2004	2003–2006	2005–2008	2007–2010	2009–2012	2011–2014	1988–1994	1999–2002	2001–2004	2003–2006
20 Years and Over, Age-Adjusted[4]												
All persons[5]	8.8	9.9	10.8	10.6	10.9	11.4	11.7	11.9	5.2	6.6	7.4	7.7
Sex												
Male	9.6	11.2	12.4	11.1	11.4	13.2	13.2	12.8	5.5	7.3	7.9	7.0
Female	8.2	8.6	9.3	10.2	10.5	9.8	10.3	11.2	5.1	5.9	6.9	8.2
Hispanic Origin												
Not Hispanic or Latino												
White only	7.7	8.5	9.0	8.9	9.2	9.6	9.1	9.6	4.8	5.5	6.1	6.2
Black or African American only	16.3	14.0	15.9	16.7	18.9	18.4	17.9	18.0	9.1	9.2	11.7	13.0
Mexican	15.6	13.9	16.1	17.1	17.7	18.9	20.5	18.0	10.7	10.8	12.7	12.9
Percent of Poverty Level[6]												
Below 100 percent	14.2	14.6	14.5	14.8	15.7	13.8	17.1	17.4	8.8	9.0	9.7	12.4
100 percent or more	8.1	9.3	10.1	10.1	10.4	10.9	10.8	11.2	4.8	6.4	7.0	7.1
100 percent to 199 percent	9.7	13.1	13.5	13.9	14.8	14.8	14.8	15.0	5.2	9.4	9.8	9.5
200 percent or more	7.8	8.2	9.1	8.9	9.3	10.0	9.4	9.7	4.7	5.5	6.1	6.3
200 percent to 399 percent	7.8	10.5	10.7	10.5	10.7	12.3	11.5	11.4	4.3	7.3	7.0	7.5
400 percent or more	7.8	6.7	8.0	7.0	7.3	7.9	7.7	8.6	5.3	4.3	5.8	5.2
20 Years and Over, Crude												
All persons[5]	8.3	9.8	10.6	10.9	11.4	12.0	12.3	12.6	4.9	6.6	7.3	7.9
Sex												
Male	8.6	10.8	11.8	11.0	11.4	13.4	13.5	13.2	4.9	7.1	7.5	6.9
Female	8.0	8.9	9.5	10.8	11.3	10.7	11.2	12.1	5.0	6.1	7.1	8.7
Hispanic Origin												
Not Hispanic or Latino												
White only	7.6	8.9	9.4	9.6	10.3	10.9	10.5	11.0	4.7	5.6	6.3	6.7
Black or African American only	13.3	12.5	14.6	15.8	17.9	17.0	17.1	17.5	7.2	8.3	10.9	12.3
Mexican	10.4	9.3	10.8	12.6	12.8	13.7	15.8	14.3	6.3	7.2	7.9	8.8
Percent of Poverty Level[6]												
Below 100 percent	11.6	13.4	12.2	12.7	13.8	11.4	14.3	15.0	7.2	8.4	8.4	10.6
100 percent or more	7.6	9.2	10.1	10.5	10.8	11.8	11.8	12.3	4.5	6.3	7.0	7.3
100 percent to 199 percent	9.1	12.9	13.3	14.9	16.3	15.8	15.8	16.8	5.2	9.3	9.6	10.2
200 percent or more	7.1	8.0	9.0	9.1	9.3	10.6	10.4	10.8	4.3	5.4	6.1	6.5
200 percent to 399 percent	6.8	10.2	10.6	11.0	11.2	13.0	12.3	12.3	3.7	7.0	7.0	7.7
400 percent or more	7.6	6.4	7.7	7.4	7.7	8.7	8.9	9.5	5.2	4.1	5.5	5.3
Age												
20 to 44 years	*2.1	4.4	4.2	3.9	3.7	3.3	3.7	4.0	*	3.2	3.1	2.8
45 to 64 years	14.0	12.8	13.5	13.7	13.8	15.3	16.2	16.6	7.9	8.3	9.3	10.1
65 years and over	19.4	20.4	24.8	24.9	26.9	28.1	26.8	26.3	12.7	13.7	16.4	17.5

NOTE: Excludes pregnant women. Fasting weights were used to obtain estimates of total, physician-diagnosed, and undiagnosed diabetes prevalence. Examination weights were used to obtain the poor glycemic control estimates. Estimates in this table may differ from other estimates based on the same data and presented elsewhere if different weights, age adjustment groups, definitions, or trend adjustments are used.
*Estimates are considered unreliable. Data preceded by an asterisk have a relative standard error (RSE) of 20 percent–30 percent. Data not shown have an RSE greater than 30 percent.
NA = Not available.
[1]Physician-diagnosed diabetes was obtained by self-report and excludes women who reported having diabetes during pregnancy.
[2]Undiagnosed diabetes is defined as a fasting plasma glucose (FPG) of at least 126 mg/dL or a hemoglobin A1c of at least 6.5% and no reported physician diagnosis. Pregnant females are excluded. Participants had fasted for at least 8 hours and less than 24 hours. Starting in 2005–2006, testing was performed at a different laboratory using different instruments than testing in earlier years. The National Health and Nutrition Examination Survey (NHANES) conducted crossover studies to evaluate the impact of these changes on FPG and A1c measurements and recommended adjustments to the FPG data. The adjustments recommended by NHANES were incorporated into the data presented here. For more information, see https://wwwn.cdc.gov/nchs/nhanes/2005-2006/GLU_D.htm. Also see Appendix II, Diabetes.
[3]Persons of Hispanic and Mexican origin may be of any race. Starting with 1999 data, race-specific estimates are tabulated according to the 1997 Revisions to the Standards for the Classification of Federal Data on Race and Ethnicity and are not strictly comparable with estimates for earlier years. The non-Hispanic race categories shown in the table conform to the 1997 Standards. Starting with 1999 data, race-specific estimates are for persons who reported only one racial group. Prior to data year 1999, estimates were tabulated according to the 1977 Standards. Estimates for single-race categories prior to 1999 included persons who reported one race, or if they reported more than one race, identified one race as best representing their race.
[4]Estimates are age-adjusted to the year 2000 standard population using three age groups: 20–44 years, 45–64 years, and 65 years and over. Age-adjusted estimates in this table may differ from other age-adjusted estimates based on the same data and presented elsewhere if different age groups are used in the adjustment procedure.
[5]Includes all other races and Hispanic origins not shown separately.
[6]Percent of poverty level was calculated by dividing family income by the U.S. Department of Health and Human Services' poverty guideline specific to family size, as well as the appropriate year, and state. Persons with unknown percent of poverty level are excluded (6 percent in 2011–2014).

Table 3-6. Diabetes Prevalence and Glycemic Control Among Adults 20 Years of Age and Over, by Sex, Age, Race and Hispanic Origin, Selected Years 1988–1994 Through 2011–2014—Continued

(Percent.)

Age, race, sex, and Hispanic origin[1]	Physician-diagnosed diabetes[2]				Undiagnosed diabetes[3]							
	2005–2008	2007–2010	2009–2012	2011–2014	1988–1994	1999–2002	2001–2004	2003–2006	2005–2008	2007–2010	2009–2012	2011–2014
20 Years and Over, Age-Adjusted[4]												
All persons[5]	7.9	8.1	8.4	9.0	3.6	3.2	3.4	3.0	3.1	3.3	3.3	2.9
Sex												
Male	7.4	8.8	9.0	9.4	4.1	3.9	4.5	4.1	4.0	4.4	4.2	3.3
Female	8.2	7.4	7.8	8.7	3.2	2.7	2.4	2.0	2.2	2.4	2.5	2.4
Hispanic Origin												
Not Hispanic or Latino												
White only	6.6	6.7	6.6	7.6	2.9	3.0	2.9	2.7	2.6	2.8	2.5	2.0
Black or African American only	13.2	13.2	13.3	13.4	7.2	4.8	4.2	3.8	5.7	5.1	4.7	4.6
Mexican	12.6	13.4	13.9	13.0	5.0	3.1	3.5	4.2	5.1	5.5	6.6	5.1
Percent of Poverty Level[6]												
Below 100 percent	12.0	10.1	12.1	13.4	*5.4	5.6	4.8	*	*3.7	3.7	5.0	3.9
100 percent or more	7.3	7.6	7.8	8.5	3.3	2.9	3.1	3.0	3.1	3.3	3.0	2.7
100 percent to 199 percent	10.2	11.0	11.4	10.5	4.4	*3.6	3.7	4.4	4.6	3.8	3.4	4.5
200 percent or more	6.6	6.8	6.5	7.7	3.1	2.7	2.9	2.6	2.7	3.2	2.9	2.1
200 percent to 399 percent	7.8	8.9	8.4	8.6	3.6	3.2	3.6	*3.1	*2.9	3.3	3.1	2.8
400 percent or more	5.1	4.9	*5.2	7.2	2.5	2.3	*2.3	*	*2.2	3.0	2.5	*1.4
20 Years and Over, Crude												
All persons[5]	8.2	8.5	8.9	9.6	3.4	3.2	3.3	3.0	3.2	3.5	3.5	3.0
Sex												
Male	7.5	8.9	9.1	9.7	3.7	3.7	4.3	4.0	3.9	4.5	4.4	3.5
Female	9.0	8.2	8.7	9.5	3.1	2.8	2.4	2.1	2.4	2.5	2.6	2.5
Hispanic Origin												
Not Hispanic or Latino												
White only	7.3	7.6	7.6	8.7	2.9	3.2	3.1	3.0	3.0	3.2	2.8	2.3
Black or African American only	12.8	12.3	12.5	13.0	6.1	4.2	3.7	3.5	5.1	4.6	4.6	4.6
Mexican	8.9	9.4	10.1	10.1	4.1	2.0	*2.9	*3.8	3.9	4.3	5.7	4.2
Percent of Poverty Level[6]												
Below 100 percent	10.3	8.3	9.8	11.2	4.4	5.1	3.9	*	*3.5	3.1	4.5	3.7
100 percent or more	7.7	8.3	8.6	9.4	3.1	2.9	3.1	3.1	3.2	3.6	3.3	2.9
100 percent to 199 percent	11.2	11.7	12.3	12.1	3.9	*3.6	3.7	4.7	5.1	4.1	3.5	4.7
200 percent or more	6.7	7.2	7.3	8.4	2.8	2.6	2.9	2.7	2.7	3.4	3.2	2.3
200 percent to 399 percent	8.1	9.4	9.0	9.3	3.1	*3.1	3.6	*3.2	*3.1	3.5	3.3	3.0
400 percent or more	5.4	5.4	*5.8	7.7	*2.5	2.3	*2.3	*2.2	2.3	3.2	*3.1	*1.8
Age												
20 to 44 years	2.6	2.1	2.1	2.6	1.1	*	*1.1	*1.1	*1.1	1.1	1.6	1.4
45 to 64 years	10.6	11.4	11.4	12.3	6.0	4.5	4.2	3.5	3.2	3.9	4.8	4.3
65 years and over	18.3	19.3	21.2	21.9	6.7	6.7	8.5	7.4	8.6	8.8	5.5	4.3

NOTE: Excludes pregnant women. Fasting weights were used to obtain estimates of total, physician-diagnosed, and undiagnosed diabetes prevalence. Examination weights were used to obtain the poor glycemic control estimates. Estimates in this table may differ from other estimates based on the same data and presented elsewhere if different weights, age adjustment groups, definitions, or trend adjustments are used.

*Estimates are considered unreliable. Data preceded by an asterisk have a relative standard error (RSE) of 20 percent–30 percent. Data not shown have an RSE greater than 30 percent.

NA = Not available.

[1]Physician-diagnosed diabetes was obtained by self-report and excludes women who reported having diabetes during pregnancy.

[2]Undiagnosed diabetes is defined as a fasting plasma glucose (FPG) of at least 126 mg/dL or a hemoglobin A1c of at least 6.5% and no reported physician diagnosis. Pregnant females are excluded. Participants had fasted for at least 8 hours and less than 24 hours. Starting in 2005–2006, testing was performed at a different laboratory using different instruments than testing in earlier years. The National Health and Nutrition Examination Survey (NHANES) conducted crossover studies to evaluate the impact of these changes on FPG and A1c measurements and recommended adjustments to the FPG data. The adjustments recommended by NHANES were incorporated into the data presented here. For more information, see https://www.cdc.gov/nchs/nhanes/2005-2006/GLU_D.htm. Also see Appendix II, Diabetes.

[3]Persons of Hispanic and Mexican origin may be of any race. Starting with 1999 data, race-specific estimates are tabulated according to the 1997 Revisions to the Standards for the Classification of Federal Data on Race and Ethnicity and are not strictly comparable with estimates for earlier years. The non-Hispanic race categories shown in the table conform to the 1997 Standards. Starting with 1999 data, race-specific estimates are for persons who reported only one racial group. Prior to data year 1999, estimates were tabulated according to the 1977 Standards. Estimates for single-race categories prior to 1999 included persons who reported one race, or if they reported more than one race, identified one race as best representing their race.

[4]Estimates are age-adjusted to the year 2000 standard population using three age groups: 20–44 years, 45–64 years, and 65 years and over. Age-adjusted estimates in this table may differ from other age-adjusted estimates based on the same data and presented elsewhere if different age groups are used in the adjustment procedure.

[5]Includes all other races and Hispanic origins not shown separately.

[6]Percent of poverty level was calculated by dividing family income by the U.S. Department of Health and Human Services' poverty guideline specific to family size, as well as the appropriate year, and state. Persons with unknown percent of poverty level are excluded (6 percent in 2011–2014).

Table 3-6. Diabetes Prevalence and Glycemic Control Among Adults 20 Years of Age and Over, by Sex, Age, Race and Hispanic Origin, Selected Years 1988–1994 Through 2011–2014—*Continued*

(Percent.)

Age, race, sex, and Hispanic origin[1]	Poor glycemic control (A1c greater than 9%) among persons with physician-diagnosed diabetes							
	1988–1994	1999–2002	2001–2004	2003–2006	2005–2008	2007–2010	2009–2012	2011–2014
20 Years and Over, Age-Adjusted[4]								
All persons[5]	26.3	24.7	17.4	18.8	20.3	18.3	21.3	20.6
Sex								
Male	22.4	27.7	22.5	20.7	21.6	20.8	26.2	24.1
Female	29.4	*20.3	11.6	17.1	19.2	15.8	16.5	18.0
Hispanic Origin								
Not Hispanic or Latino								
White only	23.7	*22.9	*18.1	*14.9	*15.2	*11.2	*	*16.6
Black or African American only	38.9	25.4	*15.5	25.7	31.8	30.4	28.8	23.9
Mexican	29.8	28.0	23.7	*26.3	*25.5	*24.3	32.5	27.6
Percent of Poverty Level[6]								
Below 100 percent	37.2	30.6	*17.8	*19.9	23.2	22.9	23.6	27.3
100 percent or more	22.8	*22.6	*18.1	19.8	20.0	17.2	21.2	18.3
100 percent to 199 percent	*	*	*	*19.2	*22.0	*	*20.0	21.7
200 percent or more	21.2	*25.6	*22.6	20.8	19.4	18.0	*22.0	*16.6
200 percent to 399 percent	*24.2	*27.0	*22.9	*19.1	*16.3	*20.2	*21.4	*13.5
400 percent or more	*	*	*	*	*22.4	*	*	*
20 Years and Over, Crude								
All persons[5]	23.3	18.4	14.5	13.0	13.9	12.5	13.8	15.6
Sex								
Male	20.2	20.2	17.5	14.8	14.9	14.0	14.8	15.4
Female	25.8	16.7	11.6	11.5	12.9	11.0	12.8	15.7
Hispanic Origin								
Not Hispanic or Latino								
White only	20.6	13.6	11.5	8.7	10.5	9.5	9.5	12.0
Black or African American only	34.2	25.4	20.0	21.0	21.0	19.0	19.6	19.0
Mexican	29.2	26.8	23.0	24.0	21.7	19.6	23.5	22.9
Percent of Poverty Level[6]								
Below 100 percent	30.2	25.6	16.3	17.6	20.3	18.5	19.8	23.2
100 percent or more	21.4	15.9	13.9	12.2	12.8	11.1	11.9	13.6
100 percent to 199 percent	24.2	*14.9	*10.6	*11.5	*11.8	9.8	12.4	13.9
200 percent or more	20.0	16.4	15.5	12.5	13.3	11.8	11.7	13.4
200 percent to 399 percent	*21.2	*17.5	15.6	*10.7	*11.2	12.4	12.3	13.1
400 percent or more	*18.3	*	15.5	14.8	*15.6	*11.2	*11.1	*13.8
Age								
20 to 44 years	29.5	*32.7	*20.0	25.2	28.1	24.9	30.1	26.2
45 to 64 years	26.0	19.9	19.5	16.6	15.4	14.1	14.4	17.8
65 years and over	18.0	*10.2	*6.3	*4.1	6.2	6.8	8.0	9.2

NOTE: Excludes pregnant women. Fasting weights were used to obtain estimates of total, physician-diagnosed, and undiagnosed diabetes prevalence. Examination weights were used to obtain the poor glycemic control estimates. Estimates in this table may differ from other estimates based on the same data and presented elsewhere if different weights, age adjustment groups, definitions, or trend adjustments are used.
*Estimates are considered unreliable. Data preceded by an asterisk have a relative standard error (RSE) of 20 percent–30 percent. Data not shown have an RSE greater than 30 percent.
NA = Not available.
[1]Physician-diagnosed diabetes was obtained by self-report and excludes women who reported having diabetes during pregnancy.
[4]Estimates are age-adjusted to the year 2000 standard population using three age groups: 20–44 years, 45–64 years, and 65 years and over. Age-adjusted estimates in this table may differ from other age-adjusted estimates based on the same data and presented elsewhere if different age groups are used in the adjustment procedure.
[5]Includes all other races and Hispanic origins not shown separately.
[6]Percent of poverty level was calculated by dividing family income by the U.S. Department of Health and Human Services' poverty guideline specific to family size, as well as the appropriate year, and state. Persons with unknown percent of poverty level are excluded (6 percent in 2011–2014).

Table 3-7. End-Stage Renal Disease Patients, by Selected Characteristics, Selected Years, 2000–2012
(Number, rate per million population.)

Characteristic	Incidence				Prevalence			
	Number of new patients				Number of patients alive on December 31			
	2000	2010	2011	2012	2000	2010	2011	2012
Total.........................	91,241	113,380	111,209	112,596	378,074	577,675	597,620	620,136
Age								
Under 20 years..........................	1,148	1,167	1,172	1,113	6,039	7,015	7,066	7,020
20 to 44 years............................	12,687	13,050	12,734	12,836	86,043	96,067	96,936	98,142
45 to 64 years............................	31,736	43,456	43,294	44,120	154,117	259,855	268,220	275,940
65 to 74 years............................	23,148	27,100	26,318	27,409	75,480	119,941	127,391	136,859
75 years and over	22,522	28,607	27,691	27,118	56,395	94,797	98,007	102,175
Sex								
Male.......................................	48,769	64,553	63,600	64,524	206,248	327,379	339,676	353,372
Female	42,472	48,827	47,609	48,072	171,826	250,296	257,944	266,764
Race[1]								
White..	59,472	75,214	73,229	74,667	231,829	353,938	364,579	377,797
Black or African American................	26,204	31,828	31,530	31,148	123,654	185,683	192,745	199,632
American Indian or Alaska Native.........	*	1,233	1,234	1,260	*	7,571	7,840	8,080
Asian or Pacific Islander	3,460	5,105	5,216	5,521	16,064	30,483	32,456	34,627
Hispanic Origin[1]								
Hispanic....................................	10,053	15,251	15,582	15,399	40,627	85,228	90,856	95,819
Not Hispanic[2]	81,188	98,129	95,627	97,197	337,447	492,447	506,764	524,317
Primary Diagnosis								
Diabetes....................................	40,489	50,020	49,151	49,258	133,128	217,165	225,110	234,160
Hypertension...............................	24,490	32,317	31,506	32,293	92,817	143,951	149,710	156,595
Glomerulonephritis......................	9,958	9,311	9,218	8,988	75,477	98,822	101,103	103,312
Cystic kidney..............................	2,140	2,582	2,476	2,495	17,685	27,492	28,407	29,389
Other urologic	1,610	526	429	533	7,996	7,499	7,287	7,253
Other cause................................	8,486	13,662	13,633	12,157	33,250	54,967	57,266	58,717
Unknown cause............................	3,712	4,262	4,026	3,469	15,539	24,232	24,733	24,923
Missing disease	356	700	770	3,403	2,182	3,547	4,004	5,787

Characteristic	New patients per million population				Patients alive on December 31 per million population			
	2000	2010	2011	2012	2000	2010	2011	2012
Total.........................	323.3	366.5	356.9	358.6	1,333.2	1,860.7	1,910.8	1,968.2
Age								
Under 20 years..........................	14.2	14.0	14.1	13.4	74.7	84.5	85.4	85.2
20 to 44 years............................	121.8	125.6	121.7	121.7	825.8	921.5	923.2	927.4
45 to 64 years............................	508.3	531.4	522.8	532.4	2,428.5	3,157.8	3,238.2	3,329.3
65 to 74 years............................	1,259.1	1,239.8	1,170.4	1,142.7	4,105.7	5,409.7	5,482.5	5,532.9
75 years and over	1,349.7	1,536.3	1,466.1	1,415.3	3,357.6	5,054.8	5,151.9	5,294.9
Sex								
Male.......................................	352.2	424.4	414.9	417.6	1,482.0	2,144.2	2,207.4	2,278.2
Female	295.5	310.5	300.7	301.5	1,189.9	1,586.3	1,623.5	1,667.5
Race[1]								
White..	257.9	306.0	296.5	300.8	1,001.9	1,436.7	1,472.4	1,518.1
Black or African American................	713.4	754.2	738.4	720.9	3,342.9	4,374.5	4,487.7	4,593.7
American Indian or Alaska Native.........	*	288.3	284.5	286.4	*	1,758.1	1,795.0	1,824.2
Asian or Pacific Islander	290.9	298.3	296.4	305.2	1,320.9	1,756.7	1,819.1	1,888.6
Hispanic Origin[1,2]								
Hispanic....................................	281.8	300.5	300.3	290.3	1,116.0	1,660.8	1,732.0	1,787.6
Not Hispanic[3]	329.3	379.4	368.2	372.5	1,365.2	1,900.2	1,946.8	2,005.2
Primary Diagnosis								
Diabetes....................................	143.4	161.7	157.7	156.9	469.4	699.5	719.7	743.1
Hypertension...............................	86.7	104.4	101.1	102.8	327.3	463.6	478.6	497.0
Glomerulonephritis......................	35.2	30.1	29.5	28.6	266.1	318.3	323.2	327.8
Cystic kidney..............................	7.5	8.3	7.9	7.9	62.3	88.5	90.8	93.2
Other urologic	5.7	1.7	1.3	1.6	28.1	24.1	23.2	23.0
Other cause................................	30.0	44.1	43.7	38.7	117.2	177.0	183.1	186.3
Unknown cause............................	13.1	13.7	12.9	11.0	54.7	78.0	79.0	79.1
Missing disease	1.2	2.2	2.4	10.8	7.6	11.4	12.8	18.3

*Data are considered unreliable and are not shown.
[1]The race groups White, Black, American Indian or Alaska Native, and Asian or Pacific Islander, include persons of Hispanic and non-Hispanic origin. Persons of Hispanic origin may be of any race.
[2]Not Hispanic includes unknown ethnicity.
[3]Includes other races besides White and Black.

Table 3-8. Severe Headache or Migraine, Low Back Pain, and Neck Pain Among Adults 18 Years of Age and Over, by Selected Characteristics, 1997, 2000, 2010, 2015, and 2016

(Percent of adults with pain in the last 3 months; data are based on household interviews of a sample of the civilian noninstitutionalized population.)

Characteristic	Severe headache or migraine[1]					Low back pain[1]					Neck pain[1]				
	1997	2000	2010	2015	2016	1997	2000	2010	2015	2016	1997	2000	2010	2015	2016
18 years and over, age-adjusted[2,3]	15.8	14.7	16.6	15.4	15.5	28.2	27.3	28.4	29.1	28.4	14.7	14.4	15.4	15.7	15.0
18 years and over, crude[3]	16.0	14.8	16.4	15.0	15.0	28.1	27.2	28.8	29.8	29.0	14.6	14.4	15.8	16.1	15.4
Age															
18 to 44 years	18.7	17.2	20.4	17.9	17.9	26.1	24.6	25.2	23.9	24.4	13.3	12.6	13.1	12.9	12.1
18 to 24 years	18.7	16.1	19.6	15.4	15.1	21.9	20.9	19.4	16.2	18.3	9.8	8.7	8.3	7.8	9.1
25 to 44 years	18.7	17.6	20.7	18.8	18.9	27.3	25.8	27.2	26.7	26.6	14.3	13.9	14.8	14.8	13.1
45 to 64 years	15.8	14.8	15.6	15.9	15.6	31.3	30.4	32.4	35.4	33.2	17.0	17.7	20.0	20.1	19.6
45 to 54 years	17.8	16.3	16.7	17.6	17.8	31.3	29.4	31.3	34.6	32.1	17.3	17.8	19.1	19.8	19.9
55 to 64 years	12.7	12.3	14.1	14.2	13.3	31.2	32.0	33.8	36.1	34.3	16.6	17.6	21.0	20.5	19.3
65 years and over	7.0	7.0	6.4	6.4	7.0	29.5	30.0	31.8	34.4	32.5	15.0	14.0	14.8	16.6	15.8
65 to 74 years	8.2	7.9	7.4	7.3	8.0	30.2	29.6	32.5	34.0	32.8	15.0	13.9	15.5	16.9	16.2
75 years and over	5.4	6.0	5.1	5.1	5.4	28.6	30.6	30.9	34.9	32.2	15.0	14.2	14.0	16.2	15.2
Sex[2]															
Male	9.9	8.9	11.0	9.7	10.3	26.5	25.5	26.3	27.6	26.7	12.6	12.1	13.1	13.9	13.0
Female	21.4	20.3	22.1	20.9	20.5	29.6	28.8	30.3	30.4	29.9	16.6	16.5	17.6	17.4	16.8
Sex and Age															
Male															
18 to 44 years	11.9	10.4	13.5	11.0	12.2	24.8	23.4	23.2	22.3	22.6	11.6	10.6	11.0	11.2	10.7
45 to 54 years	10.3	9.1	10.4	10.7	11.0	29.4	27.4	29.6	34.1	30.5	13.9	14.8	16.3	17.4	16.1
55 to 64 years	8.8	7.6	9.6	10.5	9.0	30.7	29.6	32.8	35.5	35.5	14.6	15.1	17.6	19.1	17.3
65 to 74 years	5.0	5.1	5.5	5.0	4.6	29.0	27.5	28.4	31.7	30.6	13.6	12.0	12.8	14.4	13.7
75 years and over	*2.4	4.5	4.0	3.4	4.0	22.5	26.3	27.4	32.1	27.8	12.6	12.4	13.0	14.9	14.0
Female															
18 to 44 years	25.4	23.9	27.3	24.7	23.5	27.3	25.7	27.1	25.5	26.3	14.9	14.6	15.2	14.6	13.4
45 to 54 years	24.9	23.2	22.9	24.2	24.4	33.1	31.3	33.0	35.2	33.7	20.6	20.7	21.8	22.0	23.7
55 to 64 years	16.3	16.7	18.2	17.6	17.3	31.7	34.2	34.7	36.7	33.2	18.4	19.8	24.1	21.8	21.1
65 to 74 years	10.7	10.1	9.1	9.3	11.0	31.1	31.2	36.1	35.9	34.7	16.1	15.5	17.8	19.0	18.4
75 years and over	7.4	6.9	5.8	6.3	6.5	32.4	33.2	33.2	36.9	35.3	16.5	15.2	14.6	17.0	16.0
Race[2,4]															
White only	15.9	15.0	16.7	15.5	16.0	28.7	28.0	29.1	29.9	29.0	15.1	15.0	16.0	16.3	15.9
Black or African American only	16.7	13.9	18.2	16.3	14.6	26.9	24.3	27.2	28.1	27.8	13.3	10.7	13.3	13.8	12.5
American Indian or Alaska Native only	18.9	21.1	18.8	18.7	16.4	33.3	31.4	33.6	34.1	34.7	16.2	19.6	16.9	20.4	15.1
Asian only	11.7	12.0	10.1	11.3	9.9	21.0	19.0	19.1	19.3	18.8	9.2	11.0	9.6	11.5	8.1
Native Hawaiian or Other Pacific Islander only	NA	*	*	*	*	NA	*	*	*	25.0	NA	*	*	*	11.8
2 or more races	NA	19.9	21.5	20.7	22.5	NA	41.8	35.6	33.7	34.8	NA	22.1	22.0	19.0	21.9
Hispanic Origin and Race[2,4]															
Hispanic or Latino	15.5	13.5	16.2	14.9	15.3	26.4	25.0	27.4	27.4	27.4	13.9	13.4	15.1	14.2	15.8
Mexican	14.6	12.3	15.7	14.1	14.3	25.2	21.5	26.5	26.4	25.2	12.9	11.6	14.7	12.9	13.3
Not Hispanic or Latino	15.9	15.0	16.8	15.6	15.6	28.4	27.7	28.7	29.4	28.5	14.9	14.7	15.5	16.1	14.9
White only	16.1	15.4	17.0	16.0	16.4	29.1	28.4	29.7	30.5	29.6	15.4	15.4	16.3	17.1	16.1
Black or African American only	16.8	13.8	18.4	16.1	14.4	26.9	24.2	27.1	27.9	27.4	13.3	10.6	13.3	13.6	12.0
Education[5,6]															
25 years and over															
No high school diploma or GED	19.2	17.9	18.2	19.4	19.4	33.6	32.4	34.5	34.6	35.4	16.5	15.9	18.9	18.1	20.6
High school diploma or GED	16.0	14.8	17.4	14.9	17.0	30.2	29.4	31.9	34.8	32.9	15.5	15.4	16.8	17.3	16.4
Some college or more	13.8	13.4	15.1	14.9	14.4	26.9	26.3	28.0	29.3	27.9	14.6	15.0	15.8	16.5	14.8
Percent of Poverty Level[2,7]															
Below 100 percent	23.3	19.9	22.7	21.8	21.6	35.4	32.4	34.9	36.8	36.4	18.6	16.5	20.2	19.9	20.7
100 percent to 199 percent	18.9	17.7	19.5	19.0	20.0	30.8	30.6	32.5	33.8	34.4	16.1	15.3	17.7	18.3	19.2
200 percent to 399 percent	15.5	15.4	16.6	15.5	14.9	27.9	27.4	28.5	28.7	27.2	14.8	14.7	15.2	14.9	14.4
400 percent or more	12.4	11.8	13.3	11.9	12.4	24.8	24.5	24.7	25.1	24.6	12.8	13.4	13.1	14.3	12.4
Hispanic Origin and Race and Percent of Poverty Level[2,4,7]															
Hispanic or Latino															
Below 100 percent	18.9	18.1	19.6	19.9	20.2	29.5	28.4	29.0	33.4	34.2	16.4	15.6	17.4	17.8	21.8
100 percent to 199 percent	15.7	12.9	15.1	14.2	15.5	26.8	24.8	27.2	25.9	31.1	12.9	13.3	15.7	15.9	18.2

NA = Not available.
* = Estimates are considered unreliable. Starting with 2016 data, the reliability of survey percentage estimates was assessed using new multistep National Center for Health Statistics data presentation standards for proportions. Prior to 2016 data, the reliability of estimates for earlier years was evaluated based on relative standard errors (RSE). Data preceded by an asterisk have an RSE of 20%–30%. Data not shown have an RSE greater than 30%.
[1]In three separate questions, respondents were asked, "During the past 3 months, did you have a severe headache or migraine? ... low back pain? ... neck pain?" Respondents were instructed to report pain that had lasted a whole day or more, and not to report fleeting or minor aches or pains. Persons may be represented in more than one column.
[2]Estimates are age-adjusted to the year 2000 standard population using five age groups: 18–44 years, 45–54 years, 55–64 years, 65–74 years, and 75 years and over. Age-adjusted estimates in this table may differ from other age-adjusted estimates based on the same data and presented elsewhere if different age groups are used in the adjustment procedure.
[3]Includes all other races not shown separately, unknown education level, and unknown disability status.
[4]The race groups White, Black, American Indian or Alaska Native, Asian, Native Hawaiian or Other Pacific Islander, and 2 or more races include persons of Hispanic and non-Hispanic origin. Persons of Hispanic origin may be of any race. Starting with 1999 data, race-specific estimates are tabulated according to the 1997 Revisions to the Standards for the Classification of Federal Data on Race and Ethnicity and are not strictly comparable with estimates for earlier years. The five single-race categories and multiple-race categories shown in the table conform to the 1997 Standards. Starting with 1999 data, race-specific estimates are for persons who reported only one racial group; the category 2 or more races includes persons who reported more than one racial group. Prior to 1999, data were tabulated according to the 1977 Standards with four racial groups, and the Asian only category included Native Hawaiian or Other Pacific Islander. Estimates for single-race categories prior to 1999 included persons who reported one race, or if they reported more than one race, identified one race as best representing their race. Starting with 2003 data, race responses of other race and unspecified multiple race were treated as missing, and then race was imputed if these were the only race responses. Almost all persons with a race response of other race were of Hispanic origin.
[5]Estimates are for persons aged 25 and over and are age-adjusted to the year 2000 standard population using five age groups: 25–44 years, 45–54 years, 55–64 years, 65–74 years, and 75 years and over.
[6]GED is General Educational Development high school equivalency diploma.
[7]Percent of poverty level is based on family income and family size and composition using U.S. Census Bureau poverty thresholds. Missing family income data were imputed for 1997 and beyond.

Table 3-8. Severe Headache or Migraine, Low Back Pain, and Neck Pain Among Adults 18 Years of Age and Over, by Selected Characteristics, 1997, 2000, 2010, 2015, and 2016—*Continued*

(Percent of adults with pain in the last 3 months; data are based on household interviews of a sample of the civilian noninstitutionalized population.)

Characteristic	Severe headache or migraine[1]					Low back pain[1]					Neck pain[1]				
	1997	2000	2010	2015	2016	1997	2000	2010	2015	2016	1997	2000	2010	2015	2016
200 percent to 399 percent	14.0	13.6	16.5	13.6	14.8	25.0	23.5	27.5	25.0	23.9	13.8	13.6	12.9	11.4	13.3
400 percent or more	13.0	9.6	14.0	12.9	12.1	21.6	24.1	25.6	27.5	22.7	12.1	11.6	15.3	12.0	12.0
Not Hispanic or Latino															
White only															
Below 100 percent	26.1	21.3	24.8	25.5	24.2	38.9	36.6	40.5	42.0	40.8	20.5	18.7	23.7	23.6	23.9
100 percent to 199 percent	20.4	20.3	22.0	22.8	24.2	33.3	34.6	35.9	38.6	37.8	18.0	17.6	19.9	21.5	22.5
200 percent to 399 percent	16.3	16.5	16.9	16.4	15.8	29.1	28.5	30.5	30.9	29.5	15.9	16.0	16.8	16.8	16.3
400 percent or more	12.5	12.3	13.8	11.8	13.4	25.4	25.2	25.2	25.9	25.7	13.1	14.0	13.6	15.1	13.4
Black or African American only															
Below 100 percent	22.7	21.1	24.0	19.8	18.7	34.5	27.5	32.5	33.1	32.0	17.9	13.7	18.6	17.3	15.6
100 percent to 199 percent	17.6	16.3	19.6	16.4	17.1	27.7	26.2	31.2	33.7	32.9	14.0	11.1	14.4	15.1	14.5
200 percent to 399 percent	14.0	11.4	17.6	15.7	13.8	24.3	23.8	23.7	24.9	24.8	10.2	9.8	11.7	12.0	10.5
400 percent or more	12.9	8.2	12.2	13.6	9.2	21.5	20.3	21.0	22.2	22.0	11.9	8.1	8.5	11.8	8.7
Disability Measure[2,8]															
A lot of difficulty or cannot do at all	NA	NA	37.6	36.3	38.3	NA	NA	55.1	54.0	58.7	NA	NA	36.7	31.6	35.4
Some difficulty	NA	NA	27.7	21.6	22.3	NA	NA	38.9	38.9	39.3	NA	NA	20.9	22.5	22.3
No difficulty	NA	NA	13.0	10.4	10.9	NA	NA	20.6	21.5	20.6	NA	NA	11.5	10.7	10.4
Geographic Region[2]															
Northeast	14.5	12.7	15.4	14.6	13.9	27.1	26.0	28.0	28.8	26.8	14.0	13.5	14.9	15.8	13.7
Midwest	15.6	15.1	16.8	15.9	16.4	28.7	28.2	28.1	29.0	29.2	15.3	14.5	16.0	14.9	14.9
South	17.1	14.9	18.2	15.8	16.0	27.5	26.5	28.3	28.6	28.3	13.9	13.7	14.6	14.9	14.9
West	15.3	15.9	15.1	15.2	15.1	30.0	28.6	29.3	29.9	29.0	16.1	16.5	16.5	17.5	16.1
Location of Residence[2,9]															
Within MSA	15.2	14.4	16.3	15.1	14.9	27.0	26.6	27.5	28.2	27.7	14.2	14.3	14.9	15.3	14.6
Outside MSA	18.1	16.1	18.6	17.9	19.2	32.5	29.6	33.8	34.5	32.9	16.4	14.9	18.1	18.2	17.2

NA = Not available.

[1]In three separate questions, respondents were asked, "During the past 3 months, did you have a severe headache or migraine? ... low back pain? ... neck pain?" Respondents were instructed to report pain that had lasted a whole day or more, and not to report fleeting or minor aches or pains. Persons may be represented in more than one column.

[2]Estimates are age-adjusted to the year 2000 standard population using five age groups: 18–44 years, 45–54 years, 55–64 years, 65–74 years, and 75 years and over. Age-adjusted estimates in this table may differ from other age-adjusted estimates based on the same data and presented elsewhere if different age groups are used in the adjustment procedure.

[8]Functional limitation is defined by the reported level of difficulty in six functioning domains: seeing (even if wearing glasses), hearing (even if wearing hearing aids), mobility (walking or climbing stairs), communication (understanding or being understood by others), cognition (remembering or concentrating), and self-care (such as washing all over or dressing). Respondents with answers to one or more of the six questions were included in one of three mutually exclusive categories. Those responding "A lot of difficulty" or "Cannot do at all/unable to do" to at least one question were classified in the "A lot of difficulty/cannot do" category. Of the remaining, those responding "Some difficulty" to at least one question were classified in the "Some difficulty" category, and those responding "No difficulty" to at least one question were classified in the "No difficulty" category. Those responding "Don't know" or "Refused" to all six questions were excluded. During 2010–2016, 1%–8% of respondents were missing data and excluded.

[9]MSA is metropolitan statistical area. Starting with 2016 data, MSA status is determined using 2010 Census data and the 2010 standards for defining MSAs.

Table 3-9. Joint Pain Among Adults 18 Years of Age and Over, by Selected Characteristics, Selected Years, 2002–2010

(Percent.)

Characteristic	Any joint pain[1]			Knee pain[1]			Shoulder pain[1]			Finger pain[1]			Hip pain[1]		
	2002	2005	2010	2002	2005	2010	2002	2005	2010	2002	2005	2010	2002	2005	2010
18 years and over, age-adjusted[2,3]	29.5	30.7	32.1	16.5	18.2	19.6	8.6	9.2	9.0	7.5	7.4	7.1	6.6	7.1	7.0
18 years and over, crude[3]	29.5	31.1	33.3	16.5	18.5	20.3	8.7	9.3	9.4	7.5	7.6	7.5	6.6	7.2	7.3
Age															
18 to 44 years	19.3	19.1	20.6	10.5	11.6	12.6	4.9	4.9	5.2	3.4	2.8	3.1	3.2	3.2	3.2
18 to 24 years	14.2	14.0	15.2	8.3	8.8	9.8	3.4	2.4	3.5	2.0	*1.0	1.7	1.6	2.1	*1.5
25 to 44 years	21.0	20.9	22.6	11.2	12.6	13.6	5.4	5.8	5.8	3.9	3.5	3.6	3.8	3.6	3.8
45 to 64 years	37.5	39.9	42.9	20.4	23.2	26.1	12.3	12.9	13.2	11.0	11.2	10.5	9.1	9.7	10.0
45 to 54 years	34.3	35.8	39.3	18.4	20.6	23.5	10.5	11.5	12.0	9.1	9.2	8.4	7.8	7.6	9.0
55 to 64 years	42.3	45.7	47.3	23.4	26.9	29.3	15.1	14.9	14.8	13.9	14.0	13.2	11.0	12.6	11.3
65 years and over	47.2	50.9	49.6	28.6	30.2	30.5	14.1	16.0	13.6	13.9	15.2	14.2	12.9	14.6	13.5
65 to 74 years	46.0	49.3	49.5	27.6	29.7	30.2	14.0	15.7	13.5	14.4	14.9	15.3	12.6	13.7	13.3
75 years and over	48.7	52.6	49.8	29.7	30.8	30.9	14.1	16.2	13.7	13.3	15.4	12.8	13.3	15.7	13.7
Sex[2]															
Male	28.0	28.9	30.8	15.2	16.8	18.7	8.4	9.3	9.3	5.8	6.0	5.8	5.1	5.4	5.3
Female	30.7	32.2	33.2	17.6	19.4	20.3	8.8	9.0	8.6	8.9	8.7	8.2	8.0	8.6	8.6
Sex and Age[2]															
Male															
18 to 44 years	20.1	19.3	21.6	10.7	12.0	12.9	5.5	5.4	6.1	3.0	2.6	3.0	2.5	2.4	2.0
45 to 54 years	31.1	33.4	37.3	16.2	18.9	22.3	9.5	11.4	12.2	6.6	7.5	7.3	5.6	5.7	6.8
55 to 64 years	37.3	40.7	42.5	20.1	23.1	27.4	13.7	14.7	15.3	10.5	10.4	9.9	8.0	9.5	8.7
65 to 74 years	41.7	45.1	42.9	24.1	25.1	25.3	13.3	15.7	11.8	11.2	11.4	10.9	10.5	10.8	10.3
75 years and over	43.9	47.0	46.6	25.7	25.7	28.7	11.4	15.1	13.1	10.0	12.1	9.5	10.1	12.7	12.9
Female															
18 to 44 years	18.4	18.9	19.7	10.2	11.2	12.2	4.2	4.5	4.3	3.8	3.0	3.1	3.9	4.0	4.5
45 to 54 years	37.3	38.2	41.3	20.5	22.3	24.8	11.4	11.5	11.8	11.5	10.9	9.4	9.9	9.5	11.1
55 to 64 years	46.8	50.4	51.8	26.4	30.5	31.0	16.3	15.1	14.3	17.0	17.4	16.2	13.7	15.4	13.7
65 to 74 years	49.6	52.9	55.2	30.5	33.6	34.4	14.7	15.7	15.0	17.1	17.9	19.0	14.2	16.2	15.8
75 years and over	51.6	56.2	51.9	32.1	34.0	32.4	15.7	16.9	14.1	15.3	17.5	15.1	15.2	17.5	14.3
Race[2,4]															
White only	29.8	31.3	32.6	16.3	18.5	19.7	8.8	9.5	9.1	7.6	7.8	7.4	6.9	7.4	7.2
Black or African American only	30.8	28.5	32.0	20.2	18.2	21.0	8.3	7.6	8.9	6.5	4.6	5.6	5.6	6.1	6.0
American Indian or Alaska Native only	36.7	34.8	38.1	24.5	15.0	26.9	*11.3	*8.1	10.1	*12.9	*13.0	*7.2	*10.4	*	*9.9
Asian only	18.1	18.5	20.4	8.5	10.2	12.8	3.9	5.3	6.9	*3.2	4.1	3.3	*2.3	*2.1	*2.4
Native Hawaiian or Other Pacific Islander only	*	*	*	*	*	*	*	*	*	*	*	*	*	*	*
2 or more races	42.7	46.2	43.5	28.1	28.6	27.1	15.4	18.9	13.9	12.8	10.5	12.2	10.0	13.7	11.7
Hispanic Origin and Race[2,4]															
Hispanic or Latino	23.4	24.2	25.4	13.6	14.9	15.5	7.6	8.2	7.4	6.8	6.0	6.0	3.8	4.1	4.3
Mexican	24.6	23.8	25.0	14.1	14.9	15.4	8.3	8.5	7.3	7.8	7.0	6.3	4.0	4.1	3.9
Not Hispanic or Latino	30.4	31.7	33.3	17.0	18.9	20.3	8.9	9.4	9.3	7.6	7.6	7.3	6.9	7.4	7.3
White only	30.8	32.8	34.3	16.9	19.4	20.7	9.1	9.8	9.5	7.8	8.2	7.7	7.3	7.8	7.7
Black or African American only	30.8	28.5	32.1	20.1	18.1	21.0	8.3	7.6	8.9	6.5	4.7	5.6	5.7	6.2	6.1
Education[5,6]															
25 years and over															
No high school diploma or GED	33.0	33.3	33.8	19.5	20.7	22.0	10.8	11.7	10.9	9.5	8.8	8.5	7.3	8.5	7.9
High school diploma or GED	32.9	33.1	36.8	18.6	19.7	22.7	10.2	10.5	10.9	8.3	8.8	9.1	7.3	7.5	9.0
Some college or more	31.1	33.2	34.0	16.9	19.2	20.1	8.8	9.7	9.1	8.2	8.1	7.4	7.5	7.8	7.3
Percent of Poverty Level[2,7]	Percent of adults reporting joint pain in past 30 days														
Below 100 percent	31.7	33.7	35.6	19.9	21.4	22.9	11.2	11.2	11.1	9.8	8.0	9.1	8.5	8.9	9.7
100 percent to 199 percent	31.7	31.9	34.0	19.0	19.8	21.9	10.4	10.5	10.9	8.9	8.2	8.3	7.5	8.1	8.5
200 percent to 399 percent	30.1	31.0	32.2	16.4	18.4	19.3	8.8	9.2	9.0	7.9	7.9	7.2	6.8	6.9	6.8
400 percent or more	27.6	29.3	30.5	14.9	16.6	18.1	7.3	8.1	7.7	6.2	6.6	6.0	5.8	6.3	5.7
Hispanic Origin and Race and Percent of Poverty Level[2,4,7]															
Hispanic or Latino															
Below 100 percent	26.8	24.5	25.3	16.1	15.7	15.9	11.5	10.5	7.6	8.6	6.4	6.4	5.9	4.4	5.6
100 percent to 199 percent	24.5	24.1	25.4	14.4	15.2	16.1	8.2	8.3	8.0	8.2	5.7	5.2	3.9	3.9	4.5
200 percent to 399 percent	21.6	23.6	24.8	11.7	13.1	14.5	5.7	8.2	6.8	6.2	6.5	6.8	3.2	4.2	3.1
400 percent or more	21.9	24.7	27.4	12.3	15.6	16.3	4.9	*6.4	7.4	*5.3	*5.1	5.8	*1.8	*4.3	*5.2

* = Figure does not meet standards of reliability or precision. Data preceded by an asterisk have a relative standard error (RSE) of 20 percent to 30 percent. Data not shown have an RSE of greater than 30 percent.
[1] Starting with 2002 data, respondents were asked, "During the past 30 days, have you had any symptoms of pain, aching, or stiffness in or around a joint?" Respondents were instructed not to include the back or neck. To facilitate their responses, respondents were shown a card illustrating the body joints. Respondents reporting more than one type of joint pain were included in each response category. This table shows the most commonly reported joints.
[2] Estimates are age adjusted to the year 2000 standard population using five age groups: 18 to 44 years, 45 to 54 years, 55 to 64 years, 65 to 74 years, and 75 years and over. Age-adjusted estimates in this table may differ from other age-adjusted estimates based on the same data and presented elsewhere if different age groups are used in the adjustment procedure.
[3] Includes all other races not shown separately, unknown education level, and unknown disability status.
[4] The race groups White, Black, American Indian or Alaska Native, Asian, Native Hawaiian or Other Pacific Islander, and two or more races, include persons of Hispanic and non-Hispanic origin. Persons of Hispanic origin may be of any race.
[5] Estimates are for persons 25 years of age and over and are age-adjusted to the year 2000 standard population using five age groups: 25 to 44 years, 45 to 54 years, 55 to 64 years, 65 to 74 years, and 75 years and over.
[6] GED is General Educational Development high school equivalency diploma.
[7] Percent of poverty level is based on family income and family size and composition using U.S. Census Bureau poverty thresholds.

Table 3-9. Joint Pain Among Adults 18 Years of Age and Over, by Selected Characteristics, Selected Years, 2002–2010—Continued

(Percent.)

Characteristic	Any joint pain[1]			Knee pain[1]			Shoulder pain[1]			Finger pain[1]			Hip pain[1]		
	2002	2005	2010	2002	2005	2010	2002	2005	2010	2002	2005	2010	2002	2005	2010
Not Hispanic or Latino															
White only															
Below 100 percent	34.2	39.3	40.1	21.3	24.7	25.2	12.4	13.4	12.6	10.9	9.9	11.1	9.9	11.6	12.0
100 percent to 199 percent	34.9	36.2	38.7	20.3	22.8	24.8	11.6	12.0	12.2	9.9	9.6	9.8	9.1	9.8	10.6
200 percent to 399 percent	32.0	33.6	34.8	17.0	20.1	20.9	9.6	10.1	10.0	8.5	8.9	7.8	7.5	7.8	7.8
400 percent or more	28.2	30.1	31.8	15.1	17.0	18.8	7.6	8.4	8.0	6.5	7.0	6.3	6.2	6.8	6.0
Black or African American only															
Below 100 percent	31.6	33.0	37.6	20.8	22.5	25.1	9.1	9.0	11.9	7.9	5.7	7.8	8.1	7.7	9.0
100 percent to 199 percent	34.0	28.6	33.0	23.2	18.3	22.6	10.9	8.3	10.0	7.4	6.0	6.2	6.4	6.3	5.9
200 percent to 399 percent	29.1	27.2	30.8	19.1	16.6	19.8	7.4	7.2	7.8	6.0	3.9	4.3	4.7	6.0	5.2
400 percent or more	29.8	25.8	26.8	18.2	15.8	15.7	*8.0	*5.7	6.5	*4.8	*2.8	*4.2	*4.5	*5.5	4.7
Disability Measure[2,8]															
Any basic actions difficulty or complex activity limitation	52.5	54.8	54.6	32.1	35.7	35.9	17.8	18.8	16.8	14.5	14.2	12.8	13.8	14.6	14.2
Any basic actions difficulty	54.0	56.7	56.2	33.4	37.3	37.3	18.3	19.5	17.2	14.9	14.8	13.3	14.4	15.2	14.6
Any complex activity limitation	56.4	57.8	56.5	35.2	38.2	37.5	22.0	23.5	20.6	17.8	16.9	15.0	17.8	19.7	18.7
No disability	19.6	20.3	21.5	9.4	10.4	11.6	4.6	4.8	4.9	4.0	4.1	4.2	3.1	3.3	3.1
Geographic Region[2]															
Northeast	27.5	28.6	28.9	15.8	16.7	17.9	7.9	8.1	8.3	6.6	6.2	5.5	5.7	6.4	5.5
Midwest	32.1	34.8	35.7	18.4	21.6	22.3	8.6	10.1	10.0	7.5	8.5	7.9	6.9	7.9	8.5
South	29.3	29.8	32.4	16.7	17.9	19.8	9.1	8.9	9.0	7.6	7.3	7.4	7.0	7.1	7.2
West	28.4	29.2	30.6	14.6	16.3	17.9	8.6	9.6	8.5	8.0	7.5	7.1	6.4	6.6	6.3
Location of Residence[2]															
Within MSA[9]	28.3	29.2	31.1	16.0	17.2	19.0	8.1	8.4	8.3	7.2	7.0	7.0	6.2	6.5	6.5
Outside MSA[9]	33.9	36.3	37.4	18.7	22.3	23.0	10.8	12.2	12.3	8.4	9.1	7.9	8.0	9.3	9.4

* = Figure does not meet standards of reliability or precision. Data preceded by an asterisk have a relative standard error (RSE) of 20 percent to 30 percent. Data not shown have an RSE of greater than 30 percent.
[1]Starting with 2002 data, respondents were asked, "During the past 30 days, have you had any symptoms of pain, aching, or stiffness in or around a joint?" Respondents were instructed not to include the back or neck. To facilitate their responses, respondents were shown a card illustrating the body joints. Respondents reporting more than one type of joint pain were included in each response category. This table shows the most commonly reported joints.
[2]Estimates are age adjusted to the year 2000 standard population using five age groups: 18 to 44 years, 45 to 54 years, 55 to 64 years, 65 to 74 years, and 75 years and over. Age-adjusted estimates in this table may differ from other age-adjusted estimates based on the same data and presented elsewhere if different age groups are used in the adjustment procedure.
[8]Any basic actions difficulty or complex activity limitation is defined as having one or more of the following limitations or difficulties: movement difficulty, emotional difficulty, sensory (seeing or hearing) difficulty, cognitive difficulty, self-care (activities of daily living or instrumental activities of daily living) limitation, social limitation, or work limitation.
[9]MSA = metropolitan statistical area.

Table 3-10. Basic Actions Difficulty and Complex Activity Limitation Among Adults 18 Years of Age and Over, by Selected Characteristics, Selected Years, 1997–2013

(Number, percent.)

Characteristic	18 years and over					18 to 64 years					65 years and over				
	1997	2000	2005	2010[1]	2013[1]	1997	2000	2005	2010[1]	2013[1]	1997	2000	2005	2010[1]	2013[1]
Number in Millions															
At least one basic actions difficulty or complex activity limitation[2,3]	60.9	59.0	66.5	73.7	75.4	41.3	39.3	45.4	50.7	49.8	19.6	19.7	21.1	23.0	25.6
At least one basic actions difficulty[2]	56.7	55.2	62.4	69.2	70.9	38.1	36.4	42.1	47.2	46.3	18.6	18.7	20.3	22.0	24.6
At least one complex activity limitation[3]	29.0	27.2	31.3	35.0	37.5	18.1	16.7	19.9	22.9	23.9	11.0	10.5	11.5	12.1	13.6
Percent with At Least One Basic Actions Difficulty or Complex Activity Limitation[2,3]															
Total, age-adjusted[4,5]	32.5	29.9	31.0	31.9	31.4	X	X	X	X	X	X	X	X	X	X
Total, crude[4]	31.8	29.5	31.2	32.8	32.9	25.8	23.5	25.3	27.1	26.6	62.2	60.8	62.4	61.7	61.1
Percent with At Least One Basic Actions Difficulty[2]															
Total, age-adjusted[4,5]	30.1	27.9	29.1	29.9	29.5	X	X	X	X	X	X	X	X	X	X
Total, crude[4]	29.4	27.5	29.3	30.8	30.9	23.6	21.7	23.5	25.1	24.7	58.8	58.1	60.1	59.3	58.9
Sex															
Male	25.6	23.8	25.2	26.3	26.3	20.7	18.9	20.3	21.4	21.0	54.5	53.4	55.2	53.8	52.8
Female	32.9	31.0	33.1	35.1	35.2	26.4	24.3	26.6	28.8	28.3	61.9	61.5	63.7	63.6	63.7
Race[6]															
White only	29.6	28.1	29.7	31.2	31.4	23.5	21.8	23.5	25.1	24.7	58.5	58.0	60.0	59.2	58.4
Black or African American only	31.4	27.2	30.4	32.3	33.6	26.9	22.7	26.1	28.4	29.0	64.4	60.6	63.2	62.9	63.8
American Indian or Alaska Native only	43.8	36.8	25.6	41.6	41.6	41.9	34.1	25.2	38.5	30.4	66.0	70.2	*	74.0	74.3
Asian only	15.5	15.5	15.7	17.5	17.6	13.0	12.6	11.8	12.8	12.3	46.4	44.7	46.2	50.1	53.4
Native Hawaiian or Other Pacific Islander only	NA	*	*	*	*	NA	*	*	*	*	NA	*	*	*	*
Two or more races	NA	38.0	40.0	36.3	34.7	NA	34.4	34.9	33.9	30.8	NA	70.7	90.4	65.4	71.6
Hispanic Origin and Race[6]															
Hispanic or Latino	23.8	19.6	21.6	24.7	23.3	21.0	16.6	18.7	21.2	19.9	54.6	57.5	56.2	61.5	56.9
Not Hispanic or Latino	30.0	28.5	30.4	31.8	32.3	23.9	22.4	24.3	25.9	25.7	59.0	58.2	60.3	59.1	59.1
White only	30.3	29.1	31.1	32.4	33.0	23.8	22.5	24.5	26.0	25.9	58.7	58.2	60.3	59.0	58.7
Black or African American only	31.5	27.3	30.7	32.6	34.1	27.0	22.9	26.3	28.6	29.5	64.4	60.4	63.5	63.2	63.7
Percent of Poverty Level[7]															
Below 100 percent	41.9	38.4	40.2	40.6	43.7	36.2	31.9	34.9	36.3	38.9	74.1	71.6	73.1	72.7	75.0
100 percent to 199 percent	38.2	37.1	38.4	38.7	39.4	29.2	26.5	29.6	30.5	30.6	66.6	69.4	68.5	69.5	70.2
200 percent to 399 percent	28.4	28.2	29.7	31.1	30.2	22.0	22.1	22.8	24.1	22.7	56.1	53.9	59.0	58.9	59.5
400 percent or more	21.0	19.4	21.4	23.0	22.4	18.2	16.8	18.1	19.3	18.0	45.5	44.7	48.2	47.0	45.4
Location of Residence															
Within MSA[8]	27.7	25.9	27.5	29.2	29.3	22.3	20.3	22.1	23.6	23.3	56.6	56.7	58.3	59.2	58.3
Outside MSA[8]	35.6	33.6	36.3	39.3	40.0	28.6	26.8	29.5	33.8	33.2	65.8	62.6	65.5	59.9	61.3
Percent with At Least One Complex Activity Limitation[3]															
Total, age-adjusted[4,5]	15.6	13.7	14.5	14.9	15.2	X	X	X	X	X	X	X	X	X	X
Total, crude[4]	15.1	13.4	14.6	15.5	16.0	11.2	9.8	11.0	12.1	12.4	35.1	32.0	33.6	32.3	32.0
Sex															
Male	13.7	12.0	12.9	14.0	14.8	10.6	9.4	10.1	11.3	12.0	31.9	28.1	29.4	30.1	29.1
Female	16.5	14.7	16.1	16.8	17.0	11.9	10.3	11.8	12.9	12.9	37.4	34.9	36.7	34.0	34.3
Race[6]															
White only	15.0	13.6	14.4	15.2	16.0	10.9	9.8	10.7	11.7	12.2	34.3	31.5	33.1	31.7	31.4
Black or African American only	19.0	15.0	17.1	19.7	19.0	15.2	11.7	14.0	17.0	15.9	47.1	40.4	40.9	39.9	39.7
American Indian or Alaska Native only	23.7	20.6	14.2	15.4	22.2	22.1	17.8	13.0	14.5	19.4	*42.6	*54.9	*	*	42.7
Asian only	5.7	4.7	6.6	7.7	7.4	4.9	3.6	4.7	5.0	4.7	*14.8	*15.5	*20.8	26.7	26.0
Native Hawaiian or Other Pacific Islander only	NA	*	*	*	*	NA	*	*	*	*	NA	*	*	*	*
Two or more races	NA	22.5	26.2	19.6	19.7	NA	20.3	21.8	17.0	17.8	NA	*42.2	69.7	53.6	37.9
Hispanic Origin and Race[6]															
Hispanic or Latino	11.9	9.1	9.8	10.4	10.5	9.8	7.3	7.6	7.9	8.3	33.9	32.4	35.0	37.6	32.9
Not Hispanic or Latino	15.5	14.0	15.3	16.3	16.9	11.4	10.2	11.5	12.9	13.3	35.1	32.0	33.5	31.9	31.9
White only	15.4	14.1	15.2	16.1	17.1	11.1	10.1	11.3	12.5	13.2	34.4	31.5	32.9	31.1	31.4
Black or African American only	18.8	15.1	17.3	20.0	19.4	15.0	11.7	14.1	17.3	16.3	46.8	40.3	40.9	40.0	39.7
Percent of Poverty Level[7]															
Below 100 percent	30.0	26.0	27.3	27.5	29.6	25.2	22.0	23.4	24.0	26.1	56.9	46.7	51.5	54.5	52.7
100 percent to 199 percent	23.3	22.0	22.7	23.7	23.9	16.7	15.1	17.2	18.4	17.9	43.9	42.8	41.3	43.7	45.1
200 percent to 399 percent	13.3	12.8	14.0	14.5	14.9	9.3	9.2	9.9	10.8	10.7	30.6	27.5	31.8	29.3	31.6
400 percent or more	7.3	6.4	7.3	7.7	7.8	5.8	5.0	5.5	5.8	6.0	20.2	19.6	21.5	19.8	17.2
Location of Residence															
Within MSA[8]	14.1	12.1	13.2	14.2	14.8	10.6	8.9	9.9	10.9	11.5	32.7	29.8	31.7	31.6	31.2
Outside MSA[8]	19.0	18.2	20.0	22.2	22.3	13.6	13.4	15.4	18.8	18.2	42.8	38.8	39.7	35.2	35.3

NA = Not available.

X = Not applicable.

* = Figure does not meet standards of reliability or precision. Data preceded by an asterisk have a relative standard error (RSE) of 20 percent to 30 percent. Data not shown have an RSE of greater than 30 percent.

[1] Starting with 2007 data, the hearing question, a component of the basic actions difficulty measure, was revised. Consequently, data for basic actions difficulty prior to 2007 are not comparable with 2007 data and beyond.

[2] A basic actions difficulty is defined as having one or more of the following difficulties: movement, emotional, sensory (seeing or hearing), or cognitive.

[3] A complex activity limitation is defined as having one or more of the following limitations: self-care (activities of daily living or instrumental activities of daily living), social, or work.

[4] Includes all other races not shown separately.

[5] Estimates are for persons 25 years of age and over and are age-adjusted to the year 2000 standard population using five age groups: 25 to 44 years, 45 to 54 years, 55 to 64 years, 65 to 74 years, and 75 years and over.

[6] The race groups, White, Black, American Indian or Alaska Native, Asian, Native Hawaiian or Other Pacific Islander, and 2 or more races, include persons of Hispanic and non-Hispanic origin. Persons of Hispanic origin may be of any race.

[7] Percent of poverty level is based on family income and family size and composition using U.S. Census Bureau poverty thresholds.

[8] MSA = metropolitan statistical area.

Table 3-11. Selected Vision and Hearing Limitations Among Adults 18 Years of Age and Over, by Selected Characteristics, Selected Years, 1997–2016

(Percent; data are based on household interviews of a sample of the civilian noninstitutionalized population.)

Characteristic	Any trouble seeing, even with glasses or contacts[1]						Any hearing trouble (a little, moderate, a lot, or deaf)[2]					
	1997	2000	2005	2010	2015	2016	2007	2010	2011	2012	2015	2016
Percent of Adults												
18 years and over, age-adjusted[3,4]	10.0	9.0	9.2	9.1	9.0	10.0	14.7	15.6	15.3	15.1	14.2	14.1
18 years and over, crude[4]	9.8	8.9	9.3	9.4	9.4	10.4	14.9	16.2	16.0	16.0	15.3	15.4
Age												
18 to 44 years	6.2	5.3	5.5	6.2	5.6	6.7	6.0	6.7	6.2	6.2	5.8	5.4
18 to 24 years	5.4	4.2	5.0	5.8	4.9	7.0	4.1	5.4	4.1	4.3	4.5	3.7
25 to 44 years	6.5	5.7	5.7	6.3	5.8	6.6	6.6	7.2	6.9	6.8	6.2	6.1
45 to 64 years	12.0	10.7	11.2	11.6	11.6	12.8	17.6	18.9	18.9	19.2	16.2	17.0
45 to 54 years	12.2	10.9	11.0	10.7	11.2	13.6	14.7	15.6	15.4	16.0	12.8	13.6
55 to 64 years	11.6	10.5	11.5	12.7	12.1	12.0	21.5	23.2	23.0	22.9	19.9	20.4
65 years and over	18.1	17.4	17.4	13.9	14.9	15.1	36.9	37.5	37.9	35.9	36.9	36.4
65 to 74 years	14.2	13.6	13.2	12.2	11.9	14.1	29.8	31.2	30.2	29.4	30.2	30.0
75 years and over	23.1	21.9	22.0	16.1	19.1	16.6	45.0	45.2	47.4	44.4	46.5	45.7
Sex[3]												
Male	8.8	7.9	7.9	7.9	7.4	8.4	18.3	18.9	18.7	18.2	17.4	17.0
Female	11.1	10.1	10.5	10.3	10.6	11.6	11.5	12.7	12.3	12.3	11.4	11.6
Sex and Age												
Male												
18 to 44 years	5.3	4.4	4.5	5.2	4.0	5.2	6.8	7.7	7.2	6.9	6.4	6.5
45 to 54 years	10.1	8.8	8.8	9.1	8.9	11.2	18.7	18.2	18.3	18.7	16.1	15.1
55 to 64 years	10.5	9.5	10.5	10.7	10.2	10.2	28.4	30.1	30.0	29.1	25.7	25.3
65 to 74 years	13.2	12.8	11.4	10.5	10.0	12.4	39.4	41.0	38.7	39.3	40.8	39.7
75 years and over	21.4	20.7	20.4	15.7	18.8	15.7	54.6	53.1	56.5	52.1	54.5	53.0
Female												
18 to 44 years	7.1	6.2	6.5	7.1	7.1	8.1	5.1	5.8	5.1	5.4	5.2	4.4
45 to 54 years	14.2	12.8	13.2	12.3	13.4	16.0	11.0	13.0	12.5	13.3	9.7	12.1
55 to 64 years	12.6	11.5	12.4	14.6	13.8	13.6	15.0	16.7	16.4	17.1	14.5	16.0
65 to 74 years	15.0	14.4	14.8	13.6	13.5	15.6	21.8	22.8	22.8	20.8	21.0	21.6
75 years and over	24.2	22.7	23.0	16.4	19.4	17.3	38.8	39.9	41.1	39.1	40.8	40.5
Race[3,5]												
White only	9.7	8.8	9.1	8.8	9.0	9.8	15.6	16.5	16.2	16.0	15.2	15.2
Black or African American only	12.8	10.6	10.9	12.1	10.3	12.2	8.5	10.3	10.0	10.0	8.8	9.3
American Indian or Alaska Native only	19.2	16.6	*14.9	15.0	*10.9	12.3	17.9	21.1	16.0	13.0	22.8	18.8
Asian only	6.2	6.3	5.5	5.3	6.3	7.8	8.0	8.0	9.1	9.7	9.1	7.5
Native Hawaiian or Other Pacific Islander only	NA	*	*	*	*	9.4	*	*	*	*	*	*
Two or more races	NA	16.2	16.4	13.1	12.4	14.9	24.4	23.3	21.2	19.3	17.6	15.6
Hispanic Origin and Race[3,5]												
Hispanic or Latino	10.0	9.7	9.6	9.2	9.3	10.2	10.9	10.9	11.8	11.3	9.3	11.2
Mexican	10.2	8.3	9.9	9.0	9.3	11.1	11.8	11.5	13.2	12.4	10.5	12.1
Not Hispanic or Latino	10.0	9.1	9.2	9.2	9.0	10.1	15.2	16.2	15.8	15.7	14.9	14.7
White only	9.8	8.9	9.1	8.9	9.1	9.8	16.5	17.5	17.0	16.9	16.3	16.3
Black or African American only	12.8	10.6	10.9	12.2	10.2	12.1	8.4	10.3	10.0	9.9	8.7	9.1
Education[6,7]												
25 years of age and over												
No high school diploma or GED	15.0	12.2	13.5	14.1	13.4	14.4	17.9	19.7	18.7	17.2	17.1	17.0
High school diploma or GED	10.6	9.5	10.3	10.5	9.5	11.5	17.2	18.1	19.2	18.3	16.3	17.1
Some college or more	8.9	8.9	8.6	8.0	8.9	9.2	15.4	16.2	15.5	15.9	15.2	14.8
Percent of Poverty Level[3,8]												
Below 100 percent	17.0	12.9	15.3	14.8	14.2	16.8	16.2	16.7	16.7	16.6	15.4	16.0
100 percent to 199 percent	12.9	11.6	11.5	12.2	11.8	13.3	15.5	17.2	16.2	16.0	15.8	15.2
200 percent to 399 percent	9.1	8.8	8.9	9.0	9.4	9.5	15.1	15.7	16.2	15.6	14.9	14.0
400 percent or more	7.3	7.1	6.9	6.4	6.3	7.4	13.6	14.5	13.5	13.7	12.6	13.3
Hispanic Origin and Race and Percent of Poverty Level[3,5,8]												
Hispanic or Latino												
Below 100 percent	12.8	11.0	13.6	10.8	15.1	15.5	12.7	9.1	11.0	12.2	9.7	13.0
100 percent to 199 percent	11.2	9.4	8.8	10.8	10.1	10.8	9.7	11.8	12.7	11.3	10.8	9.7
200 percent to 399 percent	8.1	9.2	8.2	8.9	7.2	9.2	9.8	10.3	11.8	10.8	8.2	11.2
400 percent or more	*8.1	10.5	8.0	5.3	5.2	6.6	13.3	12.4	11.6	11.0	8.0	12.9

NA = Not available.

* = Estimates are considered unreliable. Starting with 2016 data, the reliability of survey percentage estimates was assessed using new multistep National Center for Health Statistics data presentation standards for proportions. Prior to 2016 data, the reliability of estimates for earlier years was evaluated based on relative standard errors (RSE). Data preceded by an asterisk have an RSE of 20%–30%. Data not shown have an RSE greater than 30%.

[1]Respondents were asked, "Do you have any trouble seeing, even when wearing glasses or contact lenses?" Respondents were also asked, "Are you blind or unable to see at all?" In this analysis, any trouble seeing and blind are combined into one category.
[2]Starting in 2007, respondents were asked questions about their hearing WITHOUT the use of hearing aids or other listening devices: "Is your hearing excellent, good, a little trouble hearing, moderate trouble, a lot of trouble, or are you deaf?" Hearing limitation questions differed slightly on the National Health Interview Survey across the years for which data are shown.
[3]Estimates are age-adjusted to the year 2000 standard population using five age groups: 18–44 years, 45–54 years, 55–64 years, 65–74 years, and 75 years and over. Age-adjusted estimates in this table may differ from other age-adjusted estimates based on the same data and presented elsewhere if different age groups are used in the adjustment procedure.
[4]Includes all other races not shown separately and unknown education level.
[5]The race groups White, Black, American Indian or Alaska Native, Asian, Native Hawaiian or Other Pacific Islander, and 2 or more races include persons of Hispanic and non-Hispanic origin. Persons of Hispanic origin may be of any race. Starting with 1999 data, race-specific estimates are tabulated according to the 1997 Revisions to the Standards for the Classification of Federal Data on Race and Ethnicity and are not strictly comparable with estimates for earlier years. The five single-race categories and multiple-race categories shown in the table conform to the 1997 Standards. Starting with 1999 data, race-specific estimates are for persons who reported only one racial group; the category 2 or more races includes persons who reported more than one racial group. Prior to 1999, data were tabulated according to the 1977 Standards with four racial groups, and the Asian only category included Native Hawaiian or Other Pacific Islander. Estimates for single-race categories prior to 1999 included persons who reported one race, or if they reported more than one race, identified one race as best representing their race. Starting with 2003 data, race responses of other race and unspecified multiple race were treated as missing, and then race was imputed if these were the only race responses. Almost all persons with a race response of other race were of Hispanic origin.
[6]Estimates are for persons aged 25 and over and are age-adjusted to the year 2000 standard population using five age groups: 25–44 years, 45–54 years, 55–64 years, 65–74 years, and 75 years and over.
[7]GED is General Educational Development high school equivalency diploma.
[8]Percent of poverty level is based on family income and family size and composition using U.S. Census Bureau poverty thresholds. Missing family income data were imputed for 1997 and beyond.

Table 3-11. Selected Vision and Hearing Limitations Among Adults 18 Years of Age and Over, by Selected Characteristics, Selected Years, 1997–2016—Continued

(Percent; data are based on household interviews of a sample of the civilian noninstitutionalized population.)

Characteristic	Moderate, a lot of trouble, or deaf[2]						A lot of trouble hearing or deaf[2]					
	2007	2010	2011	2012	2015	2016	2007	2010	2011	2012	2015	2016
Percent of Adults												
18 years and over, age-adjusted[3,4]	5.6	5.7	5.7	5.4	5.2	5.4	2.3	2.1	2.2	2.0	2.0	2.2
18 years and over, crude[4]	5.7	5.9	5.9	5.7	5.6	5.8	2.3	2.2	2.2	2.0	2.1	2.3
Age												
18 to 44 years	1.3	1.7	1.5	1.6	1.1	1.3	0.4	0.5	0.6	0.4	0.4	0.4
18 to 24 years	*	*1.2	*0.7	*1.2	*0.8	0.7	*	*	*	*	*	0.2
25 to 44 years	1.6	1.8	1.8	1.7	1.2	1.5	0.5	0.5	0.7	0.5	0.4	0.5
45 to 64 years	6.0	6.1	6.1	5.8	4.9	5.3	2.0	1.9	1.9	1.7	1.5	1.8
45 to 54 years	4.1	4.8	4.7	4.6	3.3	4.5	1.2	1.2	1.5	1.3	1.1	1.6
55 to 64 years	8.5	7.8	7.7	7.1	6.5	6.1	3.0	2.7	2.4	2.0	1.9	1.9
65 years and over	18.6	17.7	18.0	16.3	18.1	17.5	8.7	7.6	7.7	7.0	7.4	7.8
65 to 74 years	11.9	12.9	12.6	10.7	12.5	12.2	4.7	4.6	4.6	4.0	4.2	3.9
75 years and over	26.3	23.7	24.6	23.6	26.0	25.2	13.3	11.1	11.6	11.1	11.9	13.3
Sex[3]												
Male	7.7	7.4	7.5	7.2	6.8	7.0	3.1	2.8	2.7	2.6	2.6	2.7
Female	3.9	4.3	4.1	3.9	3.8	4.0	1.6	1.6	1.7	1.5	1.5	1.7
Sex and Age												
Male												
18 to 44 years	1.6	1.9	1.8	1.8	1.1	1.5	*0.5	*0.7	*0.6	*0.5	*0.3	0.4
45 to 54 years	5.3	5.7	6.1	5.6	4.6	5.4	1.5	*1.1	*1.8	1.6	*1.6	1.9
55 to 64 years	12.9	11.5	11.2	10.3	9.6	8.8	4.7	3.9	3.2	2.8	2.9	2.5
65 to 74 years	17.7	17.9	17.3	16.1	17.6	17.8	7.0	6.7	6.0	5.9	5.8	5.6
75 years and over	34.8	29.7	32.2	31.8	33.1	31.5	16.9	14.5	14.7	14.2	15.8	16.1
Female												
18 to 44 years	1.0	1.4	1.3	1.3	1.1	1.0	*0.3	*0.3	0.5	0.4	*0.5	0.3
45 to 54 years	2.9	3.9	3.3	3.7	2.1	3.7	*1.0	*1.3	1.1	*1.1	*0.7	1.5
55 to 64 years	4.3	4.4	4.3	4.1	3.7	3.6	*1.3	1.6	1.6	1.3	*1.0	1.2
65 to 74 years	6.9	8.6	8.5	5.9	8.0	7.3	2.8	2.9	3.3	*2.2	2.9	2.5
75 years and over	20.9	19.7	19.3	18.1	21.0	20.7	11.1	8.9	9.5	9.0	9.1	11.3
Race[3,5]												
White only	6.0	6.1	6.1	5.8	5.5	5.8	2.4	2.3	2.3	2.1	2.1	2.3
Black or African American only	2.7	3.3	3.1	2.7	2.6	3.2	1.2	1.1	1.2	1.1	0.9	1.2
American Indian or Alaska Native only	*8.8	*7.1	*6.2	*	10.0	8.4	*3.8	*	*	*	*6.3	*
Asian only	2.8	2.6	3.6	3.4	3.5	2.6	*	*1.0	*1.8	*1.2	*1.4	1.4
Native Hawaiian or Other Pacific Islander only	*	*	*	*	*	*	*	*	*	*	*	*
Two or more races	11.5	8.7	*6.7	*5.4	7.9	7.2	*4.9	*	*	*	*	2.1
Hispanic Origin and Race[3,5]												
Hispanic or Latino	4.3	3.5	3.6	4.1	2.8	3.9	2.5	1.4	1.4	2.0	1.3	1.7
Mexican	4.4	3.5	3.9	4.5	3.2	4.3	2.5	*1.5	1.6	*2.0	1.5	1.9
Not Hispanic or Latino	5.8	6.0	5.9	5.5	5.5	5.6	2.3	2.2	2.3	2.0	2.0	2.2
White only	6.3	6.5	6.4	6.0	5.9	6.2	2.5	2.4	2.4	2.1	2.2	2.4
Black or African American only	2.7	3.3	3.1	2.8	2.6	3.1	1.2	1.1	1.2	1.1	*0.9	1.2
Education[6,7]												
25 years of age and over												
No high school diploma or GED	7.6	8.1	7.4	5.7	6.3	6.5	4.1	3.2	3.1	2.5	2.9	3.5
High school diploma or GED	6.4	6.5	7.5	6.8	6.4	7.1	2.8	2.5	2.8	2.6	2.8	3.0
Some college or more	6.1	6.0	5.5	5.7	5.5	5.5	1.9	2.0	2.0	1.9	1.8	2.0
Percent of Poverty Level[3,8]												
Below 100 percent	6.8	6.8	6.1	6.1	5.6	6.8	3.4	2.7	2.7	2.7	2.3	3.6
100 percent to 199 percent	5.8	6.6	6.1	5.9	6.0	5.9	2.8	2.5	2.5	2.3	2.6	2.5
200 percent to 399 percent	5.8	5.6	6.3	5.4	5.8	5.6	2.4	2.1	2.4	1.9	2.2	2.3
400 percent or more	5.3	5.0	4.9	4.9	4.2	4.6	1.6	1.8	1.7	1.7	1.4	1.5
Hispanic Origin and Race and Percent of Poverty Level[3,5,8]												
Hispanic or Latino												
Below 100 percent	*6.1	*3.5	3.3	4.5	3.0	6.0	*	*	*1.3	*1.8	*1.7	3.6
100 percent to 199 percent	*3.1	4.3	3.7	3.6	3.8	3.4	*2.1	*2.3	*1.8	*	*1.8	1.1
200 percent to 399 percent	*3.9	*2.6	3.2	4.1	*1.8	3.5	*	*	*1.3	*2.0	*	0.9
400 percent or more	*5.6	*3.2	*4.6	*4.9	*2.2	4.0	*	*	*	*	*	2.5

* = Estimates are considered unreliable. Starting with 2016 data, the reliability of survey percentage estimates was assessed using new multistep National Center for Health Statistics data presentation standards for proportions. Prior to 2016 data, the reliability of estimates for earlier years was evaluated based on relative standard errors (RSE). Data preceded by an asterisk have an RSE of 20%–30%. Data not shown have an RSE greater than 30%.

[2] Starting in 2007, respondents were asked questions about their hearing WITHOUT the use of hearing aids or other listening devices: "Is your hearing excellent, good, a little trouble hearing, moderate trouble, a lot of trouble, or are you deaf?" Hearing limitation questions differed slightly on the National Health Interview Survey across the years for which data are shown.

[3] Estimates are age-adjusted to the year 2000 standard population using five age groups: 18–44 years, 45–54 years, 55–64 years, 65–74 years, and 75 years and over. Age-adjusted estimates in this table may differ from other age-adjusted estimates based on the same data and presented elsewhere if different age groups are used in the adjustment procedure.

[4] Includes all other races not shown separately and unknown education level.

[5] The race groups White, Black, American Indian or Alaska Native, Asian, Native Hawaiian or Other Pacific Islander, and 2 or more races include persons of Hispanic and non-Hispanic origin. Persons of Hispanic origin may be of any race. Starting with 1999 data, race-specific estimates are tabulated according to the 1997 Revisions to the Standards for the Classification of Federal Data on Race and Ethnicity and are not strictly comparable with estimates for earlier years. The five single-race categories and multiple-race categories shown in the table conform to the 1997 Standards. Starting with 1999 data, race-specific estimates are for persons who reported only one racial group; the category 2 or more races includes persons who reported more than one racial group. Prior to 1999, data were tabulated according to the 1977 Standards with four racial groups, and the Asian only category included Native Hawaiian or Other Pacific Islander. Estimates for single-race categories prior to 1999 included persons who reported one race, or if they reported more than one race, identified one race as best representing their race. Starting with 2003 data, race responses of other race and unspecified multiple race were treated as missing, and then race was imputed if these were the only race responses. Almost all persons with a race response of other race were of Hispanic origin.

[6] Estimates are for persons aged 25 and over and are age-adjusted to the year 2000 standard population using five age groups: 25–44 years, 45–54 years, 55–64 years, 65–74 years, and 75 years and over.

[7] GED is General Educational Development high school equivalency diploma.

[8] Percent of poverty level is based on family income and family size and composition using U.S. Census Bureau poverty thresholds. Missing family income data were imputed for 1997 and beyond.

Table 3-11. Selected Vision and Hearing Limitations Among Adults 18 Years of Age and Over, by Selected Characteristics, Selected Years, 1997–2016—*Continued*

(Percent; data are based on household interviews of a sample of the civilian noninstitutionalized population.)

Characteristic	Any trouble seeing, even with glasses or contacts[1]						Any hearing trouble (a little, moderate, a lot, or deaf)[2]					
	1997	2000	2005	2010	2015	2016	2007	2010	2011	2012	2015	2016
Not Hispanic or Latino												
White only												
Below 100 percent	17.9	13.1	16.2	16.8	14.8	18.0	20.9	21.7	20.5	21.1	20.3	19.8
100 percent to 199 percent	13.1	12.0	12.7	12.6	12.9	14.3	18.8	20.8	18.6	19.5	19.7	19.9
200 percent to 399 percent	9.2	9.2	9.0	8.8	10.3	9.8	17.2	17.9	18.2	17.8	17.8	16.6
400 percent or more	7.3	7.0	6.9	6.7	6.4	7.4	14.3	15.4	14.6	14.6	13.8	14.5
Black or African American only												
Below 100 percent	17.9	13.6	16.0	15.8	13.6	16.8	9.3	11.6	13.9	12.9	10.9	12.4
100 percent to 199 percent	16.0	12.9	11.3	14.9	12.4	16.6	9.8	11.1	12.0	10.3	9.8	9.7
200 percent to 399 percent	9.3	7.7	9.7	12.0	9.5	9.0	7.8	10.4	8.8	8.9	7.7	7.8
400 percent or more	7.7	8.3	6.4	6.6	6.1	8.3	7.1	7.7	6.1	8.2	7.0	7.4
Geographic Region[3]												
Northeast	8.6	7.4	8.1	7.8	7.9	8.9	13.3	13.9	13.0	12.7	12.4	11.5
Midwest	9.5	9.6	9.7	9.1	9.3	10.5	16.0	17.5	16.4	17.1	16.0	16.3
South	11.4	9.2	9.8	10.6	9.4	10.1	14.0	16.0	15.9	15.0	13.9	13.9
West	9.7	9.9	8.6	8.0	8.9	10.3	15.5	14.4	15.1	15.1	14.4	14.5
Location of Residence[3,9]												
Within MSA	9.5	8.5	8.6	8.6	8.7	9.7	14.0	14.7	14.6	14.5	13.5	13.3
Outside MSA	12.0	11.1	11.7	11.6	11.0	12.1	18.0	20.1	19.1	18.0	18.6	19.2

[1]Respondents were asked, "Do you have any trouble seeing, even when wearing glasses or contact lenses?" Respondents were also asked, "Are you blind or unable to see at all?" In this analysis, any trouble seeing and blind are combined into one category.
[2]Starting in 2007, respondents were asked questions about their hearing WITHOUT the use of hearing aids or other listening devices: "Is your hearing excellent, good, a little trouble hearing, moderate trouble, a lot of trouble, or are you deaf?" Hearing limitation questions differed slightly on the National Health Interview Survey across the years for which data are shown.
[3]Estimates are age-adjusted to the year 2000 standard population using five age groups: 18–44 years, 45–54 years, 55–64 years, 65–74 years, and 75 years and over. Age-adjusted estimates in this table may differ from other age-adjusted estimates based on the same data and presented elsewhere if different age groups are used in the adjustment procedure.
[9]MSA is metropolitan statistical area. Starting with 2016 data, MSA status is determined using 2010 Census data and the 2010 standards for defining MSAs.

Table 3-11. Selected Vision and Hearing Limitations Among Adults 18 Years of Age and Over, by Selected Characteristics, Selected Years, 1997–2016—*Continued*

(Percent; data are based on household interviews of a sample of the civilian noninstitutionalized population.)

Characteristic	Moderate, a lot of trouble, or deaf[2]						A lot of trouble hearing or deaf[2]					
	2007	2010	2011	2012	2015	2016	2007	2010	2011	2012	2015	2016
Not Hispanic or Latino												
White only												
Below 100 percent	8.8	9.2	8.2	8.3	8.0	9.1	4.3	3.7	3.6	3.6	3.2	4.7
100 percent to 199 percent	7.2	8.3	7.3	7.3	7.6	8.0	3.3	3.0	2.8	2.7	3.2	3.3
200 percent to 399 percent	6.4	6.5	7.2	6.2	6.9	6.7	2.6	2.3	2.8	2.0	2.6	2.8
400 percent or more	5.6	5.4	5.2	5.2	4.5	4.9	1.7	2.0	1.8	1.8	1.4	1.5
Black or African American only												
Below 100 percent	*2.8	4.0	3.6	4.1	2.3	3.8	*	*1.5	*1.6	*2.1	*	1.7
100 percent to 199 percent	*3.1	3.0	3.4	3.1	3.3	3.0	*	*0.7	*1.5	*1.2	*	1.0
200 percent to 399 percent	*2.2	3.6	2.7	*2.1	2.7	2.8	*	*	*1.0	*	*	1.3
400 percent or more	*	*2.8	*3.1	*	*2.0	3.1	*	*	*	*	*	0.8
Geographic Region[3]												
Northeast	5.2	4.4	4.9	4.1	3.9	4.3	1.7	1.4	2.3	1.6	1.4	1.7
Midwest	6.1	6.3	6.0	5.8	5.8	6.3	2.3	2.3	1.9	2.0	2.2	2.3
South	5.4	6.3	5.9	5.8	5.3	5.5	2.5	2.6	2.4	2.2	2.1	2.3
West	5.9	5.3	5.7	5.4	5.4	5.0	2.4	1.9	2.1	1.9	1.9	2.1
Location of Residence[3,9]												
Within MSA	5.3	5.4	5.3	5.2	4.9	4.9	2.1	1.9	2.0	1.9	1.9	1.9
Outside MSA	7.2	7.5	7.5	6.4	6.6	7.8	3.3	3.0	3.0	2.4	2.6	3.6

* = Estimates are considered unreliable. Starting with 2016 data, the reliability of survey percentage estimates was assessed using new multistep National Center for Health Statistics data presentation standards for proportions. Prior to 2016 data, the reliability of estimates for earlier years was evaluated based on relative standard errors (RSE). Data preceded by an asterisk have an RSE of 20%–30%. Data not shown have an RSE greater than 30%

[2]Starting in 2007, respondents were asked questions about their hearing WITHOUT the use of hearing aids or other listening devices: "Is your hearing excellent, good, a little trouble hearing, moderate trouble, a lot of trouble, or are you deaf?" Hearing limitation questions differed slightly on the National Health Interview Survey across the years for which data are shown.

[3]Estimates are age-adjusted to the year 2000 standard population using five age groups: 18–44 years, 45–54 years, 55–64 years, 65–74 years, and 75 years and over. Age-adjusted estimates in this table may differ from other age-adjusted estimates based on the same data and presented elsewhere if different age groups are used in the adjustment procedure.

[9]MSA is metropolitan statistical area. Starting with 2016 data, MSA status is determined using 2010 Census data and the 2010 standards for defining MSAs.

Table 3-12. Respondent-Assessed Fair-Poor Health Status, by Selected Characteristics, Selected Years, 1991–2016

(Percent.)

Characteristic	1991[1]	1995[1]	2000	2005	2006	2007	2008	2009	2010	2011	2012	2013	2014	2015	2016
Percent of Persons with Fair or Poor Health[2]															
All ages, age-adjusted[3,4]	10.4	10.6	9.0	9.2	9.2	9.5	9.5	9.4	9.6	9.8	9.5	9.4	8.9	9.2	9.0
All ages, crude[4]	10.0	10.1	8.9	9.3	9.5	9.8	9.9	9.9	10.1	10.4	10.3	10.2	9.8	10.1	9.9
Age															
Under 18 years	2.6	2.6	1.7	1.8	1.9	1.7	1.8	1.8	2.0	2.0	2.1	1.7	1.6	1.8	1.6
Under 6 years	2.7	2.7	1.5	1.6	1.9	1.5	1.2	1.3	1.8	1.5	1.5	1.6	1.3	1.2	1.2
6 to 17 years	2.6	2.5	1.8	1.9	1.9	1.7	2.1	2.0	2.2	2.2	2.4	1.8	1.8	2.1	1.8
18 to 44 years	6.1	6.6	5.1	5.5	5.7	5.9	6.3	6.3	6.3	6.5	6.4	6.2	6.1	6.3	6.1
18 to 24 years	4.8	4.5	3.3	3.3	3.7	3.3	4.0	3.6	3.9	4.2	3.8	3.6	3.7	3.8	3.9
25 to 44 years	6.4	7.2	5.7	6.3	6.3	6.8	7.2	7.2	7.2	7.3	7.4	7.2	7.0	7.2	6.9
45 to 54 years	13.4	13.4	11.9	11.6	12.9	13.3	12.9	13.1	13.3	14.1	14.2	14.1	12.8	13.5	13.4
55 to 64 years	20.7	21.4	17.9	18.3	18.8	17.9	18.8	19.1	19.4	19.1	19.3	19.2	18.4	18.7	17.7
65 years and over	29.0	28.3	26.9	26.6	24.8	26.8	24.9	24.0	24.4	24.7	22.7	23.1	21.7	21.8	21.6
65 to 74 years	26.0	25.6	22.5	23.4	21.9	23.4	21.8	19.9	21.2	21.5	19.6	19.7	19.5	19.0	18.8
75 years and over	33.6	32.2	32.1	30.2	28.1	30.7	28.4	28.9	28.3	28.6	26.6	27.6	24.9	25.8	25.7
Sex[3]															
Male	10.0	10.1	8.8	8.8	9.0	9.1	9.1	9.1	9.2	9.4	9.2	9.0	8.7	8.9	8.7
Female	10.8	11.1	9.3	9.5	9.5	9.9	9.8	9.7	10.0	10.1	9.9	9.8	9.2	9.5	9.2
Race[3,5]															
White only	9.6	9.7	8.2	8.6	8.6	8.8	8.9	8.7	8.8	9.0	8.8	8.7	8.3	8.5	8.3
Black or African American only	16.8	17.2	14.6	14.3	14.4	14.2	14.6	14.2	14.9	15.0	14.9	14.3	13.6	13.6	13.5
American Indian or Alaska Native only	18.3	18.7	17.2	13.2	12.1	17.1	14.5	16.3	17.8	14.4	16.5	15.3	14.1	16.6	17.6
Asian only	7.8	9.3	7.4	6.8	6.9	7.1	6.7	8.4	8.1	8.7	7.9	7.7	7.3	7.8	6.9
Native Hawaiian or Other Pacific Islander only	NA	NA	*	*	*	*	*	*	*	*	*	*	*	*	12.7
Two or more races	NA	NA	16.2	14.5	13.1	16.8	12.9	15.3	15.6	14.2	13.0	13.9	12.8	14.4	12.6
Black or African American; White	NA	NA	*14.5	8.3	*15.0	*16.6	20.2	18.0	*16.7	16.7	16.3	*19.0	11.9	*13.7	8.5
American Indian and Alaska Native; White	NA	NA	18.7	17.2	13.9	19.2	14.6	15.2	19.0	16.5	14.4	16.2	17.6	18.2	15.6
Hispanic Origin and Race[3,5]															
Hispanic or Latino	15.6	15.1	12.8	13.3	13.0	13.0	12.8	13.3	13.1	13.2	13.3	12.7	12.2	12.7	12.4
Mexican	17.0	16.7	12.8	14.3	14.1	13.2	13.4	13.7	13.7	14.0	13.6	13.3	13.0	12.7	12.7
Not Hispanic or Latino	10.0	10.1	8.7	8.7	8.8	9.1	9.1	8.9	9.2	9.4	9.1	9.0	8.5	8.7	8.5
White only	9.1	9.1	7.9	8.0	8.0	8.3	8.4	8.0	8.2	8.4	8.1	8.2	7.7	7.9	7.6
Black or African American only	16.8	17.3	14.6	14.4	14.4	14.1	14.6	14.2	14.9	15.0	15.0	14.2	13.6	13.4	13.4
Percent of Poverty Level[3,6]															
Below 100 percent	22.8	23.7	19.6	20.4	20.3	21.0	21.8	21.8	20.9	21.5	21.6	21.8	19.8	21.2	20.6
100 percent to 199 percent	14.7	15.5	14.1	14.4	14.4	15.3	15.4	14.9	15.2	15.0	14.9	14.4	14.2	14.9	15.0
200 percent to 399 percent	7.9	7.9	8.4	8.3	8.1	9.0	8.7	8.6	8.3	8.7	8.4	8.2	7.9	8.4	8.1
400 percent or more	4.9	4.7	4.5	4.7	4.5	4.7	4.4	4.3	4.3	4.3	3.9	4.0	3.9	4.0	4.2
Hispanic Origin and Race and Percent of Poverty Level[3,5,6]															
Hispanic or Latino															
Below 100 percent	23.6	22.7	18.7	20.2	20.6	21.0	21.0	22.1	19.2	21.0	20.9	20.3	18.7	21.3	20.4
100 percent to 199 percent	18.0	16.9	15.3	15.3	14.4	15.1	14.6	16.2	15.6	14.4	14.5	14.3	14.1	14.4	14.1
200 percent to 399 percent	10.3	10.1	10.3	10.3	10.5	10.5	10.7	9.7	10.3	10.8	10.0	10.3	9.4	9.7	9.5
400 percent or more	6.6	4.0	5.5	7.6	5.7	7.2	5.6	5.6	6.4	5.0	6.7	5.3	5.5	5.7	6.5
Not Hispanic or Latino															
White only															
Below 100 percent	21.9	22.8	18.8	20.1	19.5	20.9	22.1	20.5	20.9	21.2	21.1	22.2	20.3	20.7	19.7
100 percent to 199 percent	14.0	14.8	13.4	13.8	14.2	15.2	15.7	14.6	14.8	15.0	15.3	14.4	14.1	15.0	15.4
200 percent to 399 percent	7.5	7.3	7.9	7.9	7.5	8.4	8.3	8.1	7.7	8.1	7.7	7.7	7.4	8.0	7.7
400 percent or more	4.7	4.6	4.2	4.3	4.2	4.3	4.1	4.0	4.0	4.1	3.5	3.8	3.5	3.7	3.7
Black or African American only															
Below 100 percent	25.8	27.7	23.8	23.3	23.0	22.6	25.1	25.2	23.9	24.7	25.0	24.8	21.8	23.3	23.2
100 percent to 199 percent	17.0	19.3	18.2	17.6	16.9	17.7	18.1	16.6	18.3	18.5	16.9	17.5	16.8	17.0	17.1
200 percent to 399 percent	12.0	11.4	11.7	11.2	11.0	11.3	11.2	11.0	11.2	10.7	11.9	9.8	9.8	9.8	9.9
400 percent or more	5.9	6.5	7.3	7.1	7.0	7.2	6.9	5.9	6.8	6.9	6.6	5.0	5.7	6.3	6.9

NA = Not available.

* = Estimates are considered unreliable. Starting with 2016 data, the reliability of survey percentage estimates was assessed using new multistep National Center for Health Statistics data presentation standards for proportions. Prior to 2016 data, the reliability of estimates for earlier years was evaluated based on relative standard errors (RSE). Data preceded by an asterisk have an RSE of 20%–30%. Data not shown have an RSE greater than 30%.

[1] Data prior to 1997 are not strictly comparable with data for later years due to the 1997 questionnaire redesign.
[2] See the CDC Web site for more information.
[3] Estimates are age-adjusted to the year 2000 standard population using six age groups: under 18 years, 18–44 years, 45–54 years, 55–64 years, 65–74 years, and 75 years and over. The disability measure is age-adjusted using the five adult age groups.
[4] Includes all other races not shown separately and unknown disability status.
[5] The race groups White, Black, American Indian or Alaska Native, Asian, Native Hawaiian or Other Pacific Islander, and 2 or more races include persons of Hispanic and non-Hispanic origin. Persons of Hispanic origin may be of any race. Starting with 1999 data, race-specific estimates are tabulated according to the 1997 Revisions to the Standards for the Classification of Federal Data on Race and Ethnicity and are not strictly comparable with estimates for earlier years. The five single-race categories and multiple-race categories shown in the table conform to the 1997 Standards. Starting with 1999 data, race-specific estimates are for persons who reported only one racial group; the category 2 or more races includes persons who reported more than one racial group. Prior to 1999, data were tabulated according to the 1977 Standards with four racial groups, and the Asian only category included Native Hawaiian or Other Pacific Islander. Estimates for single-race categories prior to 1999 included persons who reported one race, or if they reported more than one race, identified one race as best representing their race. Starting with 2003 data, race responses of other race and unspecified multiple race were treated as missing, and then race was imputed if these were the only race responses. Almost all persons with a race response of other race were of Hispanic origin.
[6] Percent of poverty level is based on family income and family size and composition using U.S. Census Bureau poverty thresholds. Missing family income data were imputed for 1991 and beyond.

Table 3-12. Respondent-Assessed Fair-Poor Health Status, by Selected Characteristics, Selected Years, 1991–2016—*Continued*

(Percent.)

Characteristic	1991[1]	1995[1]	2000	2005	2006	2007	2008	2009	2010	2011	2012	2013	2014	2015	2016
Level of Difficulty[3,7]															
A lot of difficulty or cannot do at all	NA	NA	NA	NA	NA	NA	NA	NA	47.3	48.1	52.9	44.1	43.0	44.0	52.1
Some difficulty	NA	NA	NA	NA	NA	NA	NA	NA	17.1	20.2	17.0	15.7	13.4	14.8	15.5
No difficulty	NA	NA	NA	NA	NA	NA	NA	NA	5.2	5.1	5.1	4.6	4.8	4.4	5.5
Geographic Region[3]															
Northeast	8.3	9.1	7.6	7.5	8.2	8.4	8.0	8.4	7.9	8.4	8.0	8.2	7.2	8.2	7.9
Midwest	9.1	9.7	8.0	8.3	8.8	8.6	8.8	8.6	9.0	8.8	9.1	8.8	8.5	8.8	8.6
South	13.1	12.3	10.7	11.0	10.4	11.0	11.0	10.9	11.1	11.2	10.8	10.6	10.2	10.0	10.1
West	9.7	10.1	8.8	8.6	8.5	9.0	9.0	8.8	9.2	9.5	9.1	9.1	8.6	9.1	8.4
Location of Residence[3,8]															
Within MSA	9.9	10.1	8.5	8.7	8.7	9.0	9.1	9.1	9.2	9.4	9.0	9.1	8.5	8.8	8.6
Outside MSA	11.9	12.6	11.1	11.2	11.7	12.0	11.7	11.2	11.9	11.7	12.3	11.4	11.4	11.8	11.4

NA = Not available.

[1] Data prior to 1997 are not strictly comparable with data for later years due to the 1997 questionnaire redesign.

[3] Estimates are age-adjusted to the year 2000 standard population using six age groups: under 18 years, 18–44 years, 45–54 years, 55–64 years, 65–74 years, and 75 years and over. The disability measure is age-adjusted using the five adult age groups.

[7] Functional limitation is defined by the reported level of difficulty in six functioning domains: seeing (even if wearing glasses), hearing (even if wearing hearing aids), mobility (walking or climbing stairs), communication (understanding or being understood by others), cognition (remembering or concentrating), and self-care (such as washing all over or dressing). Respondents with answers to one or more of the six questions were included in one of three mutually exclusive categories. Those responding "A lot of difficulty" or "Cannot do at all/unable to do" to at least one question were classified in the "A lot of difficulty/cannot do" category. Of the remaining, those responding "Some difficulty" to at least one question were classified in the "Some difficulty" category, and those responding "No difficulty" to at least one question were classified in the "No difficulty" category. Those responding "Don't know" or "Refused" to all six questions were excluded. During 2010–2016, 1%–8% of respondents were missing data and excluded. Different questions about vision and hearing limitations were used in separate tables on trends in vision limitations and hearing limitations.

[8] MSA = metropolitan statistical area. Starting with 2016 data, MSA status is determined using 2010 Census data and the 2010 standards for defining MSAs.

Table 3-13. Serious Psychological Distress in the Past 30 Days Among Adults 18 Years of Age and Over, by Selected Characteristics, Annual Average, Selected Years, 1997–1998 Through 2015–2016

(Percent of persons with serious psychological distress[1].)

Characteristic	1997–1998	1999–2000	2000–2001	2001–2002	2002–2003	2003–2004	2004–2005	2006–2007	2007–2008	2008–2009	2009–2010	2010–2011	2011–2012	2013–2014[2]	2014–2015[2]	2015–2016[2]
18 years and over, age-adjusted[3,4]	3.2	2.6	3.0	3.1	3.1	3.1	3.0	2.8	2.9	3.2	3.2	3.3	3.1	3.4	3.3	3.6
18 years and over, crude[4]	3.2	2.6	3.0	3.1	3.1	3.1	3.0	2.9	2.9	3.2	3.3	3.4	3.2	3.5	3.4	3.6
Age																
18 to 44 years	2.9	2.3	2.7	2.9	2.9	2.9	2.8	2.5	2.7	3.1	3.1	2.9	2.8	3.1	3.3	3.5
18 to 24 years	2.7	2.2	2.6	2.8	2.8	2.8	2.5	2.0	2.3	2.5	2.4	2.4	2.3	2.5	3.2	3.9
25 to 44 years	3.0	2.4	2.8	3.0	2.9	2.9	2.9	2.7	2.8	3.3	3.4	3.1	3.0	3.4	3.3	3.3
45 to 64 years	3.7	3.2	3.6	3.9	4.0	3.9	3.7	3.7	3.6	3.7	4.1	4.5	4.2	4.5	4.1	4.4
45 to 54 years	3.9	3.5	3.7	4.2	4.2	3.9	3.9	3.7	3.6	3.9	4.1	4.2	4.0	4.6	3.9	4.5
55 to 64 years	3.4	2.6	3.4	3.4	3.6	3.9	3.4	3.8	3.6	3.6	4.0	4.7	4.4	4.5	4.3	4.3
65 years and over	3.1	2.4	2.7	2.4	2.3	2.4	2.5	2.1	2.4	2.4	2.1	2.4	2.3	2.5	2.2	2.3
65 to 74 years	2.5	2.3	2.8	2.4	2.3	2.3	2.2	2.1	2.4	2.2	2.0	2.6	2.5	2.7	2.4	2.4
75 years and over	3.8	2.5	2.5	2.4	2.3	2.5	2.9	2.0	2.4	2.6	2.3	2.1	1.9	2.2	1.9	2.3
Sex[3]																
Male	2.5	2.0	2.4	2.4	2.3	2.3	2.3	2.1	2.2	2.7	2.8	2.8	2.5	2.9	2.7	2.9
Female	3.8	3.1	3.5	3.8	3.9	3.9	3.7	3.4	3.5	3.6	3.7	3.7	3.7	3.9	3.9	4.2
Race[3,5]																
White only	3.1	2.5	2.9	3.0	3.0	3.1	2.9	2.7	2.9	3.2	3.2	3.2	3.1	3.4	3.3	3.6
Black or African American only	4.0	2.9	3.1	3.5	3.4	3.4	3.6	3.2	3.2	3.7	3.8	3.7	3.3	3.5	3.4	3.6
American Indian or Alaska Native only	7.8	*7.2	*7.4	8.1	*7.1	*5.5	*3.5	*3.9	*	*3.8	*5.2	5.6	6.5	*5.4	*11.8	9.2
Asian only	2.0	*1.4	*2.0	*1.8	*1.9	*1.8	1.7	2.0	*1.0	*1.1	1.6	1.7	1.9	1.9	1.9	2.1
Native Hawaiian or Other Pacific Islander only	- - -	*	*	*	*	*	*	*	*	*	*	*	*	*	*	2.1
Two or more races	- - -	4.8	5.5	5.0	7.3	9.1	7.9	6.5	5.9	*4.9	5.2	5.6	6.7	8.6	8.4	6.7
Hispanic Origin and Race[3,5]																
Hispanic or Latino	5.0	3.5	4.0	4.0	3.9	3.9	3.7	3.4	3.6	3.4	3.6	4.0	3.8	4.5	4.4	3.7
Mexican	5.2	2.9	3.4	3.8	3.7	3.6	3.6	3.2	3.3	2.9	2.8	3.6	3.4	4.6	4.3	3.6
Not Hispanic or Latino	3.0	2.5	2.9	3.1	3.1	3.1	3.0	2.8	2.8	3.1	3.2	3.2	3.1	3.3	3.2	3.6
White only	2.9	2.4	2.9	3.0	3.0	3.0	2.9	2.7	2.9	3.2	3.1	3.2	3.1	3.2	3.1	3.7
Black or African American only	3.9	2.9	3.1	3.5	3.4	3.4	3.6	3.2	3.1	3.7	3.8	3.7	3.3	3.4	3.4	3.6
Percent of Poverty Level[3,6]																
Below 100 percent	9.1	6.8	7.7	8.4	8.6	8.8	8.6	7.2	8.3	9.0	8.4	8.2	8.2	9.1	8.3	9.3
100 percent to 199 percent	5.0	4.4	5.0	5.2	5.2	5.2	5.0	5.0	4.7	4.9	4.8	5.0	4.9	5.5	5.3	5.8
200 percent to 399 percent	2.5	2.3	2.7	2.8	2.6	2.5	2.5	2.1	2.4	2.7	2.8	2.9	2.6	2.6	2.8	3.0
400 percent or more	1.3	1.2	1.2	1.3	1.3	1.2	1.1	1.2	1.1	1.1	1.2	1.2	1.1	1.2	1.3	1.5
Hispanic Origin and Race and Percent of Poverty Level[3,5,6]																
Hispanic or Latino																
Below 100 percent	8.6	6.1	6.9	7.5	7.6	7.4	6.6	6.0	7.0	6.7	6.4	7.5	7.4	8.2	7.4	6.8
100 percent to 199 percent	5.4	3.8	4.4	4.1	3.8	3.7	3.9	2.9	4.5	4.5	4.1	4.3	3.9	5.0	5.1	4.1
200 percent to 399 percent	3.4	2.1	3.0	3.5	3.0	2.5	2.6	2.8	2.2	1.8	2.6	3.1	2.3	3.2	3.0	2.6
400 percent or more	*	2.3	*1.6	*	*	*1.8	*1.9	*2.2	*1.6	*1.0	*1.5	*1.4	*1.4	*1.8	2.7	2.4
Not Hispanic or Latino																
White only																
Below 100 percent	9.6	7.8	8.9	9.2	9.6	10.4	10.2	8.8	10.7	11.2	10.1	9.6	9.4	10.7	9.8	12.1
100 percent to 199 percent	5.2	4.9	5.5	5.9	6.1	6.1	5.6	6.0	5.4	5.7	5.5	5.6	5.8	6.5	6.0	7.6
200 percent to 399 percent	2.5	2.3	2.9	2.9	2.7	2.6	2.6	2.1	2.6	3.1	3.2	3.2	2.8	2.7	2.9	3.1
400 percent or more	1.3	1.1	1.2	1.3	1.3	1.2	1.1	1.1	1.0	1.0	1.1	1.1	1.0	1.2	1.2	1.6
Black or African American only																
Below 100 percent	8.7	6.0	6.3	7.2	7.1	7.4	7.6	6.2	6.2	8.0	8.3	7.7	7.3	7.4	6.9	7.6
100 percent to 199 percent	4.3	3.6	4.3	4.9	4.5	4.1	4.8	4.3	3.6	3.1	3.5	4.4	3.5	3.5	3.2	3.9
200 percent to 399 percent	2.2	*1.7	1.9	2.3	2.0	1.9	2.1	2.0	2.4	2.9	2.5	1.9	2.0	2.3	2.6	2.8
400 percent or more	*	*1.0	*	*	*1.2	*	*	*	*	*	*1.6	*1.5	*1.0	*0.7	*1.0	1.1
Geographic Region[3]																
Northeast	2.7	1.9	2.5	2.8	3.0	2.9	2.5	2.6	2.6	2.9	3.1	3.0	2.7	2.8	2.7	3.1
Midwest	2.6	2.5	2.8	2.9	2.7	2.7	2.7	2.9	2.7	3.2	3.3	3.1	3.0	3.5	3.3	3.6
South	3.8	2.9	3.2	3.5	3.5	3.5	3.7	3.1	3.3	3.5	3.5	3.6	3.5	3.7	3.4	3.6
West	3.3	2.8	3.2	3.0	3.0	3.0	2.8	2.5	2.7	2.8	2.9	3.3	3.1	3.4	3.7	3.8
Location of Residence[3,7]																
Within MSA	3.0	2.3	2.8	3.0	2.9	2.9	2.8	2.6	2.7	3.0	3.1	3.1	3.0	3.3	3.2	3.3
Outside MSA	3.9	3.5	3.6	3.8	3.9	3.8	4.0	3.7	3.7	4.0	4.1	4.0	4.1	4.3	4.3	5.1

NA = Not available.

* = Estimates are considered unreliable. Starting with 2015–2016 data, the reliability of survey percentage estimates was assessed using new multistep National Center for Health Statistics data presentation standards for proportions. Prior to 2015–2016 data, the reliability of estimates for earlier years was evaluated based on relative standard errors (RSE). Data preceded by an asterisk have an RSE of 20%–30%. Data not shown have an RSE greater than 30%.

[1]Serious psychological distress is measured by a six-question scale that asks respondents how often they experienced each of the six symptoms of psychological distress in the past 30 days. Respondents must have answered all six questions to have a computed K6 score. Only those with K6 scores were included in this analysis.

[2]Starting in 2013 (shown in spreadsheet version), the six psychological distress questions were moved to the adult selected items section of the sample adult questionnaire. Observed differences between 2012 and earlier estimates and 2013 and later estimates may be partially or fully attributable to this change in question placement within the sample adult questionnaire.

[3]Estimates are age-adjusted to the year 2000 standard population using five age groups: 18–44 years, 45–54 years, 55–64 years, 65–74 years, and 75 years and over.

[4]Includes all other races not shown separately.

[5]The race groups White, Black, American Indian or Alaska Native, Asian, Native Hawaiian or Other Pacific Islander, and 2 or more races include persons of Hispanic and non-Hispanic origin. Persons of Hispanic origin may be of any race. Starting with 1999 data, race-specific estimates are tabulated according to the 1997 Revisions to the Standards for the Classification of Federal Data on Race and Ethnicity and are not strictly comparable with estimates for earlier years. The five single-race categories and multiple-race categories shown in the table conform to the 1997 Standards. Starting with 1999 data, race-specific estimates are for persons who reported only one racial group; the category 2 or more races includes persons who reported more than one racial group. Prior to 1999, data were tabulated according to the 1977 Standards with four racial groups, and the Asian only category included Native Hawaiian or Other Pacific Islander. Estimates for single-race categories prior to 1999 included persons who reported one race, or if they reported more than one race, identified one race as best representing their race. Starting with 2003 data, race responses of other race and unspecified multiple race were treated as missing, and then race was imputed if these were the only race responses. Almost all persons with a race response of other race were of Hispanic origin.

[6]Percent of poverty level is based on family income and family size and composition using U.S. Census Bureau poverty thresholds. Missing family income data were imputed for 1997 and beyond.

[7]MSA = metropolitan statistical area. Starting with 2016 data, MSA status is determined using 2010 Census data and the 2010 standards for defining MSAs.

Table 3-14. Children Under 18 Years of Age Who Suffer from Asthma, by Selected Characteristics, Annual Average, Selected Years, 1997–1999 Through 2011–2013

(Percent of children.)

Characteristic	Current asthma[1]									Asthma attack in the past 12 months[2]								
	1997–1999	2000–2002	2003–2005	2006–2008	2007–2009	2008–2010	2009–2011	2010–2012	2011–2013	1997–1999	2000–2002	2003–2005	2006–2008	2007–2009	2008–2010	2009–2011	2010–2012	2011–2013
Children Under 18 Years[3]	NA	NA	8.7	9.3	9.4	9.5	9.5	9.4	9.0	5.4	5.7	5.4	5.5	5.4	5.6	5.6	5.5	5.3
Age																		
0 to 4 years...	NA	NA	6.1	6.2	6.4	6.2	6.4	6.1	5.5	4.3	4.7	4.2	4.3	4.3	4.4	4.5	4.2	3.6
5 to 17 years.......................................	NA	NA	9.6	10.5	10.6	10.8	10.7	10.7	10.4	5.7	6.1	5.8	5.9	5.9	6.1	6.0	6.1	5.9
5 to 9 years.......................................	NA	NA	9.1	10.6	10.2	10.7	10.2	10.3	9.8	5.6	6.3	6.1	6.8	6.2	6.5	6.2	6.6	6.2
10 to 17 years...................................	NA	NA	9.9	10.4	10.8	10.9	11.1	10.9	10.8	5.8	5.9	5.7	5.4	5.7	5.8	5.8	5.7	5.7
Sex																		
Male	NA	NA	9.9	10.7	10.8	11.1	10.7	10.2	9.8	6.2	6.6	6.3	6.2	6.2	6.5	6.3	6.3	5.9
Female	NA	NA	7.3	7.8	7.9	7.8	8.3	8.5	8.2	4.5	4.7	4.4	4.7	4.6	4.6	4.8	4.8	4.7
Hispanic Origin and Race[4]																		
Race[4]																		
White only...	NA	NA	7.7	8.2	8.0	8.2	8.1	8.1	7.8	5.0	5.2	4.9	4.9	4.7	4.9	4.8	4.9	4.7
Black or African American only	NA	NA	13.0	14.6	16.0	16.0	16.4	16.0	15.3	7.0	8.0	7.6	8.1	8.6	8.7	8.8	8.9	8.5
American Indian or Alaska Native only .	NA	NA	12.2	*10.4	*10.8	*10.3	*6.6	9.4	9.5	6.4	*8.7	*6.1	*	*	*	*3.5	*5.5	*5.8
Asian only	NA	NA	4.8	5.8	6.3	6.7	7.7	6.8	5.6	4.3	4.7	3.3	3.9	4.1	4.8	5.2	4.4	3.2
Native Hawaiian or Other Pacific Islander only	NA	NA	*	*	*	*	*	*	*	NA	*	*	*	*	*	*	*	*
Two or more races	NA	NA	13.5	13.6	13.9	12.8	13.3	12.7	13.1	NA	7.3	8.8	8.2	9.3	9.0	8.0	7.1	7.1
Hispanic Origin																		
Hispanic or Latino	NA	NA	7.6	8.3	7.9	7.5	8.5	8.8	8.6	4.8	4.2	4.6	5.0	4.6	4.4	4.7	4.9	4.6
Not Hispanic or Latino	NA	NA	8.9	9.6	9.8	10.0	9.8	9.6	9.2	5.5	6.0	5.6	5.6	5.7	5.9	5.8	5.7	5.5
White only.......................................	NA	NA	7.9	8.2	8.2	8.5	8.2	8.0	7.7	5.1	5.5	5.0	4.9	4.8	5.1	5.0	5.0	4.8
Black or African American only	NA	NA	13.0	14.6	16.0	16.2	16.4	16.1	15.2	7.0	7.9	7.5	8.0	8.5	8.8	8.8	9.0	8.5
Percent of Poverty Level[5]																		
Below 100 percent	NA	NA	10.4	11.7	12.2	12.4	12.7	12.5	12.4	6.1	7.1	6.5	6.8	6.9	7.4	7.5	7.5	7.2
100 percent to 199 percent.................	NA	NA	8.6	9.9	9.8	9.9	9.9	9.9	9.2	5.3	5.4	5.2	5.8	5.7	6.0	5.9	6.0	5.2
200 percent to 399 percent.................	NA	NA	8.3	8.8	8.2	8.2	8.3	8.7	8.3	5.0	5.3	5.2	4.9	4.7	4.6	4.6	4.7	4.7
400 percent or more	NA	NA	7.9	7.6	8.4	8.2	7.8	7.0	6.7	5.2	5.5	4.9	4.8	5.0	5.0	4.7	4.4	4.3
Health Insurance Status at the Time of Interview[6]																		
Insured...	NA	NA	9.0	9.7	9.7	9.8	9.7	9.6	9.2	5.6	5.9	5.6	5.7	5.6	5.8	5.7	5.7	5.4
Private...	NA	NA	8.0	8.3	8.4	8.4	8.2	8.1	7.7	5.0	5.3	5.0	5.0	5.1	5.1	4.9	4.8	4.6
Medicaid	NA	NA	11.4	12.4	12.1	12.0	12.0	11.9	11.4	7.7	7.7	7.1	7.0	6.7	7.0	6.9	7.0	6.4
Uninsured	NA	NA	5.6	6.0	6.3	6.6	6.8	6.7	6.9	3.9	4.3	3.3	3.7	3.5	3.6	3.6	4.0	4.3

NA = Not available.
* = Figure does not meet standards of reliability or precision. Data preceded by an asterisk have a relative standard error (RSE) of 20 percent to 30 percent. Data not shown have an RSE of greater than 30 percent.
[1]Based on parent or knowledgeable adult responding to both questions, "Has a doctor or other health professional ever told you that your child had asthma?" and "Does your child still have asthma?"
[2]Based on parent or knowledgeable adult responding to both questions, "Has a doctor or other health professional ever told you that your child had asthma?" and "During the past 12 months, did your child have an episode of asthma or an asthma attack?"
[3]Includes all other races not shown separately, unknown poverty level, and unknown health insurance status.
[4]The race groups White, Black, American Indian or Alaska Native, Asian, Native Hawaiian or Other Pacific Islander, and two or more races, include persons of Hispanic and non-Hispanic origin. Persons of Hispanic origin may be of any race.
[5]Percent of poverty level is based on family income and family size and composition using U.S. Census Bureau poverty thresholds. Missing family income data were imputed for 1997 and beyond.
[6]Health insurance categories are mutually exclusive. Persons who reported both Medicaid and private coverage are classified as having private coverage. Starting with 1997 data, state-sponsored health plan coverage is included as Medicaid coverage. Starting with 1999 data, coverage by the Children's Health Insurance Program (CHIP) is included as Medicaid coverage. In addition to private and Medicaid, the insured category also includes military, other government, and Medicare coverage. Persons not covered by private insurance, Medicaid, CHIP, state-sponsored or other government-sponsored health plans, Medicare, or military plans are considered to have no health insurance coverage. Persons with only Indian Health Service coverage are considered to have no health insurance coverage.

Table 3-15. Hypertension Among Persons 20 Years of Age and Over, by Selected Characteristics, Selected Years, 1988–1994 Through 2013–2016

(Percent; data are based on interviews and physical examinations of a sample of the civilian noninstitutionalized population.)

Sex, age, race and Hispanic origin[1], and percent of poverty level	Hypertension (systolic pressure of at least 140 mm Hg or diastolic pressure of at least 90 mm Hg or taking antihypertensive medication)[2,3]			Uncontrolled high blood pressure (systolic pressure of at least 140 mm Hg or diastolic pressure of at least 90 mm Hg) among persons with hypertension[4]		
	1988–1994	2001–2004	2013–2016	1988–1994	2001–2004	2013–2016
20 Years and Over, Age-Adjusted[5]						
Both Sexes[6]	25.5	30.9	30.5	77.2	66.0	55.4
Male	26.4	30.3	31.5	83.2	68.3	60.9
Female	24.4	31.0	29.3	68.5	57.6	46.7
Not Hispanic or Latino						
White only	24.4	29.4	29.2	76.6	66.1	51.9
White only, male	25.6	29.3	31.1	82.6	67.8	57.5
White only, female	23.0	29.0	27.0	67.0	52.7	37.1
Black or African American only	38.1	43.1	42.4	77.5	67.9	61.2
Black or African American only, male	37.5	41.5	41.8	84.0	70.8	65.3
Black or African American only, female	38.3	44.3	42.9	71.1	65.4	57.7
Asian only	NA	NA	27.0	NA	NA	68.8
Asian only, male	NA	NA	30.2	NA	NA	73.5
Asian only, female	NA	NA	24.4	NA	NA	61.3
Hispanic Origin	NA	NA	29.0	NA	NA	59.7
Male	NA	NA	27.9	NA	NA	69.3
Female	NA	NA	29.8	NA	NA	45.6
	26.1	27.8	29.1	85.7	74.0	60.8
Mexican origin, male	26.9	26.1	27.9	87.9	76.4	69.6
Mexican origin, female	25.0	29.7	30.1	77.6	63.8	44.8
Percent of Poverty Level[7]						
Below 100 percent	31.7	35.5	35.2	75.0	66.1	55.4
100 percent to 199 percent	26.6	34.0	33.7	76.0	70.1	59.0
200 percent to 399 percent	24.7	31.4	30.9	76.2	67.8	53.8
400 percent or more	22.6	27.9	26.7	81.5	60.8	52.7
20 Years and Over, Crude						
Both Sexes[6]	24.1	30.8	33.4	73.9	63.0	48.8
Male	23.8	29.0	33.1	79.3	62.1	52.0
Female	24.4	32.5	33.6	68.8	63.7	45.9
Not Hispanic or Latino						
White only	24.4	31.4	34.7	72.7	61.7	45.8
White only, male	24.3	29.9	35.1	78.0	59.4	48.4
White only, female	24.6	32.9	34.3	67.8	63.8	43.3
Black or African American only	31.8	39.4	42.4	75.9	64.9	54.7
Black or African American only, male	31.1	36.7	40.5	83.3	68.7	58.8
Black or African American only, female	32.5	41.6	44.0	70.0	61.9	51.4
Asian only	NA	NA	25.9	NA	NA	60.2
Asian only, male	NA	NA	27.8	NA	NA	64.5
Asian only, female	NA	NA	24.2	NA	NA	55.9
Hispanic Origin	NA	NA	23.5	NA	NA	54.3
Male	NA	NA	21.9	NA	NA	59.7
Female	NA	NA	25.2	NA	NA	49.5
	16.2	17.3	23.4	83.8	71.7	55.5
Mexican male	16.4	15.8	22.3	86.5	73.6	62.2
Mexican female	15.9	19.0	24.6	80.6	69.8	48.9
Percent of Poverty Level[7]						
Below 100 percent	25.7	28.3	32.4	74.0	67.3	50.7
100 percent to 199 percent	26.7	34.6	36.6	75.1	64.5	50.1
200 percent to 399 percent	22.4	31.5	33.5	73.4	63.4	47.5
400 percent or more	22.0	28.4	31.0	74.3	59.2	46.4
Male						
20 to 44 years	10.9	12.3	12.8	90.5	71.0	70.0
20 to 34 years	7.1	7.0	7.7	92.6	87.1	76.2
35 to 44 years	17.1	19.2	21.6	89.0	63.2	66.2

NA = Not available.

[1]Persons of Hispanic and Mexican origin may be of any race. Starting with 1999 data, race-specific estimates are tabulated according to the 1997 Revisions to the Standards for the Classification of Federal Data on Race and Ethnicity and are not strictly comparable with estimates for earlier years. The non-Hispanic race categories shown in the table conform to the 1997 Standards. Starting with 1999 data, race-specific estimates are for persons who reported only one racial group. Prior to data year 1999, estimates were tabulated according to the 1977 Standards. Estimates for single-race categories prior to 1999 included persons who reported one race, or if they reported more than one race, identified one race as best representing their race.

[2]Hypertension is defined as having measured high blood pressure or taking antihypertensive medication. High blood pressure is defined as having measured systolic pressure of at least 140 mm Hg or diastolic pressure of at least 90 mm Hg. Those with high blood pressure also may be taking prescribed medicine for high blood pressure. Those taking antihypertensive medication may not have measured high blood pressure but are still classified as having hypertension. Pregnant women were excluded. In 2017, a revised set of practice guidelines for defining high blood pressure was released but has not been widely adopted. Therefore, the high blood pressure cutoffs used to define hypertension and uncontrolled high blood pressure in Health, United States continue to use the original definition of 140 mm Hg/90 mm Hg.

[3]Respondents were asked, "Are you now taking prescribed medicine for your high blood pressure?"

[4]Uncontrolled high blood pressure among persons with hypertension is defined as having measured high blood pressure among those with measured high blood pressure or reporting taking antihypertensive medication. High blood pressure is defined as having measured systolic pressure of at least 140 mm Hg or diastolic pressure of at least 90 mm Hg. Pregnant women were excluded. In 2017, a revised set of practice guidelines for defining high blood pressure was released but has not been widely adopted. Therefore, the high blood pressure cutoffs used to define hypertension and uncontrolled high blood pressure in Health, United States continue to use the original definition of 140 mm Hg/90 mm Hg.

[5]Estimates are age-adjusted to the year 2000 standard population using five age groups: 20–34 years, 35–44 years, 45–54 years, 55–64 years, and 65 years and over. Age-adjusted estimates in this table may differ from other age-adjusted estimates based on the same data and presented elsewhere if different age groups are used in the adjustment procedure.

[6]Includes persons of all races and Hispanic origins, not just those shown separately.

[7]Percent of poverty level was calculated by dividing family income by the U.S. Department of Health and Human Services' poverty guideline specific to family size, as well as the appropriate year, and state. Persons with unknown percent of poverty level are excluded (7% in 2013–2016).

Table 3-15. Hypertension Among Persons 20 Years of Age and Over, by Selected Characteristics, Selected Years, 1988–1994 Through 2013–2016—*Continued*

(Percent; data are based on interviews and physical examinations of a sample of the civilian noninstitutionalized population.)

Sex, age, race and Hispanic origin[1], and percent of poverty level	Hypertension (systolic pressure of at least 140 mm Hg or diastolic pressure of at least 90 mm Hg or taking antihypertensive medication)[2,3]			Uncontrolled high blood pressure (systolic pressure of at least 140 mm Hg or diastolic pressure of at least 90 mm Hg) among persons with hypertension[4]		
	1988–1994	2001–2004	2013–2016	1988–1994	2001–2004	2013–2016
45 to 64 years.........................	34.2	39.9	43.7	73.1	61.1	49.6
45 to 54 years.........................	29.2	35.9	35.8	76.2	64.9	55.4
55 to 64 years.........................	40.6	47.5	52.2	70.3	55.5	45.3
65 to 74 years.........................	54.4	61.7	61.1	74.3	49.5	43.1
75 years and over.........................	60.4	67.1	67.4	82.5	68.3	50.3
Female						
20 to 44 years.........................	6.5	7.7	9.4	63.4	51.0	39.4
20 to 34 years.........................	2.9	*2.7	3.5	82.2	*50.2	*
35 to 44 years.........................	11.2	14.0	17.7	56.8	51.2	34.5
45 to 64 years.........................	32.8	42.6	38.8	62.1	60.9	39.3
45 to 54 years.........................	23.9	35.2	27.6	58.5	66.1	45.2
55 to 64 years.........................	42.6	54.4	51.2	64.3	55.6	35.8
65 to 74 years.........................	56.2	72.9	67.4	68.7	67.2	46.3
75 years and over.........................	73.6	82.0	78.7	81.9	72.4	62.0

* = Estimates are considered unreliable. Starting with 2013–2016 data, the reliability of survey percentage estimates was assessed using new multistep National Center for Health Statistics data presentation standards for proportions. Prior to 2013–2016 data, the reliability of estimates for earlier years was evaluated based on relative standard errors (RSE). Data preceded by an asterisk have an RSE of 20%–30%. Data not shown have an RSE greater than 30%.

[1]Persons of Hispanic and Mexican origin may be of any race. Starting with 1999 data, race-specific estimates are tabulated according to the 1997 Revisions to the Standards for the Classification of Federal Data on Race and Ethnicity and are not strictly comparable with estimates for earlier years. The non-Hispanic race categories shown in the table conform to the 1997 Standards. Starting with 1999 data, race-specific estimates are for persons who reported only one racial group. Prior to data year 1999, estimates were tabulated according to the 1977 Standards. Estimates for single-race categories prior to 1999 included persons who reported one race, or if they reported more than one race, identified one race as best representing their race.

[2]Hypertension is defined as having measured high blood pressure or taking antihypertensive medication. High blood pressure is defined as having measured systolic pressure of at least 140 mm Hg or diastolic pressure of at least 90 mm Hg. Those with high blood pressure also may be taking prescribed medicine for high blood pressure. Those taking antihypertensive medication may not have measured high blood pressure but are still classified as having hypertension. Pregnant women were excluded. In 2017, a revised set of practice guidelines for defining high blood pressure was released but has not been widely adopted. Therefore, the high blood pressure cutoffs used to define hypertension and uncontrolled high blood pressure in Health, United States continue to use the original definition of 140 mm Hg/90 mm Hg.

[3]Respondents were asked, "Are you now taking prescribed medicine for your high blood pressure?"

[4]Uncontrolled high blood pressure among persons with hypertension is defined as having measured high blood pressure among those with measured high blood pressure or reporting taking antihypertensive medication. High blood pressure is defined as having measured systolic pressure of at least 140 mm Hg or diastolic pressure of at least 90 mm Hg. Pregnant women were excluded. In 2017, a revised set of practice guidelines for defining high blood pressure was released but has not been widely adopted. Therefore, the high blood pressure cutoffs used to define hypertension and uncontrolled high blood pressure in Health, United States continue to use the original definition of 140 mm Hg/90 mm Hg.

Table 3-16. Cholesterol Among Persons 20 Years of Age and Over, by Selected Characteristics, Selected Years, 1988–1994 Through 2013–2016

(Percent, number; data are based on interviews and laboratory data of a sample of the civilian noninstitutionalized population.)

Sex, age, race and Hispanic origin[1], and percent of poverty level	1988–1994	1999–2002	2003–2006	2009–2012	2011–2014	2013–2016
PERCENT OF POPULATION WITH HYPERCHOLESTEROLEMIA (SERUM TOTAL CHOLESTEROL GREATER THAN OR EQUAL TO 240 MG/DL OR TAKING CHOLESTEROL-LOWERING MEDICATIONS)[2]						
20 Years and Over, Age-Adjusted[3]						
Both Sexes[4]	22.8	25.0	27.7	27.8	27.8	27.1
Male	21.1	25.3	27.7	27.9	28.4	29.1
Female	24.0	24.3	27.4	27.5	27.3	25.3
Not Hispanic or Latino						
White only	22.9	25.8	28.5	28.2	28.7	28.0
White only, male	21.1	26.0	28.7	28.1	29.4	30.0
White only, female	24.2	25.1	28.2	28.2	28.0	26.1
Black or African American only	21.3	21.3	23.2	25.9	25.2	24.2
Black or African American only, male	18.6	20.1	22.8	25.6	24.5	25.0
Black or African American only, female	23.1	22.0	23.3	26.3	25.7	23.7
Asian only	NA	NA	NA	NA	26.0	25.7
Asian only, male	NA	NA	NA	NA	27.4	27.3
Asian only, female	NA	NA	NA	NA	24.6	24.4
Hispanic or Latino	NA	NA	NA	28.3	26.3	24.8
Male	NA	NA	NA	29.4	26.6	26.8
Female	NA	NA	NA	27.1	25.8	22.8
	20.0	20.6	24.2	26.7	24.8	24.7
Mexican origin, male	19.9	21.6	24.2	27.2	26.6	28.2
Mexican origin, female	19.8	19.3	24.1	26.2	22.7	21.1
Percent of Poverty Level[5]						
Below 100 percent	23.0	25.0	27.9	28.7	29.2	26.0
100 percent to 199 percent	22.1	25.9	27.6	27.1	25.4	26.5
200 percent to 399 percent	23.1	26.5	27.5	28.1	29.0	28.8
400 percent or more	21.7	23.1	27.9	27.4	28.1	27.3
20 Years and Over, Crude						
Both Sexes[4]	21.5	25.0	28.0	29.5	29.8	29.4
Male	19.6	25.1	27.5	28.8	29.5	30.6
Female	23.2	24.8	28.5	30.1	30.1	28.4
Not Hispanic or Latino						
White only	22.3	26.9	30.3	32.2	33.1	32.7
White only, male	20.0	26.8	29.7	30.9	32.6	33.8
White only, female	24.5	27.0	30.8	33.4	33.5	31.6
Black or African American only	18.1	19.3	21.7	25.0	24.8	24.1
Black or African American only, male	16.0	18.5	21.3	24.4	24.0	24.3
Black or African American only, female	19.7	19.9	21.9	25.5	25.4	23.8
Asian only	NA	NA	NA	NA	24.7	24.7
Asian only, male	NA	NA	NA	NA	25.9	26.0
Asian only, female	NA	NA	NA	NA	23.7	23.5
Hispanic or Latino	NA	NA	NA	22.7	21.2	21.0
Male	NA	NA	NA	23.5	21.3	22.9
Female	NA	NA	NA	21.9	21.1	19.1
	15.6	15.5	19.0	20.7	19.1	20.7
Mexican origin, male	16.2	17.0	19.3	21.9	21.2	24.3
Mexican origin, female	14.9	13.8	18.7	19.4	16.8	17.0
Percent of Poverty Level[5]						
Below 100 percent	19.4	21.6	24.1	24.1	25.3	23.8
100 percent to 199 percent	21.3	25.4	28.3	28.2	27.4	28.5
200 percent to 399 percent	21.3	26.2	28.1	30.5	31.6	30.8
400 percent or more	21.9	24.2	28.7	31.6	32.2	31.5
Male						
20 to 44 years	13.1	16.1	16.5	12.6	12.3	13.1
20 to 34 years	8.2	10.4	10.2	6.6	6.7	7.6
35 to 44 years	21.0	23.1	25.2	21.2	21.1	22.4
45 to 64 years	30.1	36.0	35.7	39.8	39.3	39.5
45 to 54 years	29.6	34.1	32.4	35.7	32.9	31.2
55 to 64 years	30.8	39.1	41.6	44.5	46.0	48.3
65 to 74 years	27.4	36.3	49.4	50.7	55.8	56.7
75 years and over	24.4	29.0	37.1	51.2	54.4	56.4

NA = Not available.

[1]Persons of Hispanic and Mexican origin may be of any race. Starting with 1999 data, race-specific estimates are tabulated according to the 1997 Revisions to the Standards for the Classification of Federal Data on Race and Ethnicity and are not strictly comparable with estimates for earlier years. The non-Hispanic race categories shown in the table conform to the 1997 Standards. Starting with 1999 data, race-specific estimates are for persons who reported only one racial group. Prior to data year 1999, estimates were tabulated according to the 1977 Standards. Estimates for single-race categories prior to 1999 included persons who reported one race, or if they reported more than one race, identified one race as best representing their race.
[2]Hypercholesterolemia is defined as measured serum total cholesterol greater than or equal to 240 mgdL (6.20 mmol/L) or reporting taking cholesterol-lowering medications. Respondents were asked, "Are you now following this advice [from a doctor or health professional] to take prescribed medicine [to lower your cholesterol]?"
[3]Estimates are age-adjusted to the year 2000 standard population using five age groups: 20–34 years, 35–44 years, 45–54 years, 55–64 years, and 65 years and over. Age-adjusted estimates may differ from other age-adjusted estimates based on the same data and presented elsewhere if different age groups are used in the adjustment procedure.
[4]Includes persons of all races and Hispanic origins, not just those shown separately.
[5]Percent of poverty level was calculated by dividing family income by the U.S. Department of Health and Human Services' poverty guidelines specific to family size, as well as the appropriate year, and state. Persons with unknown percent of poverty level are excluded (7% in 2013–2016).

Table 3-16. Cholesterol Among Persons 20 Years of Age and Over, by Selected Characteristics, Selected Years, 1988–1994 Through 2013–2016—Continued

(Percent, number; data are based on interviews and laboratory data of a sample of the civilian noninstitutionalized population.)

Sex, age, race and Hispanic origin[1], and percent of poverty level	1988–1994	1999–2002	2003–2006	2009–2012	2011–2014	2013–2016
Female						
20 to 44 years	9.9	11.4	12.9	9.4	9.0	8.2
20 to 34 years	7.3	9.1	10.8	6.3	6.1	6.1
35 to 44 years	13.5	14.4	15.8	14.0	13.2	11.2
45 to 64 years	36.4	31.7	37.3	42.4	40.6	35.7
45 to 54 years	28.2	27.2	29.6	31.2	31.2	29.9
55 to 64 years	45.8	39.2	49.2	55.3	51.2	42.1
65 to 74 years	46.9	51.9	55.3	57.7	58.1	58.5
75 years and over	41.2	44.0	47.3	53.3	59.1	56.9
PERCENT OF POPULATION WITH HIGH CHOLESTEROL (SERUM TOTAL CHOLESTEROL GREATER THAN OR EQUAL TO 240 MG/DL)[6]						
20 Years and Over, Age-Adjusted[3]						
Both Sexes[4]	20.8	17.3	16.3	12.9	11.9	11.7
Male	19.0	16.4	15.1	11.7	10.8	11.0
Female	22.0	17.8	17.1	14.0	12.7	12.2
Not Hispanic or Latino						
White only	20.8	17.5	16.9	13.2	12.4	12.1
White only, male	18.8	16.5	15.5	11.6	11.2	10.9
White only, female	22.2	18.1	18.0	14.7	13.3	13.2
Black or African American only	19.5	15.5	12.2	10.0	8.6	8.9
Black or African American only, male	16.9	12.4	10.9	9.0	7.7	9.1
Black or African American only, female	21.4	17.7	13.3	10.8	9.4	8.7
Asian only	NA	NA	NA	NA	10.9	11.3
Asian only, male	NA	NA	NA	NA	10.6	11.8
Asian only, female	NA	NA	NA	NA	11.0	11.0
Hispanic or Latino	NA	NA	NA	14.4	13.0	11.5
Male	NA	NA	NA	14.7	13.1	12.7
Female	NA	NA	NA	13.9	12.7	10.2
	18.7	15.8	16.1	13.2	11.2	11.2
Mexican origin, male	18.5	17.4	17.6	13.5	12.8	13.9
Mexican origin, female	18.7	13.8	14.4	12.8	9.3	8.4
Percent of Poverty Level[5]						
Below 100 percent	20.6	18.3	18.1	13.4	12.3	10.9
100 percent to 199 percent	20.6	19.1	16.7	13.2	11.3	11.5
200 percent to 399 percent	20.8	18.9	15.8	13.2	13.0	12.9
400 percent or more	19.5	14.4	15.9	12.3	11.5	11.7
20 Years and Over, Crude						
Both Sexes[4]	19.6	17.3	16.4	13.4	12.1	11.8
Male	17.7	16.5	15.2	11.8	10.7	10.7
Female	21.3	18.0	17.5	14.9	13.5	12.9
Not Hispanic or Latino						
White only	20.3	18.0	17.4	14.2	12.9	12.5
White only, male	18.0	16.9	15.7	11.8	10.8	10.4
White only, female	22.5	19.1	18.9	16.5	14.9	14.5
Black or African American only	16.7	14.4	11.7	9.9	8.6	9.0
Black or African American only, male	14.7	12.2	10.8	8.8	7.4	9.0
Black or African American only, female	18.2	16.1	12.5	10.6	9.5	9.0
Asian only	NA	NA	NA	NA	10.9	11.2
Asian only, male	NA	NA	NA	NA	10.9	11.7
Asian only, female	NA	NA	NA	NA	10.9	10.8
Hispanic or Latino	NA	NA	NA	13.2	12.1	11.2
Male	NA	NA	NA	14.1	12.7	13.1
Female	NA	NA	NA	12.3	11.6	9.4
	14.9	12.9	14.2	12.0	10.6	11.1
Mexican origin, male	15.4	15.0	15.7	13.0	12.3	14.3
Mexican origin, female	14.3	10.7	12.6	10.9	8.8	7.8
Percent of Poverty Level[5]						
Below 100 percent	17.6	16.4	16.8	12.0	11.3	10.3
100 percent to 199 percent	19.8	18.2	16.0	12.9	11.1	11.2
200 percent to 399 percent	19.3	18.7	15.8	13.9	13.4	12.8
400 percent or more	19.9	15.5	17.1	13.6	12.5	12.7

NA = Not available.

[1]Persons of Hispanic and Mexican origin may be of any race. Starting with 1999 data, race-specific estimates are tabulated according to the 1997 Revisions to the Standards for the Classification of Federal Data on Race and Ethnicity and are not strictly comparable with estimates for earlier years. The non-Hispanic race categories shown in the table conform to the 1997 Standards. Starting with 1999 data, race-specific estimates are for persons who reported only one racial group. Prior to data year 1999, estimates were tabulated according to the 1977 Standards. Estimates for single-race categories prior to 1999 included persons who reported one race, or if they reported more than one race, identified one race as best representing their race.
[3]Estimates are age-adjusted to the year 2000 standard population using five age groups: 20–34 years, 35–44 years, 45–54 years, 55–64 years, and 65 years and over. Age-adjusted estimates may differ from other age-adjusted estimates based on the same data and presented elsewhere if different age groups are used in the adjustment procedure.
[4]Includes persons of all races and Hispanic origins, not just those shown separately.
[5]Percent of poverty level was calculated by dividing family income by the U.S. Department of Health and Human Services' poverty guidelines specific to family size, as well as the appropriate year, and state. Persons with unknown percent of poverty level are excluded (7% in 2013–2016).
[6]High cholesterol is defined as serum total cholesterol greater than or equal to 240 mg/dL (6.20 mmol/L), regardless of whether the respondent reported taking cholesterol-lowering medications.

Table 3-16. Cholesterol Among Persons 20 Years of Age and Over, by Selected Characteristics, Selected Years, 1988–1994 Through 2013–2016—*Continued*

(Percent, number; data are based on interviews and laboratory data of a sample of the civilian noninstitutionalized population.)

Sex, age, race and Hispanic origin[1], and percent of poverty level	1988–1994	1999–2002	2003–2006	2009–2012	2011–2014	2013–2016
Male						
20 to 44 years	12.5	14.2	14.1	10.0	10.0	10.4
20 to 34 years	8.2	9.8	9.5	6.0	6.0	6.7
35 to 44 years	19.4	19.7	20.5	15.8	16.2	16.6
45 to 64 years	27.2	22.2	19.1	16.2	13.6	13.9
45 to 54 years	26.6	23.6	20.8	18.0	15.7	15.8
55 to 64 years	28.0	19.9	16.0	14.1	11.5	11.8
65 to 74 years	21.9	13.7	10.9	8.1	7.6	6.4
75 years and over	20.4	10.2	9.6	*5.5	*3.6	2.9
Female						
20 to 44 years	9.4	10.4	11.3	7.6	7.2	6.7
20 to 34 years	7.3	8.9	10.3	5.7	5.4	5.6
35 to 44 years	12.3	12.4	12.7	10.4	9.8	8.3
45 to 64 years	33.4	23.0	23.9	22.4	19.9	18.6
45 to 54 years	26.7	21.4	19.7	18.7	18.0	18.8
55 to 64 years	40.9	25.6	30.5	26.6	22.1	18.3
65 to 74 years	41.3	32.3	24.2	19.6	15.8	18.4
75 years and over	38.2	26.5	18.6	16.2	16.1	13.8
MEAN SERUM TOTAL CHOLESTEROL LEVEL, MG/DL						
20 Years and Over, Age-Adjusted[3]						
Both Sexes[4]	206	203	200	195	192	191
Male	204	202	198	192	189	188
Female	207	204	202	198	195	193
Not Hispanic or Latino						
White only	206	204	201	196	193	192
White only, male	205	202	198	192	189	188
White only, female	208	205	203	199	196	194
Black or African American only	205	199	194	190	186	184
Black or African American only, male	202	195	193	188	183	183
Black or African American only, female	207	202	195	192	189	185
Asian only	NA	NA	NA	NA	191	191
Asian only, male	NA	NA	NA	NA	189	190
Asian only, female	NA	NA	NA	NA	192	192
Hispanic or Latino	NA	NA	NA	197	194	192
Male	NA	NA	NA	196	193	192
Female	NA	NA	NA	196	195	191
Mexican origin, male	206	202	202	196	192	191
Mexican origin, female	206	204	203	197	194	193
	206	199	200	194	191	190
Percent of Poverty Level[5]						
Below 100 percent	205	201	203	196	191	187
100 percent to 199 percent	205	204	201	194	191	191
200 percent to 399 percent	207	205	199	195	193	191
400 percent or more	205	202	201	196	194	193
20 Years and Over, Crude						
Both Sexes[4]	204	203	200	196	192	191
Male	202	202	198	193	188	188
Female	206	204	202	199	196	194
Not Hispanic or Latino						
White only	206	205	202	197	194	192
White only, male	203	203	198	193	188	187
White only, female	208	206	205	202	199	197
Black or African American only	200	197	193	190	186	184
Black or African American only, male	198	194	192	187	183	183
Black or African American only, female	201	199	194	191	189	185
Asian only	NA	NA	NA	NA	191	191
Asian only, male	NA	NA	NA	NA	190	190
Asian only, female	NA	NA	NA	NA	192	192
Hispanic or Latino	NA	NA	NA	195	193	191
Male	NA	NA	NA	197	193	193
Female	NA	NA	NA	194	193	190

NA = Not available.

[1]Persons of Hispanic and Mexican origin may be of any race. Starting with 1999 data, race-specific estimates are tabulated according to the 1997 Revisions to the Standards for the Classification of Federal Data on Race and Ethnicity and are not strictly comparable with estimates for earlier years. The non-Hispanic race categories shown in the table conform to the 1997 Standards. Starting with 1999 data, race-specific estimates are for persons who reported only one racial group. Prior to data year 1999, estimates were tabulated according to the 1977 Standards. Estimates for single-race categories prior to 1999 included persons who reported one race, or if they reported more than one race, identified one race as best representing their race.
[3]Estimates are age-adjusted to the year 2000 standard population using five age groups: 20–34 years, 35–44 years, 45–54 years, 55–64 years, and 65 years and over. Age-adjusted estimates may differ from other age-adjusted estimates based on the same data and presented elsewhere if different age groups are used in the adjustment procedure.
[4]Includes persons of all races and Hispanic origins, not just those shown separately.
[5]Percent of poverty level was calculated by dividing family income by the U.S. Department of Health and Human Services' poverty guidelines specific to family size, as well as the appropriate year, and state. Persons with unknown percent of poverty level are excluded (7% in 2013–2016).

Table 3-16. Cholesterol Among Persons 20 Years of Age and Over, by Selected Characteristics, Selected Years, 1988–1994 Through 2013–2016—*Continued*

(Percent, number; data are based on interviews and laboratory data of a sample of the civilian noninstitutionalized population.)

Sex, age, race and Hispanic origin[1], and percent of poverty level	1988–1994	1999–2002	2003–2006	2009–2012	2011–2014	2013–2016
Mexican origin, male...	199	197	198	196	192	191
Mexican origin, female..	199	200	200	198	194	194
	198	194	196	193	189	188
Percent of Poverty Level[5]						
Below 100 percent	200	198	200	192	189	186
100 percent to 199 percent...................................	202	202	199	193	190	190
200 percent to 399 percent...................................	205	204	199	196	193	190
400 percent or more...	206	204	203	199	196	195
Male						
20 to 44 years..	194	196	196	191	188	187
20 to 34 years..	186	188	186	182	179	179
35 to 44 years..	206	207	209	204	202	200
45 to 64 years..	216	213	206	200	196	196
45 to 54 years..	216	215	208	203	200	201
55 to 64 years..	216	212	202	198	192	192
65 to 74 years..	212	202	191	184	180	176
75 years and over	205	195	187	173	168	168
Female						
20 to 44 years..	189	191	192	187	184	181
20 to 34 years..	184	185	188	180	179	177
35 to 44 years..	195	198	197	196	193	188
45 to 64 years..	225	215	213	212	209	207
45 to 54 years..	217	211	208	209	207	207
55 to 64 years..	235	221	219	216	210	206
65 to 74 years..	233	224	214	206	200	202
75 years and over	229	217	206	201	199	196

[1]Persons of Hispanic and Mexican origin may be of any race. Starting with 1999 data, race-specific estimates are tabulated according to the 1997 Revisions to the Standards for the Classification of Federal Data on Race and Ethnicity and are not strictly comparable with estimates for earlier years. The non-Hispanic race categories shown in the table conform to the 1997 Standards. Starting with 1999 data, race-specific estimates are for persons who reported only one racial group. Prior to data year 1999, estimates were tabulated according to the 1977 Standards. Estimates for single-race categories prior to 1999 included persons who reported one race, or if they reported more than one race, identified one race as best representing their race.
[5]Percent of poverty level was calculated by dividing family income by the U.S. Department of Health and Human Services' poverty guidelines specific to family size, as well as the appropriate year, and state. Persons with unknown percent of poverty level are excluded (7% in 2013–2016).

Table 3-17. Mean Macronutrient Intake Among Persons 20 Years of Age and Over, by Sex and Age, Selected Years, 1988–1994 Through 2011–2014

(Number, percent.)

Characteristic	1988–1994	1999–2002	2003–2006	2007–2010	2009–2012	2011–2014
Percent kcal from carbohydrates						
Both sexes, age-adjusted[1]	49.8	50.7	48.9	49.5	49.5	48.6
Both sexes, crude	49.8	50.7	48.9	49.4	49.4	48.5
20-44 years	49.2	51.3	49.3	50.1	49.9	48.8
45-64 years	49.7	49.3	47.5	48.2	48.5	47.9
65-74 years	51.1	50.5	49.2	49.0	49.0	48.2
75 years and over	53.0	52.6	51.5	51.1	51.0	50.5
Male, age-adjusted[1]	48.5	49.5	47.8	48.0	48.1	47.5
Male, crude	48.4	49.4	47.7	47.9	48.0	47.4
20-44 years	48.1	50.2	48.4	48.7	48.5	47.5
45-64 years	48.3	48.0	46.3	46.4	47.2	47.2
65-74 years	49.4	49.4	47.6	47.5	47.0	46.6
75 years and over	50.9	51.0	50.3	50.4	50.3	49.0
Female, age-adjusted[1]	51.0	51.9	49.9	50.8	50.8	49.7
Female, crude	51.0	51.9	49.9	50.7	50.7	49.6
20-44 years	50.3	52.5	50.2	51.4	51.3	50.0
45-64 years	51.0	50.6	48.7	49.8	49.8	48.6
65-74 years	52.5	51.4	50.6	50.4	50.9	49.6
75 years and over	54.2	53.7	52.4	51.6	51.6	51.6
Percent kcal from protein						
Both sexes, age-adjusted[1]	15.5	15.3	15.6	15.8	15.7	15.8
Both sexes, crude	15.4	15.3	15.6	15.8	15.7	15.8
20-44 years	15.0	14.9	15.3	15.6	15.6	15.7
45-64 years	15.9	15.6	16.0	16.0	15.8	15.8
65-74 years	16.2	16.3	15.9	16.2	16.4	16.3
75 years and over	16.0	15.4	15.6	15.8	15.8	15.7
Male, age-adjusted[1]	15.5	15.4	15.6	16.0	16.0	16.1
Male, crude	15.4	15.4	15.6	16.0	16.0	16.1
20-44 years	15.0	15.0	15.4	15.8	15.8	16.1
45-64 years	15.9	15.7	15.8	16.3	16.0	16.0
65-74 years	15.9	16.3	16.0	16.3	16.6	16.6
75 years and over	16.3	15.7	15.8	15.9	16.0	16.1
Female, age-adjusted[1]	15.5	15.2	15.6	15.6	15.5	15.5
Female, crude	15.4	15.2	15.6	15.6	15.5	15.6
20-44 years	14.9	14.8	15.2	15.4	15.3	15.3
45-64 years	15.9	15.5	16.1	15.8	15.5	15.7
65-74 years	16.5	16.3	15.9	16.1	16.2	16.1
75 years and over	15.9	15.3	15.5	15.7	15.6	15.3
Percent kcal from total fat						
Both sexes, age-adjusted[1]	33.5	33.0	33.7	33.1	32.9	33.6
Both sexes, crude	33.5	33.0	33.7	33.2	33.0	33.7
20-44 years	34.0	32.4	33.1	32.3	32.3	33.2
45-64 years	33.4	33.9	34.6	34.1	33.5	34.0
65-74 years	32.3	33.4	34.3	34.1	33.7	34.4
75 years and over	32.0	32.8	33.1	33.3	33.3	33.7
Male, age-adjusted[1]	33.8	33.0	33.5	33.1	33.0	33.6
Male, crude	33.9	33.0	33.6	33.2	33.0	33.6
20-44 years	34.1	32.2	32.6	32.2	32.2	33.0
45-64 years	33.9	34.0	34.8	34.3	33.8	34.1
65-74 years	33.0	33.4	34.5	34.4	34.1	34.5
75 years and over	33.0	33.2	33.3	33.2	33.1	34.1
Female, age-adjusted[1]	33.2	33.1	33.8	33.1	32.8	33.7
Female, crude	33.2	33.1	33.9	33.2	32.9	33.7
20-44 years	33.9	32.6	33.6	32.4	32.4	33.5
45-64 years	32.9	33.9	34.4	33.9	33.2	33.9
65-74 years	31.6	33.3	34.1	33.9	33.3	34.2
75 years and over	31.5	32.6	32.9	33.4	33.5	33.4
Percent kcal from saturated fat						
Both sexes, age-adjusted[1]	11.2	10.7	11.2	10.8	10.6	10.8
Both sexes, crude	11.2	10.7	11.2	10.9	10.6	10.8
20-44 years	11.5	10.8	11.1	10.6	10.5	10.7
45-64 years	11.1	10.8	11.4	11.1	10.8	10.8
65-74 years	10.7	10.5	11.2	11.1	10.7	10.8
75 years and over	10.7	10.3	11.0	10.9	10.8	11.1
Male, age-adjusted[1]	11.3	10.7	11.1	10.8	10.6	10.8
Male, crude	11.4	10.7	11.1	10.9	10.6	10.8
20-44 years	11.5	10.8	11.0	10.6	10.4	10.6
45-64 years	11.2	10.7	11.3	11.2	10.9	10.9
65-74 years	10.9	10.6	11.2	11.0	10.8	11.0
75 years and over	11.2	10.7	11.2	10.9	10.7	11.1
Female, age-adjusted[1]	11.1	10.7	11.2	10.9	10.6	10.8
Female, crude	11.1	10.7	11.3	10.9	10.6	10.8
20-44 years	11.4	10.8	11.2	10.7	10.5	10.8
45-64 years	10.9	10.9	11.5	11.0	10.6	10.7
65-74 years	10.4	10.4	11.3	11.2	10.7	10.6
75 years and over	10.5	10.1	10.8	11.0	10.9	11.0

[1]Age adjusted to the 2000 standard population using four age groups: 20 to 44 years, 45 to 64 years, 65 to 74 years, and 75 years and over. Age-adjusted estimates in this table may differ from other age-adjusted estimates based on the same data and presented elsewhere if different age groups are used in the adjustment procedure.

Table 3-18. Participation in Leisure-Time Aerobic and Muscle-Strengthening Activities That Meet the 2008 Federal Physical Activity Guidelines for Adults 18 Years of Age and Over, by Selected Characteristics, 2000 and 2016

(Percent; data are based on household interviews of a sample of the civilian noninstitutionalized population.)

| | 2008 Physical Activity Guidelines for Americans[1] | | | | | | | |
| Characteristic | Met both aerobic activity and muscle-strengthening guidelines | | Met neither aerobic activity nor muscle-strengthening guideline | | Met aerobic activity guideline | | Met muscle-strengthening guideline | |
	2000	2016	2000	2016	2000	2016	2000	2016
18 years and over, age-adjusted[2,3]	15.0	22.7	54.7	43.8	42.2	52.7	18.0	26.2
18 years and over, crude[3]	15.1	21.9	54.6	44.6	42.4	51.9	18.1	25.5
Age								
18 to 44 years	18.9	28.0	49.1	37.9	47.7	59.1	22.1	30.9
18 to 24 years	23.8	30.7	44.5	34.5	52.2	62.2	27.2	34.3
25 to 44 years	17.3	27.0	50.6	39.1	46.3	58.1	20.5	29.8
45 to 64 years	12.8	19.0	57.6	46.6	39.7	49.8	15.5	22.7
45 to 54 years	14.5	20.8	55.4	45.5	42.1	51.2	17.0	24.3
55 to 64 years	10.1	17.1	61.0	47.8	36.1	48.3	13.1	21.1
65 years and over	6.8	12.7	67.0	56.7	30.1	38.5	9.8	17.5
65 to 74 years	8.4	15.7	60.3	50.8	36.8	44.7	11.3	20.1
75 years and over	4.9	8.4	75.0	65.4	22.1	29.5	8.0	13.6
Sex[2]								
Male	17.9	26.6	49.6	39.7	47.4	56.3	20.8	30.6
Female	12.3	18.9	59.4	47.7	37.6	49.4	15.4	22.0
Sex and Age								
Male								
18 to 44 years	23.0	33.5	43.0	33.1	53.6	63.2	26.3	37.2
45 to 54 years	16.0	22.6	52.7	42.8	45.2	53.6	18.0	26.4
55 to 64 years	11.3	18.7	58.7	46.0	38.9	49.8	13.8	22.9
65 to 74 years	9.4	19.0	55.3	46.7	41.8	49.0	12.2	23.2
75 years and over	7.1	11.0	66.7	59.7	30.7	35.3	10.1	15.8
Female								
18 to 44 years	15.0	22.6	55.0	42.7	42.0	55.2	17.9	24.8
45 to 54 years	13.1	19.0	57.9	48.1	39.1	48.9	16.1	22.3
55 to 64 years	9.0	15.7	63.1	49.5	33.5	46.9	12.4	19.5
65 to 74 years	7.7	12.8	64.3	54.3	32.6	41.0	10.5	17.5
75 years and over	3.6	6.6	80.0	69.5	16.8	25.3	6.7	11.9
Race[2,4]								
White only	15.7	23.5	53.1	42.6	44.1	54.1	18.5	26.8
Black or African American only	12.2	20.9	64.6	51.7	31.7	44.6	16.0	24.6
American Indian or Alaska Native only	*10.6	15.0	67.1	55.2	29.7	41.8	13.9	18.2
Asian only	14.1	16.9	55.0	44.1	41.7	52.1	17.2	20.7
Native Hawaiian or Other Pacific Islander only	*	24.0	*	46.4	*	50.3	*	27.1
Two or more races	19.0	24.7	52.8	38.2	43.9	55.3	22.2	31.1
Hispanic Origin and Race[2,4]								
Hispanic or Latino	9.2	17.0	66.5	52.5	30.8	44.5	11.9	20.1
Mexican	8.1	15.6	67.0	52.8	30.0	44.5	11.3	18.4
Not Hispanic or Latino	15.8	23.9	53.2	42.0	43.7	54.5	18.8	27.4
White only	16.5	25.2	51.4	39.9	45.7	56.7	19.3	28.6
Black or African American only	12.2	20.9	64.6	51.9	31.7	44.4	16.0	24.8
Education[5,6]								
No high school diploma or GED	4.3	9.0	74.0	63.6	23.9	32.6	6.6	12.8
High school diploma or GED	9.5	13.4	61.7	55.6	35.7	41.0	12.1	16.9
Some college or more	18.9	26.7	47.1	37.9	49.4	58.6	22.4	30.2
Percent of Poverty Level[2,7]								
Below 100 percent	9.3	13.9	68.0	56.7	29.3	40.0	12.3	17.3
100 percent to 199 percent	9.0	14.8	65.5	56.0	32.0	40.5	11.5	18.4
200 percent to 399 percent	13.2	20.3	56.8	46.1	39.9	50.5	16.5	23.8
400 percent or more	20.5	30.6	45.0	33.4	52.0	63.2	23.4	34.1

* = Estimates are considered unreliable. Starting with 2016 data, the reliability of survey percentage estimates was assessed using new multistep National Center for Health Statistics data presentation standards for proportions. Prior to 2016 data, the reliability of estimates for earlier years was evaluated based on relative standard errors (RSE). Data preceded by an asterisk have an RSE of 20%–30%. Data not shown have an RSE greater than 30%.

[1]Starting with Health, United States, 2010, measures of physical activity shown in this table changed to reflect the federal 2008 Physical Activity Guidelines for Americans (available from: https://health.gov/paguidelines/pdf/paguide.pdf). This table presents four measures of physical activity that are of interest to the public health community: the percentage of adults who met the federal 2008 guidelines for both aerobic activity and muscle strengthening; the percentage who met neither the aerobic-activity guidelines nor the muscle-strengthening guidelines; the percentage who met the aerobic-activity guidelines; and the percentage who met the muscle-strengthening guidelines. Persons who met neither the aerobic-activity nor the muscle-strengthening guidelines were unable to be active, were completely inactive, or had some aerobic or muscle-strengthening activities but amounts were insufficient to meet the guidelines. The percentage of persons who met the aerobic-activity guidelines includes those who may or may not have also met the muscle-strengthening guidelines. Similarly, the percentage of persons who met the muscle-strengthening guidelines includes those who may or may not have also met the aerobic-activity guidelines. The federal 2008 guidelines recommend that for substantial health benefits adults perform at least 150 minutes (2 hours and 30 minutes) a week of moderate-intensity, or 75 minutes (1 hour and 15 minutes) a week of vigorous-intensity aerobic physical activity, or an equivalent combination of moderate- and vigorous-intensity aerobic activity. Aerobic activity should be performed in episodes of at least 10 minutes, and preferably should be spread throughout the week. The 2008 guidelines also recommend that adults perform muscle-strengthening activities that are moderate or high intensity and involve all major muscle groups on 2 or more days a week, because these activities provide additional health benefits.
[2]Estimates are age-adjusted to the year 2000 standard population using five age groups: 18–44 years, 45–54 years, 55–64 years, 65–74 years, and 75 years and over. Age-adjusted estimates in this table may differ from other age-adjusted estimates based on the same data and presented elsewhere if different age groups are used in the adjustment procedure.
[3]Includes all other races not shown separately, unknown education level, and unknown disability status.
[4]The race groups White, Black, American Indian or Alaska Native, Asian, Native Hawaiian or Other Pacific Islander, and 2 or more races include persons of Hispanic and non-Hispanic origin. Persons of Hispanic origin may be of any race. Starting with 1999 data, race-specific estimates are tabulated according to the 1997 Revisions to the Standards for the Classification of Federal Data on Race and Ethnicity and are not strictly comparable with estimates for earlier years. The five single-race categories and multiple-race categories shown in the table conform to the 1997 Standards. Starting with 1999 data, race-specific estimates are for persons who reported only one racial group; the category 2 or more races includes persons who reported more than one racial group. Prior to 1999, data were tabulated according to the 1977 Standards with four racial groups, and the Asian only category included Native Hawaiian or Other Pacific Islander. Estimates for single-race categories prior to 1999 included persons who reported one race, or if they reported more than one race, identified one race as best representing their race. Starting with 2003 data, race responses of other race and unspecified multiple race were treated as missing, and then race was imputed if these were the only race responses. Almost all persons with a race response of other race were of Hispanic origin.
[5]Estimates are for persons 25 years of age and over and are age-adjusted to the year 2000 standard population using five age groups: 25–44 years, 45–54 years, 55–64 years, 65–74 years, and 75 years and over.
[6]GED is General Educational Development high school equivalency diploma.
[7]Percent of poverty level is based on family income and family size and composition using U.S. Census Bureau poverty thresholds. Missing family income data were imputed for 1997 and beyond.

Table 3-18. Participation in Leisure-Time Aerobic and Muscle-Strengthening Activities That Meet the 2008 Federal Physical Activity Guidelines for Adults 18 Years of Age and Over, by Selected Characteristics, 2000 and 2016—Continued

(Percent; data are based on household interviews of a sample of the civilian noninstitutionalized population.)

	2008 Physical Activity Guidelines for Americans[1]							
	Met both aerobic activity and muscle-strengthening guidelines		Met neither aerobic activity nor muscle-strengthening guideline		Met aerobic activity guideline		Met muscle-strengthening guideline	
Characteristic	2000	2016	2000	2016	2000	2016	2000	2016
Hispanic Origin and Race and Percent of Poverty Level[2,4,7]								
Hispanic or Latino								
Below 100 percent	4.4	11.5	75.2	59.8	22.1	37.2	7.2	14.6
100 percent to 199 percent	5.0	13.4	72.2	60.9	25.8	37.1	7.1	15.4
200 percent to 399 percent	10.2	18.3	63.1	51.4	33.0	46.2	14.0	20.8
400 percent or more	19.6	25.2	52.8	37.0	45.1	57.8	21.7	30.5
Not Hispanic or Latino								
White only								
Below 100 percent	11.7	17.0	63.5	53.3	34.0	43.6	14.7	20.0
100 percent to 199 percent	10.3	15.1	62.6	53.2	34.8	43.2	12.9	18.6
200 percent to 399 percent	13.9	21.4	54.7	43.7	42.3	52.8	16.9	25.0
400 percent or more	21.0	32.0	43.7	31.6	53.4	65.1	23.8	35.3
Black or African American only								
Below 100 percent	9.5	10.8	72.1	63.2	25.4	34.2	12.1	14.1
100 percent to 199 percent	9.5	15.6	69.2	58.8	28.0	36.8	12.3	20.2
200 percent to 399 percent	11.8	21.8	64.3	47.6	31.4	48.2	16.2	26.1
400 percent or more	17.6	33.4	54.9	40.9	40.3	55.6	22.4	36.8
Disability Measure[2,8]								
A lot of difficulty or cannot do at all	NA	9.6	NA	62.2	NA	30.4	NA	17.0
Some difficulty	NA	18.9	NA	46.7	NA	49.4	NA	22.8
No difficulty	NA	25.9	NA	39.2	NA	57.9	NA	28.9
Geographic Region[2]								
Northeast	17.0	23.9	51.8	44.1	45.3	52.3	20.0	27.6
Midwest	16.4	23.4	53.4	42.0	43.5	53.9	19.3	27.4
South	12.1	20.1	59.7	48.0	37.3	48.8	15.1	23.5
West	16.7	25.1	50.1	39.2	46.9	57.8	19.7	28.0
Location of residence[2,9]								
Within MSA	15.7	23.8	54.1	42.7	42.9	53.7	18.6	27.4
Outside MSA	12.3	15.5	56.9	50.8	39.9	46.4	15.5	18.4

NA = Not available.

[1]Starting with *Health, United States, 2010,* measures of physical activity shown in this table changed to reflect the federal 2008 Physical Activity Guidelines for Americans (available from: https://health.gov/paguidelines/pdf/paguide.pdf). This table presents four measures of physical activity that are of interest to the public health community: the percentage of adults who met the federal 2008 guidelines for both aerobic activity and muscle strengthening; the percentage who met neither the aerobic-activity guidelines nor the muscle-strengthening guidelines; the percentage who met the aerobic-activity guidelines; and the percentage who met the muscle-strengthening guidelines. Persons who met neither the aerobic-activity nor the muscle-strengthening guidelines were unable to be active, were completely inactive, or had some aerobic or muscle-strengthening activities but amounts were insufficient to meet the guidelines. The percentage of persons who met the aerobic-activity guidelines includes those who may or may not have also met the muscle-strengthening guidelines. Similarly, the percentage of persons who met the muscle-strengthening guidelines includes those who may or may not have also met the aerobic-activity guidelines. The federal 2008 guidelines recommend that for substantial health benefits adults perform at least 150 minutes (2 hours and 30 minutes) a week of moderate-intensity, or 75 minutes (1 hour and 15 minutes) a week of vigorous-intensity aerobic physical activity, or an equivalent combination of moderate- and vigorous-intensity aerobic activity. Aerobic activity should be performed in episodes of at least 10 minutes, and preferably should be spread throughout the week. The 2008 guidelines also recommend that adults perform muscle-strengthening activities that are moderate or high intensity and involve all major muscle groups on 2 or more days a week, because these activities provide additional health benefits.
[2]Estimates are age-adjusted to the year 2000 standard population using five age groups: 18–44 years, 45–54 years, 55–64 years, 65–74 years, and 75 years and over. Age-adjusted estimates in this table may differ from other age-adjusted estimates based on the same data and presented elsewhere if different age groups are used in the adjustment procedure.
[4]The race groups White, Black, American Indian or Alaska Native, Asian, Native Hawaiian or Other Pacific Islander, and 2 or more races include persons of Hispanic and non-Hispanic origin. Persons of Hispanic origin may be of any race. Starting with 1999 data, race-specific estimates are tabulated according to the 1997 Revisions to the Standards for the Classification of Federal Data on Race and Ethnicity and are not strictly comparable with estimates for earlier years. The five single-race categories and multiple-race categories shown in the table conform to the 1997 Standards. Starting with 1999 data, race-specific estimates are for persons who reported only one racial group; the category 2 or more races includes persons who reported more than one racial group. Prior to 1999, data were tabulated according to the 1977 Standards with four racial groups, and the Asian only category included Native Hawaiian or Other Pacific Islander. Estimates for single-race categories prior to 1999 included persons who reported one race, or if they reported more than one race, identified one race as best representing their race. Starting with 2003 data, race responses of other race and unspecified multiple race were treated as missing, and then race was imputed if these were the only race responses. Almost all persons with a race response of other race were of Hispanic origin.
[7]Percent of poverty level is based on family income and family size and composition using U.S. Census Bureau poverty thresholds. Missing family income data were imputed for 1997 and beyond.
[8]Functional limitation is defined by the reported level of difficulty in six functioning domains: seeing (even if wearing glasses), hearing (even if wearing hearing aids), mobility (walking or climbing stairs), communication (understanding or being understood by others), cognition (remembering or concentrating), and self-care (such as washing all over or dressing). Respondents with answers to one or more of the six questions were included in one of three mutually-exclusive categories. Those responding "A lot of difficulty" or "Cannot do at all/unable to do" to at least one question were classified in the "A lot of difficulty/cannot do" category. Of the remaining, those responding "Some difficulty" to at least one question were classified in the "Some difficulty" category, and those responding "No difficulty" to at least one question were classified in the "No difficulty" category. Those responding "Don't know" or "Refused" to all six questions were excluded. During 2010–2016, 1%–8% of respondents were missing data and excluded.
[9]MSA = MSA is metropolitan statistical area. Starting with 2016 data, MSA status is determined using 2010 Census data and the 2010 standards for defining MSAs.

Table 3-19. Healthy Weight, Overweight, and Obesity Among Persons 20 Years of Age and Over, by Selected Characteristics, Selected Years, 1988–1994 Through 2013–2016

(Percent; data are based on measured height and weight of a sample of the civilian noninstitutionalized population.)

Sex, age, race and Hispanic origin[1], and percent of poverty level	Healthy weight (BMI from 18.5 to 24.9)[2]								
	1988–1994	1999–2002	2001–2004	2003–2006	2005–2008	2007–2010	2009–2012	2011–2014	2013–2016
20 Years and Over, Age-Adjusted[3]									
Both Sexes[4]	41.6	33.0	32.3	31.6	30.8	29.8	29.6	28.9	27.7
Male	37.9	30.2	28.3	26.6	26.1	25.7	26.2	26.0	24.2
Female	45.0	35.7	36.1	36.5	35.2	33.7	32.8	31.7	31.0
Not Hispanic or Latino									
White only	43.1	34.6	33.9	33.2	32.1	31.4	31.2	30.0	28.8
White only, male	37.3	29.6	28.0	26.8	26.0	25.5	26.2	25.6	23.6
White only, female	48.7	39.5	39.8	39.6	37.8	36.9	36.0	34.3	33.8
Black or African American	33.9	27.6	24.2	22.7	23.3	22.7	21.7	22.0	22.5
Black or African American only, male	40.1	34.7	30.8	27.0	26.7	28.5	28.0	29.0	28.4
Black or African American only, female	29.2	21.6	18.9	19.2	20.4	17.9	16.4	16.0	17.6
Asian	NA	NA	NA	NA	NA	NA	NA	55.7	53.8
Asian only, male	NA	NA	NA	NA	NA	NA	NA	50.2	47.4
Asian only, female	NA	NA	NA	NA	NA	NA	NA	60.5	59.3
Hispanic or Latino	NA	NA	NA	NA	NA	21.1	21.0	20.9	18.8
Male	NA	NA	NA	NA	NA	19.0	19.3	20.9	18.8
Female	NA	NA	NA	NA	NA	23.5	22.9	19.5	17.5
Mexican origin	30.1	26.9	25.9	24.4	22.7	19.6	19.0	22.3	20.4
Mexican origin, male	30.2	26.5	25.3	23.8	21.8	18.5	17.5	17.7	15.9
Mexican origin, female	29.8	27.5	26.5	25.1	24.1	21.3	20.9	16.5	16.9
								19.1	15.0
Percent of Poverty Level[5]									
Below 100 percent	37.5	32.7	34.3	32.1	29.1	27.3	27.3	28.1	26.4
100 percent to 199 percent	39.3	30.5	31.9	31.3	28.3	27.6	26.5	24.6	24.4
200 percent to 399 percent	41.8	29.6	29.4	29.7	30.0	29.7	30.0	27.5	26.0
400 percent or more	45.5	36.5	35.1	33.7	33.5	32.1	32.0	33.4	31.6
20 Years and Over, Crude									
Both Sexes[4]	42.6	32.9	32.2	31.4	30.5	29.6	29.2	28.6	27.4
Male	39.4	30.4	28.4	26.6	26.1	25.8	26.2	26.2	24.4
Female	45.7	35.4	35.8	35.9	34.8	33.2	31.9	31.0	30.3
Not Hispanic or Latino									
White only	43.6	34.0	33.2	32.3	31.3	30.4	30.0	29.0	27.8
White only, male	38.2	29.2	27.4	26.2	25.4	24.8	25.6	25.1	23.2
White only, female	48.8	38.7	38.8	38.2	36.9	35.7	34.2	32.8	32.1
Black or African American	35.9	28.2	24.8	22.7	23.5	23.0	21.7	21.9	22.8
Black or African American only, male	41.5	35.9	31.5	27.1	27.4	29.4	28.5	29.3	29.2
Black or African American only, female	31.2	21.8	19.3	19.2	20.3	17.6	16.1	15.8	17.6
Asian	NA	NA	NA	NA	NA	NA	NA	55.8	53.7
Asian only, male	NA	NA	NA	NA	NA	NA	NA	50.7	47.4
Asian only, female	NA	NA	NA	NA	NA	NA	NA	60.3	59.2
Hispanic or Latino	NA	NA	NA	NA	NA	22.3	22.1	21.7	19.6
Male	NA	NA	NA	NA	NA	20.3	20.5	20.2	18.0
Female	NA	NA	NA	NA	NA	24.6	23.8	23.1	21.3
Mexican origin	34.0	29.4	28.0	25.5	23.7	20.8	19.9	18.4	16.6
Mexican origin, male	35.2	29.4	28.1	25.2	22.8	19.5	17.9	17.0	17.4
Mexican origin, female	32.5	29.5	28.0	25.8	24.7	22.3	22.2	19.9	15.8
Percent of Poverty Level[5]									
Below 100 percent	39.8	34.5	36.2	33.2	30.9	29.2	29.2	29.8	27.5
100 percent to 199 percent	41.5	31.5	32.6	31.7	28.8	28.0	26.8	25.2	25.1
200 percent to 399 percent	42.9	29.7	29.3	29.6	30.0	29.5	29.6	27.4	26.0
400 percent or more	44.6	35.3	33.5	32.1	31.8	30.5	30.3	31.3	29.8
Male									
20 to 34 years	51.1	40.3	38.3	35.9	38.0	37.5	37.5	37.6	34.6
35 to 44 years	33.4	29.0	26.5	24.1	20.9	19.8	21.0	20.5	19.3
45 to 54 years	33.6	24.0	21.2	20.8	21.7	21.8	20.0	18.7	18.5
55 to 64 years	28.6	23.8	22.2	19.3	18.5	19.4	21.9	22.7	22.3
65 to 74 years	30.1	22.8	23.1	21.2	20.2	21.6	22.4	22.2	19.3
75 years and over	40.9	32.0	32.1	33.1	28.1	25.4	28.2	28.1	24.3
Female									
20 to 34 years	57.9	42.5	44.2	45.1	40.5	41.1	40.8	38.1	37.5
35 to 44 years	47.1	37.1	38.3	37.6	36.2	34.4	35.2	32.5	31.3
45 to 54 years	37.2	33.1	31.0	31.1	32.1	30.7	27.3	27.8	29.3
55 to 64 years	31.5	27.6	29.2	29.5	29.9	26.7	23.8	24.2	23.8
65 to 74 years	37.0	26.4	27.0	28.5	28.8	23.9	23.5	26.9	23.9
75 years and over	43.0	36.9	34.6	35.4	36.3	35.4	35.3	32.9	31.0

NOTE: Percentages do not sum to 100 because the percentage of persons with BMI less than 18.5 is not shown. Additionally, the percentage of persons with obesity is embedded in the percent overweight or obese and can be further partitioned into Grades 1, 2, and 3 obesity. Age of the participant (in years) is at the time of screening. Height is measured without shoes. Estimates exclude pregnant women.

NA = Not available.

[1]Persons of Hispanic and Mexican origin may be of any race. Starting with 1999 data, race-specific estimates are tabulated according to the 1997 Revisions to the Standards for the Classification of Federal Data on Race and Ethnicity and are not strictly comparable with estimates for earlier years. The non-Hispanic race categories shown in the table conform to the 1997 Standards. Starting with 1999 data, race-specific estimates are for persons who reported only one racial group. Prior to data year 1999, estimates were tabulated according to the 1977 Standards. Estimates for single-race categories prior to 1999 included persons who reported one race, or if they reported more than one race, identified one race as best representing their race.

[2]Body mass index (BMI) equals weight in kilograms divided by height in meters squared. The National Health and Nutrition Examination Survey (NHANES) variable Body Mass Index is rounded to one decimal place and is used to assign persons to BMI categories. Estimates in this table may differ from other estimates where BMI is directly calculated using the NHANES measured weight and measured height variables.

[3]Estimates are age-adjusted to the year 2000 standard population using five age groups: 20–34 years, 35–44 years, 45–54 years, 55–64 years, and 65 years and over. Age-adjusted estimates in this table may differ from other age-adjusted estimates based on the same data and presented elsewhere if different age groups are used in the adjustment procedure.

[4]Includes all other races and origins not shown separately.

[5]Percent of poverty level was calculated by dividing family income by the U.S. Department of Health and Human Services' poverty guideline specific to family size, as well as the appropriate year, and state. Persons with unknown percent of poverty level are excluded (7% in 2013–2016).

Table 3-19. Healthy Weight, Overweight, and Obesity Among Persons 20 Years of Age and Over, by Selected Characteristics, Selected Years, 1988–1994 Through 2013–2016—Continued

(Percent; data are based on measured height and weight of a sample of the civilian noninstitutionalized population.)

Sex, age, race and Hispanic origin[1], and percent of poverty level	Overweight (includes obesity; BMI greater than or equal to 25.0)[2]								
	1988–1994	1999–2002	2001–2004	2003–2006	2005–2008	2007–2010	2009–2012	2011–2014	2013–2016
20 Years and Over, Age-Adjusted[3]									
Both Sexes[4]	56.0	65.1	66.0	66.7	67.5	68.5	68.7	69.5	70.9
Male	60.9	68.8	70.5	72.1	72.9	73.3	72.9	73.0	74.6
Female	51.4	61.6	61.6	61.3	62.5	63.9	64.6	66.2	67.4
Not Hispanic or Latino									
White only	54.4	63.3	64.3	64.8	66.0	66.8	67.0	68.5	69.8
White only, male	61.6	69.4	71.0	71.8	72.9	73.6	73.2	73.7	75.3
White only, female	47.5	57.2	57.6	57.9	59.6	60.3	60.9	63.5	64.6
Black or African American	63.7	70.5	74.0	76.1	75.1	75.5	76.5	76.3	76.1
Black or African American only, male	57.8	62.6	67.0	71.6	71.7	70.0	70.2	69.6	70.6
Black or African American only, female	68.2	77.2	79.6	79.8	78.0	80.0	81.8	82.0	80.6
Asian	NA	NA	NA	NA	NA	NA	NA	40.3	42.7
Asian only, male	NA	NA	NA	NA	NA	NA	NA	46.9	49.9
Asian only, female	NA	NA	NA	NA	NA	NA	NA	34.4	36.6
Hispanic or Latino	NA	NA	NA	NA	NA	78.4	78.3	78.4	80.4
Male	NA	NA	NA	NA	NA	80.6	80.2	79.6	81.8
Female	NA	NA	NA	NA	NA	75.7	76.3	77.1	78.8
Mexican origin	68.9	72.3	73.8	75.0	76.5	79.9	80.3	81.6	83.8
Mexican origin, male	68.9	73.2	74.6	75.8	77.7	81.3	81.9	82.7	82.9
Mexican origin, female	68.9	71.2	73.0	73.9	74.8	78.0	78.3	80.3	84.5
Percent of Poverty Level[5]									
Below 100 percent	59.6	64.7	63.4	65.7	67.7	69.7	70.0	69.1	71.6
100 percent to 199 percent	58.0	67.3	66.2	66.5	69.6	70.5	71.7	73.9	73.5
200 percent to 399 percent	56.0	68.6	68.8	69.0	68.7	68.6	68.3	71.6	72.9
400 percent or more	52.4	62.2	63.7	64.7	65.3	66.9	66.8	65.6	67.4
20 Years and Over, Crude									
Both Sexes[4]	54.9	65.2	66.1	66.9	67.8	68.7	69.1	69.8	71.1
Male	59.4	68.6	70.4	72.1	72.8	73.2	72.9	72.8	74.3
Female	50.7	62.0	61.9	61.9	63.0	64.5	65.5	67.0	68.1
Not Hispanic or Latino									
White only	53.8	63.9	65.1	65.8	66.9	67.8	68.3	69.6	70.9
White only, male	60.6	69.9	71.6	72.5	73.4	74.2	73.8	74.2	75.6
White only, female	47.4	58.2	58.7	59.4	60.7	61.7	62.9	65.2	66.3
Black or African American	61.8	70.0	73.3	76.0	74.9	75.2	76.4	76.3	75.7
Black or African American only, male	56.7	61.7	66.3	71.6	71.1	69.1	69.6	69.1	69.8
Black or African American only, female	66.0	76.9	79.1	79.7	78.1	80.2	82.1	82.3	80.5
Asian	NA	NA	NA	NA	NA	NA	NA	40.0	42.6
Asian only, male	NA	NA	NA	NA	NA	NA	NA	46.3	49.5
Asian only, female	NA	NA	NA	NA	NA	NA	NA	34.5	36.5
Hispanic or Latino	NA	NA	NA	NA	NA	77.1	77.2	77.5	79.6
Male	NA	NA	NA	NA	NA	79.3	78.9	78.8	81.3
Female	NA	NA	NA	NA	NA	74.6	75.3	76.3	77.8
Mexican origin	64.8	69.8	71.6	73.9	75.5	78.8	79.3	81.0	83.0
Mexican origin, male	63.9	70.1	71.8	74.6	76.8	80.2	81.4	82.3	82.4
Mexican origin, female	65.9	69.3	71.4	73.0	73.9	77.1	76.9	79.5	83.6
Percent of Poverty Level[5]									
Below 100 percent	56.8	62.5	61.4	64.4	65.9	67.8	68.0	67.1	70.4
100 percent to 199 percent	55.7	66.2	65.3	66.0	69.1	70.1	71.4	73.1	72.7
200 percent to 399 percent	54.9	68.5	69.0	69.0	68.7	68.8	68.8	71.8	72.9
400 percent or more	53.3	63.7	65.5	66.5	67.2	68.5	68.6	67.7	69.2
Male									
20 to 34 years	47.5	57.4	59.0	61.6	60.5	61.1	60.9	60.4	63.0
35 to 44 years	65.5	70.5	72.9	75.2	78.8	80.2	78.9	79.3	80.6
45 to 54 years	66.1	75.7	78.5	78.5	76.8	76.8	79.3	80.8	80.8
55 to 64 years	70.5	75.4	77.3	79.7	80.5	79.8	77.4	76.7	76.7
65 to 74 years	68.5	76.2	76.1	78.0	79.1	77.5	76.9	76.1	79.0
75 years and over	56.5	67.4	66.8	65.8	70.8	73.2	70.4	71.0	74.9
Female									
20 to 34 years	37.0	52.9	51.6	50.9	55.6	55.4	55.2	58.5	59.6
35 to 44 years	49.6	60.6	60.1	60.7	62.1	63.9	62.4	65.6	67.7
45 to 54 years	60.3	65.1	67.4	67.3	65.8	66.2	70.5	71.4	69.5
55 to 64 years	66.3	72.2	69.9	69.6	69.4	72.2	75.1	74.3	74.5
65 to 74 years	60.3	70.9	71.5	70.5	69.6	74.2	73.8	71.2	75.6
75 years and over	52.3	59.9	63.7	62.6	61.3	63.2	62.4	64.6	67.4

NOTE: Percentages do not sum to 100 because the percentage of persons with BMI less than 18.5 is not shown. Additionally, the percentage of persons with obesity is embedded in the percent overweight or obese and can be further partitioned into Grades 1, 2, and 3 obesity. Age of the participant (in years) is at the time of screening. Height is measured without shoes. Estimates exclude pregnant women.
NA = Not available.
[1] Persons of Hispanic and Mexican origin may be of any race. Starting with 1999 data, race-specific estimates are tabulated according to the 1997 Revisions to the Standards for the Classification of Federal Data on Race and Ethnicity and are not strictly comparable with estimates for earlier years. The non-Hispanic race categories shown in the table conform to the 1997 Standards. Starting with 1999 data, race-specific estimates are for persons who reported only one racial group. Prior to data year 1999, estimates were tabulated according to the 1977 Standards. Estimates for single-race categories prior to 1999 included persons who reported one race, or if they reported more than one race, identified one race as best representing their race.
[2] Body mass index (BMI) equals weight in kilograms divided by height in meters squared. The National Health and Nutrition Examination Survey (NHANES) variable Body Mass Index is rounded to one decimal place and is used to assign persons to BMI categories. Estimates in this table may differ from other estimates where BMI is directly calculated using the NHANES measured weight and measured height variables.
[3] Estimates are age-adjusted to the year 2000 standard population using five age groups: 20–34 years, 35–44 years, 45–54 years, 55–64 years, and 65 years and over. Age-adjusted estimates in this table may differ from other age-adjusted estimates based on the same data and presented elsewhere if different age groups are used in the adjustment procedure.
[4] Includes all other races and origins not shown separately.
[5] Percent of poverty level was calculated by dividing family income by the U.S. Department of Health and Human Services' poverty guideline specific to family size, as well as the appropriate year, and state. Persons with unknown percent of poverty level are excluded (7% in 2013–2016).

Table 3-19. Healthy Weight, Overweight, and Obesity Among Persons 20 Years of Age and Over, by Selected Characteristics, Selected Years, 1988–1994 Through 2013–2016—*Continued*

(Percent; data are based on measured height and weight of a sample of the civilian noninstitutionalized population.)

Sex, age, race and Hispanic origin[1], and percent of poverty level	Obesity (BMI greater than or equal to 30.0)[2]								
	1988–1994	1999–2002	2001–2004	2003–2006	2005–2008	2007–2010	2009–2012	2011–2014	2013–2016
20 Years and Over, Age-Adjusted[3]									
Both Sexes[4]	22.9	30.4	31.4	33.4	34.0	34.7	35.3	36.4	38.8
Male	20.2	27.5	29.5	32.4	32.7	33.9	34.6	34.5	36.8
Female	25.5	33.2	33.2	34.3	35.4	35.5	35.9	38.1	40.7
Not Hispanic or Latino									
White only	21.6	29.4	30.5	32.0	32.8	33.3	33.4	34.6	37.4
White only, male	20.2	28.0	30.2	32.4	32.6	34.1	34.4	34.0	37.0
White only, female	22.9	30.7	30.7	31.6	33.1	32.5	32.3	35.3	37.9
Black or African American	30.7	39.2	42.0	45.5	45.0	47.0	48.8	48.0	47.9
Black or African American only, male	20.9	27.8	30.8	35.7	37.5	38.3	38.1	37.9	38.0
Black or African American only, female	38.3	48.6	51.1	53.4	51.0	54.0	57.5	56.5	56.0
Asian	NA	NA	NA	NA	NA	NA	NA	11.8	12.5
Asian only, male	NA	NA	NA	NA	NA	NA	NA	11.3	10.9
Asian only, female	NA	NA	NA	NA	NA	NA	NA	11.9	13.6
Hispanic or Latino	NA	NA	NA	NA	NA	38.9	40.9	42.6	44.8
Male	NA	NA	NA	NA	NA	35.7	38.6	39.1	40.4
Female	NA	NA	NA	NA	NA	42.1	43.1	45.6	48.9
Mexican origin	29.3	32.7	34.1	35.3	37.3	40.3	43.2	46.4	47.9
Mexican origin, male	23.8	27.8	29.1	29.5	32.0	36.3	40.2	43.3	44.0
Mexican origin, female	35.2	38.0	39.4	41.8	43.3	44.6	46.3	49.6	51.7
Percent of Poverty Level[5]									
Below 100 percent	28.1	34.7	33.7	35.0	35.9	37.2	38.3	39.2	42.2
100 percent to 199 percent	26.1	34.1	33.6	35.9	38.0	37.3	40.1	42.6	42.7
200 percent to 399 percent	22.7	32.1	33.3	35.7	35.7	36.8	37.0	38.8	41.6
400 percent or more	18.7	25.5	27.3	28.9	29.4	31.3	30.2	29.7	34.0
20 Years and Over, Crude									
Both Sexes[4]	22.3	30.5	31.5	33.5	34.3	34.9	35.5	36.5	38.9
Male	19.5	27.5	29.5	32.4	32.8	33.9	34.6	34.5	36.6
Female	25.0	33.4	33.3	34.6	35.6	35.9	36.4	38.5	41.0
Not Hispanic or Latino									
White only	21.3	29.8	30.9	32.4	33.2	33.8	34.1	35.3	37.9
White only, male	19.8	28.4	30.5	32.6	33.1	34.4	34.7	34.3	36.9
White only, female	22.7	31.3	31.2	32.2	33.3	33.2	33.5	36.2	38.8
Black or African American	29.5	39.1	41.9	45.3	44.7	46.9	48.7	48.2	47.6
Black or African American only, male	20.7	27.5	30.7	35.8	37.2	38.1	37.9	37.6	37.5
Black or African American only, female	36.7	48.7	51.1	53.2	51.0	54.2	57.6	56.9	56.1
Asian	NA	NA	NA	NA	NA	NA	NA	11.8	12.7
Asian only, male	NA	NA	NA	NA	NA	NA	NA	11.7	11.7
Asian only, female	NA	NA	NA	NA	NA	NA	NA	11.9	13.6
Hispanic or Latino	NA	NA	NA	NA	NA	38.0	40.1	42.3	44.8
Male	NA	NA	NA	NA	NA	34.8	38.2	39.7	41.2
Female	NA	NA	NA	NA	NA	41.5	42.1	45.0	48.4
Mexican origin	26.4	31.0	32.7	34.5	36.2	39.5	42.5	45.9	47.7
Mexican origin, male	20.6	26.0	27.8	29.0	30.9	35.6	40.2	43.5	44.4
Mexican origin, female	33.3	37.0	38.5	41.2	42.9	44.2	45.2	48.6	51.3
Percent of Poverty Level[5]									
Below 100 percent	25.9	33.0	33.0	34.6	35.4	36.5	37.0	38.1	41.2
100 percent to 199 percent	24.3	32.8	32.6	35.0	37.0	36.8	40.0	41.9	41.6
200 percent to 399 percent	22.0	31.8	33.2	35.5	35.6	36.8	37.1	38.8	41.6
400 percent or more	19.3	27.2	28.6	30.7	31.7	32.4	31.7	31.1	34.6
Male									
20 to 34 years	14.1	21.7	23.2	26.2	25.4	27.1	28.9	28.5	30.7
35 to 44 years	21.3	28.5	33.8	37.0	35.9	37.2	38.1	39.8	43.1
45 to 54 years	23.2	30.6	31.8	34.6	35.9	36.6	38.1	36.6	38.0
55 to 64 years	27.2	35.5	36.0	39.3	40.4	37.3	38.1	38.1	39.3
65 to 74 years	24.1	31.9	32.1	33.0	36.2	41.5	36.4	36.2	40.2
75 years and over	13.2	18.0	19.9	24.0	25.6	26.6	27.4	26.8	28.0
Female									
20 to 34 years	18.5	28.3	28.6	28.4	31.4	30.4	30.0	33.4	34.8
35 to 44 years	25.5	32.1	33.3	36.1	36.7	37.1	36.0	39.1	43.4
45 to 54 years	32.4	36.9	38.0	40.0	39.1	36.9	38.3	41.7	42.9
55 to 64 years	33.7	42.1	39.0	41.0	42.3	43.4	42.9	44.4	48.2
65 to 74 years	26.9	39.3	37.9	36.4	35.6	40.3	44.2	40.7	43.5
75 years and over	19.2	23.6	23.2	24.2	25.9	28.7	29.8	30.5	32.7

NOTE: Percentages do not sum to 100 because the percentage of persons with BMI less than 18.5 is not shown. Additionally, the percentage of persons with obesity is embedded in the percent overweight or obese and can be further partitioned into Grades 1, 2, and 3 obesity. Age of the participant (in years) is at the time of screening. Height is measured without shoes. Estimates exclude pregnant women.
NA = Not available.

[1] Persons of Hispanic and Mexican origin may be of any race. Starting with 1999 data, race-specific estimates are tabulated according to the 1997 Revisions to the Standards for the Classification of Federal Data on Race and Ethnicity and are not strictly comparable with estimates for earlier years. The non-Hispanic race categories shown in the table conform to the 1997 Standards. Starting with 1999 data, race-specific estimates are for persons who reported only one racial group. Prior to data year 1999, estimates were tabulated according to the 1977 Standards. Estimates for single-race categories prior to 1999 included persons who reported one race, or if they reported more than one race, identified one race as best representing their race.
[2] Body mass index (BMI) equals weight in kilograms divided by height in meters squared. The National Health and Nutrition Examination Survey (NHANES) variable Body Mass Index is rounded to one decimal place and is used to assign persons to BMI categories. Estimates in this table may differ from other estimates where BMI is directly calculated using the NHANES measured weight and measured height variables.
[3] Estimates are age-adjusted to the year 2000 standard population using five age groups: 20–34 years, 35–44 years, 45–54 years, 55–64 years, and 65 years and over. Age-adjusted estimates in this table may differ from other age-adjusted estimates based on the same data and presented elsewhere if different age groups are used in the adjustment procedure.
[4] Includes all other races and origins not shown separately.
[5] Percent of poverty level was calculated by dividing family income by the U.S. Department of Health and Human Services' poverty guideline specific to family size, as well as the appropriate year, and state. Persons with unknown percent of poverty level are excluded (7% in 2013–2016).

Table 3-19. Healthy Weight, Overweight, and Obesity Among Persons 20 Years of Age and Over, by Selected Characteristics, Selected Years, 1988–1994 Through 2013–2016—*Continued*

(Percent; data are based on measured height and weight of a sample of the civilian noninstitutionalized population.)

Sex, age, race and Hispanic origin[1], and percent of poverty level	Grade 1 Obesity (BMI from 30.0 to 34.9)[2]								
	1988–1994	1999–2002	2001–2004	2003–2006	2005–2008	2007–2010	2009–2012	2011–2014	2013–2016
20 Years and Over, Age-Adjusted[3]									
Both Sexes[4]	14.8	17.9	19.3	19.8	19.5	19.9	20.4	20.6	21.2
Male	14.9	18.2	20.3	21.8	21.6	22.3	22.3	22.0	23.1
Female	14.7	17.6	18.2	17.9	17.5	17.6	18.5	19.3	19.4
Not Hispanic or Latino									
White only	14.0	17.6	19.2	19.3	18.8	19.2	19.5	19.6	20.5
White only, male	14.9	18.9	21.0	21.6	21.4	22.7	22.5	21.4	23.0
White only, female	13.2	16.2	17.4	17.0	16.4	15.9	16.5	17.9	18.0
Black or African American	17.3	19.0	21.9	23.1	22.8	23.0	24.3	23.5	22.6
Black or African American only, male	14.2	16.1	18.8	22.4	23.3	20.8	19.9	22.0	21.9
Black or African American only, female	19.6	21.6	24.5	23.8	22.3	24.8	27.7	24.9	23.3
Asian	NA	NA	NA	NA	NA	NA	NA	9.3	10.0
Asian only, male	NA	NA	NA	NA	NA	NA	NA	9.4	9.4
Asian only, female	NA	NA	NA	NA	NA	NA	NA	8.9	10.4
Hispanic or Latino	NA	NA	NA	NA	NA	23.7	25.2	25.6	25.7
Male	NA	NA	NA	NA	NA	23.9	26.8	27.2	26.2
Female	NA	NA	NA	NA	NA	23.5	23.6	24.1	24.9
Mexican origin	20.3	21.1	22.0	22.8	23.0	24.8	26.2	26.9	26.6
Mexican origin, male	18.9	19.5	21.9	22.0	21.9	24.7	28.3	29.7	28.2
Mexican origin, female	22.0	22.9	22.2	23.6	24.1	24.9	24.0	23.8	24.9
Percent of Poverty Level[5]									
Below 100 percent	16.6	17.3	17.7	19.3	18.6	19.8	21.1	20.7	20.9
100 percent to 199 percent	16.1	17.7	18.2	20.6	21.4	19.8	20.1	21.7	22.3
200 percent to 399 percent	14.5	19.8	21.7	21.6	20.0	20.2	21.7	22.7	22.7
400 percent or more	13.3	16.6	18.1	18.0	18.0	19.4	18.7	18.2	20.0
20 Years and Over, Crude									
Both Sexes[4]	14.4	17.9	19.3	19.8	19.6	20.0	20.5	20.7	21.3
Male	14.3	18.1	20.3	21.8	21.6	22.3	22.4	22.0	22.9
Female	14.5	17.7	18.3	18.0	17.7	17.9	18.7	19.4	19.8
Not Hispanic or Latino									
White only	13.8	17.8	19.4	19.5	19.2	19.6	20.0	20.2	21.0
White only, male	14.6	19.1	21.2	21.8	21.7	22.8	22.9	22.0	23.2
White only, female	13.2	16.6	17.7	17.3	16.7	16.6	17.3	18.5	19.0
Black or African American	16.6	19.0	22.0	22.9	22.4	22.8	24.0	23.3	22.4
Black or African American only, male	14.0	15.8	18.7	22.2	22.9	20.6	19.6	21.4	21.3
Black or African American only, female	18.7	21.7	24.7	23.5	22.1	24.6	27.6	24.9	23.3
Asian	NA	NA	NA	NA	NA	NA	NA	9.4	10.2
Asian only, male	NA	NA	NA	NA	NA	NA	NA	9.8	9.9
Asian only, female	NA	NA	NA	NA	NA	NA	NA	9.0	10.5
Hispanic or Latino	NA	NA	NA	NA	NA	22.9	24.7	25.4	25.4
Male	NA	NA	NA	NA	NA	22.9	26.2	27.2	26.3
Female	NA	NA	NA	NA	NA	22.9	23.2	23.7	24.4
Mexican origin	18.1	20.2	21.2	22.2	22.0	24.1	26.2	26.9	26.3
Mexican origin, male	15.8	18.2	20.7	21.6	20.7	23.8	28.1	29.4	27.9
Mexican origin, female	20.7	22.4	21.7	22.9	23.7	24.5	24.1	24.1	24.7
Percent of Poverty Level[5]									
Below 100 percent	15.2	16.4	17.5	19.1	18.0	19.2	20.4	19.5	20.0
100 percent to 199 percent	15.2	17.5	18.1	20.4	21.1	19.8	20.2	21.5	22.0
200 percent to 399 percent	14.0	19.6	21.7	21.5	20.0	20.3	21.8	22.6	22.8
400 percent or more	13.5	17.4	18.7	18.6	18.8	19.9	19.8	19.0	20.2
Male									
20 to 34 years	9.8	13.7	15.4	18.1	16.8	19.0	19.6	16.7	17.5
35 to 44 years	14.7	19.3	23.7	24.9	23.4	23.2	22.7	23.9	25.9
45 to 54 years	17.3	17.8	21.4	22.4	22.6	22.6	24.4	25.8	26.2
55 to 64 years	20.6	25.3	25.3	27.0	28.1	25.2	25.6	25.1	23.9
65 to 74 years	19.4	22.1	21.2	20.5	23.3	26.1	21.9	22.5	26.2
75 years and over	10.9	15.7	16.6	18.5	19.0	20.6	21.1	20.3	21.0
Female									
20 to 34 years	10.8	15.9	16.9	14.2	14.6	14.0	14.4	14.7	15.0
35 to 44 years	13.9	14.8	17.9	19.7	17.8	17.0	19.3	21.9	20.3
45 to 54 years	17.5	19.4	20.3	18.4	17.3	18.6	19.0	19.7	19.3
55 to 64 years	20.0	21.6	18.2	19.8	21.8	22.5	22.7	21.7	23.2
65 to 74 years	16.0	23.4	21.9	20.3	18.6	19.4	21.1	21.9	24.9
75 years and over	14.4	14.1	14.8	18.2	19.7	19.8	19.1	19.9	20.4

NOTE: Percentages do not sum to 100 because the percentage of persons with BMI less than 18.5 is not shown. Additionally, the percentage of persons with obesity is embedded in the percent overweight or obese and can be further partitioned into Grades 1, 2, and 3 obesity. Age of the participant (in years) is at the time of screening. Height is measured without shoes. Estimates exclude pregnant women.

NA = Not available.

[1]Persons of Hispanic and Mexican origin may be of any race. Starting with 1999 data, race-specific estimates are tabulated according to the 1997 Revisions to the Standards for the Classification of Federal Data on Race and Ethnicity and are not strictly comparable with estimates for earlier years. The non-Hispanic race categories shown in the table conform to the 1997 Standards. Starting with 1999 data, race-specific estimates are for persons who reported only one racial group. Prior to data year 1999, estimates were tabulated according to the 1977 Standards. Estimates for single-race categories prior to 1999 included persons who reported one race, or if they reported more than one race, identified one race as best representing their race.

[2]Body mass index (BMI) equals weight in kilograms divided by height in meters squared. The National Health and Nutrition Examination Survey (NHANES) variable Body Mass Index is rounded to one decimal place and is used to assign persons to BMI categories. Estimates in this table may differ from other estimates where BMI is directly calculated using the NHANES measured weight and measured height variables.

[3]Estimates are age-adjusted to the year 2000 standard population using five age groups: 20–34 years, 35–44 years, 45–54 years, 55–64 years, and 65 years and over. Age-adjusted estimates in this table may differ from other age-adjusted estimates based on the same data and presented elsewhere if different age groups are used in the adjustment procedure.

[4]Includes all other races and origins not shown separately.

[5]Percent of poverty level was calculated by dividing family income by the U.S. Department of Health and Human Services' poverty guideline specific to family size, as well as the appropriate year, and state. Persons with unknown percent of poverty level are excluded (7% in 2013–2016).

Table 3-19. Healthy Weight, Overweight, and Obesity Among Persons 20 Years of Age and Over, by Selected Characteristics, Selected Years, 1988–1994 Through 2013–2016—Continued

(Percent; data are based on measured height and weight of a sample of the civilian noninstitutionalized population.)

Sex, age, race and Hispanic origin[1], and percent of poverty level	Grade 2 Obesity (BMI from 35.0 to 39.9)[2]								
	1988–1994	1999–2002	2001–2004	2003–2006	2005–2008	2007–2010	2009–2012	2011–2014	2013–2016
20 Years and Over, Age-Adjusted[3]									
Both Sexes[4]	5.2	7.6	7.2	8.2	8.7	8.9	8.6	8.8	9.9
Male	3.5	5.9	6.0	7.1	7.0	7.4	7.9	7.6	8.3
Female	6.8	9.2	8.3	9.3	10.6	10.3	9.2	9.9	11.4
Not Hispanic or Latino									
White only	4.9	7.4	6.7	7.8	8.6	8.6	8.2	8.5	9.4
White only, male	3.5	5.8	6.0	7.2	7.0	7.3	7.9	7.8	8.4
White only, female	6.3	9.0	7.4	8.4	10.2	9.9	8.6	9.1	10.5
Black or African American	7.8	11.2	10.8	12.0	11.7	12.0	12.0	12.3	13.5
Black or African American only, male	4.1	8.3	7.6	7.6	7.8	10.2	10.8	8.9	8.8
Black or African American only, female	10.7	13.6	13.2	15.4	14.8	13.4	12.8	15.1	17.2
Asian	NA	NA	NA	NA	NA	NA	NA	1.9	2.1
Asian only, male	NA	NA	NA	NA	NA	NA	NA	*	1.2
Asian only, female	NA	NA	NA	NA	NA	NA	NA	*2.1	2.9
Hispanic or Latino	NA	NA	NA	NA	NA	9.8	10.2	10.6	11.3
Male	NA	NA	NA	NA	NA	7.8	7.8	7.3	8.5
Female	NA	NA	NA	NA	NA	12.0	12.5	13.5	13.8
Mexican origin	6.1	7.4	7.6	8.0	9.2	9.8	11.0	12.4	12.3
Mexican origin, male	3.8	5.4	4.8	5.1	6.3	7.2	7.7	8.3	9.2
Mexican origin, female	8.4	9.4	10.4	11.2	12.7	12.9	14.6	16.6	15.5
Percent of Poverty Level[5]									
Below 100 percent	6.8	9.6	8.4	8.6	10.5	10.0	9.6	10.1	11.0
100 percent to 199 percent	6.5	9.7	8.5	9.0	9.8	9.4	10.2	11.0	10.1
200 percent to 399 percent	5.2	7.5	7.9	8.8	9.0	10.3	9.4	9.4	11.3
400 percent or more	3.6	5.7	5.2	6.7	7.3	7.6	7.1	6.5	8.1
20 Years and Over, Crude									
Both Sexes[4]	5.1	7.7	7.2	8.2	8.8	8.8	8.6	8.8	9.9
Male	3.5	6.0	6.0	7.0	7.0	7.3	7.8	7.5	8.2
Female	6.6	9.3	8.4	9.4	10.5	10.3	9.4	10.1	11.5
Not Hispanic or Latino									
White only	4.8	7.5	6.9	8.0	8.7	8.7	8.4	8.5	9.4
White only, male	3.4	5.9	6.1	7.4	7.2	7.4	7.8	7.6	8.2
White only, female	6.2	9.1	7.7	8.5	10.0	9.9	8.9	9.4	10.6
Black or African American	7.6	11.1	10.4	11.7	11.6	11.9	12.1	12.5	13.4
Black or African American only, male	4.2	8.2	7.4	7.5	7.7	10.2	11.1	9.1	8.8
Black or African American only, female	10.4	13.5	12.9	15.3	14.8	13.3	12.9	15.4	17.3
Asian	NA	NA	NA	NA	NA	NA	NA	1.9	2.2
Asian only, male	NA	NA	NA	NA	NA	NA	NA	*	1.4
Asian only, female	NA	NA	NA	NA	NA	NA	NA	*2.1	2.9
Hispanic or Latino	NA	NA	NA	NA	NA	9.7	9.9	10.3	11.2
Male	NA	NA	NA	NA	NA	7.6	7.8	7.6	9.0
Female	NA	NA	NA	NA	NA	12.0	12.2	13.1	13.4
Mexican origin	5.6	6.8	7.0	7.6	8.9	9.7	10.6	11.7	12.2
Mexican origin, male	3.7	5.1	4.6	4.7	5.6	7.0	7.8	8.6	9.7
Mexican origin, female	7.9	8.8	9.8	11.2	12.9	13.0	13.7	15.2	14.9
Percent of Poverty Level[5]									
Below 100 percent	6.3	9.5	8.3	8.4	10.3	9.7	9.4	10.1	10.8
100 percent to 199 percent	6.2	8.9	7.9	8.7	9.3	9.2	10.1	10.8	9.9
200 percent to 399 percent	5.1	7.5	7.9	8.8	8.9	10.1	9.3	9.4	11.3
400 percent or more	3.8	6.4	5.7	7.4	8.2	7.9	7.4	6.5	8.2
Male									
20 to 34 years	2.9	4.1	4.3	4.5	4.4	4.7	6.3	7.0	7.0
35 to 44 years	*3.5	5.9	6.7	7.9	7.6	8.8	9.7	10.3	10.9
45 to 54 years	*3.5	8.5	6.5	8.3	9.3	8.9	8.2	6.1	6.6
55 to 64 years	5.5	*7.4	7.6	8.4	6.6	6.7	7.1	6.8	9.0
65 to 74 years	*3.8	6.9	8.5	10.3	10.2	11.8	10.8	8.9	10.1
75 years and over	*	*	*2.7	*3.9	*5.0	4.6	*4.7	*4.9	*
Female									
20 to 34 years	5.1	8.0	6.1	7.9	10.1	8.6	7.9	9.6	10.7
35 to 44 years	7.1	9.4	7.6	9.2	12.5	12.6	8.4	8.1	11.0
45 to 54 years	8.4	10.4	10.6	12.4	12.3	10.6	10.7	11.5	12.6
55 to 64 years	9.4	10.9	11.0	11.4	10.3	11.5	11.1	11.2	12.3
65 to 74 years	6.7	9.8	10.2	9.6	10.3	11.7	12.3	12.4	13.0
75 years and over	3.7	7.2	*6.0	*3.9	3.5	5.5	6.6	7.4	8.8

NOTE: Percentages do not sum to 100 because the percentage of persons with BMI less than 18.5 is not shown. Additionally, the percentage of persons with obesity is embedded in the percent overweight or obese and can be further partitioned into Grades 1, 2, and 3 obesity. Age of the participant (in years) is at the time of screening. Height is measured without shoes. Estimates exclude pregnant women.

NA = Not available.

* = Estimates are considered unreliable. Starting with 2013–2016 data, the reliability of survey percentage estimates was assessed using new multistep National Center for Health Statistics data presentation standards for proportions. Prior to 2013–2016 data, the reliability of estimates for earlier years was evaluated based on relative standard errors (RSE). Data preceded by an asterisk have an RSE of 20%–30%. Data not shown have an RSE greater than 30%.

[1]Persons of Hispanic and Mexican origin may be of any race. Starting with 1999 data, race-specific estimates are tabulated according to the 1997 Revisions to the Standards for the Classification of Federal Data on Race and Ethnicity and are not strictly comparable with estimates for earlier years. The non-Hispanic race categories shown in the table conform to the 1997 Standards. Starting with 1999 data, race-specific estimates are for persons who reported only one racial group. Prior to data year 1999, estimates were tabulated according to the 1977 Standards. Estimates for single-race categories prior to 1999 included persons who reported one race, or if they reported more than one race, identified one race as best representing their race.

[2]Body mass index (BMI) equals weight in kilograms divided by height in meters squared. The National Health and Nutrition Examination Survey (NHANES) variable Body Mass Index is rounded to one decimal place and is used to assign persons to BMI categories. Estimates in this table may differ from other estimates where BMI is directly calculated using the NHANES measured weight and measured height variables.

[3]Estimates are age-adjusted to the year 2000 standard population using five age groups: 20–34 years, 35–44 years, 45–54 years, 55–64 years, and 65 years and over. Age-adjusted estimates in this table may differ from other age-adjusted estimates based on the same data and presented elsewhere if different age groups are used in the adjustment procedure.

[4]Includes all other races and origins not shown separately.

[5]Percent of poverty level was calculated by dividing family income by the U.S. Department of Health and Human Services' poverty guideline specific to family size, as well as the appropriate year, and state. Persons with unknown percent of poverty level are excluded (7% in 2013–2016).

Table 3-19. Healthy Weight, Overweight, and Obesity Among Persons 20 Years of Age and Over, by Selected Characteristics, Selected Years, 1988–1994 Through 2013–2016—Continued

(Percent; data are based on measured height and weight of a sample of the civilian noninstitutionalized population.)

Sex, age, race and Hispanic origin[1], and percent of poverty level	Grade 3 Obesity (BMI greater than or equal to 40.0)[2]								
	1988–1994	1999–2002	2001–2004	2003–2006	2005–2008	2007–2010	2009–2012	2011–2014	2013–2016
20 Years and Over, Age-Adjusted[3]									
Both Sexes[4]	2.9	4.9	5.0	5.4	5.8	6.0	6.3	6.9	7.7
Male	1.7	3.3	3.2	3.5	4.2	4.2	4.4	4.9	5.5
Female	4.0	6.4	6.6	7.2	7.3	7.6	8.2	8.9	9.8
Not Hispanic or Latino									
White only	2.7	4.4	4.6	4.9	5.3	5.4	5.6	6.5	7.5
White only, male	*1.8	3.3	3.2	3.5	4.1	4.0	4.0	4.7	5.6
White only, female	3.5	5.5	5.8	6.3	6.5	6.7	7.2	8.2	9.4
Black or African American	5.6	8.9	9.4	10.4	10.5	11.9	12.6	12.1	11.8
Black or African American only, male	2.5	3.4	4.4	5.6	6.5	7.3	7.4	7.0	7.2
Black or African American only, female	8.0	13.4	13.4	14.2	13.8	15.8	16.9	16.5	15.5
Asian	NA	NA	NA	NA	NA	NA	NA	*	0.4
Asian only, male	NA	NA	NA	NA	NA	NA	NA	*	0.4
Asian only, female	NA	NA	NA	NA	NA	NA	NA	*	0.3
Hispanic or Latino	NA	NA	NA	NA	NA	5.3	5.5	6.4	7.9
Male	NA	NA	NA	NA	NA	4.0	4.0	4.7	5.7
Female	NA	NA	NA	NA	NA	6.6	7.0	8.1	10.2
Mexican origin	2.9	4.2	4.5	4.6	5.2	5.6	5.9	7.1	8.9
Mexican origin, male	*	*2.9	*2.4	*2.4	3.7	4.4	4.2	5.3	6.6
Mexican origin, female	4.9	5.7	6.8	6.9	6.5	6.8	7.7	9.2	11.3
Percent of Poverty Level[5]									
Below 100 percent	4.7	7.8	7.6	7.0	6.9	7.5	7.5	8.5	10.3
100 percent to 199 percent	3.6	6.7	6.9	6.3	6.9	8.1	9.8	9.8	10.2
200 percent to 399 percent	3.0	4.8	3.7	5.2	6.7	6.3	6.0	6.7	7.6
400 percent or more	1.9	3.2	4.0	4.2	4.1	4.4	4.3	5.0	5.9
20 Years and Over, Crude									
Both Sexes[4]	2.8	4.9	5.0	5.4	5.8	6.0	6.4	7.0	7.6
Male	1.7	3.4	3.3	3.5	4.2	4.3	4.4	4.9	5.5
Female	3.8	6.4	6.7	7.2	7.4	7.7	8.2	9.0	9.7
Not Hispanic or Latino									
White only	2.6	4.5	4.6	4.9	5.4	5.5	5.7	6.6	7.4
White only, male	*1.8	3.4	3.3	3.5	4.1	4.1	4.0	4.7	5.5
White only, female	3.3	5.6	5.9	6.3	6.6	6.8	7.3	8.3	9.2
Black or African American	5.3	8.9	9.5	10.6	10.7	12.2	12.7	12.3	11.8
Black or African American only, male	2.6	3.5	4.7	6.1	6.6	7.2	7.3	7.1	7.4
Black or African American only, female	7.6	13.4	13.5	14.4	14.2	16.3	17.2	16.7	15.5
Asian	NA	NA	NA	NA	NA	NA	NA	*	0.4
Asian only, male	NA	NA	NA	NA	NA	NA	NA	*	0.4
Asian only, female	NA	NA	NA	NA	NA	NA	NA	*	0.3
Hispanic or Latino	NA	NA	NA	NA	NA	5.4	5.4	6.6	8.2
Male	NA	NA	NA	NA	NA	4.3	4.1	5.0	5.9
Female	NA	NA	NA	NA	NA	6.5	6.8	8.1	10.6
Mexican origin	2.7	4.1	4.5	4.7	5.3	5.7	5.7	7.3	9.2
Mexican origin, male	*1.1	*2.7	*2.4	*2.7	*4.6	4.9	4.3	*5.6	6.9
Mexican origin, female	4.7	5.7	7.0	7.0	6.3	6.6	7.4	9.3	11.6
Percent of Poverty Level[5]									
Below 100 percent	4.3	7.1	7.2	7.1	7.1	7.5	7.2	8.5	10.4
100 percent to 199 percent	3.0	6.4	6.6	5.9	6.6	7.9	9.6	9.6	9.8
200 percent to 399 percent	2.9	4.7	3.6	5.2	6.7	6.3	5.9	6.7	7.5
400 percent or more	2.0	3.5	4.3	4.7	4.7	4.6	4.6	5.5	6.2
Male									
20 to 34 years	*1.3	3.9	3.5	3.6	4.1	3.4	3.0	4.7	6.2
35 to 44 years	*	*3.2	*3.4	4.2	4.9	5.2	5.6	5.6	6.3
45 to 54 years	*	*4.2	*3.9	*3.9	4.1	5.1	*5.5	*4.6	5.2
55 to 64 years	*	*2.8	*3.1	3.9	5.7	5.4	*5.4	*6.2	6.4
65 to 74 years	*	*	*2.4	*2.1	*2.8	*3.6	*	*4.7	3.9
75 years and over	*	*	*	*	*	*	*	*	1.9
Female									
20 to 34 years	2.6	4.5	5.6	6.3	6.7	7.7	7.7	9.1	9.1
35 to 44 years	4.5	7.9	7.7	7.2	6.5	7.5	8.3	9.0	12.1
45 to 54 years	6.4	7.2	7.0	9.2	9.5	7.7	8.6	10.5	11.0
55 to 64 years	4.2	9.5	9.8	9.8	10.2	9.4	9.1	11.5	12.7
65 to 74 years	4.2	6.2	5.9	*6.4	6.8	9.2	10.7	6.5	5.6
75 years and over	*	*	*	*2.1	*2.6	*3.4	*4.1	*3.3	3.4

NOTE: Percentages do not sum to 100 because the percentage of persons with BMI less than 18.5 is not shown. Additionally, the percentage of persons with obesity is embedded in the percent overweight or obese and can be further partitioned into Grades 1, 2, and 3 obesity. Age of the participant (in years) is at the time of screening. Height is measured without shoes. Estimates exclude pregnant women.
NA = Not available.
* = Estimates are considered unreliable. Starting with 2013–2016 data, the reliability of survey percentage estimates was assessed using new multistep National Center for Health Statistics data presentation standards for proportions. Prior to 2013–2016 data, the reliability of estimates for earlier years was evaluated based on relative standard errors (RSE). Data preceded by an asterisk have an RSE of 20%–30%. Data not shown have an RSE greater than 30%.
[1]Persons of Hispanic and Mexican origin may be of any race. Starting with 1999 data, race-specific estimates are tabulated according to the 1997 Revisions to the Standards for the Classification of Federal Data on Race and Ethnicity and are not strictly comparable with estimates for earlier years. The non-Hispanic race categories shown in the table conform to the 1997 Standards. Starting with 1999 data, race-specific estimates are for persons who reported only one racial group. Prior to data year 1999, estimates were tabulated according to the 1977 Standards. Estimates for single-race categories prior to 1999 included persons who reported one race, or if they reported more than one race, identified one race as best representing their race.
[2]Body mass index (BMI) equals weight in kilograms divided by height in meters squared. The National Health and Nutrition Examination Survey (NHANES) variable Body Mass Index is rounded to one decimal place and is used to assign persons to BMI categories. Estimates in this table may differ from other estimates where BMI is directly calculated using the NHANES measured weight and measured height variables.
[3]Estimates are age-adjusted to the year 2000 standard population using five age groups: 20–34 years, 35–44 years, 45–54 years, 55–64 years, and 65 years and over. Age-adjusted estimates in this table may differ from other age-adjusted estimates based on the same data and presented elsewhere if different age groups are used in the adjustment procedure.
[4]Includes all other races and origins not shown separately.
[5]Percent of poverty level was calculated by dividing family income by the U.S. Department of Health and Human Services' poverty guideline specific to family size, as well as the appropriate year, and state. Persons with unknown percent of poverty level are excluded (7% in 2013–2016).

Table 3-20. Obesity Among Children and Adolescents 2 to 19 Years of Age, by Selected Characteristics, Selected Years, 1988–1994 Through 2013–2016

(Percent; data are based on measured height and weight of a sample of the civilian noninstitutionalized population.)

Sex, age, race and Hispanic origin[1], and percent of poverty level	1988–1994	1999–2002	2001–2004	2003–2006	2005–2008	2007–2010	2009–2012	2011–2014	2013–2016
2 to 19 years									
Both sexes[2]	10.0	14.8	16.3	16.3	16.2	16.8	16.9	17.0	17.8
Not Hispanic or Latino									
White only	9.2	12.6	15.1	14.7	14.1	14.6	14.0	14.7	14.7
Black or African American only	12.5	18.2	18.8	20.7	20.7	22.1	22.1	19.5	20.4
Asian only	NA	NA	NA	NA	NA	NA	NA	8.6	9.8
Hispanic or Latino	NA	NA	NA	NA	NA	21.1	21.8	21.9	23.6
Mexican origin	14.3	20.0	19.4	20.9	21.7	21.0	21.9	22.2	24.2
Boys	10.2	15.5	17.3	17.0	16.8	18.2	17.6	16.9	18.1
Not Hispanic or Latino									
White only	9.7	13.2	16.4	15.6	14.5	15.8	14.4	14.3	15.3
Black or African American only	10.6	16.0	16.0	17.4	17.8	20.6	21.9	18.4	17.9
Asian only	NA	NA	NA	NA	NA	NA	NA	11.8	11.9
Hispanic or Latino	NA	NA	NA	NA	NA	23.9	23.7	22.4	24.3
Mexican origin	14.8	23.0	22.0	23.2	24.6	24.4	24.1	21.8	24.2
Girls	9.8	14.1	15.2	15.5	15.5	15.4	16.1	17.1	17.5
Not Hispanic or Latino									
White only	8.6	12.0	13.8	13.7	13.6	13.3	13.6	15.1	14.1
Black or African American only	14.5	20.5	21.8	24.1	23.6	23.5	22.3	20.7	23.0
Asian only	NA	NA	NA	NA	NA	NA	NA	*5.3	7.4
Hispanic or Latino	NA	NA	NA	NA	NA	18.1	19.8	21.4	22.9
Mexican origin	13.8	16.9	16.5	18.4	18.5	17.4	19.6	22.7	24.2
Percent of Poverty Level[3]									
Below 100 percent	12.6	17.6	17.9	18.9	19.9	20.8	20.9	19.4	21.0
100 percent to 199 percent	10.2	15.3	16.7	17.4	18.2	18.3	18.5	20.3	20.7
200 percent to 399 percent	9.4	14.0	17.8	17.1	16.0	16.7	15.9	16.4	16.9
400 percent or more	*4.7	12.6	11.2	11.0	11.6	11.9	11.5	11.4	12.2
2 to 5 years									
Both sexes[2]	7.2	10.3	12.4	12.5	10.5	11.1	10.2	8.9	11.6
Not Hispanic or Latino									
White only	5.2	8.7	10.2	10.8	9.3	9.0	6.4	*5.2	9.9
Black or African American only	7.8	8.8	11.0	14.9	14.0	15.0	14.7	10.4	11.6
Asian only	NA	NA	NA	NA	NA	NA	NA	*	*
Hispanic or Latino	NA	NA	NA	NA	NA	15.3	16.5	15.6	16.5
Mexican origin	12.3	13.1	17.7	16.7	14.1	14.6	15.7	15.3	15.1
Boys	6.2	10.0	13.1	12.8	9.8	11.9	12.0	9.2	11.5
Not Hispanic or Latino									
White only	*4.5	*8.2	*11.5	11.1	*7.4	8.8	*9.3	*	9.3
Black or African American only	7.9	*8.0	9.7	13.3	13.7	15.7	*14.3	*9.0	12.4
Asian only	NA	NA	NA	NA	NA	NA	NA	*	*
Hispanic or Latino	NA	NA	NA	NA	NA	17.7	17.9	16.7	16.7
Mexican origin	12.4	14.1	19.8	18.8	17.1	19.1	17.6	*14.5	13.1
Girls	8.2	10.6	11.7	12.2	11.2	10.2	8.4	8.6	11.7
Not Hispanic or Latino									
White only	5.9	*9.0	*9.1	10.4	11.3	*9.2	*	*4.4	10.4
Black or African American only	7.6	9.6	12.2	16.6	14.3	*14.2	15.3	11.9	11.0
Asian only	NA	NA	NA	NA	NA	NA	NA	*	*
Hispanic or Latino	NA	NA	NA	NA	NA	12.7	14.9	14.6	16.3
Mexican origin	12.3	*12.2	*15.7	14.5	10.8	*9.9	*13.8	*16.1	17.1
Percent of Poverty Level[3]									
Below 100 percent	9.7	10.9	14.4	14.3	12.3	13.2	12.3	11.6	13.5
100 percent to 199 percent	7.3	*13.8	13.3	12.7	10.0	11.8	11.6	10.2	12.6
200 percent to 399 percent	5.6	*7.6	13.6	11.9	11.6	13.9	11.0	*7.7	10.4
400 percent or more	*	*	*	*10.0	*	*	*5.8	*5.0	8.2

NOTE: Obesity in youth is defined as body mass index (BMI) at or above the sex- and age-specific 95th percentile of the 2000 Centers for Disease Control and Prevention (CDC) Growth Charts. See: Kuczmarski RJ, Ogden CL, Guo SS, Grummer-Strawn LM, Flegal KM, Mei Z, et al. 2000 CDC Growth Charts for the United States: Methods and development. Vital Health Stat 11(246). 2002. Available from: https://www.cdc.gov/nchs/data/series/sr_11/sr11_246.pdf. BMI equals weight in kilograms divided by height in meters squared. The National Health and Nutrition Examination Survey variable Body Mass Index is used to assign persons to BMI categories. Age is at the time of examination. Height is measured without shoes. Data on both age and height were collected during a standardized physical examination conducted in mobile examination centers. Estimates exclude pregnant females. Crude percentages, not age-adjusted percentages, are shown.

NA = Not available.

* = Estimates are considered unreliable. Starting with 2013–2016 data, the reliability of survey percentage estimates was assessed using new multistep National Center for Health Statistics data presentation standards for proportions. Prior to 2013–2016 data, the reliability of estimates for earlier years was evaluated based on relative standard errors (RSE). Data preceded by an asterisk have an RSE of 20%–30%. Data not shown have an RSE greater than 30%.

[1]Persons of Hispanic and Mexican origin may be of any race. Starting with 1999 data, race-specific estimates are tabulated according to the 1997 Revisions to the Standards for the Classification of Federal Data on Race and Ethnicity and are not strictly comparable with estimates for earlier years. The non-Hispanic race categories shown in the table conform to the 1997 Standards. Starting with 1999 data, race-specific estimates are for persons who reported only one racial group. Prior to data year 1999, estimates were tabulated according to the 1977 Standards. Estimates for single-race categories prior to 1999 included persons who reported one race, or if they reported more than one race, identified one race as best representing their race.

[2]Includes persons of all races and Hispanic origins, not just those shown separately.

[3]Percent of poverty level was calculated by dividing family income by the U.S. Department of Health and Human Services' poverty guideline specific to family size, as well as the appropriate year and state. Persons with unknown percent of poverty level are excluded (6% in 2013–2016).

Table 3-20. Obesity Among Children and Adolescents 2 to 19 Years of Age, by Selected Characteristics, Selected Years, 1988–1994 Through 2013–2016—Continued

(Percent; data are based on measured height and weight of a sample of the civilian noninstitutionalized population.)

Sex, age, race and Hispanic origin[1], and percent of poverty level	1988–1994	1999–2002	2001–2004	2003–2006	2005–2008	2007–2010	2009–2012	2011–2014	2013–2016
6 to 11 years									
Both sexes[2]	11.3	15.9	17.5	17.0	17.4	18.8	17.9	17.5	17.9
Not Hispanic or Latino									
White only	10.2	13.6	16.3	15.0	15.6	16.4	13.5	13.6	14.0
Black or African American only	14.6	19.8	20.9	21.3	20.0	23.9	26.1	21.4	19.8
Asian only	NA	NA	NA	NA	NA	NA	NA	*9.8	12.9
Hispanic or Latino	NA	NA	NA	NA	NA	23.8	24.4	25.0	25.3
Mexican origin	16.4	21.8	21.3	23.7	24.9	23.3	24.0	25.3	27.0
Boys	11.6	16.9	18.7	18.0	18.7	20.7	18.3	17.6	19.6
Not Hispanic or Latino									
White only	10.7	14.0	16.9	15.5	16.5	18.6	12.9	13.0	17.3
Black or African American only	12.3	17.0	17.2	18.6	18.7	23.3	27.6	21.2	15.5
Asian only	NA	NA	NA	NA	NA	NA	NA	*14.7	*
Hispanic or Latino	NA	NA	NA	NA	NA	26.0	26.4	25.8	26.1
Mexican origin	17.5	26.5	25.6	27.5	28.4	24.3	25.0	25.3	28.3
Girls	11.0	14.7	16.3	15.8	16.0	16.9	17.4	17.5	16.1
Not Hispanic or Latino									
White only	*9.8	13.1	15.6	14.4	14.5	14.0	14.2	14.4	10.4
Black or African American only	17.0	22.8	24.8	24.0	21.3	24.5	24.8	21.6	24.1
Asian only	NA	NA	NA	NA	NA	NA	NA	*	*
Hispanic or Latino	NA	NA	NA	NA	NA	21.5	22.3	24.1	24.5
Mexican origin	15.3	17.1	16.5	19.7	21.2	22.4	23.1	25.3	25.8
Percent of Poverty Level[3]									
Below 100 percent	11.4	19.1	20.0	22.0	21.5	22.2	24.6	21.5	20.8
100 percent to 199 percent	11.1	16.4	18.4	19.2	22.2	20.7	18.5	20.4	20.8
200 percent to 399 percent	11.7	15.3	18.2	16.7	16.8	18.9	15.8	15.7	17.1
400 percent or more	*	*12.9	11.4	*9.2	*9.5	*12.5	*12.2	*12.2	12.2
12 to 19 years									
Both sexes[2]	10.5	16.0	17.0	17.6	17.9	18.2	19.4	20.5	20.6
Not Hispanic or Latino									
White only	10.3	13.7	16.3	16.0	15.1	15.9	17.8	19.6	17.2
Black or African American only	13.4	21.1	20.6	22.9	24.2	24.1	22.9	22.6	25.0
Asian only	NA	NA	NA	NA	NA	NA	NA	9.4	8.8
Hispanic or Latino	NA	NA	NA	NA	NA	22.5	22.9	22.8	25.9
Mexican origin	13.8	22.3	18.6	21.1	23.8	23.1	23.8	23.5	26.6
Boys	11.3	16.7	17.9	18.2	18.7	19.4	20.0	20.1	20.0
Not Hispanic or Latino									
White only	11.6	14.6	17.9	17.3	16.1	17.1	17.9	18.7	16.3
Black or African American only	10.7	18.8	17.6	18.4	19.1	21.2	22.0	20.9	22.0
Asian only	NA	NA	NA	NA	NA	NA	NA	12.9	9.1
Hispanic or Latino	NA	NA	NA	NA	NA	26.0	25.1	22.7	26.7
Mexican origin	14.1	24.7	20.0	22.1	26.2	27.9	27.0	22.8	26.4
Girls	9.7	15.3	16.0	16.8	17.0	16.9	18.9	21.0	21.2
Not Hispanic or Latino									
White only	8.9	12.6	14.6	14.5	14.0	14.6	17.8	20.4	18.1
Black or African American only	16.3	23.5	23.8	27.7	29.5	27.1	23.7	24.4	28.2
Asian only	NA	NA	NA	NA	NA	NA	NA	*5.7	8.4
Hispanic or Latino	NA	NA	NA	NA	NA	18.7	20.6	22.8	25.0
Mexican origin	*13.4	19.6	17.1	19.9	21.3	18.0	20.2	24.2	26.8
Percent of Poverty Level[3]									
Below 100 percent	15.8	19.8	18.2	19.3	23.1	24.3	23.2	22.4	25.7
100 percent to 199 percent	11.2	15.1	17.0	18.4	19.8	20.1	22.5	25.7	24.3
200 percent to 399 percent	9.4	15.7	19.0	19.3	17.2	16.3	17.9	19.7	19.3
400 percent or more	*	13.9	13.2	12.6	14.0	14.0	13.8	*13.7	13.7

NOTE: Obesity in youth is defined as body mass index (BMI) at or above the sex- and age-specific 95th percentile of the 2000 Centers for Disease Control and Prevention (CDC) Growth Charts. See: Kuczmarski RJ, Ogden CL, Guo SS, Grummer-Strawn LM, Flegal KM, Mei Z, et al. 2000 CDC Growth Charts for the United States: Methods and development. Vital Health Stat 11(246). 2002. Available from: https://www.cdc.gov/nchs/data/series/sr_11/sr11_246.pdf. BMI equals weight in kilograms divided by height in meters squared. The National Health and Nutrition Examination Survey variable Body Mass Index is used to assign persons to BMI categories. Age is at the time of examination. Height is measured without shoes. Data on both age and height were collected during a standardized physical examination conducted in mobile examination centers. Estimates exclude pregnant females. Crude percentages, not age-adjusted percentages, are shown.
NA = Not available.
* = Estimates are considered unreliable. Starting with 2013–2016 data, the reliability of survey percentage estimates was assessed using new multistep National Center for Health Statistics data presentation standards for proportions. Prior to 2013–2016 data, the reliability of estimates for earlier years was evaluated based on relative standard errors (RSE). Data preceded by an asterisk have an RSE of 20%–30%. Data not shown have an RSE greater than 30%.
[1] Persons of Hispanic and Mexican origin may be of any race. Starting with 1999 data, race-specific estimates are tabulated according to the 1997 Revisions to the Standards for the Classification of Federal Data on Race and Ethnicity and are not strictly comparable with estimates for earlier years. The non-Hispanic race categories shown in the table conform to the 1997 Standards. Starting with 1999 data, race-specific estimates are for persons who reported only one racial group. Prior to data year 1999, estimates were tabulated according to the 1977 Standards. Estimates for single-race categories prior to 1999 included persons who reported one race, or if they reported more than one race, identified one race as best representing their race.
[2] Includes persons of all races and Hispanic origins, not just those shown separately.
[3] Percent of poverty level was calculated by dividing family income by the U.S. Department of Health and Human Services' poverty guideline specific to family size, as well as the appropriate year and state. Persons with unknown percent of poverty level are excluded (6% in 2013–2016).

Table 3-21. Untreated Dental Caries, by Selected Characteristics, Selected Years, 1988–1994 Through 2011–2014

(Percent.)

Sex, race and Hispanic origin[1], and percent of poverty level	Age 5–19 years		Age 20–44 years		Age 45-64 years		Age 65 years and over	
	1988–1994	2011–2014	1988–1994	2011–2014	1988–1994	2011–2014	1988–1994	2011–2014
Total[2]	24.3	18.6	29.5	31.6	25.4	27.2	27.1	21.8
Sex								
Male	23.6	19.7	32.8	32.8	28.5	31.8	31.2	24.7
Female	25.0	17.4	26.4	30.3	22.6	22.9	24.1	19.4
Race and Hispanic Origin								
Not Hispanic or Latino								
White only	19.4	16.7	24.8	27.1	21.7	23.4	24.6	18.6
Black or African American only	33.9	23.4	49.2	46.1	46.2	45.4	51.2	40.7
Mexican origin	37.9	23.8	40.0	40.0	41.4	40.8	46.3	46.3
Percent of Poverty Level[3]								
Below 100 percent	39.0	24.7	47.8	47.0	49.5	54.2	46.8	44.0
100 percent to 199 percent	29.6	22.3	43.7	40.8	42.5	45.0	37.6	36.8
200 percent to 399 percent	16.6	16.0	24.5	28.1	25.0	29.2	24.1	18.3
400 percent or more	*10.4	9.1	12.5	14.8	13.0	12.6	15.6	*9.5
Race and Hispanic Origin, and Percent of Poverty Level[3]								
Not Hispanic or Latino								
White only								
Below 100% of poverty level	33.8	24.5	42.9	47.4	47.6	52.2	38.5	46.7
100% or more of poverty level	17.3	14.8	22.7	23.0	19.7	20.9	23.9	17.2
Black or African American only				56.0		71.7		52.9
Below 100% of poverty level	37.4	27.5	60.0	41.3	62.9	37.9	56.3	38.6
100% or more of poverty level	31.2	19.3	44.8	44.4	41.2	49.9	47.8	58.7
Mexican origin				35.8		38.5		42.3
Below 100% of poverty level	47.5	23.1	52.7	38.0	52.7	*45.7	62.8	*56.7
100% or more of poverty level	28.0	23.7	31.2	35.1	34.5	43.4	35.4	*45.0

NOTE: Root caries are not included. Persons without at least one primary or one permanent tooth or one root tip were classified as edentulous and were excluded from this analysis. The majority of edentulous persons are 65 years of age and over. Estimates of edentulism among persons 65 years of age and over are 46 percent in 1971–1974, 33 percent in 1988–1994, and 23 percent in 2005–2008. For estimates prior to 2005–2008, only dental caries in primary teeth was evaluated for children 2–5 years of age. Caries in both permanent and primary teeth was evaluated for children 6–11 years of age. For children 12–19 years of age and adults, only dental caries in permanent teeth was evaluated. Starting with 2005–2006 data, dental caries data were collected using a simplified examination process that used health technologists to screen for caries instead of using dentists to conduct a comprehensive caries exam. In addition, dental caries data were not collected on children younger than 5 years of age. Because of this change in the examination process and because 2005–2008 dental caries data are based on both primary and permanent teeth, regardless of age, data for 2005–2008 need to be interpreted with caution, especially when comparing with earlier data.
* = Figure does not meet standards of reliability or precision. Data preceded by an asterisk have a relative standard error (RSE) of 20 percent to 30 percent. Data not shown have an RSE of greater than 30 percent.
[1]Persons of Mexican origin may be of any race.
[2]Includes persons of all races and Hispanic origins, not just those shown separately, and those with unknown percent of poverty level.
[3]Percent of poverty level is based on family income and family size. Persons with unknown percent of poverty level are excluded (6 percent in 2011–2014).

Table 3-22. Selected Health Conditions and Risk Factors, Selected Years, 1988–1994 Through 2015–2016

(Percent; data are based on interviews, physical examinations, and laboratory data of a sample of the civilian noninstitutionalized population.)

Health condition	1988–1994	1999–2000	2001–2002	2003–2004	2005–2006	2007–2008	2009–2010	2011–2012	2013–2014	2015–2016
Diabetes[1]										
Total, age-adjusted[2]	8.8	9.0	10.6	10.9	10.4	11.4	11.5	11.9	11.9	NA
Total, crude	8.3	8.6	10.3	10.9	10.9	11.9	12.1	12.5	12.7	NA
Hypercholesterolemia[3]										
Total, age-adjusted[4]	22.8	25.5	24.6	27.9	27.4	27.6	27.2	28.2	27.4	26.9
Total, crude	21.5	24.5	24.2	27.9	28.1	28.8	28.6	30.4	29.3	29.6
High Cholesterol[5]										
Total, age-adjusted[4]	20.8	18.3	16.5	16.9	15.6	14.2	13.2	12.7	11.1	12.2
Total, crude	19.6	17.7	16.4	17.0	15.9	14.6	13.6	13.1	11.1	12.5
Hypertension[6]										
Total, age-adjusted[4]	25.5	30.0	29.7	32.1	30.5	31.2	30.0	30.0	30.8	30.2
Total, crude	24.1	28.9	28.9	32.5	31.7	32.6	31.9	32.5	33.5	33.2
Uncontrolled High Blood Pressure Among Persons with Hypertension[7]										
Total, age-adjusted[4]	77.2	71.9	68.3	63.8	63.0	56.2	55.7	54.6	51.3	59.7
Total, crude	73.9	69.1	65.4	60.8	56.6	51.8	46.7	48.0	46.1	51.5
Overweight (Includes Obesity)[8]										
Total, age-adjusted[4]	56.0	64.5	65.6	66.4	66.9	68.1	68.8	68.6	70.4	71.3
Total, crude	54.9	64.1	65.6	66.5	67.3	68.3	69.2	69.0	70.7	71.6
Obesity[9]										
Total, age-adjusted[4]	22.9	30.5	30.5	32.3	34.4	33.7	35.7	34.9	37.8	39.7
Total, crude	22.3	30.3	30.6	32.3	34.7	33.9	35.9	35.1	37.9	39.8
Untreated Dental Caries[10]										
Total, age-adjusted[4]	27.7	24.4	21.3	29.8	24.4	21.7	NA	25.5	31.5	NA
Total, crude	28.2	25.0	21.7	30.2	24.5	21.8	NA	25.5	31.3	NA
Percent of Persons Under 20 Years of Age										
Obesity[11]										
2 to 5 years	7.2	10.3	10.6	14.0	11.0	10.1	12.1	8.4	9.4	13.9
6 to 11 years	11.3	15.1	16.3	18.8	15.1	19.6	18.0	17.7	17.4	18.4
12 to 19 years	10.5	14.8	16.7	17.4	17.8	18.1	18.4	20.5	20.6	20.6
Untreated Dental Caries[10]										
5 to 19 years	24.3	23.6	21.2	25.6	16.2	16.9	14.6	17.5	19.6	NA

NA = Not available.

[1]Includes physician-diagnosed and undiagnosed diabetes. Estimates were obtained using fasting weights. Physician-diagnosed diabetes was obtained by self-report and excludes women who reported having diabetes only during pregnancy. Undiagnosed diabetes is defined as a fasting plasma glucose (FPG) of at least 126 mg/dL or a hemoglobin A1c of at least 6.5% among those with no reported physician diagnosis. Pregnant women were excluded. Adjustments to FPG recommended by the National Health and Examination Nutrition Survey (NHANES) for trend analysis were incorporated into the data presented here. For more information, see https://wwwn.cdc.gov/nchs/nhanes/2005-2006/GLU_D.htm.
[2]Estimates are age-adjusted to the year 2000 standard population using three age groups: 20–44 years, 45–64 years, and 65 years and over. Age-adjusted estimates in this table may differ from other age-adjusted estimates based on the same data presented elsewhere if different age groups are used in the adjustment procedure.
[3]Hypercholesterolemia is defined as measured serum total cholesterol greater than or equal to 240 mg/dL (6.20 mmol/L) or reporting taking cholesterol-lowering medication. Respondents were asked, "Are you now following this advice [from a doctor or health professional] to take prescribed medicine [to lower your cholesterol]?"
[4]Estimates are age-adjusted to the year 2000 standard population using five age groups: 20–34 years, 35–44 years, 45–54 years, 55–64 years, and 65 years and over. Age-adjusted estimates in this table may differ from other age-adjusted estimates based on the same data and presented elsewhere if different age groups are used in the adjustment procedure.
[5]High total cholesterol is defined as measured serum total cholesterol greater than or equal to 240 mg/dL (6.20 mmol/L), regardless of whether the respondent reported taking cholesterol-lowering medications.
[6]Hypertension is defined as having measured high blood pressure or taking antihypertensive medication. High blood pressure is defined as having measured systolic pressure of at least 140 mm Hg or diastolic pressure of at least 90 mm Hg. Those with high blood pressure may also be taking prescribed medicine for high blood pressure. For antihypertensive medication use, respondents were asked, "Are you now taking prescribed medicine for your high blood pressure?" Pregnant women were excluded. In 2017, a revised set of practice guidelines for defining high blood pressure was released but has not been widely adopted. Therefore, the high blood pressure cutoffs used to define hypertension and uncontrolled high blood pressure in *Health, United States* continue to use the original definition of 140 mm Hg/90 mm Hg.
[7]Uncontrolled high blood pressure among persons with hypertension is defined as having measured high blood pressure among those with measured high blood pressure or reporting taking antihypertensive medication. High blood pressure is defined as having measured systolic pressure of at least 140 mm Hg or diastolic pressure of at least 90 mm Hg. Pregnant women were excluded. In 2017, a revised set of practice guidelines for defining high blood pressure was released but has not been widely adopted. Therefore, the high blood pressure cutoffs used to define hypertension and uncontrolled high blood pressure in *Health, United States* continue to use the original definition of 140 mm Hg/90 mm Hg.
[8]Overweight or obesity in adults is defined as body mass index (BMI) greater than or equal to 25.0 based on the NHANES variable Body Mass Index. Pregnant women were excluded.
[9]Obesity in adults is defined as BMI greater than or equal to 30.0, based on the NHANES variable Body Mass Index. Pregnant women were excluded. See Appendix II, Body mass index (BMI).
[10]Untreated dental caries refers to decay on the crown or enamel surface of a tooth (i.e., coronal caries) that has not been treated or filled. The presence of caries was evaluated in primary and permanent teeth for persons aged 5 and over. The third molars were not included. Persons without at least one natural tooth (primary or permanent) were excluded. Over time, there have been changes in the NHANES oral health examination process, ages examined, and methodology.
[11]Obesity in youth is defined as BMI at or above the sex- and age-specific 95th percentile of the 2000 CDC growth charts. See: Kuczmarski RJ, Ogden CL, Guo SS, Grummer-Strawn LM, Flegal KM, Mei Z, et al. 2000 CDC growth charts for the United States: Methods and development. National Center for Health Statistics. Vital Health Stat 11(246). 2002. Available from: https://www.cdc.gov/nchs/data/series/sr_11/sr11_246.pdf. Pregnant girls were excluded.

Table 3-23. Health Risk Behaviors Among Students in Grades 9 to 12, by Sex, Grade Level, Race, and Hispanic Origin, Selected Years, 1991–2015

(Percent.)

Sex, grade level, race, and Hispanic origin	Seriously considered suicide[1]			In a physical fight[1]			Carried a weapon[2,3]		
	1991	1999	2015	1991	1999	2015	1991	1999	2015
Total	29.0	19.3	17.7	42.5	35.7	22.6	26.1	17.3	16.2
Male									
Total	20.8	13.7	12.2	50.2	44.0	28.4	40.6	28.6	24.3
9th grade	17.6	11.9	10.7	57.8	49.5	32.5	44.4	28.7	24.6
10th grade	19.5	13.7	10.8	50.2	46.0	29.4	41.5	30.7	25.5
11th grade	25.3	13.7	13.3	51.0	38.9	27.1	44.0	26.9	23.0
12th grade	20.7	15.6	14.0	42.3	39.0	22.9	33.1	27.3	23.4
Not Hispanic or Latino									
White	21.7	12.5	11.5	49.1	43.2	26.6	41.2	28.6	28.0
Black or African American	13.3	11.7	11.0	58.4	44.4	38.6	43.4	23.1	17.6
Hispanic or Latino	18.0	13.6	12.4	48.5	50.5	27.3	40.0	29.5	20.2
Female									
Total	37.2	24.9	23.4	34.4	27.3	16.5	10.9	6.0	7.5
9th grade	40.3	24.4	26.5	42.9	32.5	22.6	10.4	6.5	6.6
10th grade	39.7	30.1	25.7	35.4	29.4	17.6	11.1	7.1	7.2
11th grade	38.4	23.0	22.1	34.5	23.4	12.8	12.9	5.2	8.0
12th grade	30.7	21.2	18.6	25.4	21.9	12.0	9.5	4.8	8.0
Not Hispanic or Latina									
White	38.6	23.2	22.8	32.2	22.3	13.5	7.5	3.6	8.1
Black or African American	29.4	18.8	18.7	43.8	38.6	25.4	23.6	11.7	6.2
Hispanic or Latina	34.6	26.1	25.6	34.8	29.7	18.6	12.9	8.4	7.1

Sex, grade level, race, and Hispanic origin	Ever had sexual intercourse			Did not use a condom at last sex[4]			Physically forced to have sex		
	1991	1999	2015	1991	1999	2015	1991	1999	2015
Total	54.1	49.9	41.2	53.8	42.0	43.1	NA	8.8	6.7
Male									
Total	57.4	52.2	43.2	45.5	34.5	38.5	NA	5.2	3.1
9th grade	45.6	44.5	27.3	44.1	30.5	36.7	NA	5.6	2.1
10th grade	50.9	51.1	37.9	43.1	30.0	34.4	NA	4.6	3.9
11th grade	64.5	51.4	51.2	43.2	30.7	37.5	NA	5.0	2.8
12th grade	68.3	63.9	59.0	49.3	44.1	42.6	NA	5.6	3.5
Not Hispanic or Latino									
White	52.7	45.4	39.5	44.8	37.0	41.9	NA	3.5	2.0
Black or African American	88.1	75.7	58.8	43.0	24.7	26.4	NA	9.7	4.4
Hispanic or Latino	64.1	62.9	45.1	53.0	33.9	37.5	NA	5.9	4.0
Female									
Total	50.8	47.7	39.2	62.0	49.3	48.0	NA	12.5	10.3
9th grade	32.2	32.5	20.7	49.7	36.9	43.3	NA	10.4	9.4
10th grade	45.3	42.6	33.5	63.6	44.7	46.0	NA	12.4	7.9
11th grade	60.2	53.8	48.2	59.3	50.0	47.1	NA	14.5	12.0
12th grade	65.1	65.8	57.2	67.4	58.9	51.2	NA	12.8	11.9
Not Hispanic or Latina									
White	47.1	44.8	40.3	62.0	52.4	44.1	NA	10.1	9.9
Black or African American	75.9	66.9	37.4	60.6	35.5	53.3	NA	13.5	10.3
Hispanic or Latina	43.3	45.5	39.8	73.1	57.0	51.7	NA	15.1	10.1

NOTE: Only youths attending school participated in the survey. Persons of Hispanic origin may be of any race.
NA = Data not available.
[1] During the last 12 months.
[2] During the last 30 days.
[3] Such as a gun, knife, or club.
[4] Among students who are sexually active.

Table 3-23. Health Risk Behaviors Among Students in Grades 9 to 12, by Sex, Grade Level, Race, and Hispanic Origin, Selected Years, 1991–2015—_Continued_

(Percent.)

Sex, grade level, race, and Hispanic origin	Did not eat breakfast on all 7 days[5,6]			Got fewer than 8 hours of sleep[5,7]		
	1991	1999	2015	1991	1999	2015
Total...	NA	NA	63.7	NA	NA	72.7
Male						
Total...	NA	NA	59.5	NA	NA	69.9
9th grade...	NA	NA	53.4	NA	NA	60.7
10th grade...	NA	NA	57.7	NA	NA	66.2
11th grade...	NA	NA	62.9	NA	NA	77.1
12th grade...	NA	NA	65.3	NA	NA	77.4
Not Hispanic or Latino						
White...	NA	NA	56.7	NA	NA	68.9
Black or African American...............................	NA	NA	69.2	NA	NA	74.4
Hispanic or Latino...	NA	NA	60.5	NA	NA	67.1
Female						
Total...	NA	NA	67.9	NA	NA	75.6
9th grade...	NA	NA	68.1	NA	NA	70.9
10th grade...	NA	NA	68.9	NA	NA	76.9
11th grade...	NA	NA	67.6	NA	NA	77.0
12th grade...	NA	NA	67.1	NA	NA	77.8
Not Hispanic or Latina						
White...	NA	NA	65.2	NA	NA	75.1
Black or African American...............................	NA	NA	75.3	NA	NA	79.4
Hispanic or Latina...	NA	NA	69.9	NA	NA	73.2

NOTE: Only youths attending school participated in the survey. Persons of Hispanic origin may be of any race.
NA = Data not available.
[5]Percent is 100 minus percent presented in MMWR Youth Risk Behavior Surveillance Summaries.
[6]During the past 7 days. Data prior to 2011 are not available.
[7]On an average school night. Data prior to 2007 are not available.

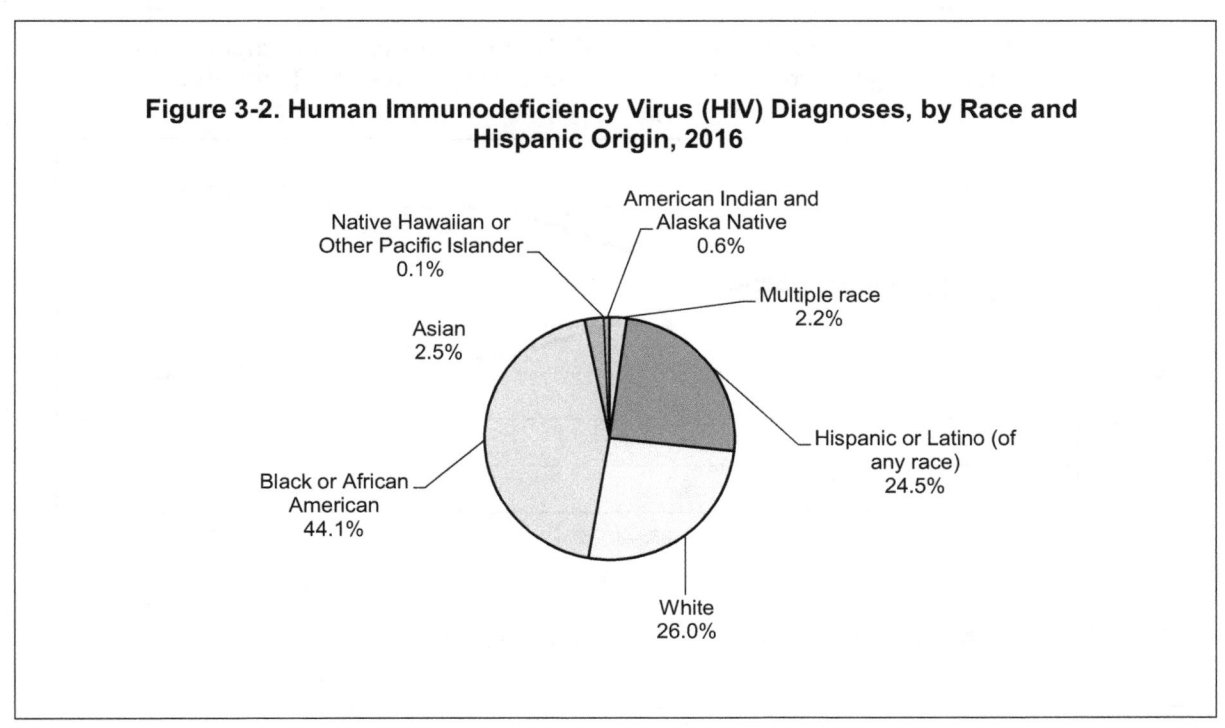

Figure 3-2. Human Immunodeficiency Virus (HIV) Diagnoses, by Race and Hispanic Origin, 2016

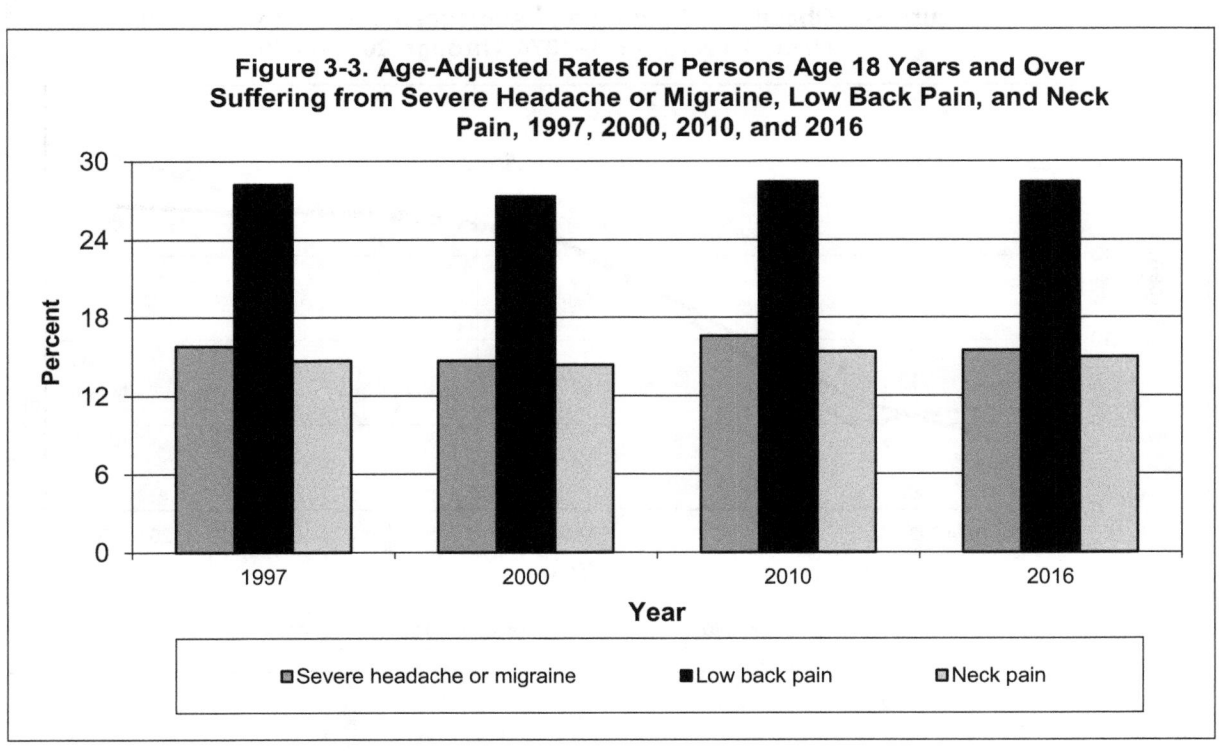

Figure 3-3. Age-Adjusted Rates for Persons Age 18 Years and Over Suffering from Severe Headache or Migraine, Low Back Pain, and Neck Pain, 1997, 2000, 2010, and 2016

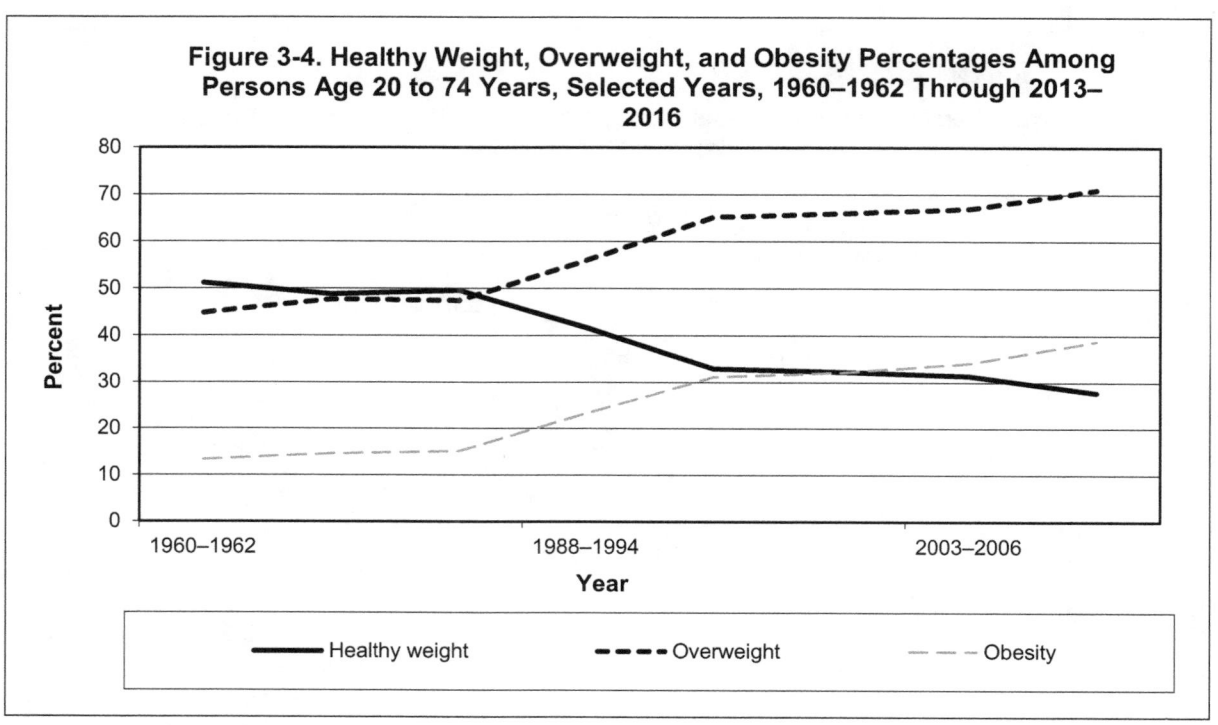

Figure 3-4. Healthy Weight, Overweight, and Obesity Percentages Among Persons Age 20 to 74 Years, Selected Years, 1960–1962 Through 2013–2016

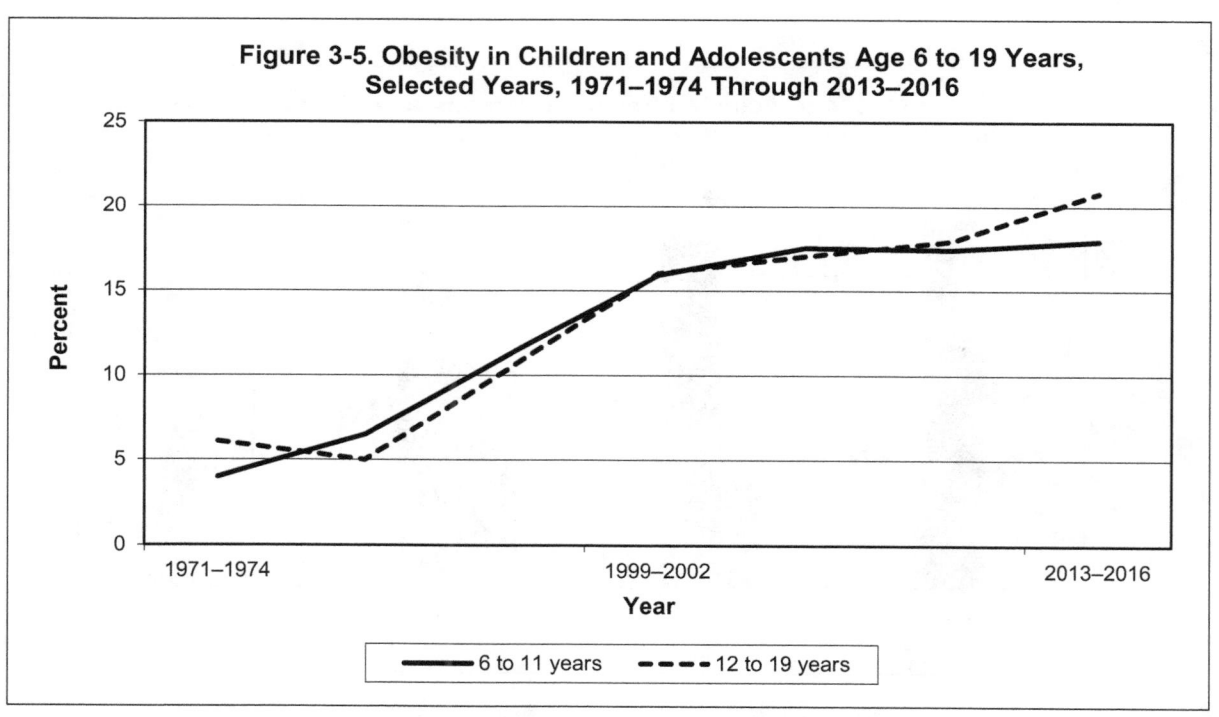

Figure 3-5. Obesity in Children and Adolescents Age 6 to 19 Years, Selected Years, 1971–1974 Through 2013–2016

USE OF ADDICTIVE SUBSTANCES

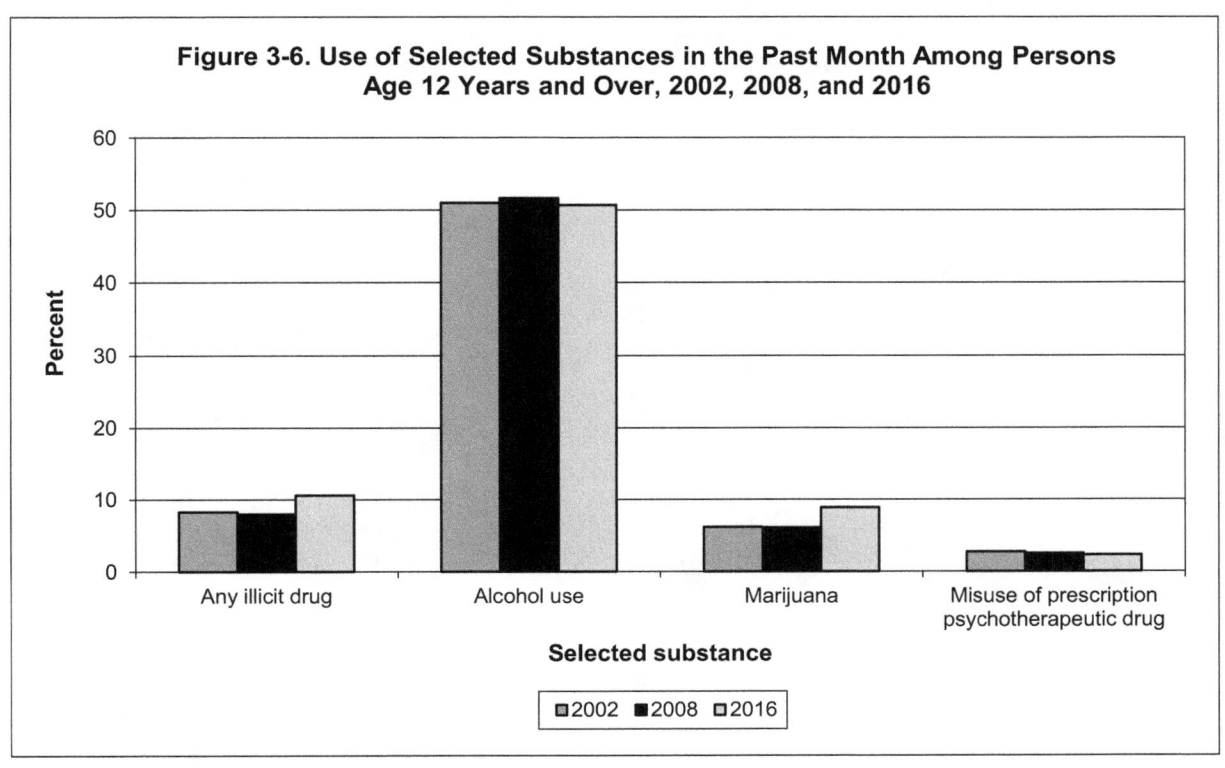

Figure 3-6. Use of Selected Substances in the Past Month Among Persons Age 12 Years and Over, 2002, 2008, and 2016

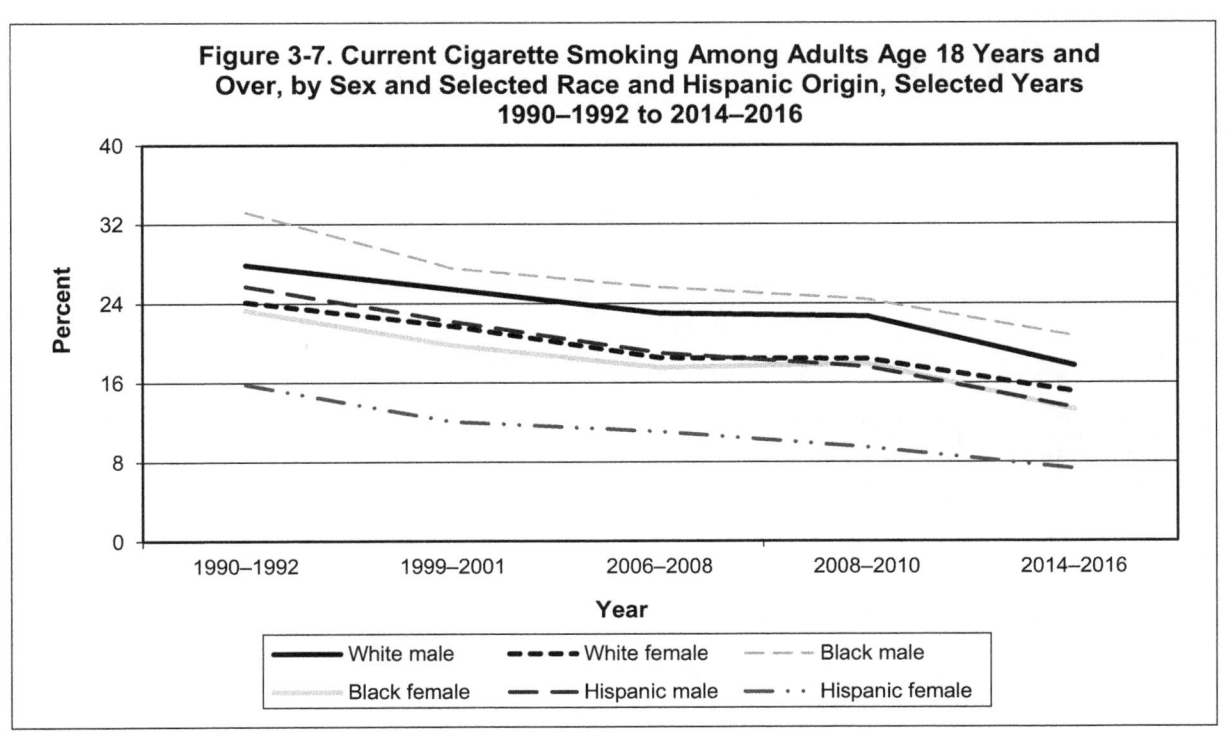

Figure 3-7. Current Cigarette Smoking Among Adults Age 18 Years and Over, by Sex and Selected Race and Hispanic Origin, Selected Years 1990–1992 to 2014–2016

Table 3-24. Use of Selected Substances in the Past Month Among Persons 12 Years of Age and Over, by Age, Sex, Race, and Hispanic Origin, Selected Years, 2002–2016

(Percent; Data are based on household interviews of a sample of the civilian noninstitutionalized population aged 12 and over.)

Age, sex, race, and Hispanic origin	Any illicit drug[1]			Marijuana			Misuse of prescription psychotherapeutic drugs[2]		
	2002	2009	2016	2002	2009	2016	2002	2009	2016
Age, 12 Years and Over............................	NA	NA	10.6	6.2	6.7	8.9	NA	NA	2.3
12 to 13 years...................................	NA	NA	2.0	1.4	0.8	0.8	NA	NA	0.7
14 to 15 years...................................	NA	NA	6.7	7.6	6.3	5.3	NA	NA	1.5
16 to 17 years...................................	NA	NA	14.5	15.7	14.1	12.9	NA	NA	2.4
18 to 25 years...................................	NA	NA	23.2	17.3	18.2	20.8	NA	NA	4.6
26 to 34 years...................................	NA	NA	16.8	7.7	9.6	14.5	NA	NA	3.6
35 years and over	NA	NA	7.1	3.1	3.4	5.6	NA	NA	1.6
Sex									
Male..	NA	NA	12.8	8.1	8.7	11.3	NA	NA	2.3
Female...	NA	NA	8.5	4.4	4.8	6.7	NA	NA	2.3
Age and Sex									
12 to 17 years...................................	NA	NA	7.9	8.2	7.4	6.5	NA	NA	1.6
Male..	NA	NA	7.9	9.1	8.4	6.8	NA	NA	1.2
Female	NA	NA	7.8	7.2	6.3	6.1	NA	NA	2.0
Hispanic Origin and Race[3]									
Not Hispanic or Latino									
White only......................................	NA	NA	10.8	6.5	6.8	9.0	NA	NA	2.7
Black or African American only	NA	NA	12.5	7.4	7.9	11.1	NA	NA	1.6
American Indian or Alaska Native only	NA	NA	15.7	6.7	10.7	13.6	NA	NA	1.9
Native Hawaiian or Other Pacific Islander only..	NA	NA	9.8	4.4	4.3	8.6	NA	NA	1.5
Asian only......................................	NA	NA	4.1	1.8	2.4	3.3	NA	NA	0.5
Two or more races	NA	NA	20.2	9.0	12.3	17.7	NA	NA	3.7
Hispanic or Latino..............................	NA	NA	9.2	4.3	5.8	7.7	NA	NA	1.8

Age, sex, race, and Hispanic origin	Alcohol use			Binge alcohol use[4]			Heavy alcohol use[5]		
	2002	2008	2016	2002	2008	2016	2002	2008	2016
Age, 12 Years and Over............................	51.0	51.9	50.7	NA	NA	24.2	NA	NA	6.0
12 to 13 years...................................	4.3	3.5	1.4	NA	NA	0.3	NA	NA	0.0
14 to 15 years...................................	16.6	13.1	7.9	NA	NA	3.7	NA	NA	0.5
16 to 17 years...................................	32.6	26.5	17.7	NA	NA	10.2	NA	NA	1.7
18 to 25 years...................................	60.5	61.8	57.1	NA	NA	38.4	NA	NA	10.1
26 to 34 years...................................	61.4	64.2	64.1	NA	NA	37.2	NA	NA	9.4
35 years and over	52.1	52.7	52.5	NA	NA	21.3	NA	NA	5.2
Sex									
Male..	57.4	57.5	55.3	31.2	31.6	28.9	10.8	10.3	8.3
Female...	44.9	46.5	46.4	NA	NA	19.8	NA	NA	3.9
Age and Sex									
12 to 17 years...................................	17.6	14.8	9.2	NA	NA	4.9	NA	NA	0.8
Male..	17.4	15.3	8.8	11.4	9.7	4.4	3.1	2.4	0.9
Female	17.9	14.4	9.6	NA	NA	5.4	NA	NA	0.6
Hispanic Origin and Race[3]									
Not Hispanic or Latino									
White only......................................	55.0	56.8	56.3	NA	NA	25.4	NA	NA	7.2
Black or African American only	39.9	42.6	41.2	NA	NA	22.7	NA	NA	4.1
American Indian or Alaska Native only	44.7	37.1	34.4	NA	NA	21.6	NA	NA	5.7
Native Hawaiian or Other Pacific Islander only..	*	*	38.1	NA	NA	16.8	NA	NA	4.1
Asian only......................................	37.1	37.3	35.5	NA	NA	12.9	NA	NA	1.9
Two or more races	49.9	47.8	47.3	NA	NA	23.2	NA	NA	6.0
Hispanic or Latino..............................	42.8	41.7	42.5	NA	NA	24.9	NA	NA	4.5

NA = Not available.

0.0 = Quantity more than zero but less than 0.05.

* = Estimates are considered unreliable. Data not shown if the relative standard error is greater than 17.5% of the log transformation of the proportion, the minimum effective sample size is less than 68, the minimum nominal sample size is less than 100, or the prevalence is close to 0% or 100%.

[1]Any illicit drug includes marijuana, cocaine (including crack), heroin, hallucinogens (including LSD, PCP, peyote, mescaline, psilocybin mushrooms, "Ecstasy," ketamine, DMT/AMT/"Foxy," and Salvia divinorum), and prescription psychotherapeutic drugs (including pain relievers, tranquilizers, stimulants, and sedatives).

[2]Misuse of prescription psychotherapeutic drugs is defined as use in any way not directed by a doctor, including use without a prescription of one's own; use in greater amounts, more often, or longer than told to take a drug; or use in any other way not directed by a doctor.

[3]Persons of Hispanic origin may be of any race. Data on race and Hispanic origin were collected using the 1997 Revisions to the Standards for the Classification of Federal Data on Race and Ethnicity. Single-race categories shown include persons who reported only one racial group. The category 2 or more races includes persons who reported more than one racial group.

[4]Binge alcohol use for men is defined as drinking five or more drinks on the same occasion on at least 1 day in the past 30 days. Starting in 2015, binge alcohol use for women is defined as drinking four or more drinks on the same occasion on at least 1 day in the past 30 days. Occasion is defined as at the same time or within a couple of hours of each other.

[5]Heavy use of alcohol is defined as binge drinking on 5 or more days in the past month. Starting in 2015, the binge drinking definition for women was lowered to four or more drinks on the same occasion. This change affected the comparability of estimates of heavy use of alcohol by women prior to 2015 with more recent years. By definition, all heavy alcohol users are also binge alcohol users.

Table 3-24. Use of Selected Substances in the Past Month Among Persons 12 Years of Age and Over, by Age, Sex, Race, and Hispanic Origin, Selected Years, 2002–2016—*Continued*

(Percent; Data are based on household interviews of a sample of the civilian noninstitutionalized population aged 12 and over.)

Age, sex, race, and Hispanic origin	Any tobacco[6]			Cigarettes			Cigars		
	2002	2008	2016	2002	2008	2016	2002	2008	2016
Age, 12 Years and Over	30.4	27.7	23.5	26.0	23.3	19.1	5.4	5.3	4.6
12 to 13 years	3.8	2.3	0.8	3.2	1.4	0.4	0.7	0.7	0.1
14 to 15 years	13.4	9.9	3.9	11.2	7.6	2.2	3.8	3.1	1.3
16 to 17 years	29.0	21.9	11.0	24.9	17.1	7.4	9.3	7.8	3.9
18 to 25 years	45.3	41.6	30.0	40.8	35.8	23.5	11.0	11.5	8.8
26 to 34 years	38.2	39.6	32.9	32.7	33.9	27.5	6.6	7.5	6.5
35 years and over	27.9	24.5	22.8	23.4	20.4	18.5	4.1	3.7	3.7
Sex									
Male	37.0	33.5	29.3	28.7	25.3	21.2	9.4	8.8	7.4
Female	24.3	22.3	18.1	23.4	21.5	17.1	1.7	2.0	1.9
Age and Sex									
12 to 17 years	15.2	11.8	5.3	13.0	9.0	3.4	4.5	4.0	1.8
Male	16.0	13.8	6.6	12.3	9.3	3.8	6.2	5.3	2.6
Female	14.4	9.6	4.0	13.6	8.7	3.1	2.7	2.7	1.0
Hispanic Origin and Race[3]									
Not Hispanic or Latino									
White only	32.0	29.7	26.0	26.9	24.6	20.7	5.5	5.3	4.6
Black or African American only	28.8	26.2	24.2	25.3	22.4	19.3	6.8	7.2	7.6
American Indian or Alaska Native only	44.3	41.8	37.9	37.1	33.1	31.3	5.2	6.9	4.0
Native Hawaiian or Other Pacific Islander only	28.8	*	20.6	*	15.4	16.7	4.1	*	1.8
Asian only	18.6	11.9	8.9	17.7	10.9	8.2	1.1	1.5	1.1
Two or more races	38.1	36.6	33.4	35.0	30.6	27.8	5.5	7.8	7.5
Hispanic or Latino	25.2	23.1	16.8	23.0	21.2	14.7	5.0	4.7	3.1

* = Estimates are considered unreliable. Data not shown if the relative standard error is greater than 17.5% of the log transformation of the proportion, the minimum effective sample size is less than 68, the minimum nominal sample size is less than 100, or the prevalence is close to 0% or 100%.
[3]Persons of Hispanic origin may be of any race. Data on race and Hispanic origin were collected using the 1997 Revisions to the Standards for the Classification of Federal Data on Race and Ethnicity. Single-race categories shown include persons who reported only one racial group. The category 2 or more races includes persons who reported more than one racial group.
[6]Any tobacco product includes cigarettes, smokeless tobacco (such as snuff, dip, chewing tobacco, or "snus"), cigars, or pipe tobacco.

Table 3-25. Heavier Drinking and Drinking Five or More Drinks in a Day Among Adults 18 Years of Age and Over, by Selected Characteristics, Selected Years, 1997–2013

(Percent.)

Characteristic	Heavier drinker[1]				Five or more drinks in a day on at least 1 day in the past year[1]				Five or more drinks in a day on at least 12 days in the past year[1]			
	1997	2000	2010	2013	1997	2000	2010	2013	1997	2000	2010	2013
BOTH SEXES												
18 years and over, age-adjusted[2]	4.9	4.3	5.2	5.3	21.1	19.2	23.8	23.6	9.7	8.7	10.1	9.5
18 years and over, crude	5.0	4.3	5.2	5.3	21.5	19.3	23.2	22.6	9.8	8.7	9.9	9.2
Age												
All persons												
18 to 44 years	5.2	4.7	5.7	5.2	29.2	26.9	32.5	31.9	13.2	12.2	13.7	12.5
18 to 24 years	5.3	5.8	6.2	5.2	31.8	30.3	34.0	31.3	15.2	15.5	16.2	12.8
25 to 44 years	5.2	4.3	5.5	5.1	28.5	25.8	31.9	32.2	12.6	11.1	12.7	12.4
45 to 64 years	5.5	4.6	5.4	6.0	15.9	14.4	19.0	18.6	7.6	6.4	8.1	8.0
45 to 54 years	5.5	4.4	5.9	5.9	19.0	16.4	22.9	21.7	8.7	7.0	9.3	9.3
55 to 64 years	5.4	5.0	4.7	6.1	11.1	11.3	14.1	15.1	5.8	5.4	6.7	6.6
65 years and over	3.1	2.6	3.7	4.3	4.9	3.8	5.5	6.4	2.2	1.8	2.6	3.0
65 to 74 years	3.9	3.1	4.4	5.4	6.7	5.2	7.9	9.1	3.0	2.5	3.5	4.2
75 years and over	2.1	2.0	2.8	2.9	2.4	2.1	2.7	2.6	1.1	*0.9	*1.4	*1.4
Race[2,3]												
White only	5.2	4.5	5.6	5.7	22.9	20.8	26.3	26.0	10.3	9.2	11.1	10.5
Black or African American only	4.0	3.5	4.1	3.5	11.7	11.6	14.0	14.4	6.5	6.5	6.1	5.7
American Indian or Alaska Native only	*	*	*	*7.8	29.2	23.7	15.3	23.3	17.4	*12.1	*9.5	*12.4
Asian only	*1.9	*2.3	*1.3	*2.5	11.4	8.8	12.1	11.7	*4.8	3.6	4.3	4.2
Native Hawaiian or Other Pacific Islander only	NA	*	*	*	NA	*	*	*	NA	*	*	*
Two or more races	NA	*7.5	*5.9	*6.5	NA	28.0	25.7	26.3	NA	15.9	12.5	10.9
Hispanic Origin and Race[2,3]												
Hispanic or Latino	3.9	3.2	2.8	3.3	20.4	17.3	19.7	20.9	11.2	9.0	9.2	9.0
Mexican	4.4	3.8	3.1	3.8	21.2	19.9	21.4	21.8	12.6	10.8	10.1	10.0
Not Hispanic or Latino	5.1	4.5	5.6	5.6	21.3	19.7	24.7	24.2	9.5	8.8	10.3	9.6
White only	5.4	4.7	6.2	6.2	23.5	21.5	27.9	27.5	10.3	9.3	11.5	11.0
Black or African American only	3.9	3.4	4.2	3.5	11.6	11.5	13.9	14.3	6.5	6.5	6.1	5.5
Percent of Poverty Level[2,4]												
Below 100 percent	4.8	4.3	4.7	4.9	17.3	15.0	17.6	19.1	9.7	8.6	8.5	9.1
100 percent to 199 percent	4.9	4.2	4.9	4.5	18.4	15.7	20.9	20.3	9.8	8.0	9.8	8.4
200 percent to 399 percent	4.9	4.2	4.8	5.2	21.0	18.7	23.3	23.4	9.8	8.9	10.1	10.0
400 percent or more	5.1	4.4	6.0	5.9	24.3	22.1	28.1	26.7	9.7	8.9	10.9	9.9
Disability Measure[2,5]												
Any basic actions difficulty or complex activity limitation	5.7	5.2	5.5	4.9	20.2	18.8	21.9	20.7	10.2	9.3	9.5	8.6
Any basic actions difficulty	5.8	5.3	5.5	4.9	20.6	19.1	22.3	21.1	10.5	9.4	9.7	8.6
Any complex activity limitation	4.5	4.3	5.5	3.7	16.4	14.3	16.2	16.1	8.8	7.3	7.8	7.0
No disability	4.9	4.1	5.3	5.6	21.8	19.7	25.0	24.9	9.6	8.7	10.4	9.9
MALE												
18 years and over, age-adjusted[2]	6.1	5.1	5.7	5.7	30.7	28.3	32.4	32.1	15.8	14.4	15.6	15.1
18 years and over, crude	6.1	5.2	5.7	5.7	31.7	29.0	32.2	31.3	16.3	14.7	15.6	14.7
Age												
All persons												
18 to 44 years	6.5	5.6	6.1	5.5	40.6	37.8	42.5	41.4	21.1	19.6	20.6	19.1
18 to 24 years	6.0	6.3	6.0	5.4	40.6	38.0	39.9	37.7	22.9	22.9	21.5	17.9
25 to 44 years	6.6	5.3	6.2	5.6	40.6	37.7	43.5	42.8	20.6	18.5	20.2	19.6
45 to 64 years	6.6	5.5	5.8	6.3	25.3	23.5	27.3	27.0	12.7	11.3	13.2	13.0
45 to 54 years	6.6	5.7	5.9	6.4	29.4	26.3	32.0	30.3	14.5	12.3	14.5	14.3
55 to 64 years	6.6	5.4	5.7	6.3	18.9	19.0	21.4	23.5	10.0	9.8	11.6	11.5
65 years and over	3.7	3.1	4.0	5.2	9.3	7.4	9.8	11.4	4.7	3.7	4.7	6.0
65 to 74 years	4.8	3.9	4.4	6.3	12.2	9.5	13.5	15.2	6.1	4.9	6.3	7.6
75 years and over	*2.1	*2.0	*3.5	*3.4	5.1	4.4	4.6	5.4	*2.5	*2.0	*2.5	*3.4
Race[2,3]												
White only	6.3	5.1	6.1	6.0	32.8	29.9	35.3	34.9	16.7	14.9	17.1	16.5
Black or African American only	5.3	5.4	4.6	4.2	18.4	19.8	20.2	21.0	11.0	12.4	9.8	9.6
American Indian or Alaska Native only	*	*	*	*	45.7	29.2	*20.5	34.7	30.4	*14.0	*15.7	*19.4
Asian only	*2.3	*3.5	*1.4	*	17.8	14.1	17.2	17.0	*7.5	*5.9	6.8	6.5
Native Hawaiian or Other Pacific Islander only	NA	*	*	*	NA	*	*	*	NA	*	*	*
Two or more races	NA	*12.1	*8.4	*6.3	NA	39.2	37.6	34.8	NA	23.7	20.3	15.7
Hispanic Origin and Race[2,3]												
Hispanic or Latino	5.7	5.2	3.9	4.9	30.9	27.9	28.8	31.1	18.8	15.9	14.6	15.3
Mexican	6.9	6.6	4.4	5.4	34.2	32.2	32.2	33.4	21.9	19.1	16.3	17.3

NA = Not available.

* = Figure does not meet standards of reliability or precision. Data preceded by an asterisk have a relative standard error (RSE) of 20 percent to 30 percent. Data not shown have an RSE of greater than 30 percent.

[1] Heavier drinking is based on self-reported responses to questions about average alcohol consumption and is defined as more than 14 drinks per week for men and more than seven drinks per week for women on average. Respondents were also asked, "In the past year, on how many days did you have five or more drinks of any alcoholic beverage?"

[2] Estimates are age adjusted to the year 2000 standard population using four age groups: 18 to 24 years, 25 to 44 years, 45 to 64 years, and 65 years and over. Age-adjusted estimates in this table may differ from other age-adjusted estimates based on the same data and presented elsewhere if different age groups are used in the adjustment procedure.

[3] The race groups White, Black, American Indian or Alaska Native, Asian, Native Hawaiian or Other Pacific Islander, and two or more races, include persons of Hispanic and non-Hispanic origin. Persons of Hispanic origin may be of any race.

[4] Percent of poverty level is based on family income and family size and composition using U.S. Census Bureau poverty thresholds. Missing family income data were imputed for 1997 and beyond.

[5] Any basic actions difficulty or complex activity limitation is defined as having one or more of the following limitations or difficulties: movement difficulty, emotional difficulty, sensory (seeing or hearing) difficulty, cognitive difficulty, self-care (activities of daily living or instrumental activities of daily living) limitation, social limitation, or work limitation.

Table 3-25. Heavier Drinking and Drinking Five or More Drinks in a Day Among Adults 18 Years of Age and Over, by Selected Characteristics, Selected Years, 1997–2013—*Continued*

(Percent.)

Characteristic	Heavier drinker[1]				Five or more drinks in a day on at least 1 day in the past year[1]				Five or more drinks in a day on at least 12 days in the past year[1]			
	1997	2000	2010	2013	1997	2000	2010	2013	1997	2000	2010	2013
Not Hispanic or Latino	6.1	5.2	6.0	5.8	30.7	28.6	33.3	32.3	15.5	14.3	15.9	15.0
White only	6.4	5.2	6.5	6.3	33.3	30.6	36.9	36.1	16.6	15.0	17.6	16.8
Black or African American only	5.3	5.4	4.7	4.1	18.4	19.7	20.3	20.6	11.1	12.3	9.9	9.2
Percent of Poverty Level[2,4]												
Below 100 percent	6.8	6.4	6.5	6.8	26.9	24.8	26.0	27.3	16.5	15.7	14.1	15.5
100 percent to 199 percent	7.1	5.8	5.8	5.6	27.3	23.6	29.1	28.9	16.4	13.3	14.8	13.5
200 percent to 399 percent	6.6	5.3	5.8	6.1	30.4	27.4	31.8	31.0	16.0	14.7	16.4	15.6
400 percent or more	5.0	4.4	5.4	5.3	33.6	31.3	36.4	35.1	15.4	14.4	15.8	15.0
Disability Measure[2,5]												
Any basic actions difficulty or complex activity limitation	7.2	6.8	6.6	5.8	29.4	28.9	30.6	29.0	17.0	16.5	14.8	14.0
Any basic actions difficulty	7.5	6.8	6.7	5.8	30.4	29.8	31.8	30.2	17.7	16.8	15.5	14.6
Any complex activity limitation	5.4	5.8	6.6	4.3	23.1	20.5	21.1	21.3	14.2	11.9	11.3	10.7
No disability	5.8	4.8	5.4	5.7	31.5	28.5	33.5	33.3	15.6	14.1	15.9	15.4
FEMALE												
18 years and over, age-adjusted[2]	3.9	3.5	4.8	4.9	12.2	10.8	15.6	15.7	3.9	3.4	4.8	4.3
18 years and over, crude	3.9	3.5	4.8	4.9	12.1	10.6	14.9	14.6	3.9	3.3	4.6	4.1
Age												
All persons												
18 to 44 years	4.0	3.8	5.2	4.8	18.3	16.5	22.6	22.8	5.5	5.2	6.9	6.1
18 to 24 years	4.5	5.2	6.4	5.0	23.0	22.8	28.1	25.0	7.6	8.3	10.9	7.7
25 to 44 years	3.9	3.4	4.8	4.7	16.9	14.5	20.6	22.1	4.9	4.2	5.4	5.5
45 to 64 years	4.4	3.8	4.9	5.7	7.2	6.0	11.1	10.6	2.9	1.9	3.4	3.4
45 to 54 years	4.5	3.2	5.9	5.4	9.2	7.1	14.3	13.6	3.3	2.1	4.3	4.6
55 to 64 years	4.4	4.6	3.8	6.0	4.1	4.4	7.3	7.4	2.1	1.5	2.3	2.0
65 years and over	2.6	2.2	3.4	3.7	1.6	1.2	2.3	2.4	*0.4	*0.4	*	*0.7
65 to 74 years	3.1	2.5	4.5	4.6	2.3	1.7	*3.1	3.8	*	*	*	*1.2
75 years and over	2.0	1.9	2.3	2.5	*0.7	*	*1.4	*0.7	*	*	*	*
Race[2,3]												
White only	4.2	4.0	5.2	5.3	13.5	12.1	17.4	17.5	4.2	3.7	5.2	4.8
Black or African American only	2.9	2.0	3.8	3.0	6.5	5.2	9.0	9.2	2.9	1.9	3.1	2.6
American Indian or Alaska Native only	*	*	*	*4.0	18.1	*19.0	*11.7	*13.3	*	*	*	*
Asian only	*	*	*	*2.3	*5.2	*3.7	7.3	7.0	*	*	*	*2.2
Native Hawaiian or Other Pacific Islander only	NA	*	*	*	NA	*	*	*	NA	*	*	*
Two or more races	NA	*	*	*	NA	17.0	16.4	18.8	NA	*8.2	*6.3	*6.4
Hispanic Origin and Race[2,3]												
Hispanic or Latina	2.2	1.2	1.7	1.9	9.7	6.8	10.3	10.8	3.5	2.1	3.6	2.8
Mexican	*1.9	*1.1	*1.7	2.1	8.2	7.1	10.4	10.4	3.2	*2.2	3.7	2.7
Not Hispanic or Latina	4.1	3.8	5.3	5.4	12.6	11.5	16.6	16.7	4.0	3.6	5.0	4.6
White only	4.4	4.3	5.9	6.1	14.2	13.0	19.1	19.4	4.3	4.0	5.6	5.3
Black or African American only	2.9	2.0	3.8	3.1	6.2	5.2	8.9	9.2	2.9	1.9	3.0	2.6
Percent of Poverty Level[2,4]												
Below 100 percent	3.6	2.8	3.4	3.5	10.8	8.2	11.3	13.2	5.1	3.6	4.2	4.4
100 percent to 199 percent	3.1	2.9	4.1	3.6	10.5	9.0	13.5	13.3	4.0	3.5	5.1	4.1
200 percent to 399 percent	3.3	3.2	3.9	4.4	12.1	10.7	15.3	15.9	4.0	3.5	4.2	4.4
400 percent or more	5.2	4.5	6.7	6.6	14.2	12.6	19.2	17.8	3.4	3.3	5.6	4.6
Disability Measure[2,5]												
Any basic actions difficulty or complex activity limitation	4.5	4.1	4.7	4.3	13.1	11.3	15.2	14.5	5.0	4.1	5.4	4.5
Any basic actions difficulty	4.5	4.2	4.7	4.3	13.2	11.6	15.4	14.9	5.1	4.1	5.4	4.5
Any complex activity limitation	3.7	*3.2	4.6	3.2	10.8	9.1	12.3	11.5	4.2	*3.1	5.0	3.7
No disability	3.9	3.5	5.1	5.4	12.0	10.9	16.1	16.3	3.6	3.3	4.7	4.3

NA = Not available.

* = Figure does not meet standards of reliability or precision. Data preceded by an asterisk have a relative standard error (RSE) of 20 percent to 30 percent. Data not shown have an RSE of greater than 30 percent.

[1]Heavier drinking is based on self–reported responses to questions about average alcohol consumption and is defined as more than 14 drinks per week for men and more than seven drinks per week for women on average. Respondents were also asked, "In the past year, on how many days did you have five or more drinks of any alcoholic beverage?"

[2]Estimates are age adjusted to the year 2000 standard population using four age groups: 18 to 24 years, 25 to 44 years, 45 to 64 years, and 65 years and over. Age-adjusted estimates in this table may differ from other age–adjusted estimates based on the same data and presented elsewhere if different age groups are used in the adjustment procedure.

[3]The race groups White, Black, American Indian or Alaska Native, Asian, Native Hawaiian or Other Pacific Islander, and two or more races, include persons of Hispanic and non–Hispanic origin. Persons of Hispanic origin may be of any race.

[4]Percent of poverty level is based on family income and family size and composition using U.S. Census Bureau poverty thresholds. Missing family income data were imputed for 1997 and beyond.

[5]Any basic actions difficulty or complex activity limitation is defined as having one or more of the following limitations or difficulties: movement difficulty, emotional difficulty, sensory (seeing or hearing) difficulty, cognitive difficulty, self–care (activities of daily living or instrumental activities of daily living) limitation, social limitation, or work limitation.

Table 3-26. Age-Adjusted Prevalence of Current Cigarette Smoking Among Adults 25 Years of Age and Over, by Sex, Race, and Education Level, Selected Years, 1974–2016

(Percent; data are based on household interviews of a sample of the civilian noninstitutionalized population.)

Sex, race, and education level	1974[1]	1979[1]	1985[2]	1990[1]	1995[1]	2000	2005	2006	2007
25 YEARS AND OVER, AGE-ADJUSTED[2,3]									
All Persons[4]	36.9	33.1	30.0	25.4	24.5	22.6	20.3	20.3	19.3
No high school diploma or GED	43.7	40.7	40.8	36.7	35.6	31.6	28.2	28.8	26.9
High school diploma or GED	36.2	33.6	32.0	29.1	29.1	29.2	27.0	26.5	26.6
Some college, no bachelor's degree	35.9	33.2	29.5	23.4	22.6	21.7	21.8	22.1	20.1
Bachelor's degree or higher	27.2	22.6	18.5	13.9	13.6	10.9	9.1	8.2	9.0
All Males[4]	42.9	37.3	32.8	28.2	26.4	24.7	22.7	22.9	21.4
No high school diploma or GED	52.3	47.6	45.7	42.0	39.7	36.0	31.7	31.6	30.8
High school diploma or GED	42.4	38.9	35.5	33.1	32.7	32.1	29.9	29.7	29.4
Some college, no bachelor's degree	41.8	36.5	32.9	25.9	23.7	23.3	24.9	25.2	21.6
Bachelor's degree or higher	28.3	22.7	19.6	14.5	13.8	11.6	9.7	9.2	10.4
White Males[4,5]	41.9	36.7	31.7	27.6	25.9	24.7	22.4	22.7	21.6
No high school diploma or GED	51.5	47.6	45.0	41.8	38.7	38.2	31.6	31.4	30.8
High school diploma or GED	42.0	38.5	34.8	32.9	32.9	32.4	30.0	29.2	29.9
Some college, no bachelor's degree	41.6	36.4	32.2	25.4	23.3	23.5	24.5	25.8	21.8
Bachelor's degree or higher	27.8	22.5	19.1	14.4	13.4	11.3	9.3	8.9	10.5
Black or African American Males[4,5]	53.4	44.4	42.1	34.5	31.6	26.4	26.5	25.4	23.7
No high school diploma or GED	58.1	49.7	50.5	41.6	41.9	38.2	35.9	35.2	30.4
High school diploma or GED	*50.7	48.6	41.8	37.4	36.6	29.0	30.1	31.3	29.6
Some college, no bachelor's degree	*45.3	39.2	41.8	28.1	26.4	19.9	27.4	21.0	23.6
Bachelor's degree or higher	*41.4	*36.8	*32.0	*20.8	*17.3	14.6	10.0	12.9	*13.5
All Females[4]	32.0	29.5	27.5	22.9	22.9	20.5	18.0	17.9	17.2
No high school diploma or GED	36.6	34.8	36.5	31.8	31.7	27.1	24.6	26.0	22.7
High school diploma or GED	32.2	29.8	29.5	26.1	26.4	26.6	24.1	23.4	23.8
Some college, no bachelor's degree	30.1	30.0	26.3	21.0	21.6	20.4	19.1	19.6	18.9
Bachelor's degree or higher	25.9	22.5	17.1	13.3	13.3	10.1	8.5	7.2	7.7
White Females[4,5]	31.7	29.7	27.3	23.3	23.1	21.0	18.6	18.5	18.0
No high school diploma or GED	36.8	35.8	36.7	33.4	32.4	28.4	24.6	25.9	23.8
High school diploma or GED	31.9	29.9	29.4	26.5	26.8	27.8	25.9	24.6	25.2
Some college, no bachelor's degree	30.4	30.7	26.7	21.2	22.2	21.1	19.5	20.5	19.6
Bachelor's degree or higher	25.5	21.9	16.5	13.4	13.5	10.2	9.1	7.7	8.2
Black or African American Females[4,5]	35.6	30.3	32.0	22.4	25.7	21.6	17.5	19.1	16.6
No high school diploma or GED	36.1	31.6	39.4	26.3	32.3	31.1	27.8	31.2	23.1
High school diploma or GED	40.9	32.6	32.1	24.1	27.8	25.4	18.2	18.6	19.8
Some college, no bachelor's degree	32.3	*28.9	23.9	22.7	20.8	20.4	17.5	18.9	17.2
Bachelor's degree or higher	*36.3	*43.3	26.6	17.0	17.3	10.8	*6.6	*8.5	*6.0

* = Estimates are considered unreliable. Starting with 2016 data, the reliability of survey percentage estimates was assessed using new multistep National Center for Health Statistics data presentation standards for proportions. Prior to 2016 data, the reliability of estimates for earlier years was evaluated based on relative standard errors (RSE). Data preceded by an asterisk have an RSE of 20%–30%.
[1]Data prior to 1997 are not strictly comparable with data for later years due to the 1997 questionnaire redesign.
[2]Estimates are age-adjusted to the year 2000 standard population using four age groups: 25–34 years, 35–44 years, 45–64 years, and 65 years and over. For age groups where smoking was 0% or 100%, the age-adjustment procedure was modified to substitute the percentage smoking from the next-lower education group.
[3]Starting with 1993 data current cigarette smokers were defined as ever smoking 100 cigarettes in their lifetime and smoking now every day or some days.
[4]Includes unknown education level. Education categories shown are for 1997 and subsequent years. GED is General Educational Development high school equivalency diploma. In 1974–1995, the following categories based on number of years of school completed were used: less than 12 years, 12 years, 13–15 years, and 16 years or more.
[5]The race groups White and Black include persons of Hispanic and non-Hispanic origin. Starting with 1999 data, race-specific estimates are tabulated according to the 1997 Revisions to the Standards for the Classification of Federal Data on Race and Ethnicity and are not strictly comparable with estimates for earlier years. The single-race categories shown in the table conform to the 1997 Standards. Starting with 1999 data, race-specific estimates are for persons who reported only one racial group. Prior to 1999, data were tabulated according to the 1977 Standards. Estimates for single-race categories prior to 1999 included persons who reported one race, or if they reported more than one race, identified one race as best representing their race. Starting with 2003 data, race responses of other race and unspecified multiple race were treated as missing, and then race was imputed if these were the only race responses. Almost all persons with a race response of other race were of Hispanic origin.

Table 3-26. Age-Adjusted Prevalence of Current Cigarette Smoking Among Adults 25 Years of Age and Over, by Sex, Race, and Education Level, Selected Years, 1974–2016—Continued

(Percent; data are based on household interviews of a sample of the civilian noninstitutionalized population.)

Sex, race, and education level	2008	2009	2010	2011	2012	2013	2014	2015	2016
25 YEARS AND OVER, AGE-ADJUSTED[2,3]									
All Persons[4]	20.5	20.4	19.2	19.0	18.3	17.8	17.1	15.6	16.0
No high school diploma or GED	29.8	28.9	26.9	27.2	26.3	25.8	24.4	25.6	26.0
High school diploma or GED	28.1	28.7	27.0	27.4	26.3	25.6	25.9	22.9	23.6
Some college, no bachelor's degree	22.1	21.4	21.3	20.7	19.6	19.5	18.6	17.9	18.0
Bachelor's degree or higher	8.5	9.0	8.3	7.5	7.8	7.7	7.0	5.9	6.5
All Males[4]	22.6	22.4	21.0	21.2	20.6	20.3	19.1	17.1	18.1
No high school diploma or GED	32.5	32.3	29.7	31.6	30.3	31.6	27.7	28.6	30.6
High school diploma or GED	31.4	31.4	29.3	29.8	29.6	28.8	28.2	24.3	26.2
Some college, no bachelor's degree	24.3	23.0	23.2	22.6	21.0	20.4	20.2	18.7	18.6
Bachelor's degree or higher	9.1	9.6	8.7	7.9	8.5	8.7	7.9	6.6	7.8
White Males[4,5]	22.6	22.7	21.0	21.3	20.5	20.1	18.6	16.9	17.8
No high school diploma or GED	33.1	32.2	29.4	32.0	29.6	30.2	26.0	27.1	30.2
High school diploma or GED	31.9	32.4	29.6	29.9	29.8	28.4	27.9	25.3	26.0
Some college, no bachelor's degree	23.7	22.4	23.4	22.4	20.3	20.3	20.3	18.0	18.0
Bachelor's degree or higher	9.1	9.6	8.8	7.9	8.9	8.8	7.4	6.6	7.5
Black or African American Males[4,5]	25.9	23.7	23.9	23.9	23.3	23.1	22.9	20.9	21.7
No high school diploma or GED	35.0	39.1	34.4	32.3	34.1	41.5	38.7	38.1	38.5
High school diploma or GED	28.3	26.0	28.8	29.4	28.0	31.9	28.7	22.1	25.9
Some college, no bachelor's degree	29.5	26.5	24.2	24.7	24.9	18.0	18.8	23.0	22.4
Bachelor's degree or higher	*10.0	9.9	8.1	7.9	*7.3	7.7	9.8	*6.9	8.2
All Females[4]	18.4	18.5	17.5	16.8	16.1	15.5	15.2	14.3	14.0
No high school diploma or GED	27.0	24.8	23.7	22.7	22.2	19.8	21.2	22.6	21.1
High school diploma or GED	25.0	26.1	24.9	24.7	22.6	22.0	23.5	21.2	20.9
Some college, no bachelor's degree	20.1	20.0	19.6	19.0	18.4	18.8	17.3	17.2	17.5
Bachelor's degree or higher	8.1	8.4	7.9	7.1	7.2	6.8	6.2	5.3	5.3
White Females[4,5]	19.4	19.0	18.3	17.6	16.9	16.2	16.0	15.3	14.7
No high school diploma or GED	28.4	24.4	24.0	22.7	22.4	19.0	21.0	23.8	20.9
High school diploma or GED	27.1	26.5	25.8	26.8	24.0	23.5	25.4	22.7	22.6
Some college, no bachelor's degree	21.6	21.2	21.0	20.0	19.0	19.8	18.3	18.6	18.5
Bachelor's degree or higher	8.5	9.1	8.7	7.5	7.7	7.3	6.6	5.9	5.4
Black or African American Females[4,5]	17.5	19.3	17.0	16.1	15.2	15.3	14.0	13.9	14.0
No high school diploma or GED	28.9	31.0	25.8	29.6	25.8	26.5	22.5	24.0	28.0
High school diploma or GED	20.0	27.3	22.9	16.9	17.0	17.0	15.9	18.0	14.6
Some college, no bachelor's degree	15.9	16.2	15.0	15.0	16.9	15.3	14.4	14.5	13.6
Bachelor's degree or higher	*9.3	*7.3	*6.6	7.2	7.4	7.1	6.9	*4.5	7.7

* = Estimates are considered unreliable. Starting with 2016 data, the reliability of survey percentage estimates was assessed using new multistep National Center for Health Statistics data presentation standards for proportions. Prior to 2016 data, the reliability of estimates for earlier years was evaluated based on relative standard errors (RSE). Data preceded by an asterisk have an RSE of 20%–30%.

[2]Estimates are age-adjusted to the year 2000 standard population using four age groups: 25–34 years, 35–44 years, 45–64 years, and 65 years and over. For age groups where smoking was 0% or 100%, the age-adjustment procedure was modified to substitute the percentage smoking from the next-lower education group.

[3]Starting with 1993 data (shown in spreadsheet version), current cigarette smokers were defined as ever smoking 100 cigarettes in their lifetime and smoking now every day or some days.

[4]Includes unknown education level. Education categories shown are for 1997 and subsequent years. GED is General Educational Development high school equivalency diploma. In 1974–1995, the following categories based on number of years of school completed were used: less than 12 years, 12 years, 13–15 years, and 16 years or more.

[5]The race groups White and Black include persons of Hispanic and non-Hispanic origin. Starting with 1999 data, race-specific estimates are tabulated according to the 1997 Revisions to the Standards for the Classification of Federal Data on Race and Ethnicity and are not strictly comparable with estimates for earlier years. The single-race categories shown in the table conform to the 1997 Standards. Starting with 1999 data, race-specific estimates are for persons who reported only one racial group. Prior to 1999, data were tabulated according to the 1977 Standards. Estimates for single-race categories prior to 1999 included persons who reported one race, or if they reported more than one race, identified one race as best representing their race. Starting with 2003 data, race responses of other race and unspecified multiple race were treated as missing, and then race was imputed if these were the only race responses. Almost all persons with a race response of other race were of Hispanic origin.

Table 3-27. Current Cigarette Smoking Among Adults, by Sex, Race, Hispanic Origin, Age, and Education Level, Average Annual, Selected Years 1990–1992 Through 2014–2016

(Percent; data are based on household interviews of a sample of the civilian noninstitutionalized population.)

Characteristic	Male						Female					
	1990–1992[1]	1999–2001	2006–2008	2008–2010	2013–2015	2014–2016	1990–1992[1]	1999–2001	2006–2008	2008–2010	2013–2015	2014–2016
18 Years and Over, Age-Adjusted[2,3]												
All persons[4]	27.9	25.0	22.8	22.4	18.8	17.8	23.7	21.1	18.0	18.0	14.8	14.2
Race[5]												
White only	27.4	25.1	22.9	22.6	18.7	17.7	24.3	22.2	18.9	18.8	15.7	15.1
Black or African American only	33.9	27.2	24.8	23.7	21.2	20.7	23.1	19.7	17.2	17.5	13.8	13.3
American Indian or Alaska Native only	34.2	30.3	31.5	25.1	20.6	19.2	36.7	34.7	22.2	21.0	19.8	21.2
Asian only	24.8	20.3	15.6	15.3	13.4	13.3	6.3	6.7	4.4	5.5	4.4	4.4
Native Hawaiian or Other Pacific Islander only	NA	*	*	*	*	*	NA	*	*	*	*	*
2 or more races	NA	34.4	25.1	27.7	27.2	26.8	NA	30.7	24.6	20.9	21.2	20.2
American Indian or Alaska Native; White	NA	38.7	34.6	34.6	30.5	29.7	NA	38.9	28.6	26.5	27.6	24.9
Hispanic Origin and Race[5]												
Hispanic or Latino	25.7	22.2	18.6	17.3	14.4	13.5	15.8	12.1	9.5	9.6	7.2	7.3
Mexican	26.2	21.9	18.7	17.5	14.6	14.2	14.8	10.6	8.8	8.4	6.7	7.1
Not Hispanic or Latino	28.1	25.5	23.7	23.4	19.8	18.8	24.4	22.3	19.4	19.5	16.4	15.7
White only	27.7	25.5	24.0	23.9	19.9	18.8	25.2	23.5	20.9	20.9	17.9	17.2
Black or African American only	33.9	27.2	25.1	24.0	21.4	21.0	23.2	19.7	17.2	17.7	14.0	13.5
18 Years and Over, Crude												
All persons[4]	28.4	25.5	23.1	22.7	18.7	17.7	23.6	21.0	17.9	17.8	14.6	14.0
Race[5]												
White only	27.8	25.4	23.0	22.7	18.4	17.4	24.1	21.7	18.5	18.4	15.3	14.6
Black or African American only	33.2	27.5	25.6	24.4	21.4	20.8	23.3	19.8	17.5	17.9	13.9	13.3
American Indian or Alaska Native only	35.5	31.8	30.7	25.6	20.5	19.5	37.3	36.9	23.0	21.6	20.3	22.0
Asian only	24.9	21.4	16.5	15.7	13.8	13.5	6.3	6.9	4.6	5.6	4.4	4.3
Native Hawaiian or Other Pacific Islander only	NA	*	*	*	*	7.9	NA	*	*	*	*	*
2 or more races	NA	35.9	27.0	29.2	27.1	26.5	NA	31.5	25.3	21.9	20.6	19.8
American Indian or Alaska Native; White	NA	41.1	33.5	33.9	28.0	28.8	NA	40.1	30.0	27.5	27.6	24.5
Hispanic Origin and Race[5]												
Hispanic or Latino	26.5	23.2	19.6	18.4	15.0	14.1	16.6	12.6	9.7	9.8	7.2	7.2
Mexican	27.1	22.8	19.4	18.6	15.0	15.0	15.0	11.0	8.8	8.5	6.6	6.8
Not Hispanic or Latino	28.5	25.8	23.7	23.4	19.4	18.4	24.2	21.9	19.1	19.0	15.9	15.2
White only	28.0	25.5	23.7	23.6	19.2	18.1	24.8	22.7	20.1	20.0	17.0	16.2
Black or African American only	33.3	27.5	26.0	24.7	21.6	21.1	23.3	19.8	17.6	18.0	14.1	13.5
Age and Hispanic Origin and Race[5]												
18 to 24 Years												
Hispanic or Latino	19.3	22.6	18.4	19.3	13.6	13.8	12.8	12.9	8.0	8.0	5.0	5.1
Not Hispanic or Latino												
White only	28.9	32.7	29.1	28.2	21.9	18.1	28.7	30.8	24.1	21.2	18.4	16.5
Black or African American only	17.7	21.9	23.6	18.4	14.2	13.6	10.8	13.0	13.5	14.9	10.1	8.6
25 to 34 Years												
Hispanic or Latino	29.9	23.2	20.4	20.1	18.7	16.7	19.2	12.5	9.5	9.6	7.0	6.0
Not Hispanic or Latino												
White only	32.7	30.8	31.6	30.8	24.4	23.4	30.9	27.4	26.7	26.5	21.4	19.6
Black or African American only	34.6	23.3	28.5	25.7	27.2	26.8	29.2	16.9	16.2	19.1	15.7	15.0
35 to 44 Years												
Hispanic or Latino	32.1	25.3	20.5	18.2	13.9	13.5	19.9	14.1	10.2	10.4	7.7	8.3
Not Hispanic or Latino												
White only	32.3	29.6	25.9	26.5	22.9	22.6	27.3	28.3	24.1	24.7	20.9	20.7
Black or African American only	44.1	32.0	20.9	23.2	22.2	21.9	31.3	27.5	19.4	19.0	16.4	16.0
45 to 64 Years												
Hispanic or Latino	26.6	24.7	21.4	19.2	15.0	14.3	17.1	13.5	12.5	12.2	9.5	9.5
Not Hispanic or Latino												
White only	28.4	25.1	23.5	24.1	20.1	19.1	26.1	22.1	20.7	21.0	19.1	18.7
Black or African American only	38.0	34.0	31.8	31.7	24.0	22.5	26.1	23.6	23.2	21.6	16.3	15.4

NA = Not available.

* = Estimates are considered unreliable. Starting with 2016 data, the reliability of survey percentage estimates was assessed using new multistep National Center for Health Statistics data presentation standards for proportions. Prior to 2016 data, the reliability of estimates for earlier years was evaluated based on relative standard errors (RSE). Data preceded by an asterisk have an RSE of 20%–30%. Data not shown have an RSE greater than 30%.

[1]Data prior to 1997 are not strictly comparable with data for later years due to the 1997 questionnaire redesign.

[2]Estimates are age-adjusted to the year 2000 standard population using five age groups: 18–24 years, 25–34 years, 35–44 years, 45–64 years, and 65 years and over. For age groups where smoking is 0% or 100%, the age-adjustment procedure was modified to substitute the percentage smoking from the previous 3-year period.

[3]Starting with 1993 data, current cigarette smokers were defined as ever smoking 100 cigarettes in their lifetime and smoking now every day or some days.

[4]Includes all other races not shown separately, unknown education level, and unknown disability measure.

[5]The race groups White, Black, American Indian or Alaska Native, Asian, Native Hawaiian or Other Pacific Islander, and 2 or more races include persons of Hispanic and non-Hispanic origin. Persons of Hispanic origin may be of any race. Starting with 1999 data, race-specific estimates are tabulated according to the 1997 Revisions to the Standards for the Classification of Federal Data on Race and Ethnicity and are not strictly comparable with estimates for earlier years. The five single-race categories and multiple-race categories shown in the table conform to the 1997 Standards. Starting with 1999–2001 data, race-specific estimates are for persons who reported only one racial group; the category 2 or more races includes persons who reported more than one racial group. Prior to 1999, data were tabulated according to the 1977 Standards with four racial groups, and the Asian only category included Native Hawaiian or Other Pacific Islander. Estimates for single-race categories prior to 1999 included persons who reported one race, or if they reported more than one race, identified one race as best representing their race. Starting with 2003 data, race responses of other race and unspecified multiple race were treated as missing, and then race was imputed if these were the only race responses. Almost all persons with a race response of other race were of Hispanic origin.

Table 3-27. Current Cigarette Smoking Among Adults, by Sex, Race, Hispanic Origin, Age, and Education Level, Average Annual, Selected Years 1990–1992 Through 2014–2016—Continued

(Percent; data are based on household interviews of a sample of the civilian noninstitutionalized population.)

Characteristic	Male						Female					
	1990–1992[1]	1999–2001	2006–2008	2008–2010	2013–2015	2014–2016	1990–1992[1]	1999–2001	2006–2008	2008–2010	2013–2015	2014–2016
65 Years and Over												
Hispanic or Latino	16.1	12.6	9.4	8.2	9.9	8.3	6.6	5.9	4.7	5.5	4.1	4.9
Not Hispanic or Latino												
White only	14.2	10.0	10.5	9.8	9.6	9.3	12.3	9.8	8.6	9.5	8.0	7.8
Black or African American only	25.2	17.6	16.3	13.7	15.0	16.7	10.7	11.0	7.8	9.8	8.1	9.1
Percent of Poverty Level[2,6]												
Below 100 percent	40.5	36.5	32.1	32.5	31.8	30.3	30.7	29.1	28.1	28.6	24.6	24.0
100 percent to 199 percent	35.0	32.8	29.4	29.3	26.0	25.1	26.9	25.6	22.4	22.8	19.8	19.6
200 percent to 399 percent	26.5	27.3	24.8	24.3	19.6	19.0	22.6	22.3	18.5	18.5	14.7	14.5
400 percent or more	22.5	18.8	17.0	16.0	11.9	11.4	19.0	15.9	12.5	11.8	8.5	7.9
Hispanic Origin and Race and Percent of Poverty Level[2,5,6]												
Hispanic or Latino												
Below 100 percent	29.2	25.3	20.8	20.2	18.0	16.6	16.3	14.4	11.9	11.4	10.3	10.2
100 percent to 199 percent	29.5	22.0	18.4	17.8	14.7	14.0	16.0	11.8	8.3	8.7	7.3	7.1
200 percent to 399 percent	23.7	23.6	19.7	16.6	14.2	13.9	15.9	12.0	8.6	10.2	5.8	6.1
400 percent or more	19.7	18.1	15.7	15.1	11.0	9.8	13.6	9.4	9.9	7.9	5.5	5.6
Not Hispanic or Latino												
White only												
Below 100 percent	44.2	40.7	38.6	40.6	41.2	39.1	37.8	38.3	38.0	39.4	36.8	37.0
100 percent to 199 percent	36.3	37.5	35.0	35.3	33.3	31.3	31.1	32.0	30.7	30.7	28.6	28.0
200 percent to 399 percent	26.4	28.5	27.0	27.4	21.0	20.6	23.7	24.8	22.1	21.9	18.5	18.6
400 percent or more	22.5	19.1	17.4	16.3	12.5	11.8	19.5	17.1	13.6	13.1	9.7	8.8
Black or African American only												
Below 100 percent	43.5	40.6	38.2	36.5	35.8	35.2	28.9	27.7	27.0	29.1	23.8	22.4
100 percent to 199 percent	36.0	33.9	30.9	30.4	25.5	26.7	20.3	21.3	18.6	19.6	15.0	15.7
200 percent to 399 percent	31.4	24.9	21.8	20.7	20.3	19.1	21.4	17.3	13.5	13.2	9.6	9.1
400 percent or more	24.3	17.9	18.4	15.6	10.3	10.7	19.2	12.6	10.3	8.2	6.3	6.7
Level of Difficulty[2,7]												
A lot of difficulty or cannot do at all	NA	NA	NA	NA	29.4	28.0	NA	NA	NA	NA	25.3	24.0
Some difficulty	NA	NA	NA	NA	23.5	22.0	NA	NA	NA	NA	18.9	18.5
No difficulty	NA	NA	NA	NA	16.0	15.1	NA	NA	NA	NA	11.7	11.1
No disability	NA	NA	NA	NA			NA	NA	NA	NA		
Education, Hispanic Origin, and Race[5,8]												
25 years and over, age-adjusted[9]												
No high school diploma or GED												
Hispanic or Latino	30.2	24.3	19.5	18.5	17.2	16.7	15.8	12.1	8.6	8.6	7.2	7.6
Not Hispanic or Latino												
White only	46.1	43.5	42.0	45.1	42.2	41.9	40.4	39.3	42.9	44.0	41.5	43.5
Black or African American only	45.4	40.0	35.9	37.2	40.5	39.3	31.3	29.4	28.7	29.9	26.0	26.2
High school diploma or GED												
Hispanic or Latino	29.6	24.1	21.7	20.3	15.2	14.2	18.4	12.5	10.7	11.4	8.0	8.3
Not Hispanic or Latino												
White only	32.9	31.8	32.7	34.4	30.5	30.2	28.4	29.2	28.8	30.3	29.2	28.8
Black or African American only	38.2	31.4	29.5	27.8	28.3	26.8	25.4	23.0	19.8	23.7	16.9	16.3
Some college or more												
Hispanic or Latino	20.4	17.1	15.8	12.9	10.8	9.8	14.3	11.1	10.3	9.9	7.5	7.2
Not Hispanic or Latino												
White only	19.3	17.6	16.2	15.9	13.4	12.9	18.1	16.7	14.7	15.5	13.0	12.3
Black or African American only	25.6	19.2	19.3	19.8	15.3	16.1	22.8	16.9	13.7	12.7	11.5	11.2

NA = Not available.

[1] Data prior to 1997 are not strictly comparable with data for later years due to the 1997 questionnaire redesign.

[2] Estimates are age-adjusted to the year 2000 standard population using five age groups: 18–24 years, 25–34 years, 35–44 years, 45–64 years, and 65 years and over. For age groups where smoking is 0% or 100%, the age-adjustment procedure was modified to substitute the percentage smoking from the previous 3-year period.

[3] The race groups White, Black, American Indian or Alaska Native, Asian, Native Hawaiian or Other Pacific Islander, and 2 or more races include persons of Hispanic and non-Hispanic origin. Persons of Hispanic origin may be of any race. Starting with 1999 data, race-specific estimates are tabulated according to the 1997 Revisions to the Standards for the Classification of Federal Data on Race and Ethnicity and are not strictly comparable with estimates for earlier years. The five single-race categories and multiple-race categories shown in the table conform to the 1997 Standards. Starting with 1999–2001 data, race-specific estimates are for persons who reported only one racial group; the category 2 or more races includes persons who reported more than one race, or if they reported more than one race, identified one race as best representing their race. Prior to 1999, data were tabulated according to the 1977 Standards with four racial groups, and the Asian only category included Native Hawaiian or Other Pacific Islander. Estimates for single-race categories prior to 1999 included persons who reported one race, or if they reported more than one race, identified one race as best representing their race. Starting with 2003 data, race responses of other race and unspecified multiple race were treated as missing, and then race was imputed if these were the only race responses. Almost all persons with a race response of other race were of Hispanic origin.

[6] Percent of poverty level is based on family income and family size and composition using U.S. Census Bureau poverty thresholds. Missing family income data were imputed for 1990 and beyond.

[7] Functional limitation is defined by the reported level of difficulty in six functioning domains: seeing (even if wearing glasses), hearing (even if wearing hearing aids), mobility (walking or climbing stairs), communication (understanding or being understood by others), cognition (remembering or concentrating), and self-care (such as washing all over or dressing). Respondents with answers to one or more of the six questions were included in one of three mutually exclusive categories. Those responding "A lot of difficulty" or "Cannot do at all/unable to do" to at least one question were classified in the "A lot of difficulty/cannot do" category. Of the remaining, those responding "Some difficulty" to at least one question were classified in the "Some difficulty" category, and those responding "No difficulty" to at least one question were classified in the "No difficulty" category. Those responding "Don't know" or "Refused" to all six questions were excluded. During 2010 2016, 1% 8% of respondents were missing data and excluded.

[8] Education categories shown are for 1997 and subsequent years. GED is General Educational Development high school equivalency diploma. In years prior to 1997, the following categories based on number of years of school completed were used: less than 12 years, 12 years, and 13 years or more.

[9] Estimates are age adjusted to the year 2000 standard using four age groups: 25 to 34 years, 35 to 44 years, 45 to 64 years, and 65 years and over.

Table 3-28. Current Cigarette Smoking Among Adults 18 Years of Age and Over, by Sex, Race, and Age, Selected Years, 1965–2016

(Percent; data are based on household interviews of a sample of the civilian noninstitutionalized population.)

Sex, race, and age	1965[1]	1974[1]	1983[1]	1985[1]	1990[1]	1995[1]	2000	2005	2006	2007	2008	2009	2010	2011	2012	2013	2014	2015	2016
18 Years and Over, Age-Adjusted[2,3]																			
All persons	41.9	37.0	31.9	29.9	25.3	24.6	23.1	20.8	20.8	19.7	20.6	20.6	19.3	19.0	18.2	17.9	17.0	15.3	15.7
Male	51.2	42.8	34.8	32.2	28.0	26.5	25.2	23.4	23.6	22.0	22.8	23.2	21.2	21.2	20.6	20.5	19.0	16.8	17.7
Female	33.7	32.2	29.4	27.9	22.9	22.7	21.1	18.3	18.1	17.5	18.5	18.1	17.5	16.8	15.9	15.5	15.1	13.8	13.7
White male[4]	50.4	41.7	34.2	31.3	27.6	26.2	25.4	23.3	23.5	22.2	23.0	23.6	21.4	21.4	20.7	20.5	18.8	16.8	17.5
Black or African American male[4]	58.8	53.6	41.7	40.2	32.8	29.4	25.7	25.9	26.1	23.4	24.7	23.1	23.3	23.2	22.0	21.8	21.7	20.3	20.3
White female[4]	33.9	32.0	29.6	27.9	23.5	23.4	22.0	19.1	18.8	18.5	19.5	18.7	18.3	17.7	16.9	16.3	16.0	14.8	14.4
Black or African American female[4]	31.8	35.6	31.3	30.9	20.8	23.5	20.7	17.1	18.5	15.6	17.4	18.5	16.6	15.2	14.2	14.9	13.4	13.2	13.2
18 Years and Over, Crude																			
All persons	42.4	37.1	32.1	30.1	25.5	24.7	23.2	20.9	20.8	19.8	20.6	20.6	19.3	19.0	18.1	17.8	16.8	15.1	15.5
Male	51.9	43.1	35.1	32.6	28.4	27.0	25.6	23.9	23.9	22.3	23.1	23.5	21.5	21.6	20.5	20.5	18.8	16.7	17.5
Female	33.9	32.1	29.5	27.9	22.8	22.6	20.9	18.1	18.0	17.4	18.3	17.9	17.3	16.5	15.8	15.3	14.8	13.6	13.5
White male[4]	51.1	41.9	34.5	31.7	28.0	26.6	25.7	23.6	23.6	22.3	23.1	23.6	21.4	21.6	20.3	20.3	18.5	16.5	17.2
Black or African American male[4]	60.4	54.3	40.6	39.9	32.5	28.5	26.2	26.5	27.0	24.6	25.3	23.7	24.3	23.8	22.0	21.9	21.8	20.6	20.0
White female[4]	34.0	31.7	29.4	27.7	23.4	23.1	21.4	18.7	18.4	18.1	19.1	18.3	17.9	17.2	16.6	15.9	15.5	14.3	14.0
Black or African American female[4]	33.7	36.4	32.2	31.0	21.2	23.5	20.8	17.3	18.8	15.9	17.8	18.8	17.0	15.3	14.7	15.1	13.5	13.1	13.2
All Males																			
18 to 44 years	57.9	47.9	37.7	35.2	31.4	29.9	29.2	27.1	26.7	25.8	25.6	26.9	23.9	23.6	24.0	22.9	21.7	18.5	19.1
18 to 24 years	54.1	42.1	32.9	28.0	26.6	27.8	28.1	28.0	28.5	25.4	23.6	28.0	22.8	21.0	20.1	21.9	18.5	15.0	14.7
25 to 34 years	60.7	50.5	38.8	38.2	31.6	29.5	28.9	27.7	27.4	28.8	28.5	27.6	26.1	27.5	28.0	24.4	23.7	21.3	20.7
35 to 44 years	58.2	51.0	41.0	37.6	34.5	31.5	30.2	26.0	24.8	23.2	24.3	25.4	22.5	21.2	22.8	22.1	22.0	18.3	20.6
45 to 64 years	51.9	42.6	35.9	33.4	29.3	27.1	26.4	25.2	24.5	22.6	24.8	24.5	23.2	24.4	20.2	21.9	19.4	17.9	19.3
45 to 54 years	55.9	46.8	39.0	34.9	32.1	27.2	28.8	28.1	26.6	24.8	26.4	27.3	25.2	27.0	21.4	21.4	19.9	18.3	19.1
55 to 64 years	46.6	37.7	32.6	31.9	25.9	26.9	22.6	21.1	21.5	19.6	22.6	20.8	20.7	21.4	18.8	22.6	18.8	17.5	19.7
65 years and over	28.5	24.8	22.0	19.6	14.6	14.9	10.2	8.9	12.6	9.3	10.5	9.5	9.7	8.9	10.6	10.6	9.8	9.7	10.1
White Male[4]																			
18 to 44 years	57.1	46.8	37.5	34.6	31.3	30.1	30.2	27.7	27.1	26.6	26.7	28.1	24.6	24.3	24.8	23.4	21.7	18.9	19.4
18 to 24 years	53.0	40.8	32.5	28.4	27.4	28.4	30.4	29.7	28.9	26.5	25.2	30.0	23.8	22.1	21.9	23.5	20.0	15.6	15.5
25 to 34 years	60.1	49.5	38.6	37.3	31.6	29.9	29.7	27.7	27.9	29.0	29.5	28.4	26.6	28.6	28.4	24.6	23.4	20.9	20.9
35 to 44 years	57.3	50.1	40.8	36.6	33.5	31.2	30.6	26.3	25.3	24.4	24.9	26.3	23.1	21.4	23.3	21.9	21.2	19.1	20.6
45 to 64 years	51.3	41.2	35.0	32.1	28.7	26.3	25.8	24.5	23.4	22.1	24.0	24.0	22.5	24.0	19.4	21.7	19.0	17.3	18.8
45 to 54 years	55.3	45.0	38.0	33.7	31.3	25.9	28.0	27.4	25.7	24.4	26.1	27.1	24.5	26.6	20.7	21.2	19.7	17.8	18.7
55 to 64 years	46.1	36.6	31.9	30.5	25.6	27.0	22.5	20.4	20.4	19.1	21.2	20.1	20.1	20.8	17.9	22.2	18.2	16.9	18.8
65 years and over	27.7	24.3	20.6	18.9	13.7	14.1	9.8	7.9	12.6	8.9	9.9	9.3	9.6	8.6	10.3	10.0	9.4	9.3	9.1
Black or African American Male[4]																			
18 to 44 years	66.3	58.1	39.4	39.6	32.9	26.4	25.5	25.1	26.2	24.2	22.0	22.5	22.6	22.7	21.3	20.9	22.2	20.2	19.5
18 to 24 years	62.8	54.9	34.2	27.2	21.3	*	20.9	21.6	31.2	21.4	*17.0	18.9	18.8	18.4	13.2	*13.2	*13.9	*15.9	10.6
25 to 34 years	68.4	58.5	39.9	45.6	33.8	25.1	23.2	29.8	26.3	32.3	25.9	24.1	25.7	25.0	24.9	24.8	28.0	26.0	23.2
35 to 44 years	67.3	61.5	44.5	45.0	42.0	36.3	30.7	23.3	22.2	17.4	21.8	24.0	22.6	24.3	24.7	24.0	24.0	17.9	23.3
45 to 64 years	57.9	57.8	44.9	46.1	36.7	33.9	32.2	32.4	32.6	28.3	33.6	28.9	31.8	28.9	24.6	25.7	24.0	22.8	21.1
45 to 54 years	62.4	63.6	47.8	47.7	42.0	36.9	35.6	33.9	32.0	29.3	31.7	28.1	33.2	29.2	23.3	25.7	22.5	20.5	21.8
55 to 64 years	51.8	50.1	41.1	44.4	30.2	29.1	26.3	29.8	33.5	26.8	36.6	30.1	29.6	28.4	26.4	25.6	25.9	25.5	20.3
65 years and over	36.4	29.7	38.9	27.7	21.5	28.5	14.2	16.8	16.0	14.3	17.5	14.0	10.0	13.7	17.4	15.5	13.9	16.0	19.1
All Females																			
18 to 44 years	42.1	37.5	33.8	31.4	25.6	25.6	24.5	21.2	20.6	19.5	20.6	20.0	19.1	18.8	16.9	16.6	16.6	14.5	13.8
18 to 24 years	38.1	34.1	35.5	30.4	22.5	21.8	24.9	20.7	19.3	19.1	19.0	15.6	17.4	16.4	14.5	15.4	14.8	11.0	11.5
25 to 34 years	43.7	38.8	32.6	32.0	28.2	26.4	22.3	21.5	21.5	19.6	21.4	21.8	20.6	19.5	19.4	17.9	17.5	15.0	13.9
35 to 44 years	43.7	39.8	33.8	31.5	24.8	27.1	26.2	21.3	20.6	19.6	20.9	21.2	19.0	19.9	16.1	16.3	17.0	16.5	15.4
45 to 64 years	32.0	33.4	31.0	29.9	24.8	24.0	21.7	18.8	19.3	19.5	20.5	19.5	19.1	18.5	18.9	18.1	16.8	16.1	16.8
45 to 54 years	37.5	36.0	34.1	32.4	28.5	24.3	22.2	20.9	22.5	22.1	23.7	22.3	21.3	21.6	21.3	20.6	18.7	18.4	18.5
55 to 64 years	25.0	30.4	28.0	27.4	20.5	23.7	20.9	16.1	14.9	16.2	16.3	16.1	16.5	15.0	16.2	15.2	14.8	13.7	15.0
65 years and over	9.6	12.0	13.1	13.5	11.5	11.5	9.3	8.3	8.3	7.6	8.3	9.5	9.3	7.1	7.5	7.5	7.5	7.3	7.7
White Female[4]																			
18 to 44 years	42.2	37.3	34.2	31.6	26.5	26.6	26.5	22.6	22.2	21.2	22.1	21.2	20.5	20.3	18.6	17.8	17.8	15.7	14.6
18 to 24 years	38.4	34.0	36.5	31.8	25.4	24.9	28.5	22.6	20.7	21.6	20.1	16.7	18.4	18.4	16.9	17.0	16.5	11.2	12.5
25 to 34 years	43.4	38.6	32.2	32.0	28.5	27.3	24.9	23.1	23.7	21.4	23.1	22.7	22.0	20.6	20.7	19.2	18.6	16.3	14.2
35 to 44 years	43.9	39.3	34.8	31.0	25.0	27.0	26.6	22.2	21.7	20.7	22.6	22.9	20.5	21.5	17.6	17.0	18.0	18.3	16.7
45 to 64 years	32.7	33.0	30.6	29.7	25.4	24.3	21.4	18.9	18.8	19.6	20.9	19.4	19.5	19.0	19.4	18.4	17.6	17.1	17.4
45 to 54 years	38.2	34.9	33.3	32.4	29.1	24.6	21.9	21.0	22.1	22.2	24.2	22.4	22.4	22.5	22.7	21.2	19.9	20.2	19.6
55 to 64 years	25.7	30.6	28.1	27.2	21.2	23.8	20.6	16.2	14.4	16.2	16.8	15.8	15.9	15.1	15.8	15.5	15.3	14.0	15.3
65 years and over	9.8	12.3	13.2	13.3	11.5	11.7	9.1	8.4	8.4	8.0	8.6	9.6	9.4	7.0	7.5	7.9	7.6	7.5	7.6
Black or African American Female[4]																			
18 to 44 years	42.9	41.1	34.6	33.5	22.8	24.0	20.8	16.9	17.3	14.2	18.0	18.3	17.1	15.0	12.3	15.1	13.9	13.3	13.0
18 to 24 years	37.1	35.6	32.0	23.7	10.0	*8.8	14.2	14.2	14.8	*8.7	16.6	13.3	14.2	9.1	*7.4	11.8	*9.3	*8.6	7.6
25 to 34 years	47.8	42.2	38.0	36.2	29.1	26.7	15.5	16.9	14.9	17.6	20.1	19.3	17.5	17.3	16.4	15.1	14.9		14.5
35 to 44 years	42.8	46.4	32.7	40.2	25.5	31.9	30.2	19.0	21.0	17.7	19.6	20.0	17.2	17.4	11.2	16.4	16.4	15.4	15.5
45 to 64 years	25.7	38.9	36.3	33.4	22.6	27.5	25.6	21.0	25.5	22.6	21.3	22.7	19.8	18.3	20.4	18.8	15.0	14.5	15.6
45 to 54 years	32.3	46.2	43.6	36.4	26.5	28.3	26.5	22.2	29.3	26.3	24.9	23.5	20.4	20.1	22.2	15.7	14.7		15.8
55 to 64 years	16.5	29.3	28.0	29.8	17.6	26.3	24.2	19.1	19.5	17.0	15.9	21.4	18.9	16.0	20.8	14.8	14.2	14.3	15.5
65 years and over	7.1	*8.9	*13.1	14.5	11.1	*13.1	10.2	10.0	9.3	6.4	8.1	11.5	9.4	9.1	9.1	6.5	8.1	9.7	8.7

* = Estimates are considered unreliable. Starting with 2016 data, the reliability of survey percentage estimates was assessed using new multistep National Center for Health Statistics data presentation standards for proportions. Prior to 2016 data, the reliability of estimates for earlier years was evaluated based on relative standard errors (RSE). Data preceded by an asterisk have an RSE of 20%–30%.

[1] Data prior to 1997 are not strictly comparable with data for later years due to the 1997 questionnaire redesign.

[2] Estimates are age-adjusted to the year 2000 standard population using five age groups: 18–24 years, 25–34 years, 35–44 years, 45–64 years, and 65 years and over. Age-adjusted estimates in this table may differ from other age-adjusted estimates based on the same data and presented elsewhere if different age groups are used in the adjustment procedure.

[3] Starting with 1993 data (shown in spreadsheet version), current cigarette smokers were defined as ever smoking 100 cigarettes in their lifetime and smoking now every day or some days.

[4] The race groups White and Black include persons of Hispanic and non-Hispanic origin. Starting with 1999 data, race-specific estimates are tabulated according to the 1997 Revisions to the Standards for the Classification of Federal Data on Race and Ethnicity and are not strictly comparable with estimates for earlier years. The single-race categories shown in the table conform to the 1997 Standards. Starting with 1999 data, race-specific estimates are for persons who reported only one racial group. Prior to 1999, data were tabulated according to the 1977 Standards. Estimates for single-race categories prior to 1999 included persons who reported one race, or if they reported more than one race, identified one race as best representing their race. Starting with 2003 data, race responses of other race and unspecified multiple race were treated as missing, and then race was imputed if these were the only race responses. Almost all persons with a race response of other race were of Hispanic origin.

Table 3-29. Use of Selected Substances in the Past 30 Days Among 12th Graders, 10th Graders, and 8th Graders, by Sex and Race, Selected Years, 1980–2016

(Percent; data are based on a survey of 12th graders, 10th graders, and 8th graders in the coterminous United States.)

Substance, grade in school, sex, and race	1980	1985	1990	1995	2000	2005	2006	2007	2008	2009	2010	2011	2012	2013	2014	2015	2016
Cigarettes																	
All 12th graders	30.5	30.1	29.4	33.5	31.4	23.2	21.6	21.6	20.4	20.1	19.2	18.7	17.1	16.3	13.6	11.4	10.5
Male	26.8	28.2	29.1	34.5	32.8	24.8	22.4	23.1	21.5	22.1	21.9	21.5	19.3	18.4	15.2	13.0	12.7
Female	33.4	31.4	29.2	32.0	29.7	20.7	20.1	19.6	19.1	17.6	15.7	15.1	14.5	13.2	11.6	9.1	8.1
White	31.0	31.7	32.5	37.3	36.6	27.0	24.7	25.2	24.1	23.7	22.2	22.2	20.1	18.5	16.5	13.4	13.0
Black or African American	25.2	18.7	12.0	15.0	13.6	10.0	11.0	10.6	10.1	9.3	10.7	8.7	8.4	10.8	7.5	6.4	5.5
All 10th graders	NA	NA	NA	27.9	23.9	14.9	14.5	14.0	12.3	13.1	13.6	11.8	10.8	9.1	7.2	6.3	4.9
Male	NA	NA	NA	27.7	23.8	14.5	13.4	14.6	12.7	13.7	15.0	13.4	12.0	10.5	7.7	6.1	5.0
Female	NA	NA	NA	27.9	23.6	15.1	15.5	13.3	11.9	12.5	12.1	10.0	9.6	7.5	6.6	6.3	4.4
White	NA	NA	NA	31.2	27.3	17.0	16.3	16.1	14.1	14.6	14.8	13.7	12.2	10.4	8.5	7.3	6.3
Black or African American	NA	NA	NA	12.2	11.3	7.7	8.5	5.8	7.1	6.4	7.0	7.2	6.2	4.2	4.2	3.5	1.8
All 8th graders	NA	NA	NA	19.1	14.6	9.3	8.7	7.1	6.8	6.5	7.1	6.1	4.9	4.5	4.0	3.6	2.6
Male	NA	NA	NA	18.8	14.3	8.7	8.1	7.5	6.7	6.7	7.4	6.2	4.6	4.0	3.5	3.3	2.5
Female	NA	NA	NA	19.0	14.7	9.7	8.9	6.4	6.7	6.0	6.8	5.7	4.9	4.7	4.2	3.7	2.6
White	NA	NA	NA	21.7	16.4	9.5	9.1	7.1	7.3	7.3	7.9	6.5	5.0	4.3	4.6	3.8	3.0
Black or African American	NA	NA	NA	8.2	8.4	6.7	5.4	4.8	4.4	4.5	4.0	4.2	3.8	3.3	2.0	2.4	1.8
E-Cigarettes																	
All 12th graders	NA	NA	NA	NA	NA	NA	NA	NA	NA	NA	NA	NA	NA	NA	17.1	16.2	12.4
Male	NA	NA	NA	NA	NA	NA	NA	NA	NA	NA	NA	NA	NA	NA	20.1	21.5	16.7
Female	NA	NA	NA	NA	NA	NA	NA	NA	NA	NA	NA	NA	NA	NA	13.7	10.9	8.3
White	NA	NA	NA	NA	NA	NA	NA	NA	NA	NA	NA	NA	NA	NA	19.5	19.0	15.2
Black or African American	NA	NA	NA	NA	NA	NA	NA	NA	NA	NA	NA	NA	NA	NA	7.1	7.4	5.3
All 10th graders	NA	NA	NA	NA	NA	NA	NA	NA	NA	NA	NA	NA	NA	NA	16.2	14.0	10.3
Male	NA	NA	NA	NA	NA	NA	NA	NA	NA	NA	NA	NA	NA	NA	19.2	15.9	10.9
Female	NA	NA	NA	NA	NA	NA	NA	NA	NA	NA	NA	NA	NA	NA	13.1	12.0	9.1
White	NA	NA	NA	NA	NA	NA	NA	NA	NA	NA	NA	NA	NA	NA	16.8	15.7	12.1
Black or African American	NA	NA	NA	NA	NA	NA	NA	NA	NA	NA	NA	NA	NA	NA	9.8	8.3	5.3
All 8th graders	NA	NA	NA	NA	NA	NA	NA	NA	NA	NA	NA	NA	NA	NA	8.7	9.5	6.2
Male	NA	NA	NA	NA	NA	NA	NA	NA	NA	NA	NA	NA	NA	NA	9.8	10.2	6.8
Female	NA	NA	NA	NA	NA	NA	NA	NA	NA	NA	NA	NA	NA	NA	7.1	8.6	5.6
White	NA	NA	NA	NA	NA	NA	NA	NA	NA	NA	NA	NA	NA	NA	7.3	8.8	6.4
Black or African American	NA	NA	NA	NA	NA	NA	NA	NA	NA	NA	NA	NA	NA	NA	5.1	6.9	3.5
Marijuana																	
All 12th graders	33.7	25.7	14.0	21.2	21.6	19.8	18.3	18.8	19.4	20.6	21.4	22.6	22.9	22.7	21.2	21.3	22.5
Male	37.8	28.7	16.1	24.6	24.7	23.6	19.7	22.3	22.2	24.3	25.2	26.4	26.5	26.4	24.3	23.1	25.0
Female	29.1	22.4	11.5	17.2	18.3	15.8	16.4	15.0	16.2	16.8	16.9	18.4	18.8	18.7	17.9	19.2	19.7
White	34.2	26.4	15.6	21.5	22.0	21.7	19.2	19.9	20.4	21.2	21.6	22.9	22.3	21.3	21.4	20.6	21.7
Black or African American	26.5	21.7	5.2	17.8	17.5	15.1	16.7	15.4	17.1	20.6	19.7	22.2	22.4	25.7	20.7	20.9	23.5
All 10th graders	NA	NA	NA	17.2	19.7	15.2	14.2	14.2	13.8	15.9	16.7	17.6	17.0	18.0	16.6	14.8	14.0
Male	NA	NA	NA	19.2	23.3	16.7	15.7	15.8	15.2	18.7	20.1	20.8	19.8	20.6	17.4	15.6	14.2
Female	NA	NA	NA	15.0	16.2	13.4	12.6	12.5	12.3	13.2	13.3	14.5	14.4	15.3	15.7	13.7	13.7
White	NA	NA	NA	17.7	20.1	15.7	14.7	14.8	13.5	15.6	15.9	16.9	16.6	16.5	15.8	13.7	14.6
Black or African American	NA	NA	NA	15.1	17.0	13.5	14.2	11.0	12.3	15.1	15.9	20.0	17.6	20.7	17.4	17.5	14.3
All 8th graders	NA	NA	NA	9.1	9.1	6.6	6.5	5.7	5.8	6.5	8.0	7.2	6.5	7.0	6.5	6.5	5.4
Male	NA	NA	NA	9.8	10.2	7.6	6.7	6.2	6.6	7.5	9.2	8.5	7.0	6.7	6.9	6.6	5.7
Female	NA	NA	NA	8.2	7.8	5.7	6.0	4.9	4.8	5.3	6.8	5.7	6.0	7.2	5.9	6.2	5.0
White	NA	NA	NA	9.0	8.3	6.0	5.7	5.1	4.9	5.9	7.1	5.9	4.7	4.8	4.7	4.5	3.8
Black or African American	NA	NA	NA	7.0	8.5	8.2	6.7	6.0	6.2	7.2	8.2	8.0	7.1	9.3	6.5	7.9	6.6
Cocaine																	
All 12th graders	5.2	6.7	1.9	1.8	2.1	2.3	2.5	2.0	1.9	1.3	1.3	1.1	1.1	1.1	1.0	1.1	0.9
Male	6.0	7.7	2.3	2.2	2.7	2.6	3.0	2.4	2.3	1.5	1.9	1.5	1.5	1.4	1.5	1.4	1.2
Female	4.3	5.6	1.3	1.3	1.6	1.8	2.1	1.5	1.3	0.9	0.7	0.7	0.6	0.5	0.5	0.8	0.4
White	5.4	7.0	1.8	1.7	2.2	2.3	2.6	2.3	2.0	1.2	1.2	1.2	1.0	0.7	0.8	1.0	0.6
Black or African American	2.0	2.7	0.5	0.4	1.0	0.5	1.0	0.5	0.5	0.2	0.9	0.8	0.5	0.6	1.4	0.4	0.4
All 10th graders	NA	NA	NA	1.7	1.8	1.5	1.5	1.3	1.2	0.9	0.9	0.7	0.8	0.8	0.6	0.8	0.4
Male	NA	NA	NA	1.8	2.1	1.9	1.6	1.4	1.4	1.0	1.1	0.8	0.8	1.2	0.8	0.9	0.5
Female	NA	NA	NA	1.5	1.4	1.2	1.3	1.1	1.0	0.8	0.5	0.5	0.7	0.5	0.4	0.6	0.3
White	NA	NA	NA	1.7	1.7	1.5	1.5	1.2	1.0	0.7	0.7	0.5	0.5	0.6	0.5	0.7	0.3
Black or African American	NA	NA	NA	0.4	0.4	0.8	0.7	0.4	0.7	0.5	0.6	0.6	1.2	0.9	0.5	0.7	0.4
All 8th graders	NA	NA	NA	1.2	1.2	1.0	1.0	0.9	0.8	0.8	0.8	0.6	0.8	0.5	0.5	0.5	0.3
Male	NA	NA	NA	1.1	1.3	0.9	1.0	0.7	0.9	0.8	0.6	0.7	0.5	0.4	0.5	0.5	0.4
Female	NA	NA	NA	1.2	1.1	1.0	0.9	1.0	0.7	0.7	0.6	0.7	0.4	0.5	0.4	0.4	0.2
White	NA	NA	NA	1.0	1.1	0.9	0.8	0.6	0.6	0.6	0.5	0.5	0.3	0.4	0.2	0.3	0.2
Black or African American	NA	NA	NA	0.4	0.5	0.3	0.4	0.6	0.4	0.7	0.3	0.5	0.5	0.5	0.5	0.5	0.3
Inhalants																	
All 12th graders	1.4	2.2	2.7	3.2	2.2	2.0	1.5	1.2	1.4	1.2	1.4	1.0	0.9	1.0	0.7	0.7	0.8
Male	1.8	2.8	3.5	3.9	2.9	2.4	1.5	1.5	1.6	1.2	2.1	1.1	0.9	1.2	1.0	0.8	0.7
Female	1.0	1.7	2.0	2.5	1.7	1.6	1.4	0.9	1.2	1.0	0.7	0.9	0.8	0.7	0.5	0.6	0.8
White	1.4	2.4	3.0	3.7	2.1	2.1	1.5	1.2	1.5	1.1	1.1	0.9	0.6	0.6	0.6	0.5	0.6
Black or African American	1.0	0.8	1.5	1.1	2.1	1.4	1.2	0.9	1.0	1.1	1.5	1.3	0.9	1.3	1.4	0.8	1.2

NA = Not available.

Table 3-29. Use of Selected Substances in the Past 30 Days Among 12th Graders, 10th Graders, and 8th Graders, by Sex and Race, Selected Years, 1980–2016—*Continued*

(Percent; data are based on a survey of 12th graders, 10th graders, and 8th graders in the coterminous United States.)

Substance, grade in school, sex, and race	1980	1985	1990	1995	2000	2005	2006	2007	2008	2009	2010	2011	2012	2013	2014	2015	2016
All 10th graders	NA	NA	NA	3.5	2.6	2.2	2.3	2.5	2.1	2.2	2.0	1.7	1.4	1.3	1.1	1.2	1.0
Male	NA	NA	NA	3.8	3.0	1.9	2.2	2.7	1.9	1.8	1.6	1.5	1.2	1.4	0.9	1.1	0.9
Female	NA	NA	NA	3.2	2.2	2.5	2.4	2.4	2.3	2.6	2.4	2.0	1.6	1.3	1.2	1.2	1.0
White	NA	NA	NA	3.9	2.8	2.2	2.4	2.6	1.6	1.9	1.7	1.4	1.1	1.0	0.9	0.8	1.0
Black or African American	NA	NA	NA	1.2	1.5	1.4	1.8	1.5	1.9	1.3	1.8	1.6	1.2	1.9	1.4	1.4	0.8
All 8th graders	NA	NA	NA	6.1	4.5	4.2	4.1	3.9	4.1	3.8	3.6	3.2	2.7	2.3	2.2	2.0	1.8
Male	NA	NA	NA	5.6	4.1	3.1	3.6	3.4	2.9	3.3	2.8	2.5	1.9	1.6	1.6	1.8	1.4
Female	NA	NA	NA	6.6	4.8	5.3	4.7	4.3	5.3	4.3	4.4	3.9	3.4	2.9	2.6	2.1	2.1
White	NA	NA	NA	7.0	4.8	4.0	4.2	3.6	3.8	3.7	3.2	2.7	2.1	1.7	1.7	1.6	1.5
Black or African American	NA	NA	NA	2.3	2.3	2.9	2.7	2.8	2.8	3.4	2.2	2.8	3.0	2.4	2.4	2.1	1.9
MDMA (Ecstasy)[1]																	
All 12th graders	NA	NA	NA	NA	3.6	1.0	1.3	1.6	1.8	1.8	1.4	2.3	0.9	1.5	1.5	1.1	0.9
Male	NA	NA	NA	NA	4.1	1.0	1.5	1.5	2.3	2.4	1.5	2.8	1.2	2.1	2.2	1.2	1.1
Female	NA	NA	NA	NA	3.1	1.0	1.1	1.6	1.2	1.2	1.2	1.8	0.6	0.9	0.9	1.0	0.6
White	NA	NA	NA	NA	3.9	1.0	1.4	1.7	1.7	1.7	0.9	2.1	0.9	1.5	0.7	1.0	0.9
Black or African American	NA	NA	NA	NA	1.9	0.9	0.6	0.8	1.1	1.8	1.1	1.1	0.4	0.7	2.6	1.2	0.7
All 10th graders	NA	NA	NA	NA	2.6	1.0	1.2	1.2	1.1	1.3	1.9	1.6	1.0	1.2	1.1	0.9	0.5
Male	NA	NA	NA	NA	2.5	1.0	1.5	1.3	1.6	1.6	2.3	1.7	1.1	1.5	1.4	1.0	0.6
Female	NA	NA	NA	NA	2.5	0.9	0.8	1.1	0.7	1.0	1.5	1.3	1.0	1.0	0.9	0.6	0.3
White	NA	NA	NA	NA	2.5	1.0	1.3	1.4	1.0	1.0	1.5	1.1	1.0	0.9	1.3	0.8	0.5
Black or African American	NA	NA	NA	NA	1.8	0.3	1.0	0.4	0.1	0.6	1.1	1.1	1.1	0.4	1.3	0.7	0.5
All 8th graders	NA	NA	NA	NA	1.4	0.6	0.7	0.6	0.8	0.6	1.1	0.6	0.5	0.5	0.7	0.5	0.3
Male	NA	NA	NA	NA	1.6	0.8	0.5	0.7	0.7	0.5	1.2	0.7	0.4	0.4	1.0	0.4	0.3
Female	NA	NA	NA	NA	1.2	0.4	0.8	0.6	0.9	0.6	1.1	0.5	0.6	0.5	0.5	0.5	0.3
White	NA	NA	NA	NA	1.4	0.6	0.5	0.5	0.7	0.6	1.0	0.4	0.4	0.3	0.6	0.4	0.2
Black or African American	NA	NA	NA	NA	0.8	0.9	0.7	0.8	0.3	0.1	0.5	0.2	0.5	0.6	0.7	0.3	0.4
Alcohol[2]																	
All 12th graders	72.0	65.9	57.1	51.3	50.0	47.0	45.3	44.4	43.1	43.5	41.2	40.0	41.5	39.2	37.4	35.3	33.2
Male	77.4	69.8	61.3	55.7	54.0	50.7	47.3	47.1	45.8	47.8	44.2	42.1	43.8	41.8	37.4	36.0	34.5
Female	66.8	62.1	52.3	47.0	46.1	43.3	43.0	41.4	40.9	38.9	37.9	37.5	38.8	36.3	37.1	35.0	32.0
White	75.8	70.2	62.2	54.8	55.3	52.2	49.1	49.4	47.8	46.6	44.1	43.4	44.3	42.8	42.1	39.7	38.2
Black or African American	47.7	43.6	32.9	37.4	29.3	28.8	29.5	27.9	29.3	32.2	30.8	29.4	29.8	27.0	24.9	23.2	20.2
All 10th graders	NA	NA	NA	38.8	41.0	33.2	33.8	33.4	28.8	30.4	28.9	27.2	27.6	25.7	23.5	21.5	19.9
Male	NA	NA	NA	39.7	43.3	32.8	33.8	33.4	28.6	31.0	30.1	28.2	28.0	26.0	23.0	20.6	18.6
Female	NA	NA	NA	37.8	38.6	33.9	33.8	33.3	29.0	29.8	27.7	26.0	27.1	25.3	23.9	22.5	20.9
White	NA	NA	NA	41.3	44.3	36.7	36.0	35.7	30.5	32.4	29.2	28.9	29.2	26.9	25.9	23.6	22.3
Black or African American	NA	NA	NA	24.9	24.7	20.8	22.4	21.0	20.4	20.1	21.3	20.3	20.1	17.7	15.5	14.8	13.1
All 8th graders	NA	NA	NA	24.6	22.4	17.1	17.2	15.9	15.9	14.9	13.8	12.7	11.0	10.2	9.0	9.7	7.3
Male	NA	NA	NA	25.0	22.5	16.2	16.3	15.6	15.4	14.7	13.2	12.1	10.3	9.3	8.2	9.1	6.7
Female	NA	NA	NA	24.0	22.0	17.9	17.6	16.0	16.4	14.9	14.3	12.8	11.5	11.2	9.5	9.9	7.8
White	NA	NA	NA	25.4	23.9	17.3	16.5	14.7	15.8	15.1	12.8	11.8	9.6	9.4	8.7	9.2	7.2
Black or African American	NA	NA	NA	17.3	15.1	13.9	12.4	12.3	13.5	11.1	12.7	10.5	9.4	9.9	7.9	8.5	5.4
Binge Drinking[3]	Percent having 5 or more drinks in a row in the last 2 weeks																
All 12th graders	41.2	36.7	32.2	29.8	30.0	27.1	25.4	25.9	24.6	25.2	23.2	21.6	23.7	22.1	19.4	17.2	15.5
Male	52.1	45.3	39.1	36.9	36.7	32.6	28.9	30.7	28.4	30.5	28.0	25.5	27.2	26.1	22.3	19.3	17.2
Female	30.5	28.2	24.4	23.0	23.5	21.6	21.5	21.5	21.3	20.2	18.4	17.6	19.7	18.1	16.6	14.9	13.5
White	44.6	40.1	36.2	32.9	34.4	31.8	28.9	30.5	29.3	28.7	26.5	25.3	26.2	25.0	22.5	19.8	18.2
Black or African American	17.0	16.7	11.6	15.5	11.0	10.9	11.9	11.0	10.8	13.7	12.6	10.0	13.0	12.0	10.6	9.1	7.4
All 10th graders	NA	NA	NA	22.0	24.1	19.0	19.9	19.6	16.0	17.5	16.3	14.7	15.6	13.7	12.6	10.9	9.7
Male	NA	NA	NA	24.1	27.6	19.9	21.0	20.9	16.6	18.8	17.9	16.5	16.4	14.7	13.1	11.3	9.6
Female	NA	NA	NA	19.7	20.6	17.9	18.9	18.3	15.4	16.1	14.6	12.7	14.8	12.5	12.2	10.6	9.8
White	NA	NA	NA	24.1	26.6	21.5	21.8	21.7	17.4	18.4	16.0	16.1	16.5	14.7	14.1	12.1	11.0
Black or African American	NA	NA	NA	9.6	10.6	8.4	9.9	10.0	9.6	10.0	11.5	7.3	9.3	7.9	7.2	6.6	5.1
All 8th graders	NA	NA	NA	12.3	11.7	8.4	8.7	8.3	8.1	7.8	7.2	6.4	5.1	5.1	4.1	4.6	3.4
Male	NA	NA	NA	12.5	11.7	8.2	8.6	8.2	8.1	7.8	6.5	6.1	4.6	4.5	3.5	4.6	3.2
Female	NA	NA	NA	12.1	11.3	8.6	8.5	8.2	8.0	7.7	7.8	6.5	5.5	5.7	4.6	4.6	3.6
White	NA	NA	NA	12.6	12.5	8.4	8.4	7.7	8.0	7.4	6.7	5.8	3.9	4.6	3.7	4.2	3.0
Black or African American	NA	NA	NA	7.8	6.2	5.8	5.5	5.7	5.7	4.8	5.9	4.4	4.2	4.8	4.1	4.1	2.7

NA = Not available.

[1]Starting in 2014, a revised question on the use of MDMA (ecstasy) including "Molly," a nickname for MDMA, was added to the questionnaire for each grade. Data reported here for 2014 and later are only for the revised question which includes "Molly."
[2]In 1993, the alcohol question was changed to indicate that a drink meant more than a few sips.
[3]Five or more alcoholic drinks in a row at least once in the prior 2-week period.

AMBULATORY CARE

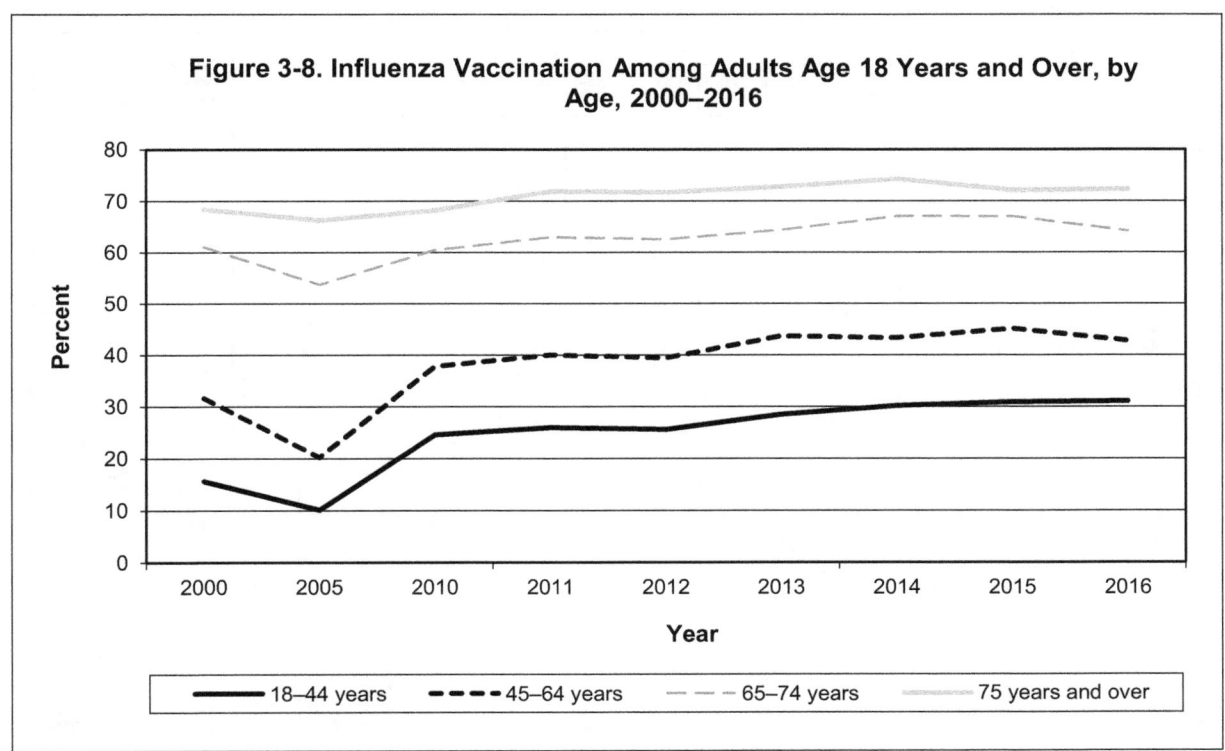

Figure 3-8. Influenza Vaccination Among Adults Age 18 Years and Over, by Age, 2000–2016

Table 3-30. No Usual Source of Health Care Among Children Under 18 Years of Age, by Selected Characteristics, Annual Average, Selected Years, 1993–1994 Through 2015–2016

(Percent; data are based on household interviews of a sample of the civilian noninstitutionalized population.)

Characteristic	Under 18 years					Under 6 years					6 to 17 years				
	1993–1994[1]	1999–2000	2009–2010	2014–2015	2015–2016	1993–1994[1]	1999–2000	2009–2010	2014–2015	2015–2016	1993–1994[1]	1999–2000	2009–2010	2014–2015	2015–2016
Percent of Children without a Usual Source of Health Care[2]															
All Children[3]	7.7	6.9	5.4	4.0	4.6	5.2	4.6	4.1	2.7	3.3	9.0	8.0	6.2	4.6	5.2
Sex															
Male	8.1	6.7	5.5	3.9	4.4	5.3	4.5	4.2	2.4	3.0	9.6	7.8	6.1	4.6	5.1
Female	7.3	7.1	5.4	4.1	4.8	5.0	4.7	4.0	3.0	3.7	8.5	8.2	6.2	4.6	5.4
Race[4]															
White only	7.0	6.3	5.3	3.7	4.3	4.7	4.4	3.8	2.4	3.0	8.3	7.2	6.1	4.3	4.9
Black or African American only	10.3	7.7	5.6	4.8	5.4	7.6	4.4	4.3	4.0	4.7	11.9	9.1	6.3	5.1	5.7
American Indian or Alaska Native only	*9.3	*9.4	*	*	*	*	*	*	*	*	*8.7	*9.4	*9.2	*	*
Asian only	9.7	10.0	6.1	5.0	4.7	*3.4	*5.8	*3.9	*4.2	3.6	13.5	12.2	7.3	5.4	5.2
Native Hawaiian or Other Pacific Islander only	NA	*	*	*	*	NA	*	*	*	*	NA	*	*	*	*
Two or more races	NA	*4.9	4.6	4.8	5.3	NA	*	*4.2	*3.3	3.1	NA	*7.2	*4.9	5.8	6.7
Hispanic Origin and Race[4]															
Hispanic or Latino	14.3	14.2	9.5	6.2	6.6	9.3	9.0	5.8	3.9	4.6	17.7	17.2	11.8	7.5	7.5
Not Hispanic or Latino	6.7	5.5	4.3	3.3	3.9	4.4	3.6	3.5	2.3	2.9	7.8	6.3	4.7	3.7	4.4
White only	5.7	4.7	3.8	2.6	3.4	3.7	3.3	2.9	1.7	2.4	6.7	5.4	4.1	3.0	3.9
Black or African American only	10.2	7.6	5.4	4.5	5.4	7.7	4.5	4.3	3.8	4.7	11.6	9.0	6.0	4.8	5.7
Percent of Poverty Level[5]															
Below 100 percent	13.9	13.1	8.3	6.5	7.2	9.4	7.6	6.6	4.4	5.2	16.8	16.2	9.3	7.6	8.3
100 percent to 199 percent	9.8	10.6	7.5	5.4	6.3	6.7	7.5	4.8	3.7	4.9	11.6	12.2	9.0	6.2	7.0
200 percent to 399 percent	3.7	4.8	4.7	3.4	4.0	1.9	3.2	*3.1	2.3	2.9	4.5	5.6	5.5	3.9	4.6
400 percent or more	3.7	2.6	2.1	1.4	1.9	*1.6	1.5	*1.9	*0.8	1.0	5.0	3.0	2.2	1.7	2.2
Hispanic Origin and Race and Percent of Poverty Level[4,5]															
Hispanic or Latino															
Below 100 percent	19.6	19.4	10.7	7.6	7.9	12.7	11.6	7.1	*4.8	5.9	24.8	24.5	13.4	9.3	9.0
100 percent to 199 percent	15.3	17.1	10.6	6.9	6.9	9.9	11.3	6.3	*4.0	5.6	18.9	20.4	13.2	8.3	7.5
200 percent to 399 percent	5.2	8.3	8.5	5.0	6.5	*	*5.0	*4.1	*3.5	3.3	6.7	10.1	10.9	5.8	8.1
400 percent or more	*	*3.8	*3.6	*2.4	2.3	*	*	*	*	1.4	*	*5.0	*4.1	*3.0	2.8
Not Hispanic or Latino															
White only															
Below 100 percent	10.2	10.7	6.1	4.9	6.7	6.5	*6.3	*5.0	*	5.1	12.7	13.1	*6.8	*5.4	7.7
100 percent to 199 percent	8.7	7.8	5.7	4.0	5.7	6.3	5.7	*4.0	*3.2	3.8	10.1	8.8	6.6	4.5	6.8
200 percent to 399 percent	3.3	4.0	3.7	2.6	2.9	1.6	2.7	*	*1.3	2.1	4.0	4.6	4.2	3.3	3.4
400 percent or more	4.0	2.3	2.1	1.1	1.7	*1.7	*1.5	*1.9	*	0.9	5.4	2.6	2.1	1.4	2.0
Black or African American only															
Below 100 percent	13.7	9.4	6.3	5.0	6.0	10.9	*4.7	*6.2	*4.8	5.4	15.5	11.8	6.4	5.1	6.4
100 percent to 199 percent	9.1	9.7	6.2	5.3	6.8	*6.0	*6.4	*	*	*	10.8	11.2	8.1	6.1	7.1
200 percent to 399 percent	5.0	5.0	5.1	*4.1	5.1	*	*	*	*	*	6.2	5.7	5.4	*4.2	5.7
400 percent or more	*	*3.5	*	*	1.2	*	*	*	*	*	*	*4.0	*	*	1.5
Health Insurance Status at the Time of Interview[6]															
Insured	5.0	3.9	3.4	2.8	3.4	3.3	2.6	2.8	2.1	2.6	5.9	4.5	3.7	3.1	3.8
Private	3.8	3.4	2.6	2.1	2.6	1.9	2.2	1.7	1.5	1.9	4.6	3.9	3.0	2.3	2.9
Medicaid	8.9	5.3	4.4	3.7	4.6	6.4	3.5	3.7	2.8	3.6	11.3	6.7	4.9	4.3	5.1
Uninsured	23.5	29.3	28.8	27.9	27.9	18.0	20.8	21.4	20.3	22.6	26.0	32.9	31.5	30.3	29.7
Health Insurance Status Prior to Interview[6]															
Insured continuously all 12 months	4.6	3.6	3.2	2.5	3.2	3.1	2.3	2.7	1.9	2.5	5.5	4.2	3.4	2.8	3.5
Uninsured for any period up to 12 months	15.3	15.0	11.7	13.5	14.8	10.9	12.5	10.4	10.8	11.6	18.1	16.4	12.4	14.8	16.3
Uninsured more than 12 months	27.6	35.8	36.2	34.9	38.2	21.4	26.8	27.5	*23.5	32.8	30.0	39.1	38.5	37.5	39.7
Percent of Poverty Level and Health Insurance Status Prior to Interview[5,6]															
Below 100 percent															
Insured continuously all 12 months	8.6	5.7	4.5	4.0	4.9	5.8	*2.7	4.1	2.9	3.7	10.7	7.5	4.7	4.5	5.5
Uninsured for any period up to 12 months	21.7	19.8	*14.7	20.8	21.9	18.0	*16.0	*14.0	*	*	23.7	21.9	*15.2	21.5	24.5
Uninsured more than 12 months	31.2	42.7	43.0	47.9	41.6	25.5	31.0	41.9	*	*	33.4	47.1	43.3	49.8	*

NA = Not available.
* = Estimates are considered unreliable. Starting with 2015–2016 data, the reliability of survey percentage estimates was assessed using new multistep National Center for Health Statistics data presentation standards for proportions. Prior to 2015–2016 data, the reliability of estimates for earlier years was evaluated based on relative standard errors (RSE). Data preceded by an asterisk have an RSE of 20%–30%. Data not shown have an RSE greater than 30%.
[1]Data prior to 1997 are not strictly comparable with data for later years due to the 1997 questionnaire redesign.
[2]Persons who report the emergency department as their usual source of care are defined as having no usual source of care.
[3]Includes all other races not shown separately and unknown health insurance status.
[4]The race groups White, Black, American Indian or Alaska Native, Asian, Native Hawaiian or Other Pacific Islander, and 2 or more races include persons of Hispanic and non-Hispanic origin. Persons of Hispanic origin may be of any race. Starting with 1999 data, race-specific estimates are tabulated according to the 1997 Revisions to the Standards for the Classification of Federal Data on Race and Ethnicity and are not strictly comparable with estimates for earlier years. The five single-race categories and multiple-race categories shown in the table conform to the 1997 Standards. Starting with 1999 data, race-specific estimates are for persons who reported only one racial group; the category 2 or more races includes persons who reported more than one racial group. Prior to 1999, data were tabulated according to the 1977 Standards with four racial groups, and the Asian only category included Native Hawaiian or Other Pacific Islander. Estimates for single-race categories prior to 1999 included persons who reported one race, or if they reported more than one race, identified one race as best representing their race. Starting with 2003 data, race responses of other race and unspecified multiple race were treated as missing, and then race was imputed if these were the only race responses. Almost all persons with a race response of other race were of Hispanic origin.
[5]Percent of poverty level is based on family income and family size and composition using U.S. Census Bureau poverty thresholds. Missing family income data were imputed starting in 1993.
[6]Health insurance categories are mutually exclusive. Persons who reported both Medicaid and private coverage are classified as having private coverage. Medicaid includes other public assistance through 1996. Starting with 1997 data, state-sponsored health plan coverage is included as Medicaid coverage. Starting with 1999 data, coverage by the Children's Health Insurance Program (CHIP) is included with Medicaid coverage. In addition to private and Medicaid, the insured category also includes military, other government, and Medicare coverage. Persons not covered by private insurance, Medicaid, CHIP, public assistance (through 1996), state-sponsored or other government-sponsored health plans (starting in 1997), Medicare, or military plans are considered to have no health insurance coverage. Persons with only Indian Health Service coverage are considered to have no health insurance coverage. Health insurance status was unknown for 8%–9% of children in 1993–1996 and about 1% in 1997–2016.

Table 3-30. No Usual Source of Health Care Among Children Under 18 Years of Age, by Selected Characteristics, Annual Average, Selected Years, 1993–1994 Through 2015–2016—*Continued*

(Percent; data are based on household interviews of a sample of the civilian noninstitutionalized population.)

Characteristic	Under 18 years					Under 6 years					6 to 17 years				
	1993–1994[1]	1999–2000	2009–2010	2014–2015	2015–2016	1993–1994[1]	1999–2000	2009–2010	2014–2015	2015–2016	1993–1994[1]	1999–2000	2009–2010	2014–2015	2015–2016
100 to 199 percent															
Insured continuously all 12 months	5.6	5.2	3.8	3.0	4.0	3.7	3.7	*3.2	2.4	3.4	6.7	6.0	4.3	3.3	4.2
Uninsured for any period up to 12 months	14.5	15.4	12.4	14.8	17.0	*9.7	*14.4	*9.3	*11.3	11.8	18.0	15.9	14.0	16.6	19.5
Uninsured more than 12 months	27.6	34.4	36.7	34.6	41.8	21.4	26.4	*22.7	*	*	30.2	37.4	40.3	36.0	41.4
200 to 399 percent															
Insured continuously all 12 months	2.8	3.2	3.1	2.3	3.0	1.5	2.1	*	1.9	2.3	3.4	3.7	3.5	2.5	3.3
Uninsured for any period up to 12 months	9.1	11.1	10.3	9.4	11.0	*	*8.4	*8.7	*	10.2	11.6	12.7	11.1	*11.4	11.3
Uninsured more than 12 months	18.2	27.1	30.5	26.5	33.1	*9.7	*20.3	*	*	*	21.0	29.4	34.4	30.1	37.4
400 percent or more															
Insured continuously all 12 months	3.1	2.0	1.8	1.2	1.6	*	*1.2	*1.6	*	0.8	4.3	2.4	1.9	1.5	1.9
Uninsured for any period up to 12 months	*	*10.3	*	*	*	*	*	*	*	*	*	*	*	*	*
Uninsured more than 12 months	*	*30.0	*19.8	*	*	*	*	*	*	*	*	*33.3	*	*	*
Geographic Region															
Northeast	4.1	2.8	2.7	1.7	2.2	2.9	2.3	*2.6	*1.4	2.8	4.8	3.0	2.7	1.8	1.8
Midwest	5.2	5.3	4.3	3.5	4.0	4.1	3.7	3.6	2.7	2.8	5.9	6.0	4.6	3.8	4.6
South	10.9	8.5	6.2	4.5	5.6	7.3	5.8	4.4	3.0	4.1	12.7	9.8	7.1	5.3	6.3
West	8.6	9.7	7.4	5.1	5.3	5.3	5.7	4.9	3.1	3.1	10.6	11.7	8.7	6.1	6.4
Location of Residence															
Within MSA[7]	7.7	6.8	5.5	4.0	4.7	5.0	4.7	4.2	2.7	3.2	9.2	7.8	6.2	4.7	5.4
Outside MSA[7]	7.8	7.4	5.0	3.8	4.0	6.0	4.2	3.3	3.1	4.1	8.7	8.7	5.8	4.1	3.9

* = Estimates are considered unreliable. Starting with 2015–2016 data, the reliability of survey percentage estimates was assessed using new multistep National Center for Health Statistics data presentation standards for proportions. Prior to 2015–2016 data, the reliability of estimates for earlier years was evaluated based on relative standard errors (RSE). Data preceded by an asterisk have an RSE of 20%–30%. Data not shown have an RSE greater than 30%.
[1]Data prior to 1997 are not strictly comparable with data for later years due to the 1997 questionnaire redesign.
[7]MSA is metropolitan statistical area. Starting with 2016 data, MSA status is determined using 2010 Census data and the 2010 standards for defining MSAs.

Table 3-31. No Usual Source of Health Care Among Adults 18 to 64 Years of Age, by Selected Characteristics, Annual Average, Selected Years, 1993–1994 Through 2015–2016

(Percent; Data are based on household interviews of a sample of the civilian noninstitutionalized population.)

Characteristic	1993 to 1994[1]	1995 to 1996[1]	1997 to 1998	1999 to 2000	2001 to 2002	2003 to 2004	2004 to 2005	2005 to 2006	2006 to 2007	2007 to 2008	2008 to 2009	2009 to 2010	2010 to 2011	2011 to 2012	2012 to 2013	2014 to 2015	2015 to 2016
PERCENT OF ADULTS WITHOUT A USUAL SOURCE OF HEALTH CARE[2]																	
Total, 18 to 64 years[3]	18.9	16.9	17.7	17.8	16.4	17.3	18.4	18.5	18.5	19.5	20.3	19.6	19.5	19.7	18.2	17.3	16.8
Age																	
18 to 44 years	21.7	19.6	21.1	21.6	20.6	21.7	23.5	23.5	23.6	25.0	26.0	25.2	25.0	25.4	23.8	22.5	22.1
18 to 24 years	26.6	22.6	27.0	27.2	27.2	28.0	29.8	28.7	28.6	29.6	29.8	28.1	27.8	28.7	26.3	24.2	24.2
19 to 25 years	28.0	24.2	28.6	29.0	28.5	29.7	31.8	30.9	30.0	32.0	33.1	30.9	30.3	30.8	28.5	26.9	26.4
25 to 44 years	20.3	18.8	19.3	19.9	18.5	19.5	21.3	21.8	21.8	23.4	24.7	24.1	23.9	24.2	22.8	21.9	21.3
45 to 64 years	12.8	11.3	11.2	10.9	9.2	10.4	10.7	11.2	11.0	11.6	12.3	11.8	12.0	12.0	10.8	10.2	9.7
45 to 54 years	14.1	12.2	12.6	12.0	10.3	11.7	12.3	13.3	13.1	13.6	14.7	14.0	14.2	14.0	12.8	12.1	11.5
55 to 64 years	11.1	9.8	9.0	9.2	7.6	8.7	8.4	8.3	8.3	9.0	9.3	9.0	9.6	9.6	8.6	8.1	7.7
Sex																	
Male	23.9	21.4	23.6	24.1	21.6	22.5	23.9	23.9	23.9	25.3	25.9	24.6	24.4	24.5	23.1	22.3	21.4
Female	14.1	12.6	12.0	11.8	11.4	12.4	13.0	13.3	13.1	13.8	14.8	14.7	14.8	15.1	13.6	12.4	12.3
Race[4]																	
White only	18.4	16.5	17.0	16.7	15.4	17.0	18.1	18.3	18.0	18.9	19.7	18.9	18.9	19.2	17.8	17.0	16.4
Black or African American only	20.0	18.3	19.4	19.2	16.9	18.4	19.8	19.8	20.5	21.5	22.4	22.5	21.9	21.4	19.9	18.0	17.2
American Indian or Alaska Native only	19.7	16.5	21.3	19.2	16.3	21.5	21.9	24.4	24.4	24.8	26.7	22.4	23.6	26.6	23.4	20.1	16.4
Asian only	24.8	21.5	21.7	22.1	20.1	19.3	17.9	17.3	17.8	19.4	20.8	20.8	20.8	19.9	18.1	17.5	17.5
Native Hawaiian or Other Pacific Islander only	NA	NA	NA	*	*	*	*	*	*	*	*	*	*	*	*	*	24.3
Two or more races	NA	NA	NA	21.0	20.1	18.4	20.9	20.4	21.4	26.1	27.5	24.4	22.3	23.5	23.9	23.1	24.4
American Indian or Alaska Native; White	NA	NA	NA	25.8	18.1	17.8	21.4	19.3	20.9	25.9	27.1	23.9	19.0	19.7	24.2	23.9	22.5
Hispanic Origin and Race[4]																	
Hispanic or Latino	30.3	27.4	30.4	32.6	32.5	32.9	35.1	34.3	32.5	32.8	33.3	33.3	33.6	32.6	28.9	26.2	24.7
Mexican	32.4	29.8	35.9	36.5	36.5	36.4	39.3	39.0	36.6	36.1	35.7	35.2	35.6	34.5	30.6	27.5	26.4
Not Hispanic or Latino	17.7	15.7	16.2	15.8	14.0	14.9	15.6	15.9	16.0	17.1	17.9	17.0	16.8	17.1	16.1	15.4	15.1
White only	17.1	15.0	15.4	14.9	13.1	14.0	14.8	15.2	15.1	16.0	16.8	15.8	15.5	16.0	15.0	14.6	14.3
Black or African American only	19.7	18.1	19.3	19.2	16.8	18.1	19.2	18.9	20.2	21.4	22.2	22.1	21.6	21.3	19.6	18.0	17.3
Percent of Poverty Level[5]																	
Below 100 percent	29.5	26.1	29.1	29.6	29.3	28.9	32.1	30.6	30.4	32.7	33.8	32.8	32.1	32.9	30.6	27.3	25.7
100 percent to 199 percent	25.4	22.9	25.6	27.1	25.6	26.6	27.8	28.6	29.1	30.3	30.5	30.4	30.2	29.4	26.6	24.2	23.7
200 percent to 399 percent	15.6	13.4	16.6	17.2	16.0	17.3	17.8	18.5	18.9	19.7	20.5	19.3	19.3	19.3	17.9	18.1	17.8
400 percent or more	13.4	13.8	11.6	11.6	9.6	10.1	10.4	10.4	10.2	10.6	10.8	9.7	9.6	10.1	9.7	9.9	10.2
Hispanic Origin and Race and Percent of Poverty Level[4,5]																	
Hispanic or Latino																	
Below 100 percent	40.0	34.3	42.8	44.4	46.3	42.8	46.7	46.7	43.7	44.1	45.5	44.3	42.9	43.5	40.1	35.4	32.2
100 percent to 199 percent	36.9	32.9	35.4	40.6	40.0	39.7	41.8	42.1	40.6	40.7	39.7	40.4	40.0	37.7	34.3	30.1	28.0
200 percent to 399 percent	20.7	19.5	23.6	26.9	27.9	28.2	31.2	29.5	28.0	27.9	29.1	28.9	29.4	28.8	24.2	23.3	22.8
400 percent or more	13.8	16.3	14.4	16.1	13.7	16.4	16.4	15.9	16.9	16.6	14.0	13.4	15.4	15.1	13.2	13.1	15.2
Not Hispanic or Latino																	
White only																	
Below 100 percent	28.2	23.6	25.0	24.2	23.4	23.0	26.2	25.0	25.2	27.8	28.8	27.5	27.0	28.9	26.9	24.2	23.2
100 percent to 199 percent	23.3	20.7	22.4	23.0	20.7	22.0	23.5	24.5	24.9	26.0	26.6	26.0	25.7	25.5	23.4	22.2	22.1
200 percent to 399 percent	14.8	12.5	15.4	15.3	13.6	15.4	15.3	16.2	16.7	17.7	18.6	17.2	16.9	16.8	16.3	16.4	16.2
400 percent or more	13.4	13.7	11.3	11.2	9.1	9.4	9.8	10.0	9.5	9.9	10.3	9.1	8.8	9.5	9.1	9.4	9.4
Black or African American only																	
Below 100 percent	24.7	21.9	23.9	23.7	22.8	24.3	29.5	26.5	27.1	29.4	30.1	30.3	29.9	28.3	27.4	24.8	23.4
100 percent to 199 percent	22.3	22.1	25.3	24.4	20.4	22.8	22.6	23.4	25.7	27.6	28.5	29.6	28.2	27.3	23.7	20.3	20.8
200 percent to 399 percent	16.5	14.5	17.6	18.2	16.2	16.3	16.2	18.0	19.7	19.9	20.1	18.1	18.5	19.7	17.3	17.8	17.2
400 percent or more	11.7	12.6	11.2	12.0	9.6	11.3	10.3	9.1	10.2	11.2	10.5	10.6	10.1	9.7	9.5	9.0	9.0
Health Insurance Status at the Time of Interview[6]																	
Insured	13.3	11.4	11.4	10.9	9.1	9.4	9.7	9.9	10.1	10.4	10.6	10.2	10.5	10.9	10.5	11.2	11.8
Private	13.1	11.3	11.5	11.1	9.0	9.5	9.6	9.8	10.0	10.3	10.6	10.1	10.1	10.6	10.5	11.1	11.6
Medicaid	16.3	13.0	10.3	9.9	11.1	9.9	11.6	11.5	11.7	12.1	12.5	12.3	13.1	13.2	11.9	13.1	14.0
Uninsured	43.1	41.8	46.7	49.2	49.1	50.2	53.0	52.8	52.1	54.1	55.6	54.2	54.1	54.2	52.5	52.6	51.6

NA = Not available.

* = Estimates are considered unreliable. Starting with 2015–2016 data, the reliability of survey percentage estimates was assessed using new multistep National Center for Health Statistics data presentation standards for proportions. Prior to 2015–2016 data, the reliability of estimates for earlier years was evaluated based on relative standard errors (RSE). Data preceded by an asterisk have an RSE of 20%–30%. Data not shown have an RSE greater than 30%.

[1]Data prior to 1997 are not strictly comparable with data for later years due to the 1997 questionnaire redesign.

[2]Persons who report the emergency department as their usual source of care are defined as having no usual source of care.

[3]Includes all other races not shown separately and unknown health insurance status.

[4]The race groups White, Black, American Indian or Alaska Native, Asian, Native Hawaiian or Other Pacific Islander, and 2 or more races include persons of Hispanic and non-Hispanic origin. Persons of Hispanic origin may be of any race. Starting with 1999 data, race-specific estimates are tabulated according to the 1997 Revisions to the Standards for the Classification of Federal Data on Race and Ethnicity and are not strictly comparable with estimates for earlier years. The five single-race categories and multiple-race categories shown in the table conform to the 1997 Standards. Starting with 1999 data, race-specific estimates are for persons who reported only one racial group; the category 2 or more races includes persons who reported more than one racial group. Prior to 1999, data were tabulated according to the 1977 Standards with four racial groups, and the Asian only category included Native Hawaiian or Other Pacific Islander. Estimates for single-race categories prior to 1999 included persons who reported one race, or if they reported more than one race, identified one race as best representing their race. Starting with 2003 data, race responses of other race and unspecified multiple race were treated as missing, and then race was imputed if these were the only race responses. Almost all persons with a race response of other race were of Hispanic origin.

[5]Percent of poverty level is based on family income and family size and composition using U.S. Census Bureau poverty thresholds. Missing family income data were imputed starting in 1993.

[6]Health insurance categories are mutually exclusive. Persons who reported both Medicaid and private coverage are classified as having private coverage. Medicaid includes other public assistance through 1996. Starting with 1997 data, state-sponsored health plan coverage is included as Medicaid coverage. Starting with 1999 data, coverage by the Children's Health Insurance Program (CHIP) is included with Medicaid coverage. In addition to private and Medicaid, the insured category also includes military, other government, and Medicare coverage. Persons not covered by private insurance, Medicaid, CHIP, public assistance (through 1996), state-sponsored or other government-sponsored health plans (starting in 1997), Medicare, or military plans are considered to have no health insurance coverage. Persons with only Indian Health Service coverage are considered to have no health insurance coverage. Health insurance status was unknown for 8%–9% of children in 1993–1996 and about 1% in 1997–2016.

Table 3-31. No Usual Source of Health Care Among Adults 18 to 64 Years of Age, by Selected Characteristics, Annual Average, Selected Years, 1993–1994 Through 2015–2016—*Continued*

(Percent; Data are based on household interviews of a sample of the civilian noninstitutionalized population.)

Characteristic	1993 to 1994[1]	1995 to 1996[1]	1997 to 1998	1999 to 2000	2001 to 2002	2003 to 2004	2004 to 2005	2005 to 2006	2006 to 2007	2007 to 2008	2008 to 2009	2009 to 2010	2010 to 2011	2011 to 2012	2012 to 2013	2014 to 2015	2015 to 2016
Health Insurance Status Prior to Interview[6]																	
Insured continuously all 12 months	12.7	10.8	10.6	10.3	8.3	8.7	8.9	9.0	9.1	9.5	9.8	9.3	9.6	10.0	9.5	10.0	10.9
Uninsured for any period up to 12 months	30.9	29.6	30.7	31.2	33.3	32.1	33.4	33.6	35.1	36.7	36.5	33.6	33.2	34.1	32.5	32.4	32.5
Uninsured more than 12 months	46.9	44.8	51.4	54.8	54.6	55.0	58.0	57.9	56.1	57.2	59.5	58.3	57.8	57.9	56.4	56.9	57.5
Percent of Poverty Level and Health Insurance Status Prior to Interview[5,6]																	
Below 100 percent																	
Insured continuously all 12 months	16.7	13.3	13.1	11.6	11.5	11.2	12.0	11.6	12.7	13.5	13.0	13.4	14.0	14.3	13.4	14.3	15.5
Uninsured for any period up to 12 months	33.6	28.5	33.0	31.9	36.5	36.2	36.5	34.5	37.4	38.9	37.8	36.6	35.6	38.7	38.3	34.6	34.4
Uninsured more than 12 months	50.1	46.1	54.3	57.1	58.8	57.2	63.2	62.6	61.1	63.4	65.3	62.6	61.3	62.3	58.8	56.1	58.7
100 percent to 199 percent																	
Insured continuously all 12 months	14.7	12.2	13.0	12.3	11.0	10.5	10.4	10.5	11.9	13.0	12.5	11.9	12.8	13.0	11.9	12.0	13.5
Uninsured for any period up to 12 months	30.9	31.1	31.1	34.6	35.1	34.2	37.8	36.6	35.9	37.1	38.1	37.0	35.9	35.0	30.0	31.9	36.1
Uninsured more than 12 months	47.6	43.8	51.1	54.9	54.5	55.1	57.0	58.4	56.8	58.3	58.5	58.2	57.9	56.8	57.4	58.6	57.4
200 percent to 399 percent																	
Insured continuously all 12 months	11.7	9.4	10.6	10.6	8.3	9.4	9.4	9.5	9.4	9.9	10.6	10.0	10.0	10.4	9.7	10.8	11.9
Uninsured for any period up to 12 months	29.2	28.3	30.1	29.0	32.0	30.9	31.3	33.4	36.3	37.0	37.6	33.7	33.2	34.2	32.8	32.9	31.9
Uninsured more than 12 months	44.5	44.7	50.9	53.6	53.4	54.2	55.5	55.3	54.2	54.1	56.6	55.4	55.3	56.1	55.1	57.2	57.0
400 percent or more																	
Insured continuously all 12 months	11.8	11.8	9.5	9.3	7.2	7.5	7.7	7.8	7.5	7.6	7.9	7.3	7.4	8.0	7.7	7.9	8.5
Uninsured for any period up to 12 months	31.5	32.3	28.6	30.2	30.7	27.5	28.6	29.1	30.3	33.8	31.2	24.6	25.6	25.9	27.5	29.8	26.7
Uninsured more than 12 months	36.5	45.5	44.6	51.8	47.0	51.6	54.2	51.5	47.9	48.1	53.8	52.5	52.9	52.7	47.4	51.7	54.7
Level of Difficulty[7]																	
A lot of difficulty or cannot do at all	NA	NA	NA	NA	NA	NA	NA	NA	NA	NA	NA	15.4	16.8	17.0	15.8	14.3	11.9
Some difficulty	NA	NA	NA	NA	NA	NA	NA	NA	NA	NA	NA	19.0	19.1	19.3	17.3	16.7	16.5
No difficulty	NA	NA	NA	NA	NA	NA	NA	NA	NA	NA	NA	20.5	20.3	20.7	19.4	18.5	17.4
Geographic Region																	
Northeast	14.7	13.4	13.3	12.8	11.9	12.1	12.2	13.1	12.5	12.9	14.0	13.9	13.1	12.8	12.2	11.5	10.9
Midwest	16.2	14.7	15.1	17.0	14.1	14.7	15.8	16.2	16.6	17.3	17.5	16.7	17.1	18.0	16.5	16.3	16.5
South	21.8	18.7	20.7	19.7	18.3	19.7	21.4	21.4	21.4	22.5	23.5	22.3	22.2	22.3	20.4	19.6	19.5
West	21.1	19.9	20.2	20.1	19.9	21.0	21.1	20.5	20.0	21.8	22.9	22.4	22.8	22.6	20.9	18.7	17.4
Location of Residence																	
Within MSA[8]	19.3	17.3	17.9	18.1	16.6	17.6	18.7	18.9	18.7	19.5	20.3	19.8	19.8	19.9	18.4	17.5	17.0
Outside MSA[8]	17.5	15.4	17.0	16.8	15.4	16.2	16.7	16.5	16.9	19.4	20.4	18.4	17.8	18.4	17.1	16.0	15.7

NA = Not available.

[1]Data prior to 1997 are not strictly comparable with data for later years due to the 1997 questionnaire redesign.

[5]Percent of poverty level is based on family income and family size and composition using U.S. Census Bureau poverty thresholds. Missing family income data were imputed starting in 1993.

[6]Health insurance categories are mutually exclusive. Persons who reported both Medicaid and private coverage are classified as having private coverage. Medicaid includes other public assistance through 1996. Starting with 1997 data, state-sponsored health plan coverage is included as Medicaid coverage. Starting with 1999 data, coverage by the Children's Health Insurance Program (CHIP) is included with Medicaid coverage. In addition to private and Medicaid, the insured category also includes military, other government, and Medicare coverage. Persons not covered by private insurance, Medicaid, CHIP, public assistance (through 1996), state-sponsored or other government-sponsored health plans (starting in 1997), Medicare, or military plans are considered to have no health insurance coverage. Persons with only Indian Health Service coverage are considered to have no health insurance coverage. Health insurance status was unknown for 8%–9% of children in 1993–1996 and about 1% in 1997–2016.

[7]Functional limitation is defined by the reported level of difficulty in six functioning domains: seeing (even if wearing glasses), hearing (even if wearing hearing aids), mobility (walking or climbing stairs), communication (understanding or being understood by others), cognition (remembering or concentrating), and self-care (such as washing all over or dressing). Respondents with answers to one or more of the six questions were included in one of three mutually exclusive categories. Those responding "A lot of difficulty" or "Cannot do at all/unable to do" to at least one question were classified in the "A lot of difficulty/cannot do" category. Of the remaining, those responding "Some difficulty" to at least one question were classified in the "Some difficulty" category, and those responding "No difficulty" to at least one question were classified in the "No difficulty" category. Those responding "Don't know" or "Refused" to all six questions were excluded. During 2010 2016, 1% 8% of respondents were missing data and excluded.

[8]MSA is metropolitan statistical area. Starting with 2016 data, MSA status is determined using 2010 Census data and the 2010 standards for defining MSAs.

Table 3-32. Delay or Nonreceipt of Needed Medical Care, Nonreceipt of Needed Prescription Drugs, or Nonreceipt of Needed Dental Care During the Past 12 Months Due to Cost, by Selected Characteristics, Selected Years 1997–2016

(Percent; data are based on household interviews of a sample of the civilian noninstitutionalized population.)

Characteristic	Delay or nonreceipt of needed medical care due to cost[1]					Delay or nonreceipt of needed prescription drugs due to cost[2]					Delay or nonreceipt of needed dental care due to cost[3]				
	1997	2005	2010	2015	2016	1997	2005	2010	2015	2016	1997	2005	2010	2015	2016
TOTAL[4]	8.3	8.5	10.9	7.3	7.2	4.8	7.2	8.3	5.2	5.1	8.6	10.7	13.5	9.4	8.9
Age															
Under 19 years	4.5	4.3	4.5	2.8	2.6	2.1	3.0	2.8	1.6	1.7	6.0	7.3	6.6	4.1	3.8
Under 18 years	4.4	4.2	4.4	2.7	2.4	2.2	2.9	2.7	1.6	1.6	6.0	7.3	6.6	4.1	3.9
Under 6 years	3.3	3.3	3.7	2.2	1.7	1.6	2.5	2.5	1.4	1.3	3.9	3.7	3.9	1.9	2.2
6 to 17 years	4.9	4.7	4.8	2.9	2.8	2.4	3.1	2.8	1.7	1.8	6.8	8.4	7.5	4.9	4.4
18 to 64 years	10.7	11.0	14.7	9.8	9.8	6.3	9.4	11.2	6.9	6.7	10.6	13.0	17.3	11.8	11.0
18 to 44 years	11.0	11.3	14.5	9.5	9.2	6.9	9.8	11.2	6.2	5.8	11.7	14.1	17.9	11.6	9.9
18 to 24 years	10.2	11.3	13.5	7.5	7.7	6.7	9.6	9.7	4.5	4.5	11.6	13.7	17.4	9.4	6.8
25 to 34 years	11.4	11.8	15.3	10.3	9.7	6.9	10.2	12.0	6.6	5.4	12.3	15.1	18.3	12.4	11.3
35 to 44 years	11.0	10.8	14.4	10.1	9.8	7.1	9.6	11.3	6.9	7.3	11.2	13.3	17.8	12.4	10.6
19 to 25 years	11.1	12.5	14.8	8.4	8.0	7.7	10.3	10.9	5.5	5.0	13.1	14.8	18.9	10.9	7.9
45 to 64 years	10.1	10.6	14.9	10.3	10.5	5.1	8.7	11.3	8.0	7.8	8.4	11.5	16.5	12.1	12.6
45 to 54 years	10.6	10.8	15.0	10.3	11.0	5.6	9.2	11.5	8.0	9.4	9.4	12.1	17.8	12.1	13.1
55 to 64 years	9.3	10.4	14.6	10.2	10.1	4.2	8.0	11.0	8.0	6.2	7.0	10.7	14.9	12.2	12.1
65 years and over	4.6	4.6	5.0	4.1	3.8	2.8	5.1	4.7	3.9	4.3	3.5	5.2	6.9	7.0	7.0
65 to 74 years	5.0	5.4	6.3	4.9	4.4	3.4	6.4	6.3	4.8	5.2	4.2	6.2	9.0	7.8	7.9
75 years and over	4.1	3.7	3.4	3.0	2.9	2.0	3.6	2.8	2.8	3.0	2.6	4.0	4.3	5.8	5.7
18 TO 64 YEARS															
Sex															
Male	9.3	10.0	13.5	8.9	9.1	5.1	7.2	8.8	5.4	5.3	8.8	10.8	15.2	10.0	9.5
Female	12.0	12.1	15.7	10.7	10.4	7.4	11.4	13.5	8.4	7.9	12.4	15.2	19.4	13.6	12.5
Race[5]															
White only	10.8	11.1	14.5	9.9	9.9	5.9	9.1	10.8	6.5	6.7	10.6	12.8	17.1	11.7	11.2
Black or African American only	10.8	12.0	17.4	11.0	10.7	9.5	11.6	15.6	10.1	8.5	10.8	15.2	20.7	13.6	12.1
American Indian or Alaska Native only	14.5	13.2	*15.7	9.8	9.7	*10.1	*14.1	18.6	*13.4	5.6	18.8	19.2	23.1	17.7	12.9
Asian only	6.3	5.0	8.0	4.8	4.6	*2.8	*3.5	4.2	3.4	2.2	7.8	6.8	8.7	7.4	5.8
Native Hawaiian or Other Pacific Islander only	NA	*	*	*	16.3	NA	*	*	*	*	NA	*	*	*	*
Two or more races	NA	19.9	24.0	15.2	14.7	NA	22.9	16.6	10.9	9.1	NA	23.0	25.6	14.3	14.5
Hispanic Origin and Race[5]															
Hispanic or Latino	10.5	11.5	15.4	10.8	9.4	6.7	11.2	13.0	8.3	7.6	11.5	15.5	21.6	14.5	13.9
Mexican origin	9.7	11.4	15.6	11.0	9.4	6.5	12.0	13.5	8.6	7.1	11.3	16.3	22.0	16.0	15.4
Not Hispanic or Latino	10.7	11.0	14.5	9.6	9.8	6.3	9.0	10.9	6.6	6.5	10.5	12.6	16.6	11.3	10.4
White only	10.9	11.1	14.3	9.7	10.0	5.9	8.7	10.3	6.1	6.4	10.5	12.3	16.2	11.1	10.4
Black or African American only	10.8	12.0	17.5	11.1	10.8	9.5	11.4	15.6	10.2	8.7	10.8	15.3	20.8	13.7	12.0
Education[6]															
No high school diploma or GED	16.2	16.2	20.6	14.0	14.2	11.5	16.4	18.1	13.9	13.4	14.5	20.3	26.3	20.3	20.3
High school diploma or GED	11.1	11.7	16.1	11.4	11.3	7.0	10.5	13.8	9.2	9.1	11.4	14.6	20.1	14.2	13.7
Some college or more	9.2	9.8	13.4	9.2	9.1	4.3	7.1	9.2	5.6	5.2	8.8	10.4	14.4	10.2	9.7
Percent of Poverty Level[7]															
Below 100 percent	19.6	20.0	23.4	16.6	15.2	14.8	19.5	21.5	12.9	12.7	19.4	24.4	30.4	21.2	18.5
100 percent to 199 percent	17.9	18.9	24.0	15.9	16.3	11.6	16.3	18.4	12.7	11.7	18.3	21.0	29.2	20.9	19.7
200 percent to 399 percent	10.5	11.8	15.2	10.8	10.6	5.5	9.5	11.4	7.0	7.2	10.2	13.7	17.3	12.9	11.5
400 percent or more	4.6	5.0	6.8	4.2	4.9	1.7	3.3	3.9	2.3	2.3	4.5	5.9	7.0	4.0	4.8
Hispanic Origin and Race and Percent of Poverty Level[5,7]															
Hispanic or Latino															
Below 100 percent	14.6	14.8	19.0	16.0	13.0	10.6	17.3	18.9	13.1	12.7	16.1	23.5	30.5	20.9	19.3
100 percent to 199 percent	12.2	14.5	18.6	12.5	11.4	8.1	13.0	14.7	10.8	9.5	13.5	18.2	25.2	18.8	18.3
200 percent to 399 percent	8.0	9.6	13.9	8.9	8.6	4.4	9.1	11.5	6.3	6.3	9.2	12.5	18.1	12.1	11.8
400 percent or more	5.1	6.2	7.7	5.6	4.7	*	*4.2	4.6	*2.1	2.3	4.5	5.8	9.1	4.8	6.6

NA = Not available.

* = Estimates are considered unreliable. Starting with 2015–2016 data, the reliability of survey percentage estimates was assessed using new multistep National Center for Health Statistics data presentation standards for proportions. Prior to 2015–2016 data, the reliability of estimates for earlier years was evaluated based on relative standard errors (RSE). Data preceded by an asterisk have an RSE of 20%–30%. Data not shown have an RSE greater than 30%.

[1]Based on persons responding to the question, "During the past 12 months was there any time when person needed medical care but did not get it because person couldn't afford it?" and "During the past 12 months has medical care been delayed because of worry about the cost?"

[2]Based on persons responding to the question, "During the past 12 months was there any time when person needed prescription medicine but didn't get it because person couldn't afford it?"

[3]Based on persons responding to the question, "During the past 12 months was there any time when person needed dental care (including checkups) but didn't get it because person couldn't afford it?"

[4]Includes all other races not shown separately and unknown health insurance status.

[5]The race groups White, Black, American Indian or Alaska Native, Asian, Native Hawaiian or Other Pacific Islander, and 2 or more races include persons of Hispanic and non-Hispanic origin. Persons of Hispanic origin may be of any race. Starting with 1999 data, race-specific estimates are tabulated according to the 1997 Revisions to the Standards for the Classification of Federal Data on Race and Ethnicity and are not strictly comparable with estimates for earlier years. The five single-race categories and multiple-race categories shown in the table conform to the 1997 Standards. Starting with 1999 data, race-specific estimates are for persons who reported only one racial group; the category 2 or more races includes persons who reported more than one racial group. Prior to 1999, data were tabulated according to the 1977 Standards with four racial groups, and the Asian only category included Native Hawaiian or Other Pacific Islander. Estimates for single-race categories prior to 1999 included persons who reported one race, or if they reported more than one race, identified one race as best representing their race. Starting with 2003 data, race responses of other race and unspecified multiple race were treated as missing, and then race was imputed if these were the only race responses. Almost all persons with a race response of other race were of Hispanic origin.

[6]Estimates are for persons aged 25–64. GED is General Educational Development high school equivalency diploma.

[7]Percent of poverty level is based on family income and family size and composition using U.S. Census Bureau poverty thresholds. Missing family income data were imputed starting in 1993.

Table 3-32. Delay or Nonreceipt of Needed Medical Care, Nonreceipt of Needed Prescription Drugs, or Nonreceipt of Needed Dental Care During the Past 12 Months Due to Cost, by Selected Characteristics, Selected Years 1997–2016—Continued

(Percent; data are based on household interviews of a sample of the civilian noninstitutionalized population.)

Characteristic	Delay or nonreceipt of needed medical care due to cost[1]					Delay or nonreceipt of needed prescription drugs due to cost[2]					Delay or nonreceipt of needed dental care due to cost[3]				
	1997	2005	2010	2015	2016	1997	2005	2010	2015	2016	1997	2005	2010	2015	2016
Not Hispanic or Latino															
White only															
Below 100 percent	24.3	23.6	26.1	19.0	17.5	17.3	20.5	24.6	12.9	12.8	23.4	25.1	31.8	22.9	18.4
100 percent to 199 percent	20.9	21.8	27.6	18.7	20.2	12.4	18.2	19.9	13.5	14.3	20.6	22.9	31.7	23.3	22.8
200 percent to 399 percent	11.4	13.1	16.0	11.7	12.0	5.4	10.0	11.3	6.7	7.5	10.6	14.4	18.0	13.5	11.9
400 percent or more	4.6	5.0	6.9	4.3	5.1	1.7	3.2	3.8	2.4	2.4	4.5	5.9	6.9	4.1	4.8
Black or African American only															
Below 100 percent	16.1	20.1	24.4	15.2	14.6	14.9	21.7	21.1	13.8	14.0	14.8	25.5	29.7	19.6	17.8
100 percent to 199 percent	14.3	16.2	22.9	14.0	15.4	13.9	14.3	21.3	14.3	11.5	16.4	19.0	28.2	18.7	16.2
200 percent to 399 percent	8.8	9.2	14.6	11.2	9.5	7.0	7.9	13.7	9.9	8.8	8.6	12.0	16.1	13.8	11.9
400 percent or more	4.6	5.5	8.1	4.7	5.2	*2.9	*4.1	5.6	*	1.7	4.3	*7.0	9.1	*3.7	4.0
Health Insurance Status at the Time of Interview[8]															
Insured	6.8	6.8	9.1	7.2	7.4	3.7	6.0	7.3	5.4	5.3	7.2	8.7	11.8	9.4	9.1
Private	6.0	5.9	8.2	6.2	6.6	2.9	4.7	6.0	4.0	4.0	6.2	6.7	9.2	6.9	6.6
Medicaid	11.9	12.0	12.5	10.5	9.7	11.1	14.0	13.5	10.7	9.4	14.8	21.8	24.2	18.9	17.6
Uninsured	27.6	29.5	34.5	28.1	27.4	18.0	23.1	25.7	17.3	16.5	26.1	30.7	37.7	28.2	26.0
Health Insurance Status Prior to Interview															
Insured continuously all 12 months	5.5	5.5	7.6	5.7	6.1	2.8	5.0	6.2	4.4	4.6	6.0	7.5	10.5	8.2	8.1
Uninsured for any period up to 12 months	28.7	31.7	35.1	30.7	31.9	17.7	23.5	25.1	19.6	18.0	25.2	30.3	33.6	27.6	25.8
Uninsured more than 12 months	30.6	31.1	35.9	28.9	27.8	18.9	24.5	26.2	17.4	17.1	28.0	32.1	39.4	29.6	27.3
Percent of Poverty Level and Health Insurance Status Prior to Interview[5,6]															
Below 100 percent															
Insured continuously all 12 months	9.4	9.4	10.1	9.1	8.9	8.1	10.8	11.4	8.2	8.9	10.7	15.0	20.7	15.6	14.5
Uninsured for any period up to 12 months	31.9	37.3	36.7	34.6	34.7	25.5	31.8	35.7	28.1	21.4	31.6	38.1	39.0	34.2	28.0
Uninsured more than 12 months	32.4	32.4	38.5	32.6	29.7	21.6	29.3	31.5	20.0	22.9	29.4	34.4	42.3	32.4	28.8
100 percent to 199 percent															
Insured continuously all 12 months	9.5	9.6	12.5	9.4	10.1	6.0	9.7	11.9	8.8	8.6	11.0	12.9	19.7	16.0	15.1
Uninsured for any period up to 12 months	33.6	35.1	38.5	34.0	35.5	20.5	28.4	26.5	22.3	21.0	28.2	35.0	38.9	33.6	31.3
Uninsured more than 12 months	30.0	32.7	37.4	28.1	30.0	19.5	24.2	26.1	20.0	18.3	29.3	31.4	40.7	30.8	32.1
200 percent to 399 percent															
Insured continuously all 12 months	6.1	6.6	9.5	7.0	7.3	2.9	6.0	7.4	4.9	5.5	6.8	8.8	11.6	9.5	9.0
Uninsured for any period up to 12 months	27.1	31.4	33.7	30.1	31.2	14.0	21.5	23.2	16.6	16.5	21.6	27.0	32.5	25.6	24.4
Uninsured more than 12 months	31.3	29.7	32.4	26.4	24.9	17.3	21.6	23.7	13.8	12.7	26.5	31.5	36.1	27.7	22.8
400 percent or more															
Insured continuously all 12 months	3.1	3.1	4.6	3.0	3.7	0.8	2.1	2.9	1.7	1.7	3.1	4.0	5.2	3.1	3.9
Uninsured for any period up to 12 months	20.8	23.9	30.7	22.8	25.6	10.7	13.9	14.0	12.9	12.9	19.3	23.4	21.6	15.9	18.2
Uninsured more than 12 months	25.5	27.6	31.8	27.2	22.2	13.5	20.7	16.3	*	*	23.6	29.6	34.6	*20.0	*
Level of difficulty[8]															
A lot of difficulty or cannot do at all	NA	NA	25.4	22.3	24.2	NA	NA	31.6	24.4	20.6	NA	NA	36.1	29.8	25.8
Some difficulty	NA	NA	22.1	15.3	15.3	NA	NA	18.2	10.4	11.3	NA	NA	23.6	17.1	18.3
No difficulty	NA	NA	12.5	7.8	7.8	NA	NA	7.8	4.1	3.5	NA	NA	14.3	7.9	7.0
Geographic Region															
Northeast	8.8	8.7	10.2	7.7	6.8	4.9	7.2	7.7	5.2	4.3	8.9	10.6	12.9	9.1	8.2
Midwest	10.5	10.6	14.8	9.9	10.1	5.9	9.0	11.6	6.5	6.2	9.7	11.9	16.0	10.9	9.3
South	11.8	12.6	16.5	11.0	11.7	7.3	11.3	13.5	8.4	8.6	10.9	14.7	19.6	13.0	12.5
West	10.8	11.1	15.1	9.5	8.9	6.3	8.2	10.0	6.2	5.9	13.1	13.6	18.4	12.9	12.5
Location of Residence															
Within MSA[9]	10.2	10.6	14.2	9.6	9.5	5.9	8.8	10.8	6.7	6.2	10.0	12.7	17.0	11.4	10.7
Outside MSA[9]	12.5	12.8	17.4	11.0	11.7	7.9	11.8	13.6	8.3	9.5	12.9	14.6	19.1	14.5	13.2

NA = Not available.

* = Estimates are considered unreliable. Starting with 2015–2016 data, the reliability of survey percentage estimates was assessed using new multistep National Center for Health Statistics data presentation standards for proportions. Prior to 2015–2016 data, the reliability of estimates for earlier years was evaluated based on relative standard errors (RSE). Data preceded by an asterisk have an RSE of 20%–30%. Data not shown have an RSE greater than 30%.

[1]Based on persons responding to the question, "During the past 12 months was there any time when person needed medical care but did not get it because person couldn't afford it?" and "During the past 12 months has medical care been delayed because of worry about the cost?"

[2]Based on persons responding to the question, "During the past 12 months was there any time when person needed prescription medicine but didn't get it because person couldn't afford it?"

[3]Based on persons responding to the question, "During the past 12 months was there any time when person needed dental care (including checkups) but didn't get it because person couldn't afford it?"

[5]The race groups White, Black, American Indian or Alaska Native, Asian, Native Hawaiian or Other Pacific Islander, and 2 or more races include persons of Hispanic and non-Hispanic origin. Persons of Hispanic origin may be of any race. Starting with 1999 data, race-specific estimates are tabulated according to the 1997 Revisions to the Standards for the Classification of Federal Data on Race and Ethnicity and are not strictly comparable with estimates for earlier years. The five single-race categories and multiple-race categories shown in the table conform to the 1997 Standards. Starting with 1999 data, race-specific estimates are for persons who reported only one racial group; the category 2 or more races includes persons who reported more than one racial group. Prior to 1999, data were tabulated according to the 1977 Standards with four racial groups, and the Asian only category included Native Hawaiian or Other Pacific Islander. Estimates for single-race categories prior to 1999 included persons who reported one race, or if they reported more than one race, identified one race as best representing their race. Starting with 2003 data, race responses of other race and unspecified multiple race were treated as missing, and then race was imputed if these were the only race responses. Almost all persons with a race response of other race were of Hispanic origin.

[6]Estimates are for persons aged 25–64. GED is General Educational Development high school equivalency diploma.

[8]Functional limitation is defined by the reported level of difficulty in six functioning domains: seeing (even if wearing glasses), hearing (even if wearing hearing aids), mobility (walking or climbing stairs), communication (understanding or being understood by others), cognition (remembering or concentrating), and self-care (such as washing all over or dressing). Respondents with answers to one or more of the six questions were included in one of three mutually exclusive categories. Those responding "A lot of difficulty" or "Cannot do at all/unable to do" to at least one question were classified in the "A lot of difficulty/cannot do" category. Of the remaining, those responding "Some difficulty" to at least one question were classified in the "Some difficulty" category, and those responding "No difficulty" to at least one question were classified in the "No difficulty" category. Those responding "Don't know" or "Refused" to all six questions were excluded. During 2010 2016, 1% 8% of respondents were missing data and excluded.

[9]MSA is metropolitan statistical area. Starting with 2016 data, MSA status is determined using 2010 Census data and the 2010 standards for defining MSAs.

Table 3-33. Reduced Access to Medical Care During the Past 12 Months Due to Cost, 25 Largest States, Selected Annual Averages, 1997–1998 Through 2010–2011

(Percent for the 25 states with the largest populations in 2010–2011.)

State	Did not get or delayed medical care due to cost[1]			Did not get prescription drugs due to cost[2]			Did not get dental care[3]		
	1997–1998	2000–2001	2010–2011	1997–1998	2000–2001	2010–2011	1997–1998	2000–2001	2010–2011
United States	7.9	7.5	10.6	4.5	5.3	8.0	8.1	8.4	13.2
Alabama	7.6	7.7	11.9	6.8	8.3	12.3	8.7	10.3	15.0
Arizona	8.0	7.4	14.4	4.1	4.6	11.1	9.4	8.4	20.6
California	6.8	6.6	10.4	3.9	4.7	7.2	8.3	8.1	15.0
Colorado	6.4	8.1	12.2	3.1	5.5	6.9	8.9	11.5	13.5
Florida	9.8	9.6	13.2	4.8	5.8	10.1	7.2	8.4	17.4
Georgia	8.0	7.7	12.1	4.2	4.0	9.7	5.8	5.3	13.8
Illinois	6.1	6.5	8.7	3.0	4.2	6.0	5.7	6.8	9.9
Indiana	9.0	8.6	12.0	5.1	6.8	11.9	7.2	6.9	12.2
Louisiana	9.8	11.1	11.4	8.7	9.8	12.0	11.3	16.4	18.0
Maryland	8.0	7.4	8.5	5.8	5.2	5.7	9.8	7.8	9.1
Massachusetts	5.1	4.3	5.1	*1.7	4.2	4.7	5.0	5.2	7.9
Michigan	7.2	7.0	11.4	3.8	5.1	9.8	7.5	7.9	15.9
Minnesota	8.1	7.0	10.3	3.6	3.9	6.0	8.7	8.3	10.7
Missouri	7.1	6.4	12.4	4.3	5.2	8.4	7.3	7.1	14.7
New Jersey	7.2	6.1	7.1	3.8	3.5	4.7	7.3	5.9	9.9
New York	6.4	5.8	6.9	2.8	3.8	5.4	5.6	7.5	7.8
North Carolina	7.8	7.9	11.3	4.0	5.8	7.9	8.2	7.9	12.4
Ohio	9.2	7.6	10.5	5.0	5.1	8.1	8.8	8.1	10.5
Pennsylvania	5.9	5.9	9.1	4.3	3.5	7.0	7.4	6.0	11.4
South Carolina	7.6	6.3	11.2	5.2	4.4	8.4	5.7	5.2	11.3
Tennessee	10.0	8.6	13.1	8.0	8.5	10.7	10.5	10.4	15.3
Texas	7.9	8.1	12.0	4.7	6.6	9.9	8.8	10.4	16.4
Virginia	6.2	7.2	9.3	4.1	5.2	6.9	8.3	7.4	9.6
Washington	8.6	9.2	13.0	4.8	6.8	8.3	11.6	11.9	17.6
Wisconsin	6.5	5.9	8.2	3.0	4.0	5.0	5.5	6.6	10.6

* = Figure does not meet standards of reliability or precision. Data preceded by an asterisk have a relative standard error (RSE) of 20 percent to 30 percent.
[1]Based on persons responding to the question, "During the past 12 months was there any time when person needed medical care but did not get it because person couldn't afford it?" and "During the past 12 months has medical care been delayed because of worry about the cost?"
[2]Based on persons responding to the question, "During the past 12 months was there any time when you needed prescription medicine but didn't get it because you couldn't afford it?"
[3]Based on persons responding to the question, "During the past 12 months was there any time when you needed dental care (including check ups) but didn't get it because you couldn't afford it?"

Table 3-34. No Health Care Visits[1] to an Office or Clinic Within the Past 12 Months Among Children Under 18 Years of Age, by Selected Characteristics, Selected Annual Averages, 1997–1998 Through 2015–2016

(Percent; Data are based on household interviews of a sample of the civilian noninstitutionalized population.)

Characteristic	Under 18 years					Under 6 years					6 to 17 years				
	1997–1998	2005–2006	2009–2010	2014–2015	2015–2016	1997–1998	2005–2006	2009–2010	2014–2015	2015–2016	1997–1998	2005–2006	2009–2010	2014–2015	2015–2016
ALL CHILDREN[2]	12.8	11.7	9.6	8.5	8.6	5.7	6.1	4.9	5.1	5.2	16.3	14.4	12.1	10.2	10.3
Sex															
Male	12.9	12.0	9.8	8.5	8.4	4.9	6.2	5.0	5.0	4.8	16.8	14.7	12.4	10.2	10.1
Female	12.7	11.4	9.4	8.5	8.9	6.5	6.1	4.8	5.2	5.7	15.8	14.0	11.8	10.2	10.6
Race[3]															
White only	12.2	11.3	9.4	8.2	8.4	5.5	6.3	4.5	5.0	4.9	15.5	13.8	11.8	9.7	10.1
Black or African American only	14.3	11.7	10.1	9.8	10.6	6.5	4.6	6.4	6.1	8.0	18.1	15.1	12.1	11.6	11.9
American Indian or Alaska Native only	13.8	*15.7	*12.4	15.6	15.3	*	*	*	*	*	*17.6	*17.7	*14.7	20.0	19.7
Asian only	16.3	17.5	12.7	9.6	7.7	*5.6	10.5	*4.8	*6.0	3.7	22.1	20.8	17.0	11.5	9.6
Native Hawaiian or Other Pacific Islander only	NA	*	*	*	*	NA	*	*	*	*	NA	*	*	*	*
Two or more races	NA	10.4	8.3	6.5	5.5	NA	*	*5.7	*	3.2	NA	14.8	10.1	9.2	6.9
Hispanic Origin and Race[3]															
Hispanic or Latino	19.3	17.4	13.5	11.3	10.7	9.7	9.6	7.7	5.9	6.0	25.3	21.9	17.2	14.2	13.1
Not Hispanic or Latino	11.6	10.3	8.5	7.6	8.0	4.8	5.1	4.0	4.8	5.0	14.9	12.6	10.7	8.9	9.4
White only	10.7	9.4	7.7	6.8	7.4	4.3	5.0	3.1	4.6	4.4	13.7	11.4	9.8	7.9	8.8
Black or African American only	14.5	11.7	10.3	9.7	10.5	6.5	*4.4	6.4	6.2	8.0	18.3	15.1	12.4	11.3	11.8
Percent of Poverty Level[4]															
Below 100 percent	17.6	14.2	12.4	10.3	10.9	8.1	7.7	6.9	6.7	6.7	23.6	18.2	16.0	12.3	13.2
100 percent to 199 percent	16.2	14.9	12.7	10.4	10.3	7.2	8.4	6.4	5.9	7.5	20.8	18.2	16.2	12.6	11.7
200 percent to 399 percent	11.7	11.1	9.0	8.8	9.0	4.9	6.1	4.2	5.3	4.7	14.8	13.4	11.4	10.5	11.1
400 percent or more	7.4	7.8	5.3	5.2	5.3	3.0	2.8	*2.3	2.6	2.6	9.5	10.0	6.7	6.3	6.4
Hispanic Origin and Race and Percent of Poverty Level[3,4]															
Hispanic or Latino															
Below 100 percent	23.2	20.0	14.6	11.1	11.7	11.7	11.5	9.0	6.8	6.1	31.1	25.6	18.5	13.7	14.5
100 percent to 199 percent	20.9	19.1	15.7	13.3	11.5	9.7	10.1	9.5	6.5	8.7	28.1	24.4	19.4	16.5	12.7
200 percent to 399 percent	15.7	14.6	10.9	11.3	11.1	8.0	8.1	*4.2	5.9	4.8	19.7	17.9	14.6	14.1	14.5
400 percent or more	7.8	10.9	8.5	6.2	5.7	*	*	*	*	*	9.3	14.1	11.3	8.9	7.6
Not Hispanic or Latino															
White only															
Below 100 percent	14.0	9.4	9.4	8.3	8.4	*5.6	*5.6	*	*6.6	*	19.7	11.8	13.1	9.2	10.1
100 percent to 199 percent	14.1	13.2	11.7	8.7	10.2	6.0	8.5	*3.6	6.5	7.3	18.0	15.4	16.1	9.8	11.7
200 percent to 399 percent	10.9	9.7	8.2	7.5	8.1	4.3	5.8	4.2	4.8	4.5	13.9	11.4	10.1	8.9	9.9
400 percent or more	7.2	7.1	4.6	4.8	5.1	*2.8	*2.2	*	*2.5	2.2	9.1	9.2	5.7	5.8	6.3
Black or African American only															
Below 100 percent	15.8	12.1	11.2	10.5	13.0	7.6	*	*6.4	*7.1	9.7	20.5	16.4	14.2	12.4	14.8
100 percent to 199 percent	16.4	13.1	11.3	9.1	9.2	*7.7	*	*	*	*	20.4	16.2	13.1	11.4	10.3
200 percent to 399 percent	13.3	11.7	9.4	10.6	9.8	*4.9	*	*	*	*	16.7	14.8	10.8	11.6	11.5
400 percent or more	8.3	*7.4	6.9	*6.5	7.5	*	*	*	*	*	10.7	*9.9	*8.4	*6.7	7.0
Health Insurance Status at the Time of Interview[5]															
Insured	10.4	9.5	7.7	7.5	7.6	4.5	4.9	4.3	4.8	4.8	13.4	11.9	9.6	8.9	9.0
Private	10.4	9.4	7.0	7.2	6.9	4.3	4.4	3.5	4.0	3.7	13.1	11.6	8.6	8.6	8.3
Medicaid	10.1	9.5	8.8	7.9	8.5	5.0	5.8	5.3	5.4	5.9	14.4	12.2	11.1	9.3	10.0
Uninsured	28.8	31.7	31.0	27.1	28.4	14.6	20.6	14.4	13.1	15.7	34.9	35.6	37.3	31.6	32.7
Health Insurance Status Prior to Interview[5]															
Insured continuously all 12 months	10.3	9.5	7.4	7.3	7.5	4.4	4.9	4.1	4.7	4.7	13.2	11.9	9.2	8.7	8.8
Uninsured for any period up to 12 months	15.9	15.8	16.3	14.6	14.4	7.7	9.3	7.7	*8.1	8.3	20.9	18.8	20.9	17.8	17.1
Uninsured more than 12 months	34.9	39.0	38.6	35.1	41.9	19.9	28.0	22.8	*18.2	26.3	40.2	42.2	42.9	39.0	46.3
Percent of Poverty Level and Health Insurance Status Prior to Interview[4,5]															
Below 100 percent															
Insured continuously all 12 months	12.6	10.4	9.1	8.8	9.3	5.7	5.8	5.8	6.1	5.7	17.6	13.5	11.4	10.3	11.3

NA = Not available.

* = Estimates are considered unreliable. Starting with 2015–2016 data, the reliability of survey percentage estimates was assessed using new multistep National Center for Health Statistics data presentation standards for proportions. Prior to 2015–2016 data, the reliability of estimates for earlier years was evaluated based on relative standard errors (RSE). Data preceded by an asterisk have an RSE of 20%–30%. Data not shown have an RSE greater than 30%.

[1]Respondents were asked how many times a doctor or other health care professional was seen in the past 12 months at a doctor's office, clinic, or some other place. Excluded are visits to emergency rooms, hospitalizations, home visits, and telephone calls. Starting with 2000 data, dental visits were also excluded.

[2]Includes all other races not shown separately and unknown health insurance status.

[3]The race groups White, Black, American Indian or Alaska Native, Asian, Native Hawaiian or Other Pacific Islander, and 2 or more races include persons of Hispanic and non-Hispanic origin. Persons of Hispanic origin may be of any race. Starting with 1999 data, race-specific estimates are tabulated according to the 1997 Revisions to the Standards for the Classification of Federal Data on Race and Ethnicity and are not strictly comparable with estimates for earlier years. The five single-race categories and multiple-race categories shown in the table conform to the 1997 Standards. Starting with 1999 data, race-specific estimates are for persons who reported only one racial group; the category 2 or more races includes persons who reported more than one racial group. Prior to 1999, data were tabulated according to the 1977 Standards with four racial groups, and the Asian only category included Native Hawaiian or Other Pacific Islander. Estimates for single-race categories prior to 1999 included persons who reported one race, or if they reported more than one race, identified one race as best representing their race. Starting with 2003 data, race responses of other race and unspecified multiple race were treated as missing, and then race was imputed if these were the only race responses. Almost all persons with a race response of other race were of Hispanic origin.

[4]Percent of poverty level is based on family income and family size and composition using U.S. Census Bureau poverty thresholds. Missing family income data were imputed starting in 1993.

[5]Health insurance categories are mutually exclusive. Persons who reported both Medicaid and private coverage are classified as having private coverage. Medicaid includes other public assistance through 1996. Starting with 1997 data, state-sponsored health plan coverage is included as Medicaid coverage. Starting with 1999 data, coverage by the Children's Health Insurance Program (CHIP) is included with Medicaid coverage. Persons not covered by private insurance, Medicaid, CHIP, public assistance (through 1996), state-sponsored or other government-sponsored health plans (starting in 1997), Medicare, or military plans are considered to have no health insurance coverage. Persons with only Indian Health Service coverage are considered to have no health insurance coverage.

Table 3-34. No Health Care Visits[1] to an Office or Clinic Within the Past 12 Months Among Children Under 18 Years of Age, by Selected Characteristics, Selected Annual Averages, 1997–1998 Through 2015–2016—Continued

(Percent; Data are based on household interviews of a sample of the civilian noninstitutionalized population.)

Characteristic	Under 18 years					Under 6 years					6 to 17 years				
	1997–1998	2005–2006	2009–2010	2014–2015	2015–2016	1997–1998	2005–2006	2009–2010	2014–2015	2015–2016	1997–1998	2005–2006	2009–2010	2014–2015	2015–2016
Uninsured for any period up to 12 months	19.9	17.5	14.8	18.4	14.9	*9.9	*	*6.6	*	*	26.1	21.6	20.0	20.4	16.9
Uninsured more than 12 months	39.9	44.6	46.2	36.2	47.5	24.9	*32.3	*32.8	*	*	45.2	48.4	50.2	40.1	*
100 percent to 199 percent															
Insured continuously all 12 months	12.6	11.5	9.0	8.3	8.5	4.8	6.7	5.1	4.9	7.0	16.7	14.2	11.3	10.0	9.3
Uninsured for any period up to 12 months	15.6	17.7	18.7	15.8	13.9	*8.7	*10.8	*9.6	*8.0	*	20.2	20.4	23.3	19.7	16.3
Uninsured more than 12 months	33.7	39.2	39.7	39.0	42.4	21.3	26.0	*22.4	*31.0	*	37.9	42.9	44.3	40.3	48.6
200 percent to 399 percent															
Insured continuously all 12 months	10.5	9.8	7.6	7.9	8.0	4.5	5.2	3.7	5.2	4.4	13.2	12.0	9.5	9.3	9.7
Uninsured for any period up to 12 months	12.8	14.6	14.7	11.5	16.2	*	*	*	*	*	17.2	17.3	17.9	14.7	20.2
Uninsured more than 12 months	29.9	31.6	32.1	31.1	39.5	*11.8	*	*	*	*	36.5	33.2	36.9	36.0	43.6
400 percent or more															
Insured continuously all 12 months	7.0	7.4	4.9	4.9	5.0	2.9	2.5	*2.3	2.6	2.5	8.8	9.5	6.1	5.9	6.1
Uninsured for any period up to 12 months	*10.8	*	*15.5	*10.7	*	*	*	*	*	*	*15.1	*	*21.9	*	*
Uninsured more than 12 months	*28.8	*35.6	*	*	*	*	*	*	*	*	*37.7	*38.3	*	*	*
Geographic Region															
Northeast	7.0	6.8	5.6	5.1	4.8	3.1	4.0	3.3	*3.2	3.7	8.9	8.1	6.7	6.0	5.4
Midwest	12.2	9.8	8.6	7.5	7.6	5.9	5.2	3.5	4.9	3.6	15.3	12.0	11.2	8.8	9.4
South	14.3	12.4	9.9	9.2	10.5	5.6	6.2	5.2	6.0	7.3	18.5	15.5	12.4	10.7	12.1
West	16.3	16.5	12.9	10.5	9.4	7.9	8.8	6.9	5.0	4.6	20.7	20.3	16.1	13.3	11.8
Location of Residence															
Within MSA[6]	12.3	11.4	9.4	8.2	8.4	5.4	5.9	4.7	5.1	5.0	15.9	14.1	11.9	9.8	10.0
Outside MSA[6]	14.6	12.9	10.8	10.2	10.3	6.9	7.4	6.0	5.3	6.5	17.9	15.4	13.1	12.6	12.1

* = Estimates are considered unreliable. Starting with 2015–2016 data, the reliability of survey percentage estimates was assessed using new multistep National Center for Health Statistics data presentation standards for proportions. Prior to 2015–2016 data, the reliability of estimates for earlier years was evaluated based on relative standard errors (RSE). Data preceded by an asterisk have an RSE of 20%–30%. Data not shown have an RSE greater than 30%.

[1]Respondents were asked how many times a doctor or other health care professional was seen in the past 12 months at a doctor's office, clinic, or some other place. Excluded are visits to emergency rooms, hospitalizations, home visits, and telephone calls. Starting with 2000 data, dental visits were also excluded.

[6]MSA is metropolitan statistical area. Starting with 2016 data, MSA status is determined using 2010 Census data and the 2010 standards for defining MSAs.

Table 3-35. Health Care Visits[1] to Doctors' Offices, Emergency Departments, and Home Visits within the Past 12 Months, by Selected Characteristics, Selected Years, 1997–2016

(Percent distribution of health care visits to doctors' offices, emergency departments, and home visits during a 12-month period; data are based on household interviews of a sample of the civilian noninstitutionalized population.)

Characteristic	None					1 to 3 visits					4 to 9 visits					10 or more visits				
	1997	2005	2010	2015	2016	1997	2005	2010	2015	2016	1997	2005	2010	2015	2016	1997	2005	2010	2015	2016
Total, age-adjusted[2,3]	16.5	15.5	15.6	15.0	14.6	46.2	45.9	45.4	48.4	49.5	23.6	25.1	25.8	23.7	23.2	13.7	13.6	13.2	12.8	12.7
Total, crude[2]	16.5	15.4	15.4	14.6	14.1	46.5	45.9	45.2	47.8	48.9	23.5	25.1	26.0	24.1	23.8	13.5	13.6	13.5	13.5	13.3
Age																				
Under 18 years	11.8	10.2	8.1	7.9	8.3	54.1	56.0	55.6	59.7	60.4	25.2	26.5	28.2	25.7	24.2	8.9	7.4	8.2	6.7	7.0
Under 6 years	5.0	5.1	3.7	4.7	4.9	44.9	47.4	48.9	52.2	52.5	37.0	38.0	36.8	35.7	34.6	13.0	9.5	10.6	7.5	7.9
6 to 17 years	15.3	12.6	10.4	9.5	10.0	58.7	60.1	59.1	63.3	64.3	19.3	20.9	23.6	20.9	19.1	6.8	6.3	6.9	6.4	6.6
18 to 44 years	21.7	22.9	24.2	23.3	22.0	46.7	45.8	43.9	46.9	48.6	19.0	19.2	20.6	18.7	17.9	12.6	12.0	11.3	11.1	11.5
18 to 24 years	22.0	24.2	25.9	24.5	22.8	46.8	44.4	43.4	47.2	50.2	20.0	19.6	21.1	19.6	16.4	11.2	11.8	9.6	8.8	10.6
25 to 44 years	21.6	22.5	23.6	22.9	21.7	46.7	46.3	44.1	46.8	48.1	18.7	19.1	20.5	18.3	18.4	13.0	12.1	11.9	11.9	11.9
45 to 64 years	16.9	14.0	14.8	13.7	12.8	42.9	42.9	42.8	45.5	45.6	24.7	26.8	26.1	24.5	25.1	15.5	16.3	16.4	16.3	16.5
45 to 54 years	17.9	15.8	17.6	16.1	15.2	43.3	44.8	43.5	47.0	46.4	23.4	24.3	23.9	23.3	22.5	14.8	15.0	15.0	13.6	15.9
55 to 64 years	15.3	11.4	11.1	11.2	10.3	41.3	40.2	41.9	43.8	44.8	26.7	30.3	28.8	25.9	27.7	16.7	18.2	18.2	19.1	17.1
65 years and over	8.9	5.6	5.3	5.5	6.4	34.7	30.7	33.8	35.5	37.2	32.5	37.5	36.7	33.9	35.0	23.8	26.2	24.2	25.1	21.4
65 to 74 years	9.8	5.9	6.3	6.4	6.8	36.9	34.4	36.1	37.9	39.7	31.6	35.8	35.7	33.7	34.6	21.6	23.9	21.9	22.0	18.9
75 years and over	7.7	5.2	4.1	4.2	5.8	31.8	26.4	31.0	32.0	33.6	33.8	39.5	38.0	34.2	35.7	26.6	28.8	27.0	29.6	25.0
Sex[2]																				
Male	21.3	20.4	20.4	19.5	18.6	47.1	46.7	46.4	49.8	50.1	20.6	22.2	22.7	20.3	21.1	11.0	10.7	10.5	10.5	10.3
Female	11.8	10.7	10.9	10.8	10.6	45.4	45.1	44.4	47.1	49.1	26.5	27.9	28.8	26.9	25.2	16.3	16.3	15.9	15.2	15.1
Race[3,4]																				
White only	16.0	15.1	15.3	14.8	14.3	46.1	45.6	44.9	47.8	48.9	23.9	25.4	26.1	24.0	23.6	14.0	13.9	13.7	13.4	13.1
Black or African American only	16.8	15.9	15.7	14.5	14.6	46.1	47.4	47.2	50.2	51.3	23.2	23.8	24.7	24.1	22.4	13.9	12.9	12.4	11.2	11.7
American Indian or Alaska Native only	17.1	20.4	19.4	20.6	19.0	38.0	36.4	40.3	39.0	41.2	24.2	29.8	28.1	23.3	22.2	20.7	13.4	12.2	17.1	17.7
Asian only	22.8	21.5	20.4	18.2	16.6	49.1	49.3	49.9	54.7	56.0	19.7	20.8	22.1	18.7	19.2	8.3	8.4	7.6	8.5	8.2
Native Hawaiian and Other Pacific Islander only	NA	*	*	*	19.9	NA	*	*	*	62.0	NA	*	*	*	11.6	NA	*	*	*	*
Two or more races	NA	15.4	13.9	17.3	14.5	NA	37.3	42.3	41.5	45.2	NA	27.6	25.2	25.0	23.6	NA	19.7	18.6	16.2	16.6
Hispanic Origin and Race[3,4]																				
Hispanic or Latino	24.9	23.9	23.5	22.3	19.4	42.3	42.1	43.2	45.9	48.0	20.3	22.2	22.6	21.9	21.2	12.5	11.8	10.7	9.9	11.4
Mexican	28.9	26.6	25.2	24.8	20.9	40.8	41.5	43.3	44.8	50.1	18.5	20.8	21.4	20.7	18.2	11.8	11.1	10.1	9.7	10.8
Not Hispanic or Latino	15.4	13.9	14.0	13.4	13.4	46.7	46.5	45.8	49.0	49.8	24.0	25.7	26.5	24.1	23.8	13.9	13.9	13.7	13.5	13.1
White only	14.7	13.0	13.2	12.7	12.7	46.6	46.4	45.3	48.1	48.9	24.4	26.2	27.1	24.7	24.6	14.3	14.5	14.4	14.5	13.8
Black or African American only	16.9	15.9	15.6	14.7	14.6	46.1	47.4	47.3	50.5	51.4	23.1	23.8	24.9	23.8	22.4	13.8	12.9	12.2	11.0	11.6
Percent of Poverty Level[3,5]																				
Below 100 percent	20.6	20.7	20.4	19.0	17.6	37.8	37.3	37.5	39.9	41.0	22.7	24.7	25.1	23.9	23.6	18.9	17.3	17.0	17.1	17.9
100 percent to 199 percent	20.1	20.2	20.8	18.4	17.6	43.3	42.0	42.1	45.1	45.6	21.7	23.4	23.1	22.9	22.3	14.9	14.4	13.9	13.6	14.5
200 percent to 399 percent	16.4	15.9	16.2	15.9	15.7	47.2	47.3	46.3	49.5	49.8	23.6	24.0	25.4	22.8	22.7	12.8	12.8	12.1	11.8	11.9
400 percent or more	12.8	11.0	10.2	11.2	10.9	49.8	49.2	49.4	51.8	53.8	24.9	27.0	27.6	24.7	23.8	12.5	12.8	12.7	12.3	11.5
Hispanic Origin and Race and Percent of Poverty Level[3,4,5]																				
Hispanic or Latino																				
Below 100 percent	30.2	27.9	28.7	26.3	22.2	34.8	37.2	36.5	38.3	40.3	19.9	20.2	22.5	22.7	22.3	15.0	14.6	12.3	12.7	15.2
100 percent to 199 percent	28.7	27.6	27.7	25.1	20.3	39.7	38.8	42.7	45.1	47.6	20.4	22.6	19.9	21.0	20.2	11.2	11.1	9.8	8.8	12.0
200 percent to 399 percent	20.7	22.7	21.6	22.2	20.2	47.4	44.9	45.0	49.5	49.6	19.8	23.1	23.1	20.2	21.0	12.1	9.2	10.3	8.2	9.1
400 percent or more	15.2	13.4	11.3	13.3	13.8	50.4	50.4	51.1	50.2	53.0	22.6	23.0	26.1	25.1	22.7	11.8	13.2	11.5	11.4	10.5
Not Hispanic or Latino																				
White only																				
Below 100 percent	17.0	16.4	15.0	15.2	14.2	38.3	36.1	37.0	38.3	39.0	23.9	28.0	27.4	25.6	26.1	20.9	19.5	20.6	20.9	20.6
100 percent to 199 percent	17.3	17.5	18.4	15.7	16.1	44.1	41.8	40.4	43.6	42.9	22.2	24.0	24.7	23.7	24.4	16.3	16.8	16.5	17.0	16.5
200 percent to 399 percent	15.4	13.8	14.7	13.7	14.2	46.9	47.3	46.0	48.6	48.8	24.3	24.7	26.3	24.0	23.6	13.4	14.2	13.0	13.7	13.4
400 percent or more	12.5	10.3	9.9	10.6	10.3	49.1	48.9	48.2	51.1	52.4	25.5	27.6	28.4	25.2	24.8	13.0	13.1	13.5	13.2	12.4
Black or African American only																				
Below 100 percent	17.4	17.8	18.4	16.2	17.8	38.5	40.1	39.8	42.9	41.1	23.4	24.8	25.0	25.1	24.6	20.7	17.3	16.8	15.7	16.5
100 percent to 199 percent	18.8	16.1	17.6	16.4	15.4	43.7	47.0	45.7	47.6	48.1	22.9	24.3	24.3	24.2	23.8	14.5	12.6	12.5	12.6	12.6
200 percent to 399 percent	16.6	17.2	15.1	15.6	14.7	49.7	49.0	49.0	54.0	53.6	22.9	22.9	25.7	22.3	21.6	10.8	10.9	10.2	8.0	10.1
400 percent or more	14.0	12.1	10.0	11.7	9.5	54.3	52.0	58.2	55.9	62.8	22.7	24.7	22.5	23.2	19.8	9.0	11.2	9.3	9.2	7.9

NA = Not available.
* = Estimates are considered unreliable. Starting with 2015–2016 data, the reliability of survey percentage estimates was assessed using new multistep National Center for Health Statistics data presentation standards for proportions. Prior to 2015–2016 data, the reliability of estimates for earlier years was evaluated based on relative standard errors (RSE). Data preceded by an asterisk have an RSE of 20%–30%. Data not shown have an RSE greater than 30%.
[1] This table presents a summary measure of the number of visits to hospital emergency departments, home visits by a nurse or other health care professional, and visits to doctor offices, clinics, or some other place during a 12-month period.
[2] Includes all other races not shown separately, unknown health insurance status, and unknown disability status.
[3] Estimates are age-adjusted to the year 2000 standard population using six age groups: under 18 years, 18–44 years, 45–54 years, 55–64 years, 65–74 years, and 75 years and over. The disability measure is age-adjusted using the five adult age groups.
[4] The race groups White, Black, American Indian or Alaska Native, Asian, Native Hawaiian or Other Pacific Islander, and 2 or more races include persons of Hispanic and non-Hispanic origin. Persons of Hispanic origin may be of any race. Starting with 1999 data, race-specific estimates are tabulated according to the 1997 Revisions to the Standards for the Classification of Federal Data on Race and Ethnicity and are not strictly comparable with estimates for earlier years. The five single-race categories and multiple-race categories shown in the table conform to the 1997 Standards. Starting with 1999 data, race-specific estimates are for persons who reported only one racial group; the category 2 or more races includes persons who reported more than one racial group. Prior to 1999, data were tabulated according to the 1977 Standards with four racial groups, and the Asian only category included Native Hawaiian or Other Pacific Islander. Estimates for single-race categories prior to 1999 included persons who reported one race, or if they reported more than one race, identified one race as best representing their race. Starting with 2003 data, race responses of other race and unspecified multiple race were treated as missing, and then race was imputed if these were the only race responses. Almost all persons with a race response of other race were of Hispanic origin.
[5] Percent of poverty level is based on family income and family size and composition using U.S. Census Bureau poverty thresholds. Missing family income data were imputed starting in 1993.

Table 3-35. Health Care Visits[1] to Doctors' Offices, Emergency Departments, and Home Visits within the Past 12 Months, by Selected Characteristics, Selected Years, 1997–2016—Continued

(Percent distribution of health care visits to doctors' offices, emergency departments, and home visits during a 12-month period; data are based on household interviews of a sample of the civilian noninstitutionalized population.)

Characteristic	None 1997	2005	2010	2015	2016	1 to 3 visits 1997	2005	2010	2015	2016	4 to 9 visits 1997	2005	2010	2015	2016	10 or more visits 1997	2005	2010	2015	2016
Health Insurance Status at the Time of Interview[6,7]																				
Under 65 years																				
Insured	14.3	12.4	12.3	13.3	12.8	49.0	49.6	48.5	51.7	52.6	23.6	25.0	26.1	23.3	22.4	13.1	13.0	13.1	11.7	12.2
Private	14.7	12.8	12.4	13.7	12.9	50.6	51.5	51.0	53.8	55.4	23.1	24.5	25.5	22.7	21.7	11.6	11.2	11.1	9.9	10.0
Medicaid	9.8	9.9	10.9	12.4	12.5	35.5	37.8	38.2	43.4	43.5	26.5	26.8	28.0	25.4	23.7	28.2	25.5	23.0	18.8	20.3
Uninsured	33.7	37.5	37.2	39.8	40.4	42.8	42.0	42.2	41.4	41.8	15.3	14.7	15.2	13.7	12.2	8.2	5.8	5.4	5.1	5.6
Health Insurance Status Prior to Interview[6,7]																				
Under 65 years																				
Insured continuously all 12 months	14.1	12.3	12.1	12.9	12.5	49.2	49.8	48.6	52.0	52.8	23.6	25.0	26.2	23.4	22.5	13.0	12.9	13.0	11.7	12.2
Uninsured for any period up to 12 months	18.9	18.9	18.5	21.5	24.2	46.0	44.9	47.8	46.9	47.2	20.8	22.5	22.0	20.0	18.0	14.4	13.7	11.6	11.6	10.5
Uninsured more than 12 months	39.0	43.5	43.8	48.7	49.9	41.4	40.0	39.7	37.8	38.0	13.2	12.3	12.6	10.4	9.1	6.4	4.2	3.9	3.1	3.0
Percent of Poverty Level and Health Insurance Status Prior to Interview (Under 65 Years)[4,5,6]																				
Below 100 percent																				
Insured continuously all 12 months	13.8	12.6	12.7	14.3	13.1	39.7	40.4	39.5	42.3	44.5	25.2	26.2	27.5	25.9	23.2	21.4	20.8	20.3	17.5	19.2
Uninsured for any period up to 12 months	19.7	18.9	16.9	21.8	21.7	37.6	37.4	43.0	45.6	43.9	21.9	23.7	25.0	19.0	20.4	20.9	20.0	15.1	13.7	14.0
Uninsured more than 12 months	41.2	46.0	45.0	48.8	55.3	39.9	35.2	38.1	36.9	30.3	12.2	14.4	13.6	10.6	12.5	6.6	4.3	3.3	*3.8	1.9
100 percent to 199 percent																				
Insured continuously all 12 months	16.0	14.8	14.8	13.3	14.1	46.4	45.7	44.4	49.1	48.1	21.9	24.3	24.8	23.8	22.6	15.8	15.2	16.0	13.8	15.1
Uninsured for any period up to 12 months	18.8	19.2	21.0	25.6	22.6	45.1	44.7	46.0	41.9	44.4	21.0	22.1	20.6	19.4	20.1	15.0	14.0	12.4	13.0	12.9
Uninsured more than 12 months	38.7	43.5	43.2	48.8	45.6	41.0	39.2	39.4	37.6	43.3	14.0	12.9	12.4	11.1	7.2	6.3	4.4	5.0	*	4.0
200 percent to 399 percent																				
Insured continuously all 12 months	15.1	13.3	13.6	14.0	13.7	49.4	50.7	49.4	53.5	52.8	23.4	23.7	25.3	22.0	22.0	12.1	12.3	11.7	10.5	11.5
Uninsured for any period up to 12 months	17.9	19.9	18.8	19.8	29.5	49.3	45.7	49.7	49.0	46.1	20.0	22.3	19.7	21.1	15.7	12.8	12.2	11.8	10.0	8.7
Uninsured more than 12 months	37.0	42.0	43.8	50.7	48.2	43.8	44.0	40.7	38.5	39.9	12.6	10.3	13.3	8.7	8.1	6.6	3.7	*2.2	*2.2	3.9
400 percent or more																				
Insured continuously all 12 months	12.4	10.6	9.7	11.4	10.5	52.2	52.1	51.8	54.3	56.4	23.9	25.9	26.8	23.5	22.7	11.5	11.4	11.6	10.8	10.3
Uninsured for any period up to 12 months	17.2	16.1	16.6	16.6	21.2	50.0	51.9	53.5	54.1	56.2	24.2	22.8	23.9	20.2	16.3	*8.5	9.2	*6.0	9.0	6.3
Uninsured more than 12 months	35.1	39.3	39.2	39.3	49.9	44.1	46.6	46.0	41.1	40.5	15.1	9.6	*8.8	*	8.3	*5.7	*	*	*	1.3
Respondent-Assessed Health Status[3]																				
Fair or poor	7.8	9.0	8.4	8.0	8.3	23.3	21.5	24.0	25.3	25.3	29.0	28.1	30.2	28.7	28.2	39.9	41.3	37.3	38.0	38.2
Good to excellent	17.2	16.1	16.3	15.7	15.2	48.4	48.2	47.5	50.6	51.8	23.3	24.8	25.5	23.3	22.9	11.1	10.8	10.7	10.3	10.1
Level of difficulty (age 18 years and over)[3,8]																				
A lot of difficulty or cannot do at all	NA	NA	*9.7	7.2	5.9	NA	NA	20.5	29.4	21.6	NA	NA	27.2	25.2	25.1	NA	NA	42.6	38.2	47.3
Some difficulty	NA	NA	14.2	15.4	13.9	NA	NA	37.8	38.3	42.3	NA	NA	28.1	27.8	25.2	NA	NA	19.9	18.5	18.6
No difficulty	NA	NA	20.2	19.9	18.7	NA	NA	46.6	49.7	51.0	NA	NA	23.1	20.9	21.3	NA	NA	10.1	9.5	9.0
Geographic Region[3]																				
Northeast	13.2	11.3	12.6	10.9	11.2	45.9	46.8	46.3	50.9	50.5	26.0	27.0	26.4	24.2	25.1	14.9	14.9	14.7	14.0	13.2
Midwest	15.9	13.8	13.4	14.5	12.8	47.7	47.2	46.8	48.9	51.2	22.8	25.2	26.4	23.3	22.9	13.6	13.9	13.3	13.3	13.1
South	17.2	16.0	16.1	15.9	17.1	46.1	45.7	44.2	47.2	48.0	23.3	25.1	26.6	24.4	23.0	13.5	13.3	13.2	12.5	11.8
West	19.1	20.0	19.1	17.1	14.8	44.8	44.2	45.2	48.3	49.6	22.8	23.3	23.5	22.5	22.2	13.3	12.5	12.2	12.1	13.4
Location of Residence[3,9]																				
Within MSA	16.2	15.5	15.6	14.9	14.2	46.4	46.2	45.8	49.0	50.1	23.7	24.9	25.6	23.4	23.1	13.7	13.3	13.0	12.6	12.6
Outside MSA	17.3	15.3	15.9	15.7	16.4	45.4	44.5	42.7	44.5	45.7	23.3	25.6	27.0	25.1	24.0	13.9	14.6	14.4	14.7	13.9

NA = Not available.

* = Estimates are considered unreliable. Starting with 2015–2016 data, the reliability of survey percentage estimates was assessed using new multistep National Center for Health Statistics data presentation standards for proportions. Prior to 2015–2016 data, the reliability of estimates for earlier years was evaluated based on relative standard errors (RSE). Data preceded by an asterisk have an RSE of 20%–30%. Data not shown have an RSE greater than 30%.

[1]This table presents a summary measure of the number of visits to hospital emergency departments, home visits by a nurse or other health care professional, and visits to doctor offices, clinics, or some other place during a 12-month period.

[2]Estimates are age-adjusted to the year 2000 standard population using six age groups: under 18 years, 18–44 years, 45–54 years, 55–64 years, 65–74 years, and 75 years and over. The disability measure is age-adjusted using the five adult age groups.

[4]The race groups White, Black, American Indian or Alaska Native, Asian, Native Hawaiian or Other Pacific Islander, and 2 or more races include persons of Hispanic and non-Hispanic origin. Persons of Hispanic origin may be of any race. Starting with 1999 data, race-specific estimates are tabulated according to the 1997 Revisions to the Standards for the Classification of Federal Data on Race and Ethnicity and are not strictly comparable with estimates for earlier years. The five single-race categories and multiple-race categories shown in the table conform to the 1997 Standards. Starting with 1999 data, race-specific estimates are for persons who reported only one racial group; the category 2 or more races includes persons who reported more than one racial group. Prior to 1999, data were tabulated according to the 1977 Standards with four racial groups, and the Asian only category included Native Hawaiian or Other Pacific Islander. Estimates for single-race categories prior to 1999 included persons who reported one race, or if they reported more than one race, identified one race as best representing their race. Starting with 2003 data, race responses of other race and unspecified multiple race were treated as missing, and then race was imputed if these were the only race responses. Almost all persons with a race response of other race were of Hispanic origin.

[5]Percent of poverty level is based on family income and family size and composition using U.S. Census Bureau poverty thresholds. Missing family income data were imputed starting in 1993.

[6]Estimates for persons under age 65 are age-adjusted to the year 2000 standard population using four age groups: under 18 years, 18–44 years, 45–54 years, and 55–64 years.

[7]Health insurance categories are mutually exclusive. Persons who reported both Medicaid and private coverage are classified as having private coverage. Medicaid includes other public assistance through 1996. Starting with 1997 data, state-sponsored health plan coverage is included as Medicaid coverage. Starting with 1999 data, coverage by the Children's Health Insurance Program (CHIP) is included with Medicaid coverage. Persons not covered by private insurance, Medicaid, CHIP, public assistance (through 1996), state-sponsored or other government-sponsored health plans (starting in 1997), Medicare, or military plans are considered to have no health insurance coverage. Persons with only Indian Health Service coverage are considered to have no health insurance coverage.

[8]Functional limitation is defined by the reported level of difficulty in six functioning domains: seeing (even if wearing glasses), hearing (even if wearing hearing aids), mobility (walking or climbing stairs), communication (understanding or being understood by others), cognition (remembering or concentrating), and self-care (such as washing all over or dressing). Respondents with answers to one or more of the six questions were included in one of three mutually exclusive categories. Those responding "A lot of difficulty" or "Cannot do at all/unable to do" to at least one question were classified in the "A lot of difficulty/cannot do" category. Of the remaining, those responding "Some difficulty" to at least one question were classified in the "Some difficulty" category, and those responding "No difficulty" to at least one question were classified in the "No difficulty" category. Those responding "Don't know" or "Refused" to all six questions were excluded. During 2010–2016, 1%–8% of respondents were missing data and excluded.

[9]MSA = metropolitan statistical area. Starting with 2016 data, MSA status is determined using 2010 Census data and the 2010 standards for defining MSAs.

Table 3-36. Vaccination Coverage Among Children 19 to 35 Months of Age for Selected Diseases, by Race, Hispanic Origin, Poverty Level, and Location of Residence in Metropolitan Statistical Area, Selected Years, 1995–2016

(Percent; Data are based on telephone interviews of a sample of the civilian noninstitutionalized population, supplemented by a survey of interview participants' immunization providers.)

| Vaccination and year | Race and Hispanic origin[1] | | | | | | | | Poverty level[2] | | Location of residence | | |
| | | Not Hispanic or Latino | | | | | | | | | Inside MSA[3] | | |
	All	White	Black or African American	American Indian or Alaska Native	Asian[4]	Native Hawaiian or Other Pacific Islander[4]	Two or more races	Hispanic or Latino	Below poverty level	At or above poverty level	Central city	Remaining area	Outside MSA[3]
Combined Series (4:3:1:3*:3:1:4)[5]													
2009	44.3	45.2	39.6	*	38.6	*	40.7	45.9	41.3	45.7	44.8	44.6	42.4
2010	56.6	56.9	54.5	64.1	59.3	*	61.3	55.5	52.8	58.7	56.5	57.2	55.2
2011	68.5	68.8	63.7	65.9	70.8	*	70.9	69.5	63.6	71.6	69.5	67.9	67.4
2012	68.4	69.3	64.8	*	71.6	*	71.5	67.8	63.4	71.6	67.6	69.4	68.0
2013	70.4	72.1	65.0	70.1	72.7	*	71.8	69.3	64.4	73.8	68.8	72.5	69.1
2014	71.6	72.6	65.4	*	69.5	*	68.5	74.3	65.7	75.4	70.8	72.7	71.2
2015	72.2	72.7	69.1	68.2	77.9	*	73.7	71.7	68.7	74.7	72.5	72.5	70.2
2016	70.7	72.2	64.1	68.5	72.3	*	71.5	71.0	66.0	72.5	71.3	71.1	67.0
DTP/DT/DTaP (4 Doses or More)[6]													
1998	83.9	86.6	77.3	82.9	89.1	NA	NA	80.5	79.5	86.1	81.6	85.4	85.1
1999	83.3	85.5	79.0	80.2	86.8	NA	NA	80.2	78.5	85.4	82.1	84.3	83.3
2000	81.7	84.4	76.1	77.8	84.5	*	81.5	78.6	76.2	83.5	79.9	82.8	82.9
2001	82.1	83.5	76.5	76.9	83.6	*	81.2	82.5	76.5	83.6	80.5	83.4	82.2
2002	81.6	84.4	75.8	*	88.0	*	77.6	79.2	75.4	83.5	79.3	84.0	80.2
2003	84.8	87.5	79.9	80.1	88.5	*	83.5	81.9	79.7	86.8	84.1	86.2	82.9
2004	85.5	87.7	79.5	76.7	89.6	*	86.0	84.1	81.2	87.4	83.9	87.2	84.5
2005	85.7	87.1	84.0	*	88.8	*	86.3	83.6	81.8	87.4	84.8	87.0	84.7
2006	85.2	86.6	81.2	82.7	86.0	86.2	83.8	84.5	81.0	86.8	84.4	86.3	84.5
2007	84.5	85.3	82.3	86.4	87.5	*	84.2	83.8	81.1	85.9	84.5	85.1	82.9
2008	84.6	85.0	80.1	82.0	92.3	*	87.6	84.9	79.9	86.8	85.0	85.3	81.8
2009	83.9	85.8	78.6	82.1	86.6	93.1	81.8	82.9	80.1	85.7	83.8	84.2	84.2
2010	84.4	84.5	83.7	81.8	88.3	*	82.8	84.4	80.8	86.1	84.0	85.0	83.7
2011	84.6	85.0	81.3	72.7	92.0	93.0	87.1	84.1	81.0	86.8	86.1	83.8	82.2
2012	82.5	83.6	79.6	88.2	88.1	*	85.6	80.8	78.5	85.0	82.4	83.4	80.5
2013	83.1	85.3	74.7	78.1	89.0	*	83.1	82.3	77.8	86.0	81.8	84.7	82.4
2014	84.2	85.5	79.1	*	87.4	*	79.6	85.4	79.1	87.4	83.6	85.3	83.1
2015	84.6	85.2	82.0	79.6	90.0	*	82.5	84.5	80.2	87.1	85.4	84.3	82.7
2016	83.4	84.8	76.8	83.5	86.4	83.2	83.6	83.3	79.2	85.1	83.3	84.8	78.8
Polio (3 Doses or More)													
1998	90.8	92.2	87.8	85.1	93.4	NA	NA	88.9	89.9	91.7	89.3	91.3	92.9
1999	89.6	90.3	87.0	88.2	90.1	NA	NA	89.4	87.4	90.5	88.7	90.1	89.7
2000	89.5	90.6	86.6	90.8	92.7	91.2	91.2	87.9	86.9	89.9	88.1	90.1	91.1
2001	89.4	90.1	85.2	87.5	89.6	*	86.5	90.7	87.4	90.1	87.9	90.2	90.6
2002	90.2	91.2	87.4	*	91.6	95.3	86.9	90.4	88.3	90.6	88.7	91.4	90.4
2003	91.6	93.0	89.2	91.3	91.3	90.2	91.0	90.1	89.1	92.5	90.7	92.1	91.9
2004	91.6	92.1	90.4	86.5	92.8	*	91.9	91.2	89.8	92.2	91.3	91.5	92.1
2005	91.7	91.4	91.0	*	92.9	*	93.8	92.3	89.7	92.4	90.6	92.6	92.2
2006	92.8	93.3	90.4	91.0	92.4	96.0	91.7	93.3	92.1	93.1	92.6	93.1	93.2
2007	92.6	92.6	91.1	94.8	95.0	87.4	92.3	93.0	91.9	92.8	92.0	92.7	93.8
2008	93.6	93.6	91.5	90.6	96.5	*	94.3	94.3	91.8	94.4	93.7	94.0	92.5
2009	92.8	93.3	90.9	92.2	94.0	97.3	92.8	92.5	92.0	93.3	93.5	92.1	92.1
2010	93.3	93.2	94.0	94.6	92.8	95.1	90.2	93.8	92.4	93.6	92.7	94.1	93.1
2011	93.9	93.9	93.9	88.1	96.5	96.6	93.5	93.8	93.6	94.2	94.3	93.4	94.2
2012	92.8	93.0	92.9	95.2	92.3	*	93.3	92.5	91.8	93.4	92.6	92.9	92.8
2013	92.7	93.7	91.2	92.2	95.5	*	90.8	91.6	89.2	94.4	91.9	93.2	93.4
2014	93.3	93.3	92.0	93.8	93.2	93.8	94.0	93.8	92.0	94.5	92.7	94.2	92.7

NOTE: Vaccine coverage is based on provider-reported vaccination data. Complex statistical methods were used to adjust vaccination estimates to account for refusals, households without telephones, and children whose vaccination histories could not be verified through their providers. Starting in 2011, the NIS sampling frame was expanded from a single-landline frame to dual-landline and cellular telephone sampling frames. Additional information on childhood immunizations is available from: https://www.cdc.gov/vaccines/schedules/index.html.

NA = Not available.

* = Estimates are considered unreliable. For data prior to 2007, percentages are not shown if the unweighted sample size for the numerator was less than 30, or the confidence interval half-width divided by the estimate was greater than 50%, or the confidence interval half-width was greater than 10. Starting with 2007 data, percentages are not shown if the unweighted sample size for the denominator was less than 30, or the confidence interval half-width divided by the estimate was greater than 58.8%, or the confidence interval half-width was greater than 10.

[1]Persons of Hispanic origin may be of any race. Starting with 2000 data, estimates were tabulated using the 1997 Revisions to the Standards for the Classification of Federal Data on Race and Ethnicity. Estimates for earlier years were tabulated using the 1977 Standards on Race and Ethnicity.

[2]Poverty level is based on family income and family size using U.S. Census Bureau poverty thresholds. In 2016, 3.7% of the 14,988 children with provider-reported vaccination history data, 6.3% of Hispanic, 2.4% of non-Hispanic White, and 6.5% of non-Hispanic Black children, were missing information about poverty level and were omitted from the estimates of vaccination coverage by poverty level (unweighted percentages).

[3]MSA = metropolitan statistical area.

[4]Prior to data year 2000, the category Asian included Native Hawaiian and Other Pacific Islander.

[5]The combined 7-vaccine series consists of 4 or more doses of either the diphtheria, tetanus toxoids, and pertussis vaccine (DTP), the diphtheria and tetanus toxoids vaccine (DT), and the diphtheria, tetanus toxoids, and acellular pertussis vaccine (DTaP); 3 or more doses of any poliovirus vaccine; 1 or more doses of a measles-containing vaccine (MCV); 3 or more doses or 4 or more doses of Haemophilus influenza type b vaccine (Hib) depending on Hib vaccine product type (full series Hib); 3 or more doses of hepatitis B vaccine; 1 or more doses of varicella vaccine; and 4 or more doses of pneumococcal conjugate vaccine (PCV). The vaccine shortage that ended in September 2004 might have reduced coverage with the fourth dose of PCV among children in the 2007 National Immunization Survey (NIS)–Child. See footnote 8 for additional information on (Hib) vaccination.

[6]Includes the diphtheria, tetanus toxoids, and pertussis vaccine (DTP), the diphtheria and tetanus toxoids vaccine (DT), and the diphtheria, tetanus toxoids, and acellular pertussis vaccine (DTaP).

Table 3-36. Vaccination Coverage Among Children 19 to 35 Months of Age for Selected Diseases, by Race, Hispanic Origin, Poverty Level, and Location of Residence in Metropolitan Statistical Area, Selected Years, 1995–2016—Continued

(Percent; Data are based on telephone interviews of a sample of the civilian noninstitutionalized population, supplemented by a survey of interview participants' immunization providers.)

| Vaccination and year | All | Race and Hispanic origin[1] | | | | | | | Poverty level[2] | | Location of residence | | |
| | | Not Hispanic or Latino | | | | | | Hispanic or Latino | Below poverty level | At or above poverty level | Inside MSA[3] | | Outside MSA[3] |
		White	Black or African American	American Indian or Alaska Native	Asian[4]	Native Hawaiian or Other Pacific Islander[4]	Two or more races				Central city	Remaining area	
2015	93.7	93.1	93.3	91.8	96.9	92.8	92.4	94.5	91.8	94.6	93.9	94.0	91.7
2016	91.9	92.5	90.3	92.4	94.7	91.3	89.4	91.7	90.6	92.5	92.0	92.2	90.8
Measles, Mumps, Rubella[7]													
1998	92.0	93.1	88.8	91.4	92.2	NA	NA	91.0	90.1	93.1	91.3	92.4	92.4
1999	91.5	92.4	89.8	91.7	92.7	NA	NA	90.2	90.0	92.4	91.3	92.1	90.4
2000	90.5	91.6	87.7	89.4	89.3	94.5	88.1	90.0	88.9	90.9	89.7	91.0	90.8
2001	91.4	91.8	89.4	93.2	90.1	*	89.2	92.1	89.1	91.9	90.9	92.0	90.8
2002	91.6	92.6	90.3	84.3	94.6	94.3	89.1	90.5	90.2	91.9	90.2	93.3	90.2
2003	93.0	93.2	92.1	91.8	96.0	*	93.7	92.7	92.0	93.4	93.2	93.1	92.3
2004	93.0	93.5	90.7	88.8	94.1	*	93.5	93.2	91.3	93.5	92.8	93.5	92.4
2005	91.5	91.4	91.9	89.7	91.9	90.3	93.7	91.1	89.3	92.1	91.6	91.8	90.4
2006	92.3	92.8	90.9	89.3	94.7	94.3	91.0	92.0	91.1	93.1	92.5	92.5	91.5
2007	92.3	92.1	91.5	96.2	93.9	87.6	94.6	92.6	91.3	92.6	91.8	92.8	92.3
2008	92.1	91.3	92.0	95.8	94.7	97.0	94.0	92.8	92.3	92.0	92.6	92.3	90.4
2009	90.0	90.8	88.2	94.9	90.7	96.9	88.5	89.3	88.8	90.6	91.1	88.6	88.6
2010	91.5	90.6	92.1	93.4	91.7	96.9	89.7	92.9	91.3	91.4	92.4	90.5	91.4
2011	91.6	91.1	90.8	94.8	93.9	98.7	91.1	92.4	91.3	91.7	92.0	91.2	91.5
2012	90.8	90.9	90.9	92.0	89.8	*	92.3	90.7	89.9	91.4	90.1	91.0	92.4
2013	91.9	91.5	90.9	96.3	96.7	90.4	91.5	92.1	90.5	92.5	91.5	92.4	91.3
2014	91.5	91.2	90.3	96.5	95.7	95.7	90.5	91.9	89.5	92.8	91.9	91.2	91.2
2015	91.9	91.8	90.7	88.5	92.5	92.0	93.0	92.3	90.3	92.9	92.4	91.7	90.7
2016	91.1	91.6	89.4	91.3	93.6	86.1	91.0	90.6	89.0	92.1	91.3	91.7	88.5
Hib (full series)[8]													
2009	54.8	55.3	51.2	*	54.6	*	53.7	55.4	51.4	56.5	55.5	54.9	53.0
2010	66.8	67.5	65.4	77.1	69.5	*	70.1	64.8	61.3	69.7	66.5	68.4	63.4
2011	80.4	81.0	74.6	73.7	83.5	*	82.0	81.6	75.5	83.4	81.4	80.3	77.8
2012	80.9	82.2	77.5	84.7	86.1	*	82.5	79.5	76.4	84.0	80.5	81.8	79.9
2013	82.0	84.2	74.9	82.9	82.0	*	84.9	80.9	75.8	85.3	80.6	84.3	79.7
2014	82.0	83.8	75.2	83.8	83.1	*	78.7	82.8	76.3	85.5	81.4	82.7	81.6
2015	82.7	83.0	78.9	81.4	87.0	*	82.4	83.0	78.1	85.5	82.3	83.6	80.9
2016	81.8	83.0	75.6	82.9	83.5	*	83.0	82.1	77.4	83.6	81.5	83.2	78.2
Hepatitis A (2 Doses or More)													
2008	40.4	NA	NA	NA	NA	NA	NA	NA	NA	NA	NA	NA	NA
2009	46.6	46.2	41.3	33.2	50.9	*	47.8	49.3	47.3	46.2	48.2	46.9	42.0
2010	49.7	45.8	48.6	*	50.8	*	49.8	57.0	51.0	49.1	52.4	48.8	45.1
2011	52.2	50.0	50.9	*	56.9	*	50.2	56.3	50.7	53.4	55.0	50.9	47.6
2012	53.0	52.6	52.0	*	57.5	*	49.4	54.4	49.4	55.4	54.7	53.0	48.2
2013	54.7	53.4	49.1	*	67.3	*	57.8	56.6	53.5	56.1	55.5	55.2	50.1
2014	57.5	55.4	56.7	*	67.7	*	53.7	61.6	54.0	59.2	58.9	58.1	51.2
2015	59.6	58.7	59.3	61.3	67.8	*	54.1	60.9	56.0	61.7	60.5	59.6	55.7
2016	60.6	60.0	53.9	69.8	69.7	*	57.4	63.6	56.9	61.9	62.1	60.5	55.6
Hepatitis B (3 Doses or More)													
1998	87.0	88.3	83.7	81.6	89.0	NA	NA	85.7	85.3	87.7	85.3	88.3	87.4
1999	88.1	88.9	86.5	*	88.2	NA	NA	87.3	86.5	89.0	87.0	89.1	88.0
2000	90.3	91.4	88.8	91.9	89.5	93.1	92.6	88.2	87.3	91.4	89.4	90.3	92.3
2001	88.9	89.6	85.0	86.6	88.8	93.9	88.0	89.8	86.5	89.5	87.5	90.0	88.9

NOTE: Vaccine coverage is based on provider-reported vaccination data. Complex statistical methods were used to adjust vaccination estimates to account for refusals, households without telephones, and children whose vaccination histories could not be verified through their providers. Starting in 2011, the NIS sampling frame was expanded from a single-landline frame to dual-landline and cellular telephone sampling frames. Additional information on childhood immunizations is available from: https://www.cdc.gov/vaccines/schedules/index.html.

NA = Not available.

* = Estimates are considered unreliable. For data prior to 2007, percentages are not shown if the unweighted sample size for the numerator was less than 30, or the confidence interval half-width divided by the estimate was greater than 50%, or the confidence interval half-width was greater than 10. Starting with 2007 data, percentages are not shown if the unweighted sample size for the denominator was less than 30, or the confidence interval half-width divided by the estimate was greater than 58.8%, or the confidence interval half-width was greater than 10.

[1]Persons of Hispanic origin may be of any race. Starting with 2000 data, estimates were tabulated using the 1997 Revisions to the Standards for the Classification of Federal Data on Race and Ethnicity. Estimates for earlier years were tabulated using the 1977 Standards on Race and Ethnicity.

[2]Poverty level is based on family income and family size using U.S. Census Bureau poverty thresholds. In 2016, 3.7% of the 14,988 children with provider-reported vaccination history data, 6.3% of Hispanic, 2.4% of non-Hispanic White, and 6.5% of non-Hispanic Black children, were missing information about poverty level and were omitted from the estimates of vaccination coverage by poverty level (unweighted percentages).

[3]MSA = metropolitan statistical area.

[4]Prior to data year 2000, the category Asian included Native Hawaiian and Other Pacific Islander.

[7]Includes children who may have been vaccinated with at least 1 dose of measles, mumps, rubella, and varicella vaccine.

[8]Haemophilus influenzae type b vaccine (Hib) full series includes primary series and the booster dose. Before January 2009, NIS did not distinguish between Hib vaccine product types; therefore, children who received 3 doses of a vaccine product that requires 4 doses were misclassified as fully vaccinated. In addition, there was a Hib vaccine shortage during December 2007–September 2009. For more information, see: CDC. Changes in measurement of Haemophilus influenzae serotype b (Hib) vaccination coverage—National Immunization Survey, United States, 2009. MMWR Morb Mortal Wkly Rep 59(33):1069–72. Available from: https://www.cdc.gov/mmwr/preview/mmwrhtml/mm5933a3.htm?s_cid=mm5933a3_e%0d%0a.

Table 3-36. Vaccination Coverage Among Children 19 to 35 Months of Age for Selected Diseases, by Race, Hispanic Origin, Poverty Level, and Location of Residence in Metropolitan Statistical Area, Selected Years, 1995–2016—Continued

(Percent; Data are based on telephone interviews of a sample of the civilian noninstitutionalized population, supplemented by a survey of interview participants' immunization providers.)

| Vaccination and year | | Race and Hispanic origin[1] | | | | | | | Poverty level[2] | | Location of residence | | |
| | | Not Hispanic or Latino | | | | | | | | | Inside MSA[3] | | |
	All	White	Black or African American	American Indian or Alaska Native	Asian[4]	Native Hawaiian or Other Pacific Islander[4]	Two or more races	Hispanic or Latino	Below poverty level	At or above poverty level	Central city	Remaining area	Outside MSA[3]
2002	89.9	90.9	88.0	*	93.8	94.1	83.7	89.5	87.7	90.3	88.5	91.1	89.5
2003	92.4	93.2	91.6	90.3	93.6	*	93.3	91.2	91.1	93.2	91.6	92.8	92.9
2004	92.4	93.0	90.8	91.2	93.0	*	94.4	91.9	91.4	92.8	91.6	92.7	93.1
2005	92.9	93.1	92.7	90.1	92.7	*	94.4	92.7	91.4	93.5	91.8	93.9	93.4
2006	93.3	93.8	91.5	95.1	91.5	97.0	91.7	93.6	92.9	93.5	92.9	94.0	92.9
2007	92.7	92.5	91.2	96.7	93.8	*	92.1	93.6	92.1	92.9	92.2	92.8	93.5
2008	93.5	93.4	92.1	91.5	97.5	*	94.9	93.7	91.4	94.4	93.4	94.1	92.6
2009	92.4	92.3	91.6	92.5	93.1	96.2	93.3	92.6	92.3	92.7	92.8	91.8	91.8
2010	91.8	91.4	92.1	97.2	91.7	96.7	89.9	92.5	91.5	92.0	91.2	92.0	92.7
2011	91.1	90.3	92.1	92.6	95.5	91.1	90.7	91.5	91.8	91.2	91.0	90.7	92.5
2012	89.7	89.3	89.7	94.0	93.2	*	92.2	89.4	89.4	89.8	89.5	89.6	90.7
2013	90.8	91.0	91.1	96.1	92.0	94.9	90.7	89.7	88.3	92.0	89.6	91.8	91.4
2014	91.6	90.7	92.3	98.5	92.9	95.2	92.9	91.9	91.3	92.0	90.5	92.5	91.9
2015	92.6	92.0	93.3	92.4	95.5	94.1	91.4	93.2	92.5	92.7	92.9	92.5	92.1
2016	90.5	91.3	90.0	91.0	93.8	86.0	88.8	89.1	90.5	90.5	90.9	89.9	91.2
Varicella[8]													
1998	43.2	41.9	42.4	28.0	52.6	NA	NA	46.9	40.5	44.1	45.1	45.2	34.3
1999	57.5	56.0	57.6	*	64.0	NA	NA	60.5	55.4	58.2	58.9	60.5	47.2
2000	67.8	66.3	67.6	65.8	76.3	*	69.7	70.2	63.5	69.2	69.0	69.8	60.2
2001	76.3	74.7	75.7	69.1	82.3	*	75.3	80.3	74.0	77.1	78.0	78.2	68.4
2002	80.6	79.4	82.7	70.8	87.2	*	79.2	81.8	78.9	80.9	81.0	82.5	74.8
2003	84.8	83.8	85.4	81.4	91.1	*	86.1	85.7	84.4	85.0	85.9	85.8	80.2
2004	87.5	86.5	86.3	84.0	91.1	*	89.4	89.1	86.4	87.5	87.5	88.5	84.8
2005	87.9	86.1	90.6	82.2	91.9	*	90.1	89.2	87.3	87.7	88.4	88.2	85.7
2006	89.2	88.7	89.1	85.4	92.7	90.4	91.2	89.6	88.6	90.0	90.0	90.0	86.1
2007	90.0	89.2	89.8	94.9	93.7	88.6	91.6	90.6	89.2	90.1	90.1	90.4	88.7
2008	90.7	89.8	90.4	93.8	94.2	92.3	90.9	91.8	90.1	91.1	91.9	90.4	88.4
2009	89.6	89.2	88.2	89.2	89.5	97.5	90.6	90.7	89.0	90.2	90.6	88.5	88.5
2010	90.4	88.9	91.5	95.7	92.5	92.7	88.9	92.3	89.6	90.6	90.8	90.1	90.0
2011	90.8	89.6	91.2	90.1	93.5	99.0	91.9	92.0	90.2	90.9	90.9	91.0	89.8
2012	90.2	89.8	90.4	92.5	91.9	*	90.9	90.9	89.7	90.6	90.1	90.0	91.3
2013	91.2	90.0	92.1	95.4	96.0	88.7	91.0	92.0	90.3	91.6	91.1	91.6	90.3
2014	91.0	90.3	90.1	95.7	95.3	94.9	90.0	92.1	89.9	91.9	91.4	91.1	89.8
2015	91.8	91.2	91.8	87.8	93.4	91.8	92.1	92.7	90.6	92.5	92.5	91.5	89.9
2016	90.6	90.8	89.9	90.9	94.2	86.7	89.3	90.2	89.3	91.2	91.2	90.7	88.0
PCV (4 doses or more)[9]													
2005	53.7	57.3	46.2	*	56.2	*	54.2	50.5	44.6	57.1	51.7	57.7	48.4
2006	68.4	70.9	60.5	62.7	64.8	*	71.3	67.4	61.8	71.1	68.9	70.5	61.8
2007	75.3	76.6	70.3	80.4	75.0	*	74.1	75.4	72.8	76.3	74.8	77.3	71.0
2008	80.1	81.4	76.4	70.6	82.3	*	85.4	78.6	74.2	82.8	80.7	81.4	75.1
2009	80.4	83.4	73.2	76.2	72.5	*	73.1	80.6	74.8	83.2	79.7	81.8	81.8
2010	83.3	84.2	79.7	85.3	78.9	*	83.0	83.9	78.7	85.6	82.6	84.3	82.6
2011	84.4	85.3	81.3	75.3	84.9	93.1	84.0	84.6	80.6	86.9	85.0	84.6	82.3
2012	81.9	83.5	77.1	*	80.7	*	84.1	82.1	76.7	85.3	80.4	84.0	80.8
2013	82.0	84.1	76.1	79.0	85.6	*	83.0	80.4	74.5	86.1	80.7	84.1	79.9
2014	82.9	84.5	78.0	*	80.9	93.1	82.1	83.2	76.9	86.9	81.4	84.5	82.9

NOTE: Vaccine coverage is based on provider-reported vaccination data. Complex statistical methods were used to adjust vaccination estimates to account for refusals, households without telephones, and children whose vaccination histories could not be verified through their providers. Starting in 2011, the NIS sampling frame was expanded from a single-landline frame to dual-landline and cellular telephone sampling frames. Additional information on childhood immunizations is available from: https://www.cdc.gov/vaccines/schedules/index.html.

NA = Not available.

* = Estimates are considered unreliable. For data prior to 2007, percentages are not shown if the unweighted sample size for the numerator was less than 30, or the confidence interval half-width divided by the estimate was greater than 50%, or the confidence interval half-width was greater than 10. Starting with 2007 data, percentages are not shown if the unweighted sample size for the denominator was less than 30, or the confidence interval half-width divided by the estimate was greater than 58.8%, or the confidence interval half-width was greater than 10.

[1]Persons of Hispanic origin may be of any race. Starting with 2000 data, estimates were tabulated using the 1997 Revisions to the Standards for the Classification of Federal Data on Race and Ethnicity. Estimates for earlier years were tabulated using the 1977 Standards on Race and Ethnicity.

[2]Poverty level is based on family income and family size using U.S. Census Bureau poverty thresholds. In 2016, 3.7% of the 14,988 children with provider-reported vaccination history data, 6.3% of Hispanic, 2.4% of non-Hispanic White, and 6.5% of non-Hispanic Black children, were missing information about poverty level and were omitted from the estimates of vaccination coverage by poverty level (unweighted percentages).

[3]MSA = metropolitan statistical area.

[4]Prior to data year 2000, the category Asian included Native Hawaiian and Other Pacific Islander.

[8]Haemophilus influenzae type b vaccine (Hib) full series includes primary series and the booster dose. Before January 2009, NIS did not distinguish between Hib vaccine product types; therefore, children who received 3 doses of a vaccine product that requires 4 doses were misclassified as fully vaccinated. In addition, there was a Hib vaccine shortage during December 2007–September 2009. For more information, see: CDC. Changes in measurement of Haemophilus influenzae serotype b (Hib) vaccination coverage—National Immunization Survey, United States, 2009. MMWR Morb Mortal Wkly Rep 59(33):1069–72. Available from: https://www.cdc.gov/mmwr/preview/mmwrhtml/mm5933a3.htm?s_cid=mm5933a3_e%0d%0a.

[9]PCV is pneumococcal conjugate vaccine. Recommended in 2000. Data collection for PCV began in July 2001. Data for 4 doses of PCV are not available prior to 2005.

Table 3-36. Vaccination Coverage Among Children 19 to 35 Months of Age for Selected Diseases, by Race, Hispanic Origin, Poverty Level, and Location of Residence in Metropolitan Statistical Area, Selected Years, 1995–2016—*Continued*

(Percent; Data are based on telephone interviews of a sample of the civilian noninstitutionalized population, supplemented by a survey of interview participants' immunization providers.)

| Vaccination and year | | Race and Hispanic origin[1] | | | | | | | | Poverty level[2] | | Location of residence | | |
| | | | Not Hispanic or Latino | | | | | | | | | Inside MSA[3] | | |
Vaccination and year	All	White	Black or African American	American Indian or Alaska Native	Asian[4]	Native Hawaiian or Other Pacific Islander[4]	Two or more races	Hispanic or Latino	Below poverty level	At or above poverty level	Central city	Remaining area	Outside MSA[3]
2015	84.1	85.0	81.4	77.1	85.0	*	83.7	84.0	78.9	87.2	83.9	85.5	80.4
2016	81.8	84.1	74.5	80.1	81.0	82.9	82.9	81.4	76.8	84.2	82.5	82.1	78.4
Rotavirus vaccine[10]													
2009	43.9	46.4	38.0	*	41.7	*	38.4	43.7	37.7	47.1	44.6	46.6	35.6
2010	59.2	60.2	52.7	*	62.6	*	57.7	60.5	51.5	62.9	59.2	62.2	51.6
2011	67.3	68.3	62.5	57.7	66.9	*	67.8	68.3	61.1	71.1	68.9	67.4	62.7
2012	68.6	70.5	60.4	*	69.9	*	69.3	70.0	63.0	72.5	68.8	70.5	62.5
2013	72.6	74.8	62.1	*	74.9	*	72.8	73.7	64.3	76.9	72.4	74.7	66.7
2014	71.7	74.8	61.6	*	72.4	*	73.9	71.3	62.8	76.9	71.2	73.2	68.4
2015	73.2	74.6	69.7	*	75.6	*	70.6	72.9	66.8	76.8	72.7	75.1	68.6
2016	74.1	77.3	67.2	*	71.8	*	73.4	73.0	65.5	78.2	74.9	74.2	70.3

Vaccination and year (percent of children age 19 to 35 months)	Poverty level[2]					
	Not Hispanic or Latino				Hispanic or Latino	
	White		Black or African American			
Vaccination and year (percent of children age 19 to 35 months)	Below poverty level	At or above poverty level	Below poverty level	At or above poverty level	Below poverty level	At or above poverty level
Combined 7-Vaccine Series[5]						
2009	43.2	45.6	37.8	43.5	43.5	48.5
2010	48.7	59.0	53.4	56.3	55.0	55.2
2011	59.8	71.8	61.0	68.0	67.9	71.1
2012	58.2	72.1	62.7	68.5	68.1	68.3
2013	61.3	74.9	60.4	69.1	68.6	70.2
2014	61.2	75.4	61.5	71.0	71.8	79.4
2015	64.1	75.4	65.8	73.2	72.9	70.1
2016	61.2	74.6	65.0	64.4	70.8	68.9

NOTE: Vaccine coverage is based on provider-reported vaccination data. Complex statistical methods were used to adjust vaccination estimates to account for refusals, households without telephones, and children whose vaccination histories could not be verified through their providers. Starting in 2011, the NIS sampling frame was expanded from a single-landline frame to dual-landline and cellular telephone sampling frames. Additional information on childhood immunizations is available from: https://www.cdc.gov/vaccines/schedules/index.html.

* = Estimates are considered unreliable. For data prior to 2007, percentages are not shown if the unweighted sample size for the numerator was less than 30, or the confidence interval half-width divided by the estimate was greater than 50%, or the confidence interval half-width was greater than 10. Starting with 2007 data, percentages are not shown if the unweighted sample size for the denominator was less than 30, or the confidence interval half-width divided by the estimate was greater than 58.8%, or the confidence interval half-width was greater than 10.

[1] Persons of Hispanic origin may be of any race. Starting with 2000 data, estimates were tabulated using the 1997 Revisions to the Standards for the Classification of Federal Data on Race and Ethnicity. Estimates for earlier years were tabulated using the 1977 Standards on Race and Ethnicity.

[2] Poverty level is based on family income and family size using U.S. Census Bureau poverty thresholds. In 2016, 3.7% of the 14,988 children with provider-reported vaccination history data, 6.3% of Hispanic, 2.4% of non-Hispanic White, and 6.5% of non-Hispanic Black children, were missing information about poverty level and were omitted from the estimates of vaccination coverage by poverty level (unweighted percentages).

[3] MSA = metropolitan statistical area.

[4] Prior to data year 2000, the category Asian included Native Hawaiian and Other Pacific Islander.

[5] The combined 7-vaccine series consists of 4 or more doses of either the diphtheria, tetanus toxoids, and pertussis vaccine (DTP), the diphtheria and tetanus toxoids vaccine (DT), and the diphtheria, tetanus toxoids, and acellular pertussis vaccine (DTaP); 3 or more doses of any poliovirus vaccine; 1 or more doses of a measles-containing vaccine (MCV); 3 or more doses or 4 or more doses of Haemophilus influenzae type b vaccine (Hib) depending on Hib vaccine product type (full series Hib); 3 or more doses of hepatitis B vaccine; 1 or more doses of varicella vaccine; and 4 or more doses of pneumococcal conjugate vaccine (PCV). The vaccine shortage that ended in September 2004 might have reduced coverage with the fourth dose of PCV among children in the 2007 National Immunization Survey (NIS)–Child. See footnote 8 for additional information on (Hib) vaccination.

[10] Rotavirus vaccine includes 2 or more or 3 or more doses, depending on the product type received. Recommended in 2006. Data collection for rotavirus began in 2009.

Table 3-37. Vaccination Coverage Among Adolescents 13 to 17 Years of Age for Selected Diseases, by Selected Characteristics, 2006–2016

(Percent; Data are based on telephone interviews of a sample of the civilian noninstitutionalized population, supplemented by a survey of interview participants' immunization providers.)

Vaccination coverage, 2016	2008	2010	2011	2012	2013	2014	2015	2016
Percent of Adolescents, 13 to 17 Years								
Measles, mumps, rubella (2 doses or more)	89.3	90.5	90.5	91.4	89.6	90.7	90.7	90.9
Hepatitis B (3 doses or more)...	87.9	91.6	92.3	92.8	91.3	91.4	91.1	91.4
Varicella vaccine (2 doses or more) among those with no history of varicella[1]...........	34.1	58.1	68.3	74.9	78.5	81.0	83.1	85.6
Tdap (1 dose or more)[2]...	40.8	68.7	78.2	84.6	84.7	87.6	86.4	88.0
Meningococcal conjugate vaccine (MenACWY) (1 dose or more)[3]............	41.8	62.7	70.5	74.0	76.6	79.3	81.3	82.2
Human papillomavirus (HPV) (3 doses or more among females)[4]..............	17.9	32.0	34.8	33.4	36.8	39.7	41.9	43.0
Human papillomavirus (HPV) (3 doses or more among males)[4]................	X	X	1.3	6.8	13.4	21.6	28.1	31.5

	Race and Hispanic origin[5]					Poverty level[6]		Location of residence		
	Not Hispanic or Latino							Inside MSA[7]		
Vaccination coverage, 2016	White	Black or African American	American Indian or Alaska Native	Asian	Hispanic or Latino	Below poverty level	At or above poverty level	Central city	Remaining area	Outside MSA[7]
Percent of Adolescents, 13 to 17 Years										
Measles, mumps, rubella (2 doses or more)	91.8	91.6	90.5	90.3	88.9	90.5	91.1	91.1	90.9	90.3
Hepatitis B (3 doses or more)...	92.4	92.3	94.4	88.4	89.2	90.2	91.9	90.9	92.0	91.1
Varicella vaccine (2 doses or more) among those with no history of varicella[1]...........	86.1	87.0	79.5	84.4	84.2	85.0	85.9	86.2	86.0	81.7
Tdap (1 dose or more)[2]...	89.3	89.6	89.7	83.7	85.4	86.7	88.4	88.4	87.8	87.7
Meningococcal conjugate vaccine (MenACWY) (1 dose or more)[3]............	81.2	85.5	78.4	82.7	83.8	82.9	82.0	83.5	83.3	74.1
Human papillomavirus (HPV) (3 doses or more among females)[4]..............	40.4	43.3	46.9	55.0	45.9	48.0	42.4	47.7	41.5	34.1
Human papillomavirus (HPV) (3 doses or more among males)[4]................	29.6	30.1	17.0	34.3	37.2	36.0	30.3	35.3	30.5	23.4

NOTE: Starting in 2014, the National Interview Survey–Teen (NIS–Teen) implemented a new definition of adequate provider data. Data for 2013 shown in this table were revised based on the 2014 definition. In general, 2013 NIS–Teen vaccination coverage estimates using the revised adequate provider data definition were different, and generally lower, than original 2013 NIS–Teen estimates. Thus, data for 2013 and beyond are not directly comparable with data for earlier years.

X = Not applicable.

[1]Denominator is comprised of adolescents aged 13–17 with no history of varicella disease. History of varicella disease was obtained by parent or guardian report or by provider records. Historically, report of varicella disease has been considered valid evidence of immunity under the Advisory Committee on Immunization Practices guidelines.

[2]Tdap refers to tetanus toxoid-diphtheria vaccine (Td) or tetanus toxoid, reduced diphtheria toxoid, and acellular pertussis vaccine (Tdap) or tetanus-unknown type vaccine received at or after age 10 years. Tdap vaccines were licensed by the U.S. Food and Drug Administration (FDA) in May and June of 2005. For the initial recommendations on Tdap vaccination, see: Broder KR, Cortese MM, Iskander JK, Kretsinger K, Slade BA, Brown KH, et al. Preventing tetanus, diphtheria, and pertussis among adolescents: Use of tetanus toxoid, reduced diphtheria toxoid and acellular pertussis vaccines. Recommendations of the Advisory Committee on Immunization Practices (ACIP). MMWR Recomm Rep 55(RR-3):1–34. 2006. Available from: https://www.cdc.gov/mmwr/preview/mmwrhtml/rr5503a1.htm.

[3]Includes persons receiving MenACWY or meningococcal-unknown type vaccine. Meningococcal vaccine was licensed for use by the FDA in January 2005. For the initial recommendations on meningococcal vaccination, see: Bilukha OO, Rosenstein N, National Center for Infectious Diseases, Centers for Disease Control and Prevention. Prevention and control of meningococcal disease: Recommendations of the Advisory Committee on Immunization Practices (ACIP). MMWR Recomm Rep 54(RR–7):1–21. 2005. Available from: https://www.cdc.gov/mmwr/preview/mmwrhtml/rr5407a1.htm.

[4]For 2008, refers to HPV vaccine quadrivalent. For 2009–2014, refers to HPV vaccine quadrivalent or bivalent. For 2015 and beyond, refers to HPV vaccine 9-valent, quadrivalent, or bivalent, when specific vaccines were licensed and recommended for use among adolescents. Quadrivalent HPV vaccine was licensed by the FDA in June 2006. For the initial recommendations on HPV vaccination, see: Markowitz LE, Dunne EF, Saraiya M, Lawson HW, Chesson H, Unger ER, et al. Quadrivalent human papillomavirus vaccine: Recommendations of the Advisory Committee on Immunization Practices (ACIP). MMWR Recomm Rep 56(RR-2):1–24. 2007. Available from: https://www.cdc.gov/mmwr/preview/mmwrhtml/rr5602a1.htm?s_cid=rr5602a1_e. HPV vaccine was recommended for males in October 2011. See: CDC. Recommendations on the use of quadrivalent human papillomavirus vaccine in males–Advisory Committee on Immunization Practices (ACIP). 2011. MMWR Morb Mortal Wkly Rep 60(50):1705–8. 2011. Available from: https://www.cdc.gov/mmwr/preview/mmwrhtml/mm6050a3.htm.

[5]Persons of Hispanic origin may be of any race. Estimates were tabulated using the 1997 Revisions to the Standards for the Classification of Federal Data on Race and Ethnicity. Data for Native Hawaiian or Other Pacific Islander persons and persons of multiple races were not included because of small sample sizes.

[6]Poverty level is based on family income and family size using U.S. Census Bureau poverty thresholds. In 2016, 3.5% of the 20,475 adolescents with provider-reported vaccination history data, 5.8% of Hispanic, 2.9% of non-Hispanic White, and 4.8% of non-Hispanic Black adolescents, were missing information about poverty level and were omitted from the estimates of vaccination coverage by poverty level (unweighted percentages).

[7]MSA is metropolitan statistical area.

Table 3-38. Influenza Vaccination[1] Among Adults 18 Years of Age and Over, by Selected Characteristics, Selected Years, 1989–2016

(Percent; data are based on household interviews of a sample of the civilian noninstitutionalized population.)

Characteristic	1989	1995	2000	2005	2006	2007	2008	2009	2010	2011	2012	2013	2014	2015	2016
Percent receiving influenza vaccination during past 12 months[1]															
18 years and over, age-adjusted[2,3]	9.6	23.7	28.7	21.6	27.5	29.9	32.2	34.2	35.3	37.2	36.8	39.9	41.0	41.7	40.9
18 years and over, crude[3]	9.1	23.0	28.4	21.4	27.6	30.1	32.6	34.7	35.8	37.9	37.7	41.0	42.2	43.2	42.2
Age															
18 to 44 years	3.3	12.0	15.6	10.1	14.6	16.5	18.8	22.2	24.6	26.0	25.6	28.5	30.2	30.9	31.1
45 to 64 years	8.8	24.5	31.6	20.2	29.2	32.5	35.9	36.8	37.8	40.0	39.4	43.7	43.3	45.1	42.8
65 years and over	30.4	58.2	64.4	59.7	64.3	66.7	67.2	66.8	63.9	66.9	66.5	67.9	70.1	69.1	67.5
65 to 74 years	28.0	54.9	61.1	53.7	60.1	61.6	60.9	61.5	60.5	63.0	62.6	64.4	67.1	67.0	64.2
75 years and over	34.2	63.0	68.4	66.3	69.2	72.6	74.3	73.2	68.2	71.9	71.7	72.8	74.3	72.1	72.3
Sex															
Male	8.5	21.5	26.7	18.4	24.8	27.1	28.9	31.2	31.3	34.1	33.4	37.0	37.9	39.2	38.7
Female	9.7	24.4	30.0	24.2	30.1	32.9	36.2	37.9	40.0	41.5	41.7	44.7	46.1	46.8	45.4
Race[4]															
White only	9.6	23.7	30.1	22.5	28.6	31.4	33.8	35.9	36.9	39.0	38.7	42.2	43.4	44.2	43.1
Black or African American only	6.4	19.0	19.8	15.5	21.1	22.5	25.8	27.6	28.1	30.8	30.6	33.0	34.1	35.7	35.6
American Indian or Alaska Native only	10.9	*16.5	31.1	16.2	26.7	30.8	26.9	26.9	36.3	38.1	37.2	37.9	42.6	39.3	43.8
Asian only	4.3	20.0	27.0	16.9	26.4	27.9	31.7	36.2	38.6	39.1	40.9	43.9	45.0	47.0	46.4
Native Hawaiian or Other Pacific Islander only	NA	NA	*	*	*	*	*	*	*	*	*	*	*	*	31.8
Two or more races	NA	NA	25.3	15.9	23.7	25.4	29.3	25.2	28.9	30.8	30.1	34.7	34.3	40.8	36.2
Hispanic Origin and Race[4]															
Hispanic or Latino	5.9	16.1	17.7	12.0	16.0	19.2	20.8	23.7	26.5	28.9	28.1	28.9	31.0	31.2	32.6
Mexican	5.2	16.0	16.6	10.9	15.2	18.2	19.2	22.7	25.1	27.6	26.8	29.2	31.2	30.4	33.2
Not Hispanic or Latino	9.4	23.7	29.8	22.8	29.3	31.8	34.5	36.4	37.3	39.4	39.4	43.1	44.2	45.4	44.0
White only	9.9	24.6	31.4	24.3	30.8	33.6	36.2	38.1	38.8	41.0	40.9	44.9	46.0	46.9	45.5
Black or African American only	6.4	19.2	19.9	15.6	21.6	22.3	25.7	27.8	28.0	30.9	30.9	33.2	34.4	36.0	35.6
Percent of Poverty Level[5]															
Below 100 percent	8.9	20.6	23.1	16.9	21.3	22.7	24.8	25.9	25.0	28.1	29.2	30.1	32.0	33.6	34.4
100 percent to 199 percent	11.5	23.4	28.1	22.0	26.7	28.3	30.2	31.0	31.3	32.7	32.3	35.5	36.7	37.0	36.4
200 percent to 399 percent	8.0	22.8	29.6	22.9	27.8	29.5	32.2	34.1	34.8	38.0	36.8	40.1	40.8	41.2	42.2
400 percent or more	9.0	24.3	29.2	21.3	30.0	33.6	36.4	39.8	42.7	44.1	44.5	48.6	49.7	50.4	47.1
Hispanic Origin and Race and Percent of Poverty Level[4,5]															
Hispanic or Latino															
Below 100 percent	5.1	13.3	14.5	9.5	13.7	20.5	17.9	19.5	21.9	25.3	25.4	25.8	26.8	29.9	35.1
100 percent to 199 percent	7.5	17.8	15.8	11.9	13.7	17.9	19.6	20.3	23.3	27.2	25.7	25.4	29.6	27.7	28.0
200 percent to 399 percent	6.3	15.7	19.3	11.8	17.2	17.4	19.7	25.2	27.5	29.3	28.6	29.4	30.8	30.0	33.8
400 percent or more	6.0	19.8	22.2	15.5	20.3	22.5	26.4	32.1	36.4	36.0	35.5	37.6	39.8	40.0	34.5
Not Hispanic or Latino															
White only															
Below 100 percent	10.6	23.9	27.8	20.6	25.0	24.4	28.4	30.3	26.5	29.3	31.3	32.4	35.1	34.9	35.2
100 percent to 199 percent	13.2	25.6	33.1	27.4	32.1	33.8	35.7	36.2	35.0	34.9	35.8	40.7	41.2	41.7	40.6
200 percent to 399 percent	8.3	23.8	32.5	26.3	30.9	32.9	35.8	36.5	37.5	40.7	38.9	42.9	44.0	44.4	45.1
400 percent or more	9.4	25.5	30.5	22.4	31.5	35.7	38.1	41.4	43.8	45.9	46.2	50.4	51.3	52.2	49.1
Black or African American only															
Below 100 percent	7.5	19.8	20.0	17.0	20.0	18.9	23.4	24.5	24.0	27.5	27.7	28.3	29.4	30.2	32.1
100 percent to 199 percent	6.4	18.8	21.3	15.4	21.4	20.5	24.3	26.6	28.6	30.7	29.9	30.9	33.0	33.9	34.1
200 percent to 399 percent	6.9	20.4	19.5	15.1	21.1	24.5	25.9	28.9	27.4	31.6	31.8	35.2	34.6	36.1	37.9
400 percent or more	5.6	15.6	19.2	15.3	23.8	24.2	28.8	31.1	32.9	33.9	34.2	38.2	41.6	43.3	37.1
Level of difficulty[6]															
A lot of difficulty or cannot do at all	NA	NA	NA	NA	NA	NA	NA	NA	52.8	53.9	47.5	54.9	53.7	54.3	55.3
Some difficulty	NA	NA	NA	NA	NA	NA	NA	NA	38.6	43.9	41.0	44.8	48.2	48.1	45.7
No difficulty	NA	NA	NA	NA	NA	NA	NA	NA	31.7	33.9	33.3	36.2	38.1	39.1	38.7
Geographic Region															
Northeast	8.6	21.2	28.0	23.2	27.4	31.2	34.0	37.0	39.1	40.8	40.1	44.5	45.0	46.6	46.4
Midwest	8.8	22.7	28.5	22.6	30.5	32.6	35.4	35.9	37.6	37.9	38.4	41.4	43.6	43.1	43.8
South	9.5	24.7	28.7	20.3	26.5	29.1	31.8	34.5	35.1	38.2	37.2	40.1	41.5	42.4	39.7
West	9.4	22.3	28.1	20.2	26.3	28.2	30.1	31.8	32.6	35.4	36.0	39.4	39.7	41.8	41.2
Location of Residence															
Within MSA[7]	8.5	22.3	27.5	20.4	26.5	28.8	31.7	34.1	35.7	37.7	37.7	40.8	41.9	43.4	42.2
Outside MSA[7]	11.4	25.7	31.8	25.1	32.3	36.4	37.2	37.4	36.1	39.2	37.9	42.2	44.1	41.9	42.4

NA = Not available.

* = Estimates are considered unreliable. Starting with 2015–2016 data, the reliability of survey percentage estimates was assessed using new multistep National Center for Health Statistics data presentation standards for proportions. Prior to 2015–2016 data, the reliability of estimates for earlier years was evaluated based on relative standard errors (RSE). Data preceded by an asterisk have an RSE of 20%–30%. Data not shown have an RSE greater than 30%.
[1]Questions concerning use of influenza vaccination differed slightly on the National Health Interview Survey across the years for which data are shown.
[2]Estimates are age adjusted to the year 2000 standard population using four age groups: 18 to 49 years, 50 to 64 years, 65 to 74 years, and 75 years and over.
[3]Includes all other races not shown separately, unknown disability status, and unknown poverty level in 1989.
[4]The race groups White, Black, American Indian or Alaska Native, Asian, Native Hawaiian or Other Pacific Islander, and 2 or more races include persons of Hispanic and non-Hispanic origin. Persons of Hispanic origin may be of any race. Starting with 1999 data, race-specific estimates are tabulated according to the 1997 Revisions to the Standards for the Classification of Federal Data on Race and Ethnicity and are not strictly comparable with estimates for earlier years. The five single-race categories and multiple-race categories shown in the table conform to the 1997 Standards. Starting with 1999 data, race-specific estimates are for persons who reported only one racial group; the category 2 or more races includes persons who reported more than one racial group. Prior to 1999, data were tabulated according to the 1977 Standards with four racial groups, and the Asian only category included Native Hawaiian or Other Pacific Islander. Estimates for single-race categories prior to 1999 included persons who reported one race, or if they reported more than one race, identified one race as best representing their race. Starting with 2003 data, race responses of other race and unspecified multiple race were treated as missing, and then race was imputed if these were the only race responses. Almost all persons with a race response of other race were of Hispanic origin.
[5]Percent of poverty level is based on family income and family size and composition using U.S. Census Bureau poverty thresholds. Poverty level was unknown for 11% of persons aged 18 and over in 1989. Missing family income data were imputed for 1991 and beyond.
[6]Functional limitation is defined by the reported level of difficulty in six functioning domains: seeing (even if wearing glasses), hearing (even if wearing hearing aids), mobility (walking or climbing stairs), communication (understanding or being understood by others), cognition (remembering or concentrating), and self-care (such as washing all over or dressing). Respondents with answers to one or more of the six questions were included in one of three mutually exclusive categories. Those responding "A lot of difficulty" or "Cannot do at all/unable to do" to at least one question were classified in the "A lot of difficulty/cannot do" category. Of the remaining, those responding "Some difficulty" to at least one question were classified in the "Some difficulty" category, and those responding "No difficulty" to at least one question were classified in the "No difficulty" category. Those responding "Don't know" or "Refused" to all six questions were excluded. During 2010–2016, 1%–8% of respondents were missing data and excluded.
[7]MSA is metropolitan statistical area. Starting with 2016 data, MSA status is determined using 2010 Census data and the 2010 standards for defining MSAs.

Table 3-39. Pneumococcal Vaccination[1] Among Adults 18 Years of Age and Over, by Selected Characteristics, Selected Years, 1989–2016

(Percent; data are based on household interviews of a sample of the civilian noninstitutionalized population.)

Characteristic	1989	1995	2000	2005	2006	2007	2008	2009	2010	2011	2012	2013	2014	2015	2016
18 years and over, age-adjusted[2,3]	4.6	12.0	15.4	16.7	17.1	16.8	18.3	19.0	19.2	20.6	19.9	19.9	20.5	21.2	22.9
18 years and over, crude[3]	4.4	11.7	15.1	16.5	17.0	16.7	18.5	19.3	19.6	21.1	20.7	21.0	21.8	22.9	24.9
Age															
18 to 44 years	2.1	6.6	5.1	5.3	5.4	4.9	6.3	6.8	6.9	8.3	7.9	7.5	8.3	8.8	10.0
45 to 64 years	3.7	8.8	12.2	14.3	14.9	14.4	15.9	16.8	17.7	18.4	18.0	18.8	18.4	18.8	20.3
65 years and over	14.1	34.0	53.1	56.2	57.1	57.7	60.0	60.6	59.7	62.3	59.9	59.7	61.3	63.6	66.9
65 to 74 years	13.1	31.4	48.2	49.4	52.0	51.8	52.5	54.6	54.6	56.0	55.0	54.4	55.8	60.2	62.4
75 years and over	15.7	37.8	59.1	63.9	63.0	64.4	68.7	68.0	66.0	70.0	66.4	67.1	69.3	68.5	73.6
High-Risk Group[4]															
Total, 18 to 64 years	NA	NA	18.3	22.6	23.1	24.4	24.9	17.4	18.3	20.0	19.9	21.0	20.2	23.0	23.2
18 to 49 years	NA	NA	11.3	13.8	11.7	14.3	13.8	9.5	9.8	12.4	11.3	11.7	11.3	12.8	14.3
50 to 64 years	NA	NA	23.3	27.9	29.5	29.6	31.3	25.4	26.7	27.3	28.0	29.4	28.3	31.6	31.4
65 YEARS AND OVER															
Sex															
Male	13.9	34.6	52.1	53.4	54.3	55.1	56.4	59.2	57.6	59.5	55.8	57.1	58.4	62.9	65.8
Female	14.3	33.6	53.9	58.4	59.2	59.6	62.8	61.7	61.3	64.5	63.1	61.8	63.7	64.2	67.8
Race[5]															
White only	14.8	35.3	55.6	58.4	60.0	60.1	62.5	63.1	61.6	64.7	62.3	61.7	63.1	65.8	69.0
Black or African American only	6.4	21.9	30.6	40.2	35.5	43.7	44.1	44.2	45.5	47.5	46.0	48.4	49.2	49.9	55.0
American Indian or Alaska Native only	31.2	*	70.1	*	*57.5	*	66.9	*	*48.5	53.0	*36.3	52.9	57.1	60.3	*
Asian only	*	*23.4	40.9	35.0	35.6	33.4	45.7	44.8	47.9	40.3	41.1	45.0	47.7	49.3	53.5
Native Hawaiian or Other Pacific Islander only	NA	NA	*	*	*	*	*	*	*	*	*	*	*	*	*
Two or more races	NA	NA	55.6	64.8	63.6	55.8	*35.9	67.9	65.5	77.1	45.4	50.8	71.2	60.4	64.1
Hispanic Origin and Race[5]															
Hispanic or Latino	9.8	23.2	30.4	27.5	33.3	31.8	36.4	40.1	39.0	43.1	43.4	39.2	45.2	41.7	48.6
Mexican	12.9	*18.8	32.0	31.3	29.3	34.3	39.5	42.8	41.4	47.1	45.5	47.4	47.8	49.1	53.1
Not Hispanic or Latino	14.3	34.5	54.4	58.1	58.7	59.6	61.8	62.2	61.3	63.8	61.2	61.4	62.7	65.5	68.5
White only	15.0	35.9	56.8	60.6	62.0	62.2	64.5	64.8	63.5	66.5	64.0	63.6	64.7	68.1	71.0
Black or African American only	6.2	21.8	30.6	40.4	35.6	44.0	44.5	44.7	46.2	47.6	46.1	48.7	49.8	50.2	55.5
Percent of Poverty Level[6]															
Below 100 percent	11.2	28.7	40.6	46.7	45.4	48.7	46.5	48.5	42.6	49.6	39.5	50.5	47.3	48.7	51.5
100 percent to 199 percent	15.1	30.7	51.4	54.5	55.8	55.6	59.5	60.6	57.2	60.3	59.8	58.0	59.5	61.7	63.9
200 percent to 399 percent	15.1	36.1	55.8	60.8	59.9	58.8	61.4	62.9	62.2	63.4	63.6	61.7	64.5	64.8	66.6
400 percent or more	15.5	39.5	56.9	55.3	59.3	59.8	62.8	61.5	64.0	66.4	61.4	61.6	63.2	67.1	71.9
Hispanic Origin and Race and Percent of Poverty Level[5,6]															
Hispanic or Latino															
Below 100 percent	*	*14.1	23.8	20.9	24.5	*22.4	*25.7	32.6	30.2	34.8	30.9	35.3	34.1	31.0	42.6
100 percent to 199 percent	*11.0	*15.6	32.3	26.9	30.9	37.9	32.9	41.8	36.9	49.3	42.0	39.1	44.4	45.2	48.7
200 percent to 399 percent	*11.1	*34.4	37.6	35.2	42.3	29.6	44.8	40.0	45.8	39.2	54.5	36.1	52.1	43.9	43.8
400 percent or more	*	*55.1	*26.4	*25.2	*38.2	*33.7	42.4	49.1	43.0	49.1	46.4	49.1	54.0	44.3	62.9
Not Hispanic or Latino															
White only															
Below 100 percent	13.3	32.5	47.9	55.6	56.0	59.7	60.4	61.0	51.1	60.3	46.5	59.1	55.4	54.1	62.6
100 percent to 199 percent	16.0	33.5	56.1	60.5	61.6	60.8	66.3	66.3	61.3	64.6	66.1	63.3	64.1	67.4	67.2
200 percent to 399 percent	15.7	37.1	57.6	64.1	62.6	63.4	64.5	66.3	64.9	66.9	65.9	65.2	66.9	68.4	70.8
400 percent or more	15.9	39.3	59.5	57.4	63.0	62.4	64.1	62.9	66.0	68.6	63.5	63.2	64.5	70.2	73.6
Black or African American only															
Below 100 percent	*5.0	*22.6	28.8	42.3	38.4	40.7	37.6	33.8	34.9	39.5	36.1	48.9	46.0	53.3	40.1
100 percent to 199 percent	7.8	*20.9	28.1	36.6	36.2	41.9	43.5	46.9	46.4	45.6	44.5	46.9	49.1	46.9	63.6
200 percent to 399 percent	*5.9	*21.7	35.5	41.6	40.0	48.7	44.5	49.3	51.8	54.2	54.1	49.4	47.9	44.1	54.8
400 percent or more	*	*	*32.6	44.6	*24.7	43.6	56.5	45.8	50.1	49.1	45.4	50.3	56.0	61.8	58.6
Level of difficulty[7]															
A lot of difficulty or cannot do at all	NA	NA	NA	NA	NA	NA	NA	NA	66.0	64.5	63.7	67.2	67.3	66.4	67.6
Some difficulty	NA	NA	NA	NA	NA	NA	NA	NA	61.7	61.3	61.0	61.1	64.6	65.1	71.1
No difficulty	NA	NA	NA	NA	NA	NA	NA	NA	55.5	60.2	56.0	53.6	56.2	59.5	62.7
Geographic Region															
Northeast	10.4	28.2	51.2	55.8	53.7	54.6	60.9	58.5	56.7	60.0	58.0	59.1	59.6	60.8	66.1
Midwest	13.7	31.0	52.6	58.5	61.5	60.6	63.8	58.4	61.2	65.6	63.8	62.3	65.4	68.3	72.2
South	14.9	35.9	51.3	57.4	55.7	58.5	59.8	61.9	60.9	63.2	59.5	59.3	60.9	62.3	64.2
West	17.9	41.1	59.7	51.4	57.2	55.6	55.4	63.0	58.9	59.5	58.2	58.3	59.3	63.7	66.4
Location of Residence															
Within MSA[8]	13.1	33.8	52.4	55.1	56.6	56.5	59.1	60.0	58.8	61.7	59.3	59.0	60.7	63.4	67.2
Outside MSA[8]	16.9	34.7	55.4	59.8	58.9	61.7	63.2	62.9	63.3	64.6	62.4	62.8	64.0	64.7	65.8

NA = Not available.

* = Estimates are considered unreliable. Starting with 2015–2016 data, the reliability of survey percentage estimates was assessed using new multistep National Center for Health Statistics data presentation standards for proportions. Prior to 2015–2016 data, the reliability of estimates for earlier years was evaluated based on relative standard errors (RSE). Data preceded by an asterisk have an RSE of 20%–30%. Data not shown have an RSE greater than 30%.

[1] Questions concerning receipt of pneumococcal vaccination differed slightly on the National Health Interview Survey across the years. Data prior to 1997 are not strictly comparable with data for later years due to the 1997 questionnaire redesign.

[2] Estimates are age adjusted to the year 2000 standard population using four age groups: 18 to 44 years, 45 to 64 years, 65 to 74 years, and 75 years and over.

[3] Includes all other races not shown separately, unknown poverty level in 1989, and unknown disability status.

[4] High-risk group membership is based on recommendations of the Centers for Disease Control and Prevention's Advisory Committee on Immunization Practices (ACIP). The high-risk group includes persons who reported diabetes, cancer, or heart, lung, liver, or kidney disease. Starting with data year 2009, this definition was expanded to also include persons who reported asthma or cigarette smoking, to be consistent with the revised ACIP recommendation. Starting with data year 2012, the survey questionnaire changed and now asks respondents if a health professional had ever told them they had chronic obstructive pulmonary disease (COPD), and this information was added to the list of lung diseases used to construct the high-risk category. For more information on high-risk groups, see the 2012 (adult) and 2013 (child) ACIP recommendations. Available from: https://www.cdc.gov/mmwr/preview/mmwrhtml/mm6140a4.htm and https://www.cdc.gov/mmwr/preview/mmwrhtml/mm6225a3.htm, respectively.

[5] The race groups white, black, American Indian or Alaska Native, Asian, Native Hawaiian or Other Pacific Islander, and 2 or more races include persons of Hispanic and non-Hispanic origin. Persons of Hispanic origin may be of any race. Starting with 1999 data, race-specific estimates are tabulated according to the 1997 Revisions to the Standards for the Classification of Federal Data on Race and Ethnicity and are not strictly comparable with estimates for earlier years. The five single-race categories and multiple-race categories shown in the table conform to the 1997 Standards. Starting with 1999 data, race-specific estimates for persons who reported only one racial group; the category 2 or more races includes persons who reported more than one racial group. Prior to 1999, data were tabulated according to the 1977 Standards with four racial groups, and the Asian only category included Native Hawaiian or Other Pacific Islander. Estimates for single-race categories prior to 1999 included persons who reported one race, or if they reported more than one race, identified one race as best representing their race. Starting with 2003 data, race responses of other race and unspecified multiple race were treated as missing, and then race was imputed if these were the only race responses. Almost all persons with a race response of other race were of Hispanic origin.

[6] Percent of poverty level is based on family income and family size and composition using U.S. Census Bureau poverty thresholds. Poverty level was unknown for 11% of persons aged 18 and over in 1989. Missing family income data were imputed for 1991 and beyond.

[7] Functional limitation is defined by the reported level of difficulty in six functioning domains: seeing (even if wearing glasses), hearing (even if wearing hearing aids), mobility (walking or climbing stairs), communication (understanding or being understood by others), cognition (remembering or concentrating), and self-care (such as washing all over or dressing). Respondents with answers to one or more of the six questions were included in one of three mutually exclusive categories. Those responding "A lot of difficulty" or "Cannot do at all/unable to do" to at least one question were classified in the "A lot of difficulty/cannot do" category. Of the remaining, those responding "Some difficulty" to at least one question were classified in the "Some difficulty" category, and those responding "No difficulty" to at least one question were classified in the "No difficulty" category. Those responding "Don't know" or "Refused" to all six questions were excluded. During 2010–2016, 1%–8% of respondents were missing data and excluded.

[8] MSA is metropolitan statistical area. Starting with 2016 data, MSA status is determined using 2010 Census data and the 2010 standards for defining MSAs.

Table 3-40. Use of Mammography[1] Among Women 40 Years of Age and Over, by Selected Characteristics, Selected Years, 1987–2015

(Percent.)

Characteristic	1987	1990	1991	1993	1994	1998	1999	2000	2003	2005	2008	2010	2013	2015
40 years and over, age-adjusted[2,3]	29.0	51.7	54.7	59.7	61.0	67.0	70.3	70.4	69.5	66.6	67.1	66.5	65.7	64.0
40 years and over, crude[2]	28.7	51.4	54.6	59.7	60.9	66.9	70.3	70.4	69.7	66.8	67.6	67.1	66.8	65.3
50 years and over, age-adjusted[2,3]	27.3	49.8	54.3	59.7	60.9	69.0	72.1	73.7	72.4	68.2	70.3	68.8	69.1	67.2
50 years and over, crude[2]	27.4	49.7	54.1	59.7	60.6	68.9	71.9	73.6	72.4	68.4	70.5	69.2	69.5	67.8
Age														
40 to 49 years	31.9	55.1	55.6	59.9	61.3	63.4	67.2	64.3	64.4	63.5	61.5	62.3	59.6	58.3
50 to 64 years	31.7	56.0	60.3	65.1	66.5	73.7	76.5	78.7	76.2	71.8	74.2	72.6	71.4	71.3
65 years and over	22.8	43.4	48.1	54.2	55.0	63.8	66.8	67.9	67.7	63.8	65.5	64.4	66.9	63.3
65 to 74 years	26.6	48.7	55.7	64.2	63.0	69.4	73.9	74.0	74.6	72.5	72.6	71.9	75.3	72.2
75 years and over	17.3	35.8	37.8	41.0	44.6	57.2	58.9	61.3	60.6	54.7	57.9	55.7	56.5	51.5
Race[4]														
40 years and over, crude														
White only	29.6	52.2	55.6	60.0	60.6	67.4	70.6	71.4	70.1	67.4	67.9	67.4	66.8	65.3
Black or African American only	24.0	46.4	48.0	59.1	64.3	66.0	71.0	67.8	70.4	64.9	68.0	67.9	67.1	69.8
American Indian or Alaska Native only	*	43.2	54.5	49.8	65.8	45.2	63.0	47.4	63.1	72.8	62.7	71.2	62.6	51.5
Asian only	*	46.0	45.9	55.1	55.8	60.2	58.3	53.5	57.6	54.6	66.1	62.4	66.6	59.7
Native Hawaiian or Other Pacific Islander only	NA	NA	NA	NA	NA	NA	*	*	*	*	*	*	*	*
Two or more races	NA	NA	NA	NA	NA	NA	70.2	69.2	65.3	63.7	55.2	51.4	65.4	62.7
Hispanic Origin and Race[4]														
40 years and over, crude														
Hispanic or Latina	18.3	45.2	49.2	50.9	51.9	60.2	65.7	61.2	65.0	58.8	61.2	64.2	61.4	60.9
Not Hispanic or Latina	29.4	51.8	54.9	60.3	61.5	67.5	70.7	71.1	70.1	67.5	68.3	67.4	67.5	65.9
White only	30.3	52.7	56.0	60.6	61.3	68.0	71.1	72.2	70.5	68.3	68.7	67.8	67.6	65.8
Black or African American only	23.8	46.0	47.7	59.2	64.4	66.0	71.0	67.9	70.5	65.2	68.3	67.4	67.2	69.7
Age, Hispanic Origin, and Race[4]														
40 to 49 years														
Hispanic or Latina	*15.3	45.1	44.0	52.6	47.5	55.2	61.6	54.1	59.4	54.2	54.1	59.8	56.4	50.3
Not Hispanic or Latina														
White only	34.3	57.0	58.1	61.6	62.0	64.4	68.3	67.2	65.2	65.5	64.1	62.6	60.3	58.8
Black or African American only	27.8	48.4	48.0	55.6	67.2	65.0	69.2	60.9	68.2	62.1	59.5	63.5	59.4	67.8
50 to 64 years														
Hispanic or Latina	23.0	47.5	61.7	59.2	60.1	67.2	69.7	66.5	69.4	61.5	71.3	68.6	65.6	71.6
Not Hispanic or Latina														
White only	33.6	58.1	61.5	66.2	67.5	75.3	77.9	80.6	77.2	73.5	74.1	73.5	72.1	71.4
Black or African American only	26.4	48.4	52.4	65.5	63.6	71.2	75.0	77.7	76.2	71.6	76.7	74.0	71.7	73.5
65 years and over														
Hispanic or Latina														
Not Hispanic or Latina	*	41.1	40.9	*35.7	48.0	59.0	67.2	68.3	69.5	63.8	59.0	65.2	63.2	60.9
White only														
Black or African American only	24.0	43.8	49.1	54.7	54.9	64.3	66.8	68.3	68.1	64.7	66.1	65.0	67.3	63.9
Age and Percent of Poverty Level[5]														
40 years and over, crude														
Below 100 percent	14.6	30.8	35.2	41.1	44.2	50.1	57.4	54.8	55.4	48.5	51.4	51.4	49.9	52.2
100 percent to 199 percent	20.9	39.1	44.4	47.5	48.6	56.1	59.5	58.1	60.8	55.3	55.8	53.8	56.7	54.9
200 percent to 399 percent	29.7	53.3	57.5	63.2	65.0	67.4	69.1	68.8	69.9	67.2	64.4	66.2	66.0	63.4
400 percent or more	42.9	68.7	69.8	74.1	74.1	76.8	79.8	81.5	77.7	76.6	79.0	78.1	77.2	74.7
40 to 49 years														
Below 100 percent	18.6	32.2	33.0	36.1	43.0	44.8	51.3	47.4	50.6	42.5	46.6	48.1	43.3	45.8
100 percent to 199 percent	18.4	39.0	43.8	47.8	47.6	46.9	52.8	43.6	54.0	49.8	46.5	46.2	52.0	47.5
200 percent to 399 percent	31.2	55.2	56.3	63.0	64.5	61.8	63.0	60.2	63.0	61.8	56.8	59.2	58.5	55.6
400 percent or more	44.1	68.9	69.6	69.6	69.9	72.7	77.4	75.8	71.6	73.6	72.5	73.6	69.0	68.2
50 to 64 years														
Below 100 percent	14.6	29.9	37.3	47.3	46.2	52.7	63.3	61.7	58.3	50.4	57.5	54.7	55.0	56.9
100 percent to 199 percent	24.2	39.8	50.2	47.0	49.0	61.8	64.9	68.3	64.0	58.8	58.9	57.3	57.2	60.5
200 percent to 399 percent	29.7	56.2	60.2	66.1	69.6	71.1	74.8	75.1	74.1	70.7	69.8	70.7	69.5	69.0
400 percent or more	44.7	71.6	72.6	78.7	78.0	83.4	83.4	86.9	84.9	80.6	84.3	82.8	80.9	79.2
65 years and over														
Below 100 percent	13.1	30.8	35.2	40.4	43.9	51.9	57.6	54.8	57.0	52.3	49.1	50.6	49.8	52.7
100 percent to 199 percent	19.9	38.6	41.8	47.6	48.8	57.8	60.2	60.3	62.8	56.1	59.4	55.5	59.3	54.4
200 percent to 399 percent	27.7	47.4	55.9	60.3	61.0	69.5	70.0	71.1	72.3	68.6	65.0	67.2	68.1	63.3
400 percent or more	34.7	61.2	63.0	71.3	73.0	71.1	76.7	81.9	73.0	72.6	78.3	74.5	79.0	73.1

NA = Not available.
* = Estimates are considered unreliable. Data preceded by an asterisk have a relative standard error (RSE) of 20 percent to 30 percent. Data not shown have an RSE of greater than 30 percent.
[1]Questions concerning use of mammography differed slightly on the National Health Interview Survey across the years for which data are shown.
[2]Includes all other races not shown separately, unknown poverty level in 1987, unknown health insurance status, unknown education level, and unknown disability status.
[3]Estimates for women 40 years of age and over are age-adjusted to the year 2000 standard population using four age groups: 40 to 49 years, 50 to 64 years, 65 to 74 years, and 75 years and over. Estimates for women 50 years of age and over are age-adjusted using three age groups.
[4]The race groups White, Black, American Indian or Alaska Native, Asian, Native Hawaiian or Other Pacific Islander, and two or more races, include persons of Hispanic and non-Hispanic origin. Persons of Hispanic origin may be of any race.
[5]Percent of poverty level is based on family income and family size and composition using U.S. Census Bureau poverty thresholds. Poverty level was unknown for 11 percent of women 40 years of age and over in 1987. Missing family income data were imputed for 1997 and beyond.

Table 3-40. Use of Mammography[1] Among Women 40 Years of Age and Over, by Selected Characteristics, Selected Years, 1987–2015—*Continued*

(Percent.)

Characteristic	1987	1990	1991	1993	1994	1998	1999	2000	2003	2005	2008	2010	2013	2015
Health Insurance Status at the Time of Interview[6]														
40 to 64 years														
Insured..	NA	NA	NA	66.2	68.3	72.3	75.5	76.0	75.1	72.5	73.4	74.1	72.1	69.7
Private..	NA	NA	NA	67.1	69.4	73.4	76.3	77.1	76.3	74.5	74.2	75.6	73.4	72.2
Medicaid	NA	NA	NA	51.9	54.5	59.7	62.5	61.7	63.5	55.6	64.2	64.4	63.5	57.7
Uninsured	NA	NA	NA	36.0	34.0	40.1	44.8	40.7	41.5	38.1	39.7	36.0	37.3	30.0
Health Insurance Status Prior to Interview[6]														
40 to 64 years														
Insured continuously all 12 months..................	NA	NA	NA	66.6	68.6	73.0	76.1	76.8	75.6	73.1	74.1	74.7	72.7	70.6
Uninsured for any period up to 12 months	NA	NA	NA	49.4	49.9	47.6	57.1	53.0	56.0	51.3	55.3	57.3	54.5	50.0
Uninsured more than 12 months	NA	NA	NA	28.4	26.6	36.3	38.9	34.0	37.0	32.9	34.6	30.0	32.8	23.9
Age and Education[7]														
40 years and over, crude														
No high school diploma or GED	17.8	36.4	40.0	46.4	48.2	54.5	56.7	57.7	58.1	52.8	53.8	53.0	53.6	51.7
High school diploma or GED	31.3	52.7	55.8	59.0	61.0	66.7	69.2	69.7	67.8	64.9	65.2	64.4	63.4	60.1
Some college or more................................	37.7	62.8	65.2	69.5	69.7	72.8	77.3	76.2	75.1	72.7	73.4	72.1	71.6	70.5
40 to 49 years														
No high school diploma or GED	15.1	38.5	40.8	43.6	50.4	47.3	48.8	46.8	53.3	51.2	46.9	44.9	46.9	43.8
High school diploma or GED	32.6	53.1	52.0	56.6	55.8	59.1	60.8	59.0	60.8	58.8	57.2	58.4	51.8	47.5
Some college or more................................	39.2	62.3	63.7	66.1	68.7	68.3	74.4	70.6	68.1	68.3	66.3	66.5	64.3	64.0
50 to 64 years														
No high school diploma or GED	21.2	41.0	43.6	51.4	51.6	58.8	62.3	66.5	63.4	56.9	64.9	56.7	58.2	58.1
High school diploma or GED	33.8	56.5	60.8	62.4	67.8	73.3	77.2	76.6	71.8	70.1	70.4	69.9	66.9	67.0
Some college or more................................	40.5	68.0	72.7	78.5	74.7	79.8	81.2	84.2	82.7	77.0	78.5	77.0	75.7	75.3
65 years and over														
No high school diploma or GED	16.5	33.0	37.7	44.2	45.6	54.7	56.6	57.4	56.9	50.7	49.2	54.1	53.4	50.8
High school diploma or GED	25.9	47.5	54.0	57.4	59.1	66.8	68.4	71.8	69.7	64.3	65.7	62.5	66.5	60.0
Some college or more................................	32.3	56.7	57.9	64.8	64.3	71.3	77.1	74.1	75.1	73.0	75.6	70.9	73.6	69.8
Disability Measure[8]														
40 years and over, crude														
Any basic actions difficulty or complex activity limitation	NA	NA	NA	NA	NA	65.8	67.6	67.8	67.2	63.5	63.9	63.3	63.5	62.2
Any basic actions difficulty	NA	NA	NA	NA	NA	65.9	67.1	67.9	67.3	63.5	63.9	63.3	63.8	62.4
Any complex activity limitation	NA	NA	NA	NA	NA	61.8	64.8	64.1	62.3	59.9	60.2	58.2	58.4	56.1
No disability	NA	NA	NA	NA	NA	68.2	72.3	72.6	71.8	69.8	71.1	70.8	69.8	68.0

NA = Not available.

[1]Questions concerning use of mammography differed slightly on the National Health Interview Survey across the years for which data are shown.

[6]Health insurance categories are mutually exclusive. Persons who reported both Medicaid and private coverage are classified as having private coverage. Medicaid includes other public assistance through 1996. Starting with 1997 data, state-sponsored health plan coverage is included as Medicaid coverage. Starting with 1999 data, coverage by the Children's Health Insurance Program (CHIP) is included with Medicaid coverage. Persons not covered by private insurance, Medicaid, CHIP, public assistance (through 1996), state-sponsored or other government-sponsored health plans (starting in 1997), Medicare, or military plans are considered to have no health insurance coverage. Persons with only Indian Health Service coverage are considered to have no health insurance coverage. Health insurance status was unknown for 8 to 9 percent of children in 1993-1996 and about 1 percent in 1997-2011.

[7]Education categories shown are for 1998 and subsequent years. GED is General Educational Development high school equivalency diploma. In years prior to 1998, the following categories based on number of years in school completed were used: less than 12 years, 12 years, and 13 years or more.

[8]Any basic actions difficulty or complex activity limitation is defined as having one or more of the following limitations or difficulties: movement difficulty, emotional difficulty, sensory (seeing or hearing) difficulty, cognitive difficulty, self-care (activities of daily living or instrumental activities of daily living) limitation, social limitation, or work limitation.

Table 3-41. Percent of Women 18 Years of Age and Over Who Have Had a Pap Smear[1] Within the Last Three Years, by Selected Characteristics, Selected Years, 1987–2015

(Percent.)

Characteristic	1987	1993	1994	1998	1999	2000	2003	2005	2008	2010	2013	2015
18 years and over, age-adjusted[2,3]	74.1	77.7	76.8	79.3	80.8	81.3	79.2	77.9	75.6	73.7	70.4	70.2
18 years and over, crude[2]	74.4	77.7	76.8	79.1	80.8	81.2	79.0	77.7	75.1	73.2	69.4	69.0
Age												
18 to 44 years	83.3	84.6	82.8	84.4	86.8	84.9	83.9	83.6	81.8	80.4	77.2	76.1
18 to 20 years	59.4	66.8	62.9	59.5	65.3	59.8	63.7	61.1	57.5	52.0	38.6	34.0
21 to 44 years	86.1	86.2	84.7	87.1	89.2	87.8	86.1	86.3	84.8	84.0	81.6	81.1
21 to 24 years	85.3	86.1	85.4	84.2	85.3	84.1	82.7	84.0	80.2	81.1	74.6	69.7
25 to 44 years	86.3	86.3	84.6	87.6	89.9	88.5	86.8	86.8	85.7	84.6	83.2	83.5
45 to 64 years	70.5	77.2	77.4	81.4	81.7	84.6	81.3	80.6	78.8	76.9	73.9	75.5
45 to 54 years	75.7	82.1	81.9	83.7	83.8	86.3	83.6	83.4	81.0	79.9	78.6	79.7
55 to 64 years	65.2	70.6	71.0	78.0	78.4	82.0	77.8	76.8	76.0	73.2	68.6	71.1
65 years and over	50.8	57.6	57.3	59.8	61.0	64.5	60.8	54.9	50.0	47.1	42.7	42.3
65 to 74 years	57.9	64.7	64.9	67.0	70.0	71.6	70.1	66.3	61.6	58.0	54.5	52.9
75 years and over	40.4	48.0	47.3	51.2	50.8	56.7	51.1	42.7	37.5	34.6	27.9	28.1
Race[4]												
18 years and over, crude												
White only	74.1	77.3	76.2	78.9	80.6	81.3	78.7	77.7	74.9	72.8	68.7	68.4
Black or African American only	80.7	82.7	83.5	84.2	85.7	85.1	84.0	81.1	80.1	77.9	75.3	74.6
American Indian or Alaska Native only	85.4	78.1	73.5	74.6	92.2	76.8	84.8	75.2	69.4	73.4	70.1	60.9
Asian only	51.9	68.8	66.4	68.5	64.4	66.4	68.3	64.1	65.1	68.0	65.3	64.9
Native Hawaiian or Other Pacific Islander only.	NA	NA	NA	NA	*	*	*	*	*	*	*	*
Two or more races	NA	NA	NA	NA	86.9	80.0	81.6	86.2	77.1	70.8	70.8	72.5
Hispanic Origin and Race[4]												
18 years and over, crude	67.6	77.2	74.4	75.2	76.3	77.0	75.4	75.5	75.4	73.6	70.5	68.6
Hispanic or Latina	74.9	77.8	77.0	79.6	81.3	81.7	79.5	78.0	75.1	73.1	69.2	69.0
Not Hispanic or Latina	74.7	77.3	76.5	79.3	81.0	81.8	79.3	78.1	74.9	72.8	68.4	68.4
White only	80.9	82.7	83.8	84.2	86.0	85.1	83.8	81.2	80.0	77.4	75.1	74.6
Black or African American only												
Age, Hispanic Origin, and Race[4]												
18 to 44 years												
Hispanic or Latina	73.9	80.9	80.6	76.4	77.0	78.1	75.9	76.5	77.9	75.9	72.3	70.2
Not Hispanic or Latina												
White only	84.5	85.3	82.9	85.7	88.7	86.6	85.8	85.8	83.8	82.1	79.0	78.2
Black or African American only	89.1	88.0	89.1	88.9	90.8	88.5	88.6	86.4	83.5	84.2	82.8	82.1
45 to 64 years												
Hispanic or Latina	57.7	75.8	70.1	78.3	79.5	77.8	77.9	78.4	78.2	75.4	74.4	74.0
Not Hispanic or Latina												
White only	71.2	77.2	77.5	81.7	81.9	85.9	81.4	81.4	79.0	77.2	73.6	75.5
Black or African American only	76.2	80.3	82.2	84.1	84.6	85.7	84.7	80.5	82.1	78.2	76.0	77.4
65 years and over												
Hispanic or Latina	41.7	57.1	43.8	59.8	63.7	66.8	64.6	60.0	52.6	54.2	49.4	46.2
Not Hispanic or Latina												
White only	51.8	57.1	58.2	59.7	60.5	64.2	60.7	54.1	49.0	46.5	41.4	41.9
Black or African American only	44.8	61.2	59.5	61.7	64.5	67.2	59.6	60.1	58.7	48.0	45.8	43.5
Age and Percent of Poverty Level[5]												
18 years and over, crude												
Below 100 percent	64.3	70.3	68.8	69.8	73.6	72.0	70.5	68.7	68.9	65.1	60.6	63.2
100 percent to 199 percent	68.2	71.2	68.8	70.6	72.5	73.4	71.4	69.0	65.0	64.3	59.8	60.3
200 percent to 399 percent	77.6	80.6	80.1	79.7	80.6	80.2	78.6	77.9	72.5	71.3	68.5	66.6
400 percent or more	83.6	85.1	85.4	87.0	87.6	89.1	86.6	85.7	84.4	83.1	79.4	77.6
18 to 44 years												
Below 100 percent	77.1	77.0	78.9	77.1	79.7	77.1	77.1	76.2	76.5	73.0	69.2	69.1
100 percent to 199 percent	80.4	81.9	78.2	79.2	84.0	79.4	79.5	78.1	75.5	75.7	72.6	73.5
200 percent to 399 percent	84.8	86.6	84.5	85.3	86.7	86.1	84.0	85.5	82.6	79.8	78.6	74.7
400 percent or more	88.9	91.3	88.7	89.8	91.1	89.8	89.5	88.7	87.0	88.9	84.5	83.2
45 to 64 years												
Below 100 percent	53.6	66.5	62.0	67.6	73.1	73.6	66.0	65.9	66.2	61.7	54.9	63.7
100 percent to 199 percent	60.4	64.8	66.2	69.9	70.4	76.1	71.4	69.6	65.6	63.2	61.2	64.2
200 percent to 399 percent	71.0	79.5	80.3	79.7	79.9	80.0	80.8	79.3	75.3	75.2	73.7	73.5
400 percent or more	79.1	83.9	84.0	88.2	87.4	91.5	87.5	87.4	87.1	85.7	82.8	82.9
65 years and over												
Below 100 percent	33.2	47.4	44.0	48.2	51.9	53.7	52.6	44.4	41.6	35.1	34.1	37.1
100 percent to 199 percent	50.4	55.7	51.5	55.1	54.7	61.0	55.4	49.5	43.5	40.7	33.0	31.9
200 percent to 399 percent	58.0	59.7	63.7	64.2	64.0	65.1	62.4	56.8	45.8	47.1	39.6	41.5
400 percent or more	65.2	67.5	76.2	67.5	70.4	75.4	70.2	64.6	65.7	57.7	58.1	52.3

NA = Not available.
* = Figure does not meet standards of reliability or precision. Data not shown have an RSE of greater than 30 percent.
[1]Questions concerning use of Pap smears differed slightly on the National Health Interview Survey across the years for which data are shown.
[2]Includes all other races not shown separately, unknown poverty level in 1987, unknown health insurance status, unknown education level, and unknown disability status.
[3]Estimates are age adjusted to the year 2000 standard population using five age groups: 18 to 44 years, 45 to 54 years, 55 to 64 years, 65 to 74 years, and 75 years and over.
[4]The race groups White, Black, American Indian or Alaska Native, Asian, Native Hawaiian or Other Pacific Islander, and two or more races, include persons of Hispanic and non-Hispanic origin. Persons of Hispanic origin may be of any race.
[5]Percent of poverty level is based on family income and family size and composition. Missing family income data were imputed for 1993 and beyond.

Table 3-41. Percent of Women 18 Years of Age and Over Who Have Had a Pap Smear[1] Within the Last Three Years, by Selected Characteristics, Selected Years, 1987–2015—*Continued*

(Percent.)

Characteristic	1987	1993	1994	1998	1999	2000	2003	2005	2008	2010	2013	2015
Health Insurance Status at the Time of Interview[6]												
18 to 64 years, crude												
Insured	NA	84.7	83.8	86.0	87.2	87.8	86.4	85.6	83.4	82.8	80.0	78.2
Private	NA	84.8	83.6	86.5	87.5	88.0	87.0	86.5	84.2	84.2	81.3	79.6
Medicaid	NA	82.7	86.2	83.0	84.2	85.8	82.8	80.9	80.3	78.0	75.7	72.6
Uninsured	NA	69.4	68.6	69.6	73.3	70.4	66.6	67.7	67.1	61.9	57.6	57.3
Health Insurance Status Prior to Interview[6]												
18 to 64 years, crude												
Insured continuously all 12 months	NA	84.8	83.7	86.3	87.3	88.0	86.6	85.8	83.7	83.2	80.4	78.5
Uninsured for any period up to 12 months	NA	81.8	83.4	81.7	83.5	83.7	81.8	81.3	78.9	78.3	72.3	72.0
Uninsured more than 12 months	NA	65.1	63.6	64.0	68.8	65.1	60.2	62.0	62.1	55.2	52.7	51.0
Age and Education[7]												
25 years and over, crude												
No high school diploma or GED	57.1	61.9	60.9	65.0	66.1	69.9	64.9	64.1	60.6	56.7	56.2	55.9
High school diploma or GED	76.4	78.2	76.0	77.4	79.3	79.8	75.9	73.8	69.5	66.8	62.0	62.0
Some college or more	84.0	84.4	85.2	86.9	87.8	88.0	86.2	84.6	82.6	80.7	77.1	76.9
25 to 44 years												
No high school diploma or GED	75.1	73.6	73.6	76.8	79.0	79.6	71.7	75.5	76.2	69.1	71.7	73.3
High school diploma or GED	85.6	85.4	82.4	83.9	87.6	86.2	84.3	83.1	80.0	79.0	79.5	75.1
Some college or more	90.1	89.8	89.1	91.5	93.0	91.4	90.8	90.5	89.3	89.0	86.1	87.2
45 to 64 years												
No high school diploma or GED	58.0	65.6	66.1	69.2	71.6	75.7	71.4	69.7	70.4	63.4	63.0	60.3
High school diploma or GED	72.3	77.6	75.9	81.0	79.8	81.8	77.6	79.0	73.9	72.4	67.0	70.7
Some college or more	80.1	83.0	84.7	85.5	85.7	89.1	86.2	84.1	83.0	81.5	78.7	79.9
65 years and over												
No high school diploma or GED	44.0	50.7	47.7	52.4	51.8	56.6	52.5	46.0	36.7	37.7	33.8	32.9
High school diploma or GED	55.4	61.6	61.2	60.7	63.7	66.9	61.2	52.5	49.3	42.6	38.8	39.0
Some college or more	59.4	62.3	66.5	67.9	68.8	69.8	67.8	63.8	59.0	54.9	49.7	47.5
Disability measure[8]												
18 years and over, crude												
Any basic actions difficulty or complex activity limitation	NA	NA	NA	72.7	74.4	75.4	72.7	69.1	66.1	63.8	59.3	59.9
Any basic actions difficulty	NA	NA	NA	72.4	74.3	75.1	72.6	69.1	66.2	63.6	59.2	59.9
Any complex activity limitation	NA	NA	NA	67.9	69.3	71.0	67.6	62.2	60.1	58.5	52.8	54.6
No disability	NA	NA	NA	82.5	83.8	84.1	82.5	82.6	80.4	78.9	75.2	74.5

NA = Not available.

[1]Questions concerning use of Pap smears differed slightly on the National Health Interview Survey across the years for which data are shown.

[6]Health insurance categories are mutually exclusive. Persons who reported both Medicaid and private coverage are classified as having private coverage. Medicaid includes other public assistance through 1996. Starting with 1997 data, state-sponsored health plan coverage is included as Medicaid coverage. Starting with 1999 data, coverage by the Children's Health Insurance Program (CHIP) is included with Medicaid coverage. Persons not covered by private insurance, Medicaid, CHIP, public assistance (through 1996), state-sponsored or other government-sponsored health plans (starting in 1997), Medicare, or military plans are considered to have no health insurance coverage. Persons with only Indian Health Service coverage are considered to have no health insurance coverage. Health insurance status was unknown for 8 to 9 percent of children in 1993-1996 and about 1 percent in 1997-2011.

[7]Education categories shown are for 1998 and subsequent years. GED is General Educational Development high school equivalency diploma. In years prior to 1998, the following categories based on number of years in school completed were used: less than 12 years, 12 years, and 13 years or more.

[8]Any basic actions difficulty or complex activity limitation is defined as having one or more of the following limitations or difficulties: movement difficulty, emotional difficulty, sensory (seeing or hearing) difficulty, cognitive difficulty, self-care (activities of daily living or instrumental activities of daily living) limitation, social limitation, or work limitation.

Table 3-42. Use of Colorectal Tests or Procedures Among Adults 50 to 75 Years of Age, by Selected Characteristics, Selected Years, 2000–2015

(Percent.)

Characteristic	Any colorectal test or procedure[1,2]					Colonoscopy[2,3]				
	2000	2003	2005	2008	2015	2000	2003	2005	2008	2015
All adults, 50 to 75 years[4]	33.9	39.1	44.3	51.6	62.4	19.1	29.2	37.6	46.7	59.2
Sex										
Male	33.1	40.1	44.4	51.4	61.6	19.5	30.2	37.9	46.9	58.4
Female	34.5	38.1	44.2	51.9	63.1	18.8	28.4	37.4	46.6	60.0
Race[5]										
White only	34.9	39.8	45.6	52.8	63.7	19.7	30.0	38.9	47.8	60.7
Black or African American only	29.6	35.2	38.1	46.9	59.6	17.4	24.8	32.2	43.1	56.3
American Indian or Alaska Native only	*35.2	*37.9	*33.9	28.5	48.9	*	*	*	*26.7	45.3
Asian only	20.4	26.7	30.8	47.1	52.3	*8.6	20.0	24.4	39.3	45.8
Native Hawaiian and Other Pacific Islander only	*	*	*	*	*	*	*	*	*	*
Two or more races	37.5	40.7	33.8	38.4	52.7	*25.1	29.7	29.6	37.4	49.8
Hispanic Origin and Race[5]										
Hispanic or Latino	21.7	27.2	28.5	34.0	47.4	13.3	19.8	23.1	29.3	44.0
Mexican	19.3	22.4	24.6	27.5	41.2	11.2	14.2	18.2	21.2	37.6
Not Hispanic or Latino	34.7	40.0	45.6	53.3	64.1	19.5	30.0	38.9	48.4	61.0
White only	35.7	41.0	47.4	54.8	65.6	20.0	30.9	40.5	49.8	62.8
Black or African American only	29.7	35.3	38.0	47.4	60.3	17.5	25.0	32.0	43.5	56.9
Percent of Poverty Level[6]										
Below 100 percent	26.5	29.7	28.7	33.9	45.6	16.3	22.0	23.6	28.5	42.8
100 percent to 199 percent	29.4	31.9	38.4	42.7	51.8	17.7	23.3	31.5	38.0	48.0
200 percent to 399 percent	33.7	38.8	43.6	49.9	61.3	18.6	29.4	37.0	44.3	58.6
400 percent or more	37.1	43.8	49.6	58.9	70.0	20.5	32.7	42.8	54.5	66.8
Hispanic Origin and Race and Percent of Poverty Level[5,6]										
Hispanic or Latino										
Below 100 percent	15.3	21.4	19.3	21.1	40.4	*9.3	15.2	13.1	17.9	37.0
100 percent to 199 percent	16.8	20.5	24.6	27.7	37.7	8.6	16.0	19.4	24.4	34.0
200 percent to 399 percent	23.6	29.0	28.3	39.3	48.9	*13.7	20.7	21.6	33.8	45.0
400 percent or more	31.1	37.9	42.1	43.9	61.5	22.4	27.1	39.3	37.6	58.7
Not Hispanic or Latino										
White only										
Below 100 percent	29.6	33.9	30.6	39.8	46.1	19.3	26.8	26.8	33.2	43.7
100 percent to 199 percent	32.1	34.7	42.4	46.0	55.1	19.7	25.7	35.0	40.7	51.6
200 percent to 399 percent	35.2	40.3	47.3	51.6	64.3	19.3	31.0	40.2	45.8	62.1
400 percent or more	37.9	44.3	50.6	60.5	71.3	20.7	32.9	43.8	56.3	68.3
Black or African American only										
Below 100 percent	27.5	27.4	29.0	35.1	49.1	14.5	17.6	23.5	30.1	44.8
100 percent to 199 percent	28.7	30.0	36.2	46.7	56.2	17.2	20.0	30.3	43.2	51.8
200 percent to 399 percent	27.7	36.8	35.8	48.5	60.2	16.5	25.6	31.8	44.7	58.2
400 percent or more	33.9	43.5	48.9	54.3	71.9	20.7	33.3	40.2	50.6	68.5
Education[7]										
No high school diploma or GED	25.9	28.9	34.5	36.2	46.6	14.9	21.2	29.0	31.8	43.7
High school diploma or GED	33.1	38.3	42.1	48.5	58.2	19.0	29.3	35.7	44.6	55.2
Some college or more	37.8	43.3	48.7	57.5	67.2	20.9	32.1	41.6	52.1	63.9
Disability Measure[8]										
Any basic actions difficulty or complex activity limitation	37.8	42.0	47.7	54.2	64.9	22.1	31.9	40.1	48.5	61.8
Any basic actions difficulty	38.1	41.9	47.9	54.6	65.1	22.5	31.9	40.6	48.9	62.0
Any complex activity limitation	37.4	41.5	48.1	52.4	62.9	22.6	31.3	39.7	46.7	59.5
No disability	30.9	36.9	41.6	50.0	60.7	16.6	27.1	35.6	45.8	57.5
Geographic Region										
Northeast	34.4	43.5	50.9	54.7	66.4	19.1	33.1	44.8	51.0	64.5
Midwest	35.2	40.4	43.5	52.5	63.1	19.8	30.6	36.6	47.8	61.7
South	32.5	36.7	43.9	51.6	60.4	20.0	28.5	38.1	47.4	57.8
West	34.1	37.0	39.6	48.2	61.8	16.3	24.3	31.3	41.1	54.9
Location of Residence										
Within MSA[9]	34.1	40.3	44.7	52.4	63.2	19.0	29.9	37.9	47.6	59.8
Outside MSA[9]	33.2	34.8	42.7	48.5	58.5	19.6	26.8	36.7	43.3	56.5

* = Figure does not meet standards of reliability or precision. Data preceded by an asterisk have a relative standard error (RSE) of 20 percent to 30 percent. Data not shown have an RSE of greater than 30 percent.
[1]Includes reports of home fecal occult blood test (FOBT) in the past year, sigmoidoscopy procedure in the past 5 years with FOBT in the past 3 years, or colonoscopy in the past 10 years. Colorectal procedures are performed for diagnostic and screening purposes.
[2]Questions differed slightly on the National Health Interview Survey across the years for which data are shown.
[3]Includes any colonoscopy in the past 10 years, alone or in addition to another type of colorectal test or procedure.
[4]Includes all other races not shown separately, unknown disability status, and unknown education level.
[5]The race groups White, Black, American Indian or Alaska Native, Asian, Native Hawaiian or Other Pacific Islander, and two or more races include persons of Hispanic and non-Hispanic origin. Persons of Hispanic origin may be of any race.
[6]Based on family income and family size and composition using U.S. Census Bureau poverty thresholds. Missing family income data were imputed.
[7]GED is General Educational Development high school equivalency diploma.
[8]Any basic actions difficulty or complex activity limitation is defined as having one or more of the following limitations or difficulties: movement difficulty, emotional difficulty, sensory (seeing or hearing) difficulty, cognitive difficulty, self-care (activities of daily living or instrumental activities of daily living) limitation, social limitation, or work limitation.
[9]MSA = metropolitan statistical area.

Table 3-43. Emergency Department Visits Within the Past 12 Months Among Children Under 18 Years of Age, by Selected Characteristics, Selected Years, 1997–2016

(Percent; Data are based on household interviews of a sample of the civilian noninstitutionalized population.)

Characteristic	Under 18 years						Under 6 years						6 to 17 years					
	1997	2000	2005	2010	2015	2016	1997	2000	2005	2010	2015	2016	1997	2000	2005	2010	2015	2016
PERCENT OF CHILDREN WITH ONE OR MORE EMERGENCY DEPARTMENT VISITS[1]																		
All children[2]	19.9	20.3	20.5	22.1	16.9	17.5	24.3	25.7	26.8	27.8	21.7	22.0	17.7	17.6	17.4	19.1	14.5	15.3
Sex																		
Male	21.5	21.5	21.7	23.3	17.3	18.7	25.2	27.7	27.6	29.3	23.0	24.4	19.6	18.6	18.8	20.1	14.6	15.9
Female	18.3	19.0	19.2	20.9	16.3	16.2	23.3	23.7	25.9	26.3	20.4	19.4	15.7	16.6	15.9	18.2	14.4	14.6
Race[3]																		
White only	19.4	19.9	19.8	21.2	16.3	16.6	22.6	24.8	25.3	26.6	20.9	21.4	17.8	17.6	17.1	18.4	14.1	14.3
Black or African American only	24.0	22.7	23.8	27.6	21.6	21.8	33.1	30.8	31.6	34.0	27.4	25.4	19.4	19.0	20.0	24.2	18.8	19.9
American Indian or Alaska Native only	*24.1	38.0	*32.1	20.9	23.3	34.4	*24.3	*	67.1	*35.4	*37.2	*	*24.0	*39.0	*	*	*17.5	30.9
Asian only	12.6	12.3	14.6	15.0	9.2	8.4	20.8	*16.7	20.2	18.4	13.9	11.1	8.6	9.8	12.3	13.3	*7.0	7.1
Native Hawaiian and Other Pacific Islander only	NA	*	*	*	*	*	NA	*	*	*	*	*	NA	*	*	*	*	*
Two or more races	NA	24.2	24.8	27.2	18.6	24.3	NA	31.7	38.3	34.9	23.1	26.8	NA	18.3	17.1	21.6	*15.8	22.8
Hispanic Origin and Race[3]																		
Hispanic or Latino	21.1	18.6	19.5	23.6	18.8	17.8	25.7	23.9	28.0	30.2	25.9	22.6	18.1	15.6	14.5	19.4	15.2	15.4
Not Hispanic or Latino	19.7	20.6	20.7	21.7	16.2	17.4	24.0	26.2	26.5	27.0	20.3	21.8	17.6	18.0	18.0	19.0	14.3	15.2
White only	19.2	20.2	19.9	20.4	15.4	16.5	22.2	25.1	24.5	25.1	18.8	21.0	17.7	17.9	17.9	18.2	13.8	14.3
Black or African American only	23.6	22.7	23.8	27.2	21.3	21.9	32.7	30.9	31.8	34.4	27.2	26.3	19.2	19.0	20.0	23.3	18.4	19.6
Percent of Poverty Level[4]																		
Below 100 percent	25.1	25.0	27.3	30.6	23.1	25.1	29.5	30.7	33.5	35.4	28.8	32.8	22.2	21.7	23.5	27.6	19.9	21.0
100 percent to 199 percent	22.0	22.4	21.8	25.7	18.7	20.3	28.0	27.4	30.8	31.6	24.0	23.1	19.0	19.9	17.4	22.3	16.2	18.8
200 percent to 399 percent	18.0	19.0	18.9	18.4	14.7	15.2	21.4	25.7	25.9	22.7	20.8	19.5	16.4	15.9	15.7	16.4	11.8	13.0
400 percent or more	16.3	17.0	16.8	15.9	12.9	12.5	19.1	20.3	19.1	21.7	14.7	15.3	15.1	15.6	15.8	13.3	12.0	11.2
Hispanic Origin and Race and Percent of Poverty Level[3,4]																		
Hispanic or Latino																		
Below 100 percent	21.9	19.9	21.8	27.0	21.7	21.4	25.0	25.7	28.4	32.0	27.9	31.3	19.6	16.4	17.4	23.4	18.2	16.7
100 percent to 199 percent	20.8	18.2	17.8	23.3	18.1	17.6	28.8	20.8	26.1	31.6	24.9	18.8	15.6	16.6	13.1	18.0	15.3	17.0
200 percent to 399 percent	21.4	17.9	20.2	19.5	17.0	16.7	24.6	26.1	31.7	25.2	28.2	22.5	19.6	13.3	14.3	16.1	11.0	13.7
400 percent or more	17.7	17.6	15.3	21.4	16.0	11.6	*20.2	*22.9	23.3	28.6	*18.0	12.5	16.4	15.4	*11.5	18.0	14.9	11.1
Not Hispanic or Latino																		
White only																		
Below 100 percent	25.5	26.5	34.1	33.7	24.7	26.2	27.2	35.6	37.3	37.4	26.8	30.7	24.4	21.2	32.2	31.6	23.6	23.6
100 percent to 199 percent	22.3	24.7	22.8	26.3	17.8	22.6	25.8	29.2	30.7	29.2	21.5	26.7	20.7	22.7	19.1	24.7	15.9	20.2
200 percent to 399 percent	17.8	19.5	17.9	17.6	13.9	14.9	20.9	26.0	22.9	21.2	18.3	19.3	16.3	16.6	15.7	15.9	11.8	12.7
400 percent or more	16.5	16.9	16.8	15.5	12.7	12.6	19.0	18.5	18.7	21.0	15.0	16.1	15.4	16.2	16.0	13.2	11.7	11.1
Black or African American only																		
Below 100 percent	29.3	27.8	27.1	32.4	23.7	29.9	39.5	28.9	34.8	41.6	30.8	38.3	23.0	27.3	22.6	26.6	20.1	25.0
100 percent to 199 percent	22.5	20.8	24.1	27.5	23.5	19.1	31.7	35.3	33.3	34.5	29.3	17.7	18.5	13.8	20.3	23.7	20.6	19.9
200 percent to 399 percent	18.5	19.6	22.6	22.3	17.4	16.5	23.9	28.3	33.3	24.6	*27.1	20.2	16.3	16.2	17.8	21.4	13.8	15.1
400 percent or more	16.1	19.3	16.9	18.9	16.3	15.8	*18.8	32.8	*	*24.1	*	*	15.2	*13.9	17.4	16.1	*18.0	14.8
Health Insurance Status at the Time of Interview[5]																		
Insured	19.8	20.7	20.7	22.3	16.9	17.5	24.4	25.8	26.8	28.1	21.7	22.1	17.5	18.2	17.7	19.2	14.6	15.3
Private	17.5	18.4	17.4	17.1	12.5	13.2	20.9	22.8	21.7	21.8	16.7	15.5	15.9	16.5	15.5	14.9	10.6	12.1
Medicaid	28.2	28.6	28.5	30.0	22.8	23.4	33.0	33.2	35.5	35.5	27.3	29.7	24.1	25.5	23.6	26.4	20.4	19.8
Uninsured	20.2	17.2	18.4	19.4	14.3	16.6	23.0	24.5	26.6	24.0	*19.4	20.3	18.9	13.9	15.4	17.6	12.7	15.2
Health Insurance Status Prior to Interview[5]																		
Insured continuously all 12 months	19.6	20.2	20.5	22.2	16.8	17.4	24.1	25.3	26.7	28.1	21.4	21.9	17.3	17.8	17.3	19.1	14.6	15.1
Uninsured for any period up to 12 months	24.0	25.9	26.0	23.7	20.7	22.4	27.1	33.9	34.4	28.0	29.2	32.8	21.9	21.7	22.4	21.3	16.6	18.2
Uninsured more than 12 months	18.4	14.7	14.4	17.6	*10.4	10.4	19.3	19.1	*15.7	*21.3	*	*	18.1	13.1	14.0	16.7	*9.8	11.9
Percent of Poverty Level and Health Insurance Status Prior to Interview[4,5]																		
Below 100 percent																		
Insured continuously all 12 months	26.3	26.1	28.1	31.7	23.6	25.5	30.9	31.2	34.3	36.3	29.6	33.1	22.8	22.9	23.8	28.7	20.1	21.3
Uninsured for any period up to 12 months	26.5	30.8	31.2	30.3	23.8	32.0	29.7	34.6	39.1	34.7	*	*	24.4	28.4	*28.2	27.5	*24.7	27.0
Uninsured more than 12 months	17.5	15.6	15.7	*19.6	*	*	*16.0	*22.1	*	*	*	*	18.0	*13.2	*15.6	*16.0	*	*

NA = Not available.

* = Estimates are considered unreliable. Starting with 2016 data, the reliability of survey percentage estimates was assessed using new multistep National Center for Health Statistics data presentation standards for proportions. Prior to 2016 data, the reliability of estimates for earlier years was evaluated based on relative standard errors (RSE). Data preceded by an asterisk have an RSE of 20%–30%. Data not shown have an RSE greater than 30%.

[1] See the CDC Web site for more information.

[2] Includes all other races not shown separately and unknown health insurance status.

[3] The race groups White, Black, American Indian or Alaska Native, Asian, Native Hawaiian or Other Pacific Islander, and 2 or more races include persons of Hispanic and non-Hispanic origin. Persons of Hispanic origin may be of any race. Starting with 1999 data, race-specific estimates are tabulated according to the 1997 Revisions to the Standards for the Classification of Federal Data on Race and Ethnicity and are not strictly comparable with estimates for earlier years. The five single-race categories and multiple-race categories shown in the table conform to the 1997 Standards. Starting with 1999 data, race-specific estimates are for persons who reported only one racial group; the category 2 or more races includes persons who reported more than one racial group. Prior to 1999, data were tabulated according to the 1977 Standards with four racial groups, and the Asian only category included Native Hawaiian or Other Pacific Islander. Estimates for single-race categories prior to 1999 included persons who reported one race, or if they reported more than one race, identified one race as best representing their race. Starting with 2003 data, race responses of other race and unspecified multiple race were treated as missing, and then race was imputed if these were the only race responses. Almost all persons with a race response of other race were of Hispanic origin.

[4] Percent of poverty level is based on family income and family size and composition using U.S. Census Bureau poverty thresholds. Missing family data were imputed for 1997 and beyond.

[5] Health insurance categories are mutually exclusive. Persons who reported both Medicaid and private coverage are classified as having private coverage. Starting with 1997 data, state-sponsored health plan coverage is included as Medicaid coverage. Starting with 1999 data, coverage by the Children's Health Insurance Program (CHIP) is included with Medicaid coverage. In addition to private and Medicaid, the insured category also includes military, other government, and Medicare coverage. Persons not covered by private insurance, Medicaid, CHIP, state-sponsored or other government-sponsored health plans (starting in 1997), Medicare, or military plans are considered to have no health insurance coverage. Persons with only Indian Health Service coverage are considered to have no health insurance coverage.

Table 3-43. Emergency Department Visits Within the Past 12 Months Among Children Under 18 Years of Age, by Selected Characteristics, Selected Years, 1997–2016—*Continued*

(Percent; Data are based on household interviews of a sample of the civilian noninstitutionalized population.)

Characteristic	Under 18 years						Under 6 years						6 to 17 years					
	1997	2000	2005	2010	2015	2016	1997	2000	2005	2010	2015	2016	1997	2000	2005	2010	2015	2016
100 percent to 199 percent																		
Insured continuously all 12 months	21.8	23.8	22.1	26.2	18.5	20.0	28.0	28.2	31.0	32.4	23.4	22.9	18.6	21.4	17.4	22.4	16.1	18.5
Uninsured for any period up to 12 months	24.5	24.6	27.4	28.4	23.2	23.6	29.7	33.3	41.2	30.9	*34.5	*	21.0	20.3	21.9	27.0	*17.8	18.1
Uninsured more than 12 months	19.5	14.3	14.7	17.6	*	*	*22.5	*15.5	*	*	*	*	18.6	13.9	*14.5	*17.2	*	*
200 percent to 399 percent																		
Insured continuously all 12 months	17.7	18.9	18.8	18.4	14.7	15.4	21.2	25.0	25.5	22.8	20.1	19.6	16.1	16.1	15.6	16.3	12.1	13.3
Uninsured for any period up to 12 months	21.1	23.4	24.3	16.2	15.5	14.0	*19.5	33.0	35.1	*22.7	*25.9	*	22.1	*18.4	19.0	*12.6	*10.6	9.5
Uninsured more than 12 months	19.2	*14.7	*	*17.4	*	*	*22.7	*	*	*	*	*	17.6	*11.7	*	*18.7	*	*
400 percent or more																		
Insured continuously all 12 months	16.2	16.8	17.0	16.1	12.8	12.2	18.9	19.9	19.4	22.0	14.3	15.3	15.1	15.5	15.9	13.5	12.0	10.9
Uninsured for any period up to 12 months	*19.2	24.8	*	*	*	21.3	*	*37.0	*	*	*	*	*	*19.5	*	*	*	21.3
Uninsured more than 12 months	*	*	*	*	*	*	*	*	*	*	*	*	*	*	*	*	*	*
Geographic Region																		
Northeast	18.5	19.7	20.9	22.3	16.5	17.5	20.7	21.6	26.3	27.8	22.4	17.8	17.4	18.8	18.5	19.6	13.7	17.3
Midwest	19.5	20.3	21.8	23.3	19.1	20.2	26.0	25.6	30.1	28.8	23.5	27.1	16.4	17.8	17.8	20.7	17.1	17.0
South	21.8	21.9	21.7	23.4	17.6	16.4	25.6	28.6	27.1	30.4	23.5	21.7	19.9	18.7	18.8	19.5	14.9	13.6
West	18.5	18.0	16.7	19.1	13.7	16.7	23.5	24.7	22.9	23.3	17.2	21.0	15.9	14.7	13.8	16.8	11.9	14.6
Location of Residence																		
Within MSA[6]	19.7	19.9	20.0	21.8	16.4	16.7	23.9	24.5	25.7	27.7	21.1	20.8	17.4	17.6	17.2	18.6	14.0	14.7
Outside MSA[6]	20.8	21.9	22.4	24.2	20.0	22.2	26.2	31.3	31.8	28.6	25.6	29.3	18.6	17.8	18.2	22.1	17.3	18.6
PERCENT OF CHILDREN WITH TWO OR MORE EMERGENCY DEPARTMENT VISITS																		
All children[2]	10.8	7.0	8.2	5.8	5.6	5.4	7.2	4.5	4.2	10.8		7.0	5.8	5.6	5.4	7.2		4.5
Sex																		
Male	7.3	7.3	7.2	8.5	5.4	5.8	9.9	10.3	10.7	11.3	7.4	9.5	6.0	5.8	5.4	7.0	4.4	4.0
Female	6.9	6.7	6.5	8.3	5.3	5.2	9.4	9.6	8.9	10.3	6.5	6.9	5.7	5.3	5.3	7.3	4.7	4.3
Race[3]																		
White only	6.6	6.4	6.3	7.6	4.9	4.9	8.4	8.7	9.1	10.1	6.0	7.6	5.7	5.4	4.9	6.3	4.3	3.6
Black or African American only	9.6	10.5	9.2	12.6	7.6	8.4	14.9	16.2	12.7	15.7	10.0	12.4	6.9	7.9	7.5	11.0	6.3	6.3
American Indian or Alaska Native only	*	*	*	*	*13.5	*	*	*	*	*	*	*	*	*	*	*	*	*
Asian only	*5.7	*3.1	*4.6	7.3	*2.6	1.2	*12.9	*	*	*	*	1.1	*	*	*3.9	*7.1	*	1.3
Native Hawaiian and Other Pacific Islander only	NA	*	*	*	*	*	NA	*	*	*	*	*	NA	*	*	*	*	*
Two or more races	NA	*8.7	*8.6	10.3	6.7	9.8	NA	*14.3	*13.2	*11.7	*10.2	12.1	NA	*	*	*9.2	*	8.4
Hispanic Origin and Race[3]																		
Hispanic or Latino	8.9	7.0	7.7	8.6	6.2	5.8	11.8	9.4	12.1	11.7	8.6	9.6	7.0	5.6	5.2	6.6	5.0	3.9
Not Hispanic or Latino	6.8	7.0	6.6	8.4	5.0	5.4	9.2	10.1	9.2	10.5	6.4	7.8	5.7	5.6	5.4	7.3	4.3	4.3
White only	6.2	6.3	5.9	7.4	4.4	4.6	7.8	8.6	8.2	9.3	5.1	6.6	5.5	5.2	4.9	6.4	4.1	3.6
Black or African American only	9.3	10.6	9.1	12.3	7.4	8.7	14.6	16.6	12.4	15.8	9.8	12.8	6.8	7.9	7.5	10.4	6.2	6.6
Percent of Poverty Level[4]																		
Below 100 percent	11.1	11.9	11.2	13.4	8.9	10.4	14.5	16.4	15.9	15.3	11.8	15.6	8.9	9.4	8.4	12.1	7.4	7.6
100 percent to 199 percent	8.3	8.0	7.9	10.3	7.2	7.2	12.2	11.8	12.7	13.4	9.7	9.1	6.3	6.1	5.5	8.4	6.0	6.3
200 percent to 399 percent	6.2	5.6	5.7	6.3	3.4	3.8	7.4	8.0	7.6	7.3	4.1	6.2	5.6	4.5	4.8	5.9	3.0	2.6
400 percent or more	4.0	4.7	4.4	5.0	3.0	2.6	5.0	5.8	5.1	7.3	*3.5	4.0	3.6	4.2	4.0	3.9	2.7	2.0
Hispanic Origin and Race and Percent of Poverty Level[3,4]																		
Hispanic or Latino																		
Below 100 percent	10.4	8.2	10.0	9.9	7.0	8.3	13.9	10.9	13.8	10.9	*9.1	14.7	8.0	6.6	7.4	9.2	5.9	5.2
100 percent to 199 percent	8.2	7.4	6.1	9.4	7.3	6.5	12.0	8.5	*8.7	15.4	11.7	*	5.7	6.7	*4.7	5.5	5.5	4.8
200 percent to 399 percent	8.5	6.2	7.7	5.9	*4.0	3.2	10.0	9.2	14.2	*8.0	*5.7	6.4	*7.6	*4.5	*4.4	*4.6	*3.1	1.6
400 percent or more	*5.0	*4.0	*5.4	*6.5	*5.6	2.6	*	*	*	*	*	*	*	*	*	*5.2	*	2.4
Not Hispanic or Latino																		
White only																		
Below 100 percent	10.7	12.8	13.5	14.0	9.6	10.5	12.2	18.4	18.6	15.5	*10.1	12.2	9.8	*9.5	10.4	13.1	*9.4	9.6
100 percent to 199 percent	8.0	8.0	8.2	10.4	7.7	7.3	11.2	11.8	13.7	12.3	*8.6	7.8	6.4	6.3	*5.5	9.4	7.3	7.0
200 percent to 399 percent	6.0	5.4	5.1	5.7	2.9	3.8	6.7	7.7	6.1	*6.5	*2.8	6.1	5.6	4.4	4.6	5.4	*3.0	2.6
400 percent or more	3.7	4.5	3.7	5.0	2.6	2.5	4.6	4.5	4.1	7.6	*3.5	4.6	3.3	4.5	3.5	3.9	*2.2	1.6

NA = Not available.

* = Estimates are considered unreliable. Starting with 2016 data, the reliability of survey percentage estimates was assessed using new multistep National Center for Health Statistics data presentation standards for proportions. Prior to 2016 data, the reliability of estimates for earlier years was evaluated based on relative standard errors (RSE). Data preceded by an asterisk have an RSE of 20%–30%. Data not shown have an RSE greater than 30%.

[2]Includes all other races not shown separately and unknown health insurance status.

[3]The race groups White, Black, American Indian or Alaska Native, Asian, Native Hawaiian or Other Pacific Islander, and 2 or more races include persons of Hispanic and non-Hispanic origin. Persons of Hispanic origin may be of any race. Starting with 1999 data, race-specific estimates are tabulated according to the 1997 Revisions to the Standards for the Classification of Federal Data on Race and Ethnicity and are not strictly comparable with estimates for earlier years. The five single-race categories and multiple-race categories shown in the table conform to the 1997 Standards. Starting with 1999 data, race-specific estimates are for persons who reported only one racial group; the category 2 or more races includes persons who reported more than one racial group. Prior to 1999, data were tabulated according to the 1977 Standards with four racial groups, and the Asian only category included Native Hawaiian or Other Pacific Islander. Estimates for single-race categories prior to 1999 included persons who reported one race, or if they reported more than one race, identified one race as best representing their race. Starting with 2003 data, race responses of other race and unspecified multiple race were treated as missing, and then race was imputed if these were the only race responses. Almost all persons with a race response of other race were of Hispanic origin.

[4]Percent of poverty level is based on family income and family size and composition using U.S. Census Bureau poverty thresholds. Missing family data were imputed for 1997 and beyond.

[6]MSA is metropolitan statistical area. Starting with 2016 data, MSA status is determined using 2010 Census data and the 2010 standards for defining MSAs.

Table 3-43. Emergency Department Visits Within the Past 12 Months Among Children Under 18 Years of Age, by Selected Characteristics, Selected Years, 1997–2016—*Continued*

(Percent; Data are based on household interviews of a sample of the civilian noninstitutionalized population.)

Characteristic	Under 18 years						Under 6 years						6 to 17 years					
	1997	2000	2005	2010	2015	2016	1997	2000	2005	2010	2015	2016	1997	2000	2005	2010	2015	2016
Black or African American only																		
Below 100 percent	12.7	14.7	11.4	16.1	9.9	13.3	19.1	18.5	16.2	22.1	14.5	20.7	8.8	12.8	8.6	12.4	*7.5	8.9
100 percent to 199 percent	9.2	8.9	8.4	12.4	6.9	7.2	*13.5	17.5	*13.3	*14.6	*	*	*7.2	*4.8	*6.5	11.1	*6.5	*
200 percent to 399 percent	5.8	7.8	*7.6	9.9	*5.6	*	*8.9	*12.5	*	*10.2	*	*	*4.5	*6.0	*7.5	*9.8	*	*
400 percent or more	*	*8.9	*7.2	*3.7	*	*	*	*17.8	*	*	*	*	*	*	*	*	*	*
Health Insurance Status at the Time of Interview[5]																		
Insured	7.0	7.0	6.8	8.5	5.4	5.5	9.6	9.6	9.7	11.0	7.1	8.1	5.7	5.7	5.3	7.1	4.6	4.2
Private	5.2	5.2	5.0	5.5	3.0	2.8	6.8	7.1	6.2	7.4	3.5	3.6	4.5	4.5	4.4	4.6	2.8	2.4
Medicaid	13.1	13.1	11.1	12.8	8.8	9.0	16.2	15.9	15.8	15.3	11.5	13.4	10.4	11.2	7.7	11.2	7.4	6.6
Uninsured	7.7	6.6	7.0	8.0	*3.5	5.5	9.8	11.3	11.5	*8.5	*	*	6.8	4.5	5.4	7.8	*3.5	3.4
Health Insurance Status Prior to Interview[5]																		
Insured continuously all 12 months	6.9	6.7	6.7	8.4	5.3	5.5	9.4	9.2	9.7	10.8	6.9	8.1	5.7	5.5	5.2	7.1	4.5	4.2
Uninsured for any period up to 12 months	8.5	10.6	8.9	10.1	7.8	8.5	11.5	16.0	13.6	13.3	*10.1	*	6.6	7.7	6.9	8.4	*6.7	5.8
Uninsured more than 12 months	6.8	5.8	5.5	7.8	*	1.6	*8.6	8.9	*	*	*	*	6.2	4.7	5.3	*7.9	*	1.4
Geographic Region																		
Northeast	6.2	6.4	6.2	7.8	4.6	5.2	7.6	7.9	8.9	10.3	7.5	5.7	5.4	5.6	5.0	6.6	3.2	5.0
Midwest	6.6	6.6	6.9	9.1	5.7	6.7	10.4	9.0	9.6	11.4	6.5	10.7	4.8	5.5	5.5	8.0	5.3	4.8
South	8.0	8.5	7.9	9.1	5.9	5.6	10.1	12.6	10.8	12.9	7.6	9.1	6.9	6.6	6.3	7.1	5.1	3.8
West	7.1	5.4	5.5	7.2	4.5	4.5	10.0	8.5	9.1	7.6	6.2	6.5	5.6	3.9	3.9	7.0	3.6	3.6
Location of Residence																		
Within MSA[6]	7.2	6.6	6.7	8.3	5.0	5.2	9.6	8.9	9.5	10.6	6.6	7.8	5.9	5.5	5.2	7.0	4.2	4.0
Outside MSA[6]	6.8	8.6	7.5	9.3	7.2	7.4	9.7	15.0	11.2	12.2	9.5	10.7	5.6	5.8	5.9	7.9	6.2	5.6

* = Estimates are considered unreliable. Starting with 2016 data, the reliability of survey percentage estimates was assessed using new multistep National Center for Health Statistics data presentation standards for proportions. Prior to 2016 data, the reliability of estimates for earlier years was evaluated based on relative standard errors (RSE). Data preceded by an asterisk have an RSE of 20%–30%. Data not shown have an RSE greater than 30%.

[5]Health insurance categories are mutually exclusive. Persons who reported both Medicaid and private coverage are classified as having private coverage. Starting with 1997 data, state-sponsored health plan coverage is included as Medicaid coverage. Starting with 1999 data, coverage by the Children's Health Insurance Program (CHIP) is included with Medicaid coverage. In addition to private and Medicaid, the insured category also includes military, other government, and Medicare coverage. Persons not covered by private insurance, Medicaid, CHIP, state-sponsored or other government-sponsored health plans (starting in 1997), Medicare, or military plans are considered to have no health insurance coverage. Persons with only Indian Health Service coverage are considered to have no health insurance coverage.

[6]MSA is metropolitan statistical area. Starting with 2016 data, MSA status is determined using 2010 Census data and the 2010 standards for defining MSAs.

Table 3-44. Emergency Department Visits Within the Past 12 Months Among Adults 18 Years of Age and Over, by Selected Characteristics, Selected Years, 1997–2016

(Percent[1]; Data are based on household interviews of a sample of the civilian noninstitutionalized population.)

Characteristic	One or more emergency department visits						Two or more emergency department visits					
	1997	2000	2005	2010	2015	2016	1997	2000	2005	2010	2015	2016
18 years and over, age-adjusted[2,3]	19.6	20.2	20.5	21.4	18.8	19.4	6.7	6.9	7.1	7.8	6.9	6.8
18 years and over, crude[2]	19.6	20.1	20.4	21.3	18.8	19.4	6.7	6.8	7.0	7.7	6.9	6.8
Age												
18 to 44 years	20.7	20.5	20.8	22.0	18.6	18.8	6.8	7.0	7.1	8.4	6.9	6.5
18 to 24 years	26.3	25.7	25.3	25.4	20.5	20.6	9.1	8.8	8.9	9.6	7.5	7.2
25 to 44 years	19.0	18.8	19.2	20.7	17.9	18.1	6.2	6.4	6.5	8.0	6.7	6.2
45 to 64 years	16.2	17.6	18.2	19.2	17.4	18.1	5.6	5.6	6.4	6.7	6.1	6.6
45 to 54 years	15.7	17.9	17.6	18.6	16.4	18.4	5.5	5.8	6.1	6.6	6.0	6.7
55 to 64 years	16.9	17.0	19.0	19.8	18.4	17.8	5.7	5.3	6.8	6.8	6.2	6.4
65 years and over	22.0	23.7	23.7	23.7	21.8	23.3	8.1	8.6	8.2	7.7	8.2	8.0
65 to 74 years	20.3	21.6	20.8	20.7	18.3	20.5	7.1	7.4	7.4	6.4	6.9	6.4
75 years and over	24.3	26.2	27.1	27.4	26.7	27.4	9.3	10.0	9.1	9.4	10.0	10.3
Sex[3]												
Male	19.1	18.7	18.6	18.5	16.9	17.0	5.9	5.7	5.9	6.0	5.7	5.6
Female	20.2	21.6	22.3	24.3	20.6	21.7	7.5	7.9	8.2	9.6	8.1	8.0
Race[3,4]												
White only	19.0	19.4	19.8	20.7	18.0	18.9	6.2	6.4	6.5	7.2	6.4	6.3
Black or African American only	25.9	26.5	26.3	28.6	26.6	25.6	11.1	10.8	11.9	12.6	10.9	10.8
American Indian or Alaska Native only	24.8	30.3	31.0	22.6	28.3	26.7	13.1	*12.6	*11.1	*11.8	16.1	11.7
Asian only	11.6	13.6	15.4	13.3	9.4	11.5	*2.9	*3.8	*3.8	3.3	2.7	3.2
Native Hawaiian and Other Pacific Islander only	NA	*	*	*	*	15.2	NA	*	*	*	*	*
Two or more races	NA	32.5	25.7	29.7	27.1	23.1	NA	11.3	12.8	11.1	12.4	10.7
American Indian or Alaska Native; White	NA	33.9	29.3	31.1	29.0	29.2	NA	*9.4	*15.3	*15.2	*14.1	15.2
Hispanic Origin and Race[3,4]												
Hispanic or Latino	19.2	18.3	20.1	19.8	17.3	18.9	7.4	7.0	7.1	6.9	6.4	6.9
Mexican	17.8	17.4	17.2	18.1	16.0	18.2	6.4	7.1	5.8	6.1	6.0	6.3
Not Hispanic or Latino	19.7	20.6	20.7	21.9	19.2	19.6	6.7	6.9	7.1	8.1	7.0	6.9
White only	19.1	19.8	20.1	21.1	18.3	19.2	6.2	6.4	6.4	7.4	6.4	6.4
Black or African American only	25.9	26.5	26.2	29.0	26.5	25.8	11.0	10.8	11.9	12.7	10.8	10.8
Percent of Poverty Level[3,5]												
Below 100 percent	28.1	29.0	29.8	30.6	29.5	29.8	12.8	13.3	13.7	14.9	14.7	14.4
100 percent to 199 percent	23.8	23.9	23.2	25.6	24.1	25.5	9.3	9.6	9.6	10.5	9.9	10.2
200 percent to 399 percent	18.3	19.8	20.2	20.4	17.1	19.2	5.9	6.3	6.5	6.8	6.2	6.1
400 percent or more	15.9	16.8	16.9	17.0	14.3	13.9	3.9	4.5	4.5	4.7	3.6	3.7
Hispanic Origin and Race and Percent of Poverty Level[3,4,5]												
Hispanic or Latino												
Below 100 percent	22.1	22.4	24.0	23.6	22.6	24.8	9.8	9.7	9.2	11.5	11.5	11.1
100 percent to 199 percent	19.2	18.1	18.7	19.9	17.7	19.2	8.1	6.7	7.1	6.3	6.7	6.9
200 percent to 399 percent	18.5	17.3	18.9	18.1	13.3	19.2	6.0	7.4	5.9	5.2	4.1	6.0
400 percent or more	14.6	16.4	20.9	18.8	17.5	13.8	*3.8	*4.3	*6.9	*5.5	*4.4	4.3
Not Hispanic or Latino												
White only												
Below 100 percent	29.5	30.1	30.8	33.3	32.0	31.6	13.0	13.9	13.7	15.5	16.0	14.7
100 percent to 199 percent	24.3	25.5	24.3	26.8	26.0	28.5	9.1	10.4	9.8	11.2	10.5	11.6
200 percent to 399 percent	18.1	20.1	20.7	20.3	17.4	19.4	5.8	6.3	6.4	6.5	6.4	6.1
400 percent or more	15.8	16.3	16.2	16.9	14.0	14.2	3.8	4.1	4.0	4.9	3.5	3.6
Black or African American only												
Below 100 percent	34.6	35.4	35.4	36.9	35.8	35.3	17.5	17.4	18.3	20.2	17.1	20.6
100 percent to 199 percent	29.2	28.5	28.9	33.5	32.6	30.6	12.8	12.2	14.2	15.9	14.0	13.7
200 percent to 399 percent	20.8	23.2	21.5	25.7	22.2	22.9	8.1	8.0	8.7	10.2	8.3	7.4
400 percent or more	18.2	22.6	22.6	18.8	18.3	16.2	5.9	8.8	*9.2	*4.0	5.4	4.0
Health Insurance Status at the Time of Interview[6,7]												
18 to 64 years												
Insured	18.8	19.5	20.0	20.8	18.0	18.7	6.1	6.4	6.6	7.5	6.5	6.5
Private	16.9	17.6	17.3	17.4	14.1	14.5	4.7	5.1	4.8	5.2	3.9	3.8
Medicaid	37.6	42.2	40.1	40.2	34.9	35.4	19.7	21.0	20.1	21.1	18.0	16.8
Uninsured	20.0	19.3	19.5	21.3	18.0	17.6	7.5	6.9	8.0	8.9	6.9	6.6

NA = Not available.

* = Estimates are considered unreliable. Starting with 2016 data, the reliability of survey percentage estimates was assessed using new multistep National Center for Health Statistics data presentation standards for proportions. Prior to 2016 data, the reliability of estimates for earlier years was evaluated based on relative standard errors (RSE). Data preceded by an asterisk have an RSE of 20%–30%. Data not shown have an RSE greater than 30%.

[1]See the CDC Web site for more information.

[2]Includes all other races not shown separately and unknown health insurance status.

[3]Estimates are for persons aged 18 and over and are age-adjusted to the year 2000 standard population using five age groups: 18–44 years, 45–54 years, 55–64 years, 65–74 years, and 75 years and over.

[4]The race groups White, Black, American Indian or Alaska Native, Asian, Native Hawaiian or Other Pacific Islander, and 2 or more races include persons of Hispanic and non-Hispanic origin. Persons of Hispanic origin may be of any race. Starting with 1999 data, race-specific estimates are tabulated according to the 1997 Revisions to the Standards for the Classification of Federal Data on Race and Ethnicity and are not strictly comparable with estimates for earlier years. The five single-race categories and multiple-race categories shown in the table conform to the 1997 Standards. Starting with 1999 data, race-specific estimates are for persons who reported only one racial group; the category 2 or more races includes persons who reported more than one racial group. Prior to 1999, data were tabulated according to the 1977 Standards with four racial groups, and the Asian only category included Native Hawaiian or Other Pacific Islander. Estimates for single-race categories prior to 1999 included persons who reported one race, or if they reported more than one race, identified one race as best representing their race. Starting with 2003 data, race responses of other race and unspecified multiple race were treated as missing, and then race was imputed if these were the only race responses. Almost all persons with a race response of other race were of Hispanic origin.

[5]Percent of poverty level is based on family income and family size and composition using U.S. Census Bureau poverty thresholds. Missing family data were imputed for 1997 and beyond.

[6]Estimates for persons aged 18–64 are age-adjusted to the year 2000 standard population using three age groups: 18–44 years, 45–54 years, and 55–64 years.

[7]Health insurance categories are mutually exclusive. Persons who reported both Medicaid and private coverage are classified as having private coverage. Starting with 1997 data, state-sponsored health plan coverage is included as Medicaid coverage. Starting with 1999 data, coverage by the Children's Health Insurance Program (CHIP) is included with Medicaid coverage. In addition to private and Medicaid, the insured category also includes military, other government, and Medicare coverage. Persons not covered by private insurance, Medicaid, CHIP, state-sponsored or other government-sponsored health plans (starting in 1997), Medicare, or military plans are considered to have no health insurance coverage. Persons with only Indian Health Service coverage are considered to have no health insurance coverage.

Table 3-44. Emergency Department Visits Within the Past 12 Months Among Adults 18 Years of Age and Over, by Selected Characteristics, Selected Years, 1997–2016—*Continued*

(Percent[1]; Data are based on household interviews of a sample of the civilian noninstitutionalized population.)

Characteristic	One or more emergency department visits						Two or more emergency department visits					
	1997	2000	2005	2010	2015	2016	1997	2000	2005	2010	2015	2016
Health Insurance Status Prior to Interview[6,7]												
18 to 64 years												
Insured continuously all 12 months	18.3	19.0	19.4	20.2	17.6	18.2	5.8	6.1	6.3	7.1	6.2	6.1
Uninsured for any period up to 12 months	25.5	28.2	28.0	26.0	22.6	24.6	9.4	10.3	12.4	12.5	9.9	10.5
Uninsured more than 12 months	18.9	17.3	18.0	20.6	16.6	15.4	7.1	6.4	7.0	8.1	6.4	5.5
Percent of Poverty Level and Health Insurance Status Prior to Interview[5,6,7]												
18 to 64 years												
Below 100 percent												
Insured continuously all 12 months	30.2	31.6	33.6	35.2	31.7	30.8	14.7	15.4	15.3	18.3	16.7	14.8
Uninsured for any period up to 12 months	34.1	43.7	39.1	34.2	32.7	38.1	16.1	18.1	21.5	16.5	15.3	19.2
Uninsured more than 12 months	20.8	20.5	20.5	23.4	21.6	19.1	8.1	9.1	8.5	11.7	8.8	9.3
100 percent to 199 percent												
Insured continuously all 12 months	24.5	25.5	23.7	26.1	25.1	26.0	8.9	10.2	9.8	10.8	10.2	10.5
Uninsured for any period up to 12 months	28.7	27.7	28.4	29.7	26.7	30.2	12.3	11.7	12.7	15.6	13.8	12.1
Uninsured more than 12 months	19.0	17.4	18.5	21.2	17.4	15.2	8.3	6.4	7.7	7.8	6.6	4.3
200 to 399 percent												
Insured continuously all 12 months	17.5	19.5	19.7	19.6	15.7	18.6	5.3	6.3	6.4	6.0	5.5	5.7
Uninsured for any period up to 12 months	21.6	24.6	26.8	25.4	18.9	18.9	6.6	7.3	10.6	12.2	7.3	8.4
Uninsured more than 12 months	16.8	15.6	14.7	17.6	12.4	14.2	5.9	4.5	4.5	5.7	*5.7	4.5
400 percent or more												
Insured continuously all 12 months	14.9	15.5	15.6	15.9	13.2	12.5	3.7	3.7	3.6	4.5	3.0	3.0
Uninsured for any period up to 12 months	18.0	20.1	20.2	12.5	*14.5	13.8	*3.1	6.4	7.2	*	*	3.9
Uninsured more than 12 months	19.1	15.8	17.9	19.4	*8.7	*	*	*5.2	*7.4	*	*	1.2
Level of difficulty[3,8]												
A lot of difficulty or cannot do at all	NA	NA	NA	43.2	39.1	41.1	NA	NA	NA	25.2	21.0	20.0
Some difficulty	NA	NA	NA	26.6	23.7	24.4	NA	NA	NA	11.0	8.7	8.6
No difficulty	NA	NA	NA	17.1	13.5	14.2	NA	NA	NA	4.5	3.9	3.9
Geographic Region[3]												
Northeast	19.5	20.0	21.6	22.6	18.1	20.0	6.9	6.2	7.2	8.4	5.8	6.7
Midwest	19.3	20.1	21.6	22.3	20.5	21.1	6.2	6.9	7.2	8.2	8.1	7.5
South	20.9	21.2	20.7	22.1	19.5	19.3	7.3	7.6	7.6	8.0	7.0	7.4
West	17.7	18.6	17.8	18.9	16.6	17.9	6.0	6.3	6.0	6.7	6.4	5.5
Location of Residence[3,9]												
Within MSA	19.1	19.6	20.1	20.8	18.2	18.9	6.4	6.6	6.8	7.5	6.5	6.4
Outside MSA	21.5	22.5	22.3	25.5	22.8	23.4	7.8	7.8	8.1	9.8	9.6	9.4

NA = Not available.

* = Estimates are considered unreliable. Starting with 2016 data, the reliability of survey percentage estimates was assessed using new multistep National Center for Health Statistics data presentation standards for proportions. Prior to 2016 data, the reliability of estimates for earlier years was evaluated based on relative standard errors (RSE). Data preceded by an asterisk have an RSE of 20%–30%. Data not shown have an RSE greater than 30%.
[1]See the CDC Web site for more information.
[3]Estimates are for persons aged 18 and over and are age-adjusted to the year 2000 standard population using five age groups: 18–44 years, 45–54 years, 55–64 years, 65–74 years, and 75 years and over.
[5]Percent of poverty level is based on family income and family size and composition using U.S. Census Bureau poverty thresholds. Missing family data were imputed for 1997 and beyond.
[6]Estimates for persons aged 18–64 are age-adjusted to the year 2000 standard population using three age groups: 18–44 years, 45–54 years, and 55–64 years.
[7]Health insurance categories are mutually exclusive. Persons who reported both Medicaid and private coverage are classified as having private coverage. Starting with 1997 data, state-sponsored health plan coverage is included as Medicaid coverage. Starting with 1999 data, coverage by the Children's Health Insurance Program (CHIP) is included with Medicaid coverage. In addition to private and Medicaid, the insured category also includes military, other government, and Medicare coverage. Persons not covered by private insurance, Medicaid, CHIP, state-sponsored or other government-sponsored health plans (starting in 1997), Medicare, or military plans are considered to have no health insurance coverage. Persons with only Indian Health Service coverage are considered to have no health insurance coverage.
[8]Functional limitation is defined by the reported level of difficulty in six functioning domains: seeing (even if wearing glasses), hearing (even if wearing hearing aids), mobility (walking or climbing stairs), communication (understanding or being understood by others), cognition (remembering or concentrating), and self-care (such as washing all over or dressing). Respondents with answers to one or more of the six questions were included in one of three mutually exclusive categories. Those responding "A lot of difficulty" or "Cannot do at all/unable to do" to at least one question were classified in the "A lot of difficulty/cannot do" category. Of the remaining, those responding "Some difficulty" to at least one question were classified in the "Some difficulty" category, and those responding "No difficulty" to at least one question were classified in the "No difficulty" category. Those responding "Don't know" or "Refused" on all six questions were excluded. During 2010–2016, 1%–8% of respondents were missing data and excluded.
[9]MSA is metropolitan statistical area. Starting with 2016 data, MSA status is determined using 2010 Census data and the 2010 standards for defining MSAs.

Table 3-45. Initial Injury-Related Visits to Hospital Emergency Departments, by Sex, Age, and Intent and Mechanism of Injury, Selected Annual Averages, 2005–2006 Through 2014–2015

(Numbers in thousands; rate per 10,000 population; data are based on reporting by a sample of hospital emergency departments.)

Sex, age, and intent and mechanism of injury[1]	Initial injury-related visits in thousands									Initial injury-related visits per 10,000 persons								
	2005–2006	2007–2008	2008–2009	2009–2010	2010–2011	2011–2012	2012–2013	2013–2014	2014–2015	2005–2006	2007–2008	2008–2009	2009–2010	2010–2011	2011–2012	2012–2013	2013–2014	2014–2015
Both Sexes																		
All ages, age-adjusted[2,3]	X	X	X	X	X	X	X	X	X	1,076.4	960.9	1,040.8	1,063.2	1,084.0	1,029.7	983.4	1,047.8	1,078.1
All ages, crude[2]	31,706	28,699	31,328	32,204	33,007	31,546	30,402	32,595	33,649	1,068.6	951.3	1,029.4	1,049.7	1,067.9	1,012.6	968.9	1,030.7	1,055.1
Unintentional injuries[4]	25,658	23,670	25,725	26,523	27,275	25,955	25,078	27,422	28,849	864.7	784.6	845.3	864.5	882.4	833.2	799.2	867.1	904.6
Falls	8,100	8,144	8,900	9,393	9,932	9,225	8,760	9,693	10,060	273.0	270.0	292.4	306.2	321.3	296.1	279.2	306.5	315.4
Struck by or against objects or persons	2,935	2,746	2,916	3,055	3,166	3,106	3,149	3,154	2,982	98.9	91.0	95.8	99.6	102.4	99.7	100.4	99.7	93.5
Motor vehicle traffic	3,714	3,387	3,508	3,622	3,557	3,199	3,207	3,636	4,042	125.2	112.3	115.3	118.1	115.1	102.7	102.2	115.0	126.7
Cut or pierce	2,145	1,944	2,008	1,829	1,922	1,941	1,699	1,801	2,091	72.3	64.4	66.0	59.6	62.2	62.3	54.1	57.0	65.6
Intentional injuries	1,977	1,888	2,313	2,418	2,446	2,119	1,692	1,927	2,104	66.6	62.6	76.0	78.8	79.1	68.0	53.9	60.9	66.0
Male																		
All ages, age-adjusted[2,3]	X	X	X	X	X	X	X	X	X	1,166.1	1,039.7	1,118.0	1,143.0	1,164.5	1,094.6	1,000.4	1,083.5	1,139.7
All ages, crude[2]	16,966	15,332	16,640	17,124	17,483	16,474	15,184	16,550	17,471	1,164.2	1,033.8	1,111.8	1,133.8	1,150.5	1,077.8	985.9	1,066.0	1,115.9
Unintentional injuries[4]	13,736	12,611	13,590	14,083	14,451	13,503	12,447	13,950	15,119	942.5	850.3	908.0	932.4	951.0	883.4	808.1	898.6	965.7
Falls	3,685	3,581	3,944	4,285	4,689	4,205	3,649	4,032	4,389	252.9	241.4	263.5	283.7	308.6	275.1	236.9	259.7	280.4
Struck by or against objects or persons	1,833	1,771	1,863	1,931	2,008	1,903	1,781	1,857	1,813	125.8	119.4	124.4	127.8	132.2	124.5	115.6	119.6	115.8
Motor vehicle traffic	1,733	1,693	1,734	1,762	1,710	1,515	1,519	1,842	1,996	118.9	114.2	115.8	116.7	112.5	99.1	98.6	118.7	127.5
Cut or pierce	1,392	1,270	1,263	1,183	1,236	1,224	1,042	1,154	1,362	95.5	85.7	84.4	78.3	81.4	80.1	67.7	74.3	87.0
Intentional injuries	1,135	1,020	1,266	1,348	1,396	1,169	907	1,004	1,003	77.8	68.8	84.6	89.3	91.8	76.5	58.9	64.7	64.1
Under 18 years[2]	5,072	4,602	5,132	5,403	5,309	4,598	4,117	4,649	5,223	1,346.6	1,216.8	1,351.1	1,416.3	1,397.8	1,218.1	1,093.6	1,236.6	1,389.1
Unintentional injuries[4]	4,391	3,995	4,509	4,817	4,724	4,058	3,641	4,152	4,741	1,165.8	1,056.3	1,187.1	1,262.9	1,243.9	1,075.2	967.0	1,104.4	1,261.0
Falls	1,362	1,305	1,512	1,647	1,737	1,441	1,092	1,331	1,611	361.5	345.0	398.1	431.8	457.4	381.9	290.1	354.1	428.5
Struck by or against objects or persons	816	850	909	1,022	997	827	735	807	891	216.6	224.6	239.2	267.9	262.6	219.2	195.2	214.6	236.9
Motor vehicle traffic	357	265	305	309	301	239	198	184	213	94.8	70.0	80.3	81.0	79.1	63.2	52.6	48.9	56.6
Cut or pierce	291	264	284	248	238	273	265	261	332	77.3	69.8	74.8	64.9	62.7	72.4	70.5	69.5	88.4
Intentional injuries	190	198	194	173	167	125	*122	*189	*192	50.4	52.2	51.1	45.3	44.1	33.1	*32.5	*50.3	*51.0
18 to 24 years[2]	2,552	2,305	2,562	2,516	2,511	2,337	2,122	2,264	2,316	1,729.5	1,547.4	1,695.5	1,630.1	1,612.1	1,495.4	1,348.5	1,435.4	1,474.1
Unintentional injuries[4]	1,985	1,788	1,947	1,878	1,890	1,790	1,634	1,758	1,877	1,345.4	1,200.6	1,288.6	1,216.7	1,213.7	1,145.7	1,038.4	1,114.7	1,194.2
Falls	318	309	366	375	390	347	268	240	252	215.2	207.7	242.4	243.0	250.4	222.3	170.3	152.4	160.2
Struck by or against objects or persons	290	280	283	216	259	290	227	231	218	196.9	188.0	187.4	140.2	166.6	185.4	144.0	146.5	138.5
Motor vehicle traffic	386	366	373	406	357	331	343	371	484	261.6	245.8	247.0	263.2	229.3	211.6	217.9	235.4	308.3
Cut or pierce	265	190	215	187	192	179	152	170	179	179.5	127.8	142.6	121.4	123.5	114.5	96.8	107.8	113.7
Intentional injuries	273	308	381	389	403	318	216	250	248	185.2	206.9	252.2	252.2	258.7	203.2	137.3	158.8	157.7
25 to 44 years[2]	5,199	4,471	4,611	4,719	4,850	4,867	4,429	4,592	4,802	1,243.6	1,072.7	1,109.5	1,140.9	1,184.3	1,194.1	1,079.9	1,111.0	1,151.4
Unintentional injuries[4]	4,001	3,531	3,540	3,577	3,690	3,673	3,426	3,781	4,039	957.1	847.0	851.8	864.8	901.1	901.0	835.4	914.7	968.5
Falls	763	677	703	739	815	813	791	767	718	182.4	162.5	169.2	178.7	199.1	199.4	192.8	185.5	172.3
Struck by or against objects or persons	472	384	401	400	452	500	495	462	446	112.9	92.1	96.4	96.8	110.4	122.6	120.7	111.7	106.8
Motor vehicle traffic	629	638	578	585	591	501	509	689	722	150.5	153.0	139.1	141.5	144.3	122.8	124.1	166.7	173.1
Cut or pierce	480	426	401	380	423	464	354	385	415	114.8	102.2	96.5	91.9	103.2	113.9	86.4	93.3	99.6
Intentional injuries	436	350	495	586	589	528	424	391	358	104.4	83.9	119.2	141.6	143.8	129.5	103.4	94.6	85.9
45 to 64 years[2]	2,842	2,707	2,996	3,071	3,270	3,193	3,101	3,350	3,303	790.0	718.3	780.7	788.7	822.7	791.7	767.3	825.7	809.0
Unintentional injuries[4]	2,275	2,223	2,437	2,531	2,741	2,671	2,505	2,714	2,764	632.5	590.0	635.1	649.9	689.6	662.3	620.0	668.9	677.1
Falls	599	651	669	775	909	790	716	767	811	166.6	172.8	174.2	199.0	228.6	195.9	177.2	189.1	198.7
Struck by or against objects or persons	208	205	216	208	204	219	256	245	185	57.9	54.3	56.4	53.3	51.4	54.4	63.4	60.4	45.2
Motor vehicle traffic	262	331	375	334	334	350	389	485	440	72.9	87.9	97.7	85.9	84.0	86.7	96.3	119.6	107.8
Cut or pierce	285	309	306	297	294	231	190	231	264	79.2	81.9	79.7	76.2	73.9	57.4	47.1	56.9	64.7
Intentional injuries	205	145	168	180	219	170	130	169	196	57.1	38.4	43.9	46.2	55.2	42.1	32.1	41.7	48.0
65 years and over[2]	1,301	1,247	1,340	1,415	1,544	1,478	1,415	1,695	1,827	837.5	768.6	805.1	824.7	871.6	804.3	736.6	848.3	881.8
Unintentional injuries[4]	1,082	1,073	1,157	1,280	1,406	1,311	1,240	1,545	1,698	696.8	661.7	695.2	746.1	793.5	713.1	645.5	773.6	819.5
Falls	644	638	694	749	838	814	782	926	997	414.5	393.2	416.7	436.3	473.0	442.7	407.3	463.8	481.2
Struck by or against objects or persons	46	*52	*54	84	95	*66	*67	*112	*75	29.8	*32.3	*32.2	49.1	53.6	*36.1	*35.1	*55.9	*36.0
Motor vehicle traffic	98	93	103	127	128	*96	*79	*113	137	63.4	57.4	61.7	74.1	72.1	*52.0	*41.4	*56.5	66.1
Cut or pierce	70	81	*57	71	90	*76	*80	106	*172	45.3	50.0	*34.0	41.1	50.6	*41.4	*41.7	53.0	*82.9
Intentional injuries	*	*	*	*	*	*	*	*	*	*	*	*	*	*	*	*	*	*
Female																		
All ages, age-adjusted[2,3]	X	X	X	X	X	X	X	X	X	980.5	874.2	955.6	976.8	997.2	958.5	959.0	1,006.8	1,012.5
All ages, crude[2]	14,740	13,367	14,688	15,080	15,524	15,072	15,218	16,046	16,178	976.3	871.6	949.7	968.2	988.0	949.9	952.6	996.6	996.4
Unintentional injuries[4]	11,922	11,060	12,134	12,439	12,824	12,451	12,632	13,472	13,730	789.7	721.1	784.6	798.6	816.1	784.7	790.7	836.7	845.6
Falls	4,415	4,564	4,956	5,109	5,243	5,020	5,111	5,661	5,671	292.4	297.6	320.4	328.0	333.6	316.4	319.9	351.6	349.3

NOTE: An emergency department visit was considered injury-related if the first-listed diagnosis was injury-related (International Classification of Diseases, Ninth Revision, Clinical Modification [ICD-9-CM] codes 800–909.2, 909.4, 909.9–994.9, 995.50–995.59, and 995.80–995.85) or the first-listed external cause code (E code) was injury-related (ICD-9-CM codes E800–E869, E880–E929, and E950–E999). See: https://www.cdc.gov/nchs/injury/injury_tools.htm for codes used to classify injury-related visits in this table. Visits with a first-listed diagnosis or first-listed E code describing a complication or adverse effect of medical care were not considered injury-related. For more information on injury-related visits, see: Bergen G, Chen LH, Warner M, Fingerhut LA. *Injury in the United States: 2007 Chartbook.* Hyattsville, MD: National Center for Health Statistics. 2008. Available from: https://www.cdc.gov/nchs/data/misc/injury2007.pdf. Estimates for first- listed injury-related visits were further limited to those visits that were initial visits for the injury. This was determined using an imputed variable in 2005–2006; for 2007 and beyond, this was determined by using the initial visit episode of care information collected on the questionnaire. Limiting the estimates to initial visits decreases the total number of injury-related visits by 9% in 2005–2006, 14% in 2007–2008, 10%–13% in 2008–2009 through 2012–2013, and 6%–7% in 2013–2014 and 2014–2015. Rates were calculated using U.S. Census Bureau estimates of the civilian population of the United States, including institutionalized persons. Rates for 2005–2010 were computed using 2000-based postcensal population estimates. Rates for 2011 and beyond were computed using 2010-based postcensal population estimates. Data for additional years are available. See the Excel spreadsheet on the *Health, United States* website at: https://www.cdc.gov/nchs/hus.htm.
X = Not applicable.
* = Estimates are considered unreliable. Data preceded by an asterisk have a relative standard error (RSE) of 20%–30%. Data not shown have an RSE greater than 30%.
[1] Intent and mechanism of injury are based on the first-listed external cause-of-injury code (E code). Intentional injuries include self-inflicted injuries and assaults.
[2] Includes all injury-related visits not shown separately in table, including those with undetermined intent (1% in 2014–2015) and insufficient or no information to code cause of injury (7% in 2014–2015).
[3] Rates are age adjusted to the year 2000 standard population using six age groups: under 18 years, 18 to 24 years, 25 to 44 years, 45 to 64 years, 65 to 74 years, and 75 years and over.
[4] Includes unintentional injury-related visits with mechanism of injury not shown in table.

Table 3-45. Initial Injury-Related Visits to Hospital Emergency Departments, by Sex, Age, and Intent and Mechanism of Injury, Selected Annual Averages, 2005–2006 Through 2014–2015—*Continued*

(Numbers in thousands; rate per 10,000 population; data are based on reporting by a sample of hospital emergency departments.)

Sex, age, and intent and mechanism of injury[1]	Initial injury-related visits in thousands									Initial injury-related visits per 10,000 persons								
	2005–2006	2007–2008	2008–2009	2009–2010	2010–2011	2011–2012	2012–2013	2013–2014	2014–2015	2005–2006	2007–2008	2008–2009	2009–2010	2010–2011	2011–2012	2012–2013	2013–2014	2014–2015
Struck by or against objects or persons	1,102	976	1,053	1,124	1,158	1,204	1,368	1,297	1,169	73.0	63.6	68.1	72.2	73.7	75.9	85.7	80.6	72.0
Motor vehicle traffic	1,981	1,695	1,774	1,860	1,847	1,684	1,688	1,794	2,046	131.2	110.5	114.7	119.4	117.6	106.1	105.7	111.4	126.0
Cut or pierce	753	673	745	646	685	717	657	648	728	49.9	43.9	48.2	41.5	43.6	45.2	41.1	40.2	44.9
Intentional injuries	843	867	1,048	1,070	1,050	951	785	923	1,100	55.8	56.5	67.7	68.7	66.8	59.9	49.1	57.3	67.8
Under 18 years[2]	3,625	3,062	3,508	3,645	3,673	3,643	3,602	3,792	3,929	1,008.7	848.2	967.5	1,001.6	1,013.2	1,009.5	1,000.4	1,053.8	1,091.0
Unintentional injuries[4]	3,058	2,690	3,008	3,115	3,120	3,096	3,105	3,256	3,419	851.1	745.3	829.5	855.9	860.7	857.9	862.2	904.8	949.4
Falls	1,039	1,014	1,096	1,144	1,138	1,093	1,047	1,127	1,232	289.1	280.9	302.3	314.3	314.0	302.8	290.9	313.1	342.0
Struck by or against objects or persons	419	391	439	454	425	473	522	504	489	116.7	108.3	121.1	124.7	117.2	131.0	145.0	140.1	135.7
Motor vehicle traffic	367	282	249	285	302	275	273	262	328	102.1	78.2	68.6	78.3	83.4	76.1	75.8	72.9	91.1
Cut or pierce	160	145	154	139	158	167	*148	137	*183	44.4	40.1	42.4	38.2	43.7	46.2	*41.0	38.1	*50.9
Intentional injuries	188	163	222	207	196	193	144	*198	*244	52.3	45.1	61.4	56.8	54.1	53.6	39.9	*55.1	*67.8
18 to 24 years[2]	1,882	1,698	1,736	1,854	1,936	1,790	1,769	1,753	1,824	1,329.3	1,186.5	1,194.5	1,259.9	1,297.1	1,180.1	1,160.3	1,148.1	1,199.5
Unintentional injuries[4]	1,431	1,318	1,325	1,437	1,530	1,370	1,367	1,411	1,474	1,010.5	921.0	911.7	976.4	1,025.0	903.7	896.7	924.5	969.6
Falls	290	301	307	299	305	288	326	347	340	205.0	210.5	210.9	203.5	204.5	190.0	214.2	227.0	223.6
Struck by or against objects or persons	146	106	110	135	171	142	129	130	140	103.4	74.0	75.4	91.6	114.7	93.9	84.4	85.2	91.8
Motor vehicle traffic	397	378	360	426	460	387	372	353	357	280.6	264.5	247.5	289.8	308.1	255.4	244.3	231.1	235.0
Cut or pierce	116	89	77	*81	*94	*81	81	83	*89	82.2	61.9	53.2	*55.1	*63.3	*53.6	53.2	54.2	*58.4
Intentional injuries	176	209	232	262	251	198	151	153	201	124.2	145.8	159.7	177.9	168.4	130.8	99.2	99.9	132.4
25 to 44 years[2]	4,173	3,733	4,087	4,152	4,233	3,956	3,914	4,308	4,415	1,004.2	905.4	996.6	1,016.6	1,034.6	962.1	947.8	1,035.7	1,052.6
Unintentional injuries[4]	3,266	2,865	3,179	3,244	3,308	3,123	3,105	3,490	3,575	785.8	694.7	775.1	794.2	808.5	759.5	751.8	839.1	852.3
Falls	873	900	1,004	986	941	908	921	1,015	1,009	210.1	218.2	244.7	241.4	229.9	220.8	223.0	244.1	240.5
Struck by or against objects or persons	309	216	198	250	284	251	326	333	270	74.3	52.4	48.3	61.2	69.4	60.9	79.0	80.0	64.4
Motor vehicle traffic	719	572	621	612	616	554	529	718	814	173.1	138.8	151.3	149.9	150.5	134.8	128.0	172.5	194.1
Cut or pierce	269	214	270	230	219	227	215	226	240	64.7	51.8	65.9	56.4	53.6	55.3	52.1	54.3	57.2
Intentional injuries	313	345	396	396	408	367	310	340	416	75.4	83.6	96.5	96.9	99.8	89.3	75.0	81.8	99.2
45 to 64 years[2]	2,904	2,681	3,061	3,106	3,101	3,106	3,173	3,335	3,264	767.8	677.5	760.0	759.3	741.9	732.3	746.6	781.7	760.8
Unintentional injuries[4]	2,278	2,209	2,539	2,536	2,519	2,521	2,538	2,696	2,734	602.2	558.3	630.4	619.9	602.7	594.4	597.4	631.9	637.0
Falls	865	886	1,012	1,067	1,075	1,005	993	1,244	1,268	228.7	223.9	251.2	260.8	257.1	237.0	233.7	291.6	295.5
Struck by or against objects or persons	160	171	216	205	197	227	246	206	161	42.2	43.2	53.5	50.0	47.2	53.6	58.0	48.2	37.5
Motor vehicle traffic	359	345	399	403	345	343	388	355	385	94.8	87.3	99.0	98.4	82.6	80.8	91.2	83.1	89.6
Cut or pierce	158	163	190	159	157	169	159	158	148	41.7	41.1	47.2	38.8	37.6	39.8	37.4	37.0	34.4
Intentional injuries	149	130	161	184	182	180	*171	*200	*193	39.4	32.9	39.9	45.0	43.5	42.5	*40.2	*46.8	*45.1
65 years and over[2]	2,155	2,193	2,294	2,322	2,582	2,577	2,760	2,858	2,745	1,002.9	989.9	1,016.3	1,014.2	1,110.7	1,078.8	1,116.8	1,121.0	1,044.5
Unintentional injuries[4]	1,889	1,978	2,083	2,108	2,348	2,341	2,517	2,619	2,527	879.1	892.5	922.8	920.4	1,009.8	980.0	1,018.2	1,027.0	961.7
Falls	1,347	1,463	1,538	1,612	1,784	1,726	1,823	1,929	1,822	626.9	660.1	681.2	704.1	767.2	722.4	737.7	756.4	693.4
Struck by or against objects or persons	69	91	91	81	81	*111	*145	*125	*110	31.9	41.2	40.4	35.5	34.7	*46.3	*58.6	*48.8	*41.7
Motor vehicle traffic	139	116	146	134	124	125	127	106	162	64.5	52.5	64.7	58.3	53.5	52.2	51.2	41.7	61.5
Cut or pierce	*50	*64	*54	*37	*56	*72	*54	*44	*69	*23.3	*28.8	*23.9	*16.3	*24.2	*30.1	*21.8	*17.3	*26.2
Intentional injuries	*	*	*	*	*	*	*	*	*	*	*	*	*	*	*	*	*	*

NOTE: An emergency department visit was considered injury-related if the first-listed diagnosis was injury-related (International Classification of Diseases, Ninth Revision, Clinical Modification [ICD-9-CM] codes 800–909.2, 909.4, 909.9–994.9, 995.50–995.59, and 995.80–995.85) or the first-listed external cause code (E code) was injury-related (ICD-9-CM codes E800–E869, E880–E929, and E950–E999). See: https://www.cdc.gov/nchs/injury/injury_tools.htm for codes used to classify injury-related visits in this table. Visits with a first-listed diagnosis or first-listed E code describing a complication or adverse effect of medical care were not considered injury-related. For more information on injury-related visits, see: Bergen G, Chen LH, Warner M, Fingerhut LA. *Injury in the United States: 2007 Chartbook.* Hyattsville, MD: National Center for Health Statistics. 2008. Available from: https://www.cdc.gov/nchs/data/misc/injury2007.pdf. Estimates for first- listed injury-related visits were further limited to those visits that were initial visits for the injury. This was determined using an imputed variable in 2005–2006; for 2007 and beyond, this was determined by using the initial visit episode of care information collected on the questionnaire. Limiting the estimates to initial visits decreases the total number of injury-related visits by 9% in 2005–2006, 14% in 2007–2008, 10%–13% in 2008–2009 through 2012–2013, and 6%–7% in 2013–2014 and 2014–2015. Rates were calculated using U.S. Census Bureau estimates of the civilian population of the United States, including institutionalized persons. Rates for 2005–2010 were computed using 2000-based postcensal population estimates. Rates for 2011 and beyond were computed using 2010-based postcensal population estimates. Data for additional years are available. See the Excel spreadsheet on the *Health, United States* website at: https://www.cdc.gov/nchs/hus.htm.
* = Estimates are considered unreliable. Data preceded by an asterisk have a relative standard error (RSE) of 20%–30%. Data not shown have an RSE greater than 30%.
[1] Intent and mechanism of injury are based on the first-listed external cause-of-injury code (E code). Intentional injuries include self-inflicted injuries and assaults.
[2] Includes all injury-related visits not shown separately in table, including those with undetermined intent (1% in 2014–2015) and insufficient or no information to code cause of injury (7% in 2014–2015).
[4] Includes unintentional injury-related visits with mechanism of injury not shown in table.

Table 3-46. Visits to Physician Offices, Hospital Outpatient Departments, and Hospital Emergency Departments, by Age, Sex, and Race, Selected Years, 2000–2015

(Number; rate; data are based on reporting by a sample of office-based physicians, hospital outpatient departments, and hospital emergency departments.)

Age, sex, and race	All places[1]					Physician offices				
	2000	2005	2009	2010	2015[2]	2000	2005	2009	2010	2015[2]
	Number of visits in thousands									
Age										
Total	1,014,848	1,169,333	1,270,001	1,239,387	NA	823,542	963,617	1,037,796	1,008,802	990,808
Under 18 years	212,165	238,389	239,590	246,228	NA	163,459	185,186	183,999	191,500	149,556
18 to 44 years	315,774	324,108	341,209	342,797	NA	243,011	247,568	257,890	261,941	230,511
45 to 64 years	255,894	328,564	374,775	352,001	NA	216,783	283,180	316,395	296,385	305,071
45 to 54 years	142,233	170,674	190,701	171,039	NA	119,474	145,034	158,120	140,819	142,016
55 to 64 years	113,661	157,890	184,074	180,962	NA	97,309	138,146	158,275	155,566	163,055
65 years and over	231,014	278,272	314,428	298,362	NA	200,289	247,683	279,514	258,976	305,670
65 to 74 years	116,505	133,334	153,884	151,075	NA	102,447	119,061	137,452	132,201	159,752
75 years and over	114,510	144,938	160,544	147,287	NA	97,842	128,623	142,062	126,775	145,918
	Number of visits per 100 persons									
Total, age-adjusted[3]	374	400	414	401	NA	304	329	337	325	297
Total, crude	370	402	421	408	NA	300	331	344	332	313
Under 18 years	293	325	322	331	NA	226	253	247	257	203
18 to 44 years	291	294	309	310	NA	224	224	234	237	204
45 to 64 years	422	454	475	441	NA	358	391	401	371	366
45 to 54 years	385	405	431	388	NA	323	344	358	320	333
55 to 64 years	481	523	532	505	NA	412	458	457	434	401
65 years and over	706	792	829	767	NA	612	705	737	666	658
65 to 74 years	656	725	749	713	NA	577	647	669	624	585
75 years and over	766	865	923	831	NA	654	768	817	715	762
Sex and Age										
Male, age-adjusted[3]	325	352	358	350	NA	261	289	290	283	252
Male, crude	314	345	356	350	NA	251	283	289	283	262
Under 18 years	302	338	334	340	NA	231	265	257	262	203
18 to 44 years	203	212	201	205	NA	148	158	145	151	122
45 to 54 years	316	331	361	324	NA	260	278	296	265	251
55 to 64 years	428	468	473	460	NA	367	411	403	396	378
65 to 74 years	614	691	731	680	NA	539	619	654	597	560
75 years and over	771	833	907	871	NA	670	741	807	760	799
Female, age-adjusted[3]	420	445	469	452	NA	345	367	383	367	342
Female, crude	424	456	483	464	NA	348	377	397	379	362
Under 18 years	285	311	310	322	NA	221	240	237	252	204
18 to 44 years	377	375	416	415	NA	298	290	322	323	285
45 to 54 years	451	476	499	450	NA	384	408	417	372	411
55 to 64 years	529	574	586	546	NA	453	501	507	469	424
65 to 74 years	692	754	764	741	NA	609	671	681	647	607
75 years and over	763	886	934	804	NA	645	785	823	685	736
Race and Age[4]										
White, age-adjusted[3]	380	413	421	408	NA	315	347	351	336	293
White, crude	381	420	434	421	NA	316	355	365	349	315
Under 18 years	306	348	339	341	NA	243	280	269	270	213
18 to 44 years	301	306	312	319	NA	239	242	244	249	211
45 to 54 years	386	416	432	389	NA	330	362	369	326	310
55 to 64 years	480	534	531	505	NA	416	476	466	440	394
65 to 74 years	641	727	752	727	NA	568	656	678	642	548
75 years and over	764	854	936	838	NA	658	763	835	723	710
Black or African American, age-adjusted[3]	353	398	459	439	NA	239	270	314	316	326
Black or African American, crude	324	369	438	425	NA	214	243	296	303	316
Under 18 years	264	278	315	351	NA	167	162	198	241	167
18 to 44 years	257	295	373	339	NA	149	172	228	222	205
45 to 54 years	383	422	486	466	NA	269	297	329	339	420
55 to 64 years	495	515	645	617	NA	373	374	478	481	496
65 to 74 years	656	745	821	715	NA	512	589	667	565	743
75 years and over	745	982	908	845	NA	568	806	718	682	874

NOTE: Rates were calculated using estimates of the civilian noninstitutionalized population of the United States. Rates for 2000 were computed using 1990-based postcensal population estimates. Rates for 2001–2010 were computed using 2000-based postcensal population estimates. Rates for 2011 data and beyond were computed using 2010-based postcensal population estimates. Rates using the civilian noninstitutionalized population will be overestimated to the extent that visits by institutionalized persons are counted in the numerator (e.g., hospital emergency department visits by nursing home residents), but institutionalized persons are omitted from the denominator (the civilian noninstitutionalized population). Starting with Health, United States, 2005, data for physician offices for 2001 and beyond use a revised weighting scheme.

NA = Not available.

[1]All places includes visits to physician offices and hospital outpatient and emergency departments. See Appendix II, Emergency department; Emergency department or emergency room visit; Office visit; Outpatient department; Outpatient visit.

[2]In 2012–2015, data for All places and Physician offices exclude visits to community health centers; in 2006–2011, data for All places and Physician offices include visits to community health centers (2%–3% of visits to physician offices in 2006–2011 were to community health centers). Prior to 2006, visits to community health centers were not included in the survey.

[3]Estimates are age adjusted to the year 2000 standard population using six age groups: under 18 years, 18 to 44 years, 45 to 54 years, 55 to 64 years, 65 to 74 years, and 75 years and over.

[4]Estimates by racial group should be used with caution because information on race was collected from medical records and race is imputed for records missing that information. Information on the race imputation process used in each data year is available in the public-use file documentation. Starting with 1999 data, the instruction for the race item on the Patient Record Form was changed so that more than one race could be recorded. In previous years only one race could be recorded. Estimates for race in this table are for visits where only one race was recorded. Because of the small number of responses with more than one racial group recorded, estimates for visits with multiple races recorded are unreliable and are not presented.

Table 3-46. Visits to Physician Offices, Hospital Outpatient Departments, and Hospital Emergency Departments, by Age, Sex, and Race, Selected Years, 2000–2015—Continued

(Number; rate; data are based on reporting by a sample of office-based physicians, hospital outpatient departments, and hospital emergency departments.)

Age, sex, and race	Hospital outpatient departments					Hospital emergency departments				
	2000	2005	2009	2010	2015²	2000	2005	2009	2010	2015²
	Number of visits in thousands									
Age										
Total	83,289	90,393	96,132	100,742	NA	108,017	115,323	136,072	129,843	136,943
Under 18 years	21,076	24,288	22,418	24,913	NA	27,630	28,915	33,173	29,815	31,860
18 to 44 years	26,947	29,044	29,535	28,159	NA	45,816	47,496	53,784	52,697	54,592
45 to 64 years	20,772	23,202	29,083	27,739	NA	18,339	22,182	29,297	27,877	29,119
45 to 54 years	11,558	12,546	15,310	13,639	NA	11,201	13,094	17,271	16,581	16,070
55 to 64 years	9,214	10,656	13,774	14,100	NA	7,138	9,088	12,026	11,296	13,050
65 years and over	14,494	13,859	15,096	19,932	NA	16,232	16,730	19,818	19,454	21,372
65 to 74 years	7,515	7,517	8,036	10,675	NA	6,543	6,756	8,396	8,199	9,797
75 years and over	6,979	6,341	7,060	9,257	NA	9,690	9,974	11,423	11,255	11,575
	Number of visits per 100 persons									
Total, age-adjusted³	31	31	31	33	NA	40	40	46	43	44
Total, crude	30	31	32	33	NA	39	40	45	43	43
Under 18 years	29	33	30	33	NA	38	39	45	40	43
18 to 44 years	25	26	27	25	NA	42	43	49	48	48
45 to 64 years	34	32	37	35	NA	30	31	37	35	35
45 to 54 years	31	30	35	31	NA	30	31	39	38	38
55 to 64 years	39	35	40	39	NA	30	30	35	32	32
65 years and over	44	39	40	51	NA	50	48	52	50	46
65 to 74 years	42	41	39	50	NA	37	37	41	39	36
75 years and over	47	38	41	52	NA	65	60	66	64	60
Sex and Age										
Male, age-adjusted³	26	25	25	27	NA	38	38	42	40	40
Male, crude	25	25	26	27	NA	38	37	42	39	39
Under 18 years	29	33	30	34	NA	41	41	46	43	44
18 to 44 years	17	16	16	16	NA	38	38	40	38	39
45 to 54 years	26	24	28	24	NA	30	29	36	35	36
55 to 64 years	32	29	35	32	NA	30	28	34	32	31
65 to 74 years	38	34	37	47	NA	36	39	40	37	34
75 years and over	42	32	37	50	NA	59	60	63	60	60
Female, age-adjusted³	35	37	37	38	NA	41	42	49	47	48
Female, crude	35	37	38	39	NA	41	42	48	46	47
Under 18 years	29	33	30	33	NA	35	38	43	37	43
18 to 44 years	33	37	38	35	NA	46	48	57	57	57
45 to 54 years	36	36	41	37	NA	31	33	42	40	39
55 to 64 years	45	41	44	46	NA	31	32	35	31	33
65 to 74 years	46	47	41	54	NA	37	35	42	40	38
75 years and over	49	42	43	53	NA	69	59	68	66	61
Race and Age⁴										
White, age-adjusted³	28	28	29	31	NA	37	37	41	41	42
White, crude	28	28	29	32	NA	37	37	41	40	41
Under 18 years	27	31	29	33	NA	36	37	40	39	42
18 to 44 years	23	24	24	25	NA	39	40	43	45	45
45 to 54 years	28	26	30	28	NA	28	28	34	34	34
55 to 64 years	36	31	34	36	NA	28	27	30	29	30
65 to 74 years	38	36	35	48	NA	35	35	38	37	35
75 years and over	44	35	36	52	NA	63	56	64	62	61
Black or African American, age-adjusted³	51	58	59	51	NA	62	70	85	73	78
Black or African American, crude	48	57	58	50	NA	62	69	84	72	77
Under 18 years	40	*54	42	48	NA	57	63	75	62	70
18 to 44 years	40	46	50	37	NA	68	77	94	81	91
45 to 54 years	61	63	74	54	NA	53	62	83	73	81
55 to 64 years	70	*84	91	73	NA	52	58	76	62	57
65 to 74 years	85	*94	*81	*85	NA	59	62	73	66	57
75 years and over	85	*78	*	*74	NA	92	98	95	89	77

NOTE: Rates were calculated using estimates of the civilian noninstitutionalized population of the United States. Rates for 2000 were computed using 1990-based postcensal population estimates. Rates for 2001–2010 were computed using 2000-based postcensal population estimates. Rates for 2011 data and beyond were computed using 2010-based postcensal population estimates. Rates using the civilian noninstitutionalized population will be overestimated to the extent that visits by institutionalized persons are counted in the numerator (e.g., hospital emergency department visits by nursing home residents), but institutionalized persons are omitted from the denominator (the civilian noninstitutionalized population). Starting with Health, United States, 2005, data for physician offices for 2001 and beyond use a revised weighting scheme.

NA = Not available.

* = Estimates are considered unreliable. Data preceded by an asterisk have a relative standard error (RSE) of 20%–30%. Data not shown have an RSE greater than 30%.

²In 2012–2015, data for All places and Physician offices exclude visits to community health centers; in 2006–2011, data for All places and Physician offices include visits to community health centers (2%–3% of visits to physician offices in 2006–2011 were to community health centers). Prior to 2006, visits to community health centers were not included in the survey.

³Estimates are age adjusted to the year 2000 standard population using six age groups: under 18 years, 18 to 44 years, 45 to 54 years, 55 to 64 years, 65 to 74 years, and 75 years and over.

⁴Estimates by racial group should be used with caution because information on race was collected from medical records and race is imputed for records missing that information. Information on the race imputation process used in each data year is available in the public-use file documentation. Starting with 1999 data, the instruction for the race item on the Patient Record Form was changed so that more than one race could be recorded. In previous years only one race could be recorded. Estimates for race in this table are for visits where only one race was recorded. Because of the small number of responses with more than one racial group recorded, estimates for visits with multiple races recorded are unreliable and are not presented.

Table 3-47. Visits to Primary Care Generalist and Specialist Physicians, by Selected Characteristics and Type of Physician, Selected Years, 1980–2015

(Percent; data are based on reporting by a sample of office-based physicians.)

Age, sex, and race	Type of primary care generalist physician[1]														
	All primary care generalists					General and family practice					Internal medicine				
	1980	1990	2000	2010	2015[2]	1980	1990	2000	2010	2015[2]	1980	1990	2000	2010	2015[2]
Age															
Total	66.2	63.6	58.9	55.2	41.2	33.5	29.9	24.1	21.1	10.3	12.1	13.8	15.3	*	14.0
Under 18 years	77.8	79.5	79.7	80.9	65.5	26.1	26.5	19.9	15.3	5.5	2.0	2.9	*	*	*
18 to 44 years	65.3	65.2	62.1	62.7	50.0	34.3	31.9	28.2	27.8	11.3	8.6	11.8	12.7	11.6	11.5
45 to 64 years	60.2	55.5	51.2	46.7	34.1	36.3	32.1	26.4	23.1	11.8	19.5	18.6	20.1	18.5	17.9
45 to 54 years	60.2	55.6	52.3	48.7	34.5	37.4	32.0	27.8	26.2	10.0	17.1	17.1	18.7	15.7	18.4
55 to 64 years	60.2	55.5	49.9	44.8	33.6	35.4	32.1	24.7	20.4	13.4	21.8	20.0	21.7	21.0	17.4
65 years and over	61.6	52.6	46.5	38.3	29.7	37.5	28.1	20.2	16.4	10.3	22.7	23.3	24.5	20.5	17.8
65 to 74 years	61.2	52.7	46.6	37.3	29.1	37.4	28.1	19.7	17.5	10.9	22.1	23.0	24.5	18.2	15.9
75 years and over	62.3	52.4	46.4	39.2	30.3	37.6	28.0	20.8	15.4	9.5	23.5	23.7	24.5	22.8	19.8
Sex and Age															
Male															
Under 18 years	77.3	78.1	77.7	80.1	65.6	25.6	24.1	18.3	15.7	*	2.0	3.0	*	*	*
18 to 44 years	50.8	51.8	51.5	51.7	34.7	38.0	35.9	34.2	33.7	16.3	11.5	15.0	14.4	16.4	16.0
45 to 64 years	55.6	50.6	49.4	43.7	31.5	34.4	31.0	28.7	24.4	13.3	20.5	19.2	19.8	19.1	18.1
65 years and over	58.2	51.2	43.1	36.6	28.0	35.6	27.7	19.3	16.2	10.0	22.3	23.3	23.8	20.3	18.0
Female															
Under 18 years	78.5	81.1	82.0	81.7	65.5	26.6	29.1	21.7	14.9	*	2.0	2.8	*	*	1.7
18 to 44 years	72.1	71.3	67.2	67.9	56.4	32.5	30.0	25.3	25.0	9.2	7.3	10.3	11.9	9.4	9.6
45 to 64 years	63.4	58.8	52.5	48.9	35.8	37.7	32.8	24.9	22.2	10.7	18.9	18.2	20.2	18.1	17.7
65 years and over	63.9	53.5	48.9	39.6	31.0	38.7	28.3	20.9	16.7	10.5	22.9	23.3	25.0	20.5	17.5
Race and Age[2,3]															
White															
Under 18 years	77.6	79.2	78.5	79.6	62.6	26.4	27.1	21.2	15.6	6.5	2.0	2.3	*	*	*
18 to 44 years	64.8	64.4	61.4	61.2	49.4	34.5	31.9	29.2	27.9	11.4	8.6	10.6	11.0	11.1	11.5
45 to 64 years	59.6	54.2	49.3	45.2	31.3	36.0	31.5	27.3	22.8	11.4	19.2	17.6	17.1	17.5	15.0
65 years and over	61.4	51.9	45.1	37.6	26.6	36.6	27.5	20.3	16.6	11.5	23.3	23.1	23.0	19.7	13.1
Black or African American															
Under 18 years	79.9	85.5	87.3	88.0	*	23.7	20.2	*	*16.5	1.8	*2.2	9.8	*	*	*
18 to 44 years	68.5	68.3	65.0	72.6	*	31.7	31.9	22.0	29.4	*	9.0	18.1	20.9	*14.0	*
45 to 64 years	66.1	61.6	61.7	57.0	53.2	38.6	31.2	23.3	26.7	*	22.6	26.9	35.9	24.5	*
65 years and over	64.6	58.6	52.8	45.2	*	49.0	28.9	*18.5	*18.6	*	14.2	28.7	33.4	*25.4	*

Age, sex, and race	Type of primary care generalist physician[1]										Specialty care physicians				
	Obstetrics and gynecology					Pediatrics									
	1980	1990	2000	2010	2015[2]	1980	1990	2000	2010	2015[2]	1980	1990	2000	2010	2015[2]
Age															
Total	9.6	8.7	7.8	7.8	8.2	10.9	11.2	11.7	12.4	8.7	33.8	36.4	41.1	44.8	58.8
Under 18 years	1.3	1.2	*1.1	*1.3	1.5	48.5	48.9	57.3	63.4	55.9	22.2	20.5	20.3	19.1	34.5
18 to 44 years	21.7	20.8	20.4	22.3	26.1	0.7	0.7	*0.9	1.0	1.0	34.7	34.8	37.9	37.3	50.0
45 to 64 years	4.2	4.6	4.5	4.9	4.4	*	*	*	*	*	39.8	44.5	48.8	53.3	65.9
45 to 54 years	5.6	6.3	5.6	6.7	6.2	*	*	*	*	*	39.8	44.4	47.7	51.3	65.5
55 to 64 years	2.9	3.1	3.3	3.3	2.8	*	*	*	*	*	39.8	44.5	50.1	55.2	66.4
65 years and over	1.4	1.1	1.5	1.3	1.7	*	*	*	*	*	38.4	47.4	53.5	61.7	70.3
65 to 74 years	1.7	1.6	2.0	1.7	2.3	*	*	*	*	*	38.8	47.3	53.4	62.7	70.9
75 years and over	1.0	*0.6	*1.0	*1.0	1.0	*	*	*	*	*	37.7	47.6	53.6	60.8	69.7
Sex and Age															
Male															
Under 18 years	X	X	X	X	X	49.4	50.7	58.0	63.7	55.5	22.7	21.9	22.3	19.9	34.4
18 to 44 years	X	X	X	X	X	1.0	0.7	*1.7	*1.4	1.7	49.2	48.2	48.5	48.3	65.3
45 to 64 years	X	X	X	X	X	*	*	*	*	*	44.4	49.4	50.6	56.3	68.5
65 years and over	X	X	X	X	X	*	*	*	*	*	41.8	48.8	56.9	63.4	72.0
Female															
Under 18 years	2.5	2.3	2.1	*2.8	3.0	47.4	46.9	56.5	63.1	56.4	21.5	18.9	18.0	18.3	34.5
18 to 44 years	31.7	30.4	29.6	32.5	36.8	0.6	0.7	*	*0.9	0.8	27.9	28.7	32.8	32.1	43.6
45 to 64 years	6.7	7.7	7.3	8.5	7.4	*	*	*	*	*	36.6	41.2	47.5	51.1	64.2
65 years and over	2.1	1.8	2.6	2.4	3.0	*	*	*	*	*	36.1	46.5	51.1	60.4	69.0
Race and Age[2,3]															
White															
Under 18 years	1.1	1.0	*1.2	*1.3	1.5	48.2	48.8	54.7	61.7	51.4	22.4	20.8	21.5	20.4	37.4
18 to 44 years	21.0	21.1	20.4	21.1	25.5	0.7	0.7	*0.8	*1.1	0.9	35.2	35.6	38.6	38.8	50.6
45 to 64 years	4.1	4.8	4.7	4.7	4.9	*	*	*	*	*	40.4	45.8	50.7	54.8	68.7
65 years and over	1.4	1.2	1.5	*1.3	2.0	*	*	*	*	*	38.6	48.1	54.9	62.4	73.4
Black or African American															
Under 18 years	2.8	*3.4	*	*	*	51.2	52.1	75.0	70.2	*	20.1	14.5	*12.7	*12.0	*
18 to 44 years	27.1	17.9	20.7	28.4	*	*	*	*	*	0.9	31.5	31.7	35.0	27.4	*
45 to 64 years	4.8	3.5	*2.4	*5.6	2.7	*	*	*	*	*	33.9	38.4	38.3	43.0	46.8
65 years and over	*	*	*	*1.2	0.3	*	*	*	*	*	35.4	41.4	47.2	54.8	*

NOTE: This table presents data on visits to physician offices and excludes visits to other sites, such as hospital outpatient and emergency departments. In 1980, the survey excluded Alaska and Hawaii. Data for all other years include all 50 states and the District of Columbia. Visits with specialty of physician unknown are excluded. Starting with Health, United States, 2005, data for 2001 and later years for physician offices use a revised weighting scheme.

X = Not applicable.

* = Estimates are considered unreliable. Data preceded by an asterisk have a relative standard error (RSE) of 20%–30%. Data not shown have a RSE greater than 30%.

[1]Type of physician is based on physician's self-designated primary area of practice. Primary care generalist physicians are defined as practitioners in the fields of general and family practice, general internal medicine, general obstetrics and gynecology, and general pediatrics and exclude primary care specialists. Primary care generalists in general and family practice exclude primary care specialties, such as sports medicine and geriatrics. Primary care internal medicine physicians exclude internal medicine specialists, such as allergists, cardiologists, and endocrinologists. Primary care obstetrics and gynecology physicians exclude obstetrics and gynecology specialties, such as gynecological oncology, maternal and fetal medicine, obstetrics and gynecology critical care medicine, and reproductive endocrinology. Primary care pediatricians exclude pediatric specialists, such as adolescent medicine specialists, neonatologists, pediatric allergists, and pediatric cardiologists.

[2]In 2012 and 2013, data exclude visits to community health centers; in 2006–2011, data include visits to community health centers (2%–3% of visits to physician offices in 2006–2011 were to community health centers). Prior to 2006, visits to community health centers were not included in the survey.

[3]Estimates by racial group should be used with caution because information on race was collected from medical records. In 2013, race data were missing and imputed for 30% of visits. Information on the race imputation process used in each data year is available in the public-use file documentation. Available from: http://www.cdc.gov/nchs/ahcd.htm. Starting with 1999 data, the instruction for the race item on the Patient Record Form was changed so that more than one race could be recorded. In previous years only one racial category could be checked. Estimates for racial groups presented in this table are for visits where only one race was recorded. Because of the small number of responses with more than one racial group checked, estimates for visits with multiple races checked are unreliable and are not presented.

Table 3-48. Dental Visits in the Past Year, by Selected Characteristics, Selected Years, 1997–2016

(Percent; data are based on household interviews of a sample of the civilian noninstitutionalized population.)

Characteristic	2 years and over				2 to 17 years				18 to 64 years				65 years and over[1]			
	1997	2000	2010	2016	1997	2000	2010	2016	1997	2000	2010	2016	1997	2000	2010	2016
Total with Dental Visit[2,3]	65.1	66.2	64.7	68.7	72.7	74.1	78.9	84.6	64.1	65.1	61.1	64.4	54.8	56.6	57.7	64.3
Sex																
Male	62.9	63.5	61.7	66.3	72.3	73.7	78.3	84.3	60.4	60.7	56.8	60.9	55.4	56.1	56.2	62.1
Female	67.1	68.8	67.5	71.0	73.0	74.6	79.6	84.9	67.7	69.4	65.4	67.8	54.4	56.9	58.9	66.2
Race[4]																
White only	66.4	67.9	65.6	69.5	74.0	75.8	79.2	84.3	65.7	67.2	62.4	65.6	56.8	58.4	59.3	66.4
Black or African American only	58.9	59.5	58.8	64.7	68.8	70.0	79.0	86.6	57.0	57.1	53.1	59.1	35.4	38.2	40.6	48.4
American Indian or Alaska Native only	55.1	58.6	57.4	58.3	66.8	71.3	73.2	85.8	49.9	55.0	49.8	49.8	*	*	72.2	*
Asian only	62.5	67.1	66.5	69.0	69.9	72.8	74.8	84.0	60.3	65.6	64.6	66.2	53.9	60.6	61.9	60.4
Native Hawaiian and Other Pacific Islander only	NA	*	*	56.2	NA	*	*	*	NA	*	*	*	NA	*	*	*
Two or more races	NA	65.1	65.2	69.1	NA	71.4	77.9	83.5	NA	60.5	54.7	59.1	NA	57.4	48.1	59.2
Black or African American; White	NA	63.5	72.5	70.1	NA	65.7	78.4	82.6	NA	60.7	62.1	48.8	NA	*	*	*
American Indian or Alaska Native; White	NA	61.7	54.7	63.2	NA	63.4	70.0	78.8	NA	61.6	49.0	57.1	NA	*57.8	*54.5	62.3
Hispanic Origin and Race[4]																
Hispanic or Latino	54.0	52.3	56.5	63.4	61.0	60.6	74.8	83.7	50.8	48.6	48.5	55.3	47.8	44.5	42.1	51.8
Not Hispanic or Latino	66.4	68.2	66.2	69.8	74.7	76.8	80.1	84.9	65.7	67.5	63.4	66.4	55.2	57.2	59.0	65.4
White only	68.0	69.9	67.6	71.1	76.4	78.9	80.9	84.7	67.5	69.4	65.4	68.3	57.2	59.1	60.9	67.9
Black or African American only	58.8	59.4	58.7	64.7	68.8	70.0	79.2	87.0	56.9	57.2	53.1	59.3	35.3	38.0	40.5	47.7
Percent of Poverty Level[5]																
Below 100 percent	50.5	50.4	50.6	57.2	62.0	62.4	73.2	80.8	46.9	46.8	41.0	49.0	31.5	33.3	32.8	37.4
100 percent to 199 percent	50.8	52.2	51.6	54.9	62.5	66.1	73.4	81.3	48.3	48.4	44.1	46.4	40.8	43.0	43.8	42.8
200 percent to 399 percent	66.2	65.6	63.5	66.4	76.1	75.5	79.0	84.2	63.4	62.2	59.6	60.9	60.7	62.8	57.9	63.6
400 percent or more	78.9	79.5	79.3	81.2	85.7	85.9	88.0	90.0	77.7	78.5	77.5	79.1	74.7	73.8	77.2	81.8
Hispanic Origin and Race and Percent of Poverty Level[4,5]																
Hispanic or Latino																
Below 100 percent	45.7	43.4	50.8	61.1	55.9	54.2	74.3	83.6	39.2	36.8	34.7	46.2	33.6	31.3	32.4	46.1
100 percent to 199 percent	47.2	45.5	50.8	58.2	53.8	56.9	71.1	84.1	43.5	39.2	40.2	46.1	47.9	42.9	39.5	43.2
200 percent to 399 percent	61.2	57.2	59.1	62.9	70.5	65.6	76.5	82.3	57.5	53.7	54.1	57.5	57.0	54.8	46.0	49.3
400 percent or more	73.0	70.0	73.3	75.0	82.4	78.4	84.2	85.2	70.8	68.7	71.6	72.1	64.9	53.4	54.3	77.7
Not Hispanic or Latino																
White only																
Below 100 percent	51.7	53.6	49.3	53.8	64.4	65.0	69.1	72.0	50.6	53.3	44.4	51.2	32.0	37.2	36.4	37.9
100 percent to 199 percent	52.4	53.8	52.7	53.7	66.1	69.7	75.3	79.1	50.4	51.7	47.2	47.8	42.2	43.4	45.4	43.6
200 percent to 399 percent	67.5	67.6	64.7	67.0	77.1	78.3	79.6	83.8	65.0	64.4	61.4	61.3	61.9	63.9	59.8	66.5
400 percent or more	79.7	80.8	79.8	82.6	86.8	87.5	88.6	91.0	78.5	79.7	77.9	80.7	75.5	76.1	78.8	82.6
Black or African American only																
Below 100 percent	52.8	51.8	52.0	59.3	66.1	67.1	78.0	86.1	46.2	44.4	39.7	48.2	27.7	21.7	20.9	32.4
100 percent to 199 percent	48.7	52.4	50.0	53.2	61.2	67.3	75.9	83.1	46.3	48.0	41.5	43.5	26.9	35.2	33.6	35.4
200 percent to 399 percent	63.3	62.3	61.2	67.1	75.0	74.0	81.2	89.7	60.7	58.4	57.2	62.7	41.5	48.4	45.3	49.4
400 percent or more	74.6	72.8	77.2	79.2	81.8	74.2	87.2	91.5	73.4	73.3	75.9	77.5	66.1	60.5	69.8	76.2
Level of difficulty[6]																
A lot of difficulty or cannot do at all	X	X	X	X	X	X	X	X	NA	NA	43.4	50.3	NA	NA	40.1	50.2
Some difficulty	X	X	X	X	X	X	X	X	NA	NA	56.5	61.8	NA	NA	56.3	61.4
No difficulty	X	X	X	X	X	X	X	X	NA	NA	63.3	67.2	NA	NA	65.4	70.6
Geographic Region																
Northeast	69.6	72.3	70.1	73.9	77.5	81.1	83.8	87.6	69.6	72.1	67.9	71.4	55.5	58.1	61.5	65.7
Midwest	68.4	69.9	67.3	69.9	76.4	77.2	80.8	84.8	67.4	69.2	64.3	66.0	57.6	58.6	58.2	65.9
South	60.2	61.0	60.9	64.4	68.0	69.5	77.4	82.4	59.4	59.8	56.5	59.4	49.0	50.8	54.1	59.7
West	65.0	65.3	63.9	69.9	71.5	72.0	76.1	85.3	62.9	63.0	60.2	65.1	61.9	63.1	59.8	68.9
Location of Residence																
Within MSA[7]	66.7	67.5	65.9	69.9	73.6	74.3	79.3	84.8	65.7	66.5	62.4	65.7	57.6	58.9	59.4	66.6
Outside MSA[7]	59.1	61.2	58.4	61.3	69.3	73.3	76.4	83.4	58.0	59.7	53.8	56.1	46.1	49.3	51.3	53.9

NA = Not available.

X = Not applicable.

* = Estimates are considered unreliable. Starting with 2016 data, the reliability of survey percentage estimates was assessed using new multistep National Center for Health Statistics data presentation standards for proportions. Prior to 2016 data, the reliability of estimates for earlier years was evaluated based on relative standard errors (RSE). Data preceded by an asterisk have an RSE of 20%–30%. Data not shown have an RSE greater than 30%.

[1]Based on the 1997–2016 National Health Interview Surveys, about 19%–30% of persons aged 65 and over were edentulous (having lost all their natural teeth). In 1997–2016, about 69%–73% of older dentate persons, compared with 17%–28% of older edentate persons, had a dental visit in the past year.

[2]Respondents were asked, "About how long has it been since you last saw or talked to a dentist?"

[3]Includes all other races not shown separately and unknown disability status.

[4]The race groups White, Black, American Indian or Alaska Native, Asian, Native Hawaiian or Other Pacific Islander, and 2 or more races include persons of Hispanic and non-Hispanic origin. Persons of Hispanic origin may be of any race. Starting with 1999 data, race-specific estimates are tabulated according to the 1997 Revisions to the Standards for the Classification of Federal Data on Race and Ethnicity and are not strictly comparable with estimates for earlier years. The five single-race categories and multiple-race categories shown in the table conform to the 1997 Standards. Starting with 1999 data, race-specific estimates are for persons who reported only one racial group; the category 2 or more races includes persons who reported more than one racial group. Prior to 1999, data were tabulated according to the 1977 Standards with four racial groups, and the Asian only category included Native Hawaiian or Other Pacific Islander. Estimates for single-race categories prior to 1999 included persons who reported one race, or if they reported more than one race, identified one race as best representing their race. Starting with 2003 data, race responses of other race and unspecified multiple race were treated as missing, and then race was imputed if these were the only race responses. Almost all persons with a race response of other race were of Hispanic origin.

[5]Percent of poverty level is based on family income and family size and composition using U.S. Census Bureau poverty thresholds. Missing family income data were imputed for 1997 and beyond.

[6]Functional limitation is defined by the reported level of difficulty in six functioning domains: seeing (even if wearing glasses), hearing (even if wearing hearing aids), mobility (walking or climbing stairs), communication (understanding or being understood by others), cognition (remembering or concentrating), and self-care (such as washing all over or dressing). Respondents with answers to one or more of the six questions were included in one of three mutually-exclusive categories. Those responding "A lot of difficulty" or "Cannot do at all/unable to do" to at least one question were classified in the "A lot of difficulty/cannot do" category. Of the remaining, those responding "Some difficulty" to at least one question were classified in the "Some difficulty" category, and those responding "No difficulty" to at least one question were classified in the "No difficulty" category. Those responding "Don't know" or "Refused" to all six questions were excluded. During 2010–2016, 1%–8% of respondents were missing data and excluded.

[7]MSA = metropolitan statistical area.

Table 3-49. Prescription Drug Use in the Past 30 Days, by Sex, Age, Race and Hispanic Origin, Selected Years, 1988–1994 Through 2011–2014

(Percent.)

Sex, race, Hispanic origin, and age[1]	At least one prescription drug in past 30 days				Three or more prescription drugs in past 30 days				Five or more prescription drugs in past 30 days			
	1988–1994	1999–2002	2007–2010	2011–2014	1988–1994	1999–2002	2007–2010	2011–2014	1988–1994	1999–2002	2007–2010	2011–2014
All ages, age-adjusted[2]												
Both sexes[3]	39.1	45.2	47.5	46.9	11.8	17.8	20.8	21.5	4.0	7.5	10.1	10.9
Male	32.7	39.8	42.8	42.6	9.4	14.8	19.1	19.7	2.9	6.1	9.2	9.7
Female	45.0	50.3	52.0	51.2	13.9	20.4	22.5	23.2	4.9	8.7	11.0	12.0
Not Hispanic or Latino												
White only	41.1	48.7	52.8	51.9	12.4	18.9	22.4	23.1	4.2	7.8	10.7	11.5
White only, male	34.2	43.0	47.5	46.8	9.9	15.9	20.6	21.0	3.1	6.3	9.8	10.2
White only, female	47.6	54.3	57.9	57.0	14.6	21.8	24.3	25.1	5.1	9.2	11.6	12.8
Black or African American only	36.9	40.1	42.3	44.2	12.6	16.5	20.7	22.5	3.8	7.7	10.8	12.1
Black or African American only, male	31.1	35.4	36.7	38.3	10.2	14.5	17.7	19.4	2.9	6.4	9.1	10.1
Black or African American only, female	41.4	43.8	46.8	49.0	14.3	18.1	22.9	24.9	4.5	8.7	12.0	13.7
Asian only	NA	NA	NA	34.3	NA	NA	NA	14.3	NA	NA	NA	6.2
Asian only, male	NA	NA	NA	31.9	NA	NA	NA	14.1	NA	NA	NA	6.2
Asian only, female	NA	NA	NA	36.3	NA	NA	NA	14.6	NA	NA	NA	6.1
Hispanic or Latino	NA	NA	35.2	35.7	NA	NA	15.7	16.0	NA	NA	8.4	8.4
Hispanic or Latino, male	NA	NA	31.7	32.1	NA	NA	14.0	15.0	NA	NA	7.3	7.9
Hispanic or Latina, female	NA	NA	38.8	39.2	NA	NA	17.4	17.1	NA	NA	9.5	8.8
Mexican origin	31.7	31.7	33.9	34.2	9.0	11.2	15.0	15.9	2.9	4.4	7.9	8.7
Mexican origin, male	27.5	25.8	31.0	31.8	7.0	9.5	13.4	14.9	2.0	3.5	7.2	8.2
Mexican origin, female	36.0	37.8	37.0	36.9	11.0	12.8	16.6	17.0	3.7	5.2	8.7	9.2
All ages, crude												
Both sexes[3]	37.8	45.0	48.5	48.9	11.0	17.6	21.7	23.1	3.6	7.4	10.6	11.9
Male	30.6	38.6	43.0	43.7	8.3	13.9	19.0	20.4	2.5	5.6	9.1	10.0
Female	44.6	51.1	53.8	53.9	13.6	21.1	24.2	25.8	4.7	9.1	12.1	13.6
Not Hispanic or Latino												
White only	41.4	50.7	56.2	57.0	12.5	20.6	25.8	27.7	4.2	8.7	12.6	14.3
White only, male	33.5	43.8	50.3	51.4	9.5	16.5	22.9	24.6	2.9	6.6	11.0	12.1
White only, female	48.9	57.5	61.8	62.4	15.4	24.5	28.6	30.7	5.4	10.8	14.2	16.4
Black or African American only	31.2	36.0	40.2	42.8	9.2	13.5	18.6	21.1	2.6	6.2	9.4	11.2
Black or African American only, male	25.5	30.7	33.9	36.3	7.0	10.9	15.0	17.5	1.8	4.8	7.5	8.9
Black or African American only, female	36.2	40.6	45.7	48.5	11.1	15.7	21.7	24.2	3.3	7.4	11.1	13.1
Asian only	NA	NA	NA	34.0	NA	NA	NA	13.6	NA	NA	NA	5.7
Asian only, male	NA	NA	NA	30.5	NA	NA	NA	12.6	NA	NA	NA	5.5
Asian only, female	NA	NA	NA	37.1	NA	NA	NA	14.5	NA	NA	NA	6.0
Hispanic or Latino	NA	NA	28.6	29.5	NA	NA	10.3	10.9	NA	NA	5.0	5.3
Hispanic or Latino, male	NA	NA	24.9	25.4	NA	NA	8.4	9.3	NA	NA	3.8	4.6
Hispanic or Latina, female	NA	NA	32.5	33.5	NA	NA	12.3	12.6	NA	NA	6.2	6.0
Mexican origin	24.0	23.6	26.4	27.0	4.8	6.1	9.0	9.8	1.4	2.1	4.1	4.9
Mexican origin, male	20.1	18.8	23.7	24.9	3.4	4.8	7.6	9.0	0.9	1.6	3.4	4.6
Mexican origin, female	28.1	28.9	29.4	29.3	6.4	7.5	10.6	10.8	1.9	2.7	4.9	5.4
Both sexes												
Under 18 years	20.5	23.8	24.0	21.5	2.4	4.1	3.8	3.9	*	*0.8	0.8	0.8
18-44 years	31.3	35.9	38.7	37.1	5.7	8.4	9.7	10.1	1.2	2.3	3.1	3.9
45-64 years	54.8	64.1	66.2	69.0	20.0	30.8	34.4	36.4	7.4	13.3	16.8	18.3
65 years and over	73.6	84.7	89.7	90.6	35.3	51.8	66.6	66.8	13.8	27.1	39.7	40.7
Male												
Under 18 years	20.4	25.7	24.5	21.1	2.6	4.3	4.4	4.3	*	*	0.8	0.9
18-44 years	21.5	27.1	29.5	28.8	3.6	6.7	7.1	7.5	*0.8	1.7	2.1	3.0
45-64 years	47.2	55.6	61.3	65.6	15.1	23.6	30.4	33.0	4.8	9.5	14.4	15.7
65 years and over	67.2	80.1	88.8	88.7	31.3	46.3	66.8	65.2	11.3	24.7	39.5	38.4
Female												
Under 18 years	20.6	21.7	23.5	22.0	2.3	3.9	3.1	3.5	*	*0.8	*0.7	*
18-44 years	40.7	44.6	47.6	45.3	7.6	10.2	12.2	12.6	1.7	2.8	4.0	4.8
45-64 years	62.0	72.0	70.8	72.1	24.7	37.5	38.1	39.4	9.7	16.8	19.1	20.7
65 years and over	78.3	88.1	90.4	92.1	38.2	55.9	66.4	68.1	15.6	28.9	39.8	42.6

NA = Not available.

* = Figure does not meet standards of reliability or precision. Data preceded by an asterisk have a relative standard error (RSE) of 20 to 30 percent. Data not shown have an RSE of greater than 30 percent.

[1] Persons of Hispanic and Mexican origin may be of any race. Starting with 1999 data, race-specific estimates are tabulated according to the 1997 Revisions to the Standards for the Classification of Federal Data on Race and Ethnicity and are not strictly comparable with estimates for earlier years. The non-Hispanic race categories shown in the table conform to the 1997 Standards. Starting with 1999 data, race-specific estimates are for persons who reported only one racial group. Prior to data year 1999, estimates were tabulated according to the 1977 Standards. Estimates for single-race categories prior to 1999 included persons who reported one race or, if they reported more than one race, identified one race as best representing their race.

[2] Estimates are age-adjusted to the year 2000 standard population using four age groups: under 18 years, 18–44 years, 45–64 years, and 65 years and over. Age-adjusted estimates in this table may differ from other age-adjusted estimates based on the same data and presented elsewhere if different age groups are used in the adjustment procedure.

[3] Includes persons of all races and Hispanic origins, not just those shown separately.

Table 3-50. Selected Prescription Drug Classes Used in the Past 30 Days, by Sex and Age, Selected Years, 1988–1994 Through 2011–2014

(Percent.)

Age group and Multum Lexicon Plus therapeutic class[1] (common indications for use)	Total			Male			Female		
	1988–1994	1999–2002	2011–2014	1988–1994	1999–2002	2011–2014	1988–1994	1999–2002	2011–2014
All Ages									
Antihyperlipidemic agents (high cholesterol)	1.7	6.5	14.3	1.5	7.1	15.0	1.8	5.8	13.7
Analgesics (pain relief)	7.2	9.4	9.1	5.4	7.3	7.6	9.0	11.3	10.5
Antidepressants (depression and related disorders)	1.8	6.4	10.7	1.2	4.4	7.3	2.3	8.3	13.9
Proton pump inhibitors (gastrointestinal reflux, ulcers)[2]	2.8	5.3	8.5	2.4	4.7	7.5	3.0	5.9	9.4
Beta-adrenergic blocking agents (high blood pressure, heart disease)	3.1	4.4	7.7	2.7	4.1	7.1	3.5	4.6	8.4
ACE inhibitors (high blood pressure, heart disease)	2.4	4.6	7.3	2.4	4.7	8.1	2.4	4.5	6.6
Antidiabetic agents (diabetes)	2.6	3.7	6.6	2.5	3.7	6.8	2.6	3.8	6.3
Diuretics (high blood pressure, heart disease, kidney disease)[3]	3.4	4.1	5.6	2.3	3.1	4.4	4.4	5.1	6.7
Thyroid hormones (hypothyroidism)	2.3	3.9	5.1	0.8	1.5	1.9	3.7	6.2	8.0
Bronchodilators (asthma, breathing)	2.6	3.5	4.6	2.5	3.1	4.5	2.7	3.8	4.6
Sex hormones (contraceptives, menopause, hot flashes)[4]	X	X	X	X	X	X	X	X	X
Anxiolytics, sedatives, and hypnotics (anxiety, insomnia, and related disorders)	2.8	3.3	5.3	1.9	2.6	4.4	3.6	4.0	6.2
Antihypertensive combinations (high blood pressure)	2.4	2.9	4.1	1.4	1.9	3.3	3.3	3.8	4.8
Anticonvulsants (epilepsy, seizure, and related disorders)	1.4	2.4	4.9	1.2	2.1	4.3	1.6	2.7	5.5
Calcium channel blocking agents (high blood pressure, heart disease)	3.6	4.2	4.7	3.4	3.5	4.6	3.8	4.8	4.7
Under 18 Years									
Bronchodilators (asthma, breathing)	3.0	4.0	4.4	3.3	4.4	4.9	2.7	3.6	3.9
CNS stimulants (attention deficit disorder, hyperactivity)	*0.8	2.9	3.4	*1.2	4.4	5.0	*	1.4	1.7
Penicillins (bacterial infections)	6.1	5.1	2.6	5.9	5.2	2.0	6.4	5.0	3.2
Leukotriene modifiers (asthma, allergies)	X	0.7	2.1	X	*0.9	2.5	X	*	1.7
Antihistamines (allergies)	2.0	4.4	2.0	2.1	4.9	2.3	1.9	3.9	1.8
Respiratory inhalant products (asthma, chronic obstructive pulmonary disease, and related disorders)	*0.7	1.5	1.9	*	1.7	2.4	*	1.3	*1.3
Adrenal cortical steroids (anti-inflammatory)	*0.5	0.8	1.0	*	*0.7	*1.0	*0.5	0.9	*1.1
Nasal preparations (nose symptoms)	*	1.1	1.7	*	*1.3	2.2	*	1.0	*
Antidepressants (depression and related disorders)	*	1.8	*1.3	*	2.2	*0.7	*	*1.5	*
Upper respiratory combinations (cough and cold, congestion)	2.3	2.3	*	2.6	*2.4	*	2.0	*2.2	*
Analgesics (pain relief)	1.2	1.4	1.1	*1.2	1.3	*1.0	1.4	1.6	*1.3
Dermatological agents (skin symptoms)	0.7	1.1	1.1	*	1.1	*0.9	*1.0	*1.1	1.4
18 to 44 Years									
Analgesics (pain relief)	7.2	8.0	7.0	5.1	6.0	5.3	9.1	9.9	8.8
Antidepressants (depression and related disorders)	1.6	6.0	8.8	*1.0	3.6	6.4	2.3	8.5	11.2
Sex hormones (contraceptives, menopause, hot flashes)[4]	X	X	X	X	X	X	11.5	13.5	13.4
Proton pump inhibitors (gastrointestinal reflux, ulcers)[2]	2.0	3.0	3.8	1.6	3.0	4.2	2.4	3.0	3.4
Anxiolytics, sedatives, and hypnotics (generalized anxiety and related disorders)	1.4	2.1	4.2	*1.0	*1.7	3.5	1.9	2.5	5.0
Anticonvulsants (epilepsy, seizure, and related disorders)	0.8	1.6	4.1	*0.6	1.6	4.0	1.0	*1.5	4.2
Bronchodilators (asthma, breathing)	1.4	2.2	2.9	*1.1	1.6	2.6	*1.8	2.8	3.2
Antihyperlipidemic agents (high cholesterol)	*0.4	1.3	2.3	*	2.0	2.9	*	*	1.8
Antihistamines (allergies)	2.5	3.9	1.8	1.8	3.6	*1.6	3.2	4.2	*2.0
Thyroid hormones (hypothyroidism)	1.3	1.6	2.2	*	*	*0.7	2.1	2.8	3.6
ACE inhibitors (high blood pressure, heart disease)	0.7	1.4	2.1	*0.9	1.5	2.1	*0.6	*1.2	2.2
Antidiabetic agents (diabetes)	*1.0	1.5	2.5	*	*1.5	2.1	*1.0	*1.6	2.9
Muscle relaxants (muscle spasm and related disorders)	1.0	1.3	1.7	*1.3	*1.1	1.4	*0.7	*1.4	2.1
Beta-adrenergic blocking agents (high blood pressure, heart disease)	1.1	*1.2	1.6	*0.9	*1.3	1.2	1.3	*	2.0
Nasal preparations (nose symptoms)	*0.6	1.5	1.4	*	*1.2	*0.8	*0.7	1.7	2.1
45 to 64 Years									
Antihyperlipidemic agents (high cholesterol)	4.3	13.8	25.6	4.4	17.2	28.2	4.2	10.7	23.1
Proton pump inhibitors (gastrointestinal reflux, ulcers)[2]	5.2	9.9	14.1	5.3	8.4	12.7	5.2	11.3	15.4
Antidepressants (depression and related disorders)	3.5	10.5	17.5	*2.3	7.0	12.5	4.6	13.8	22.2
Sex hormones (contraceptives, menopause, hot flashes)[4]	X	X	X	X	X	X	X	X	X
Analgesics (pain relief)	11.9	16.0	15.5	9.2	13.5	14.3	14.3	18.3	16.7
Beta-adrenergic blocking agents (high blood pressure, heart disease)	6.6	8.7	11.5	7.0	7.8	10.8	6.2	9.5	12.1
ACE inhibitors (high blood pressure, heart disease)	5.2	8.8	12.5	5.7	9.8	14.9	4.6	7.9	10.2
Antidiabetic agents (diabetes)	5.5	7.0	11.3	5.9	7.8	12.5	5.1	6.3	10.2
Thyroid hormones (hypothyroidism)	4.7	6.6	8.1	*1.2	*2.7	*2.6	8.1	10.1	13.2
Antihypertensive combinations (high blood pressure)	5.3	5.6	7.9	3.3	*3.7	7.4	7.1	7.3	8.3
Anxiolytics, sedatives, and hypnotics (generalized anxiety and related disorders)	6.0	6.2	8.6	4.3	4.9	7.7	7.5	7.4	9.4
Diuretics (high blood pressure, heart disease, kidney disease)[3]	6.1	6.6	8.6	4.8	4.8	7.2	7.3	8.3	9.9
Anticonvulsants (epilepsy, seizure, and related disorders)	2.7	4.3	7.5	*2.5	3.5	6.3	2.9	5.1	8.6
Bronchodilators (asthma, breathing)	3.4	3.8	5.2	2.9	3.1	*4.6	3.8	4.5	5.8
Calcium channel blocking agents (high blood pressure, heart disease)	7.0	6.7	6.6	8.2	5.9	7.9	5.9	7.5	5.4

X = Not applicable.

* = Figure does not meet standards of reliability or precision. Data preceded by an asterisk have a relative standard error (RSE) of 20 to 30 percent. Data not shown have an RSE of greater than 30 percent.

[1]The drug therapeutic class is based on the December 2014 Lexicon Plus, a proprietary database of Cerner Multum, Inc. Lexicon Plus is a comprehensive database of all prescription and some nonprescription drug products available in the U.S. drug market. Data on prescription drug use are collected by the National Health and Nutrition Examination Survey. Respondents were asked if they had taken a prescription drug in the past 30 days. Those who answered "yes" were asked to show the interviewer the medication containers for all prescriptions. If no container was available, the respondent was asked to verbally report the name of the medication. Each drug's complete name was recorded and classified. Data presented are based on the second level classification of prescription drugs. Up to four classes are assigned to each drug. Drugs classified into more than one class were counted in each class. Some drug classes were not available in 1988-1994 and are coded as not applicable.

[2]The drugs classes proton pump inhibitors (272) and H2 antagonists (94) have been combined because of their similar indications for use.

[3]This category includes carbonic anhydrase inhibitors which are primarily used to treat glaucoma.

[4]Although sex hormones may be used by males, most are used by females. Therefore, data for sex hormones are only presented for females.

Table 3-50. Selected Prescription Drug Classes Used in the Past 30 Days, by Sex and Age, Selected Years, 1988–1994 Through 2011–2014—Continued

(Percent.)

Age group and Multum Lexicon Plus therapeutic class[1] (common indications for use)	Total			Male			Female		
	1988–1994	1999–2002	2011–2014	1988–1994	1999–2002	2011–2014	1988–1994	1999–2002	2011–2014
65 Years and Over									
Antihyperlipidemic agents (high cholesterol)	5.9	23.4	50.3	5.3	24.3	54.4	6.4	22.7	47.1
Beta-adrenergic blocking agents (high blood pressure, heart disease)	11.8	15.9	30.5	10.4	17.5	31.4	12.8	14.8	29.8
Diuretics (high blood pressure, heart disease, kidney disease)[3]									
ACE inhibitors (high blood pressure, heart disease)	16.2	19.2	21.1	12.2	17.1	19.0	19.1	20.7	22.7
Proton pump inhibitors (gastrointestinal reflux, ulcers)[2]	7.5	14.6	23.2	7.2	14.1	19.8	7.7	15.0	25.9
Antidiabetic agents (diabetes)	9.0	12.4	19.5	9.0	12.9	22.6	9.0	12.0	17.1
Anticoagulants or antiplatelet agents (blood clot prevention)[5]	6.1	9.1	14.6	6.8	11.5	17.8	5.6	7.4	12.1
Analgesics (pain relief)	13.8	18.4	16.4	11.4	15.0	14.2	15.6	20.9	18.2
Calcium channel blocking agents (high blood pressure, heart disease)	16.1	19.1	17.8	14.5	17.4	16.7	17.3	20.4	18.7
Thyroid hormones (hypothyroidism)	7.0	14.3	15.5	3.3	6.7	7.7	9.7	19.8	21.7
Antihypertensive combinations (high blood pressure)	9.6	9.8	11.7	6.0	7.4	8.0	12.2	11.6	14.6
Antidepressants (depression and related disorders)	3.0	9.3	18.9	*2.3	7.2	12.0	3.5	10.8	24.4
Angiotensin II inhibitors (high blood pressure, heart disease)	X	4.8	12.2	...	4.1	11.8	...	5.3	12.6
Antiarrhythmic agents (heart rhythm irregularities)	23.1	16.6	8.8	21.6	17.9	8.4	24.3	15.6	9.0
65 to 74 Years									
Antihyperlipidemic agents (high cholesterol)	7.3	26.2	49.1	6.2	26.6	51.9	8.1	25.9	46.7
Beta-adrenergic blocking agents (high blood pressure, heart disease)	11.3	14.8	25.8	10.6	16.0	27.9	11.9	13.9	24.1
ACE inhibitors (high blood pressure, heart disease)	9.6	17.2	23.5	10.6	18.1	28.9	8.9	16.4	18.9
Proton pump inhibitors (gastrointestinal reflux, ulcers)[2]	7.0	14.7	20.7	6.3	13.4	18.3	7.5	15.8	22.8
Antidiabetic agents (diabetes)	8.8	12.9	19.9	8.0	13.8	22.5	9.4	12.0	17.7
Diuretics (high blood pressure, heart disease, kidney disease)[3]	14.2	15.9	17.2	10.8	14.6	14.6	17.0	16.9	19.4
Analgesics (pain relief)	13.0	18.5	16.8	10.5	14.9	15.3	15.0	21.4	18.0
Antihypertensive combinations (high blood pressure)	8.1	8.0	11.8	4.8	*6.7	8.5	10.8	9.0	14.5
Anticoagulants or antiplatelet agents (blood clot prevention)[5]	5.4	6.7	10.7	6.3	9.8	*13.8	4.6	*4.2	8.1
Antidepressants (depression and related disorders)	2.8	9.3	18.7	*2.3	5.8	12.6	3.1	12.1	23.9
Calcium channel blocking agents (high blood pressure, heart disease)	15.0	16.1	14.4	14.0	15.3	15.0	15.8	16.8	13.9
Thyroid hormones (hypothyroidism)	6.4	13.0	14.6	*3.4	*5.0	*7.3	8.9	19.7	20.8
Angiotensin II inhibitors (high blood pressure, heart disease)	X	4.2	11.1	...	*3.5	9.5	X	4.9	12.4
Antiarrhythmic agents (heart rhythm irregularities)	20.2	13.0	6.4	19.0	15.5	*5.8	21.1	10.8	6.9
75 Years and Over									
Antihyperlipidemic agents (high cholesterol)	3.8	19.9	52.1	*3.5	21.1	58.4	4.0	19.2	47.6
Beta-adrenergic blocking agents (high blood pressure, heart disease)	12.5	17.3	37.0	9.8	19.6	36.8	14.1	15.8	37.1
Diuretics (high blood pressure, heart disease, kidney disease)[3]	19.2	23.2	26.5	14.7	20.5	26.0	21.9	24.9	26.9
ACE inhibitors (high blood pressure, heart disease)	9.3	16.4	25.0	8.5	17.7	27.0	9.8	15.6	23.7
Anticoagulants or antiplatelet agents (blood clot prevention)[5]	7.2	12.0	20.1	7.8	13.9	24.1	6.9	10.9	17.4
Proton pump inhibitors (gastrointestinal reflux, ulcers)[2]	8.3	14.6	26.8	9.0	15.3	22.3	7.9	14.2	30.0
Calcium channel blocking agents (high blood pressure, heart disease)	17.8	22.8	22.6	15.3	20.5	19.4	19.2	24.2	24.9
Thyroid hormones (hypothyroidism)	7.9	15.8	16.8	3.0	9.2	8.2	10.9	20.0	22.9
Analgesics (pain relief)	15.1	18.4	16.0	13.0	15.1	12.6	16.3	20.4	18.3
Antidiabetic agents (diabetes)	9.3	11.8	18.9	10.7	11.5	22.8	8.5	12.0	16.3
Antihypertensive combinations (high blood pressure)	11.9	12.0	11.5	8.3	*8.2	7.1	14.0	14.4	14.6
Antiarrhythmic agents (heart rhythm irregularities)	27.7	21.0	12.1	26.3	21.3	12.6	28.6	20.7	11.7
Angiotensin II inhibitors (high blood pressure, heart disease)	X	5.4	13.9	X	*4.9	15.2	X	5.8	12.9
Antidepressants (depression and related disorders)	3.4	9.3	19.2	*2.3	9.2	11.0	4.0	9.4	X

X = Not applicable.

* = Figure does not meet standards of reliability or precision. Data preceded by an asterisk have a relative standard error (RSE) of 20 to 30 percent. Data not shown have an RSE of greater than 30 percent.

[1]The drug therapeutic class is based on the December 2014 Lexicon Plus, a proprietary database of Cerner Multum, Inc. Lexicon Plus is a comprehensive database of all prescription and some nonprescription drug products available in the U.S. drug market. Data on prescription drug use are collected by the National Health and Nutrition Examination Survey. Respondents were asked if they had taken a prescription drug in the past 30 days. Those who answered "yes" were asked to show the interviewer the medication containers for all prescriptions. If no container was available, the respondent was asked to verbally report the name of the medication. Each drug's complete name was recorded and classified. Data presented are based on the second level classification of prescription drugs. Up to four classes are assigned to each drug. Drugs classified into more than one class were counted in each class. Some drug classes were not available in 1988-1994 and are coded as not applicable.

[2]The drugs classes proton pump inhibitors (272) and H2 antagonists (94) have been combined because of their similar indications for use.

[3]This category includes carbonic anhydrase inhibitors which are primarily used to treat glaucoma.

[5]The drugs classes anticoagulants (82) and antiplatelet agents (83) have been combined because of their similar indications for use.

INPATIENT CARE

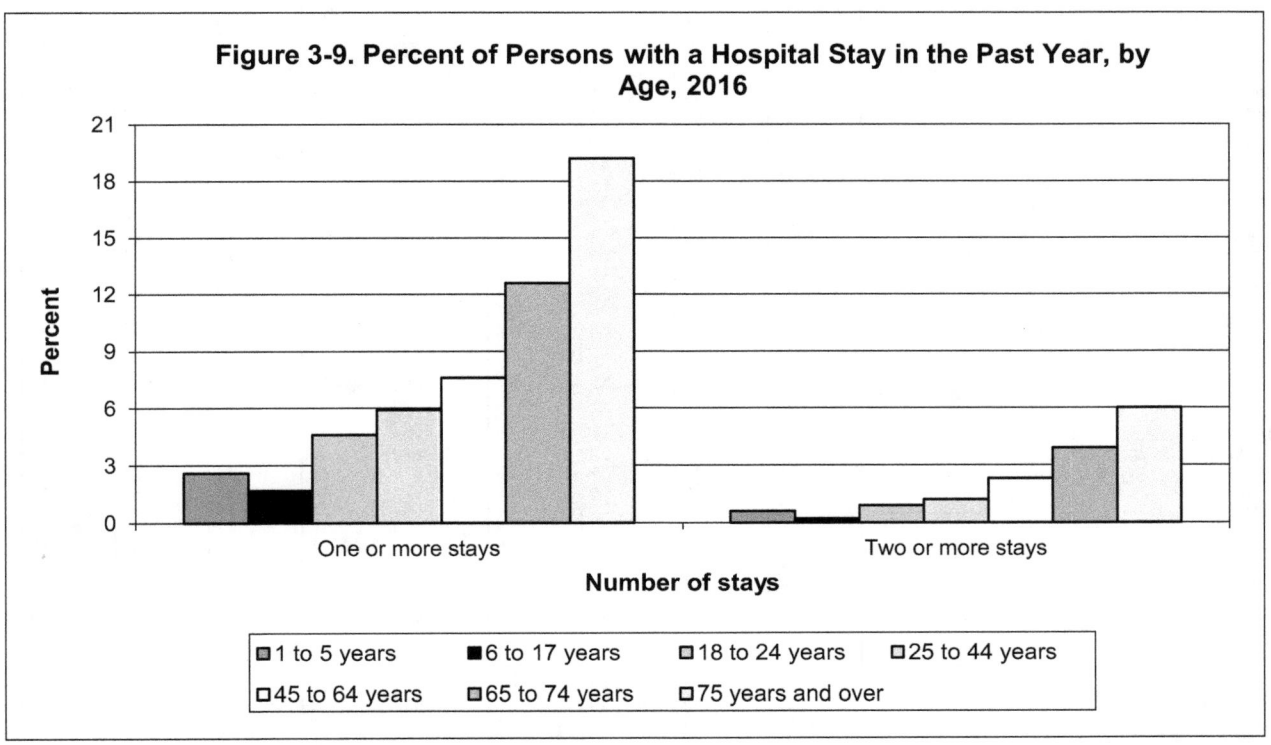

Figure 3-9. Percent of Persons with a Hospital Stay in the Past Year, by Age, 2016

Table 3-51. Persons with Hospital Stays in the Past Year, by Selected Characteristics, Selected Years, 1997–2016

(Percent.)

Characteristic	One or more hospital stays[1]					Two or more hospital stays[1]				
	1997	2000	2005	2010	2016	1997	2000	2005	2010	2016
1 year and over, age-adjusted[2,3]	7.8	7.6	7.4	7.0	6.4	1.8	1.8	1.7	1.8	1.6
1 year and over, crude[2]	7.7	7.5	7.4	7.2	6.8	1.7	1.8	1.8	1.9	1.8
Age										
1 to 17 years	2.8	2.5	2.5	2.4	2.0	0.5	0.4	0.4	0.5	0.3
1 to 5 years	3.9	3.8	3.7	3.4	2.6	0.7	0.7	0.8	0.6	0.6
6 to 17 years	2.3	1.9	2.0	1.9	1.7	0.4	0.3	0.3	0.5	0.2
18 to 44 years	7.4	7.0	6.7	6.3	5.6	1.2	1.1	1.1	1.3	1.1
18 to 24 years	7.9	7.0	6.3	5.7	4.6	1.3	1.1	1.0	1.1	0.9
25 to 44 years	7.3	7.0	6.9	6.6	5.9	1.2	1.2	1.2	1.3	1.2
45 to 64 years	8.2	8.4	8.2	8.3	7.6	2.2	2.2	2.2	2.5	2.3
45 to 54 years	6.9	7.3	7.1	7.3	6.8	1.7	1.8	1.8	2.1	2.0
55 to 64 years	10.2	10.0	9.8	9.5	8.3	2.9	2.8	2.9	2.9	2.5
65 years and over	18.0	18.2	17.8	16.1	15.3	5.4	5.8	5.4	4.9	4.7
65 to 74 years	16.1	16.1	14.5	13.6	12.6	4.8	4.9	4.5	3.8	3.9
75 years and over	20.4	20.7	21.4	19.0	19.2	6.2	6.8	6.4	6.2	6.0
75 to 84 years	19.8	20.1	19.9	18.3	17.9	6.1	6.2	6.1	6.1	5.7
85 years and over	22.8	23.4	26.6	20.8	22.8	6.2	9.0	7.4	6.6	6.7
1 to 64 Years										
Total, 1 to 64 years[2,4]	6.3	6.1	5.9	5.7	5.0	1.3	1.2	1.2	1.3	1.2
Sex										
Male, crude	4.4	4.2	4.5	4.2	4.0	0.9	1.0	1.1	1.1	1.1
1 to 17 years	2.9	2.4	2.8	2.4	2.2	0.6	0.4	0.5	0.5	0.4
18 to 44 years	3.6	3.1	3.2	2.9	2.7	0.6	0.6	0.7	0.7	0.7
45 to 64 years	6.0	7.0	6.6	6.4	5.9	1.4	1.8	1.9	1.9	1.8
65 years and over	11.1	10.2	10.3	9.3	8.6	3.0	3.0	3.4	2.8	2.6
Female, crude	8.0	7.9	7.5	7.6	6.5	1.6	1.5	1.4	1.7	1.5
1 to 17 years	2.6	2.5	2.2	2.3	1.7	0.5	0.4	0.4	0.5	0.3
18 to 44 years	11.2	10.8	10.2	9.8	8.3	1.8	1.7	1.6	1.9	1.5
45 to 64 years	7.6	7.6	7.6	8.3	7.7	2.0	1.9	1.7	2.3	2.2
65 years and over	9.4	9.8	9.3	9.7	8.1	2.9	2.7	2.4	2.9	2.4
Race[4,5]										
White only	6.2	5.9	5.9	5.6	5.0	1.2	1.1	1.1	1.3	1.1
Black or African American only	7.6	7.4	6.6	6.7	5.8	1.9	1.9	1.8	1.9	1.7
American Indian or Alaska Native only	7.6	7.0	6.9	*7.6	5.5	*	*	*2.5	*2.4	1.7
Asian only	3.9	3.9	3.9	3.6	3.0	*0.5	*0.6	*0.5	0.4	0.5
Native Hawaiian and Other Pacific Islander only	NA	*	*	*	*	NA	*	*	*	0.9
Two or more races	NA	8.8	6.0	7.7	5.9	NA	*1.6	*1.9	*2.4	1.7
Hispanic Origin and Race[4,5]										
Hispanic or Latino	6.8	5.5	5.4	5.2	4.3	1.3	0.9	1.2	1.1	0.9
Not Hispanic or Latino	6.2	6.1	6.0	5.8	5.2	1.3	1.3	1.2	1.4	1.2
White only	6.1	6.0	6.0	5.7	5.3	1.2	1.2	1.1	1.3	1.2
Black or African American only	7.5	7.4	6.6	6.7	5.8	1.9	1.9	1.7	1.9	1.7
Percent of Poverty Level[4,6]										
Below 100 percent	10.3	9.1	8.8	8.3	7.4	2.8	2.6	2.5	2.7	2.4
100 percent to 199 percent	7.3	7.3	7.4	7.0	6.4	1.7	1.9	1.9	1.9	1.9
200 percent to 399 percent	6.0	6.0	5.4	5.2	5.0	1.2	1.1	1.1	1.1	1.1
400 percent or more	4.7	5.0	4.8	4.5	3.8	0.7	0.8	0.8	0.8	0.6
Hispanic Origin and Race and Percent of Poverty Level[4,5,6]										
Hispanic or Latino										
Below 100 percent	9.1	7.4	7.6	7.3	5.9	2.0	1.6	2.0	2.0	1.4
100 percent to 199 percent	5.9	5.4	5.9	4.8	4.4	1.0	0.8	1.4	1.1	1.1
200 percent to 399 percent	5.9	4.6	4.4	4.3	3.8	1.1	0.7	0.8	0.7	0.9
400 percent or more	5.5	4.7	3.8	4.4	3.5	*1.1	*0.6	*0.6	*0.8	0.5
Not Hispanic or Latino										
White only										
Below 100 percent	10.7	9.6	9.3	8.8	8.2	3.2	2.7	2.5	2.9	2.7
100 percent to 199 percent	7.7	7.8	8.2	7.8	7.7	1.8	2.2	2.0	2.2	2.2
200 percent to 399 percent	6.1	6.1	5.8	5.5	5.6	1.2	1.1	1.1	1.2	1.3
400 percent or more	4.7	5.0	4.9	4.6	4.0	0.7	0.8	0.7	0.8	0.6

0.0 = Quantity more than zero but less than 0.05.
NA = Not available.
* = Estimates are considered unreliable. Starting with 2016 data, the reliability of survey percentage estimates was assessed using new multistep National Center for Health Statistics data presentation standards for proportions. Prior to 2016 data, the reliability of estimates for earlier years was evaluated based on relative standard errors (RSE). Data preceded by an asterisk have an RSE of 20%–30%. Data not shown have an RSE greater than 30%.
[1]These estimates exclude hospitalizations for institutionalized persons and those who died while hospitalized, because they are outside the scope of the National Health Interview Survey.
[2]Includes all other races not shown separately, unknown health insurance status, and unknown disability status.
[3]Estimates are for persons aged 1 year and over and are age-adjusted to the year 2000 standard population using six age groups: 1–17 years, 18–44 years, 45–54 years, 55–64 years, 65–74 years, and 75 years and over.
[4]Estimates are for persons aged 1–64 and are age-adjusted to the year 2000 standard population using four age groups: 1–17 years, 18–44 years, 45–54 years, and 55–64 years. The disability measure is age-adjusted using the three adult age groups.
[5]The race groups White, Black, American Indian or Alaska Native, Asian, Native Hawaiian or Other Pacific Islander, and 2 or more races include persons of Hispanic and non-Hispanic origin. Persons of Hispanic origin may be of any race. Starting with 1999 data, race-specific estimates are tabulated according to the 1997 Revisions to the Standards for the Classification of Federal Data on Race and Ethnicity and are not strictly comparable with estimates for earlier years. The five single-race categories and multiple-race categories shown in the table conform to the 1997 Standards. Starting with 1999 data, race-specific estimates are for persons who reported only one racial group; the category 2 or more races includes persons who reported more than one racial group. Prior to 1999, data were tabulated according to the 1977 Standards with four racial groups, and the Asian only category included Native Hawaiian or Other Pacific Islander. Estimates for single-race categories prior to 1999 included persons who reported one race, or if they reported more than one race, identified one race as best representing their race. Starting with 2003 data, race responses of other race and unspecified multiple race were treated as missing, and then race was imputed if these were the only race responses. Almost all persons with a race response of other race were of Hispanic origin.
[6]Percent of poverty level is based on family income and family size and composition using U.S. Census Bureau poverty thresholds. Missing family data were imputed for 1997 and beyond.

Table 3-51. Persons with Hospital Stays in the Past Year, by Selected Characteristics, Selected Years, 1997–2016—Continued

(Percent.)

Characteristic	One or more hospital stays[1]					Two or more hospital stays[1]				
	1997	2000	2005	2010	2016	1997	2000	2005	2010	2016
Black or African American only										
Below 100 percent	11.4	10.8	9.4	9.4	8.2	3.3	3.4	3.1	3.1	3.0
100 percent to 199 percent	8.0	8.5	7.7	7.7	7.0	2.1	2.3	2.0	2.3	2.6
200 percent to 399 percent	6.2	6.1	5.2	5.3	4.5	1.5	1.3	1.3	1.4	0.9
400 percent or more	4.7	5.8	5.1	4.5	4.2	*0.9	*1.3	*1.2	*1.0	1.0
Health Insurance Status at the Time of Interview[4,7]										
Insured	6.6	6.4	6.3	6.2	5.2	1.3	1.3	1.3	1.4	1.2
Private	5.6	5.5	5.2	5.0	4.3	1.0	1.0	0.9	0.9	0.8
Medicaid	16.1	15.9	14.6	12.7	9.3	4.9	4.7	4.1	4.5	3.0
Uninsured	4.8	4.5	4.4	4.0	3.6	1.0	0.9	0.9	0.9	0.7
Health Insurance Status Prior to Interview[4,7]										
18 to 64 years										
Insured continuously all 12 months	6.5	6.3	6.1	6.0	5.1	1.3	1.2	1.2	1.4	1.2
Uninsured for any period up to 12 months	8.5	8.4	9.0	7.9	6.5	1.8	1.9	2.4	1.9	1.6
Uninsured more than 12 months	3.8	3.5	3.2	3.0	2.4	0.8	0.8	0.6	0.8	0.5
Percent of Poverty Level and Health Insurance Status Prior to Interview[4,6,7]										
18 to 64 years										
Below 100 percent	12.4	10.7	10.8	10.4	8.3	3.7	3.1	3.1	3.4	2.9
Insured continuously all 12 months	13.7	13.4	13.6	10.4	8.8	3.4	*3.4	4.1	3.0	2.5
Uninsured for any period up to 12 months	4.9	5.0	3.9	4.0	3.1	1.0	*1.6	*0.8	1.3	0.6
Uninsured more than 12 months										
100 percent to 199 percent										
Insured continuously all 12 months	8.5	8.6	8.4	8.5	7.3	2.0	2.3	2.2	2.5	2.3
Uninsured for any period up to 12 months	9.3	9.1	10.7	10.1	7.2	*1.9	*2.2	3.1	1.9	1.9
Uninsured more than 12 months	3.8	3.2	3.7	2.7	2.3	*0.7	*0.7	*0.8	*0.5	0.4
200 to 399 percent										
Insured continuously all 12 months	6.3	6.4	5.8	5.6	5.2	1.3	1.2	1.1	1.2	1.1
Uninsured for any period up to 12 months	7.0	6.6	7.8	6.1	5.7	*1.5	*1.3	*1.7	*1.6	1.4
Uninsured more than 12 months	3.3	2.8	2.1	2.6	1.7	*0.7	*0.4	*	*0.7	0.5
400 percent or more										
Insured continuously all 12 months	4.9	5.1	5.0	4.7	3.8	0.7	0.8	0.8	0.8	0.6
Uninsured for any period up to 12 months	3.9	6.0	5.3	4.1	4.5	*	*	*	*	1.0
Uninsured more than 12 months	*	*2.1	*2.9	*1.8	2.7	*	*	*	*	0.2
Level of difficulty[4,8]										
A lot of difficulty or cannot do at all	NA	NA	NA	18.4	14.7	NA	NA	NA	*	7.3
Some difficulty	NA	NA	NA	8.6	7.9	NA	NA	NA	*2.2	2.0
No difficulty	NA	NA	NA	5.9	4.9	NA	NA	NA	*1.0	0.8
Geographic Region[4]										
Northeast	6.0	5.5	5.8	5.2	4.9	1.2	1.0	1.1	1.2	1.1
Midwest	6.5	6.3	6.3	6.3	5.7	1.5	1.3	1.3	1.5	1.4
South	6.8	6.6	6.3	6.0	5.3	1.4	1.5	1.4	1.5	1.3
West	5.4	5.2	4.8	4.9	4.1	0.8	0.9	0.8	1.1	0.8
Location of Residence[4]										
Within MSA[9]	6.1	5.8	5.7	5.5	4.9	1.2	1.1	1.2	1.3	1.1
Outside MSA[9]	7.0	6.9	6.8	6.9	5.9	1.6	1.5	1.4	1.6	1.5
65 Years and Over										
Total, 65 years and over[2,10]	18.1	18.3	17.8	16.2	15.8	5.4	5.8	5.4	4.9	4.9
65 to 74 years	16.1	16.1	14.5	13.6	12.6	4.8	4.9	4.5	3.8	3.9
75 years and over	20.4	20.7	21.4	19.0	19.2	6.2	6.8	6.4	6.2	6.0
Sex[10]										
Male	19.0	19.5	18.6	16.2	16.6	5.8	5.8	6.0	5.4	5.2
Female	17.5	17.4	17.3	16.2	15.0	5.1	5.7	4.9	4.6	4.6

0.0 = Quantity more than zero but less than 0.05.

NA = Not available.

* = Estimates are considered unreliable. Starting with 2016 data, the reliability of survey percentage estimates was assessed using new multistep National Center for Health Statistics data presentation standards for proportions. Prior to 2016 data, the reliability of estimates for earlier years was evaluated based on relative standard errors (RSE). Data preceded by an asterisk have an RSE of 20%–30%. Data not shown have an RSE greater than 30%.

[1]These estimates exclude hospitalizations for institutionalized persons and those who died while hospitalized, because they are outside the scope of the National Health Interview Survey.

[2]Includes all other races not shown separately, unknown health insurance status, and unknown disability status.

[4]Estimates are for persons aged 1–64 and are age-adjusted to the year 2000 standard population using four age groups: 1–17 years, 18–44 years, 45–54 years, and 55–64 years. The disability measure is age-adjusted using the three adult age groups.

[6]Percent of poverty level is based on family income and family size and composition using U.S. Census Bureau poverty thresholds. Missing family data were imputed for 1997 and beyond.

[7]Health insurance categories are mutually exclusive. Persons who reported both Medicaid and private coverage are classified as having private coverage. Starting with 1997 data, state- sponsored health plan coverage is included as Medicaid coverage. Starting with 1999 data, coverage by the Children's Health Insurance Program (CHIP) is included with Medicaid coverage. In addition to private and Medicaid, the insured category also includes military, other government, and Medicare coverage. Persons not covered by private insurance, Medicaid, CHIP, state- sponsored or other government-sponsored health plans (starting in 1997), Medicare, or military plans are considered to have no health insurance coverage. Persons with only Indian Health Service coverage are considered to have no health insurance coverage.

[8]Functional limitation is defined by the reported level of difficulty in six functioning domains: seeing (even if wearing glasses), hearing (even if wearing hearing aids), mobility (walking or climbing stairs), communication (understanding or being understood by others), cognition (remembering or concentrating), and self-care (such as washing all over or dressing). Respondents with answers to one or more of the six questions were included in one of three mutually exclusive categories. Those responding "A lot of difficulty" or "Cannot do at all/unable to do" to at least one question were classified in the "A lot of difficulty/cannot do" category. Of the remaining, those responding "Some difficulty" to at least one question were classified in the "Some difficulty" category, and those responding "No difficulty" to at least one question were classified in the "No difficulty" category. Those responding "Don't know" or "Refused" to all six questions were excluded. During 2010–2016, 1%–8% of respondents were missing data and excluded.

[9]MSA is metropolitan statistical area. Starting with 2016 data, MSA status is determined using 2010 Census data and the 2010 standards for defining MSAs.

[10]Estimates are for persons 65 years of age and over and are age adjusted to the standard population using two age groups: 65 to 74 years and 75 years and over.

Table 3-51. Persons with Hospital Stays in the Past Year, by Selected Characteristics, Selected Years, 1997–2016—Continued

(Percent.)

Characteristic	One or more hospital stays[1]					Two or more hospital stays[1]				
	1997	2000	2005	2010	2016	1997	2000	2005	2010	2016
Hispanic Origin and Race[5,10]										
Hispanic or Latino..............................	17.3	16.6	17.7	13.9	12.1	6.2	6.4	5.7	5.0	4.7
Not Hispanic or Latino	18.2	18.4	17.9	16.4	16.1	5.4	5.8	5.4	4.9	4.9
White only...............................	18.3	18.4	17.9	16.5	16.1	5.4	5.7	5.4	4.9	4.7
Black or African American only....................	18.9	19.8	19.0	16.9	17.2	5.5	7.5	6.3	5.5	6.2
Percent of Poverty Level[6,10]										
Below 100 percent	20.9	20.9	22.1	18.8	16.6	6.4	7.5	7.9	5.1	7.8
100 percent to 199 percent......................	19.6	19.2	19.2	17.2	17.9	6.5	6.6	5.9	5.2	5.9
200 percent to 399 percent......................	17.3	18.1	17.2	16.0	16.2	4.9	5.8	4.8	5.5	4.6
400 percent or more	16.6	16.0	16.1	15.0	14.0	4.7	4.2	5.1	4.1	3.9
Level of difficulty[8,10]										
A lot of difficulty or cannot do at all	NA	NA	NA	23.8	28.2	NA	NA	NA	*7.1	12.0
Some difficulty..............................	NA	NA	NA	16.7	16.4	NA	NA	NA	*4.8	5.1
No difficulty................................	NA	NA	NA	12.1	10.1	NA	NA	NA	*	2.3
Geographic Region[10]										
Northeast...................................	17.2	16.6	16.1	16.5	16.3	5.1	4.5	4.5	6.1	5.5
Midwest....................................	18.2	19.5	18.9	16.4	16.1	5.6	7.2	5.8	4.7	4.7
South......................................	19.4	19.5	19.7	16.4	16.2	6.1	6.3	6.3	4.7	4.9
West.......................................	16.5	16.4	15.0	15.3	14.3	4.4	4.4	4.3	4.5	4.4
Location of Residence[10]..................										
Within MSA[9]................................	17.8	17.8	17.4	15.9	15.6	5.2	5.4	5.2	4.8	4.7
Outside MSA[9]..............................	19.1	19.6	19.2	17.3	16.3	6.3	6.9	6.2	5.6	5.6

0.0 = Quantity more than zero but less than 0.05.
NA = Not available.
* = Estimates are considered unreliable. Starting with 2016 data, the reliability of survey percentage estimates was assessed using new multistep National Center for Health Statistics data presentation standards for proportions. Prior to 2016 data, the reliability of estimates for earlier years was evaluated based on relative standard errors (RSE). Data preceded by an asterisk have an RSE of 20%–30%. Data not shown have an RSE greater than 30%.
[1]These estimates exclude hospitalizations for institutionalized persons and those who died while hospitalized, because they are outside the scope of the National Health Interview Survey.
[5]The race groups White, Black, American Indian or Alaska Native, Asian, Native Hawaiian or Other Pacific Islander, and 2 or more races include persons of Hispanic and non-Hispanic origin. Persons of Hispanic origin may be of any race. Starting with 1999 data, race-specific estimates are tabulated according to the 1997 Revisions to the Standards for the Classification of Federal Data on Race and Ethnicity and are not strictly comparable with estimates for earlier years. The five single-race categories and multiple-race categories shown in the table conform to the 1997 Standards. Starting with 1999 data, race-specific estimates are for persons who reported only one racial group; the category 2 or more races includes persons who reported more than one racial group. Prior to 1999, data were tabulated according to the 1977 Standards with four racial groups, and the Asian only category included Native Hawaiian or Other Pacific Islander. Estimates for single-race categories prior to 1999 included persons who reported one race, or if they reported more than one race, identified one race as best representing their race. Starting with 2003 data, race responses of other race and unspecified multiple race were treated as missing, and then race was imputed if these were the only race responses. Almost all persons with a race response of other race were of Hispanic origin.
[6]Percent of poverty level is based on family income and family size and composition using U.S. Census Bureau poverty thresholds. Missing family data were imputed for 1997 and beyond.
[8]Functional limitation is defined by the reported level of difficulty in six functioning domains: seeing (even if wearing glasses), hearing (even if wearing hearing aids), mobility (walking or climbing stairs), communication (understanding or being understood by others), cognition (remembering or concentrating), and self-care (such as washing all over or dressing). Respondents with answers to one or more of the six questions were included in one of three mutually exclusive categories. Those responding "A lot of difficulty" or "Cannot do at all/unable to do" to at least one question were classified in the "A lot of difficulty/cannot do" category. Of the remaining, those responding "Some difficulty" to at least one question were classified in the "Some difficulty" category, and those responding "No difficulty" to at least one question were classified in the "No difficulty" category. Those responding "Don't know" or "Refused" to all six questions were excluded. During 2010–2016, 1%–8% of respondents were missing data and excluded.
[9]MSA is metropolitan statistical area. Starting with 2016 data, MSA status is determined using 2010 Census data and the 2010 standards for defining MSAs.
[10]Estimates are for persons 65 years of age and over and are age adjusted to the standard population using two age groups: 65 to 74 years and 75 years and over.

Table 3-52. Discharges, Days of Care, and Average Length of Stay in Nonfederal Short-Stay Hospitals, by Selected Characteristics, Selected Years, 1980 Through 2009–2010

(Rate per 10,000 population, number.)

Characteristic	1980[1]	1985[1]	1990	1995	2000	2005	2006	2007	2008[2]	2009[2]	2009–2010[2]
DISCHARGES PER 10,000 POPULATION											
Total, age-adjusted[3]	1,744.5	1,522.3	1,252.4	1,180.2	1,132.8	1,162.4	1,153.1	1,124.0	1,150.3	1,149.3	1,125.1
Total, crude	1,676.8	1,484.1	1,222.7	1,157.4	1,128.3	1,174.4	1,168.7	1,143.9	1,178.6	1,181.2	1,160.3
Age											
Under 18 years	756.5	614.0	463.5	423.7	402.6	411.0	393.9	376.7	343.3	340.2	336.2
Under 1 year	2,317.6	2,137.9	1,915.3	1,977.6	2,027.6	1,949.3	1,818.4	1,639.3	1,657.5	1,550.7	1,542.6
1 to 4 years	864.6	650.2	466.9	457.1	458.0	429.7	418.8	389.9	337.1	335.2	340.8
5 to 17 years	609.3	477.4	334.1	290.2	268.6	286.5	276.0	271.5	238.2	244.9	239.5
18 to 44 years	1,578.8	1,301.2	1,026.6	914.3	849.4	898.0	906.7	888.8	884.6	886.7	867.3
18 to 24 years	1,570.3	1,297.8	1,065.3	928.9	854.1	862.4	870.4	846.1	817.0	811.8	789.0
25 to 44 years	1,582.8	1,302.5	1,013.8	909.9	847.9	910.3	919.3	903.8	908.6	914.0	896.0
25 to 34 years	1,682.9	1,416.9	1,140.3	1,015.0	942.5	1,007.8	1,011.2	1,003.5	1,003.8	998.1	981.9
35 to 44 years	1,438.3	1,153.1	868.8	808.0	764.8	821.5	834.6	810.4	817.4	830.2	809.3
45 to 64 years	1,947.6	1,707.8	1,354.5	1,185.4	1,114.2	1,147.0	1,161.2	1,143.9	1,197.6	1,221.3	1,200.5
45 to 54 years	1,750.2	1,470.7	1,123.9	984.7	920.8	964.3	970.5	959.3	1,033.3	1,021.8	999.3
55 to 64 years	2,153.6	1,948.0	1,632.6	1,483.4	1,415.0	1,402.4	1,422.1	1,391.2	1,413.8	1,476.6	1,453.1
65 years and over	3,836.9	3,698.0	3,341.2	3,477.4	3,533.6	3,595.6	3,507.9	3,507.9	3,576.5	3,521.5	3,436.1
65 to 74 years	3,158.4	2,972.6	2,616.3	2,600.0	2,546.0	2,628.9	2,533.6	2,439.9	2,531.3	2,554.9	2,487.1
75 years and over	4,893.0	4,756.1	4,340.3	4,590.7	4,619.6	4,588.4	4,512.6	4,392.4	4,698.4	4,591.7	4,493.8
75 to 84 years	4,638.6	4,464.2	3,957.0	4,155.7	4,124.4	4,131.7	4,025.9	3,983.3	4,213.1	4,068.0	3,982.8
85 years and over	5,764.6	5,728.9	5,606.3	5,925.1	6,050.9	5,758.1	5,711.4	5,358.9	5,803.2	5,814.6	5,667.7
Sex[3]											
Male	1,543.9	1,382.5	1,130.0	1,048.5	990.8	1,013.0	1,000.5	973.8	997.3	1,004.3	975.3
Female	1,951.9	1,675.6	1,389.5	1,317.3	1,277.3	1,319.6	1,312.3	1,280.6	1,311.8	1,303.4	1,283.5
Sex and Age											
Male, all ages	1,390.4	1,240.2	1,002.2	941.7	910.6	959.0	954.9	936.7	964.9	978.8	957.4
Under 18 years	762.6	626.4	463.1	431.3	408.6	412.2	401.5	385.6	353.1	348.0	343.1
18 to 44 years	950.9	776.9	579.2	507.2	450.0	471.1	476.8	460.8	439.3	456.0	434.0
45 to 64 years	1,953.1	1,775.6	1,402.7	1,212.0	1,127.4	1,148.8	1,175.7	1,156.6	1,214.1	1,235.4	1,209.8
65 to 74 years	3,474.1	3,255.2	2,877.6	2,762.2	2,649.1	2,742.6	2,584.3	2,559.3	2,601.6	2,678.2	2,598.5
75 to 84 years	5,093.5	5,031.8	4,417.3	4,361.1	4,294.1	4,388.1	4,220.3	4,162.6	4,498.4	4,242.3	4,137.3
85 years and over	6,372.3	6,406.9	6,420.9	6,387.9	6,166.6	5,984.1	5,983.5	5,440.6	6,003.9	6,425.5	6,193.4
Female, all ages	1,944.0	1,712.2	1,431.7	1,362.9	1,336.6	1,382.2	1,375.3	1,344.0	1,385.2	1,377.2	1,357.1
Under 18 years	750.2	601.0	464.1	415.7	396.2	409.8	385.9	367.3	333.1	332.0	329.0
18 to 44 years	2,180.2	1,808.3	1,468.0	1,318.0	1,248.1	1,330.9	1,343.5	1,324.5	1,338.7	1,326.4	1,310.2
45 to 64 years	1,942.5	1,645.9	1,309.7	1,160.5	1,101.7	1,145.3	1,147.3	1,131.7	1,182.0	1,207.8	1,191.6
65 to 74 years	2,916.6	2,754.8	2,411.2	2,469.4	2,461.0	2,533.1	2,490.7	2,338.4	2,471.3	2,449.3	2,391.0
75 to 84 years	4,370.4	4,130.4	3,678.9	4,024.1	4,013.5	3,957.7	3,893.0	3,859.8	4,015.1	3,944.7	3,871.9
85 years and over	5,500.3	5,458.0	5,289.6	5,743.7	6,003.3	5,654.4	5,584.1	5,320.0	5,706.2	5,531.7	5,415.6
Geographic Region[3]											
Northeast	1,622.9	1,428.7	1,332.2	1,335.3	1,274.8	1,245.9	1,261.4	1,274.6	1,283.7	1,361.0	1,299.6
Midwest	1,925.2	1,584.7	1,287.5	1,132.8	1,109.2	1,174.9	1,168.0	1,125.5	1,172.1	1,153.7	1,146.8
South	1,814.1	1,569.4	1,325.0	1,252.4	1,209.2	1,202.5	1,198.8	1,139.9	1,179.0	1,149.3	1,136.1
West	1,519.7	1,469.6	1,006.6	967.4	894.0	1,005.9	964.1	966.0	960.2	959.2	932.7
DAYS OF CARE PER 10,000 POPULATION											
Total, age-adjusted[3]	13,027.0	10,017.9	8,189.3	6,386.2	5,576.8	5,541.7	5,474.7	5,404.1	5,577.2	5,536.3	5,369.2
Total, crude	12,166.8	9,576.6	7,840.5	6,201.7	5,546.5	5,620.9	5,577.8	5,539.4	5,773.9	5,748.1	5,598.7
Age											
Under 18 years	3,415.1	2,812.3	2,263.1	1,846.7	1,789.7	1,918.3	1,857.6	1,785.0	1,482.8	1,491.6	1,479.5
Under 1 year	13,213.9	14,141.2	11,484.7	10,834.5	11,524.0	12,131.6	11,624.2	8,466.7	9,401.0	9,277.7	9,170.4
1 to 4 years	3,333.5	2,280.4	1,700.1	1,525.6	1,482.2	1,355.3	1,405.4	1,280.3	1,018.8	1,041.0	1,111.0
5 to 17 years	2,698.5	2,049.8	1,633.2	1,240.3	1,172.1	1,300.9	1,239.1	1,406.4	984.0	1,012.6	990.5
18 to 44 years	8,323.6	6,294.7	4,676.7	3,517.2	3,093.8	3,305.0	3,360.6	3,258.0	3,180.3	3,268.3	3,147.4
18 to 24 years	7,174.6	5,287.2	4,015.9	2,987.4	2,679.5	2,819.9	2,889.4	2,738.7	2,606.0	2,755.3	2,687.1
25 to 44 years	8,861.4	6,685.2	4,895.5	3,676.4	3,225.5	3,472.8	3,524.5	3,439.7	3,383.8	3,454.9	3,316.3
25 to 34 years	8,497.5	6,688.9	4,939.7	3,536.1	3,161.7	3,434.3	3,462.2	3,423.1	3,462.0	3,482.0	3,342.6
35 to 44 years	9,386.6	6,680.4	4,844.8	3,812.3	3,281.5	3,507.9	3,581.9	3,455.2	3,308.9	3,428.0	3,289.7
45 to 64 years	15,969.5	12,015.9	9,139.3	6,574.5	5,515.4	5,717.3	5,793.0	5,868.2	6,284.3	6,184.5	6,058.0
45 to 54 years	13,167.2	9,692.8	6,996.6	5,162.0	4,374.2	4,711.2	4,667.4	4,745.9	5,185.7	4,772.0	4,719.7
55 to 64 years	18,895.4	14,369.5	11,722.6	8,671.6	7,290.8	7,124.0	7,333.6	7,371.8	7,729.7	7,993.0	7,739.0
65 years and over	40,983.5	32,279.7	28,956.1	23,736.5	21,118.9	19,882.8	19,197.5	18,951.7	20,391.2	19,933.0	19,225.8
65 to 74 years	31,470.3	24,373.3	20,878.2	16,847.0	14,389.7	13,985.3	13,170.2	13,274.8	13,911.2	13,888.2	13,504.6
75 years and over	55,788.2	43,812.7	40,090.8	32,478.1	28,518.6	25,939.4	25,413.1	24,878.5	27,347.0	26,625.9	25,602.5
75 to 84 years	51,836.2	40,521.6	35,995.1	28,947.5	25,397.8	23,155.3	22,671.7	22,658.1	24,400.0	23,644.1	22,884.1
85 years and over	69,332.0	54,782.4	53,616.9	43,305.9	37,537.8	33,071.5	32,165.5	30,124.5	34,055.6	33,588.7	31,848.6
Sex[3]											
Male	12,475.8	9,792.1	8,057.8	6,239.0	5,358.8	5,301.3	5,208.8	5,157.4	5,376.4	5,342.4	5,158.3
Female	13,662.9	10,340.4	8,404.5	6,548.8	5,809.7	5,828.7	5,764.2	5,685.1	5,832.4	5,784.1	5,630.6

[1]Comparisons of data from 1980–1985 with data from subsequent years should be made with caution because estimates of change may reflect improvements in the survey design rather than true changes in hospital use.
[2]Starting with 2008 data, the sample of nonfederal short-stay hospitals was cut in half. This smaller sample size has increased standard errors. Therefore, caution should be exercised in interpreting trends in these data.
[3]Estimates are age adjusted to the year 2000 standard population using six age groups: under 18 years, 18 to 44 years, 45 to 54 years, 55 to 64 years, 65 to 74 years, and 75 years and over.

Table 3-52. Discharges, Days of Care, and Average Length of Stay in Nonfederal Short-Stay Hospitals, by Selected Characteristics, Selected Years, 1980 Through 2009–2010—*Continued*

(Rate per 10,000 population, number.)

Characteristic	1980[1]	1985[1]	1990	1995	2000	2005	2006	2007	2008[2]	2009[2]	2009–2010[2]
Sex and Age											
Male, all ages	10,674.1	8,518.8	6,943.0	5,507.5	4,860.8	4,979.7	4,947.3	4,937.6	5,176.0	5,178.1	5,043.5
Under 18 years	3,473.1	2,942.7	2,335.7	1,998.0	1,955.7	2,006.2	1,968.0	1,858.1	1,646.9	1,526.4	1,555.6
18 to 44 years	6,102.4	4,746.6	3,517.4	2,729.7	2,175.0	2,282.7	2,375.6	2,241.8	2,045.7	2,203.9	2,036.6
45 to 64 years	15,894.9	12,290.1	9,434.2	6,822.7	5,704.4	5,773.5	6,004.3	6,103.5	6,553.3	6,443.8	6,327.1
65 to 74 years	33,697.6	26,220.5	22,515.5	17,697.4	14,897.4	14,502.6	13,262.1	13,666.7	14,473.2	14,915.8	14,462.9
75 to 84 years	54,723.3	44,087.4	38,257.8	29,642.6	26,616.7	25,106.9	23,972.7	23,894.6	26,208.6	24,959.5	24,184.6
85 years and over	77,013.1	58,609.5	60,347.3	45,263.6	37,765.3	35,179.0	32,604.0	31,480.6	37,292.7	37,649.7	35,211.1
Female, all ages	13,560.1	10,566.3	8,691.1	6,863.4	6,202.7	6,239.5	6,186.8	6,121.1	6,352.3	6,300.0	6,137.1
Under 18 years	3,354.5	2,675.5	2,186.8	1,687.9	1,615.1	1,826.1	1,741.8	1,708.3	1,310.9	1,455.1	1,399.7
18 to 44 years	10,450.7	7,792.0	5,820.3	4,297.9	4,010.8	4,341.8	4,361.5	4,292.3	4,337.0	4,354.8	4,283.0
45 to 64 years	16,037.1	11,765.5	8,865.1	6,341.7	5,336.4	5,663.9	5,592.2	5,644.3	6,028.1	5,937.5	5,801.9
65 to 74 years	29,764.7	22,949.2	19,592.7	16,162.0	13,971.3	13,549.0	13,092.4	12,942.1	13,431.6	13,007.9	12,678.4
75 to 84 years	50,133.3	38,424.7	34,628.3	28,502.5	24,601.0	21,830.1	21,782.1	21,806.2	23,144.7	22,713.5	21,949.6
85 years and over	65,990.5	53,253.6	51,000.5	42,538.6	37,444.4	32,103.5	31,960.3	29,479.5	32,492.0	31,707.4	30,236.0
Geographic Region[3]											
Northeast	14,024.4	11,143.1	10,266.8	8,389.7	7,185.9	6,636.5	6,608.5	7,284.4	7,055.4	7,512.7	7,072.6
Midwest	14,871.9	10,803.6	8,306.5	5,908.8	5,005.3	4,954.3	4,893.5	4,775.3	5,176.9	4,990.1	4,932.7
South	12,713.5	9,642.6	8,204.1	6,659.9	5,925.1	5,830.4	5,844.8	5,555.7	5,667.9	5,610.4	5,514.2
West	9,635.2	8,300.7	5,755.1	4,510.6	4,082.0	4,690.3	4,451.6	4,184.5	4,528.7	4,241.2	4,084.4
AVERAGE LENGTH OF STAY IN DAYS											
Total, age-adjusted[3]	7.5	6.6	6.5	5.4	4.9	4.8	4.7	4.8	4.8	4.8	4.8
Total, crude	7.3	6.5	6.4	5.4	4.9	4.8	4.8	4.8	4.9	4.9	4.8
Age											
Under 18 years	4.5	4.6	4.9	4.4	4.4	4.7	4.7	4.7	4.3	4.4	4.4
Under 1 year	5.7	6.6	6.0	5.5	5.7	6.2	6.4	5.2	5.7	6.0	5.9
1 to 4 years	3.9	3.5	3.6	3.3	3.2	3.2	3.4	3.3	3.0	3.1	3.3
5 to 17 years	4.4	4.3	4.9	4.3	4.4	4.5	4.5	5.2	4.1	4.1	4.1
18 to 44 years	5.3	4.8	4.6	3.8	3.6	3.7	3.7	3.7	3.6	3.7	3.6
18 to 24 years	4.6	4.1	3.8	3.2	3.1	3.3	3.3	3.2	3.2	3.4	3.4
25 to 44 years	5.6	5.1	4.8	4.0	3.8	3.8	3.8	3.8	3.7	3.8	3.7
25 to 34 years	5.0	4.7	4.3	3.5	3.4	3.4	3.4	3.4	3.4	3.5	3.4
35 to 44 years	6.5	5.8	5.6	4.7	4.3	4.3	4.3	4.3	4.0	4.1	4.1
45 to 64 years	8.2	7.0	6.7	5.5	5.0	5.0	5.0	5.1	5.2	5.1	5.0
45 to 54 years	7.5	6.6	6.2	5.2	4.8	4.9	4.8	4.9	5.0	4.7	4.7
55 to 64 years	8.8	7.4	7.2	5.8	5.2	5.1	5.2	5.3	5.5	5.4	5.3
65 years and over	10.7	8.7	8.7	6.8	6.0	5.5	5.5	5.6	5.7	5.7	5.6
65 to 74 years	10.0	8.2	8.0	6.5	5.7	5.3	5.2	5.4	5.5	5.4	5.4
75 years and over	11.4	9.2	9.2	7.1	6.2	5.7	5.6	5.7	5.8	5.8	5.7
75 to 84 years	11.2	9.1	9.1	7.0	6.2	5.6	5.6	5.7	5.8	5.8	5.7
85 years and over	12.0	9.6	9.6	7.3	6.2	5.7	5.6	5.6	5.9	5.8	5.6
Sex[3]											
Male	8.1	7.1	7.1	6.0	5.4	5.2	5.2	5.3	5.4	5.3	5.3
Female	7.0	6.2	6.0	5.0	4.5	4.4	4.4	4.4	4.4	4.4	4.4
Sex and Age											
Male, all ages	7.7	6.9	6.9	5.8	5.3	5.2	5.2	5.3	5.4	5.3	5.3
Under 18 years	4.6	4.7	5.0	4.6	4.8	4.9	4.9	4.8	4.7	4.4	4.5
18 to 44 years	6.4	6.1	6.1	5.4	4.8	4.8	5.0	4.9	4.7	4.8	4.7
45 to 64 years	8.1	6.9	6.7	5.6	5.1	5.0	5.1	5.3	5.4	5.2	5.2
65 to 74 years	9.7	8.1	7.8	6.4	5.6	5.3	5.1	5.3	5.6	5.6	5.6
75 to 84 years	10.7	8.8	8.7	6.8	6.2	5.7	5.7	5.7	5.8	5.9	5.8
85 years and over	12.1	9.1	9.4	7.1	6.1	5.9	5.4	5.8	6.2	5.9	5.7
Female, all ages	7.0	6.2	6.1	5.0	4.6	4.5	4.5	4.6	4.6	4.6	4.5
Under 18 years	4.5	4.5	4.7	4.1	4.1	4.5	4.5	4.7	3.9	4.4	4.3
18 to 44 years	4.8	4.3	4.0	3.3	3.2	3.3	3.2	3.2	3.2	3.3	3.3
45 to 64 years	8.3	7.1	6.8	5.5	4.8	4.9	4.9	5.0	5.1	4.9	4.9
65 to 74 years	10.2	8.3	8.1	6.5	5.7	5.3	5.3	5.5	5.4	5.3	5.3
75 to 84 years	11.5	9.3	9.4	7.1	6.1	5.5	5.6	5.6	5.8	5.8	5.7
85 years and over	12.0	9.8	9.6	7.4	6.2	5.7	5.7	5.5	5.7	5.7	5.6
Geographic Region[3]											
Northeast	8.6	7.8	7.7	6.3	5.6	5.3	5.2	5.7	5.5	5.5	5.4
Midwest	7.7	6.8	6.5	5.2	4.5	4.2	4.2	4.2	4.4	4.3	4.3
South	7.0	6.1	6.2	5.3	4.9	4.8	4.9	4.9	4.8	4.9	4.9
West	6.3	5.6	5.7	4.7	4.6	4.7	4.6	4.3	4.7	4.4	4.4

[1]Comparisons of data from 1980–1985 with data from subsequent years should be made with caution because estimates of change may reflect improvements in the survey design rather than true changes in hospital use.
[2]Starting with 2008 data, the sample of nonfederal short–stay hospitals was cut in half. This smaller sample size has increased standard errors. Therefore, caution should be exercised in interpreting trends in these data.
[3]Estimates are age adjusted to the year 2000 standard population using six age groups: under 18 years, 18 to 44 years, 45 to 54 years, 55 to 64 years, 65 to 74 years, and 75 years and over.

Table 3-53. Discharges in Nonfederal Short-Stay Hospitals, by Sex, Age, and Selected First-Listed Diagnosis, Selected Years, 1990 Through 2009–2010

(Numbers in thousands.)

Age and first-listed diagnosis	Both sexes 1990	1995	2009[1]	2009–2010[1]	Male 1990	1995	2009[1]	2009–2010[1]	Female 1990	1995	2009[1]	2009–2010[1]
ALL AGES[2]	30,788	30,722	36,120	35,599	12,280	12,198	14,721	14,461	18,508	18,525	21,398	21,139
Under 18 Years[2]	3,072	3,002	*2,536	*2,506	1,572	1,565	*1,327	*1,309	1,500	1,437	*1,209	*1,197
Dehydration	63	106	*73	*64	32	59	*39	*35	31	47	*34	*29
Acute bronchitis and bronchiolitis	114	170	*109	*119	67	109	*70	*73	47	61	*40	*46
Pneumonia	221	250	170	*167	126	143	*86	*84	95	107	*84	*83
Asthma	182	227	*143	*140	111	137	*92	*88	71	90	*50	*52
Appendicitis	83	69	*76	*72	50	41	*47	*45	34	28	29	*26
Injury	329	286	161	*173	210	171	*96	*104	119	115	*65	*69
Fracture	117	102	*67	*76	76	66	*42	*48	42	36	*25	*28
Complications of care and adverse effects	41	46	*43	*39	22	25	*23	*21	19	*21	*20	*18
18 to 44 Years[2]	11,138	9,996	9,963	9,746	3,120	2,761	2,588	2,465	8,018	7,235	7,375	7,280
HIV/AIDS	*20	88	23	24	*15	66	*17	17	*	22	*6	*7
Cancer, all	181	150	113	114	64	47	*35	40	116	102	77	74
Childbirth	X	X	X	X	X	X	X	X	3,815	3,574	3,862	3,851
Uterine fibroids	X	X	X	X	X	X	X	X	110	115	81	84
Diabetes	105	102	159	159	61	52	79	79	44	50	80	81
Alcohol and drug	284	363	224	215	199	255	152	147	84	107	71	69
Schizophrenia, mood disorders, delusional disorders, nonorganic psychoses	384	551	544	541	184	262	268	271	200	289	276	271
Schizophrenia	145	*181	148	140	88	*118	88	84	57	63	*61	56
Mood disorders	211	324	359	368	83	121	160	166	128	203	199	202
Heart disease	236	265	239	228	163	157	144	140	73	108	95	88
Ischemic heart disease	129	130	72	68	95	90	48	47	34	39	*25	21
Pneumonia	136	149	126	107	69	74	59	51	67	75	67	56
Asthma	106	119	90	85	27	30	*28	26	79	89	62	59
Intervertebral disc disorders	222	157	105	96	138	94	53	49	84	62	52	47
Injury	935	688	555	503	641	465	359	316	294	223	196	187
Fracture	302	250	221	203	217	176	162	142	85	74	59	61
Poisoning and toxic effects	124	118	134	125	54	59	58	55	70	59	76	70
Complications of care and adverse effects	135	146	195	187	63	64	81	74	72	82	114	113
45 to 64 Years[2]	6,244	6,168	9,686	9,585	3,115	3,053	4,781	4,710	3,129	3,115	4,906	4,874
HIV/AIDS	*3	20	*16	16	*3	15	*12	12	*	*5	*4	*4
Cancer, all	545	461	525	497	236	193	255	244	309	268	269	253
Colorectal cancer	59	29	66	60	33	17	32	30	26	13	34	29
Lung/bronchus/tracheal cancer	101	76	68	62	60	37	31	28	41	39	*37	34
Breast cancer[3]	X	X	X	X	X	X	X	X	69	61	48	47
Prostate cancer	X	X	X	X	19	32	*57	*53	X	X	X	X
Uterine fibroids	X	X	X	X	X	X	X	X	70	74	93	95
Diabetes	134	172	256	255	65	86	124	128	70	86	132	127
Alcohol and drug	100	128	191	194	77	100	138	142	23	28	53	52
Schizophrenia, mood disorders, delusional disorders, nonorganic psychoses	152	194	384	379	56	75	177	169	95	118	207	210
Schizophrenia	47	*67	119	115	19	*	*66	61	28	36	54	54
Mood disorders	91	112	241	242	32	37	98	97	58	74	142	146
Heart disease	1,100	1,152	1,204	1,162	704	749	756	730	397	403	448	432
Ischemic heart disease	739	762	579	544	502	537	393	371	237	225	187	173
Heart attack	233	256	205	210	165	188	144	147	68	68	61	63
Arrhythmias	131	131	186	197	79	75	115	121	53	56	71	76
Heart failure	122	143	271	254	68	75	161	145	54	68	111	109
Hypertension	75	82	155	143	38	37	76	69	37	45	80	74
Stroke	162	182	275	288	91	96	149	160	72	86	126	127
Pneumonia	154	163	264	261	76	75	141	135	79	88	122	126
Chronic obstructive pulmonary disease	73	154	236	231	39	72	95	94	34	82	141	137
Asthma	86	87	132	125	26	21	40	34	59	66	93	92
Osteoarthritis	87	110	476	491	36	47	211	211	51	64	265	280
Intervertebral disc disorders	145	115	167	162	82	65	85	82	63	51	81	79
Injury	334	296	441	450	178	165	229	242	157	131	211	208
Fracture	149	147	211	233	74	74	109	122	75	72	102	111
Poisoning and toxic effects	29	30	101	95	10	13	44	43	19	17	57	52
Internal organ injury	36	38	64	56	23	27	36	35	14	11	*28	*21
Complications of care and adverse effects	148	186	402	398	79	92	204	199	69	94	198	199
65 to 74 Years[2]	4,689	4,832	5,312	5,251	2,268	2,290	2,569	2,540	2,421	2,542	2,743	2,711
Septicemia	49	65	139	150	27	27	67	76	21	38	72	74
Cancer, all	436	416	326	311	222	203	178	171	214	212	147	140
Colorectal cancer	48	46	43	35	24	22	*23	20	24	24	*20	15
Lung/bronchus/tracheal cancer	77	73	61	58	50	44	*34	33	26	29	27	25
Breast cancer[3]	X	X	X	X	X	X	X	X	42	35	*21	19
Prostate cancer	X	X	X	X	40	41	*34	29	X	X	X	X
Diabetes	93	93	107	96	34	44	45	45	59	49	61	51
Schizophrenia, mood disorders, delusional disorders, nonorganic psychoses	59	80	*65	*62	20	20	*26	*21	39	60	*38	*41
Dementia and Alzheimer's disease	10	18	*14	*18	4	11	*	*	*6	7	*	*9

X = Not applicable.
* = Figure does not meet standards of reliability or precision. Data preceded by an asterisk have a relative standard error (RSE) of 20 to 30 percent. Data not shown have an RSE of greater than 30 percent.
[1]Starting with 2008 data, the sample of nonfederal short-stay hospitals was cut in half. This smaller sample size has increased standard errors. Therefore, caution should be exercised in interpreting trends in these data.
[2]Includes discharges with first-listed diagnoses not shown in table.
[3]Shown for women only.

Table 3-53. Discharges in Nonfederal Short-Stay Hospitals, by Sex, Age, and Selected First-Listed Diagnosis, Selected Years, 1990 Through 2009–2010—*Continued*

(Numbers in thousands.)

Age and first-listed diagnosis	Both sexes				Male				Female			
	1990	1995	2009[1]	2009–2010[1]	1990	1995	2009[1]	2009–2010[1]	1990	1995	2009[1]	2009–2010[1]
Heart disease	1,000	1,115	888	860	547	618	514	498	453	497	375	363
Ischemic heart disease	576	614	389	359	331	365	241	229	245	250	148	131
Heart attack	185	210	138	131	110	129	83	81	75	82	54	50
Arrhythmias	124	153	176	180	67	74	97	97	57	79	79	82
Heart failure	188	233	209	198	93	126	114	110	95	107	95	88
Hypertension	39	42	*77	61	13	14	*32	*24	26	28	*45	38
Stroke	222	250	225	231	108	141	125	124	114	109	100	107
Pneumonia	176	214	174	177	90	105	79	85	86	109	95	92
Chronic obstructive pulmonary disease	81	191	211	208	41	83	96	91	40	107	115	117
Gallstones	79	78	49	47	30	31	25	23	49	46	23	24
Kidney disease	18	31	121	121	9	16	65	70	9	15	56	51
Urinary tract infection	54	50	82	80	17	20	29	25	37	30	53	56
Hyperplasia of the prostate	X	X	X	X	113	62	*23	21	X	X	X	X
Osteoarthritis	122	154	308	339	44	53	115	133	78	101	193	206
Injury	193	176	201	203	71	67	80	75	122	109	121	128
Fracture	120	109	121	126	36	36	37	37	85	72	84	88
Hip fracture	48	44	40	39	12	15	12	12	36	29	*28	27
Complications of care and adverse effects	125	144	204	203	68	66	107	102	57	78	97	101
75 to 84 Years[2]	3,949	4,590	5,349	5,257	1,660	1,880	2,311	2,283	2,289	2,710	3,038	2,973
Septicemia	54	87	171	183	24	38	81	84	30	50	90	99
Cancer, all	300	281	236	227	158	131	108	109	142	150	128	119
Colorectal cancer	50	46	39	39	20	22	*15	17	29	24	24	22
Lung/bronchus/tracheal cancer	36	32	44	44	22	17	*21	22	*15	15	23	22
Breast cancer[3]	X	X	X	X	X	X	X	X	24	24	*10	13
Prostate cancer	X	X	X	X	37	18	*5	*6	X	X	X	X
Diabetes	44	73	100	88	17	30	39	37	27	43	*60	51
Schizophrenia, mood disorders, delusional disorders, nonorganic psychoses	39	44	*	*	*10	10	*	*	28	35	*23	*24
Dementia and Alzheimer's disease	20	46	53	58	9	19	*29	26	11	26	*25	33
Heart disease	865	1,057	1,025	976	377	471	480	466	488	585	545	510
Ischemic heart disease	382	479	358	328	177	228	189	173	205	251	169	156
Heart attack	156	188	165	149	83	91	79	70	73	97	86	78
Arrhythmias	133	175	241	223	58	83	99	92	76	92	143	131
Heart failure	261	290	296	291	108	116	132	137	153	174	164	154
Hypertension	23	31	64	50	*	*11	*21	*17	19	20	43	33
Stroke	258	297	258	260	104	129	123	116	154	169	135	144
Pneumonia	224	282	234	237	112	142	109	107	112	140	124	130
Chronic obstructive pulmonary disease	55	143	181	173	34	63	86	83	22	80	94	91
Gallstones	48	55	51	52	20	22	20	22	28	33	*31	30
Kidney disease	24	28	143	145	10	17	70	68	*14	12	73	77
Urinary tract infection	86	99	158	162	25	35	46	48	61	64	112	114
Hyperplasia of the prostate	X	X	X	X	69	41	*21	21	X	X	X	X
Osteoarthritis	69	115	205	213	25	34	80	84	44	80	125	129
Injury	259	270	306	313	58	77	104	104	201	193	202	208
Fracture	195	208	211	219	35	53	60	62	161	154	151	158
Hip fracture	115	122	83	92	20	29	20	25	95	93	63	66
Complications of care and adverse effects	81	108	159	162	38	40	81	83	43	68	78	79
85 Years and Over[2]	1,694	2,134	3,274	3,256	543	648	1,145	1,153	1,151	1,486	2,129	2,102
Septicemia	41	57	134	150	12	17	52	60	29	40	82	90
Cancer, all	77	77	94	83	31	32	43	39	45	45	51	44
Colorectal cancer	14	17	*12	10	*5	*	*	*4	9	11	*7	*6
Lung/bronchus/tracheal cancer	*6	*4	*13	*14	*	*2	*	*	*	*	*	*6
Breast cancer[3]	X	X	X	X	X	X	X	X	*9	8	*	*5
Prostate cancer	X	X	X	X	*7	*	*	*4	X	X	X	X
Diabetes	16	22	*34	34	*5	*	*13	13	11	15	*21	*21
Schizophrenia, mood disorders, delusional disorders, nonorganic psychoses	*8	16	*	*	*	*	*	*8	*7	*12	*	*
Dementia and Alzheimer's disease	15	28	42	44	*2	*6	16	18	13	22	26	26
Heart disease	335	446	611	606	112	135	236	228	223	311	376	378
Ischemic heart disease	128	144	139	142	49	48	62	60	79	96	76	82
Heart attack	60	73	88	92	23	28	37	37	37	44	51	56
Arrhythmias	51	72	127	122	16	20	37	40	35	51	90	82
Heart failure	126	181	263	259	39	52	101	98	87	129	162	161
Hypertension	*5	8	37	28	*	*	*12	*9	*4	*6	*25	19
Stroke	129	156	162	163	35	42	48	52	95	114	114	111
Pneumonia	151	194	207	204	64	73	74	80	88	121	134	124
Chronic obstructive pulmonary disease	13	39	81	83	*6	18	*28	32	*7	21	53	50

X = Not applicable.
* = Figure does not meet standards of reliability or precision. Data preceded by an asterisk have a relative standard error (RSE) of 20 to 30 percent. Data not shown have an RSE of greater than 30 percent.
[1]Starting with 2008 data, the sample of nonfederal short-stay hospitals was cut in half. This smaller sample size has increased standard errors. Therefore, caution should be exercised in interpreting trends in these data.
[2]Includes discharges with first-listed diagnoses not shown in table.
[3]Shown for women only.

Table 3-53. Discharges in Nonfederal Short-Stay Hospitals, by Sex, Age, and Selected First-Listed Diagnosis, Selected Years, 1990 Through 2009–2010—*Continued*

(Numbers in thousands.)

Age and first-listed diagnosis	Both sexes				Male				Female			
	1990	1995	2009[1]	2009–2010[1]	1990	1995	2009[1]	2009–2010[1]	1990	1995	2009[1]	2009–2010[1]
Gallstones	18	21	*24	23	*6	*7	*7	*8	13	15	*17	15
Kidney disease	14	16	90	96	8	*8	36	43	*6	*9	54	53
Urinary tract infection	65	74	195	185	20	*18	46	40	45	56	149	144
Hyperplasia of the prostate	X	X	X	X	13	9	*6	*6	X	X	X	X
Osteoarthritis	13	20	36	40	*	*6	*10	*10	8	14	26	30
Injury	164	216	300	302	37	47	78	80	127	169	223	222
Fracture	133	172	227	228	28	32	54	51	104	140	173	177
Hip fracture	82	108	123	122	19	19	29	29	63	88	94	93
Complications of care and adverse effects	29	29	75	73	11	*10	*27	30	18	19	48	43

X = Not applicable.
* = Figure does not meet standards of reliability or precision. Data preceded by an asterisk have a relative standard error (RSE) of 20 to 30 percent. Data not shown have an RSE of greater than 30 percent.
[1]Starting with 2008 data, the sample of nonfederal short-stay hospitals was cut in half. This smaller sample size has increased standard errors. Therefore, caution should be exercised in interpreting trends in these data.

Table 3-54. Discharge Rate in Nonfederal Short-Stay Hospitals, by Sex, Age, and Selected First-Listed Diagnosis, Selected Years 1990 Through 2009–2010

(Number per 10,000 population.)

Age and first-listed diagnosis	Both sexes				Male				Female			
	1990	2000	2009[1]	2009–2010[1]	1990	2000	2009[1]	2009–2010[1]	1990	2000	2009[1]	2009–2010[1]
All Ages, Age-Adjusted[2,3]	1,252.4	1,132.8	1,149.3	1,125.1	1,130.0	990.8	1,004.3	975.3	1,389.5	1,277.3	1,303.4	1,283.5
All Ages, Crude[3]	1,222.7	1,128.3	1,181.2	1,160.3	1,002.2	910.6	978.8	957.4	1,431.7	1,336.6	1,377.2	1,357.1
Under 18 Years[3]	463.5	402.6	*340.2	*336.2	463.1	408.6	*348.0	*343.1	464.1	396.2	*332.0	*329.0
Dehydration	9.5	15.7	*9.8	*8.6	9.4	17.2	*10.4	*9.1	9.7	14.2	*9.2	*8.0
Acute bronchitis and bronchiolitis	17.2	27.8	*14.7	*16.0	19.6	31.4	*18.3	*19.1	14.6	24.1	*10.9	*12.7
Pneumonia	33.3	25.2	22.7	*22.4	37.0	25.7	*22.5	*22.0	29.5	24.6	*23.0	*22.7
Asthma	27.5	29.6	*19.1	*18.7	32.7	34.8	*24.2	*23.1	22.0	24.0	*13.8	*14.2
Appendicitis	12.6	11.9	*10.2	*9.6	14.6	13.0	*12.2	*11.9	10.5	10.8	8.1	*7.2
Injury	49.7	33.6	21.6	*23.2	62.0	42.0	*25.1	*27.2	36.8	24.8	*17.9	*19.1
Fracture	17.7	13.8	*8.9	*10.2	22.3	18.3	*10.9	*12.6	12.9	9.0	*6.9	*7.8
Complications of care and adverse effects	6.2	*7.3	*5.8	*5.2	6.5	*7.9	*6.0	*5.5	5.9	*6.6	*5.5	*4.9
18 to 44 Years[3]	1,026.6	849.4	886.7	867.3	579.2	450.0	456.0	434.0	1,468.0	1,248.1	1,326.4	1,310.2
HIV/AIDS	*1.8	4.3	2.1	2.2	*2.8	5.8	*3.0	3.1	*	2.8	*1.1	*1.2
Cancer, all	16.6	10.5	10.0	10.1	11.9	7.3	*6.2	7.0	21.3	13.7	13.9	13.3
Childbirth	X	X	X	X	X	X	X	X	698.6	645.2	694.5	693.1
Uterine fibroids	X	X	X	X	X	X	X	X	20.2	21.7	14.6	15.2
Diabetes	9.7	11.5	14.1	14.2	11.3	13.0	13.9	13.9	8.1	9.9	14.4	14.5
Alcohol and drug	26.2	29.7	19.9	19.2	37.0	39.1	26.9	25.8	15.5	*20.2	12.8	12.4
Schizophrenia, mood disorders, delusional disorders,												
nonorganic psychoses	35.4	*53.6	48.5	48.2	34.1	*53.2	47.3	47.6	36.7	*53.9	49.7	48.7
Schizophrenia	13.4	*14.4	13.2	12.4	16.4	*18.6	15.5	14.8	10.5	*10.1	*10.9	10.0
Mood disorders	19.4	*35.9	31.9	32.8	15.4	*31.0	28.2	29.3	23.4	*40.9	35.8	36.3
Heart disease	21.7	21.8	21.3	20.3	30.2	26.6	25.4	24.6	13.4	17.0	17.1	15.8
Ischemic heart disease	11.9	9.9	6.4	6.0	17.7	14.2	8.4	8.3	6.3	5.6	*4.5	3.7
Pneumonia	12.5	10.9	11.2	9.5	12.8	10.0	10.4	8.9	12.2	11.9	12.0	10.1
Asthma	9.8	9.0	8.0	7.6	5.1	5.4	*4.9	4.6	14.4	12.6	11.1	10.7
Intervertebral disc disorders	20.5	12.5	9.3	8.5	25.6	14.5	9.4	8.6	15.4	10.4	9.3	8.4
Injury	86.2	45.8	49.4	44.8	119.0	62.3	63.2	55.7	53.8	29.4	35.3	33.6
Fracture	27.8	17.8	19.7	18.1	40.2	25.4	28.5	25.0	15.5	10.2	10.6	11.0
Poisoning and toxic effects	11.4	8.5	11.9	11.2	10.0	6.7	10.2	9.7	12.7	10.3	13.7	12.6
Complications of care and adverse effects	12.5	12.2	17.4	16.6	11.7	11.2	14.3	13.1	13.3	13.1	20.5	20.3
45 to 64 Years[3]	1,354.5	1,114.2	1,221.3	1,200.5	1,402.7	1,127.4	1,235.4	1,209.8	1,309.7	1,101.7	1,207.8	1,191.6
HIV/AIDS	*0.6	*3.2	*2.0	2.0	*1.2	*4.9	*3.0	3.0	*	*	*1.0	*1.1
Cancer, all	118.3	62.9	66.1	62.2	106.3	62.1	65.9	62.6	129.5	63.6	66.3	61.8
Colorectal cancer	12.7	7.9	8.3	7.5	14.8	8.9	8.2	7.8	10.8	6.9	8.3	7.2
Lung/bronchus/tracheal cancer	21.8	6.9	8.6	7.8	26.8	8.6	8.1	7.2	17.2	5.2	*9.2	8.3
Breast cancer[4]	X	X	X	X	X	X	X	X	29.0	14.2	11.8	11.5
Prostate cancer	X	X	X	X	8.5	9.6	*14.6	*13.5	X	X	X	X
Uterine fibroids	X	X	X	X	X	X	X	X	29.3	35.6	22.9	23.3
Diabetes	29.1	33.1	32.3	32.0	29.1	37.4	32.0	32.9	29.2	29.0	32.6	31.1
Alcohol and drug	21.7	23.3	24.1	24.2	34.6	33.5	35.6	36.4	9.6	13.7	13.0	12.7
Schizophrenia, mood disorders, delusional disorders,												
nonorganic psychoses	32.9	42.7	48.4	47.5	25.4	*39.6	45.7	43.5	39.8	45.6	50.9	51.3
Schizophrenia	10.1	12.8	15.1	14.4	8.4	*14.4	*17.0	15.7	11.7	11.3	13.2	13.2
Mood disorders	19.6	*26.9	30.3	30.4	14.5	*21.6	25.4	24.9	24.4	*32.0	35.1	35.6
Heart disease	238.7	203.6	151.8	145.6	316.8	264.0	195.3	187.5	166.1	146.4	110.3	105.6
Ischemic heart disease	160.3	126.4	73.1	68.2	226.1	177.3	101.4	95.4	99.2	78.2	46.0	42.3
Heart attack	50.6	38.8	25.9	26.4	74.4	58.7	37.3	37.8	28.4	19.9	15.0	15.4
Arrhythmias	28.5	25.1	23.5	24.7	35.5	31.8	29.8	31.1	22.1	18.7	17.5	18.6
Heart failure	26.4	31.4	34.2	31.8	30.7	33.5	41.5	37.3	22.4	29.3	27.3	26.6
Hypertension	16.3	19.0	19.6	17.9	16.9	17.6	19.6	17.6	15.6	20.3	19.6	18.2
Stroke	35.2	36.7	34.7	36.0	40.8	38.3	38.6	41.2	30.1	35.2	31.0	31.1
Pneumonia	33.5	35.3	33.2	32.6	34.0	34.2	36.5	34.7	33.0	36.4	30.2	30.7
Chronic obstructive pulmonary disease	15.8	30.8	29.7	28.9	17.4	30.8	24.5	24.1	14.3	30.8	34.8	33.5
Asthma	18.6	13.4	16.7	15.7	11.8	6.2	10.3	8.7	24.9	20.2	22.8	22.4
Osteoarthritis	18.9	24.0	60.0	61.5	16.3	20.8	54.6	54.1	21.2	27.0	65.1	68.4
Intervertebral disc disorders	31.5	21.2	21.0	20.3	36.8	22.5	22.1	21.2	26.5	20.0	20.0	19.4
Injury	72.5	47.9	55.6	56.4	79.9	51.2	59.3	62.2	65.6	44.7	52.0	50.8
Fracture	32.4	26.2	26.6	29.2	33.4	25.3	28.2	31.3	31.5	27.0	25.0	27.2
Poisoning and toxic effects	6.3	6.3	12.7	11.9	4.5	5.5	11.3	11.0	8.0	7.1	14.1	12.7
Internal organ injury	7.9	4.5	8.1	7.1	10.2	5.9	9.3	9.1	5.7	3.2	*6.8	*5.1
Complications of care and adverse effects	32.0	34.5	50.7	49.8	35.6	36.3	52.8	51.0	28.7	32.7	48.8	48.7
65 to 74 Years[3]	2,616.3	2,546.0	2,554.9	2,487.1	2,877.6	2,649.1	2,678.2	2,598.5	2,411.2	2,461.0	2,449.3	2,391.0
Septicemia	27.2	35.6	66.9	71.3	34.9	40.1	69.7	77.9	21.2	32.0	64.5	65.5
Cancer, all	243.1	159.0	156.6	147.5	281.4	176.4	186.0	175.3	213.0	144.7	131.4	123.6
Colorectal cancer	27.0	22.8	20.5	16.6	30.6	29.9	*24.1	20.1	24.1	16.9	*17.4	13.5
Lung/bronchus/tracheal cancer	42.9	26.1	29.2	27.3	63.9	28.2	*35.2	33.6	26.4	24.5	24.0	21.9
Breast cancer[4]	X	X	X	X	X	X	X	X	42.3	31.2	*18.8	16.7
Prostate cancer	X	X	X	X	50.6	37.1	*35.9	30.1	X	X	X	X

X = Not applicable.
* = Figure does not meet standards of reliability or precision. Data preceded by an asterisk have a relative standard error (RSE) of 20 to 30 percent. Data not shown have an RSE of greater than 30 percent.
[1]Starting with 2008 data, the sample of nonfederal short-stay hospitals was cut in half. This smaller sample size has increased standard errors. Therefore, caution should be exercised in interpreting trends in these data.
[2]Estimates are age adjusted to the year 2000 standard population using six age groups: under 18 years, 18 to 44 years, 45 to 54 years, 55 to 64 years, 65 to 74 years, and 75 years and over.
[3]Includes discharges with first-listed diagnoses not shown in table.
[4]Shown for women only.

Table 3-54. Discharge Rate in Nonfederal Short-Stay Hospitals, by Sex, Age, and Selected First-Listed Diagnosis, Selected Years 1990 Through 2009–2010—Continued

(Number per 10,000 population.)

Age and first-listed diagnosis	Both sexes				Male				Female			
	1990	2000	2009[1]	2009–2010[1]	1990	2000	2009[1]	2009–2010[1]	1990	2000	2009[1]	2009–2010[1]
Diabetes	51.8	46.4	51.3	45.4	43.6	46.8	47.1	45.7	58.3	46.2	54.9	45.2
Schizophrenia, mood disorders, delusional disorders, nonorganic psychoses	32.7	37.1	*31.0	*29.2	25.3	*34.2	*27.5	*21.6	38.6	39.6	*34.0	*35.7
Dementia and Alzheimer's disease	5.6	*11.2	*6.9	*8.3	4.9	*16.2	*	*	*6.1	*7.0	*	*7.6
Heart disease	558.1	604.8	427.2	407.4	694.2	706.4	535.4	509.0	451.3	521.0	334.4	319.8
Ischemic heart disease	321.3	307.0	187.0	170.2	419.9	396.5	251.4	233.9	243.9	233.2	131.8	115.2
Heart attack	103.3	100.3	66.3	62.0	139.8	124.7	86.9	82.8	74.6	80.2	48.6	44.1
Arrhythmias	69.1	102.6	84.6	85.1	84.7	108.3	101.4	99.4	56.9	97.9	70.2	72.7
Heart failure	105.2	131.6	100.6	93.9	118.0	136.4	119.3	112.3	95.1	127.6	84.6	78.0
Hypertension	21.8	21.5	*37.0	29.1	16.2	16.5	*33.0	*24.3	26.2	25.5	*40.4	33.2
Stroke	123.9	127.1	108.1	109.5	137.5	131.8	129.9	126.6	113.1	123.2	89.4	94.7
Pneumonia	98.1	121.3	83.5	83.8	113.6	127.7	81.9	86.8	85.9	116.1	84.9	81.2
Chronic obstructive pulmonary disease	45.3	102.3	101.5	98.5	52.6	102.6	100.1	92.8	39.6	102.0	102.7	103.4
Gallstones	44.2	33.4	23.4	22.2	38.2	30.2	26.4	23.6	48.9	36.0	20.9	21.1
Kidney disease	9.9	19.1	58.2	57.1	11.0	21.0	67.9	71.3	9.0	17.5	49.9	44.9
Urinary tract infection	30.2	25.5	39.4	38.0	21.7	19.7	29.8	25.4	36.9	30.3	47.6	49.0
Hyperplasia of the prostate	X	X	X	X	143.5	53.6	*23.7	21.6	X	X	X	X
Osteoarthritis	68.0	101.4	148.0	160.7	55.2	103.1	119.9	136.4	78.0	100.1	172.0	181.7
Injury	107.7	101.5	96.8	96.4	90.7	83.8	83.4	77.1	121.1	116.2	108.3	112.9
Fracture	67.2	63.3	58.2	59.5	45.2	46.8	38.8	38.0	84.4	76.9	74.8	77.9
Hip fracture	26.7	26.4	19.2	18.3	15.3	*20.0	12.4	12.2	35.7	31.7	*25.0	23.6
Complications of care and adverse effects	69.7	80.0	98.3	96.3	85.7	95.7	112.0	104.5	57.2	67.1	86.4	89.3
75 to 84 Years[3]	3,957.0	4,124.4	4,068.0	3,982.8	4,417.3	4,294.1	4,242.3	4,137.3	3,678.9	4,013.5	3,944.7	3,871.9
Septicemia	53.9	68.3	129.9	138.7	63.8	78.1	148.5	151.6	47.9	61.9	116.7	129.3
Cancer, all	300.3	194.0	179.8	172.3	420.8	211.0	198.9	197.3	227.6	182.9	166.3	154.3
Colorectal cancer	49.8	33.0	29.8	29.8	54.0	37.5	*27.4	30.8	47.3	30.1	31.4	29.1
Lung/bronchus/tracheal cancer	36.5	27.0	33.4	33.5	57.2	32.2	*38.4	40.5	*24.0	23.6	29.8	28.5
Breast cancer[4]	X	X	X	X	X	X	X	X	38.7	30.8	*12.5	16.5
Prostate cancer	X	X	X	X	99.2	27.4	*9.4	*11.1	X	X	X	X
Diabetes	44.3	63.4	75.7	66.9	44.8	68.1	72.0	67.5	44.0	60.3	*78.3	66.5
Schizophrenia, mood disorders, delusional disorders, nonorganic psychoses	38.8	41.4	*	*	*27.3	*30.6	*	*	45.7	48.5	*29.7	*31.3
Dementia and Alzheimer's disease	20.0	36.5	40.7	44.0	22.8	36.8	*52.4	46.2	18.3	36.3	*32.4	42.3
Heart disease	866.6	954.8	779.8	739.5	1,003.8	1,062.5	881.6	844.7	783.7	884.3	707.7	663.8
Ischemic heart disease	382.4	416.7	272.1	248.7	470.5	528.5	346.4	312.9	329.1	343.6	219.5	202.7
Heart attack	155.9	166.9	125.5	112.8	220.9	212.8	144.2	127.7	116.7	136.9	112.2	102.2
Arrhythmias	133.4	176.8	183.6	168.7	153.3	174.4	181.6	165.9	121.4	178.3	185.1	170.7
Heart failure	261.4	263.1	225.1	220.7	286.2	271.1	242.9	248.3	246.4	257.9	212.5	200.9
Hypertension	22.6	39.7	48.9	38.0	*	*28.4	*38.9	*31.7	30.7	47.1	56.0	42.5
Stroke	259.0	255.5	196.5	196.9	277.7	278.4	225.7	210.6	247.7	240.6	175.8	187.1
Pneumonia	224.6	263.5	177.7	179.3	297.8	310.8	201.0	193.3	180.4	232.6	161.3	169.3
Chronic obstructive pulmonary disease	55.4	146.2	137.5	131.4	89.4	179.6	158.7	149.9	34.8	124.3	122.5	118.0
Gallstones	47.6	39.6	38.7	39.1	51.9	41.4	36.5	39.0	45.0	38.5	*40.2	39.1
Kidney disease	24.5	37.6	108.9	110.2	27.6	48.7	129.1	123.9	*22.6	30.4	94.6	100.3
Urinary tract infection	86.0	85.6	120.1	123.0	66.6	72.5	84.6	87.6	97.8	94.2	145.2	148.5
Hyperplasia of the prostate	X	X	X	X	183.3	67.2	*39.1	38.5	X	X	X	X
Osteoarthritis	68.6	100.6	156.0	161.4	65.2	76.5	147.5	152.6	70.7	116.4	162.1	167.8
Injury	259.1	229.1	232.8	237.0	153.4	171.7	190.3	189.0	323.0	266.6	262.9	271.5
Fracture	195.8	170.2	160.4	166.2	92.6	116.4	110.4	111.8	258.1	205.4	195.7	205.3
Hip fracture	115.2	99.0	63.2	69.4	53.7	68.6	36.0	45.6	152.4	118.8	82.3	86.5
Complications of care and adverse effects	81.5	101.4	121.1	123.1	101.4	136.0	149.4	150.8	69.4	78.8	101.1	103.2
85 Years and Over[3]	5,606.3	6,050.9	5,814.6	5,667.7	6,420.9	6,166.6	6,425.5	6,193.4	5,289.6	6,003.3	5,531.7	5,415.6
Septicemia	135.6	153.9	237.5	261.4	139.0	207.3	292.9	320.8	134.3	131.9	211.8	232.8
Cancer, all	254.0	194.5	167.7	144.0	370.6	250.5	241.0	209.0	208.7	171.5	133.7	112.8
Colorectal cancer	47.6	49.7	*21.8	17.0	*59.1	*58.8	*	*20.7	43.2	45.9	*18.3	*15.2
Lung/bronchus/tracheal cancer	*19.1	12.1	*23.1	*25.0	*	*20.9	*	*	*	8.5	*	*15.2
Breast cancer[4]	X	X	X	X	X	X	X	X	*41.7	*20.5	*	*12.0
Prostate cancer	X	X	X	X	*87.8	*49.3	*	*20.0	X	X	X	X
Diabetes	53.0	65.6	*59.8	58.7	*53.5	*54.2	*70.1	69.4	52.8	70.3	*55.1	*53.6
Schizophrenia, mood disorders, delusional disorders, nonorganic psychoses	*27.9	*37.3	*	*	*	*	*	*40.6	*30.7	*43.0	*	*
Dementia and Alzheimer's disease	49.7	107.0	73.8	77.2	*28.9	94.3	88.7	96.2	57.7	112.2	66.9	68.0
Heart disease	1,107.0	1,298.2	1,085.8	1,054.7	1,320.3	1,407.4	1,323.1	1,224.2	1,024.1	1,253.4	975.9	973.4
Ischemic heart disease	423.0	427.2	246.1	246.9	581.6	534.4	349.8	323.5	361.3	383.2	198.1	210.2
Heart attack	199.8	251.1	155.6	161.0	274.2	296.0	205.0	197.1	170.9	232.7	132.7	143.6
Arrhythmias	167.2	232.4	225.0	212.3	189.6	247.1	207.0	213.2	158.5	226.4	233.3	211.9
Heart failure	416.7	480.4	466.6	451.7	460.5	455.7	565.1	528.8	399.7	490.5	421.0	414.7
Hypertension	*17.9	41.1	66.2	49.1	*	*18.3	*69.3	*47.6	*19.3	50.4	*64.8	49.8

X = Not applicable.

* = Figure does not meet standards of reliability or precision. Data preceded by an asterisk have a relative standard error (RSE) of 20 to 30 percent. Data not shown have an RSE of greater than 30 percent.

[1]Starting with 2008 data, the sample of nonfederal short-stay hospitals was cut in half. This smaller sample size has increased standard errors. Therefore, caution should be exercised in interpreting trends in these data.

[3]Includes discharges with first-listed diagnoses not shown in table.

[4]Shown for women only.

Table 3-54. Discharge Rate in Nonfederal Short-Stay Hospitals, by Sex, Age, and Selected First-Listed Diagnosis, Selected Years 1990 Through 2009–2010—Continued

(Number per 10,000 population.)

Age and first-listed diagnosis	Both sexes				Male				Female			
	1990	2000	2009[1]	2009–2010[1]	1990	2000	2009[1]	2009–2010[1]	1990	2000	2009[1]	2009–2010[1]
Stroke	427.2	373.8	288.3	284.1	408.2	396.7	270.7	278.5	434.6	364.3	296.4	286.8
Pneumonia	501.0	514.9	367.9	355.3	753.7	607.8	412.7	429.2	402.8	476.8	347.1	319.9
Chronic obstructive pulmonary disease	44.1	130.9	144.3	144.0	*72.9	150.4	*157.2	173.4	*32.9	123.0	138.4	129.8
Gallstones	60.7	39.2	*42.4	39.7	*68.2	*29.7	*40.4	*40.6	57.8	*43.1	*43.3	39.3
Kidney disease	47.1	49.5	160.2	167.4	92.4	*68.1	202.1	230.5	*29.4	*41.9	140.8	137.1
Urinary tract infection	216.5	191.5	346.0	321.9	239.3	153.1	259.5	217.0	207.6	207.2	386.1	372.1
Hyperplasia of the prostate	X	X	X	X	158.6	*69.9	*33.5	*31.8	X	X	X	X
Osteoarthritis	44.5	56.0	64.5	70.2	*	*	*57.3	*54.9	35.8	57.3	67.8	77.6
Injury	542.0	545.5	533.3	525.3	435.4	355.6	435.1	428.4	583.4	623.5	578.9	571.7
Fracture	439.0	450.9	403.5	396.6	335.7	252.4	302.1	275.7	479.2	532.4	450.4	454.6
Hip fracture	272.3	275.1	218.2	211.6	224.4	146.5	160.6	155.4	291.0	327.9	244.9	238.6
Complications of care and adverse effects	96.6	79.1	132.8	127.1	132.3	90.5	*151.7	160.0	82.7	74.4	124.1	111.4

X = Not applicable.
* = Figure does not meet standards of reliability or precision. Data preceded by an asterisk have a relative standard error (RSE) of 20 to 30 percent. Data not shown have an RSE of greater than 30 percent.
[1]Starting with 2008 data, the sample of nonfederal short-stay hospitals was cut in half. This smaller sample size has increased standard errors. Therefore, caution should be exercised in interpreting trends in these data.

Table 3-55. Discharges with at Least One Procedure in Nonfederal Short-Stay Hospitals, by Sex, Age, and Selected Procedures, Selected Years, 1990 Through 2009–2010

(Percent; rate per 10,000 population.)

Age and procedure (any listed)	Both sexes					Male					Female				
	1990	2000	2005	2009[1]	2009-2010[1]	1990	2000	2005	2009[1]	2009-2010[1]	1990	2000	2005	2009[1]	2009-2010[1]
18 Years and Over															
Hospital discharges with at least one procedure, crude (percent)[2]	67.4	62.1	62.6	63.3	63.2	65.2	59.2	59.4	60.0	59.9	68.7	63.9	64.7	65.5	65.3
Hospital discharges with at least one procedure, age-adjusted[2,3]	1,020.1	859.9	893.5	908.8		882.2	701.4	722.0	733.7		1,176.4	1,026.2	1,078.1	1,098.0	
Hospital discharges with at least one procedure, crude[2]	1,006.4	856.8	893.8	920.0	900.0	788.1	648.4	683.9	716.3	697.8	1,205.9	1,049.8	1,090.9	1,112.3	1,091.3
Operations on vessels of heart	28.3	41.2	41.2	36.0	33.1	41.9	56.9	58.5	50.2	46.7	15.8	26.7	25.0	22.6	20.2
Coronary angioplasty or arthrectomy	14.0	26.2	28.5	25.6	23.2	20.5	34.9	40.5	34.8	31.7	8.0	18.1	17.3	17.0	15.1
Coronary artery stent insertion	X	21.7	27.0	22.6	20.5	X	28.7	38.5	30.4	28.0	X	15.3	16.2	15.2	13.5
Drug-eluting stent insertion	X	X	23.9	15.8	15.0	X	X	34.1	21.0	20.4	X	X	14.4	10.9	9.9
Coronary artery bypass graft (CABG)	14.1	15.0	11.8	10.5	9.9	21.2	21.8	16.6	15.6	15.0	7.7	8.7	7.2	5.7	5.1
Cardiac catheterization	52.1	57.8	53.9	46.1	43.1	68.3	72.1	68.5	55.1	53.0	37.4	44.6	40.2	37.5	33.7
Pacemaker	8.6	8.5	9.6	9.2	8.7	10.1	8.5	10.5	9.0	9.0	7.1	8.5	8.8	9.4	8.4
Carotid (neck arteries) endarterectomy	3.6	5.9	4.6	4.0	4.1	4.1	6.6	5.7	4.6	4.7	3.1	5.3	3.6	3.5	3.5
Endoscopy of small intestine	40.8	42.5	45.8	45.7	44.6	38.6	39.1	42.3	42.3	40.7	42.8	45.6	49.1	48.9	48.3
Endoscopy of large intestine	27.9	25.0	24.0	21.9	20.6	22.5	20.2	19.7	19.1	18.0	32.8	29.4	28.0	24.4	23.1
Gall bladder removal	27.9	19.6	17.7	18.4	18.2	16.5	13.3	13.2	14.5	13.1	38.2	25.5	21.9	22.2	23.0
Laparoscopic gall bladder removal	X	14.8	13.5	14.7	14.8	X	9.2	8.8	10.4	9.6	X	20.1	17.9	18.7	19.7
Treatment of intra-abdominal scar tissue	17.0	14.4	15.3	15.1	14.7	6.5	5.7	6.5	7.8	7.8	26.6	22.4	23.5	22.0	21.3
Reduction of fracture	27.6	24.9	23.2	22.8	23.2	27.3	22.0	21.1	20.5	20.0	27.8	27.7	25.2	25.0	26.3
Excision of intervertebral disc and spinal fusion	18.7	18.2	18.4	22.3	21.8	22.3	20.0	18.8	22.5	21.4	15.4	16.4	18.0	22.2	22.1
Total hip replacement	6.4	7.3	10.5	13.8	13.9	5.4	6.8	10.1	14.0	13.6	7.3	7.7	10.9	13.5	14.1
Partial hip replacement	4.8	5.0	10.2	13.3	13.1	2.0	2.3	7.8	*11.3	10.9	7.3	7.6	12.3	15.2	15.1
Total knee replacement	6.7	13.8	23.1	28.0	28.8	4.9	11.0	16.4	20.2	21.6	8.4	16.4	29.3	35.4	35.6
CT scan	68.4	29.2	27.9	*17.1	*17.0	68.6	27.4	26.1	16.0	15.7	68.2	30.9	29.7	*18.1	*18.2
Arteriography and angiocardiography with contrast	59.7	63.0	59.9	56.4	53.8	75.6	76.2	72.1	64.9	63.4	45.2	50.7	48.5	48.3	44.8
Diagnostic ultrasound	72.3	36.9	36.0	34.7	34.9	62.1	33.1	35.2	34.0	33.9	81.7	40.4	36.7	35.4	35.9
Magnetic resonance imaging	9.5	9.2	11.2	*10.1	9.8	9.4	8.2	10.3	*9.4	9.0	9.6	10.2	12.1	*10.7	*10.6
Mechanical ventilation	17.6	23.0	27.0	32.9	32.4	18.8	23.9	29.5	34.9	34.0	16.4	22.1	24.7	31.1	30.9
18 to 44 Years															
Hospital discharges with at least one procedure, crude (percent)[2]	73.0	71.7	71.7	71.9	72.4	62.6	55.9	54.0	53.6	53.7	77.0	77.4	78.1	78.4	78.7
Hospital discharges with at least one procedure[2]	749.3	609.1	644.0	638.0	627.6	362.8	251.6	254.4	244.3	233.3	1,130.6	965.9	1,039.0	1,039.7	1,030.6
Operations on vessels of heart	3.0	3.9	4.1	*3.1	2.8	4.9	5.5	5.7	4.5	4.1	*1.2	2.3	2.4	*	*1.5
Coronary angioplasty or arthrectomy	1.9	3.0	3.0	*2.5	*2.3	3.0	4.3	4.3	*3.5	3.4	*0.8	1.6	*1.7	*	*1.2
Coronary artery stent insertion	X	2.5	3.1	*2.3	*2.0	X	3.6	4.3	*3.1	*2.9	X	1.4	*1.8	*	*1.1
Drug-eluting stent insertion	X	X	2.6	*	*1.5	X	X	3.4	*	*2.1	X	X	*1.8	*	*
Coronary artery bypass graft (CABG)	1.0	0.9	0.8	*	*0.5	*1.8	1.1	*1.1	*	*0.8	*	*0.7	*	*	*
Cardiac catheterization	9.0	8.5	7.6	7.1	6.3	12.5	11.0	9.6	8.7	8.3	5.5	5.9	5.6	5.5	4.3
Endoscopy of small intestine	13.1	10.3	13.3	15.7	14.7	13.2	10.4	11.7	12.2	11.4	13.0	10.2	14.9	19.3	18.0
Endoscopy of large intestine	6.9	5.5	6.5	7.2	6.2	5.6	4.7	5.5	*6.2	5.3	8.1	6.3	7.5	8.3	7.0
Gall bladder removal	18.7	11.9	11.5	13.5	12.8	6.2	4.3	5.1	6.5	5.1	31.0	19.4	17.9	20.6	20.7
Laparoscopic gall bladder removal	X	9.9	9.9	11.0	11.0	X	3.0	4.1	4.5	3.7	X	16.8	15.8	17.7	18.4
Treatment of intra-abdominal scar tissue	14.1	10.8	11.7	11.1	10.5	2.0	1.5	*1.8	*2.9	*2.5	26.0	20.1	21.7	19.4	18.6
Hysterectomy	X	X	X	X	X	X	X	X	X	X	63.3	55.7	51.2	37.4	38.0
Abdominal hysterectomy	X	X	X	X	X	X	X	X	X	X	47.1	34.6	31.5	22.8	21.3
Vaginal hysterectomy	X	X	X	X	X	X	X	X	X	X	15.8	19.1	15.6	*10.6	*12.3
Forceps, vacuum, and breech delivery	X	X	X	X	X	X	X	X	X	X	77.5	59.9	51.1	*45.0	*43.9
Episiotomy	X	X	X	X	X	X	X	X	X	X	293.3	160.8	90.9	52.3	53.6
Other procedures inducing or assisting delivery	X	X	X	X	X	X	X	X	X	X	387.9	384.2	396.7	418.5	422.6
Medical induction of labor	X	X	X	X	X	X	X	X	X	X	41.1	77.7	107.5	120.5	125.9
Cesarean section	X	X	X	X	X	X	X	X	X	X	167.1	149.5	220.7	232.5	233.5
Reduction of fracture	19.1	13.7	13.2	12.0	11.6	27.9	19.0	18.9	17.2	15.3	10.4	8.4	7.5	6.8	7.9
Excision of intervertebral disc and spinal fusion	17.0	14.1	11.7	11.9	10.7	21.5	16.2	13.1	11.7	10.3	12.6	12.1	10.3	12.1	11.0
CT scan	27.5	10.6	12.6	*6.5	*6.6	32.3	11.0	12.3	5.8	*6.1	22.7	10.3	12.8	*7.2	*7.1
Arteriography and angiocardiography with contrast	12.5	10.3	10.5	9.7	9.1	17.4	12.9	12.2	9.7	9.9	7.6	7.7	8.7	9.7	8.2
Diagnostic ultrasound	34.2	11.6	12.3	9.8	10.0	19.3	8.3	9.5	*7.3	7.2	48.9	14.9	15.1	12.3	12.8
Magnetic resonance imaging	4.9	3.8	4.3	*4.4	*4.1	4.9	3.6	3.8	*	*2.9	4.9	*4.0	4.8	*5.6	*5.4
Mechanical ventilation	4.6	7.0	8.8	11.0	9.9	5.4	8.2	10.1	11.9	11.2	3.8	5.8	7.5	10.1	8.6
45 to 64 Years															
Hospital discharges with at least one procedure, crude (percent)[2]	68.2	62.3	62.6	63.2	63.0	68.9	63.4	63.3	63.5	63.3	67.6	61.3	61.8	62.9	62.8
Hospital discharges with at least one procedure[2]	924.2	694.6	717.4	771.7	756.7	965.9	714.4	727.3	784.1	766.2	885.4	675.9	708.1	759.9	747.7

X = Not applicable.
* = Figure does not meet standards of reliability or precision. Data preceded by an asterisk have a relative standard error (RSE) of 20 to 30 percent. Data not shown have an RSE of greater than 30 percent.
[1]Starting with 2008 data, the sample of nonfederal short-stay hospitals was cut in half. This smaller sample size has increased standard errors. Therefore, caution should be exercised in interpreting trends in these data.
[2]Includes discharges for procedures not shown separately.
[3]Estimates are age-adjusted to the year 2000 standard population using five age groups: 18 to 44 years, 45 to 54 years, 55 to 64 years, 65 to 74 years, and 75 years and over.

Table 3-55. Discharges with at Least One Procedure in Nonfederal Short-Stay Hospitals, by Sex, Age, and Selected Procedures, Selected Years, 1990 Through 2009–2010—Continued

(Percent; rate per 10,000 population.)

Age and procedure (any listed)	Both sexes					Male					Female				
	1990	2000	2005	2009¹	2009-2010¹	1990	2000	2005	2009¹	2009-2010¹	1990	2000	2005	2009¹	2009-2010¹
Operations on vessels of heart	53.0	57.7	53.5	42.5	40.0	83.2	88.5	83.5	62.8	59.5	24.8	28.4	24.9	23.1	21.4
Coronary angioplasty or arthrectomy	29.4	37.5	38.4	31.2	28.9	45.3	55.9	59.4	46.1	42.7	14.5	20.0	18.3	17.1	15.8
Coronary artery stent insertion	X	31.1	36.7	26.9	25.4	X	46.5	57.7	39.9	37.5	X	16.5	16.7	14.6	13.8
Drug-eluting stent insertion	X	X	33.0	18.7	18.7	X	X	51.8	28.1	27.5	X	X	15.1	*9.8	10.2
Coronary artery bypass graft (CABG)	23.4	20.3	14.0	11.5	11.1	37.5	32.5	21.9	17.1	16.9	10.3	8.6	6.4	*6.1	*5.5
Cardiac catheterization	98.2	83.0	69.7	56.6	54.4	136.8	113.9	95.6	75.7	72.3	62.3	53.7	45.1	38.4	37.2
Pacemaker	7.8	4.0	3.9	3.2	3.2	10.9	5.2	4.6	*4.5	4.2	*4.9	2.8	3.2	*2.0	*2.3
Carotid (neck arteries) endarterectomy	4.0	5.2	2.9	2.6	3.1	5.2	5.2	3.7	*3.1	3.6	3.0	*5.2	2.2	*2.1	*2.7
Endoscopy of small intestine	45.0	36.4	42.5	43.5	43.2	46.3	40.7	44.7	45.3	42.2	43.8	32.3	40.3	41.9	44.2
Endoscopy of large intestine	28.5	19.3	19.4	18.9	18.0	25.4	18.1	17.4	16.7	15.9	31.4	20.4	21.2	21.0	20.0
Gall bladder removal	36.4	20.6	17.6	18.4	18.0	22.3	16.3	14.0	15.6	13.8	49.5	24.6	20.9	21.0	21.9
Laparoscopic gall bladder removal	X	15.3	13.0	15.0	14.6	X	12.1	9.0	11.8	10.6	X	18.5	16.8	18.0	18.5
Treatment of intra-abdominal scar tissue	17.1	15.0	15.6	14.6	13.8	9.5	7.0	6.2	8.5	8.2	24.2	22.6	24.5	20.4	19.1
Removal of prostate	X	X	X	X	X	35.8	15.6	14.4	*17.9	16.9	X	X	X	X	X
Transurethral prostatectomy	X	X	X	X	X	30.4	7.0	4.6	*2.7	3.3	X	X	X	X	X
Hysterectomy	X	X	X	X	X	X	X	X	X	X	76.4	78.2	63.8	54.5	54.1
Abdominal hysterectomy	X	X	X	X	X	X	X	X	X	X	58.4	53.2	39.7	33.9	32.1
Vaginal hysterectomy	X	X	X	X	X	X	X	X	X	X	17.6	21.6	19.3	14.4	15.4
Reduction of fracture	20.3	18.5	16.5	17.0	18.2	19.5	17.6	17.9	16.7	18.1	21.0	19.3	15.3	17.3	18.3
Excision of intervertebral disc and spinal fusion	26.1	25.7	26.9	31.1	30.8	29.4	27.1	27.0	30.6	31.3	23.1	24.4	26.8	31.7	30.2
Total hip replacement	6.2	8.1	10.9	18.3	18.0	5.7	9.1	12.3	20.8	19.0	6.5	7.2	9.6	15.8	17.1
Partial hip replacement	*	*1.3	9.1	*14.0	*13.8	*	*0.8	8.8	*14.1	*13.7	*	*1.7	9.5	*13.9	*13.8
Total knee replacement	6.7	12.7	25.4	36.5	37.1	5.8	8.7	17.7	27.0	27.8	*7.4	16.4	32.7	45.5	46.0
Mastectomy	X	X	X	.	X	X	X	X	X	X	21.2	10.6	8.1	8.5	9.3
CT scan	65.4	25.2	26.1	17.0	*17.1	69.9	25.9	26.7	18.0	17.4	61.2	24.5	25.5	*16.1	*16.9
Arteriography and angiocardiography with contrast	105.4	85.3	73.2	66.3	64.3	138.5	111.4	94.6	86.7	83.3	74.6	60.7	52.8	46.9	46.3
Diagnostic ultrasound	69.5	34.3	33.5	30.9	31.8	73.8	38.0	39.4	35.9	36.3	65.5	30.9	27.9	26.2	27.5
Magnetic resonance imaging	10.9	8.9	11.6	8.9	9.2	10.7	9.4	12.4	9.2	9.2	11.0	8.4	11.0	*8.6	9.2
Mechanical ventilation	17.6	21.2	24.7	32.2	32.9	18.6	22.9	28.0	33.5	34.4	16.7	19.6	21.6	30.8	31.5
65 to 74 Years															
Hospital discharges with at least one procedure, crude (percent)²	66.5	61.3	62.9	63.9	63.2	69.3	63.9	65.0	64.4	64.6	63.8	58.9	60.9	63.4	62.0
Hospital discharges with at least one procedure²	1,739.4	1,559.8	1,653.0	1,632.6	1,573.0	1,994.1	1,692.3	1,783.2	1,725.0	1,678.0	1,539.4	1,450.6	1,543.1	1,553.5	1,482.5
Operations on vessels of heart	97.0	139.8	142.1	117.4	104.2	148.9	195.3	211.0	165.8	152.6	56.3	94.1	84.0	75.9	62.4
Coronary angioplasty or arthrectomy	44.1	86.3	91.2	83.2	69.4	64.9	116.0	138.2	113.2	96.6	27.8	61.9	51.5	57.4	45.9
Coronary artery stent insertion	X	71.7	86.2	73.6	61.1	X	94.9	129.4	97.3	83.3	X	52.5	49.8	53.2	42.0
Drug-eluting stent insertion	X	X	76.8	53.5	46.1	X	X	115.7	69.1	62.5	X	X	44.0	*40.2	32.1
Coronary artery bypass graft (CABG)	52.1	53.9	47.4	34.4	34.7	83.1	79.7	68.1	52.9	55.9	27.7	32.6	30.0	*18.6	16.5
Cardiac catheterization	164.0	174.2	170.3	130.9	120.4	213.8	222.7	230.4	159.3	153.7	124.9	134.2	119.6	106.6	91.7
Pacemaker	24.6	22.5	23.7	19.6	18.6	32.1	22.8	29.0	*17.3	18.1	18.7	22.3	19.1	*21.5	19.0
Carotid (neck arteries) endarterectomy	14.6	24.1	24.0	*17.8	15.6	18.0	29.5	31.2	*21.8	21.8	11.9	19.6	18.0	*14.3	*10.3
Endoscopy of small intestine	92.8	106.6	102.5	99.4	93.2	91.5	102.4	102.6	106.7	99.0	93.7	110.0	102.4	93.2	88.2
Endoscopy of large intestine	70.3	64.8	58.3	45.7	44.3	62.5	59.7	52.1	44.9	41.6	76.5	69.0	63.6	46.4	46.7
Gall bladder removal	45.0	42.1	34.4	31.3	30.0	42.0	37.9	34.0	33.7	31.9	47.4	45.5	34.8	29.3	28.3
Laparoscopic gall bladder removal	X	29.5	23.6	21.9	22.0	X	24.4	22.4	*20.3	21.2	X	33.7	24.6	23.2	22.6
Treatment of intra-abdominal scar tissue	23.1	21.4	23.5	27.4	29.0	17.1	14.5	19.6	*20.5	24.3	27.7	27.1	26.8	*33.2	33.0
Removal of prostate	X	X	X	X	X	201.1	83.7	65.3	56.9	50.8	X	X	X	X	X
Transurethral prostatectomy	X	X	X	X	X	180.9	59.4	39.5	*23.7	24.1	X	X	X	X	X
Hysterectomy	X	X	X	X	X	X	X	X	X	X	37.4	35.9	28.0	*29.3	30.2
Abdominal hysterectomy	X	X	X	X	X	X	X	X	X	X	20.8	20.5	12.8	*12.2	15.0
Vaginal hysterectomy	X	X	X	X	X	X	X	X	X	X	16.5	14.7	14.1	*15.0	*14.1
Reduction of fracture	36.2	36.4	38.0	34.8	32.9	24.3	26.2	25.8	19.0	18.4	45.5	44.8	48.3	48.3	45.5
Excision of intervertebral disc and spinal fusion	16.3	21.1	31.1	41.7	42.1	14.2	22.5	27.6	*45.9	39.2	18.0	20.0	34.1	*38.0	*44.5
Total hip replacement	24.0	25.4	36.6	37.4	39.3	23.0	26.4	36.2	34.6	37.1	24.9	24.5	37.0	39.9	41.2
Partial hip replacement	8.9	7.6	20.1	*24.7	*25.3	*4.0	*	15.4	*20.8	*19.1	*12.7	10.5	24.1	*27.9	*30.7
Total knee replacement	33.2	65.4	99.5	104.6	108.3	26.4	64.5	71.8	76.2	84.0	38.6	66.0	122.8	128.9	129.3
Mastectomy	X	X	X	X	X	X	X	X	X	X	30.7	22.7	*11.5	*15.5	*12.9
CT scan	153.7	64.3	53.7	*30.9	*29.4	163.4	65.7	53.6	*32.6	*31.1	146.1	63.1	53.7	*29.5	*27.9
Arteriography and angiocardiography with contrast	184.5	186.2	180.8	153.6	146.5	239.0	231.9	233.2	191.5	186.7	141.7	148.5	136.6	121.2	111.9
Diagnostic ultrasound	155.2	92.7	80.9	82.7	79.8	165.2	94.1	87.0	*93.0	85.6	147.4	91.6	75.8	73.9	74.8
Magnetic resonance imaging	20.6	17.2	24.4	*18.1	*18.3	19.2	*14.6	19.9	*19.2	18.9	21.7	*19.3	28.3	*	*17.8
Mechanical ventilation	48.6	60.0	70.1	79.5	79.9	58.7	70.3	83.0	86.0	90.7	40.6	51.6	59.3	73.9	70.7
75 to 84 Years															
Hospital discharges with at least one procedure, crude (percent)²	59.0	53.6	54.9	57.1	56.4	61.7	56.3	58.1	59.6	59.0	57.0	51.8	52.5	55.2	54.5
Hospital discharges with at least one procedure²	2,332.9	2,212.3	2,269.1	2,322.2	2,247.8	2,723.9	2,416.5	2,549.4	2,528.1	2,441.4	2,096.7	2,078.8	2,078.7	2,176.6	2,108.7

X = Not applicable.

* = Figure does not meet standards of reliability or precision. Data preceded by an asterisk have a relative standard error (RSE) of 20 to 30 percent. Data not shown have an RSE of greater than 30 percent.

¹Starting with 2008 data, the sample of nonfederal short-stay hospitals was cut in half. This smaller sample size has increased standard errors. Therefore, caution should be exercised in interpreting trends in these data.

²Includes discharges for procedures not shown separately.

Table 3-55. Discharges with at Least One Procedure in Nonfederal Short-Stay Hospitals, by Sex, Age, and Selected Procedures, Selected Years, 1990 Through 2009–2010—*Continued*

(Percent; rate per 10,000 population.)

Age and procedure (any listed)	Both sexes					Male					Female				
	1990	2000	2005	2009¹	2009-2010¹	1990	2000	2005	2009¹	2009-2010¹	1990	2000	2005	2009¹	2009-2010¹
Operations on vessels of heart	69.1	143.2	142.3	138.6	126.0	107.6	202.5	199.6	208.3	189.8	45.8	104.5	103.4	89.2	80.2
Coronary angioplasty or arthrectomy	22.4	84.7	97.3	87.3	82.7	33.7	109.3	134.8	121.2	116.8	15.7	68.7	71.9	63.3	58.2
Coronary artery stent insertion	X	69.8	88.2	79.6	75.3	X	86.5	122.2	111.4	107.5	X	58.8	65.2	57.1	52.2
Drug-eluting stent insertion	X	X	75.5	55.6	54.7	X	X	104.9	77.5	77.5	X	X	55.6	*40.2	38.2
Coronary artery bypass graft (CABG)	47.0	57.7	44.4	*50.7	42.7	74.7	90.5	62.6	*86.2	*72.3	30.3	36.2	32.0	*25.7	*21.5
Cardiac catheterization	116.6	190.2	183.9	159.3	149.3	166.0	236.9	238.1	179.6	179.9	86.8	159.6	147.1	144.8	127.4
Pacemaker	50.8	58.1	67.9	59.9	60.0	70.6	72.2	91.0	79.6	84.9	38.8	48.9	52.2	46.0	42.1
Carotid (neck arteries) endarterectomy	19.8	32.8	24.4	23.3	23.7	24.2	45.5	34.1	31.6	29.6	*17.1	24.5	17.7	*17.5	19.5
Endoscopy of small intestine	171.4	189.7	182.2	167.4	166.0	188.9	193.8	202.0	162.5	164.2	160.8	187.0	168.7	170.9	167.3
Endoscopy of large intestine	131.1	123.7	106.4	93.7	87.9	126.1	113.8	109.3	89.5	83.9	134.1	130.1	104.3	96.7	90.7
Gall bladder removal	51.8	43.4	43.3	38.2	43.6	64.4	46.7	48.9	50.7	50.5	44.2	41.3	39.4	29.3	38.7
Laparoscopic gall bladder removal	X	28.9	30.5	32.3	35.9	X	29.6	30.4	40.7	39.2	X	28.5	30.5	26.4	33.6
Treatment of intra-abdominal scar tissue	34.0	28.6	27.9	28.1	30.2	28.2	26.3	*34.5	*30.0	28.7	37.5	30.2	23.4	26.7	31.3
Removal of prostate	X	X	X	X	X	273.5	98.0	65.4	*47.0	41.2	X	X	X	X	X
Transurethral prostatectomy	X	X	X	X	X	257.5	89.0	58.6	*44.0	36.6	X	X	X	X	X
Hysterectomy	X	X	X	X	X	X	X	X	X	X	28.5	25.5	16.1	*23.2	18.5
Abdominal hysterectomy	X	X	X	X	X	X	X	X	X	X	18.8	16.2	8.6	*14.7	*11.1
Vaginal hysterectomy	X	X	X	X	X	X	X	X	X	X	*9.4	8.1	7.1	*	*5.6
Reduction of fracture	86.2	80.1	70.7	61.9	68.1	43.4	57.2	41.5	*41.9	46.0	112.1	95.0	90.6	76.0	84.0
Excision of intervertebral disc and spinal fusion	12.0	17.4	16.4	36.1	36.5	*13.2	*20.4	14.3	*42.8	*39.9	11.3	15.3	17.8	31.3	34.0
Total hip replacement	30.7	26.3	44.4	47.3	49.4	*26.9	*21.3	36.6	*44.4	47.2	33.1	29.6	49.7	49.4	51.1
Partial hip replacement	43.6	36.6	39.9	41.2	37.9	*14.3	20.0	27.4	*29.9	*29.9	61.2	47.5	48.3	49.1	43.7
Total knee replacement	28.4	59.3	90.4	89.8	86.2	*19.5	48.7	83.6	80.4	80.4	33.9	66.3	95.0	96.5	90.4
Mastectomy	X	X	X	X	X	X	X	X	X	X	29.2	22.0	16.2	*8.7	*11.3
CT scan	279.7	119.2	95.8	*56.8	*55.2	307.2	127.9	92.3	*58.3	*51.0	263.0	113.5	98.1	*55.8	*58.3
Arteriography and angiocardiography with contrast	141.0	219.2	212.4	198.1	187.8	192.3	287.9	269.9	219.0	223.3	109.9	174.3	173.3	183.4	162.2
Diagnostic ultrasound	273.5	134.1	133.0	122.4	122.0	315.7	142.8	148.3	135.8	137.7	248.0	128.4	122.6	113.0	110.8
Magnetic resonance imaging	30.5	*37.3	38.4	*38.5	*37.6	43.0	*33.6	41.3	*47.9	*44.0	*23.0	*39.8	36.5	*31.9	*33.0
Mechanical ventilation	79.8	91.1	102.6	105.3	102.0	110.3	106.5	119.4	139.7	119.5	61.3	80.9	91.1	81.1	89.5
85 Years and Over															
Hospital discharges with at least one procedure, crude (percent)²	49.3	44.6	45.4	47.0	46.8	52.4	45.4	47.7	51.4	50.5	47.8	44.3	44.2	44.6	44.7
Hospital discharges with at least one procedure²	2,762.1	2,700.5	2,612.5	2,731.1	2,650.6	3,367.3	2,797.9	2,857.1	3,301.9	3,125.0	2,526.8	2,660.6	2,500.2	2,466.7	2,423.0
Operations on vessels of heart	*14.0	51.1	53.9	60.9	55.5	*	83.0	86.2	*124.2	98.6	*	38.0	39.1	*31.6	34.8
Coronary angioplasty or arthrectomy	*	36.3	45.0	*51.7	44.6	*	*52.9	*64.6	*101.8	74.6	*	29.5	35.9	*28.4	*30.2
Coronary artery stent insertion	X	31.6	43.2	45.5	40.0	X	*48.9	*62.3	*83.9	66.6	X	*24.4	34.4	*27.7	*27.2
Drug-eluting stent insertion	X	X	38.4	*27.2	22.7	X	X	*55.8	*	*36.9	X	X	30.4	*19.6	*15.8
Coronary artery bypass graft (CABG)	*	*15.1	*	*	*10.1	*	*30.1	*	*	*22.5	*	*9.0	*3.0	*	*4.2
Cardiac catheterization	*23.7	87.7	88.8	*96.7	78.5	*	122.8	122.5	*145.1	111.7	*19.0	73.2	73.3	*74.4	62.6
Pacemaker	79.5	82.9	92.7	105.3	89.3	120.4	104.3	122.7	*121.0	100.6	63.5	74.2	78.9	*98.0	84.0
Carotid (neck arteries) endarterectomy	*	*12.0	*9.2	*	*	*	*	*	*	*7.1	*	*4.8	*	*	*
Endoscopy of small intestine	228.8	262.4	251.8	192.1	192.2	288.7	245.1	217.8	224.3	228.5	205.5	269.5	267.3	177.2	174.7
Endoscopy of large intestine	180.8	158.1	139.4	99.2	98.1	188.0	133.3	104.3	131.1	128.9	178.0	168.3	155.6	84.4	83.4
Gall bladder removal	46.4	40.9	29.1	*24.7	23.0	*68.4	*42.9	*48.4	*	*30.2	37.8	*40.1	20.3	*22.7	*19.5
Laparoscopic gall bladder removal	X	*30.4	18.6	*15.6	15.4	X	*	*28.2	*	*	X	*30.5	*14.2	*13.5	*14.0
Treatment of intra-abdominal scar tissue	29.6	24.3	29.0	*28.9	23.0	*	*16.4	*20.6	*	*13.9	33.7	*27.5	*32.8	*35.2	*27.4
Removal of prostate	X	X	X	X	X	257.2	*113.0	73.0	*39.7	42.7	X	X	X	X	X
Transurethral prostatectomy	X	X	X	X	X	247.1	*110.0	67.1	*39.7	41.8	X	X	X	X	X
Hysterectomy	X	X	X	X	X	X	X	X	X	X	*	*	*5.9	*	*
Abdominal hysterectomy	X	X	X	X	X	X	X	X	X	X	*	*	*4.3	*	*
Vaginal hysterectomy	X	X	X	X	X	X	X	X	X	X	*	*	*	*	*
Reduction of fracture	196.2	200.5	160.6	182.9	180.3	150.6	93.8	75.4	147.5	132.8	213.9	244.3	199.7	199.4	203.0
Excision of intervertebral disc and spinal fusion	*	*2.3	*	*	*6.2	*	*	*	*	*	*	*	*	*	*
Total hip replacement	*27.8	*20.7	*24.8	*31.6	*25.5	*	*	*	*	*	*23.2	*26.3	*23.6	*	*21.6
Partial hip replacement	67.4	82.2	71.2	78.1	77.1	*52.9	*44.1	56.4	67.0	66.2	73.1	97.9	78.0	83.3	82.3
Total knee replacement	*12.4	*22.9	*30.2	*26.7	34.0	*	*	*27.0	*	*31.3	*	*16.2	*31.7	*31.1	35.3
Mastectomy	X	X	X	X	X	X	X	X	X	X	*28.9	*15.7	*	*	*
CT scan	378.4	158.7	123.7	*86.2	*84.9	401.2	141.4	*131.8	*79.2	*84.8	369.5	165.9	119.9	*	*85.0
Arteriography and angiocardiography with contrast	50.6	120.8	126.6	156.8	135.6	*87.6	164.4	175.2	197.2	161.9	36.2	102.8	104.3	138.2	123.0
Diagnostic ultrasound	327.7	208.5	179.3	203.3	200.6	394.5	181.4	200.7	215.6	216.3	301.7	219.6	169.6	*197.6	193.1
Magnetic resonance imaging	*18.5	*40.4	40.5	*	*35.7	*	*	*40.8	*	*35.9	*16.2	*	*40.5	*	*
Mechanical ventilation	91.5	106.0	110.0	139.1	130.3	97.9	116.5	166.1	199.1	172.2	89.1	101.7	84.3	111.3	110.2

X = Not applicable.
* = Figure does not meet standards of reliability or precision. Data preceded by an asterisk have a relative standard error (RSE) of 20 to 30 percent. Data not shown have an RSE of greater than 30 percent.
¹Starting with 2008 data, the sample of nonfederal short-stay hospitals was cut in half. This smaller sample size has increased standard errors. Therefore, caution should be exercised in interpreting trends in these data.
²Includes discharges for procedures not shown separately.

HEALTH PERSONNEL

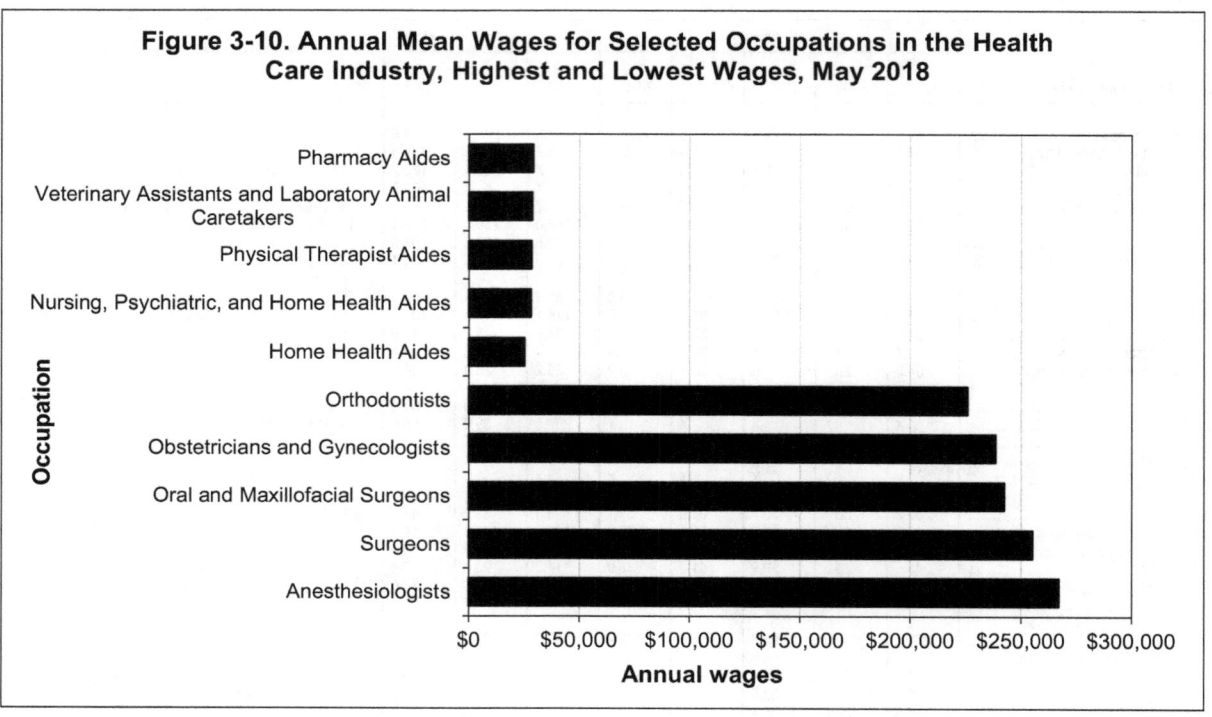

Figure 3-10. Annual Mean Wages for Selected Occupations in the Health Care Industry, Highest and Lowest Wages, May 2018

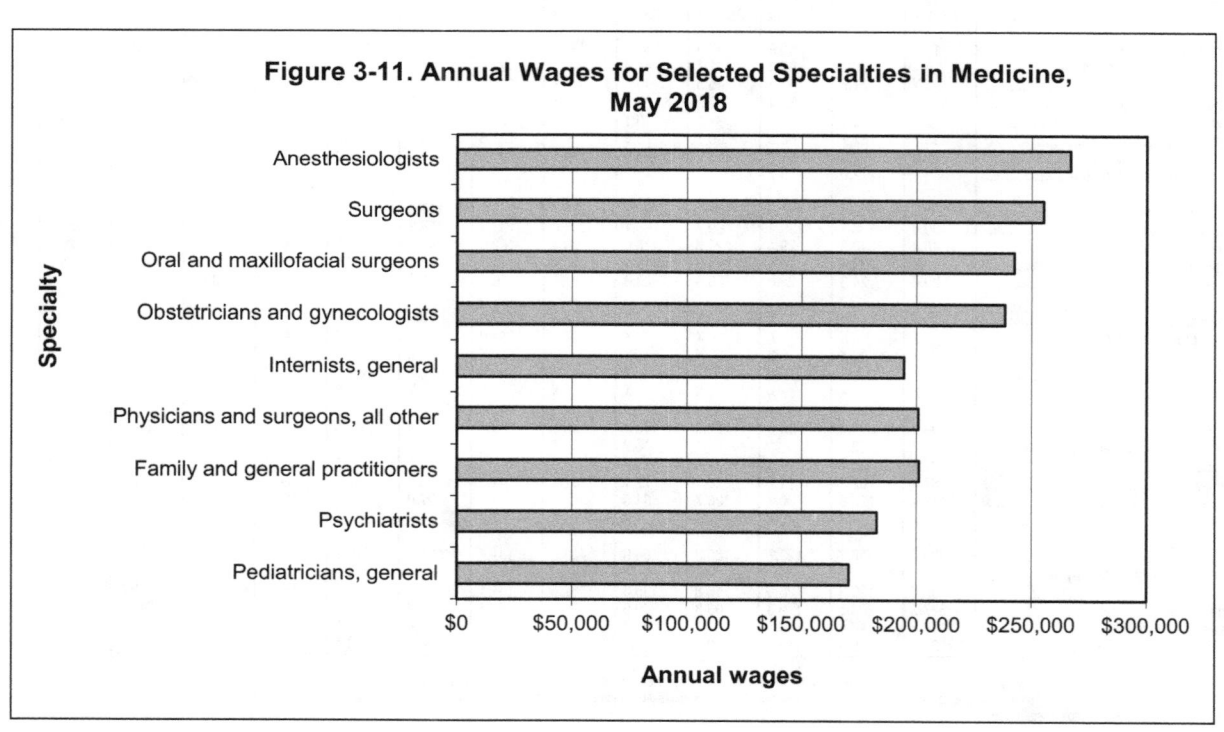

Figure 3-11. Annual Wages for Selected Specialties in Medicine, May 2018

Table 3-56. Health Care Employment and Wages, by Selected Occupations, Selected Years, 2000–2016

(Number; dollars; data are based on a semiannual survey of nonfarm establishments.)

Occupation title	Employment[1]					Mean hourly wage (dollars)[2]				
	2000	2005	2010	2015	2016	2000	2005	2010	2015	2016
Health Care Practitioners and Technical Occupations										
Audiologists	11,530	10,030	12,860	12,070	12,310	22.92	27.72	33.58	37.22	38.12
Cardiovascular technologists and technicians	40,080	43,560	48,720	51,400	53,760	16.81	19.99	24.38	26.97	27.45
Dental hygienists	148,460	161,140	177,520	200,550	204,990	24.99	29.15	33.02	34.96	35.31
Diagnostic medical sonographers	31,760	43,590	53,010	61,250	65,790	22.03	26.65	31.20	34.08	34.49
Dietetic technicians	28,010	23,780	23,890	28,950	32,240	10.98	12.20	13.86	14.03	14.12
Dietitians and nutritionists	43,030	48,850	53,510	59,740	61,430	18.76	22.09	26.13	28.08	28.69
Emergency medical technicians and paramedics	165,530	196,880	221,760	236,890	244,960	11.89	13.68	16.01	17.04	17.36
Licensed practical and licensed vocational nurses	679,470	710,020	730,290	697,250	702,400	14.65	17.41	19.88	21.17	21.56
Magnetic resonance imaging technologists	NA	NA	NA	33,460	35,850	NA	NA	NA	32.86	33.29
Medical and clinical laboratory technicians	146,060	142,330	156,480	157,610	160,190	13.93	15.95	18.36	19.91	20.05
Medical and clinical laboratory technologists	144,530	155,250	164,430	162,950	166,730	19.84	23.37	27.34	29.74	30.02
Medical records and health information technicians	143,870	160,450	176,090	189,930	200,140	11.74	13.81	16.83	19.44	19.93
Nuclear medicine technologists	18,030	18,280	21,600	19,740	19,650	21.56	29.10	33.20	36.06	36.52
Nurse anesthetists	NA	NA	NA	39,410	39,860	NA	NA	NA	77.04	78.86
Nurse midwives	NA	NA	NA	7,430	6,270	NA	NA	NA	45.01	49.23
Nurse practitioners	NA	NA	NA	136,060	150,230	NA	NA	NA	48.68	50.30
Occupational therapists	75,150	87,430	100,300	114,660	118,070	24.10	28.41	35.28	39.27	40.25
Opticians, dispensing	66,580	70,090	62,200	73,520	75,270	12.67	14.80	16.73	17.70	18.20
Pharmacists	212,660	229,740	268,030	295,620	305,510	33.39	42.62	52.59	57.34	57.82
Pharmacy technicians	190,940	266,790	333,500	379,430	398,390	10.38	12.19	14.10	15.23	15.47
Physical therapists	120,410	151,280	180,280	209,690	216,920	27.62	31.42	37.50	41.25	41.93
Physician assistants	55,490	63,350	81,420	98,470	104,050	29.17	34.17	41.89	47.73	49.08
Psychiatric technicians	53,350	62,040	72,650	58,450	61,720	12.53	14.04	15.15	17.44	17.25
Radiation therapists	13,100	14,120	16,590	16,930	17,450	25.59	30.59	37.64	40.61	40.86
Radiologic technologists[3]	172,080	184,580	216,730	195,590	200,650	17.93	22.60	26.80	28.13	28.49
Recreational therapists	26,940	23,260	20,830	17,880	18,100	14.23	16.90	19.92	22.98	23.17
Registered nurses[4]	2,189,670	2,368,070	2,655,020	2,745,910	2,857,180	22.31	27.35	32.56	34.14	34.70
Respiratory therapists	82,670	95,320	109,270	120,330	126,770	18.37	22.24	26.54	28.67	29.15
Respiratory therapy technicians	28,230	22,060	13,570	10,000	10,600	16.46	18.57	22.28	23.90	24.29
Speech-language pathologists	82,850	94,660	112,530	131,450	135,980	23.31	27.89	33.60	36.97	37.60
Health Care Support Occupations										
Dental assistants	250,870	270,720	294,030	323,110	327,290	12.86	14.41	16.41	17.75	18.22
Home health aides	561,120	663,280	982,840	820,630	814,300	8.71	9.34	10.46	11.00	11.35
Massage therapists	24,620	37,670	60,040	92,090	95,830	15.51	19.33	19.12	20.76	21.39
Medical assistants	330,830	382,720	523,260	601,240	623,560	11.46	12.58	14.31	15.34	15.79
Medical equipment preparers	32,760	41,790	47,310	50,330	52,500	10.68	12.42	14.59	16.80	17.29
Medical transcriptionists	97,330	90,380	78,780	57,830	54,070	12.37	14.36	16.12	17.17	17.86
Nursing assistants[5]	1,273,460	1,391,430	1,451,090	1,420,570	1,443,150	9.18	10.67	12.09	12.89	13.29
Occupational therapy aides	8,890	6,220	7,180	7,570	7,210	11.21	13.20	14.95	14.95	15.31
Occupational therapy assistants	15,910	22,160	27,720	35,460	38,170	16.76	19.13	24.66	28.05	28.62
Orderlies	NA	NA	NA	52,660	52,940	NA	NA	NA	13.26	13.73
Pharmacy aides	59,890	46,610	49,580	38,040	36,660	9.10	9.76	10.98	13.20	13.66
Physical therapist aides	34,620	41,930	45,900	50,540	50,030	10.06	11.01	12.02	13.19	13.41
Physical therapist assistants	44,120	58,670	65,960	81,230	85,580	16.52	18.98	23.95	26.56	27.33
Psychiatric aides	57,680	56,150	64,730	69,550	67,410	10.79	11.47	12.84	13.55	13.83

NOTE: This table excludes occupations such as dentists, physicians, and chiropractors, which have a large percentage of workers who are self-employed. Challenges in using Occupational Employment Statistics data as a time series include changes in the occupational, industrial, and geographical classification systems; changes in the way data are collected; changes in the survey reference period; and changes in mean wage estimation methodology, as well as permanent features of the methodology.

[1]Employment is the number of filled positions. This table includes both full-time and part-time wage and salary positions. Estimates do not include the self-employed, owners and partners in unincorporated firms, household workers, or unpaid family workers. Estimates were rounded to the nearest 10.

[2]The mean hourly wage rate for an occupation is the total wages that all workers in the occupation earn in an hour, divided by the total number of employees in the occupation. More information is available from: https://www.bls.gov/oes/current/oes_tec.htm.

[3]Starting with 2012 data, the radiologic technologists and technicians occupation category was split into two occupations as part of the 2010 Standard Occupational Classification (SOC) revision: Radiologic technologists (29-2034) and Magnetic resonance imaging technologists (29-2035). Thus, data prior to 2012 include radiologic technologists as well as magnetic resonance imaging technologists and are not comparable with 2012–2016 data.

[4]Starting with 2012 data, the registered nurses occupation category was split into four occupations as part of the 2010 SOC revision: Registered nurses (29-1141), plus three advanced practice nursing occupations: Nurse anesthetists (29-1151), Nurse midwives (29-1161), and Nurse practitioners (29-1171). Thus, data prior to 2012 include registered nurses as well as nurse anesthetists, nurse midwives, and nurse practitioners and are not comparable with 2012–2016 data.

[5]Starting with 2012 data, the nursing aides, orderlies, and attendants occupation category was split into two occupations as part of the 2010 SOC revision: Nursing assistants (31-1014) and Orderlies (31-1015). Thus, data prior to 2012 include nursing assistants as well as orderlies and are not comparable with 2012–2016 data.

Table 3-57. Employment and Wages in the Health Care Industry, by Selected Occupation, May 2018

(Number; dollars.)

Occupation	Employment	Median hourly wage (dollars)	Mean hourly wage (dollars)	Annual median wage (dollars)	Annual mean wage (dollars)
Healthcare Practitioners and Technical Occupations	8,646,730	31.94	39.42	66,440	82,000
Chiropractors	34,740	34.33	41.28	71,410	85,870
Dentists, General	113,000	73.00	84.54	151,850	175,840
Oral and Maxillofacial Surgeons	4,830	#	116.52	#	242,370
Orthodontists	5,350	#	108.54	#	225,760
Prosthodontists	380	84.88	92.02	176,540	191,400
Dentists, All Other Specialists	4,490	70.66	85.96	146,970	178,800
Dietitians and Nutritionists	64,670	29.02	29.43	60,370	61,210
Optometrists	37,220	53.75	57.68	111,790	119,980
Pharmacists	309,550	60.64	59.45	126,120	123,670
Anesthesiologists	31,060	#	128.38	#	267,020
Family and General Practitioners	114,130	96.68	101.82	201,100	211,780
Internists, General	37,820	93.51	94.47	194,500	196,490
Obstetricians and Gynecologists	18,590	#	114.58	#	238,320
Pediatricians, General	28,490	82.00	88.10	170,560	183,240
Psychiatrists	25,630	#	105.95	#	220,380
Surgeons	34,390	#	122.65	#	255,110
Physicians and Surgeons, All Other	389,180	96.58	98.02	200,890	203,880
Physician Assistants	114,710	52.22	52.13	108,610	108,430
Podiatrists	9,500	62.28	71.26	129,550	148,220
Therapists	687,790	37.23	38.24	77,450	79,530
Occupational Therapists	126,900	40.51	41.04	84,270	85,350
Physical Therapists	228,600	42.27	42.73	87,930	88,880
Radiation Therapists	18,260	39.58	41.70	82,330	86,730
Recreational Therapists	18,840	23.01	24.34	47,860	50,640
Respiratory Therapists	129,600	28.98	30.05	60,280	62,500
Speech-Language Pathologists	146,900	37.26	38.80	77,510	80,700
Therapists, All Other	11,950	24.51	27.73	50,980	57,680
Veterinarians	71,060	45.11	50.59	93,830	105,240
Registered Nurses	2,951,960	34.48	36.30	71,730	75,510
Nurse Anesthetists	43,520	80.75	84.03	167,950	174,790
Nurse Midwives	6,250	49.89	51.40	103,770	106,910
Nurse Practitioners	179,650	51.46	52.90	107,030	110,030
Audiologists	13,300	36.50	39.52	75,920	82,210
Miscellaneous Health Diagnosing and Treating Practitioners	36,680	35.56	41.16	73,960	85,600
Health Diagnosing and Treating Practitioners, All Other	36,680	35.56	41.16	73,960	85,600
Health Technologists and Technicians	3,110,180	21.49	23.26	44,700	48,380
Clinical Laboratory Technologists and Technicians	321,220	25.16	25.91	52,330	53,880
Dental Hygienists	215,150	35.97	36.30	74,820	75,500
Diagnostic Related Technologists and Technicians	390,630	30.60	31.38	63,650	65,260
Cardiovascular Technologists and Technicians	56,560	27.33	28.24	56,850	58,730
Diagnostic Medical Sonographers	71,130	34.86	35.51	72,510	73,860
Nuclear Medicine Technologists	18,810	36.93	37.92	76,820	78,870
Radiologic Technologists	205,590	28.62	29.59	59,520	61,540
Emergency Medical Technicians and Paramedics	257,210	16.50	18.15	34,320	37,760
Health Practitioner Support Technologists and Technicians	801,590	16.70	17.76	34,730	36,930
Dietetic Technicians	33,540	13.05	14.49	27,140	30,120
Pharmacy Technicians	417,860	15.72	16.35	32,700	34,020
Psychiatric Technicians	71,360	15.80	18.15	32,870	37,760
Respiratory Therapy Technicians	9,090	24.62	24.70	51,210	51,380
Surgical Technologists	110,160	22.74	23.58	47,300	49,040
Veterinary Technologists and Technicians	106,680	16.55	17.10	34,420	35,560
Licensed Practical and Licensed Vocational Nurses	701,690	22.23	22.62	46,240	47,050
Medical Records and Health Information Technicians	208,650	19.40	21.16	40,350	44,010
Opticians, Dispensing	72,250	17.80	19.20	37,010	39,930
Orthotists and Prosthetists	8,830	33.23	35.51	69,120	73,860
Hearing Aid Specialists	7,680	25.37	26.75	52,770	55,650
Health Technologists and Technicians, All Other	125,270	20.63	22.81	42,920	47,450
Other Healthcare Practitioners and Technical Occupations	168,630	30.01	32.01	62,420	66,590
Occupational Health and Safety Specialists and Technicians	106,410	33.35	34.43	69,370	71,610
Occupational Health and Safety Specialists	88,390	35.11	36.03	73,020	74,940
Occupational Health and Safety Technicians	18,020	24.41	26.57	50,780	55,270
Athletic Trainers	26,890	*	*	47,510	49,280
Genetic Counselors	2,640	38.64	38.88	80,370	80,860
Healthcare Practitioners and Technical Workers, All Other	32,680	26.26	30.45	54,620	63,340
Healthcare Support Occupations	4,117,450	14.30	15.57	29,740	32,380
Home Health Aides	797,670	11.63	12.18	24,200	25,330
Psychiatric Aides	56,910	14.03	14.95	29,180	31,090
Nursing assistants	1,450,960	13.72	14.22	28,540	29,580
Orderlies	50,100	13.49	14.35	28,060	29,840

= This wage is equal to or greater than $100.00 per hour or $208,000 per year.
* = Wages for some occupations that do not generally work year-round, full time, are reported either as hourly wages or annual salaries depending on how they are typically paid.

Table 3-57. Employment and Wages in the Health Care Industry, by Selected Occupation, May 2018—*Continued*

(Number; dollars.)

Occupation	Employment	Median hourly wage (dollars)	Mean hourly wage (dollars)	Annual median wage (dollars)	Annual mean wage (dollars)
Occupational Therapy Assistants	42,660	28.95	29.04	60,220	60,410
Occupational Therapy Aides	7,700	13.54	15.66	28,160	32,580
Physical Therapist Assistants	94,250	27.91	27.77	58,040	57,750
Physical Therapist Aides	47,260	12.62	13.70	26,240	28,500
Massage Therapists	105,160	19.92	22.06	41,420	45,880
Dental Assistants	341,060	18.59	19.12	38,660	39,770
Medical Assistants	673,660	16.16	16.61	33,610	34,540
Medical Equipment Preparers	55,610	17.42	18.27	36,240	37,990
Medical Transcriptionists	53,730	16.72	17.48	34,770	36,350
Pharmacy Aides	36,970	12.72	14.03	26,450	29,190
Veterinary Assistants and Laboratory Animal Caretakers	89,480	13.24	13.79	27,540	28,690
Phlebotomists	125,280	16.58	17.10	34,480	35,560
Healthcare Support Workers, All Other	88,990	18.19	18.80	37,830	39,110

Table 3-58. Employment and Wages for the Highest- and Lowest-Paying Detailed Health Sector Occupations, by Annual Mean Wage, May 2018

(Dollars; number.)

Occupation title	Annual mean wage (dollars)[1]	Mean hourly wage (dollars)	Employment
Highest-Paying Positions			
Anesthesiologists	267,020	128.38	31,060
Surgeons	255,110	122.65	34,390
Oral and Maxillofacial Surgeons	242,370	116.52	4,830
Obstetricians and Gynecologists	238,320	114.58	18,590
Orthodontists	225,760	108.54	5,350
Psychiatrists	220,380	105.95	25,630
Family and General Practitioners	211,780	101.82	114,130
Physicians and Surgeons	210,980	101.43	679,280
Physicians and Surgeons, All Other	203,880	98.02	389,180
Internists, General	196,490	94.47	37,820
Lowest-Paying Positions			
Home Health Aides	25,330	12.18	797,670
Nursing, Psychiatric, and Home Health Aides	28,180	13.55	2,355,640
Physical Therapist Aides	28,500	13.70	47,260
Veterinary Assistants and Laboratory Animal Caretakers	28,690	13.79	89,480
Pharmacy Aides	29,190	14.03	36,970
Nursing Assistants	29,580	14.22	1,450,960
Orderlies	29,840	14.35	50,100
Dietetic Technicians	30,130	14.49	33,540
Psychiatric Aides	31,090	14.95	56,910
Occupational Therapy Aides	32,580	15.66	7,700

[1]Annual wages have been calculated by multiplying the hourly mean wage by a "year-round, full-time" hours figure of 2,080 hours; for those occupations where there is not an hourly mean wage published, the annual wage has been directly calculated from the reported survey data.

Table 3-59. Industries with the Highest Levels of Employment and Highest Concentrations of Employment in Health Care and Practitioner and Technical Occupations, May 2018

(Number; dollars.)

Industry	Employment[1]	Hourly mean wage (dollars)	Annual mean wage (dollars)[2]
Industries with the Highest Levels of Employment in Health Care and Practitioner and Technical Occupations			
Healthcare Practitioners and Technical Occupations	8,646,730	39.42	82,000
Health Diagnosing and Treating Practitioners	5,367,930	49.02	101,960
Healthcare Support Occupations	4,117,450	15.57	32,380
Health Technologists and Technicians	3,110,180	23.26	48,380
Registered Nurses	2,951,960	36.30	75,510
Industries with the Highest Concentrations of Employment in Health Care and Practitioner and Technical Occupations			
General Medical and Surgical Hospitals	3,129,490	56.42	79,040
Other Ambulatory Health Care Services	166,930	54.26	42,670
Specialty (except Psychiatric and Substance Abuse) Hospitals	135,860	51.90	82,740
Offices of Physicians	1,120,400	43.25	127,330
Outpatient Care Centers	370,070	40.13	84,460

[1]Estimates do not include self-employed workers.
[2]Annual wages have been calculated by multiplying the hourly mean wage by a "year-round, full-time" hours figure of 2,080 hours; for those occupations where there is not an hourly mean wage published, the annual wage has been directly calculated from the reported survey data.

Table 3-60. States with the Highest Level of Employment and Highest Concentration of Jobs in Health Care Practitioner and Technical Occupations, May 2016

(Number, dollar.)

State	Employment[1]	Employment per thousand jobs	Location quotient[2]	Hourly mean wage (dollars)	Annual mean wage (dollars)[3]
States with the Highest Employment Level in This Occupation					
California	838,440	49.30	0.83	$47.55	$98,910
Texas	679,150	56.06	0.94	37.54	78,070
New York	545,670	58.14	0.97	43.53	90,540
Florida	532,310	61.83	1.04	36.38	75,680
Pennsylvania	408,340	69.83	1.17	36.47	75,860
States with the Highest Concentration of Jobs and Location Quotients in This Occupation					
West Virginia	59,000	84.69	1.42	$32.91	$68,460
South Dakota	31,250	74.00	1.24	34.32	71,380
Mississippi	79,780	70.99	1.19	30.86	64,190
Delaware	31,680	70.63	1.18	42.08	87,520
Pennsylvania	408,340	69.83	1.17	36.47	75,860

[1]Estimates for detailed occupations do not sum to the totals because the totals include occupations not shown separately. Estimates do not include self-employed workers.
[2]The location quotient is the ratio of the area concentration of occupational employment to the national average concentration. A location quotient greater than one indicates the occupation has a higher share of employment than average, and a location quotient less than one indicates the occupation is less prevalent in the area than average.
[3]Annual wages have been calculated by multiplying the hourly mean wage by a "year-round, full-time" hours figure of 2,080 hours; for those occupations where there is not an hourly mean wage published, the annual wage has been directly calculated from the reported survey data.

Table 3-61. Top Paying Metropolitan Areas for Health Care Practitioner and Technical Occupations, May 2016

(Number, dollar.)

Metropolitan area	Employment[1]	Employment per thousand jobs	Location quotient[2]	Hourly mean wage (dollars)	Annual mean wage (dollars)[3]
San Jose-Sunnyvale-Santa Clara, CA	45,320	40.49	0.68	$55.98	$116,440
Salinas, CA	7,330	40.80	0.68	$54.57	$113,510
Santa Cruz-Watsonville, CA	4,710	48.07	0.80	$54.19	$112,720
San Francisco-Redwood City-South San Francisco, CA Metropolitan Division	112,170	46.37	0.78	54.08	112,490
Yuba City, CA	2,890	65.21	1.09	52.30	108,780
Rochester, MN	NR	NR	NR	51.77	107,690
Santa Maria-Santa Barbara, CA	8,640	46.21	0.77	51.16	106,420
Sacramento--Roseville--Arden-Arcade, CA	50,490	51.28	0.86	51.03	106,140
Napa, CA	4,930	65.31	1.09	50.84	105,750
Bend-Redmond, OR	5,360	64.41	1.08	49.44	102,830

NR = Not released.
[1]Estimates for detailed occupations do not sum to the totals because the totals include occupations not shown separately. Estimates do not include self-employed workers.
[2]The location quotient is the ratio of the area concentration of occupational employment to the national average concentration. A location quotient greater than one indicates the occupation has a higher share of employment than average, and a location quotient less than one indicates the occupation is less prevalent in the area than average.
[3]Annual wages have been calculated by multiplying the hourly mean wage by a "year-round, full-time" hours figure of 2,080 hours; for those occupations where there is not an hourly mean wage published, the annual wage has been directly calculated from the reported survey data.

Table 3-62. Top Paying Nonmetropolitan Areas for Health Care Practitioner and Technical Occupations, May 2018

(Number, dollar.)

Metropolitan area	Employment[1]	Employment per thousand jobs	Location quotient[2]	Hourly mean wage (dollars)	Annual mean wage (dollars)[3]
Alaska nonmetropolitan area	4,450	41.97	0.70	$53.29	$110,840
West Central New Hampshire nonmetropolitan area	8,250	80.80	1.35	47.72	99,260
Eastern Sierra-Mother Lode Region of California nonmetropolitan area	2,890	49.06	0.82	47.48	98,760
North Valley-Northern Mountains Region of California nonmetropolitan area	4,430	44.71	0.75	45.57	94,780
Coast Oregon nonmetropolitan area	5,880	52.01	0.87	44.49	92,530

[1]Estimates for detailed occupations do not sum to the totals because the totals include occupations not shown separately. Estimates do not include self-employed workers.
[2]The location quotient is the ratio of the area concentration of occupational employment to the national average concentration. A location quotient greater than one indicates the occupation has a higher share of employment than average, and a location quotient less than one indicates the occupation is less prevalent in the area than average.
[3]Annual wages have been calculated by multiplying the hourly mean wage by a "year-round, full-time" hours figure of 2,080 hours; for those occupations where there is not an hourly mean wage published, the annual wage has been directly calculated from the reported survey data.

HEALTH EXPENDITURES

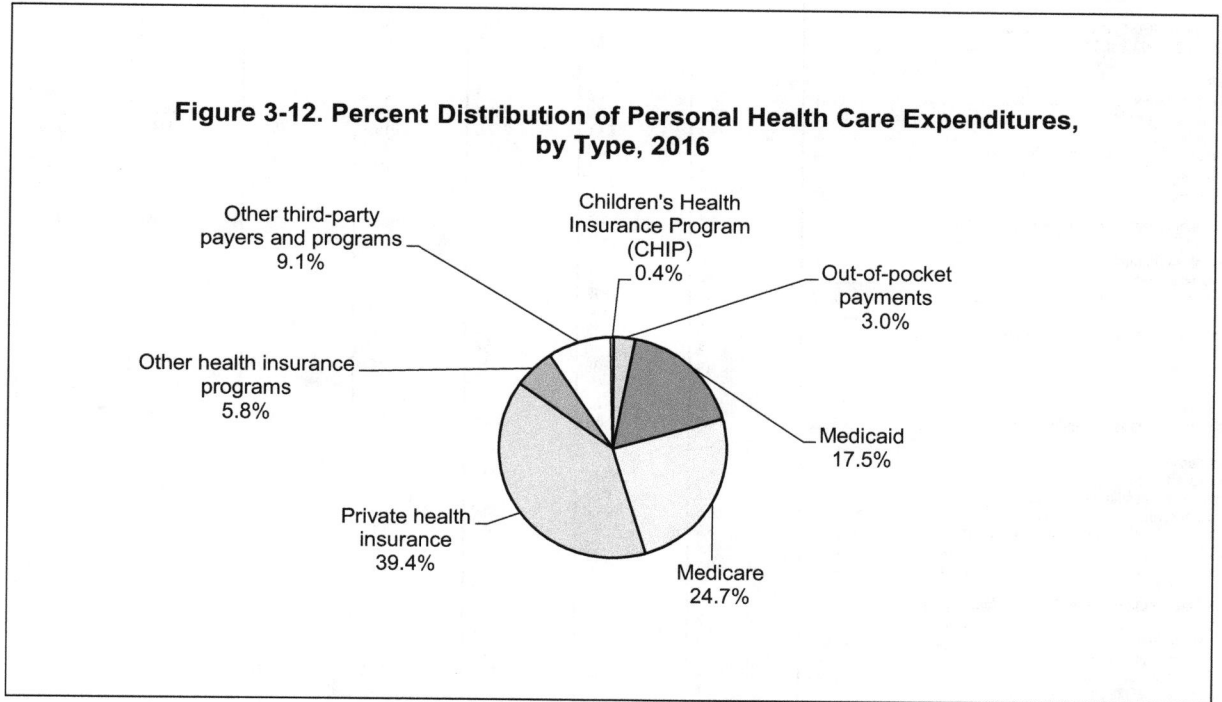

Figure 3-12. Percent Distribution of Personal Health Care Expenditures, by Type, 2016

Other third-party payers and programs
9.1%

Children's Health Insurance Program (CHIP)
0.4%

Out-of-pocket payments
3.0%

Other health insurance programs
5.8%

Medicaid
17.5%

Private health insurance
39.4%

Medicare
24.7%

Table 3-63. Gross Domestic Product, National Health Expenditures, Per Capita Amounts, Percent Distribution, and Average Annual Percent Change, Selected Years, 1960–2016

(Number; dollars; data are compiled from various sources by the Centers for Medicare & Medicaid Services.)

Gross domestic product and national health expenditures	1960	1970	1980	1990	2000	2009	2015	2016
Gross domestic product (GDP), in billions....................	543	1,076	2,863	5,980	10,285	14,419	18,121	18,625
Price deflator for GDO (2009 = 100.0)[1]	17.5	22.8	44.5	66.8	81.9	100.0	110.0	111.4
Amount (in Billions)								
National health expenditures.....................	27.2	74.6	255.3	721.4	1,369.1	2,495.4	3,200.8	3,337.2
Health consumption expenditures..................	24.7	67.0	235.5	674.1	1,285.8	2,356.5	3,047.1	3,179.8
Personal health care.................	23.3	63.1	217.0	615.3	1,161.5	2,114.6	2,715.5	2,834.0
Administration and net cost of private health insurance	1.1	2.6	12.1	38.7	81.2	167.7	249.9	263.7
Public health.........................	0.4	1.4	6.4	20.0	43.0	74.2	81.7	82.2
Investment[2].......................	2.5	7.5	19.9	47.3	83.3	139.0	153.7	157.4
Chain-weighted national health expenditure deflator (2009 = 100.0)[1]	NA	NA	NA	NA	NA	100.0	111.3	112.8
Per Capita Amount (in Dollars)								
National health expenditures.....................	146	355	1,108	2,843	4,855	8,143	9,994	10,348
Health consumption expenditures..................	133	319	1,022	2,657	4,560	7,690	9,514	9,860
Personal health care.................	125	300	942	2,425	4,119	6,901	8,479	8,788
Administration and net cost of private health insurance	6	13	52	153	288	547	780	818
Public health.........................	2	6	28	79	153	242	255	255
Investment[2].......................	13	36	86	187	295	453	480	488
Percent								
National health expenditures as percent of GDP	5.0	6.9	8.9	12.1	13.3	17.3	17.7	17.9
Percent Distribution								
National health expenditures.....................	100.0	100.0	100.0	100.0	100.0	100.0	100.0	100.0
Health consumption expenditures..................	90.8	89.9	92.2	93.4	93.9	94.4	95.2	95.3
Personal health care.................	85.5	84.6	85.0	85.3	84.8	84.7	84.8	84.9
Administration and net cost of private health insurance	3.9	3.5	4.7	5.4	5.9	6.7	7.8	7.9
Public health.........................	1.4	1.8	2.5	2.8	3.1	3.0	2.6	2.5
Investment[2].......................	9.2	10.1	7.8	6.6	6.1	5.6	4.8	4.7
Average Annual Percent Change from Previous Year Shown								
GDP	X	7.1	11.1	7.6	5.6	3.8	3.9	2.8
National health expenditures.....................	X	10.6	13.9	10.9	6.6	6.9	4.2	4.3
Health consumption expenditures..................	X	10.5	14.2	11.1	6.7	7.0	4.4	4.4
Personal health care.................	X	10.5	13.9	11.0	6.6	6.9	4.3	4.4
Administration and net cost of private health insurance	X	9.4	19.6	12.4	7.7	8.4	6.9	5.5
Public health.........................	X	13.8	16.8	12.0	8.0	6.2	1.6	0.6
Investment[2].......................	X	11.6	10.3	9.1	5.8	5.8	1.7	2.4
National health expenditures.....................	X	9.3	12.9	9.9	5.5	5.9	3.5	3.5
Health consumption expenditures..................	X	9.2	13.2	10.0	5.6	6.0	3.6	3.6
Personal health care.................	X	9.2	12.9	9.9	5.4	5.9	3.5	3.6
Administration and net cost of private health insurance	X	8.1	18.5	11.3	6.6	7.4	6.1	4.8
Public health.........................	X	12.5	15.7	10.9	6.8	5.3	0.9	−0.1
Investment[2].......................	X	10.3	9.3	8.0	4.7	4.9	0.9	1.7

NOTE: Dollar amounts shown are in current dollars. Percentages are calculated using unrounded data. Estimates may not add to totals because of rounding. Census resident population is used to calculate per capita. For more information on national health expenditure categories, sources, and methods, see "National Health Expenditure Accounts: Methodology Paper, 2016."
NA = Not available.
X = Not applicable.
[1]Year 2009 = 100. For more information on the detailed price series recommended for deflating each category of spending, see "National Health Expenditure Accounts Methodology Paper, 2016." Available from: https://www.cms.gov/Research-Statistics-Data-and-Systems/Statistics-Trends-and-Reports/NationalHealthExpendData/downloads/dsm-16.pdf.
[2]Investment consists of research and structures and equipment.

Table 3-64. National Health Expenditures, Average Annual Percent Change and Percent Distribution, by Type of Expenditure, Selected Years, 1960–2016

(Dollars; percent; data are compiled from various sources by the Centers for Medicare & Medicaid Services.)

Type of national health expenditure	1960	1970	1980	1990	2000	2009	2015	2016
Amount (in Billions of Dollars)								
National health expenditures	27.2	74.6	255.3	721.4	1,369.1	2,495.4	3,200.8	3,337.2
Health consumption expenditures	24.7	67.0	235.5	674.1	1,285.8	2,356.5	3,047.1	3,179.8
Personal health care	23.3	63.1	217.0	615.3	1,161.5	2,114.6	2,715.5	2,834.0
Hospital care	9.0	27.2	100.5	250.4	415.5	779.6	1,033.4	1,082.5
Professional services	7.9	19.8	64.5	207.3	386.9	667.8	837.7	881.2
Physician and clinical services	5.6	14.3	47.7	158.4	288.2	497.7	631.0	664.9
Other professional services	0.4	0.7	3.5	17.3	36.6	67.0	87.8	92.0
Dental services	2.0	4.7	13.3	31.6	62.1	103.1	118.9	124.4
Other health, residential, and personal care	0.4	1.3	8.4	23.8	63.9	123.4	164.8	173.5
Home health care[1]	0.1	0.2	2.4	12.5	32.3	67.7	88.8	92.4
Nursing care facilities and continuing care retirement communities[1]	0.8	4.0	15.3	44.7	85.0	135.2	158.1	162.7
Retail outlet sales of medical products	5.0	10.6	25.9	76.5	177.8	340.9	432.7	441.7
Prescription drugs	2.7	5.5	12.0	40.3	121.0	252.7	324.5	328.6
Durable medical equipment	0.7	1.7	4.1	13.8	25.2	37.8	48.6	51.0
Other nondurable medical products	1.6	3.3	9.8	22.4	31.6	50.3	59.6	62.2
Government administration[2]	0.1	0.7	2.8	7.2	17.1	29.5	42.1	43.8
Net cost of health insurance[3]	1.0	1.9	9.3	31.6	64.2	138.2	207.7	219.8
Government public health activities[4]	0.4	1.4	6.4	20.0	43.0	74.2	81.7	82.2
Investment	2.5	7.5	19.9	47.3	83.3	139.0	153.7	157.4
Research[5]	0.7	2.0	5.4	12.7	25.5	45.4	46.5	47.7
Structures and equipment	1.8	5.6	14.4	34.6	57.8	93.6	107.2	109.7
Average Annual Percent Change from Previous Year Shown								
National health expenditures	X	10.6	13.9	10.9	6.6	6.9	4.2	4.3
Health consumption expenditures	X	10.5	14.2	11.1	6.7	7.0	4.4	4.4
Personal health care	X	10.5	13.9	11.0	6.6	6.9	4.3	4.4
Hospital care	X	11.7	14.4	9.6	5.2	7.2	4.8	4.7
Professional services	X	9.6	13.2	12.4	6.4	6.3	3.9	5.2
Physician and clinical services	X	9.9	13.5	12.7	6.2	6.3	4.0	5.4
Other professional services	X	6.3	21.1	17.4	7.8	6.9	4.6	4.7
Dental services	X	9.0	10.7	9.0	7.0	5.8	2.4	4.6
Other health, residential, and personal care	X	11.5	23.9	11.0	10.4	7.6	4.9	5.3
Home health care[1]	X	14.5	30.7	18.1	9.9	8.6	4.6	4.0
Nursing care facilities and continuing care retirement communities[1]	X	17.4	13.7	11.4	6.6	5.3	2.6	2.9
Retail outlet sales of medical products	X	7.7	10.4	11.4	8.8	7.5	4.1	2.1
Prescription drugs	X	7.5	8.4	12.8	11.6	8.5	4.3	1.3
Durable medical equipment	X	9.0	7.7	13.0	6.2	4.6	4.3	4.9
Other nondurable medical products	X	7.4	14.6	8.6	3.5	5.3	2.9	4.4
Government administration[2]	X	30.0	13.2	10.0	9.0	6.3	6.1	4.0
Net cost of health insurance[3]	X	6.4	22.0	13.0	7.4	8.9	7.0	5.8
Government public health activities[4]	X	13.8	16.8	12.0	8.0	6.2	1.6	0.6
Investment	X	11.6	10.3	9.1	5.8	5.8	1.7	2.4
Research[5]	X	10.9	10.0	8.9	7.2	6.6	0.4	2.6
Structures and equipment	X	11.9	10.4	9.2	5.3	5.5	2.3	2.3
Percent Distribution								
National health expenditures	100.0	100.0	100.0	100.0	100.0	100.0	100.0	100.0
Health consumption expenditures	90.8	89.9	92.2	93.4	93.9	94.4	95.2	95.3
Personal health care	85.5	84.6	85.0	85.3	84.8	84.7	84.8	84.9
Hospital care	33.0	36.4	39.4	34.7	30.4	31.2	32.3	32.4
Professional services	29.1	26.5	25.3	28.7	28.3	26.8	26.2	26.4
Physician and clinical services	20.4	19.2	18.7	22.0	21.0	19.9	19.7	19.9
Other professional services	1.4	1.0	1.4	2.4	2.7	2.7	2.7	2.8
Dental services	7.3	6.3	5.2	4.4	4.5	4.1	3.7	3.7
Other health, residential, and personal care	1.6	1.7	3.3	3.3	4.7	4.9	5.1	5.2
Home health care[1]	0.2	0.3	0.9	1.7	2.4	2.7	2.8	2.8
Nursing care facilities and continuing care retirement communities[1]	3.0	5.4	6.0	6.2	6.2	5.4	4.9	4.9
Retail outlet sales of medical products	18.5	14.2	10.1	10.6	13.0	13.7	13.5	13.2
Prescription drugs	9.8	7.4	4.7	5.6	8.8	10.1	10.1	9.8
Durable medical equipment	2.7	2.3	1.6	1.9	1.8	1.5	1.5	1.5
Other nondurable medical products	6.0	4.5	3.8	3.1	2.3	2.0	1.9	1.9
Government administration[2]	0.2	1.0	1.1	1.0	1.2	1.2	1.3	1.3
Net cost of health insurance[3]	3.7	2.5	3.6	4.4	4.7	5.5	6.5	6.6
Government public health activities[4]	1.4	1.8	2.5	2.8	3.1	3.0	2.6	2.5
Investment	9.2	10.1	7.8	6.6	6.1	5.6	4.8	4.7
Research[5]	2.6	2.6	2.1	1.8	1.9	1.8	1.5	1.4
Structures and equipment	6.7	7.5	5.7	4.8	4.2	3.8	3.4	3.3
Percent Distribution								
Personal health care	100.0	100.0	100.0	100.0	100.0	100.0	100.0	100.0
Hospital care	38.6	43.1	46.3	40.7	35.8	36.9	38.1	38.2
Professional services	34.1	31.3	29.7	33.7	33.3	31.6	30.8	31.1
Physician and clinical services	23.9	22.7	22.0	25.7	24.8	23.5	23.2	23.5
Other professional services	1.7	1.2	1.6	2.8	3.2	3.2	3.2	3.2
Dental services	8.5	7.5	6.1	5.1	5.3	4.9	4.4	4.4
Other health, residential, and personal care	1.9	2.1	3.9	3.9	5.5	5.8	6.1	6.1
Home health care[1]	0.2	0.3	1.1	2.0	2.8	3.2	3.3	3.3
Nursing care facilities and continuing care retirement communities[1]	3.5	6.4	7.0	7.3	7.3	6.4	5.8	5.7
Retail outlet sales of medical products	21.7	16.8	11.9	12.4	15.3	16.1	15.9	15.6
Prescription drugs	11.5	8.7	5.6	6.5	10.4	12.0	12.0	11.6
Durable medical equipment	3.2	2.8	1.9	2.2	2.2	1.8	1.8	1.8
Other nondurable medical products	7.0	5.3	4.5	3.6	2.7	2.4	2.2	2.2

NOTE: Percentages and average annual percent change are calculated using unrounded data. For more information on national health expenditure categories, sources, and methods, see "National Health Expenditure Accounts: Methodology Paper, 2016." Available from: https://www.cms.gov/Research-Statistics-Data-and-Systems/Statistics-Trends-and- Reports/NationalHealthExpendData/downloads/dsm-16.pdf.
X = Not applicable.

[1]Includes expenditures for care in freestanding facilities only. Additional services of this type are provided in hospital-based facilities and are considered hospital care.
[2]Includes all administrative costs (federal and state and local employees' salaries; contracted employees, including fiscal intermediaries; rent and building costs; computer systems and programs; other materials and supplies; and other miscellaneous expenses) associated with insuring individuals enrolled in the following health insurance programs: Medicare, Medicaid, Children's Health Insurance Program, Department of Defense, Department of Veterans Affairs, Indian Health Service, workers' compensation, maternal and child health, vocational rehabilitation, Substance Abuse and Mental Health Services Administration, and other federal programs.
[3]Net cost of health insurance is calculated as the difference between calendar year incurred premiums earned and benefits incurred for private health insurance. This includes administrative costs, and in some cases additions to reserves, rate credits and dividends, premium taxes, and net underwriting gains or losses. Also included in this category is the difference between premiums earned and benefits incurred for the private health insurance companies that insure the enrollees of the following programs: Medicare, Medicaid, Children's Health Insurance Program, and workers' compensation (health portion only).
[4]Includes health care services delivered by government public health agencies.
[5]Research and development expenditures of drug companies and other manufacturers and providers of medical equipment and supplies are excluded. These are included in the expenditure class in which the product falls because such expenditures are covered by the payment received for that product.

Table 3-65. Personal Health Care Expenditures, by Source of Funds and Type of Expenditure, Selected Years, 1960–2016

(Number; percent; data are compiled from various sources by the Centers for Medicare & Medicaid Services.)

Type of personal health care expenditures and source of funds	1960	1970	1980	1990	2000	2009	2015	2016
Amount in Billions								
Per capita	125	300	942	2,425	4,119	6,901	8,479	8,788
Amount in Billions								
All personal health care expenditures[1]	23.3	63.1	217.0	615.3	1,161.5	2,114.6	2,715.5	2,834.0
Out-of-pocket payments	12.9	25.0	58.1	137.9	198.9	293.7	339.3	352.5
Health insurance		29.6	132.1	402.9	843.8	1,636.9	2,151.4	2,243.9
Private health insurance	5.0	14.1	61.5	204.8	405.6	734.7	943.3	993.8
Medicare	X	7.3	36.3	107.3	216.3	470.3	607.1	625.3
Medicaid	X	5.0	24.7	69.7	186.9	346.2	485.8	505.2
Federal	X	2.7	13.7	40.3	109.3	230.6	305.8	319.2
State and local	X	2.3	11.0	29.4	77.6	115.6	180.0	186.1
CHIP[2]	X	X	X	X	2.5	9.5	12.2	14.0
Federal	X	X	X	X	1.8	6.7	9.1	12.7
State and local	X	X	X	X	0.8	2.8	3.1	1.3
Other health insurance programs[3]	1.7	3.3	9.6	21.2	32.3	76.2	103.0	105.6
Other third-party payers and programs[4]	3.7	8.5	26.7	74.5	118.9	183.9	224.8	237.6
Amount in Billions								
Chain-weighted personal health care deflator (2009 = 100.0)[5]	9.3	13.5	28.5	56.3	75.7	100.0	110.7	112.0
Percent Distribution								
All sources of funds	100.0	100.0	100.0	100.0	100.0	100.0	100.0	100.0
Out-of-pocket payments	55.7	39.6	26.8	22.4	17.1	13.9	12.5	12.4
Health insurance	28.5	47.0	60.9	65.5	72.6	77.4	79.2	79.2
Private health insurance	21.3	22.3	28.4	33.3	34.9	34.7	34.7	35.1
Medicare	X	11.5	16.7	17.4	18.6	22.2	22.4	22.1
Medicaid	X	8.0	11.4	11.3	16.1	16.4	17.9	17.8
Federal	X	4.3	6.3	6.6	9.4	10.9	11.3	11.3
State and local	X	3.7	5.1	4.8	6.7	5.5	6.6	6.6
CHIP[2]	X	X	X	X	0.2	0.5	0.4	0.5
Federal	X	X	X	X	0.2	0.3	0.3	0.4
State and local	X	X	X	X	0.1	0.1	0.1	0.0
Other health insurance programs[3]	7.2	5.2	4.4	3.4	2.8	3.6	3.8	3.7
Other third-party payers and programs[4]	15.8	13.4	12.3	12.1	10.2	8.7	8.3	8.4
Amount in Billions								
Hospital expenditures[6]	9.0	27.2	100.5	250.4	415.5	779.6	1,033.4	1,082.5
Percent Distribution								
All sources of funds	100.0	100.0	100.0	100.0	100.0	100.0	100.0	100.0
Out-of-pocket payments	20.6	9.0	5.4	4.5	3.2	3.3	3.0	3.0
Health insurance	50.7	71.5	79.7	82.6	86.2	87.4	87.8	87.9
Private health insurance	35.6	32.5	36.6	38.5	33.9	36.6	38.7	39.4
Medicare	X	19.7	26.1	26.9	29.7	27.5	25.2	24.7
Medicaid	X	9.7	9.2	10.6	17.1	17.1	17.8	17.5
Federal	X	5.2	5.0	6.3	10.3	11.3	11.5	11.4
State and local	X	4.5	4.2	4.3	6.8	5.8	6.3	6.2
CHIP[2]	X	X	X	X	0.2	0.4	0.4	0.4
Federal	X	X	X	X	0.2	0.3	0.3	0.4
State and local	X	X	X	X	0.1	0.1	0.1	0.0
Other health insurance programs[3]	15.2	9.6	7.8	6.5	5.3	5.8	5.8	5.8
Other third-party payers and programs[4]	28.7	19.5	15.0	12.9	10.6	9.3	9.1	9.1
Amount in Billions								
Physician and clinical expenditures	5.6	14.3	47.7	158.4	288.2	497.7	631.0	664.9
Percent Distribution								
All sources of funds	100.0	100.0	100.0	100.0	100.0	100.0	100.0	100.0
Out-of-pocket payments	59.5	45.1	29.8	18.9	11.1	9.1	9.0	8.9
Health insurance	33.1	48.8	59.8	67.8	76.4	80.5	81.4	81.2
Private health insurance	28.7	29.4	34.8	42.1	47.0	45.9	43.0	43.2
Medicare	X	11.5	17.4	19.2	20.4	22.5	22.9	22.6
Medicaid	X	4.5	5.1	4.4	6.7	8.1	11.0	10.9
Federal	X	2.4	2.9	2.6	3.9	5.6	7.7	7.7
State and local	X	2.1	2.2	1.8	2.7	2.5	3.3	3.2
CHIP[2]	X	X	X	X	0.3	0.6	0.6	0.6
Federal	X	X	X	X	0.2	0.4	0.4	0.5
State and local	X	X	X	X	0.1	0.2	0.1	0.1
Other health insurance programs[3]	4.4	3.4	2.4	2.1	2.1	3.4	3.9	3.9
Other third-party payers and programs[4]	7.4	6.1	10.4	14.8	13.3	12.5	10.3	9.6	10.0

NOTE: Percentages may not add to totals because of rounding. Census resident population is used to calculate per capita. The Medicare and Medicaid programs began coverage in 1965. The Children's Health Insurance Program began coverage in 1997. For more information on national health expenditure sources and methods, see "National Health Expenditure Accounts: Methodology Paper, 2016." Available from: https://www.cms.gov/Research-Statistics-Data-and-Systems/Statistics-Trends-and-Reports/NationalHealthExpendData/Downloads/DSM-16.pdf.
X = Not applicable.
0.0 = Quantity more than zero but less than 0.05.
[1]Includes all expenditures other than expenses for government administration, net cost of health insurance, public health activities, research, and structures and equipment.
[2]Children's Health Insurance Program (CHIP). Medicaid CHIP expansions are included.
[3]Includes Department of Defense and Department of Veterans Affairs.
[4]Includes worksite health care, other private revenues, Indian Health Service, workers' compensation, general assistance, maternal and child health, vocational rehabilitation, other federal programs, Substance Abuse and Mental Health Services Administration, other state and local programs, and school health.
[5]The personal health care deflator is calculated as a chain-weighted price index using the Producer Price Indexes for hospitals, offices of physicians, medical and diagnostic laboratories, home health care services, and nursing care facilities; and Consumer Price Indices specific to each of the remaining personal health care components.
[6]Includes expenditures for hospital-based nursing home and home health agency care.

Table 3-65. Personal Health Care Expenditures, by Source of Funds and Type of Expenditure, Selected Years, 1960–2016—*Continued*

(Number; percent; data are compiled from various sources by the Centers for Medicare & Medicaid Services.)

Type of personal health care expenditures and source of funds	1960	1970	1980	1990	2000	2009	2015	2016
Amount in Billions								
Home health care expenditures[7]	0.1	0.2	2.4	12.5	32.3	67.7	88.8	92.4
Percent Distribution								
All sources of funds	100.0	100.0	100.0	100.0	100.0	100.0	100.0	100.0
Out-of-pocket payments	12.5	9.4	15.2	17.8	19.2	8.5	9.0	8.7
Health insurance	5.6	37.9	53.7	66.2	71.8	88.1	88.2	88.5
Private health insurance	2.5	3.0	14.7	22.8	24.0	7.5	10.6	10.4
Medicare	X	26.7	26.8	26.0	26.5	44.7	40.3	40.5
Medicaid	X	6.7	11.7	17.1	20.9	35.4	36.6	36.8
Federal	X	3.3	6.2	9.2	11.3	23.1	20.9	21.3
State and local	X	3.4	5.4	8.0	9.6	12.3	15.7	15.5
CHIP[2]	X	X	X	X	0.0	0.0	0.1	0.1
Federal	X	X	X	X	0.0	0.0	0.0	0.1
State and local	X	X	X	X	0.0	0.0	0.0	0.0
Other health insurance programs[3]	3.1	1.4	0.5	0.3	0.3	0.4	0.7	0.7
Other third-party payers and programs[4]	81.9	52.7	31.1	16.0	9.0	3.3	2.7	2.8
Amount in Billions								
Nursing care facilities and continuing care retirement communities expenditures[8]	0.8	4.0	15.3	44.7	85.0	135.2	158.1	162.7
Percent Distribution								
All sources of funds	100.0	100.0	100.0	100.0	100.0	100.0	100.0	100.0
Out-of-pocket payments	74.4	49.2	40.5	40.2	31.9	27.4	26.2	26.9
Health insurance	X	28.5	51.9	49.0	61.2	66.1	66.8	66.0
Private health insurance	X	0.2	1.3	6.2	8.8	7.3	8.8	9.1
Medicare	X	3.5	2.0	3.8	12.7	22.3	23.4	23.0
Medicaid	X	23.3	46.2	36.7	37.5	33.6	31.3	30.7
Federal	X	12.5	26.1	20.7	21.8	22.4	18.0	17.7
State and local	X	10.8	20.1	16.1	15.7	11.2	13.3	13.0
CHIP[2]	X	X	X	X	0.0	0.0	0.0	0.0
Federal	X	X	X	X	0.0	0.0	0.0	0.0
State and local	X	X	X	X	0.0	0.0	0.0	0.0
Other health insurance programs[3]	X	1.5	2.4	2.2	2.2	2.9	3.2	3.1
Other third-party payers and programs[4]	25.6	22.3	7.6	10.8	6.9	6.5	7.0	7.1
Amount in Billions								
Prescription drug expenditures	2.7	5.5	12.0	40.3	121.0	252.7	324.5	328.6
Percent Distribution								
All sources of funds	100.0	100.0	100.0	100.0	100.0	100.0	100.0	100.0
Out-of-pocket payments	96.0	82.4	71.3	56.8	27.8	19.4	14.0	13.7
Health insurance	1.5	16.5	26.9	40.2	70.3	79.2	85.4	85.7
Private health insurance	1.3	8.8	15.0	27.0	50.5	46.0	43.6	43.4
Medicare	X	X	X	0.5	1.7	21.6	28.6	29.0
Medicaid	X	7.6	11.7	12.6	16.3	8.0	9.8	10.2
Federal	X	4.1	6.8	7.2	9.3	5.4	6.5	6.7
State and local	X	3.5	4.9	5.4	7.0	2.7	3.3	3.4
CHIP[2]	X	X	X	X	0.2	0.5	0.5	0.5
Federal	X	X	X	X	0.2	0.4	0.4	0.5
State and local	X	X	X	X	0.1	0.2	0.1	0.0
Other health insurance programs[3]	0.1	0.1	0.2	0.2	1.5	3.1	2.9	2.6
Other third-party payers and programs[4]	2.5	1.1	1.8	3.0	1.9	1.4	0.6	0.6
Amount in Billions								
Dental services expenditures	2.0	4.7	13.3	31.6	62.1	103.1	118.9	124.4
Percent Distribution								
All sources of funds	100.0	100.0	100.0	100.0	100.0	100.0	100.0	100.0
Out-of-pocket payments	96.0	90.0	65.8	48.3	44.2	41.5	40.3	40.1
Health insurance	3.2	9.5	33.4	51.2	55.3	58.0	59.3	59.5
Private health insurance	1.9	4.5	28.4	47.9	50.3	48.1	46.3	46.4
Medicare	X	X	X	X	0.1	0.3	0.4	0.4
Medicaid	X	3.4	3.8	2.4	3.9	7.4	9.7	9.7
Federal	X	1.8	2.1	1.3	2.2	5.0	6.4	6.5
State and local	X	1.6	1.7	1.0	1.7	2.4	3.3	3.3
CHIP[2]	X	X	X	X	0.4	0.7	1.4	1.5
Federal	X	X	X	X	0.3	0.5	1.0	1.4
State and local	X	X	X	X	0.1	0.2	0.3	0.1
Other health insurance programs[3]	1.3	1.6	1.2	0.9	0.6	1.4	1.6	1.4
Other third-party payers and programs[4]	0.8	0.4	0.8	0.6	0.6	0.5	0.4	0.4

NOTE: Percentages may not add to totals because of rounding. Census resident population is used to calculate per capita. The Medicare and Medicaid programs began coverage in 1965. The Children's Health Insurance Program began coverage in 1997. For more information on national health expenditure sources and methods, see "National Health Expenditure Accounts: Methodology Paper, 2016." Available from: https://www.cms.gov/Research-Statistics-Data-and-Systems/Statistics-Trends-and-Reports/NationalHealthExpendData/Downloads/DSM-16.pdf.

X = Not applicable.
0.0 = Quantity more than zero but less than 0.05.
[2]Children's Health Insurance Program (CHIP). Medicaid CHIP expansions are included.
[3]Includes Department of Defense and Department of Veterans Affairs.
[4]Includes worksite health care, other private revenues, Indian Health Service, workers' compensation, general assistance, maternal and child health, vocational rehabilitation, other federal programs, Substance Abuse and Mental Health Services Administration, other state and local programs, and school health.
[7]Includes expenditures for care in freestanding facilities only. Additional services of this type are provided in hospital-based facilities and are considered hospital care.
[8]Includes expenditures for care in freestanding nursing homes. Expenditures for care in hospital-based nursing homes are included with hospital care.

Table 3-65. Personal Health Care Expenditures, by Source of Funds and Type of Expenditure, Selected Years, 1960–2016—Continued

(Number; percent; data are compiled from various sources by the Centers for Medicare & Medicaid Services.)

Type of personal health care expenditures and source of funds	1960	1970	1980	1990	2000	2009	2015	2016
Amount in Billions								
All other personal health care expenditures[9]	3.2	7.1	25.7	77.3	157.3	278.5	360.8	378.6
Percent Distribution								
All sources of funds	100.0	100.0	100.0	100.0	100.0	100.0	100.0	100.0
Out-of-pocket payments	84.6	74.2	56.9	49.7	37.6	31.6	30.2	30.2
Health insurance	4.1	9.1	25.7	33.7	45.0	52.2	54.9	55.0
Private health insurance	3.1	4.6	7.8	13.0	13.7	14.3	14.3	14.5
Medicare	X	1.0	2.8	5.5	8.1	10.3	10.1	9.8
Medicaid	X	3.0	14.8	15.0	22.8	27.0	29.7	29.9
Federal	X	1.6	8.1	8.5	13.0	18.0	17.4	17.5
State and local	X	1.4	6.7	6.4	9.8	9.0	12.4	12.4
CHIP[2]	X	X	X	X	0.2	0.4	0.5	0.5
Federal	X	X	X	X	0.1	0.3	0.4	0.5
State and local	X	X	X	X	0.1	0.1	0.1	0.0
Other health insurance programs[3]	1.1	0.5	0.3	0.2	0.2	0.2	0.3	0.3
Other third-party payers and programs[4]	11.2	16.7	17.4	16.6	17.4	16.2	14.9	14.8

NOTE: Percentages may not add to totals because of rounding. Census resident population is used to calculate per capita. The Medicare and Medicaid programs began coverage in 1965. The Children's Health Insurance Program began coverage in 1997. For more information on national health expenditure sources and methods, see "National Health Expenditure Accounts: Methodology Paper, 2016." Available from: https://www.cms.gov/Research-Statistics-Data-and-Systems/Statistics-Trends-and-Reports/NationalHealthExpendData/Downloads/DSM-16.pdf.
X = Not applicable.
0.0 = Quantity more than zero but less than 0.05.
[2]Children's Health Insurance Program (CHIP). Medicaid CHIP expansions are included.
[3]Includes Department of Defense and Department of Veterans Affairs.
[4]Includes worksite health care, other private revenues, Indian Health Service, workers' compensation, general assistance, maternal and child health, vocational rehabilitation, other federal programs, Substance Abuse and Mental Health Services Administration, other state and local programs, and school health.
[9]Includes expenditures for other professional services, other nondurable medical products, durable medical equipment, and other health, residential, and personal care, not shown separately.

Table 3-66. Cost of Hospital Discharges with Common Hospital Operating Room Procedures in Nonfederal Community Hospitals, by Age and Selected Principal Procedure, Selected Years, 2000–2014

(Dollars.)

Age and principal operating room procedure[1]	Mean inflation-adjusted cost per hospitalization: 2014 dollars[2]			Number of discharges with operating room principal procedure			Total inflation-adjusted national costs: 2014 dollars (in millions of dollars)[2]		
	2000	2010	2014	2000	2010	2014	2000	2010	2014
All Ages									
Hospital discharges with an operating room principal procedure[3]	$13,782	$19,186	$19,266	8,743,631	9,637,687	8,308,949	$119,757	$184,725	$159,951
Laminectomy (back surgery)	8,493	11,920	14,883	285,636	204,786	151,705	2,436	2,440	2,268
Heart valve procedures	44,609	56,426	51,896	79,719	98,101	110,915	3,550	5,541	5,756
Coronary artery bypass graft (CABG)	32,520	41,897	41,932	337,972	164,801	160,240	11,028	6,907	6,717
Percutaneous coronary angioplasty (PTCA) (balloon angioplasty of heart)	15,587	20,957	21,448	581,183	488,521	377,475	9,057	10,240	8,104
Insertion, revision, replacement, removal of cardiac pacemaker or cardioverter/defibrillator	28,757	38,023	34,974	66,286	122,847	78,970	1,921	4,667	2,762
Colorectal resection (removal of part of the bowel)	20,241	25,560	23,616	253,780	261,401	234,290	5,244	6,678	5,529
Appendectomy	7,616	9,934	10,657	269,089	273,753	177,550	2,027	2,719	1,897
Cholecystectomy (gall bladder removal)	10,811	13,767	13,327	389,079	379,753	300,245	4,170	5,232	4,006
Hysterectomy	6,790	9,617	10,394	580,019	354,313	184,950	3,910	3,411	1,923
Cesarean section	5,646	6,313	6,150	898,859	1,226,435	1,142,680	4,956	7,750	7,032
Treatment, fracture or dislocation of hip and femur	13,072	18,814	17,286	237,615	248,777	246,135	3,159	4,678	4,255
Arthroplasty knee (knee replacement)	14,357	17,592	16,292	318,854	693,086	723,086	4,551	12,198	11,783
Hip replacement	15,568	18,820	17,079	295,940	437,380	487,625	4,664	8,229	8,328
Spinal fusion	18,119	30,933	28,949	204,320	444,508	413,206	3,614	13,755	11,970
Under 18 Years									
Hospital discharges with an operating room principal procedure[3]	13,831	21,126	28,582	382,455	413,852	297,290	5,112	8,759	8,457
Incision and excision of CNS (a type of brain surgery)	30,026	44,269	47,633	6,352	8,925	7,870	184	396	372
Tonsillectomy and/or adenoidectomy	4,597	6,465	7,897	12,045	13,000	8,635	57	85	69
Small bowel resection (removal of part of the small bowel)	37,710	44,954	60,727	1,712	2,694	1,855	64	120	112
Appendectomy	6,833	9,206	10,336	75,481	79,575	46,745	502	733	483
Cesarean section	6,269	6,718	6,594	23,690	22,582	12,090	134	152	80
Spinal fusion	30,463	56,100	60,000	7,463	10,628	10,995	224	596	658
18 to 44 Years									
Hospital discharges with an operating room principal procedure[3]	9,107	12,588	12,289	2,806,078	2,842,807	2,339,211	25,005	35,784	28,735
Incision and excision of CNS (a type of brain surgery)	26,477	39,120	37,330	19,510	22,908	18,660	497	902	699
Laminectomy	7,643	11,222	14,038	95,687	44,303	27,800	736	498	392
Appendectomy	7,014	9,112	9,519	133,662	116,699	71,470	924	1,064	683
Cholecystectomy (gall bladder removal)	8,855	10,939	10,747	132,538	139,244	102,825	1,127	1,526	1,108
Oophorectomy (removal of one or both ovaries)	6,602	9,584	10,800	38,252	32,130	17,915	255	308	193
Ligation of fallopian tubes ("tying" of fallopian tubes)	4,882	5,546	7,516	75,221	44,524	31,045	346	247	230
Hysterectomy	6,296	8,729	9,481	291,704	149,442	72,870	1,811	1,306	691
Cesarean section	5,628	6,300	6,141	873,231	1,198,961	1,126,890	4,809	7,561	6,925
Treatment, fracture or dislocation of lower extremity (other than hip or femur)	9,702	15,136	17,248	68,015	59,800	45,040	648	904	776
Spinal fusion	17,033	29,044	27,341	73,228	89,655	64,600	1,206	2,605	1,768
45 to 64 Years									
Hospital discharges with an operating room principal procedure[3]	$15,076	$21,513	$21,420	2,435,212	3,085,028	2,636,652	$36,552	$66,262	$56,404
Laminectomy	8,567	12,311	15,482	107,720	80,487	59,585	924	990	927
Heart valve procedures	41,898	54,544	50,655	22,849	28,546	28,045	951	1,558	1,421
Coronary artery bypass graft (CABG)	30,385	40,362	39,934	139,897	73,265	67,165	4,271	2,958	2,682
Percutaneous coronary angioplasty (PTCA)	15,086	20,557	20,751	252,151	224,713	170,935	3,796	4,620	3,550
Insertion, revision, replacement, removal of cardiac pacemaker or cardioverter/defibrillator	35,219	40,063	37,584	15,957	36,456	23,770	558	1,460	893
Colorectal resection	18,207	23,500	22,622	76,604	99,837	90,725	1,422	2,349	2,050
Cholecystectomy	10,197	13,874	13,322	117,432	120,321	97,220	1,198	1,670	1,297
Oophorectomy	7,903	10,736	13,172	21,232	37,253	22,565	168	400	297
Hysterectomy	6,926	9,742	10,369	231,498	164,344	88,465	1,601	1,603	918
Arthroplasty knee (knee replacement)	14,687	17,632	16,404	95,902	291,502	303,150	1,402	5,141	4,973
Hip replacement	16,180	18,471	16,915	65,118	150,253	176,055	1,061	2,774	2,976
Spinal fusion	17,391	29,546	27,210	87,388	218,349	193,710	1,480	6,454	5,272
65 to 74 Years									
Hospital discharges with an operating room principal procedure[3]	16,890	22,719	22,079	1,511,467	1,648,763	1,623,736	25,661	37,391	35,822
Laminectomy	8,975	11,479	14,571	45,976	43,879	36,780	413	503	538
Heart valve procedures	45,656	56,733	50,565	23,236	26,078	29,145	1,052	1,481	1,473
Coronary artery bypass graft (CABG)	33,093	41,966	42,230	112,652	53,818	56,070	3,726	2,258	2,367
Percutaneous coronary angioplasty (PTCA)	15,519	21,035	21,929	166,497	125,005	99,675	2,579	2,629	2,189
Insertion, revision, replacement, removal of cardiac pacemaker or cardioverter/defibrillator	31,418	39,604	36,477	19,096	32,601	20,425	603	1,290	746
Endarterectomy (plaque removal from artery lining of brain, head, neck)	9,044	10,830	10,809	51,292	34,638	30,055	476	375	325
Colorectal resection	20,355	26,106	23,350	63,693	59,112	58,000	1,336	1,539	1,354
Cholecystectomy	11,945	15,967	15,122	65,953	52,412	48,435	801	836	733
Arthroplasty knee	14,623	17,438	16,075	110,961	232,195	264,425	1,607	4,053	4,253
Hip replacement	15,508	18,526	16,729	71,986	106,955	135,840	1,133	1,981	2,273
Spinal fusion	19,151	32,385	29,609	23,419	84,861	100,785	446	2,748	2,986
75 to 84 Years									
Hospital discharges with an operating room principal procedure[3]	17,144	22,844	22,152	1,224,573	1,189,769	1,010,816	21,299	27,126	22,392
Laminectomy	9,684	11,627	14,173	31,059	28,311	21,510	304	329	307
Heart valve procedures	47,093	58,243	52,058	21,004	26,690	30,675	1,001	1,555	1,597
Coronary artery bypass graft (CABG)	35,880	44,789	45,596	68,750	29,874	29,395	2,486	1,339	1,340
Percutaneous coronary angioplasty (PTCA)	16,431	21,714	22,467	111,169	87,441	63,865	1,838	1,899	1,437
Insertion, revision, replacement, removal of cardiac pacemaker or cardioverter/defibrillator	25,771	36,946	33,177	19,975	33,287	19,725	524	1,228	654

Note: Excludes newborn infants.

[1] Data are based on valid operating room procedures. Operating room procedures were identified using the Centers for Medicare & Medicaid Services' Diagnosis Related Groups (DRGs). For DRGs, physician panels identified International Classification of Diseases (ICD-9-CM) procedure codes, which would be performed in operating rooms in most hospitals. Operating room procedures, as defined by DRGs, are classified by the Clinical Classifications Software (CCS) into 1 of 231 clinically meaningful categories. Mean costs per hospitalization are based on the principal procedure as determined by the CCS. The number of discharges is based on the first-listed (principal) major procedure.

[2] Charges (the amount billed by the hospital) were converted to costs using cost-charge ratios from the Centers for Medicare & Medicaid Services. Costs are for the entire hospitalization including the principal procedure. Costs were adjusted to 2010 dollars for inflation using the gross domestic product deflator.

[3] Includes discharges for operating room principal procedures not shown separately.

Table 3-66. Cost of Hospital Discharges with Common Hospital Operating Room Procedures in Nonfederal Community Hospitals, by Age and Selected Principal Procedure, Selected Years, 2000–2014—Continued

(Dollars.)

Age and principal operating room procedure[1]	Mean inflation-adjusted cost per hospitalization: 2014 dollars[2]			Number of discharges with operating room principal procedure			Total inflation-adjusted national costs: 2014 dollars (in millions of dollars)[2]		
	2000	2010	2014	2000	2010	2014	2000	2010	2014
Endarterectomy (plaque removal from artery lining of brain, head, neck)	9,395	11,012	11,049	45,337	28,078	23,495	439	309	260
Colorectal resection	22,198	28,167	24,861	62,096	48,800	39,230	1,416	1,372	975
Cholecystectomy	13,689	18,110	16,705	52,448	42,922	33,660	733	777	563
Treatment, fracture or dislocation of hip and femur	12,310	17,392	16,203	73,332	66,038	63,765	930	1,150	1,034
Arthroplasty knee	14,615	17,530	16,188	79,138	133,319	123,855	1,158	2,338	2,006
Hip replacement	15,321	19,155	17,336	92,715	102,563	100,695	1,443	1,964	1,746
Spinal fusion	19,927	32,830	29,844	11,770	36,462	39,065	233	1,197	1,166
85 Years and Over									
Hospital discharges with an operating room principal procedure[3]	$15,718	$20,752	$20,304	382,341	445,658	399,570	$6,104	$9,247	$8,120
Heart valve procedures	49,507	52,561	50,551	2,985	5,639	13,005	147	297	658
Coronary artery bypass graft (CABG)	40,365	52,110	48,287	5,280	2,955	3,170	211	154	153
Percutaneous coronary angioplasty (PTCA)	18,647	22,360	22,746	16,682	23,538	20,930	308	527	476
Insertion, revision, replacement, removal of cardiac pacemaker or cardioverter/defibrillator	15,294	28,712	25,877	7,071	11,702	8,845	111	335	229
Colorectal resection	23,987	30,829	25,933	20,729	18,420	15,005	508	568	389
Cholecystectomy	16,660	19,751	18,071	15,698	16,524	13,485	265	326	243
Treatment, fracture or dislocation of hip and femur	11,986	16,550	15,737	76,900	76,798	77,365	949	1,273	1,219
Arthroplasty knee	14,819	18,543	17,068	10,122	18,713	17,250	151	347	294
Hip replacement	14,899	19,487	17,855	50,005	57,878	56,850	757	1,128	1,015
Amputation of lower extremity (amputation of leg, foot or toe)	13,752	18,157	18,145	12,855	8,243	8,315	179	150	151

Note: Excludes newborn infants.

[1]Data are based on valid operating room procedures. Operating room procedures were identified using the Centers for Medicare & Medicaid Services' Diagnosis Related Groups (DRGs). For DRGs, physician panels identified International Classification of Diseases (ICD-9-CM) procedure codes, which would be performed in operating rooms in most hospitals. Operating room procedures, as defined by DRGs, are classified by the Clinical Classifications Software (CCS) into 1 of 231 clinically meaningful categories. Mean costs per hospitalization are based on the principal procedure as determined by the CCS. The number of discharges is based on the first-listed (principal) major procedure.

[2]Charges (the amount billed by the hospital) were converted to costs using cost-charge ratios from the Centers for Medicare & Medicaid Services. Costs are for the entire hospitalization including the principal procedure. Costs were adjusted to 2010 dollars for inflation using the gross domestic product deflator.

[3]Includes discharges for operating room principal procedures not shown separately.

Table 3-67. Expenses[1] for Health Care and Prescribed Medicine, by Selected Population Characteristics, Selected Years, 1987–2014

(Number, percent, dollars; Data are based on household interviews of a sample of the civilian noninstitutionalized population and a sample of medical providers.)

Characteristic	Total expenses[1]											
	Population in millions[3]				Percent of persons with expense				Mean annual expense per person with expense (dollars)[3]			
	1997	2000	2005	2014	1987	2000	2005	2014	1987	2000	2005	2014
All Ages	271.3	278.4	296.2	318.4	84.5	83.5	84.7	85.1	3,245	3,712	4,948	5,531
Under 65 Years												
Total	237.1	243.6	258.7	270.5	83.2	81.8	82.9	83.1	2,522	2,924	3,927	4,430
Under 6 years	23.8	24.1	23.8	24.0	88.9	86.7	88.9	90.4	2,152	1,545	1,881	2,340
6 to 17 years	48.1	48.4	49.7	49.8	80.2	80.0	83.0	85.8	1,402	1,536	1,986	2,394
18 to 44 years	108.9	109.0	111.1	113.0	81.5	77.7	77.1	76.4	2,216	2,619	3,492	3,522
45 to 64 years	56.3	62.1	74.1	83.7	87.0	88.5	89.7	88.5	4,300	4,897	6,343	7,274
Sex												
Male	118.0	120.9	129.2	134.5	78.8	76.6	77.5	78.6	2,383	2,799	3,546	4,230
Female	119.1	122.7	129.6	136.0	87.5	87.0	88.4	87.6	2,643	3,033	4,259	4,607
Hispanic Origin and Race[5]												
Hispanic or Latino	29.4	32.0	41.1	52.1	71.0	69.0	69.3	73.4	2,018	1,992	2,667	2,846
Not Hispanic or Latino												
White	166.2	169.2	166.5	157.7	86.9	86.6	88.1	88.2	2,529	3,059	4,258	5,030
Black or African American	31.3	32.1	32.8	34.6	72.2	71.3	76.4	77.5	3,065	3,105	3,999	4,525
Asian	X	X	11.3	15.3	X	X	75.5	76.3	1,650	2,373	2,424	2,722
American Indian, Alaska Native, Native Hawaiian, Other Pacific Islander, and multiple race	X	X	7.0	10.8	X	X	82.0	83.7	1,707	3,058	3,619	3,830
Insurance Status[6]												
Any private insurance	174.0	181.6	180.1	179.2	86.5	85.9	87.9	87.6	2,418	2,786	3,955	4,423
Public insurance only	29.8	29.7	42.2	60.2	82.4	83.6	84.2	85.9	4,071	4,439	4,775	4,860
Uninsured all year	33.3	32.3	36.4	31.1	61.8	57.3	56.8	51.8	1,554	2,062	2,250	3,109
65 Years and Over												
Total	34.2	34.8	37.5	48.0	93.7	95.5	96.7	96.4	8,030	8,441	10,999	10,890
Sex												
Male	14.6	15.0	16.0	21.4	92.0	93.4	95.9	95.7	8,216	9,051	10,763	11,604
Female	19.6	19.8	21.5	26.6	94.9	97.1	97.2	96.9	7,902	7,997	11,172	10,323
Hispanic Origin and Race[5]												
Hispanic or Latino	1.7	1.9	2.4	3.8	82.5	92.5	92.0	92.2	7,638	7,575	9,522	9,100
Not Hispanic or Latino												
White	28.8	28.9	30.0	36.9	94.9	95.9	97.3	97.1	7,903	8,569	11,125	11,169
Black or African American	2.8	2.9	3.1	4.3	88.5	94.0	94.9	94.0	9,706	8,118	13,178	11,066
Asian	X	X	1.3	2.0	X	X	94.4	93.7	X	X	6,460	7,739
American Indian, Alaska Native, Native Hawaiian, Other Pacific Islander, and multiple race	X	X	*	*	X	X	*	*	X	X	*	*
Insurance Status[7]												
Medicare only	8.8	12.0	10.9	17.1	85.9	94.8	96.2	94.9	6,322	7,247	10,635	9,162
Medicare and private insurance	21.7	19.2	20.7	23.5	95.4	96.0	97.8	98.1	7,944	8,656	10,566	11,178
Medicare and other public coverage	3.2	3.2	5.5	6.5	94.4	96.3	95.5	95.8	12,351	11,583	13,513	14,918

NOTE: Estimates for 1987 are based on the National Medical Expenditure Survey (NMES); estimates for other years are based on the Medical Expenditure Panel Survey (MEPS). Because expenditures in NMES were based primarily on charges and those for MEPS were based on payments, NMES data were adjusted to be more comparable with MEPS by using estimated charge-to- payment ratios for 1987. Overall, this resulted in an approximate 11% reduction from the unadjusted 1987 NMES expenditure estimates. For a detailed explanation of this adjustment, see Zuvekas S, Cohen JW. A guide to comparing health care expenditures in the 1996 MEPS to the 1987 NMES. Inquiry 39(1):76–86; 2002.

X = Not applicable.

* = Estimates are considered unreliable. Data preceded by an asterisk have a relative standard error equal to or greater than 30%. Data not shown if based on fewer than 100 sample cases.

[1]Includes expenses for inpatient hospital and physician services, ambulatory physician and nonphysician services, prescribed medicines, home health services, dental services, and other medical equipment, supplies, and services that were purchased or rented during the year. Excludes expenses for over-the-counter medications, phone contacts with health providers, and premiums for health insurance.

[3]Includes persons in the civilian noninstitutionalized population for all or part of the year. Expenditures for persons in this population for only part of the year are restricted to those incurred during periods of eligibility (e.g., expenses incurred during periods of institutionalization and military service are not included in estimates).

[5]Persons of Hispanic origin may be of any race. Estimates for Asian persons as well as for American Indian, Alaska Native, Native Hawaiian, Other Pacifc Islander, and Multiple Race persons are not available for years prior to 2002 because Asian persons could not be distinguished separately and multiple race information was not collected.

[6]Any private insurance includes individuals with insurance that provided coverage for hospital and physician care at any time during the year, other than Medicare, Medicaid, or other public coverage for hospital or physician services. Public insurance only includes individuals who were not covered by private insurance at any time during the year but were covered by Medicare, Medicaid, other public coverage for hospital or physician services, and/or CHAMPUS/CHAMPVA (TRICARE) at any point during the year. Uninsured includes persons not covered by either private or public insurance throughout the entire year or period of eligibility for the survey. Individuals with Indian Health Service coverage only are considered uninsured.

[7]Populations do not add to total because uninsured persons and persons with unknown insurance status were excluded.

Table 3-67. Expenses[1] for Health Care and Prescribed Medicine, by Selected Population Characteristics, Selected Years, 1987–2014—*Continued*

(Number, percent, dollars; Data are based on household interviews of a sample of the civilian noninstitutionalized population and a sample of medical providers.)

Characteristic	Prescribed medicine expenses[2]							
	Percent of persons with expense				Mean annual expense per person with expense (dollars)[4]			
	1987	2000	2005	2014	1987	2000	2005	2014
All Ages	57.3	62.3	63.1	61.4	192	377	536	249
Under 65 Years								
Total	54.0	58.5	59.1	56.2	142	274	398	198
Under 6 years	61.8	56.9	54.5	47.8	50	51	73	27
6 to 17 years	44.3	46.2	47.1	42.6	95	96	120	63
18 to 44 years	51.3	56.0	54.9	51.5	110	208	279	158
45 to 64 years	65.3	73.3	74.8	72.9	269	516	723	316
Sex								
Male	46.5	51.3	52.0	50.3	131	240	368	212
Female	61.4	65.6	66.1	62.0	149	299	422	187
Hispanic Origin and Race[5]								
Hispanic or Latino	41.6	45.0	44.2	44.0	103	201	279	133
Not Hispanic or Latino								
White	57.7	63.8	65.5	63.1	148	294	434	236
Black or African American	44.1	47.6	51.1	51.1	126	225	334	133
Asian	X	X	42.0	39.4	X	X	225	103
American Indian, Alaska Native, Native Hawaiian, Other Pacific Islander, and multiple race	X	X	59.7	54.3	X	X	429	113
Insurance Status[6]								
Any private insurance	56.5	61.6	63.4	59.8	147	235	376	216
Public insurance only	56.5	62.4	59.4	57.5	98	392	385	95
Uninsured all year	35.1	37.6	37.3	32.6	155	453	613	359
65 Years and Over								
Total	81.6	88.3	91.1	90.5	441	857	1,153	429
Sex								
Male	78.0	83.9	89.8	90.0	411	643	899	437
Female	84.0	91.5	92.1	91.0	460	1,005	1,337	422
Hispanic Origin and Race[5]								
Hispanic or Latino	74.7	83.9	85.8	86.1	*585	721	982	244
Not Hispanic or Latino								
White	82.3	89.0	91.9	91.5	450	888	1,198	470
Black or African American	79.5	85.3	90.2	87.4	345	732	1,087	338
Asian	X	X	84.8	X	X	X	627	241
American Indian, Alaska Native, Native Hawaiian, Other Pacific Islander, and multiple race	X	X	*	*	X	X	*	*
Insurance Status[7]								
Medicare only	70.6	87.7	90.0	89.4	488	1,023	1,495	442
Medicare and private insurance	83.4	89.0	92.6	91.8	459	792	1,103	492
Medicare and other public coverage	88.2	88.5	90.3	91.8	166	678	692	182

NOTE: Estimates for 1987 are based on the National Medical Expenditure Survey (NMES); estimates for other years are based on the Medical Expenditure Panel Survey (MEPS). Because expenditures in NMES were based primarily on charges and those for MEPS were based on payments, NMES data were adjusted to be more comparable with MEPS by using estimated charge-to- payment ratios for 1987. Overall, this resulted in an approximate 11% reduction from the unadjusted 1987 NMES expenditure estimates. For a detailed explanation of this adjustment, see Zuvekas S, Cohen JW. A guide to comparing health care expenditures in the 1996 MEPS to the 1987 NMES. Inquiry 39(1):76–86; 2002.

X = Not applicable.

* = Estimates are considered unreliable. Data preceded by an asterisk have a relative standard error equal to or greater than 30%. Data not shown if based on fewer than 100 sample cases.

[1]Includes expenses for inpatient hospital and physician services, ambulatory physician and nonphysician services, prescribed medicines, home health services, dental services, and other medical equipment, supplies, and services that were purchased or rented during the year. Excludes expenses for over-the-counter medications, phone contacts with health providers, and premiums for health insurance.

[2]Includes expenses for all prescribed medications that were purchased or refilled during the survey year.

[3]Includes persons in the civilian noninstitutionalized population for all or part of the year. Expenditures for persons in this population for only part of the year are restricted to those incurred during periods of eligibility (e.g., expenses incurred during periods of institutionalization and military service are not included in estimates).

[4]Estimates of expenses were converted to 2014 dollars using the Consumer Price Index (all items).

[5]Persons of Hispanic origin may be of any race. Estimates for Asian persons as well as for American Indian, Alaska Native, Native Hawaiian, Other Pacifc Islander, and Multiple Race persons are not available for years prior to 2002 because Asian persons could not be distinguished separately and multiple race information was not collected.

[6]Any private insurance includes individuals with insurance that provided coverage for hospital and physician care at any time during the year, other than Medicare, Medicaid, or other public coverage for hospital or physician services. Public insurance only includes individuals who were not covered by private insurance at any time during the year but were covered by Medicare, Medicaid, other public coverage for hospital or physician services, and/or CHAMPUS/CHAMPVA (TRICARE) at any point during the year. Uninsured includes persons not covered by either private or public insurance throughout the entire year or period of eligibility for the survey. Individuals with Indian Health Service coverage only are considered uninsured.

[7]Populations do not add to total because uninsured persons and persons with unknown insurance status were excluded.

Table 3-68. Out-of-Pocket Health Care Expenses Among Persons with Medical Expenses, by Age, Selected Years 1987–2014

(Percent; data are based on household interviews of a sample of the civilian noninstitutionalized population and a sample of medical providers.)

Age and year	Percent of persons with expenses	Amount paid out of pocket among persons with expenses[1]						
		Total	$0	$1 to 99	$100 to 499	$500 to 999	$1,000 to 1,999	$2,000+
All Ages								
1987	84.5	100.0	10.4	18.3	35.9	15.7	10.9	8.8
1997	84.1	100.0	8.5	24.7	34.3	14.7	10.2	7.6
1998	83.8	100.0	7.7	25.0	35.0	14.5	10.2	7.6
1999	84.3	100.0	7.4	25.2	34.0	15.0	10.0	8.3
2000	83.5	100.0	6.9	25.0	33.4	15.3	10.4	8.9
2001	85.4	100.0	7.1	23.0	33.1	15.1	11.7	10.0
2002	85.2	100.0	7.8	22.1	31.6	15.5	12.3	10.8
2003	85.6	100.0	7.6	20.5	31.4	16.0	12.6	11.9
2004	84.7	100.0	8.8	20.6	30.5	15.1	12.6	12.4
2005	84.7	100.0	8.7	20.1	30.5	15.9	12.7	12.1
2006	84.6	100.0	8.7	20.0	30.7	15.9	12.9	11.7
2007	84.9	100.0	9.8	21.2	30.9	15.4	12.4	10.3
2008	84.4	100.0	9.9	21.8	30.9	15.3	11.9	10.2
2009	84.6	100.0	11.0	21.5	31.0	15.5	11.6	9.4
2010	84.6	100.0	12.6	22.1	30.4	14.4	11.2	9.3
2011	84.6	100.0	12.1	21.6	31.3	15.1	11.2	8.7
2012	84.7	100.0	12.2	23.2	31.1	14.0	10.8	8.8
2013	84.4	100.0	13.4	21.7	31.6	14.0	10.5	8.8
2014	85.1	100.0	15.0	22.6	30.2	13.6	10.2	8.4
Under 6 Years								
1987	88.9	100.0	19.2	26.1	39.5	10.0	3.1	2.1
1997	88.0	100.0	20.0	42.8	29.8	4.4	2.1	1.0
1998	87.6	100.0	17.4	46.0	30.1	4.4	1.6	0.3
1999	87.9	100.0	17.7	47.9	27.9	4.7	1.0	*0.8
2000	86.7	100.0	16.7	48.6	27.8	4.7	1.5	0.7
2001	88.8	100.0	18.5	46.6	29.3	3.8	1.3	*0.4
2002	88.8	100.0	21.5	40.4	30.4	5.6	1.4	0.8
2003	91.3	100.0	20.6	40.4	30.2	6.4	1.7	*0.6
2004	90.0	100.0	26.0	37.4	28.0	5.6	2.2	0.8
2005	88.9	100.0	27.2	35.3	27.7	6.8	2.1	0.9
2006	89.2	100.0	27.1	37.1	27.2	5.3	2.3	*1.0
2007	88.7	100.0	30.2	34.3	25.9	5.6	2.3	1.7
2008	88.8	100.0	31.4	35.2	26.1	3.8	2.5	*1.0
2009	88.7	100.0	34.2	32.6	25.0	5.4	1.9	1.0
2010	88.9	100.0	40.0	33.1	21.1	3.7	1.5	*0.7
2011	89.6	100.0	40.1	31.0	22.8	4.1	1.3	*0.7
2012	88.8	100.0	38.4	35.1	19.8	3.8	2.4	*0.5
2013	90.3	100.0	41.4	29.5	21.2	3.4	2.6	2.0
2014	90.4	100.0	46.3	27.2	20.4	3.3	1.9	*0.9
6 to 17 Years								
1987	80.2	100.0	15.5	25.6	37.4	9.7	6.2	5.6
1997	81.7	100.0	16.5	34.5	32.7	7.8	4.3	4.3
1998	80.6	100.0	16.3	34.2	33.0	9.1	4.1	3.3
1999	81.5	100.0	15.0	35.8	32.4	8.5	4.2	4.1
2000	80.0	100.0	14.7	35.0	33.4	7.7	4.3	4.9
2001	83.2	100.0	15.0	34.3	32.9	8.2	3.7	5.9
2002	83.6	100.0	16.6	34.0	32.0	8.8	3.9	4.7
2003	84.1	100.0	16.1	30.7	33.8	9.3	5.8	4.4
2004	83.9	100.0	18.7	32.3	29.9	8.9	5.2	5.0
2005	83.0	100.0	18.6	30.8	31.3	9.8	5.2	4.3
2006	83.6	100.0	19.2	31.1	30.1	9.1	4.6	6.0
2007	84.0	100.0	21.6	31.5	29.4	8.4	4.7	4.4
2008	82.5	100.0	22.4	31.7	28.2	8.4	4.2	5.2
2009	85.3	100.0	24.5	29.5	28.9	7.6	5.0	4.5
2010	84.4	100.0	28.4	29.4	26.5	7.4	3.8	4.5
2011	84.9	100.0	28.5	29.3	26.4	7.4	3.7	4.6
2012	85.7	100.0	29.0	28.1	26.8	6.3	3.8	6.0
2013	85.4	100.0	30.8	26.7	26.3	7.8	4.0	4.4
2014	85.8	100.0	34.3	27.5	22.2	6.9	4.4	4.8

NOTE: Includes persons in the civilian noninstitutionalized population for all or part of the year. Expenses for persons in this population for only part of the year are restricted to those incurred during periods of eligibility (e.g., expenses incurred during periods of institutionalization and military service are not included in estimates). Out-of-pocket expenses include expenditures for inpatient hospital and physician services, ambulatory physician and nonphysician services, prescribed medicines, home health services, dental services, and various other medical equipment, supplies, and services that were purchased or rented during the year. Out-of-pocket expenses for over-the-counter medications, phone contacts with health providers, and premiums for health insurance policies are not included in these estimates. Estimates for 1987 are based on the National Medical Expenditure Survey (NMES); estimates for other years are based on the Medical Expenditure Panel Survey (MEPS). Because expenditures in NMES were based primarily on charges and those for MEPS were based on payments, NMES data were adjusted to be more comparable with MEPS using estimated charge-to-payment ratios for 1987. Overall, this resulted in an approximate 11% reduction from the unadjusted 1987 NMES expenditure estimates. For a detailed explanation of this adjustment, see Zuvekas S, Cohen JW. A guide to comparing health care expenditures in the 1996 MEPS to the 1987 NMES. Inquiry 39(1):76–86; 2002.
*Estimates are considered unreliable. Data preceded by an asterisk have a relative standard error equal to or greater than 30 percent.
[1]Estimates of expenses were converted to 2014 dollars using the Consumer Price Index (all items).

Table 3-68. Out-of-Pocket Health Care Expenses Among Persons with Medical Expenses, by Age, Selected Years 1987–2014—Continued

(Percent; data are based on household interviews of a sample of the civilian noninstitutionalized population and a sample of medical providers.)

Age and year	Percent of persons with expenses	Amount paid out of pocket among persons with expenses[1]						
		Total	$0	$1 to 99	$100 to 499	$500 to 999	$1,000 to 1,999	$2,000+
18 to 44 Years								
1987	81.5	100.0	10.1	20.1	38.8	15.6	9.3	6.2
1997	78.3	100.0	7.3	26.7	38.8	14.8	7.9	4.5
1998	78.0	100.0	6.4	27.2	39.8	14.0	7.8	4.8
1999	78.9	100.0	6.4	27.6	39.1	14.1	7.6	5.1
2000	77.7	100.0	5.8	27.6	38.5	15.4	7.7	5.0
2001	79.3	100.0	6.0	24.6	39.1	15.6	9.6	5.1
2002	78.5	100.0	6.7	24.9	37.4	15.5	9.5	6.0
2003	79.0	100.0	6.4	23.0	38.0	16.0	10.0	6.6
2004	77.0	100.0	7.2	23.2	36.9	15.5	10.3	7.0
2005	77.1	100.0	7.0	23.5	36.8	15.6	9.7	7.3
2006	76.9	100.0	6.8	22.7	37.4	16.1	9.6	7.6
2007	77.3	100.0	7.7	25.3	36.5	14.5	9.8	6.2
2008	76.5	100.0	7.9	25.6	35.7	14.7	9.1	6.9
2009	76.2	100.0	8.5	25.0	35.7	15.1	9.5	6.3
2010	76.0	100.0	9.5	27.2	35.5	13.8	8.1	5.8
2011	75.6	100.0	8.7	26.0	37.2	13.7	8.3	6.1
2012	75.5	100.0	9.6	28.4	34.8	12.6	8.5	6.1
2013	75.4	100.0	10.6	26.9	36.9	11.9	8.2	5.5
2014	76.4	100.0	12.4	28.2	35.5	11.3	7.5	5.1
45 to 64 Years								
1987	87.0	100.0	5.6	11.5	34.1	20.6	16.1	12.1
1997	89.2	100.0	3.4	15.6	34.2	20.0	16.1	10.7
1998	89.2	100.0	2.9	16.2	34.6	19.7	15.4	11.2
1999	88.9	100.0	2.7	15.0	34.9	20.5	15.5	11.4
2000	88.5	100.0	2.6	14.7	33.2	21.0	16.1	12.4
2001	89.9	100.0	2.4	13.3	31.8	20.1	18.3	14.2
2002	90.0	100.0	2.3	13.1	29.4	21.3	18.8	15.2
2003	89.6	100.0	2.4	11.9	28.2	21.2	18.6	17.7
2004	88.9	100.0	2.7	12.0	29.0	20.9	18.2	17.3
2005	89.7	100.0	2.4	12.0	28.2	20.9	19.6	16.9
2006	89.2	100.0	2.7	11.9	28.8	20.7	18.8	17.0
2007	89.2	100.0	2.9	13.3	28.8	21.3	17.8	15.9
2008	89.1	100.0	2.8	14.3	31.2	20.4	17.3	14.0
2009	88.4	100.0	3.4	15.3	31.5	19.5	16.4	13.8
2010	89.2	100.0	4.0	15.6	31.4	19.0	16.2	13.8
2011	88.8	100.0	3.7	15.9	31.7	19.4	16.6	12.7
2012	88.9	100.0	3.8	17.6	32.8	18.0	15.6	12.1
2013	88.0	100.0	4.4	17.3	32.2	18.1	15.1	13.0
2014	88.5	100.0	5.3	18.5	32.4	18.9	14.1	10.9
65 to 74 Years								
1987	92.8	100.0	5.3	8.7	26.0	21.3	20.4	18.3
1997	94.6	100.0	3.2	10.2	29.5	22.8	17.7	16.5
1998	94.3	100.0	2.0	9.2	30.9	21.7	19.7	16.5
1999	95.3	100.0	1.4	9.0	26.4	22.5	20.5	20.2
2000	94.7	100.0	1.5	9.3	25.0	21.7	21.2	21.5
2001	95.6	100.0	1.5	8.8	25.3	21.4	21.0	22.0
2002	96.1	100.0	1.8	5.9	23.1	20.5	24.5	24.1
2003	95.3	100.0	1.7	6.1	19.6	22.2	22.9	27.6
2004	96.6	100.0	1.5	7.3	22.3	17.6	21.1	30.3
2005	95.9	100.0	1.7	6.0	22.5	20.5	22.6	26.7
2006	95.7	100.0	1.7	6.9	21.9	20.3	26.1	23.0
2007	95.8	100.0	2.7	7.5	27.6	21.5	22.0	18.7
2008	95.8	100.0	1.5	9.1	26.7	21.2	21.9	19.7
2009	95.7	100.0	2.0	10.7	27.3	24.0	20.2	15.8
2010	95.8	100.0	2.4	8.8	27.2	22.4	21.9	17.4
2011	96.2	100.0	2.6	9.4	28.8	24.4	20.0	14.7
2012	95.5	100.0	1.9	12.0	31.3	21.8	17.8	15.1
2013	94.9	100.0	2.8	11.3	30.8	22.2	18.6	14.4
2014	95.7	100.0	3.2	13.9	28.8	20.2	17.6	16.4

NOTE: Includes persons in the civilian noninstitutionalized population for all or part of the year. Expenses for persons in this population for only part of the year are restricted to those incurred during periods of eligibility (e.g., expenses incurred during periods of institutionalization and military service are not included in estimates). Out-of-pocket expenses include expenditures for inpatient hospital and physician services, ambulatory physician and nonphysician services, prescribed medicines, home health services, dental services, and various other medical equipment, supplies, and services that were purchased or rented during the year. Out-of-pocket expenses for over-the-counter medications, phone contacts with health providers, and premiums for health insurance policies are not included in these estimates. Estimates for 1987 are based on the National Medical Expenditure Survey (NMES); estimates for other years are based on the Medical Expenditure Panel Survey (MEPS). Because expenditures in NMES were based primarily on charges and those for MEPS were based on payments, NMES data were adjusted to be more comparable with MEPS using estimated charge-to-payment ratios for 1987. Overall, this resulted in an approximate 11% reduction from the unadjusted 1987 NMES expenditure estimates. For a detailed explanation of this adjustment, see Zuvekas S, Cohen JW. A guide to comparing health care expenditures in the 1996 MEPS to the 1987 NMES. Inquiry 39(1):76–86; 2002.
[1]Estimates of expenses were converted to 2014 dollars using the Consumer Price Index (all items).

Table 3-68. Out-of-Pocket Health Care Expenses Among Persons with Medical Expenses, by Age, Selected Years 1987–2014—*Continued*

(Percent; data are based on household interviews of a sample of the civilian noninstitutionalized population and a sample of medical providers.)

Age and year	Percent of persons with expenses	Amount paid out of pocket among persons with expenses[1]						
		Total	$0	$1 to 99	$100 to 499	$500 to 999	$1,000 to 1,999	$2,000+
75 Years and Over								
1987	95.1	100.0	5.6	7.1	23.1	18.7	20.1	25.4
1997	95.8	100.0	2.4	9.0	25.7	19.6	21.7	21.7
1998	96.3	100.0	3.0	8.9	25.5	18.7	22.5	21.3
1999	95.3	100.0	2.6	8.0	23.7	22.6	19.9	23.1
2000	96.5	100.0	2.6	8.7	23.7	21.0	19.9	24.1
2001	97.0	100.0	1.7	6.3	20.2	19.1	22.4	30.2
2002	96.5	100.0	2.2	5.7	18.3	18.1	23.9	31.8
2003	97.5	100.0	1.9	5.5	17.8	18.2	22.7	33.9
2004	97.7	100.0	1.8	5.7	17.7	15.9	24.6	34.3
2005	97.4	100.0	1.6	5.9	19.5	19.2	20.2	33.6
2006	97.6	100.0	1.7	5.7	21.2	20.8	25.2	25.4
2007	97.3	100.0	1.9	7.9	24.7	18.6	23.3	23.6
2008	97.6	100.0	1.9	9.4	23.7	21.3	21.9	21.9
2009	97.5	100.0	2.7	9.4	24.0	22.4	20.7	20.7
2010	97.0	100.0	3.0	9.3	26.6	19.2	22.1	19.8
2011	96.7	100.0	2.4	10.7	28.0	22.6	20.3	16.1
2012	97.4	100.0	2.3	11.5	29.7	22.7	18.6	15.3
2013	96.5	100.0	3.4	10.1	31.1	22.6	15.8	17.1
2014	97.2	100.0	2.6	9.6	29.6	20.5	19.0	18.6

NOTE: Includes persons in the civilian noninstitutionalized population for all or part of the year. Expenses for persons in this population for only part of the year are restricted to those incurred during periods of eligibility (e.g., expenses incurred during periods of institutionalization and military service are not included in estimates). Out-of-pocket expenses include expenditures for inpatient hospital and physician services, ambulatory physician and nonphysician services, prescribed medicines, home health services, dental services, and various other medical equipment, supplies, and services that were purchased or rented during the year. Out-of-pocket expenses for over-the-counter medications, phone contacts with health providers, and premiums for health insurance policies are not included in these estimates. Estimates for 1987 are based on the National Medical Expenditure Survey (NMES); estimates for other years are based on the Medical Expenditure Panel Survey (MEPS). Because expenditures in NMES were based primarily on charges and those for MEPS were based on payments, NMES data were adjusted to be more comparable with MEPS using estimated charge-to-payment ratios for 1987. Overall, this resulted in an approximate 11% reduction from the unadjusted 1987 NMES expenditure estimates. For a detailed explanation of this adjustment, see Zuvekas S, Cohen JW. A guide to comparing health care expenditures in the 1996 MEPS to the 1987 NMES. Inquiry 39(1):76–86; 2002.
[1]Estimates of expenses were converted to 2014 dollars using the Consumer Price Index (all items).

Table 3-69. Expenditures for Health Services and Supplies and Percent Distribution, by Sponsor, Selected Years, 1987–2013

(Dollars, percent.)

Type of sponsor	1987	1990	1995	2000	2009	2010	2012	2013
NATIONAL HEALTH EXPENDITURES (AMOUNT IN BILLIONS)	$519.1	$724.3	$1,027.4	$1,378.0	$2,505.8	$2,604.1	$2,817.3	$2,919.1
Business, Households, and Other Private Revenues	354.0	488.2	642.3	888.4	1,415.2			
Private business	122.3	178.3	243.7	346.5	530.3	533.7	587.3	610.9
Employer contribution to private health insurance premiums[1]	84.3	129.5	176.3	255.1	411.8	413.5	453.9	471.1
Employer contribution to Medicare hospital insurance trust fund[2]	24.6	29.4	43.1	62.3	77.9	79.7	88.0	91.7
Workers compensation and temporary disability insurance and worksite health care	13.4	19.3	24.3	29.1	40.6	40.5	45.4	48.2
Household	189.9	253.0	318.9	434.0	717.3	738.3	801.5	823.8
Employee contribution to private health insurance premiums and individual policy premiums[3]	44.0	68.5	100.3	133.6	260.7	270.8	293.8	300.2
Employee and self-employment contributions and voluntary premiums paid to Medicare hospital insurance trust fund[4]	29.5	35.7	56.0	82.6	108.4	112.1	125.5	124.8
Premiums paid by individuals to Medicare supplementary medical insurance trust fund[5]	6.2	10.2	16.4	16.3	47.2	49.2	53.4	59.4
Out-of-pocket health spending	110.2	138.6	146.2	201.5	300.9	306.2	328.8	339.4
Other private revenues	41.9	56.9	79.7	107.9	167.6	174.6	203.9	218.1
Governments	165.1	236.1	385.2	489.6	1,090.6	1,157.5	1,224.6	1,266.3
Federal government	86.2	125.3	217.3	261.9	682.8	733.1	731.5	757.5
Employer contributions to private health insurance premiums	4.9	9.9	11.4	14.3	26.8	28.5	31.0	32.4
Employer contributions to Medicare hospital insurance trust fund	1.7	2.0	2.3	2.7	3.9	4.1	4.1	4.0
Adjusted Medicare[6]	17.4	27.7	57.6	49.2	236.0	250.2	266.2	274.0
Health program expenditures (excluding Medicare)	62.2	85.8	146.0	195.8	416.1	450.3	430.2	447.1
Medicaid[7]	28.2	43.3	87.9	119.4	255.5	275.9	251.5	267.1
Other programs[8]	34.0	42.5	58.1	76.4	160.6	174.5	178.8	180.0
State and local government	78.9	110.8	167.9	227.7	407.9	424.5	493.1	508.8
Employer contributions to private health insurance premiums[9]	16.0	26.4	38.9	56.9	127.8	142.9	153.5	156.0
Employer contributions to Medicare hospital insurance trust fund	3.1	4.1	5.6	7.5	11.3	11.2	11.3	11.4
Health expenditures by program	59.8	80.3	123.3	163.4	268.8	270.4	328.3	341.5
Medicaid[7]	22.7	31.5	60.3	85.3	130.8	135.0	185.5	196.3
Other programs[10]	37.1	48.8	63.1	78.0	138.0	135.3	142.8	145.2
PERCENT DISTRIBUTION								
NATIONAL HEALTH EXPENDITURES	100.0	100.0	100.0	100.0	100.0	100.0	100.0	100.0
Business, Households, and Other Private Revenues	68.2	67.4	62.5	64.5	56.5	55.6	56.5	56.6
Private business	23.6	24.6	23.7	25.1	21.2	20.5	20.8	20.9
Employer contribution to private health insurance premiums[1]	16.2	17.9	17.2	18.5	16.4	15.9	16.1	16.1
Employer contribution to Medicare hospital insurance trust fund[2]	4.7	4.1	4.2	4.5	3.1	3.1	3.1	3.1
Workers compensation and temporary disability insurance and worksite health care	2.6	2.7	2.4	2.1	1.6	1.6	1.6	1.7
Household	36.6	34.9	31.0	31.5	28.6	28.4	28.4	28.2
Employee contribution to private health insurance premiums and individual policy premiums[3]	8.5	9.5	9.8	9.7	10.4	10.4	10.4	10.3
Employee and self-employment contributions and voluntary premiums paid to Medicare hospital insurance trust fund[4]	5.7	4.9	5.5	6.0	4.3	4.3	4.5	4.3
Premiums paid by individuals to Medicare supplementary medical insurance trust fund[5]	1.2	1.4	1.6	1.2	1.9	1.9	1.9	2.0
Out-of-pocket health spending	21.2	19.1	14.2	14.6	12.0	11.8	11.7	11.6
Other private revenues	8.1	7.9	7.8	7.8	6.7	6.7	7.2	7.5
Governments	31.8	32.6	37.5	35.5	43.5	44.4	43.5	43.4
Federal government	16.6	17.3	21.2	19.0	27.2	28.2	26.0	25.9
Employer contributions to private health insurance premiums	0.9	1.4	1.1	1.0	1.1	1.1	1.1	1.1
Employer contributions to Medicare hospital insurance trust fund	0.3	0.3	0.2	0.2	0.2	0.2	0.1	0.1
Adjusted Medicare[6]	3.4	3.8	5.6	3.6	9.4	9.6	9.4	9.4
Health program expenditures (excluding Medicare)	12.0	11.8	14.2	14.2	16.6	17.3	15.3	15.3
Medicaid[7]	5.4	6.0	8.6	8.7	10.2	10.6	8.9	9.2
Other programs[8]	6.5	5.9	5.7	5.5	6.4	6.7	6.3	6.2
State and local government	15.2	15.3	16.3	16.5	16.3	16.3	17.5	17.4
Employer contributions to private health insurance premiums[9]	3.1	3.6	3.8	4.1	5.1	5.5	5.4	5.3
Employer contributions to Medicare hospital insurance trust fund	0.6	0.6	0.5	0.5	0.5	0.4	0.4	0.4
Health expenditures by program								
Medicaid[7]	4.4	4.3	5.9	6.2	5.2	5.2	6.6	6.7
Other programs[10]	7.1	6.7	6.1	5.7	5.5	5.2	5.1	5.0

[1]Excludes Medicare Retiree Drug Subsidy (RDS) payments to private plans beginning in 2006, small-business tax credits beginning in 2010 and Early Retirement Reinsurance Program (ERRP) payments for 2010–2011.
[2]Includes one-half of self-employment contribution to the Medicare Hospital Insurance (HI) Trust Fund.
[3]Excludes government-subsidized Consolidated Omnibus Budget Reconciliation Act (COBRA) payments in 2009–2011.
[4]Includes one-half of self-employment contribution to Medicare HI Trust Fund and trust fund revenues from the income taxation of Social Security benefits.
[5]Includes premiums paid for the Pre-Existing Condition Insurance Plan (PCIP) beginning in 2010.
[6]Federal government Medicare expenditures equal Trust Fund interest income and Federal general revenue contributions to Medicare less the net change in Trust Fund balances. Includes Medicare RDS paid to private and state and local government employer plans beginning in 2006. Excludes Part D state phase-down payments to Medicare beginning in 2006 and Medicare premium buy-in programs by Medicaid for people eligible for both Medicaid and Medicare (dual eligibles).
[7]Includes Medicare Premium buy-in programs by Medicaid for people eligible for both Medicaid and Medicare (dual eligibles).
[8]Includes maternal and child health, vocational rehabilitation, Substance Abuse and Mental Health Services Administration, Indian Health Service, federal workers' compensation, and other federal programs, public health activities, Department of Defense, Department of Veterans Affairs, Children's Health Insurance Program (CHIP), and investment (research, structures and equipment). Also includes government-subsidized COBRA payments in 2009–2011, small business tax credits beginning in 2006, and ERRP payments in 2010–2011. Excludes premiums paid for the Pre-Existing Condition Insurance Plan (PCIP) premiums beginning in 2010.
[9]Excludes Medicare RDS payments to state and local government employer plans beginning in 2006 and ERRP payments in 2010–2011.
[10]Includes maternal and child health, vocational rehabilitation, general assistance, school health, CHIP, public health activities, other state and local programs, investment (research, structures and equipment). Also includes Part D state phase-down payments to Medicare beginning in 2006.

Table 3-70. Department of Veterans Affairs Health Care Expenditures and Use, and Persons Treated, by Selected Characteristics, Selected Fiscal Years, 2005–2016

(Dollars; numbers in thousands; percent; data are compiled from patient records, enrollment information, and budgetary data by the Department of Veterans Affairs.)

Type of expenditure and use	2005	2006	2007	2008	2009	2010	2011	2012	2013	2014	2015	2016
All Expenditures (Amount in Millions)[1]	30,291	31,909	34,025	38,282	42,955	47,280	50,575	51,880	54,738	58,010	64,688	69,622
Percent Distribution												
All services	100.0	100.0	100.0	100.0	100.0	100.0	100.0	100.0	100.0	100.0	100.0	100.0
Inpatient hospital	24.3	24.0	24.0	23.5	22.7	21.4	20.6	20.1	19.8	19.8	18.4	18.1
Outpatient care	53.4	55.2	53.5	53.2	53.5	52.5	52.6	53.8	53.2	55.5	59.6	60.2
Nursing home care	8.4	8.2	8.3	8.1	7.8	7.4	7.2	7.3	7.0	7.0	6.4	6.5
All other[2]	13.9	12.6	14.2	15.2	16.0	18.8	19.6	18.8	20.0	17.7	15.6	15.3
Health Care Use												
Inpatient hospital discharges[3]	614	601	607	622	640	656	653	646	632	619	592	581
Outpatient visits[4]	57,169	59,132	62,234	66,484	73,969	79,457	83,146	87,370	90,226	93,852	101,791	104,930
Nursing home discharges[5]	61	59	63	64	65	67	63	67	69	68	68	67
Inpatients[6]	488	467	477	492	512	532	540	546	545	558	566	574
Percent Distribution												
Total	100.0	100.0	100.0	100.0	100.0	100.0	100.0	100.0	100.0	100.0	100.0	100.0
Veterans with service-connected disability	37.6	38.8	39.9	41.1	42.6	43.5	44.9	46.5	48.3	50.0	52.0	53.5
Veterans without service-connected disability	61.5	60.2	59.1	58.0	56.4	55.6	54.3	52.6	50.8	49.1	47.2	45.7
Low income	39.9	37.9	36.9	35.4	34.8	34.6	33.4	32.1	30.4	28.8	28.2	27.1
Veterans receiving aid and attendance or housebound benefits or who are catastrophically disabled	12.1	11.6	11.3	11.1	10.5	10.1	9.8	9.6	9.4	9.0	8.3	8.0
Veterans receiving medical care subject to copayments[7]	8.6	9.7	9.8	10.0	9.5	9.3	9.3	9.2	9.3	9.6	9.1	9.1
Other and unknown[8]	1.0	1.0	1.0	1.6	1.6	1.6	1.7	1.7	1.7	1.6	1.5	1.5
Nonveterans	0.9	0.9	0.9	0.9	1.0	0.9	0.9	0.9	0.9	0.9	0.9	0.9
Outpatients[6]	5,077	5,180	5,221	5,291	5,439	5,631	5,789	5,903	6,009	6,176	6,296	6,383
Percent Distribution												
Total	100.0	100.0	100.0	100.0	100.0	100.0	100.0	100.0	100.0	100.0	100.0	100.0
Veterans with service-connected disability	31.6	32.4	33.8	34.7	37.1	38.6	39.8	41.7	44.0	45.8	47.6	49.3
Veterans without service-connected disability	62.7	62.0	60.8	59.7	57.2	56.4	55.1	53.3	51.1	49.0	46.9	45.0
Low income	31.8	30.3	28.9	27.2	25.9	25.7	24.9	24.0	22.6	21.3	21.0	19.9
Veterans receiving aid and attendance or housebound benefits or who are catastrophically disabled	3.5	3.4	3.5	3.5	3.4	3.4	3.3	3.2	3.2	3.1	2.9	2.9
Veterans receiving medical care subject to copayments[7]	25.4	25.7	25.5	25.2	23.8	23.0	22.3	21.4	20.7	20.1	18.8	18.2
Other and unknown[8]	2.0	2.6	3.0	3.8	4.0	4.3	4.6	4.6	4.6	4.5	4.2	4.1
Nonveterans	5.7	5.6	5.4	5.7	5.7	5.1	5.1	5.1	5.1	4.9	5.3	5.6

NOTE: Some veterans have multiple sources of health coverage, including Medicare or private insurance. Estimates in this table relate only to health care use paid for by the Veteran's Administration. At the end of FY2016, the veteran population was estimated at 20.4 million, with 47% aged 65 and over. Of all living veterans, 4% had served during World War II, 8% during the Korean conflict, 34% during the Vietnam era, 35% during the Persian Gulf War (service from August 2, 1990 to present), and 23% during peacetime. Percentages sum to more than 100% because some veterans served during more than one war.

[1]Health care expenditures exclude construction, medical administration, and miscellaneous operating expenses at Department of Veterans Affairs headquarters.

[2]Includes miscellaneous benefits and services, contract hospitals, education and training, subsidies to state veterans hospitals, nursing homes and residential rehabilitation treatment programs (formerly domiciliaries), and the Civilian Health and Medical Program of the Department of Veterans Affairs.

[3]Includes discharges from medicine, surgery, psychiatry, rehabilitation medicine, spinal cord, and neurology units, and residential rehabilitation treatment programs (formerly domiciliary care). Does not include long-term stays.

[4]Includes hospital outpatient care from the following services: physicians, laboratory, home-based primary care, and outpatient fee-basis care.

[5]Includes discharges of VA-covered state nursing home veteran patients.

[6]Includes veterans receiving services. Veterans with multiple discharges or visits are only counted once in the inpatient or outpatient category. The inpatient and outpatient totals are not additive because most inpatients are also treated as outpatients.

[7]Includes veterans who receive medical care subject to copayments according to income level, based on financial means testing.

[8]Includes expenditures for services for veterans who were prisoners of war, exposed to Agent Orange, and other. Veterans reporting Agent Orange exposure but not treated for it were means tested and placed in the low income or other group depending on income.

HEALTH INSURANCE

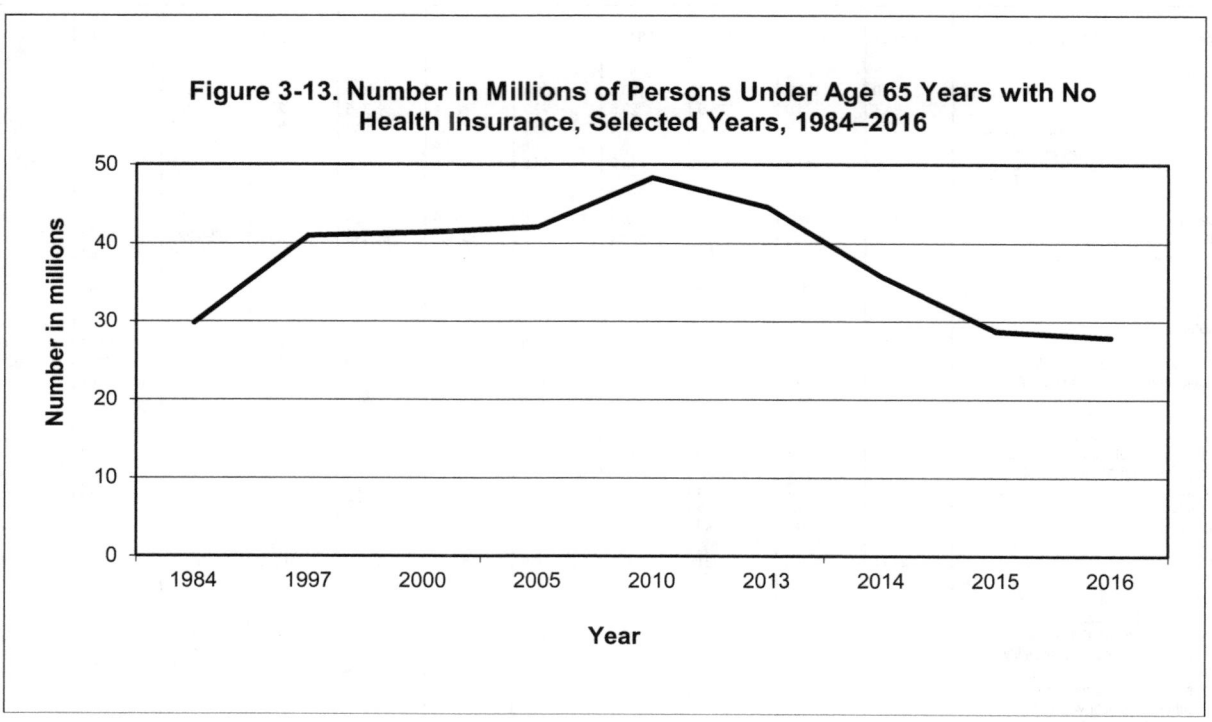

Figure 3-13. Number in Millions of Persons Under Age 65 Years with No Health Insurance, Selected Years, 1984–2016

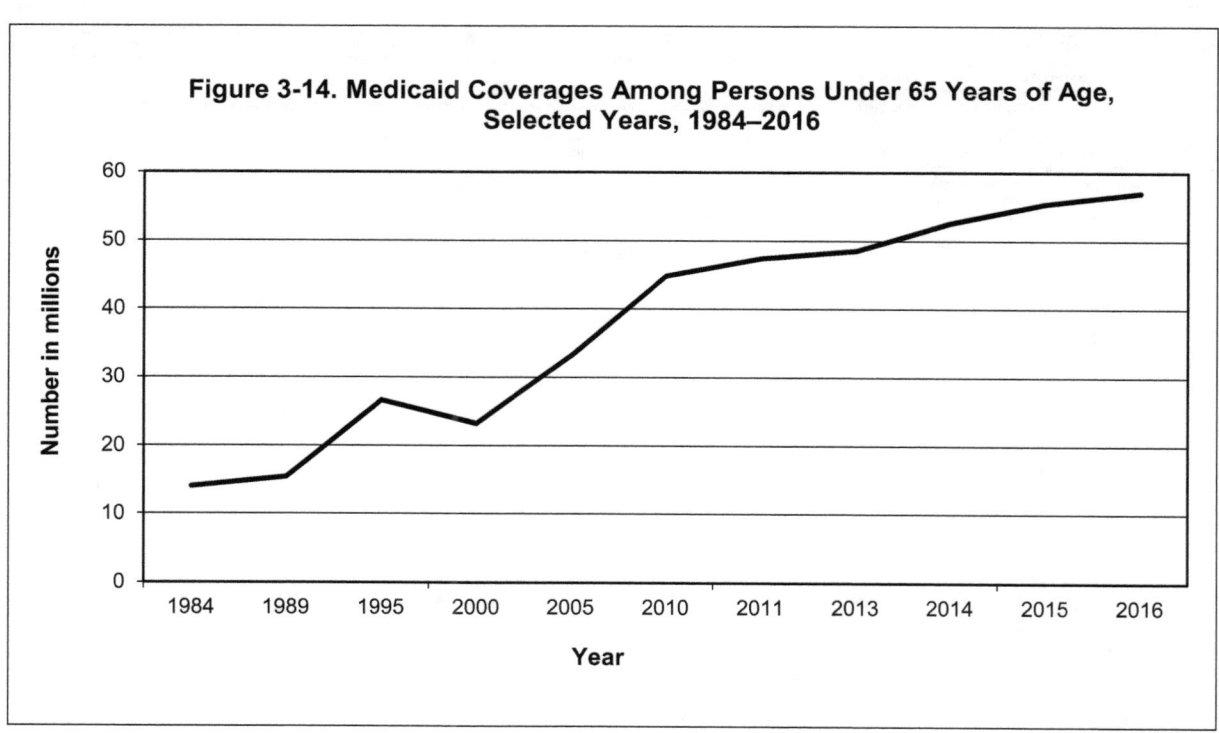

Figure 3-14. Medicaid Coverages Among Persons Under 65 Years of Age, Selected Years, 1984–2016

Table 3-71. Private Health Insurance[1] Coverage Among Persons Under 65 Years of Age, by Selected Characteristics, Selected Years, 1984–2016

(Numbers in millions; percent; data are based on household interviews of a sample of the civilian noninstitutionalized population.)

Characteristic	1984[2]	1989[2]	1995[2]	2000[3]	2005	2006	2007	2008	2009	2010	2011	2012	2013	2014	2015	2016
Total (number in millions)[4]..........	157.5	162.7	164.2	174.0	174.7	171.2	174.1	171.9	166.7	163.9	164.5	164.9	165.3	170.7	176.6	177.7
Total (percent of population)[4].......	76.8	75.9	71.3	71.5	68.2	66.3	66.8	65.6	63.3	61.7	61.8	61.8	61.8	63.7	65.5	65.7
Age																
Under 19 years...............................	72.6	71.9	65.4	66.7	62.3	59.5	59.9	58.6	56.1	54.3	53.9	53.6	53.5	54.1	55.0	54.8
Under 6 years............................	68.1	67.9	59.5	62.7	56.6	54.7	54.1	53.2	50.1	48.3	47.8	48.4	47.3	50.2	51.0	51.0
6 to 18 years.............................	74.8	73.9	68.3	68.5	64.9	61.7	62.6	61.1	59.0	57.2	56.9	56.0	56.3	55.9	56.7	56.5
Under 18 years............................	72.6	71.8	65.2	66.6	62.1	59.4	59.8	58.4	55.8	54.1	53.7	53.4	53.2	53.7	54.6	54.3
6 to 17 years............................	74.9	74.0	68.3	68.5	64.7	61.7	62.6	61.1	58.8	57.2	56.7	55.8	56.0	55.4	56.2	55.9
18 to 64 years................................	78.6	77.6	73.9	73.5	70.7	69.1	69.5	68.5	66.2	64.7	65.0	65.1	65.1	67.4	69.7	69.9
18 to 44 years............................	76.5	75.5	70.9	70.5	66.6	65.0	65.5	64.4	61.7	60.0	60.9	61.4	61.8	64.3	66.8	67.2
18 to 24 years.......................	67.4	64.5	60.8	60.3	58.0	57.0	59.0	56.2	54.4	52.3	57.2	58.1	59.0	62.0	64.8	65.7
19 to 25 years.......................	67.4	63.8	60.1	59.1	56.3	56.1	57.9	55.8	53.0	51.8	56.9	58.1	58.9	62.2	65.5	66.2
25 to 34 years.......................	77.4	75.9	70.1	70.1	65.1	63.0	63.5	62.7	60.0	58.7	58.6	58.7	59.0	62.0	65.1	65.4
35 to 44 years.......................	83.9	82.7	77.7	77.0	73.7	72.0	71.7	71.7	68.4	66.9	66.0	66.7	67.0	68.6	70.0	70.3
45 to 64 years............................	83.3	82.5	80.1	78.7	76.9	75.2	75.5	74.3	72.6	71.3	70.6	70.0	69.5	71.7	73.6	73.6
45 to 54 years.......................	83.3	83.4	80.9	80.0	77.4	75.1	75.4	74.8	72.6	70.9	70.1	69.6	69.8	71.6	74.1	73.3
55 to 64 years.......................	83.3	81.6	79.0	76.7	76.2	75.4	75.5	73.6	72.6	71.8	71.2	70.4	69.1	71.7	73.1	73.8
Sex																
Male...	77.3	76.1	71.6	71.6	68.0	65.9	66.4	65.3	62.9	61.1	61.4	61.8	61.9	63.8	65.4	66.0
Female..	76.2	75.7	70.9	71.3	68.4	66.7	67.1	65.9	63.7	62.4	62.2	61.9	61.7	63.5	65.6	65.4
Sex and Marital Status[5]																
Male																
Married....................................	85.0	84.2	80.2	81.5	79.6	78.1	78.1	77.7	75.8	75.1	74.5	74.9	74.8	77.1	78.3	78.5
Divorced, separated, widowed	65.5	64.6	62.4	62.2	56.7	55.4	55.8	56.0	52.9	50.6	50.5	51.0	50.9	54.0	56.6	56.9
Never married	71.3	68.3	65.4	63.8	60.2	57.8	59.8	57.9	54.9	52.5	55.1	54.7	55.8	58.2	60.6	61.7
Female																
Married....................................	83.8	83.5	79.3	81.0	79.3	78.6	78.4	77.7	76.7	75.6	75.1	75.0	74.3	75.9	78.0	78.6
Divorced, separated, widowed	63.1	63.6	61.7	63.2	59.9	56.3	57.0	56.3	54.2	53.9	52.6	51.8	52.1	55.1	58.1	56.4
Never married	72.2	70.0	66.2	64.2	61.5	59.0	60.8	58.8	56.4	54.1	55.9	56.2	56.2	58.4	60.4	60.0
Race[6]																
White only...................................	79.9	79.1	74.5	75.7	70.9	69.1	69.7	68.5	66.3	64.9	64.9	64.8	64.7	66.6	68.2	68.2
Black or African American only	58.1	57.7	53.0	55.9	52.9	51.3	51.8	50.0	47.4	44.8	45.9	45.8	45.4	47.1	50.6	50.9
American Indian or Alaska Native only	49.1	45.5	45.3	43.7	43.0	36.3	36.4	30.7	35.9	31.7	33.7	34.9	36.0	34.7	41.1	39.7
Asian only	69.9	71.9	68.4	72.1	72.2	72.1	73.2	74.3	71.3	68.1	65.9	67.6	69.4	72.5	73.8	75.1
Native Hawaiian or Other Pacific Islander only	NA	NA	NA	*	*	*	*	*	*	*	*	*	*	*	*	63.7
Two or more races	NA	NA	NA	61.4	57.6	54.0	52.7	58.0	47.8	52.4	52.3	52.9	50.0	55.4	55.3	57.5
Hispanic Origin and Race[6]																
Hispanic or Latino	55.7	51.5	46.4	47.8	42.4	40.0	41.7	39.9	37.3	36.8	36.4	36.7	37.3	41.2	43.8	45.3
Mexican	53.3	46.8	42.6	45.4	39.7	36.5	37.9	36.8	34.7	33.4	33.9	34.1	34.9	39.0	40.9	41.3
Puerto Rican	48.4	45.6	47.6	51.1	48.5	46.1	54.2	48.2	46.2	46.0	45.5	43.7	42.1	46.8	48.0	48.4
Cuban....................................	72.5	70.3	63.6	63.9	58.1	63.4	64.8	57.9	54.3	53.8	51.1	49.1	45.3	56.6	61.7	56.9
Other Hispanic or Latino	61.6	61.0	51.4	50.7	45.6	44.3	44.3	43.5	39.7	40.9	38.1	39.5	41.2	43.1	47.8	52.1
Not Hispanic or Latino	78.7	78.5	74.4	75.2	73.0	71.3	71.7	70.8	68.6	67.0	67.3	67.5	67.4	68.9	70.7	70.6
White only.................................	82.4	82.5	78.6	79.5	77.3	75.6	76.2	75.3	73.3	72.0	72.2	72.6	72.4	73.7	75.2	75.2
Black or African American only	58.2	57.7	53.4	56.0	53.1	52.2	52.3	50.6	48.0	45.1	46.5	46.4	45.7	48.0	51.2	51.2
Age and Percent of Poverty Level[7]																
Under 65 years																
Below 100 percent	32.2	27.0	22.6	25.2	21.4	21.4	21.4	19.2	15.3	16.0	17.2	16.5	15.5	17.4	18.6	19.8
100 percent to 199 percent	70.3	64.3	55.3	50.1	44.7	42.8	40.0	38.1	37.4	34.8	35.1	36.7	35.1	38.2	39.8	36.6
100 percent to 133 percent	59.4	52.8	41.7	39.3	36.0	33.6	29.5	27.3	26.1	24.4	24.1	26.9	25.3	26.5	30.6	28.0
134 percent to 199 percent	75.2	69.5	62.7	55.3	49.4	47.8	45.4	43.7	43.3	40.3	41.1	42.4	40.8	45.1	45.1	41.3
200 percent to 399 percent	89.3	89.2	86.4	78.1	74.8	74.9	73.2	72.3	70.6	70.7	71.1	71.3	71.3	73.6	73.4	73.7
400 percent or more	95.4	94.6	93.2	91.9	90.6	89.8	91.0	90.1	90.2	89.9	90.7	90.6	90.4	91.5	91.9	91.3
Under 19 years																
Below 100 percent	29.6	24.1	19.0	20.3	15.0	15.0	14.1	12.4	9.7	9.8	10.6	10.0	9.3	9.5	10.6	10.9
100 percent to 199 percent	73.6	68.5	55.8	49.5	41.6	38.5	35.7	34.1	34.0	31.5	31.2	32.4	29.2	30.4	30.3	26.8
100 percent to 133 percent	63.8	56.9	42.5	37.1	32.6	29.0	25.4	23.2	21.3	20.1	19.1	22.3	18.3	18.2	22.3	17.7
134 percent to 199 percent	78.4	74.0	64.4	56.1	47.0	44.6	41.7	40.1	41.3	38.1	38.0	38.4	36.2	38.6	35.5	32.1
200 percent to 399 percent	91.1	92.1	89.1	80.8	76.6	77.1	75.8	73.7	73.2	72.6	72.4	72.5	71.8	73.5	71.1	71.9
400 percent or more	96.2	96.2	93.3	93.0	92.5	91.4	93.2	92.0	91.8	91.2	92.7	91.2	92.3	92.5	92.7	90.8

NOTE: This table includes persons who had private coverage through the workplace in addition to other types of health insurance coverage. Private health insurance coverage is at the time of interview. The number of persons with private coverage was calculated by multiplying the percentage with private coverage by the number of persons under age 65 in the civilian noninstitutionalized U.S. population, which was determined from the poststratification Census control total for each survey year. Percentages of persons with private coverage were calculated with unknown values excluded from denominators.

NA = Not available.

* = Estimates are considered unreliable. Starting with 2016 data, the reliability of survey percentage estimates was assessed using new multistep National Center for Health Statistics data presentation standards for proportions. Prior to 2016 data, the reliability of estimates for earlier years was evaluated based on relative standard errors (RSE). Data not shown have an RSE greater than 30%.

[1]Any private health insurance coverage (both individual and insurance obtained through the workplace) at the time of interview; includes those who had other types of coverage in addition to their private coverage.

[2]Data prior to 1997 are not strictly comparable with data for later years due to the 1997 questionnaire redesign.

[3]Estimates for 2000–2002 were calculated using 2000-based sample weights and may differ from estimates in other reports that used 1990-based sample weights for 2000-2002 estimates.

[4]Includes all other races not shown separately, those with unknown marital status, unknown disability status, and, in 1984 and 1989, persons with unknown poverty level.

[5]Includes persons 14 to 64 years of age.

[6]The race groups White, Black, American Indian or Alaska Native, Asian, Native Hawaiian or Other Pacific Islander, and 2 or more races include persons of Hispanic and non-Hispanic origin. Persons of Hispanic origin may be of any race. Starting with 1999 data, race-specific estimates are tabulated according to the 1997 Revisions to the Standards for the Classification of Federal Data on Race and Ethnicity and are not strictly comparable with estimates for earlier years. The five single-race categories and multiple-race categories shown in the table conform to the 1997 Standards. Starting with 1999 data, race-specific estimates are for persons who reported only one racial group; the category 2 or more races includes persons who reported more than one racial group. Prior to 1999, data were tabulated according to the 1977 Standards with four racial groups, and the Asian only category included Native Hawaiian or Other Pacific Islander. Estimates for single-race categories prior to 1999 included persons who reported one race, or if they reported more than one race, identified one race as best representing their race. Starting with 2003 data, race responses of other race and unspecified multiple race were treated as missing, and then race was imputed if these were the only race responses. Almost all persons with a race response of other race were of Hispanic origin.

[7]Percent of poverty level is based on family income and family size and composition using U.S. Census Bureau poverty thresholds. Poverty level was unknown for 10%–11% of persons under age 65 in 1984 and 1989. Missing family income data were imputed for 1995 and beyond.

Table 3-71. Private Health Insurance[1] Coverage Among Persons Under 65 Years of Age, by Selected Characteristics, Selected Years, 1984–2016—*Continued*

(Numbers in millions; percent; data are based on household interviews of a sample of the civilian noninstitutionalized population.)

Characteristic	1984[2]	1989[2]	1995[2]	2000[3]	2005	2006	2007	2008	2009	2010	2011	2012	2013	2014	2015	2016
Under 18 years																
Below 100 percent	28.5	22.3	16.9	19.5	14.2	14.0	12.7	11.3	9.3	9.2	9.7	9.1	8.4	8.6	9.3	8.0
100 percent to 199 percent	73.9	68.9	56.1	49.4	41.4	38.3	35.6	34.1	34.0	31.5	31.0	32.1	28.5	30.2	30.1	26.7
100 percent to 133 percent	63.9	57.3	42.3	36.8	32.0	29.0	25.4	23.2	21.1	19.9	19.0	21.6	17.8	18.2	21.9	17.6
134 percent to 199 percent	78.6	74.5	64.9	56.2	47.0	44.4	41.5	40.1	41.3	38.3	37.7	38.4	35.3	38.3	35.3	32.0
200 percent to 399 percent	91.3	92.3	89.2	81.1	76.6	77.3	76.0	73.8	73.0	72.6	72.5	72.5	71.9	73.2	71.1	71.9
400 percent or more	96.1	96.5	93.1	93.1	92.5	91.6	93.4	92.2	91.8	91.4	92.8	91.4	92.2	92.6	92.7	90.9
18 to 64 years																
Below 100 percent	35.0	30.8	27.0	29.1	25.9	26.1	26.8	24.0	19.2	20.4	21.8	20.9	19.9	22.7	24.3	26.6
100 percent to 199 percent	68.3	61.5	54.8	50.5	46.5	45.1	42.5	40.2	39.1	36.4	37.2	38.9	38.2	42.1	44.6	41.7
100 percent to 133 percent	56.6	50.0	41.4	40.9	38.3	36.4	32.1	29.6	28.8	26.9	26.7	29.6	29.2	31.1	35.4	33.7
134 percent to 199 percent	73.3	66.6	61.5	54.9	50.7	49.4	47.5	45.7	44.3	41.3	42.8	44.2	43.2	48.2	49.8	46.0
200 percent to 399 percent	88.3	87.6	85.0	76.7	74.0	73.9	72.0	71.7	69.6	70.0	70.5	70.8	71.1	73.7	74.3	74.4
400 percent or more	95.2	94.4	93.2	91.6	90.1	89.3	90.4	89.6	89.8	89.5	90.2	90.4	89.9	91.2	91.8	91.4
Level of Difficulty[6]																
18 to 64 years																
A lot of difficulty or cannot do at all	NA	NA	NA	NA	NA	NA	NA	NA	NA	36.5	33.1	33.3	35.5	36.1	39.6	38.9
Some difficulty	NA	NA	NA	NA	NA	NA	NA	NA	NA	61.2	57.6	61.3	62.0	64.6	64.0	65.8
No difficulty	NA	NA	NA	NA	NA	NA	NA	NA	NA	69.5	69.8	67.4	69.9	71.4	73.5	74.3
Geographic Region																
Northeast	80.5	82.0	75.4	76.3	74.0	70.8	72.2	71.3	69.7	68.2	66.8	67.2	66.1	67.7	70.2	69.5
Midwest	80.6	81.5	77.3	78.8	74.6	71.7	72.0	69.9	67.5	66.7	67.9	68.4	68.0	68.7	70.1	70.8
South	74.3	71.4	66.9	66.8	62.5	61.8	62.6	62.1	59.3	57.5	57.8	57.3	57.4	59.4	62.5	61.8
West	71.9	71.2	67.5	66.5	65.6	64.6	64.0	62.8	60.6	58.9	58.4	58.5	59.6	62.9	62.6	63.9
Location of Residence																
Within MSA[9]	77.5	76.5	72.1	72.3	69.0	67.5	67.8	66.5	64.6	62.9	63.2	63.0	63.0	64.8	66.7	66.8
Outside MSA[9]	75.2	73.8	67.9	67.8	64.6	60.3	61.0	61.1	56.2	55.1	54.1	55.3	54.7	56.2	57.8	57.8

NOTE: This table includes persons who had private coverage through the workplace in addition to other types of health insurance coverage. Private health insurance coverage is at the time of interview. The number of persons with private coverage was calculated by multiplying the percentage with private coverage by the number of persons under age 65 in the civilian noninstitutionalized U.S. population, which was determined from the poststratification Census control total for each survey year. Percentages of persons with private coverage were calculated with unknown values excluded from denominators.
NA = Not available.
[1]Any private health insurance coverage (both individual and insurance obtained through the workplace) at the time of interview; includes those who had other types of coverage in addition to their private coverage.
[2]Data prior to 1997 are not strictly comparable with data for later years due to the 1997 questionnaire redesign.
[3]Estimates for 2000–2002 were calculated using 2000-based sample weights and may differ from estimates in other reports that used 1990-based sample weights for 2000-2002 estimates.
[6]Functional limitation is defined by the reported level of difficulty in six functioning domains: seeing (even if wearing glasses), hearing (even if wearing hearing aids), mobility (walking or climbing stairs), communication (understanding or being understood by others), cognition (remembering or concentrating), and self-care (such as washing all over or dressing). Respondents with answers to one or more of the six questions were included in one of three mutually exclusive categories. Those responding "A lot of difficulty" or "Cannot do at all/unable to do" to at least one question were classified in the "A lot of difficulty/cannot do" category. Of the remaining, those responding "Some difficulty" to at least one question were classified in the "Some difficulty" category, and those responding "No difficulty" to at least one question were classified in the "No difficulty" category. Those responding "Don't know" or "Refused" on all six questions were excluded. During 2010–2016, 1%–8% of respondents were missing data and excluded.
[9]MSA = metropolitan statistical area. Starting with 2016 data, MSA status is determined using 2010 Census data and the 2010 standards for defining MSAs.

Table 3-72. Private Health Insurance[1] Coverage Obtained Through the Workplace Among Persons Under 65 Years of Age, by Selected Characteristics, Selected Years, 1984–2016

(Numbers in millions; percent; data are based on household interviews of a sample of the civilian noninstitutionalized population.)

Characteristic	1984[2]	1989[2]	1995[2]	2000[3]	2005	2006	2007	2008	2009	2010	2011	2012	2013	2014	2015	2016
Total population (in millions)[4]	141.8	146.3	150.7	160.8	160.1	155.8	157.9	155.6	150.2	147.6	146.4	148.6	148.3	146.4	151.2	152.0
Total (percent of population)[4]	69.1	68.3	65.4	67.1	63.6	61.5	61.6	60.5	58.0	56.6	56.4	56.9	56.6	56.4	57.4	57.4
Age																
Under 19 years	66.4	65.6	60.5	63.1	58.7	55.6	55.8	54.5	52.0	50.9	49.9	50.1	49.6	49.6	49.8	49.7
Under 6 years	62.1	62.3	55.1	58.9	53.4	50.8	50.8	49.6	46.3	44.9	44.3	45.0	44.2	45.7	46.6	46.7
6 to 18 years	68.4	67.3	63.1	64.9	61.1	57.8	58.1	56.9	54.8	53.8	52.5	52.4	52.0	51.3	51.2	51.0
Under 18 years	66.5	65.8	60.4	63.0	58.6	55.5	55.8	54.4	51.8	50.7	49.7	49.9	49.3	49.3	49.6	49.3
6 to 17 years	68.7	67.7	63.3	65.0	61.1	57.8	58.3	56.9	54.7	53.8	52.4	52.3	51.8	51.1	51.0	50.6
18 to 64 years	70.3	69.4	67.6	68.8	65.7	63.9	63.9	62.9	60.4	58.9	59.1	59.6	59.5	59.2	60.4	60.5
18 to 44 years	69.6	68.4	65.3	66.5	62.2	60.6	60.3	59.4	56.6	54.6	55.6	56.7	56.9	57.0	58.6	59.1
18 to 24 years	58.7	55.3	53.5	55.5	52.1	51.7	52.3	49.5	47.4	45.3	51.0	52.7	53.1	53.9	55.8	57.3
19 to 25 years	59.0	55.0	53.0	54.2	50.6	50.7	51.4	48.9	45.9	44.1	50.5	52.7	53.0	54.0	56.7	57.5
25 to 34 years	71.2	69.5	65.0	66.4	61.1	59.3	59.0	58.4	55.5	53.3	53.0	53.8	53.8	54.2	56.9	57.0
35 to 44 years	77.4	76.2	72.7	73.2	69.9	67.5	67.0	67.0	64.3	62.8	61.6	62.7	63.1	62.2	62.4	62.6
45 to 64 years	71.8	71.6	72.2	72.9	70.9	68.9	69.2	68.0	65.7	64.8	63.9	63.6	62.9	62.2	62.8	62.5
45 to 54 years	74.6	74.4	74.7	75.6	72.6	70.2	70.4	69.5	67.1	65.9	64.7	64.4	64.3	63.8	65.0	64.3
55 to 64 years	69.0	68.3	68.4	68.6	68.6	67.2	67.7	66.2	64.0	63.4	62.4	62.6	61.3	60.4	60.5	60.6
Sex																
Male	69.8	68.7	65.9	67.3	63.6	61.2	61.3	60.3	57.6	56.1	56.1	57.1	56.9	56.9	57.6	57.9
Female	68.4	67.9	64.9	66.9	63.6	61.8	61.9	60.8	58.4	57.1	56.7	56.8	56.4	56.0	57.3	56.9
Sex and Marital Status[5]																
Male																
Married	77.9	76.9	74.9	77.5	75.3	73.3	73.3	72.7	70.6	70.1	69.3	69.9	69.8	69.6	70.3	69.7
Divorced, separated, widowed	58.0	57.3	56.4	57.4	51.9	51.0	50.8	51.0	48.0	45.3	45.0	46.2	45.3	45.7	45.3	47.1
Never married	61.5	58.8	58.2	58.8	54.9	52.6	53.5	51.9	48.8	46.2	48.4	49.6	50.0	50.1	51.6	52.9
Female																
Married	76.1	75.5	73.2	76.3	74.2	73.1	72.7	72.2	70.7	69.8	69.2	69.3	68.5	67.7	69.2	69.1
Divorced, separated, widowed	51.9	54.9	54.6	57.8	54.3	51.5	51.3	51.4	48.6	48.1	46.5	46.3	46.3	45.8	46.2	45.9
Never married	63.5	60.9	59.2	60.1	56.3	54.2	55.1	53.0	50.6	48.2	50.0	50.9	50.6	50.7	51.7	51.4
Race[6]																
White only	72.0	71.2	68.4	71.0	66.1	64.0	64.2	63.0	60.6	59.3	59.0	59.6	59.2	59.2	59.9	59.8
Black or African American only	52.4	52.8	49.3	53.4	50.6	48.5	49.1	47.7	45.3	42.3	43.5	43.2	42.9	42.0	44.8	44.9
American Indian or Alaska Native only	45.8	40.9	40.2	41.7	39.9	33.7	35.1	29.4	33.6	*29.4	32.4	34.0	34.2	30.9	35.9	34.5
Asian only	59.0	61.1	59.6	65.8	64.4	64.5	64.6	66.2	62.5	60.6	58.7	60.1	61.4	61.4	62.2	63.6
Native Hawaiian or Other Pacific Islander only	NA	NA	NA	*	*	*	*	*	*	*	*	*	*	*	*	56.9
Two or more races	NA	NA	NA	59.8	54.8	50.6	49.7	54.3	45.0	49.5	48.3	48.8	46.9	50.9	47.8	50.4
Hispanic Origin and Race[6]																
Hispanic or Latino	52.0	47.3	43.4	45.3	40.0	37.7	38.8	37.6	34.9	34.6	34.1	34.6	34.9	36.5	37.4	38.6
Mexican	50.5	44.2	40.9	43.6	37.6	34.9	35.7	35.2	32.6	31.6	32.0	32.5	32.5	35.1	36.2	36.5
Puerto Rican	45.9	42.3	44.5	49.4	46.2	43.5	51.2	45.9	42.9	43.6	42.8	41.6	40.8	42.6	41.6	42.6
Cuban	57.4	56.5	54.0	53.6	53.5	56.9	54.7	49.2	46.4	47.4	45.0	42.8	41.2	42.7	40.6	41.5
Other Hispanic or Latino	57.4	54.7	46.7	47.3	42.6	40.9	40.8	39.8	36.9	37.8	35.1	36.7	38.6	37.3	38.8	41.8
Not Hispanic or Latino	70.7	70.5	68.2	70.6	68.0	66.0	66.1	65.2	62.8	61.3	61.3	62.0	61.7	61.2	62.2	62.1
White only	74.0	74.1	72.1	74.5	71.9	69.9	70.2	69.0	66.8	65.7	65.5	66.6	66.1	65.5	66.3	66.3
Black or African American only	52.5	52.8	49.8	53.6	50.9	49.5	49.5	48.2	45.9	42.6	44.1	43.6	43.2	42.9	45.4	45.3
Age and Percent of Poverty Level[7]																
Under 65 years																
Below 100 percent	24.1	19.8	17.5	21.0	17.8	17.6	17.4	15.5	11.9	12.4	13.6	13.6	12.2	12.2	12.7	13.9
100 percent to 199 percent	61.7	56.1	49.3	45.4	40.1	38.3	35.5	33.8	33.3	30.2	30.4	32.2	31.0	31.0	30.2	27.5
100 percent to 133 percent	50.0	44.3	36.0	35.0	31.3	30.0	25.3	22.8	22.6	20.6	19.7	23.0	21.7	20.5	22.7	19.0
134 percent to 199 percent	66.9	61.5	56.6	50.5	44.8	42.9	40.7	39.1	39.0	35.3	36.2	37.5	36.3	37.3	34.5	32.1
200 percent to 399 percent	82.8	82.2	80.5	73.4	69.8	69.7	67.7	66.8	64.7	65.3	65.0	65.9	65.6	65.4	64.0	63.5
400 percent or more	88.8	87.8	86.7	87.9	86.1	84.7	85.5	84.6	84.1	84.2	85.0	85.1	84.6	84.5	84.8	84.2
Under 19 years																
Below 100 percent	23.6	18.6	15.1	17.1	13.3	12.7	12.1	11.3	7.9	8.2	9.1	8.7	7.8	7.2	7.8	8.0
100 percent to 199 percent	67.0	62.1	50.5	45.8	38.3	35.5	32.7	31.4	31.9	28.8	27.9	29.7	26.6	26.8	26.1	22.5
100 percent to 133 percent	56.1	49.9	37.4	33.6	29.1	27.0	22.4	21.0	19.8	17.9	16.3	20.5	16.4	15.6	19.7	13.8
134 percent to 199 percent	72.3	67.9	58.8	52.2	43.7	41.0	38.6	37.1	38.9	35.1	34.4	35.2	33.1	34.4	30.3	27.6
200 percent to 399 percent	85.7	86.0	83.9	76.9	72.4	72.5	71.2	68.3	67.7	68.7	67.0	68.0	66.7	67.6	64.4	65.0
400 percent or more	90.8	90.3	87.5	89.5	88.3	86.3	87.5	86.9	86.0	86.5	87.5	86.3	86.9	87.1	86.9	85.1

NOTE: This table includes persons who had private coverage through the workplace in addition to other types of health insurance coverage. Private health insurance coverage is at the time of interview. The number of persons with private coverage was calculated by multiplying the percentage with private coverage by the number of persons under age 65 in the civilian noninstitutionalized U.S. population, which was determined from the poststratification Census control total for each survey year. Percentages of persons with private coverage were calculated with unknown values excluded from denominators.

NA = Not available.

* = Estimates are considered unreliable. Starting with 2016 data, the reliability of survey percentage estimates was assessed using new multistep National Center for Health Statistics data presentation standards for proportions. Prior to 2016 data, the reliability of estimates for earlier years was evaluated based on relative standard errors (RSE). Data not shown have an RSE greater than 30%.

[1] Any private insurance at the time of interview that was originally obtained through a present or former employer or union, or starting with 1997 data, through the workplace, self-employment, or a professional association; includes those who had other types of coverage in addition to their private coverage. Starting in 2014, an additional question on the Health Insurance Marketplace was added to the National Health Interview Survey for those respondents who did not indicate that their health plan was obtained through a present or former employer, union, self-employment, or professional association to evaluate whether their plan was obtained through the Health Insurance Marketplace or state-based exchange. Starting in 2015, an additional category was added to the list describing how a private health plan was obtained. Individuals who selected this new category did not receive the additional question about the Health Insurance Marketplace.

[2] Data prior to 1997 are not strictly comparable with data for later years due to the 1997 questionnaire redesign.

[3] Estimates for 2000–2002 were calculated using 2000-based sample weights and may differ from estimates in other reports that used 1990-based sample weights for 2000-2002 estimates.

[4] Includes all other races not shown separately, those with unknown marital status, unknown disability status, and, in 1984 and 1989, persons with unknown poverty level.

[5] Includes persons 14 to 64 years of age.

[6] The race groups White, Black, American Indian or Alaska Native, Asian, Native Hawaiian or Other Pacific Islander, and 2 or more races include persons of Hispanic and non-Hispanic origin. Persons of Hispanic origin may be of any race. Starting with 1999 data, race-specific estimates are tabulated according to the 1997 Revisions to the Standards for the Classification of Federal Data on Race and Ethnicity and are not strictly comparable with estimates for earlier years. The five single-race categories and multiple-race categories shown in the table conform to the 1997 Standards. Starting with 1999 data, race-specific estimates are for persons who reported only one racial group; the category 2 or more races includes persons who reported more than one racial group. Prior to 1999, data were tabulated according to the 1977 Standards with four racial groups, and the Asian only category included Native Hawaiian or Other Pacific Islander. Estimates for single-race categories prior to 1999 included persons who reported one race, or if they reported more than one race, identified one race as best representing their race. Starting with 2003 data, race responses of other race and unspecified multiple race were treated as missing, and then race was imputed if these were the only race responses. Almost all persons with a race response of other race were of Hispanic origin.

[7] Percent of poverty level is based on family income and family size and composition using U.S. Census Bureau poverty thresholds. Poverty level was unknown for 10%–11% of persons under age 65 in 1984 and 1989. Missing family income data were imputed for 1995 and beyond.

Table 3-72. Private Health Insurance[1] Coverage Obtained Through the Workplace Among Persons Under 65 Years of Age, by Selected Characteristics, Selected Years, 1984–2016—*Continued*

(Numbers in millions; percent; data are based on household interviews of a sample of the civilian noninstitutionalized population.)

Characteristic	1984[2]	1989[2]	1995[2]	2000[3]	2005	2006	2007	2008	2009	2010	2011	2012	2013	2014	2015	2016
Under 18 years																
Below 100 percent	23.0	17.5	13.6	16.6	12.5	11.8	11.2	10.3	7.5	7.8	8.4	8.1	7.2	6.7	6.9	5.7
100 percent to 199 percent	67.5	62.5	50.9	45.8	38.2	35.4	32.7	31.4	32.0	28.8	27.7	29.4	26.0	26.7	26.0	22.5
100 percent to 133 percent	56.3	50.3	37.2	33.5	28.6	27.1	22.5	21.0	19.8	17.8	16.1	19.8	16.0	15.6	19.7	13.7
134 percent to 199 percent	72.8	68.4	59.6	52.4	43.9	40.8	38.5	37.1	38.9	35.2	34.1	35.2	32.4	34.3	30.1	27.7
200 percent to 399 percent	85.9	86.4	84.1	77.1	72.4	72.7	71.5	68.4	67.6	68.7	67.0	68.1	66.8	67.5	64.4	65.0
400 percent or more	90.7	90.5	87.1	89.7	88.5	86.4	87.7	87.1	86.0	86.6	87.7	86.4	86.8	87.2	87.0	85.2
18 to 64 years																
Below 100 percent	24.8	21.8	20.5	24.0	21.2	21.3	21.2	18.7	14.8	15.4	16.8	16.9	15.2	15.6	16.3	18.6
100 percent to 199 percent	58.3	52.3	48.4	45.2	41.1	39.9	37.0	35.1	34.0	30.9	31.8	33.6	33.3	33.1	32.2	30.0
100 percent to 133 percent	46.0	40.4	35.3	35.9	32.9	31.8	27.0	25.5	24.2	22.1	21.5	24.6	24.7	23.2	24.4	21.9
134 percent to 199 percent	63.6	57.5	55.0	49.5	45.3	43.9	41.8	40.1	39.0	35.3	37.2	38.7	38.0	38.6	36.6	34.4
200 percent to 399 percent	81.4	80.2	78.8	71.7	68.7	68.4	66.2	66.1	63.6	63.9	64.3	65.0	65.2	64.7	63.8	63.0
400 percent or more	88.5	87.5	86.7	87.5	85.4	84.3	84.9	83.9	83.6	83.6	84.2	84.7	84.0	83.8	84.3	83.9
Level of Difficulty[a]																
18 to 64 years																
A lot of difficulty or cannot do at all	NA	NA	NA	NA	NA	NA	NA	NA	NA	31.7	29.0	29.6	30.4	28.6	30.3	30.4
Some difficulty	NA	NA	NA	NA	NA	NA	NA	NA	NA	55.7	53.2	55.6	57.0	55.9	53.9	54.4
No difficulty	NA	NA	NA	NA	NA	NA	NA	NA	NA	63.7	63.5	61.8	63.7	63.0	64.1	65.0
Geographic Region																
Northeast	74.0	75.0	69.8	72.5	70.6	67.5	68.2	68.0	65.3	64.4	63.0	63.4	62.3	61.5	62.9	61.5
Midwest	72.0	73.3	71.2	74.9	70.1	67.0	68.0	64.7	62.0	61.8	62.2	63.8	62.6	61.5	62.7	63.2
South	66.2	63.6	61.8	62.5	58.0	57.2	57.2	56.7	54.1	52.2	52.3	52.2	52.4	52.3	54.3	53.2
West	64.7	63.9	60.4	61.1	59.7	58.1	57.3	56.8	54.5	52.7	52.3	52.8	53.6	54.7	53.5	55.5
Location of Residence																
Within MSA[9]	70.9	69.6	66.6	68.2	64.5	62.7	62.7	61.5	59.3	57.9	57.8	58.1	57.8	57.8	58.6	58.7
Outside MSA[9]	65.3	63.5	60.7	62.6	59.6	55.4	55.7	55.7	55.1	50.8	49.4	48.7	50.3	49.4	50.0	49.4

NOTE: This table includes persons who had private coverage through the workplace in addition to other types of health insurance coverage. Private health insurance coverage is at the time of interview. The number of persons with private coverage was calculated by multiplying the percentage with private coverage by the number of persons under age 65 in the civilian noninstitutionalized U.S. population, which was determined from the poststratification Census control total for each survey year. Percentages of persons with private coverage were calculated with unknown values excluded from denominators.

NA = Not available.

[1]Any private insurance at the time of interview that was originally obtained through a present or former employer or union, or starting with 1997 data, through the workplace, self-employment, or a professional association; includes those who had other types of coverage in addition to their private coverage. Starting in 2014, an additional question on the Health Insurance Marketplace was added to the National Health Interview Survey for those respondents who did not indicate that their health plan was obtained through a present or former employer, union, self-employment, or professional association to evaluate whether their plan was obtained through the Health Insurance Marketplace or state-based exchange. Starting in 2015, an additional category was added to the list describing how a private health plan was obtained. Individuals who selected this new category did not receive the additional question about the Health Insurance Marketplace.

[2]Data prior to 1997 are not strictly comparable with data for later years due to the 1997 questionnaire redesign.

[3]Estimates for 2000–2002 were calculated using 2000-based sample weights and may differ from estimates in other reports that used 1990-based sample weights for 2000-2002 estimates.

[a]Functional limitation is defined by the reported level of difficulty in six functioning domains: seeing (even if wearing glasses), hearing (even if wearing hearing aids), mobility (walking or climbing stairs), communication (understanding or being understood by others), cognition (remembering or concentrating), and self-care (such as washing all over or dressing). Respondents with answers to one or more of the six questions were included in one of three mutually exclusive categories. Those responding "A lot of difficulty" or "Cannot do at all/unable to do" to at least one question were classified in the "A lot of difficulty/cannot do" category. Of the remaining, those responding "Some difficulty" to at least one question were classified in the "Some difficulty" category, and those responding "No difficulty" to at least one question were classified in the "No difficulty" category. Those responding "Don't know" or "Refused" on all six questions were excluded. During 2010–2016, 1%–8% of respondents were missing data and excluded.

[9]MSA = metropolitan statistical area. Starting with 2016 data, MSA status is determined using 2010 Census data and the 2010 standards for defining MSAs.

Table 3-73. No Health Insurance Coverage Among Persons Under 65 Years of Age, by Selected Characteristics, Selected Years, 1984–2016

(Numbers in millions; percent; data are based on household interviews of a sample of the civilian noninstitutionalized population.)

Characteristic	1984[1]	1989[1]	1995[1]	2000[2]	2005[3]	2006[3]	2007[3]	2008[3]	2009[3]	2010[3]	2011[3]	2012[3]	2013[3]	2014[3]	2015[3]	2016[3]
Total (number in millions)[4]	29.8	33.4	37.1	41.4	42.1	43.9	43.3	44.1	46.2	48.3	45.8	45.2	44.6	35.7	28.7	27.9
Total (percent of population)[4]	14.5	15.6	16.1	17.0	16.4	17.0	16.6	16.8	17.5	18.2	17.2	16.9	16.7	13.3	10.6	10.3
Age																
Under 19 years	14.1	15.0	13.7	12.9	9.7	9.8	9.4	9.5	8.5	8.3	7.4	7.0	7.1	5.7	4.8	5.4
Under 6 years	14.9	15.1	11.8	11.8	7.7	7.5	7.3	7.6	6.6	6.3	5.0	4.6	5.0	4.1	3.3	4.1
6 to 18 years	13.8	15.0	14.6	13.4	10.6	10.9	10.4	10.5	9.4	9.2	8.5	8.1	8.0	6.5	5.5	5.9
Under 18 years	13.9	14.7	13.4	12.6	9.3	9.5	9.0	9.0	8.2	7.8	7.0	6.6	6.6	5.4	4.5	5.2
6 to 17 years	13.4	14.5	14.3	13.0	10.1	10.5	9.9	9.8	9.0	8.6	8.0	7.6	7.4	6.1	5.1	5.7
18 to 64 years	14.8	16.0	17.3	18.9	19.3	20.0	19.6	19.9	21.2	22.3	21.2	20.9	20.5	16.3	13.0	12.2
18 to 44 years	17.1	18.4	20.4	22.4	23.5	24.6	23.9	24.4	25.9	27.1	25.4	24.8	24.2	19.7	15.9	14.8
18 to 24 years	25.0	27.1	28.0	30.4	29.1	29.9	27.9	29.0	29.6	31.4	25.9	24.5	24.6	18.1	14.6	13.0
19 to 25 years	25.1	27.9	28.8	32.3	31.7	32.4	30.5	31.1	32.8	33.8	27.9	26.3	26.7	19.7	16.0	13.9
25 to 34 years	16.2	18.3	21.1	23.3	25.6	27.2	26.1	26.6	27.8	28.3	28.1	28.1	27.1	22.7	18.0	16.2
35 to 44 years	11.2	12.3	15.1	16.9	17.9	18.8	19.1	19.1	21.4	22.6	22.2	21.7	21.0	17.7	14.6	14.7
45 to 64 years	9.6	10.5	10.9	12.6	12.9	13.2	13.5	13.6	14.6	15.7	15.4	15.6	15.4	11.8	9.0	8.8
45 to 54 years	10.5	11.0	11.6	12.8	14.2	15.0	14.9	14.9	16.5	17.9	17.4	17.7	17.1	13.7	10.2	10.6
55 to 64 years	8.7	10.0	9.9	12.4	11.1	10.8	11.6	11.8	12.2	12.8	13.0	13.2	13.5	9.7	7.7	7.0
Sex																
Male	15.3	16.8	17.4	18.1	17.9	18.8	18.2	18.3	19.4	20.3	18.8	18.5	18.1	14.7	12.0	11.6
Female	13.8	14.4	14.8	15.9	15.0	15.3	15.1	15.4	15.7	16.1	15.6	15.4	15.2	11.9	9.3	9.0
Sex and Marital Status[5]																
Male																
Married	11.1	12.5	15.0	14.1	14.4	15.3	15.3	15.4	16.3	17.2	16.5	16.2	15.9	12.6	10.6	10.5
Divorced, separated, widowed	24.9	25.0	24.0	25.8	28.6	29.1	28.1	27.0	29.8	31.4	30.0	29.3	28.1	23.2	20.0	18.5
Never married	22.4	25.0	25.6	27.2	27.6	28.6	27.0	27.6	29.4	31.1	28.0	27.5	26.9	21.9	17.4	16.1
Female																
Married	11.2	11.8	13.6	13.3	13.0	13.5	13.5	13.5	14.2	14.7	14.4	14.6	14.6	11.6	8.8	8.7
Divorced, separated, widowed	19.2	19.1	18.1	21.3	22.1	23.0	22.6	22.1	22.8	23.6	24.0	24.2	22.8	17.7	13.4	13.0
Never married	16.3	18.0	17.5	21.1	20.0	20.4	19.5	20.7	21.0	21.9	20.5	19.6	19.6	15.1	12.1	10.9
Race[6]																
White only	13.6	14.5	15.5	15.4	15.9	16.7	16.3	16.7	17.1	17.6	16.7	16.7	16.3	13.3	10.7	10.2
Black or African American only	19.9	21.6	18.0	19.5	18.4	18.1	17.0	18.0	18.9	20.6	19.0	18.0	18.9	13.7	11.3	11.5
American Indian or Alaska Native only	22.5	28.4	34.3	38.4	32.2	38.0	38.8	28.4	32.5	44.0	34.2	27.0	29.4	28.3	21.4	25.4
Asian only	18.5	16.9	18.6	17.6	17.1	15.0	15.4	13.9	16.2	17.1	16.5	16.8	14.2	10.8	7.5	6.5
Native Hawaiian or Other Pacific Islander only	NA	NA	NA	*	*	*	*	*	*	*	*	*	*	*	*	9.3
Two or more races	NA	NA	NA	16.8	16.5	18.4	15.0	15.8	18.2	15.8	16.0	14.5	15.3	10.1	9.5	9.0
Hispanic Origin and Race[6]																
Hispanic or Latino	29.5	33.7	31.4	35.6	33.0	35.0	31.8	33.3	32.9	32.0	31.1	30.4	30.7	25.5	21.1	19.6
Mexican	33.8	39.9	35.6	39.9	36.0	38.6	34.7	36.1	35.0	34.8	33.0	33.2	33.4	27.2	23.5	22.3
Puerto Rican	18.3	24.7	17.6	16.4	16.3	16.8	12.8	16.8	17.8	13.7	15.8	14.4	15.6	13.0	9.6	7.6
Cuban	21.6	20.6	22.3	25.4	23.2	22.8	20.7	28.1	27.8	26.5	28.1	24.3	26.6	19.4	14.2	18.1
Other Hispanic or Latino	27.4	25.8	30.2	33.4	32.6	33.2	32.7	32.5	33.4	32.4	31.8	30.1	28.8	26.2	19.7	18.0
Not Hispanic or Latino	13.2	13.7	14.2	14.0	13.4	13.6	13.7	13.5	14.4	15.2	14.2	13.9	13.4	10.5	8.2	8.1
White only	11.9	12.1	13.0	12.5	12.0	12.5	12.6	12.5	13.2	13.7	12.9	12.7	12.2	9.7	7.5	7.3
Black or African American only	19.7	21.5	17.9	19.5	18.3	17.5	16.8	17.9	18.8	20.7	18.8	17.8	18.8	13.5	11.2	11.3
Age and Percent of Poverty Level[7]																
Under 65 years																
Below 100 percent	33.9	35.2	29.6	34.2	30.6	30.2	28.4	29.0	30.4	30.3	28.4	28.2	28.0	23.0	18.2	18.5
100 percent to 199 percent	21.8	25.6	28.3	31.0	28.6	29.6	30.0	30.6	29.8	32.4	30.0	29.3	29.3	23.4	18.3	18.0
100 percent to 133 percent	28.8	32.3	34.1	35.7	30.1	31.3	32.0	32.8	30.1	34.9	32.0	31.1	30.4	25.0	18.4	18.8
134 percent to 199 percent	18.7	22.6	25.1	28.7	27.8	28.7	29.0	29.5	29.6	31.0	28.9	28.4	28.6	22.4	18.1	17.5
200 percent to 399 percent	7.6	8.3	10.0	15.4	15.7	15.5	16.9	16.6	17.8	17.4	16.5	16.2	16.1	12.6	11.1	10.1
400 percent or more	3.2	4.2	5.4	5.9	6.3	6.5	5.6	6.2	5.8	5.6	5.2	4.9	4.8	3.8	3.3	3.7
Under 19 years																
Below 100 percent	29.0	31.7	20.4	22.6	15.2	14.2	12.7	14.0	12.2	11.3	9.4	8.3	8.9	6.7	5.4	7.6
100 percent to 199 percent	18.0	20.7	22.6	22.1	15.6	16.4	16.4	16.3	13.0	13.5	12.1	11.1	11.7	9.3	7.4	7.9
100 percent to 133 percent	24.4	27.6	26.4	26.5	15.6	17.9	17.4	17.3	12.9	15.9	12.5	9.6	11.6	9.4	7.7	7.9
134 percent to 199 percent	14.9	17.4	20.1	19.7	15.6	15.5	15.9	15.8	13.1	12.0	11.9	12.0	11.7	9.3	7.2	7.8
200 percent to 399 percent	5.1	4.9	6.7	9.6	8.2	7.8	8.5	8.0	8.0	7.4	6.8	6.8	6.7	5.7	5.4	4.7
400 percent or more	1.8	2.1	4.4	3.5	3.3	3.4	2.3	2.8	2.4	2.3	2.1	1.9	1.7	1.4	1.7	2.5

NOTE: Persons not covered by private insurance, Medicaid, Children's Health Insurance Program (CHIP), public assistance (through 1996), state-sponsored or other government-sponsored health plans (starting in 1997), Medicare, or military plans are considered to have no health insurance coverage. Persons with only Indian Health Service coverage are considered to have no health insurance coverage. Health insurance coverage is at the time of interview. The number of persons with no health insurance coverage was calculated by multiplying the percentage with no coverage by the number of persons under age 65 in the civilian noninstitutionalized U.S. population, which was determined from the poststratification Census control total for each survey year. Percentages of persons without coverage were calculated with unknown values excluded from denominators.

NA = Not available.

* = Estimates are considered unreliable. Starting with 2016 data, the reliability of survey percentage estimates was assessed using new multistep National Center for Health Statistics data presentation standards for proportions. Prior to 2016 data, the reliability of estimates for earlier years was evaluated based on relative standard errors (RSE). Data not shown have an RSE greater than 30%.

[1] Any private health insurance coverage (both individual and insurance obtained through the workplace) at the time of interview; includes those who had other types of coverage in addition to their private coverage.
[2] Data prior to 1997 are not strictly comparable with data for later years due to the 1997 questionnaire redesign.
[3] Estimates for 2000–2002 were calculated using 2000-based sample weights and may differ from estimates in other reports that used 1990-based sample weights for 2000-2002 estimates.
[4] Includes all other races not shown separately, those with unknown marital status, unknown disability status, and, in 1984 and 1989, persons with unknown poverty level.
[5] Includes persons 14 to 64 years of age.
[6] The race groups White, Black, American Indian or Alaska Native, Asian, Native Hawaiian or Other Pacific Islander, and 2 or more races include persons of Hispanic and non-Hispanic origin. Persons of Hispanic origin may be of any race. Starting with 1999 data, race-specific estimates are tabulated according to the 1997 Revisions to the Standards for the Classification of Federal Data on Race and Ethnicity and are not strictly comparable with estimates for earlier years. The five single-race categories and multiple-race categories shown in the table conform to the 1997 Standards. Starting with 1999 data, race-specific estimates are for persons who reported only one racial group; the category 2 or more races includes persons who reported more than one racial group. Prior to 1999, data were tabulated according to the 1977 Standards with four racial groups, and the Asian only category included Native Hawaiian or Other Pacific Islander. Estimates for single-race categories prior to 1999 included persons who reported one race, or if they reported more than one race, identified one race as best representing their race. Starting with 2003 data, race responses of other race and unspecified multiple race were treated as missing, and then race was imputed if these were the only race responses. Almost all persons with a race response of other race were of Hispanic origin.
[7] Percent of poverty level is based on family income and family size and composition using U.S. Census Bureau poverty thresholds. Poverty level was unknown for 10%–11% of persons under age 65 in 1984 and 1989. Missing family income data were imputed for 1995 and beyond.

Table 3-73. No Health Insurance Coverage Among Persons Under 65 Years of Age, by Selected Characteristics, Selected Years, 1984–2016—Continued

(Numbers in millions; percent; data are based on household interviews of a sample of the civilian noninstitutionalized population.)

Characteristic	1984[1]	1989[1]	1995[1]	2000[2]	2005[3]	2006[3]	2007[3]	2008[3]	2009[3]	2010[3]	2011[3]	2012[3]	2013[3]	2014[3]	2015[3]	2016[3]
Under 18 years																
Below 100 percent	28.9	31.6	20.0	22.0	14.3	13.9	11.9	13.3	11.8	10.6	8.8	7.6	8.2	6.4	4.9	7.3
100 percent to 199 percent	17.5	20.2	22.0	21.7	15.0	16.0	15.7	15.5	12.3	12.7	11.4	10.4	11.1	8.7	6.9	7.6
100 percent to 133 percent	24.0	27.1	26.1	26.4	15.1	17.5	16.5	16.4	11.8	15.1	11.5	9.0	11.2	8.9	7.3	7.9
134 percent to 199 percent	14.4	16.9	19.5	19.1	15.0	15.1	15.3	15.0	12.6	11.3	11.3	11.3	11.1	8.5	6.7	7.4
200 percent to 399 percent	4.9	4.7	6.6	9.3	7.8	7.4	8.2	7.5	7.8	7.0	6.4	6.7	6.3	5.5	5.2	4.5
400 percent or more	1.8	1.9	4.6	3.3	3.2	3.1	2.2	2.7	2.3	2.1	2.0	2.1	1.8	*1.6	1.6	2.5
18 to 64 years																
Below 100 percent	37.6	38.2	37.0	42.4	40.9	40.7	38.6	38.6	42.5	42.7	40.4	40.5	40.0	32.9	26.2	24.8
100 percent to 199 percent	24.4	28.8	32.0	36.4	35.9	36.7	37.9	38.9	38.9	42.1	39.3	38.6	37.8	30.5	23.9	23.3
100 percent to 133 percent	31.9	35.6	39.7	41.7	38.9	39.8	41.7	42.1	40.4	45.7	42.5	42.2	40.4	33.9	24.5	24.8
134 percent to 199 percent	21.1	25.9	28.2	34.0	34.4	35.1	36.1	37.3	38.1	40.3	37.6	36.5	36.4	28.7	23.6	22.5
200 percent to 399 percent	8.9	10.0	11.7	18.2	19.0	18.8	20.5	20.2	21.7	21.3	20.4	19.8	19.7	15.3	13.3	12.2
400 percent or more	3.4	4.4	5.5	6.6	7.1	7.4	6.5	7.1	6.7	6.5	6.1	5.6	5.6	4.3	3.8	4.1
Level of Difficulty[8]																
18 to 64 years																
A lot of difficulty or cannot do at all	NA	NA	NA	NA	NA	NA	NA	NA	NA	21.5	19.9	21.1	19.0	17.3	11.3	12.2
Some difficulty	NA	NA	NA	NA	NA	NA	NA	NA	NA	23.5	21.5	21.1	20.2	16.6	13.4	12.2
No difficulty	NA	NA	NA	NA	NA	NA	NA	NA	NA	21.4	20.1	21.3	20.0	16.4	12.9	11.2
Geographic Region																
Northeast	10.2	10.9	13.3	12.2	11.3	11.2	11.0	11.4	11.4	12.4	11.8	11.5	11.2	9.3	6.8	6.7
Midwest	11.3	10.7	12.2	12.3	11.9	13.4	13.0	13.9	14.6	14.1	13.4	13.6	13.1	10.3	8.2	7.8
South	17.7	19.7	19.4	20.5	21.0	21.1	20.1	20.1	21.2	21.9	20.4	20.3	19.9	16.9	14.2	14.3
West	18.2	18.8	17.9	20.7	18.4	18.8	18.9	18.8	19.4	20.6	20.0	19.0	18.9	13.3	10.1	9.3
Location of Residence																
Within MSA[9]	13.6	15.2	15.5	16.6	16.1	16.6	16.1	16.4	17.1	17.8	16.7	16.4	16.2	13.0	10.3	9.9
Outside MSA[9]	16.6	17.0	18.6	18.6	17.8	19.3	19.4	19.1	20.2	20.4	20.4	19.8	19.9	15.2	12.8	13.3

NOTE: Persons not covered by private insurance, Medicaid, Children's Health Insurance Program (CHIP), public assistance (through 1996), state-sponsored or other government-sponsored health plans (starting in 1997), Medicare, or military plans are considered to have no health insurance coverage. Persons with only Indian Health Service coverage are considered to have no health insurance coverage. Health insurance coverage is at the time of interview. The number of persons with no health insurance coverage was calculated by multiplying the percentage with no coverage by the number of persons under age 65 in the civilian noninstitutionalized U.S. population, which was determined from the poststratification Census control total for each survey year. Percentages of persons without coverage were calculated with unknown values excluded from denominators.

NA = Not available.

* = Estimates are considered unreliable. Starting with 2016 data, the reliability of survey percentage estimates was assessed using new multistep National Center for Health Statistics data presentation standards for proportions. Prior to 2016 data, the reliability of estimates for earlier years was evaluated based on relative standard errors (RSE). Data not shown have an RSE greater than 30%.

[1]Any private health insurance coverage (both individual and insurance obtained through the workplace) at the time of interview; includes those who had other types of coverage in addition to their private coverage.

[2]Data prior to 1997 are not strictly comparable with data for later years due to the 1997 questionnaire redesign.

[3]Estimates for 2000–2002 were calculated using 2000-based sample weights and may differ from estimates in other reports that used 1990-based sample weights for 2000-2002 estimates.

[8]Functional limitation is defined by the reported level of difficulty in six functioning domains: seeing (even if wearing glasses), hearing (even if wearing hearing aids), mobility (walking or climbing stairs), communication (understanding or being understood by others), cognition (remembering or concentrating), and self-care (such as washing all over or dressing). Respondents with answers to one or more of the six questions were included in one of three mutually exclusive categories. Those responding "A lot of difficulty" or "Cannot do at all/unable to do" to at least one question were classified in the "A lot of difficulty/cannot do" category. Of the remaining, those responding "Some difficulty" to at least one question were classified in the "Some difficulty" category, and those responding "No difficulty" to at least one question were classified in the "No difficulty" category. Those responding "Don't know" or "Refused" on all six questions were excluded. During 2010–2016, 1%–8% of respondents were missing data and excluded.

[9]MSA is metropolitan statistical area. Starting with 2016 data, MSA status is determined using 2010 Census data and the 2010 standards for defining MSAs.

Table 3-74. Health Insurance Coverage of Noninstitutionalized Medicare Beneficiaries 65 Years of Age and Over, by Type of Coverage and Selected Characteristics, Selected Years, 1992–2015

(Numbers in millions; percent; data are based on household interviews of a sample of noninstitutionalized Medicare beneficiaries.)

Characteristic	Medicare Advantage Plan[1]						Medicaid[2]					
	1992	1995	2000	2005	2010	2015	1992	1995	2000	2005	2010	2015
Age												
65 years and over (number in millions)	1.1	2.6	5.9	4.6	10.3	15.8	2.7	2.8	2.7	3.2	3.2	4.5
65 years and over (percent of population)	3.9	8.9	19.3	14.5	26.7	34.0	9.4	9.6	9.0	10.1	8.4	9.7
65 to 74 years	4.2	9.5	20.6	13.9	26.9	33.7	7.9	8.8	8.5	9.9	7.7	7.5
75 to 84 years	3.7	8.3	18.5	15.3	27.6	35.6	10.6	9.6	8.9	9.9	9.1	10.5
85 years and over	0.0	7.3	16.3	13.9	23.7	31.3	16.6	13.6	11.2	11.9	9.5	17.5
Sex												
Male	4.6	9.2	19.3	13.5	25.4	32.8	6.3	6.2	6.3	7.2	6.3	8.6
Female	3.4	8.6	19.3	15.2	27.8	34.9	11.6	12.0	10.9	12.3	10.1	10.5
Race and Hispanic Origin												
White, not Hispanic or Latino	3.6	8.4	18.4	13.2	23.9	31.7	5.6	5.4	5.1	6.1	5.4	7.3
Black, not Hispanic or Latino	0.0	7.9	20.7	17.1	34.3	39.7	28.5	30.3	23.6	23.6	16.8	14.8
Hispanic	0.0	15.5	27.5	27.2	47.2	49.3	39.0	40.5	28.7	29.2	18.8	18.3
Percent of Poverty Level[3]												
Below 100 percent	3.6	7.7	18.4	NA	NA	36.3	22.3	17.2	15.9	NA	NA	35.7
100 percent to less than 200 percent	3.7	9.5	23.4	NA	NA	38.9	6.7	6.3	8.4	NA	NA	14.9
200 percent or more	4.2	10.1	18.0	NA	NA	31.5	*	*	*	NA	NA	3.0
Marital Status												
Married	4.6	9.5	18.7	13.8	27.1	33.8	4.0	4.3	4.3	5.4	3.6	5.2
Widowed	2.3	7.7	19.4	15.0	25.4	32.6	14.9	15.0	13.6	14.9	12.6	14.5
Divorced	*	9.7	24.4	17.1	29.1	36.6	23.4	24.5	20.2	20.0	16.9	16.3
Never married	*	*	15.8	13.9	23.1	35.5	19.2	19.0	17.0	21.3	19.8	18.7

Characteristic	Employer-sponsored plan[4]						Medigap[5]					
	1992	1995	2000	2005	2010	2015	1992	1995	2000	2005	2010	2015
Age												
65 years and over (number in millions)	12.5	11.3	10.7	11.6	11.9	9.5	9.9	9.5	7.6	8.2	7.6	11.9
65 years and over (percent of population)	42.8	38.6	35.2	36.4	30.6	20.5	33.9	32.5	25.0	25.7	19.6	25.6
65 to 74 years	46.9	41.1	36.6	38.1	32.5	20.7	31.4	29.9	21.7	23.2	17.4	27.1
75 to 84 years	38.2	37.1	35.0	35.5	28.4	21.1	37.5	35.2	27.8	27.3	21.3	24.0
85 years and over	31.6	30.2	29.4	31.8	28.5	18.4	38.3	37.6	31.1	30.8	24.7	22.8
Sex												
Male	46.3	42.1	37.7	39.4	32.9	21.5	30.6	30.0	23.4	23.8	18.2	25.2
Female	40.4	36.0	33.4	34.2	28.9	19.7	36.2	34.4	26.2	27.1	20.8	26.0
Race and Hispanic Origin												
White, not Hispanic or Latino	45.9	41.3	38.6	39.5	33.5	22.6	37.2	36.2	28.3	29.1	23.0	29.4
Black, not Hispanic or Latino	25.9	26.7	22.0	27.9	23.7	16.9	13.6	10.2	7.5	9.5	6.7	13.2
Hispanic	20.7	16.9	15.8	18.6	14.8	10.4	15.8	10.1	11.3	11.1	6.4	10.3
Percent of Poverty Level[3]												
Below 100 percent	29.0	32.1	28.1	NA	NA	5.9	30.8	29.8	22.6	NA	NA	9.4
100 percent to less than 200 percent	37.5	32.0	27.0	NA	NA	11.9	39.3	39.1	28.4	NA	NA	20.0
200 percent or more	58.4	52.8	49.0	NA	NA	26.6	32.8	32.2	26.2	NA	NA	30.8
Marital Status												
Married	49.9	44.6	41.0	41.7	35.9	24.3	33.0	32.6	25.6	27.0	19.6	28.2
Widowed	34.1	30.3	28.7	30.4	26.3	17.4	37.5	35.2	26.7	26.2	22.0	24.6
Divorced	27.3	26.6	22.4	25.1	18.9	13.5	27.9	24.1	16.9	19.8	15.3	19.8
Never married	38.0	35.1	28.5	29.1	25.2	12.0	29.1	26.2	21.9	15.4	17.5	19.3

NOTE: Data are for noninstitutionalized Medicare beneficiaries. Insurance categories are mutually exclusive. Persons with more than one type of coverage are categorized according to the order in which the health insurance categories appear in the table. Due to changes in sampling and data collection methodologies, 2014 data are not available.
NA = Not available.
* = Estimates are considered unreliable if the sample cell size is 50 or fewer.
[1]Enrollee has a Medicare Advantage plan regardless of other insurance. Medicare Advantage plans include health maintenance organizations, preferred provider organizations, private fee-for-service plans, special needs plans, and Medicare medical savings account plans. Starting with 2013 data, the term Medicare Risk Health Maintenance Organization was replaced with Medicare Advantage plan.
[2]Enrolled in Medicaid and not enrolled in a Medicare Advantage plan.
[3]Percent of poverty level is based on family income and family size and composition using U.S. Census Bureau poverty thresholds.
[4]Private insurance plans purchased through employers (own, current, or former employer, family business, union, or former employer or union of spouse) and not enrolled in a Medicare risk HMO or Medicaid.
[5]Supplemental insurance purchased privately or through organizations such as American Association of Retired Persons or professional organizations, and not enrolled in a Medicare risk HMO, Medicaid, or employer-sponsored plan.

Table 3-74. Health Insurance Coverage of Noninstitutionalized Medicare Beneficiaries 65 Years of Age and Over, by Type of Coverage and Selected Characteristics, Selected Years, 1992–2015—*Continued*

(Numbers in millions; percent; data are based on household interviews of a sample of noninstitutionalized Medicare beneficiaries.)

Characteristic	Medicare fee-for-service only or other[6]					
	1992	1995	2000	2005	2010	2015
Age						
65 years and over (number in millions)	2.9	3.1	3.5	4.3	5.7	4.7
65 years and over (percent of population)	9.9	10.5	11.5	13.3	14.6	10.2
65 to 74 years	9.7	10.7	12.6	14.9	15.5	11.0
75 to 84 years	10.1	9.9	9.9	11.9	13.5	8.8
85 years and over	10.8	11.3	12.1	11.6	13.6	10.0
Sex						
Male	12.2	12.6	13.3	16.2	17.3	11.9
Female	8.3	8.9	10.2	11.2	12.5	8.9
Race and Hispanic Origin						
White, not Hispanic or Latino	7.7	8.7	9.6	12.2	14.2	9.0
Black, not Hispanic or Latino	26.7	25.0	26.1	21.9	18.6	15.4
Hispanic	18.3	17.1	16.7	13.9	12.7	11.7
Percent of Poverty Level[3]						
Below 100 percent	14.3	13.3	15.1	NA	NA	12.8
100 percent to less than 200 percent	12.9	13.1	12.7	NA	NA	14.3
200 percent or more	4.0	4.5	6.3	NA	NA	8.1
Marital Status						
Married	8.5	9.0	10.5	12.1	13.9	8.6
Widowed	11.2	11.9	11.6	13.5	13.7	10.9
Divorced	15.7	15.1	16.1	17.9	19.8	13.8
Never married	*	13.1	16.8	20.4	14.4	14.5

NOTE: Data are for noninstitutionalized Medicare beneficiaries. Insurance categories are mutually exclusive. Persons with more than one type of coverage are categorized according to the order in which the health insurance categories appear in the table. Due to changes in sampling and data collection methodologies, 2014 data are not available.

NA = Not available.

* = Estimates are considered unreliable if the sample cell size is 50 or fewer.

[3]Percent of poverty level is based on family income and family size and composition using U.S. Census Bureau poverty thresholds.

[6]Medicare fee-for-service only or other public plans (except Medicaid).

Table 3-75. Persons Under 65 Years of Age Without Health Insurance Coverage, by State, Territory, and Age, 2009–2016

(Percent; data are based on household interviews of a sample of the civilian noninstitutionalized population in the United States and Puerto Rico.)

Characteristic	2009	2010	2011	2012	2013	2014	2015	2016
Under 65 Years								
United States[1]	17.2	17.6	17.2	16.9	16.7	13.4	10.9	9.9
Alabama	16.0	16.9	16.3	15.4	15.9	14.0	11.9	10.8
Alaska	22.0	19.4	21.7	22.0	20.3	19.2	16.0	15.9
Arizona	19.8	19.5	19.9	20.3	20.3	16.0	13.1	11.8
Arkansas	19.3	20.2	19.7	19.0	18.8	13.8	11.0	9.4
California	20.1	20.7	20.3	20.0	19.3	14.0	9.6	8.4
Colorado	17.4	17.6	17.0	16.3	15.7	11.9	9.2	8.7
Connecticut	10.1	10.3	9.8	10.6	10.8	8.0	7.0	5.7
Delaware	11.9	11.5	10.2	9.9	11.7	8.7	6.5	6.8
District of Columbia	7.8	8.4	8.3	6.1	7.1	6.1	4.0	4.3
Florida	24.8	25.4	25.0	24.0	24.2	20.1	16.2	15.2
Georgia	21.0	21.9	21.8	20.8	21.1	17.8	15.7	14.7
Hawaii	7.9	8.7	8.4	7.7	8.3	5.7	4.5	4.1
Idaho	19.1	20.3	17.8	18.3	18.5	15.4	13.1	12.1
Illinois	14.9	15.7	14.5	14.6	14.4	11.2	8.1	7.5
Indiana	15.8	17.0	16.6	16.6	16.2	13.8	11.4	9.3
Iowa	10.1	10.8	10.4	9.7	10.2	6.7	5.7	4.7
Kansas	14.5	15.6	14.4	14.6	14.3	12.2	10.8	9.7
Kentucky	16.5	17.5	16.6	15.8	16.8	10.2	7.1	6.0
Louisiana	19.5	20.1	19.9	19.0	19.2	16.6	13.9	11.8
Maine	11.9	12.5	13.1	12.4	13.3	11.8	10.4	9.6
Maryland	12.5	12.7	11.5	11.5	11.4	9.0	7.6	6.9
Massachusetts	4.9	4.9	4.8	4.5	4.4	3.9	3.2	2.9
Michigan	14.1	14.3	13.6	13.4	12.8	9.8	7.1	6.3
Minnesota	10.2	10.1	9.9	9.4	9.5	6.8	5.2	4.9
Mississippi	20.0	20.7	20.2	19.7	19.6	16.8	14.7	13.7
Missouri	15.3	15.2	15.7	16.1	15.2	13.5	11.3	10.5
Montana	21.9	19.6	21.8	21.4	19.7	16.2	13.8	10.0
Nebraska	13.1	13.4	13.6	12.7	12.2	10.8	9.1	10.2
Nevada	24.6	25.4	24.7	25.0	23.4	17.5	14.1	12.8
New Hampshire	12.0	12.7	11.4	12.8	12.6	10.9	8.1	7.5
New Jersey	14.2	15.0	14.7	14.5	15.3	12.6	10.1	8.8
New Mexico	23.1	22.8	22.8	21.6	22.2	17.3	12.7	10.6
New York	13.0	13.5	13.0	12.5	12.4	9.9	8.1	7.0
North Carolina	18.2	19.2	18.7	18.9	18.0	15.2	13.1	12.2
North Dakota	11.4	11.5	11.5	12.4	11.9	9.2	9.4	9.4
Ohio	14.0	14.1	13.9	13.4	12.8	9.7	7.5	6.5
Oklahoma	21.3	22.0	21.3	21.1	20.4	17.7	16.5	16.0
Oregon	19.8	19.7	18.0	16.9	17.4	11.5	8.3	7.2
Pennsylvania	11.3	11.9	11.8	11.3	11.3	10.1	7.4	6.9
Rhode Island	12.8	13.7	12.6	13.3	13.9	8.3	6.1	5.0
South Carolina	19.2	20.2	19.4	19.3	18.4	16.0	12.8	11.8
South Dakota	15.6	13.6	13.4	12.3	14.3	11.6	13.1	9.7
Tennessee	16.3	16.4	17.0	16.1	16.2	13.9	12.0	10.7
Texas	26.3	26.3	25.5	24.8	24.5	21.2	19.0	18.6
Utah	15.7	17.0	16.5	15.3	14.7	13.6	11.7	9.4
Vermont	9.9	9.0	8.3	7.7	8.1	5.4	5.0	4.2
Virginia	13.3	14.5	14.1	14.2	14.1	12.4	10.7	10.2
Washington	15.3	16.1	16.0	15.7	16.1	10.5	7.5	6.9
West Virginia	16.7	17.2	18.2	16.9	16.1	10.7	6.6	6.0
Wisconsin	10.4	10.9	10.6	10.6	10.4	8.7	6.7	6.1
Wyoming	17.5	16.6	17.5	18.3	14.6	14.1	12.0	12.6
Puerto Rico[2]	9.4	9.4	8.9	8.5	7.7	7.2	6.7	7.7
Under 18 Years								
United States[1]	8.5	8.0	7.5	7.1	7.1	6.0	4.8	4.4
Alabama	6.1	5.9	5.2	4.0	4.5	3.7	2.7	2.3
Alaska	12.8	9.3	13.9	13.3	11.7	12.3	9.2	10.7
Arizona	12.1	13.0	12.8	12.8	12.1	10.0	8.7	7.5
Arkansas	6.2	6.3	5.5	5.4	5.7	4.5	4.9	3.7
California	9.4	9.0	8.0	8.0	7.3	5.4	3.3	3.0
Colorado	9.8	9.8	9.3	8.1	8.4	6.0	4.1	4.2
Connecticut	3.9	2.9	2.5	3.7	4.1	3.9	3.5	2.5

NOTE: Health insurance estimates are shown for the civilian noninstitutionalized population. Data for 2009 use Census 2000 population controls, and data for 2010 and beyond use Census 2010 population controls. Questions on health insurance coverage ask about current coverage as of the day of American Community Survey (ACS) interview. Persons were considered uninsured if they were not covered by private health insurance, Medicare, Medicaid, Medical Assistance, TRICARE or other military health care, veteran's coverage through the Veteran's Administration, or other government coverage. People with Indian Health Service coverage only are considered uninsured by ACS. Standard errors were computed with replicate weights using 80 balanced repeated replicate weights (BRR) with a Fay-modified BRR adjustment factor of 0.5. Standard errors are available in the spreadsheet version of this table. Available from: https://www.cdc.gov/nchs/hus.htm.
0.0 = Quantity is greater than zero but less than 0.05.
[1]Excludes data for Puerto Rico.
[2]Data for Puerto Rico are collected in the Puerto Rico Community Survey. Data are not collected for the other territories.

Table 3-75. Persons Under 65 Years of Age Without Health Insurance Coverage, by State, Territory, and Age, 2009–2016—Continued

(Percent; data are based on household interviews of a sample of the civilian noninstitutionalized population in the United States and Puerto Rico.)

Characteristic	2009	2010	2011	2012	2013	2014	2015	2016
Delaware	5.7	5.6	3.5	3.6	5.1	*5.0	*2.7	3.7
District of Columbia	*	*2.0	*4.1	*	*2.2	*2.6	*1.5	*
Florida	14.7	12.7	11.9	10.8	11.0	9.2	6.8	6.2
Georgia	10.7	9.8	9.5	8.9	9.5	7.5	7.0	6.4
Hawaii	2.4	3.7	3.9	2.9	3.2	2.0	*1.4	2.1
Idaho	10.7	10.6	8.5	7.6	8.3	7.2	6.0	5.3
Illinois	4.4	4.8	3.4	3.2	4.3	3.8	2.5	2.5
Indiana	8.5	8.9	8.4	8.0	8.4	7.2	7.1	5.6
Iowa	4.4	4.3	4.6	4.3	4.8	3.2	3.3	2.2
Kansas	8.1	7.7	6.1	6.9	6.6	6.1	5.2	4.7
Kentucky	5.8	5.8	5.9	5.9	5.9	4.3	4.4	3.2
Louisiana	6.4	5.6	5.7	5.3	5.6	5.0	3.5	3.3
Maine	5.7	3.8	5.5	4.2	5.1	6.1	6.2	4.7
Maryland	4.7	4.9	4.5	3.8	4.3	3.4	4.2	3.2
Massachusetts	1.7	1.4	1.6	1.3	1.5	1.6	1.2	0.9
Michigan	4.3	4.2	3.9	4.2	4.2	3.6	3.3	2.9
Minnesota	7.0	6.3	6.1	5.7	6.1	3.5	3.2	3.1
Mississippi	10.1	8.2	7.4	7.2	7.3	5.4	4.0	4.3
Missouri	7.2	6.3	6.7	7.2	7.3	6.8	5.8	4.7
Montana	13.4	12.7	12.8	10.9	10.4	8.6	7.4	4.2
Nebraska	6.3	5.2	7.3	5.4	5.9	5.0	4.7	5.4
Nevada	18.0	17.9	16.1	16.5	13.9	9.7	7.6	6.0
New Hampshire	4.6	4.9	3.2	4.2	3.5	5.2	3.2	3.1
New Jersey	6.2	6.0	5.2	5.1	5.7	4.5	3.8	3.1
New Mexico	12.0	9.9	9.1	8.1	9.0	7.6	4.4	5.6
New York	4.8	4.8	4.4	4.0	4.1	3.4	2.5	2.5
North Carolina	7.9	8.1	7.8	7.3	5.9	5.3	4.5	4.3
North Dakota	6.3	6.6	7.6	7.4	7.7	6.7	8.5	9.7
Ohio	6.4	5.9	6.1	5.4	5.1	4.9	4.3	3.4
Oklahoma	11.1	10.4	10.9	9.9	10.5	8.7	8.1	7.0
Oregon	10.8	8.8	7.0	5.6	6.3	4.3	3.4	3.2
Pennsylvania	5.0	5.2	5.4	5.1	5.0	5.4	4.0	4.7
Rhode Island	4.9	4.8	3.9	5.1	6.0	3.3	3.2	*1.7
South Carolina	9.5	9.8	8.7	7.8	7.0	5.2	4.2	3.9
South Dakota	6.8	7.2	5.6	3.9	7.2	7.2	7.2	4.3
Tennessee	5.7	5.3	5.8	5.6	5.7	5.2	4.3	3.5
Texas	16.3	14.7	13.3	12.3	12.5	11.2	9.4	9.2
Utah	10.2	11.1	11.1	9.3	9.0	9.2	7.6	5.3
Vermont	*3.3	*2.7	*	*3.0	*	*	*	*
Virginia	6.7	6.4	5.8	5.6	5.7	5.9	4.9	4.9
Washington	7.0	6.4	6.1	5.5	6.3	4.4	2.8	2.4
West Virginia	5.4	4.7	5.0	3.9	4.0	3.0	2.6	*1.4
Wisconsin	4.6	5.2	4.6	4.7	4.4	4.9	3.6	3.3
Wyoming	9.0	7.4	8.7	9.9	6.3	6.7	6.2	7.6
Puerto Rico[2]	4.2	4.5	4.0	4.3	3.5	3.1	2.7	3.1
18 to 64 Years								
United States[1]	20.6	21.4	21.0	20.6	20.3	16.2	13.1	12.0
Alabama	19.8	21.2	20.5	19.7	20.2	17.9	15.4	14.0
Alaska	25.8	23.6	24.8	25.5	23.9	22.0	18.8	18.0
Arizona	23.3	22.3	22.8	23.4	23.7	18.5	14.8	13.6
Arkansas	24.6	25.8	25.4	24.5	24.0	17.6	13.5	11.6
California	24.5	25.3	25.1	24.7	23.8	17.3	12.0	10.3
Colorado	20.3	20.5	19.9	19.4	18.5	14.0	11.0	10.3
Connecticut	12.4	13.0	12.4	13.1	13.1	9.4	8.2	6.7
Delaware	14.3	13.7	12.7	12.2	14.1	10.1	7.9	7.9
District of Columbia	9.2	9.9	9.3	7.1	8.3	7.0	4.6	4.6
Florida	28.6	29.9	29.5	28.6	28.8	23.8	19.5	18.3
Georgia	25.4	26.9	26.8	25.6	25.8	21.9	19.2	18.0
Hawaii	9.9	10.5	10.1	9.4	10.1	7.1	5.7	4.9
Idaho	22.8	24.7	22.0	23.1	23.1	19.2	16.3	15.1
Illinois	19.0	20.0	18.8	19.0	18.1	13.9	10.1	9.3
Indiana	18.8	20.3	19.8	20.0	19.2	16.4	13.1	10.8
Iowa	12.2	13.3	12.6	11.8	12.3	8.0	6.6	5.7
Kansas	17.1	18.9	17.9	17.8	17.4	14.8	13.1	11.8
Kentucky	20.6	22.0	20.7	19.5	20.8	12.4	8.2	7.0
Louisiana	24.8	25.8	25.6	24.4	24.5	21.2	18.0	15.2
Maine	14.0	15.4	15.5	15.1	15.8	13.7	11.8	11.1

NOTE: Health insurance estimates are shown for the civilian noninstitutionalized population. Data for 2009 use Census 2000 population controls, and data for 2010 and beyond use Census 2010 population controls. Questions on health insurance coverage ask about current coverage as of the day of American Community Survey (ACS) interview. Persons were considered uninsured if they were not covered by private health insurance, Medicare, Medicaid, Medical Assistance, TRICARE or other military health care, veteran's coverage through the Veteran's Administration, or other government coverage. People with Indian Health Service coverage only are considered uninsured by ACS. Standard errors were computed with replicate weights using 80 balanced repeated replicate weights (BRR) with a Fay-modified BRR adjustment factor of 0.5. Standard errors are available in the spreadsheet version of this table. Available from: https://www.cdc.gov/nchs/hus.htm.
*Estimates are considered unreliable. Data preceded by an asterisk have a relative standard error of 20 percent to 30 percent. Data not shown have an RSE greater than 30 percent.
0.0 = Quantity is greater than zero but less than 0.05.
[1]Excludes data for Puerto Rico.
[2]Data for Puerto Rico are collected in the Puerto Rico Community Survey. Data are not collected for the other territories.

Table 3-75. Persons Under 65 Years of Age Without Health Insurance Coverage, by State, Territory, and Age, 2009–2016—*Continued*

(Percent; data are based on household interviews of a sample of the civilian noninstitutionalized population in the United States and Puerto Rico.)

Characteristic	2009	2010	2011	2012	2013	2014	2015	2016
Maryland	15.4	15.5	14.0	14.3	14.0	11.0	8.8	8.3
Massachusetts	5.9	6.1	5.8	5.5	5.3	4.6	3.9	3.5
Michigan	17.8	18.1	17.3	16.8	16.0	12.1	8.5	7.5
Minnesota	11.4	11.6	11.3	10.9	10.8	8.1	5.9	5.6
Mississippi	24.3	26.0	25.6	25.0	24.6	21.4	19.0	17.6
Missouri	18.4	18.7	19.2	19.5	18.2	16.0	13.4	12.7
Montana	25.0	22.1	25.0	25.1	23.0	18.9	16.1	12.2
Nebraska	15.9	16.8	16.2	15.7	14.8	13.1	10.9	12.1
Nevada	27.3	28.4	28.1	28.4	27.1	20.4	16.5	15.3
New Hampshire	14.4	15.3	14.1	15.6	15.6	12.6	9.6	8.9
New Jersey	17.2	18.3	18.2	17.9	18.7	15.5	12.3	10.9
New Mexico	27.8	28.2	28.5	27.2	27.6	21.1	16.1	12.6
New York	16.0	16.6	16.0	15.4	15.2	12.1	10.0	8.5
North Carolina	22.2	23.5	22.9	23.3	22.6	19.0	16.3	15.1
North Dakota	13.2	13.3	12.9	14.1	13.4	10.1	9.7	9.2
Ohio	16.9	17.2	16.8	16.4	15.6	11.5	8.7	7.7
Oklahoma	25.6	26.8	25.6	25.6	24.5	21.4	19.9	19.8
Oregon	23.1	23.6	21.9	20.9	21.2	14.0	9.9	8.6
Pennsylvania	13.6	14.2	14.0	13.4	13.5	11.7	8.6	7.6
Rhode Island	15.5	16.7	15.5	16.0	16.4	9.8	7.0	6.0
South Carolina	23.0	24.2	23.5	23.6	22.5	19.9	15.9	14.7
South Dakota	19.1	16.3	16.6	15.7	17.2	13.4	15.5	12.0
Tennessee	20.4	20.7	21.2	20.0	20.1	17.1	14.9	13.4
Texas	30.9	31.5	30.9	30.4	29.7	25.6	23.1	22.7
Utah	18.6	20.1	19.3	18.4	17.7	16.0	13.8	11.6
Vermont	12.0	11.1	10.3	9.2	9.6	6.8	6.2	5.2
Virginia	15.8	17.4	17.1	17.3	17.1	14.7	12.8	12.1
Washington	18.4	19.7	19.6	19.4	19.8	12.7	9.2	8.5
West Virginia	20.5	21.5	22.7	21.2	20.2	13.3	8.0	7.5
Wisconsin	12.5	13.1	12.8	12.8	12.7	10.1	7.8	7.1
Wyoming	20.7	20.2	20.7	21.5	17.8	16.9	14.2	14.6
Puerto Rico[2]	11.5	11.3	10.9	10.0	9.2	8.7	8.2	9.2

NOTE: Health insurance estimates are shown for the civilian noninstitutionalized population. Data for 2009 use Census 2000 population controls, and data for 2010 and beyond use Census 2010 population controls. Questions on health insurance coverage ask about current coverage as of the day of American Community Survey (ACS) interview. Persons were considered uninsured if they were not covered by private health insurance, Medicare, Medicaid, Medical Assistance, TRICARE or other military health care, veteran's coverage through the Veteran's Administration, or other government coverage. People with Indian Health Service coverage only are considered uninsured by ACS. Standard errors were computed with replicate weights using 80 balanced repeated replicate weights (BRR) with a Fay-modified BRR adjustment factor of 0.5. Standard errors are available in the spreadsheet version of this table. Available from: https://www.cdc.gov/nchs/hus.htm.
0.0 = Quantity is greater than zero but less than 0.05.
[2]Data for Puerto Rico are collected in the Puerto Rico Community Survey. Data are not collected for the other territories.

Table 3-76. Medicaid Coverage Among Persons Under 65 Years of Age, by Selected Characteristics, Selected Years, 1984–2016

(Numbers in millions; percent; data are based on household interviews of a sample of the civilian noninstitutionalized population.)

Characteristic	1984[1]	1989[1]	1995[1]	2000[2]	2005[3]	2006[3]	2007[3]	2008[3]	2009[3]	2010[3]	2011[3]	2012[3]	2013[3]	2014[3]	2015[3]	2016[3]
Total (number in millions)[4]	14.0	15.4	26.6	23.2	33.2	36.2	36.2	38.4	42.4	44.8	47.4	48.1	48.5	52.6	55.4	57.0
Total (percent of population)[4]	6.8	7.2	11.5	9.5	12.9	14.0	13.9	14.7	16.1	16.9	17.8	18.0	18.1	19.6	20.6	21.1
Age																
Under 19 years	11.7	12.2	21.1	19.2	26.6	29.4	29.3	30.6	33.9	35.7	37.5	38.1	38.1	38.6	39.2	38.8
Under 6 years	15.5	15.7	29.3	24.7	34.0	36.6	36.6	38.1	41.4	43.7	46.1	45.7	45.9	43.8	44.2	44.0
6 to 18 years	9.8	10.5	17.0	16.8	23.3	26.1	25.9	27.1	30.3	31.8	33.4	34.7	34.6	36.3	36.9	36.5
Under 18 years	11.9	12.6	21.5	19.6	27.2	29.9	29.8	31.3	34.5	36.4	38.2	38.9	38.9	39.4	39.9	39.6
6 to 17 years	10.1	10.9	17.4	17.2	23.9	26.7	26.4	27.9	30.9	32.5	34.1	35.5	35.5	37.3	37.9	37.4
18 to 64 years	4.5	4.9	7.1	5.2	7.2	7.7	7.5	8.1	8.9	9.2	9.9	10.0	10.2	12.1	13.2	14.1
18 to 44 years	5.1	5.2	7.8	5.6	8.3	8.6	8.7	9.2	10.3	10.9	11.6	11.6	11.6	13.8	15.0	16.0
18 to 24 years	6.4	6.8	10.4	8.1	11.3	11.4	11.4	12.2	14.0	14.5	15.2	15.4	14.2	17.9	18.5	19.7
19 to 25 years	6.3	6.6	10.2	7.3	10.3	9.7	9.9	10.6	12.2	12.6	13.4	13.4	12.1	16.1	16.3	18.4
25 to 34 years	5.3	5.2	8.2	5.5	8.0	8.3	8.5	9.3	10.1	11.1	11.5	11.4	11.7	13.3	14.7	16.0
35 to 44 years	3.5	4.0	5.9	4.3	6.6	7.1	7.0	7.1	7.7	8.1	9.0	8.8	9.6	11.3	12.8	13.1
45 to 64 years	3.4	4.3	5.6	4.5	5.5	6.3	5.9	6.4	6.9	6.8	7.5	8.0	8.4	9.9	10.8	11.6
45 to 54 years	3.2	3.8	5.1	4.2	5.2	6.4	6.0	6.2	7.0	7.0	8.0	8.2	8.6	9.8	11.2	11.8
55 to 64 years	3.6	4.9	6.4	4.9	5.8	6.1	5.7	6.8	6.8	6.6	6.9	7.7	8.2	9.9	10.4	11.4
Sex																
Male	5.4	5.7	9.6	8.2	11.6	12.6	12.5	13.4	14.4	15.2	16.3	16.3	16.5	17.8	19.1	19.4
Female	8.1	8.6	13.4	10.8	14.3	15.5	15.2	15.9	17.8	18.5	19.3	19.7	19.8	21.4	22.0	22.7
Sex and Marital Status[5]																
Male																
Married	1.9	1.8	2.9	2.2	3.5	3.7	3.5	3.6	4.1	4.0	4.9	4.8	5.3	6.2	7.0	7.3
Divorced, separated, widowed	4.9	5.4	7.7	6.1	7.0	7.9	7.8	8.1	8.3	9.3	9.8	9.7	10.3	12.0	12.6	15.3
Never married	4.8	5.6	8.1	7.2	10.4	11.6	11.3	12.1	13.1	13.5	14.5	15.1	14.8	17.6	19.6	20.0
Female																
Married	2.6	3.0	5.2	3.1	4.7	4.6	4.7	5.2	5.3	5.7	6.4	6.2	6.9	8.1	8.8	8.8
Divorced, separated, widowed	16.0	16.1	19.0	12.7	14.6	16.2	16.3	17.2	18.7	17.6	18.0	18.8	18.8	21.6	23.3	24.5
Never married	10.7	11.9	16.5	13.2	17.3	19.0	18.1	18.7	20.9	22.2	21.9	22.6	22.2	24.9	25.7	27.8
Race[6]																
White only	4.6	5.1	8.9	7.1	11.0	11.8	11.4	12.1	13.7	14.5	15.4	15.5	15.6	16.9	17.9	18.7
Black or African American only	20.5	19.0	28.5	21.2	24.9	26.6	27.7	28.3	29.5	30.4	30.9	31.6	31.6	34.1	34.3	33.8
American Indian or Alaska Native only	*28.2	29.7	19.0	15.1	24.2	24.3	21.2	37.0	29.7	21.6	29.0	36.5	32.0	35.5	34.3	32.1
Asian only	*8.7	*8.8	10.5	7.5	8.2	9.7	8.7	9.2	9.9	12.0	14.7	13.0	13.2	14.7	16.5	15.9
Native Hawaiian or Other Pacific Islander only	NA	NA	NA	*	*	*	*	*	*	*	*	*	*	*	*	27.4
Two or more races	NA	NA	NA	19.1	22.0	24.0	27.9	24.7	30.1	27.4	27.2	29.1	30.4	30.2	31.5	30.7
Hispanic Origin and Race[6]																
Hispanic or Latino	13.3	13.5	21.9	15.5	22.9	23.1	24.7	24.9	27.6	28.6	30.1	30.5	29.5	31.3	33.5	33.6
Mexican	12.2	12.4	21.6	14.0	23.0	23.0	25.9	25.4	28.4	29.5	31.0	31.0	29.8	32.1	34.2	35.2
Puerto Rican	31.5	27.3	33.4	29.4	31.9	35.7	28.0	31.0	32.1	35.7	33.0	35.3	36.9	35.7	38.9	38.9
Cuban	*4.8	*7.7	13.4	9.2	17.7	*11.3	13.3	13.0	16.7	17.3	20.0	22.9	23.3	22.4	22.8	24.3
Other Hispanic or Latino	7.9	11.1	18.2	14.5	19.7	20.2	21.4	22.3	24.6	24.5	27.7	28.3	27.0	28.6	30.7	28.8
Not Hispanic or Latino	6.2	6.5	10.2	8.5	11.1	12.3	11.7	12.6	13.7	14.4	15.2	15.2	15.5	16.9	17.5	18.0
White only	3.7	4.1	7.1	6.1	8.5	9.5	8.5	9.2	10.4	11.0	11.8	11.5	11.9	13.0	13.6	14.2
Black or African American only	20.7	19.0	28.1	21.0	24.8	26.2	27.3	27.9	29.1	30.0	30.5	31.3	31.3	33.4	33.6	33.5
Age and Percent of Poverty Level[7]																
Under 65 years																
Below 100 percent	33.0	37.6	48.4	38.4	45.7	45.8	47.6	49.1	51.2	50.8	51.4	52.5	53.7	56.5	60.6	59.4
100 percent to 199 percent	5.3	7.5	14.4	16.2	23.4	23.8	26.1	27.4	29.0	28.5	30.6	30.1	30.8	34.0	38.1	41.4
100 percent to 133 percent	8.7	11.9	23.1	22.4	30.6	30.8	34.8	36.1	39.3	36.3	38.8	38.0	38.8	43.9	47.6	49.4
134 percent to 199 percent	3.7	5.6	9.7	13.1	19.5	20.0	21.7	22.9	23.6	24.4	26.1	25.5	26.2	28.1	32.6	36.9
200 percent to 399 percent	0.8	1.3	2.3	4.0	6.6	7.0	6.8	7.8	8.0	8.4	8.9	9.0	9.0	9.9	11.3	12.8
400 percent or more	0.2	0.5	0.4	0.9	1.5	1.7	1.5	1.6	1.7	2.0	1.7	1.7	1.9	2.2	2.2	2.7
Under 19 years																
Below 100 percent	42.0	45.8	63.5	56.9	69.4	70.4	72.7	73.4	77.5	78.4	79.9	82.1	82.1	83.3	84.8	82.1
100 percent to 199 percent	6.5	8.6	21.3	27.8	41.7	44.1	47.2	48.5	52.7	53.5	56.7	56.3	58.9	59.1	61.9	64.8
100 percent to 133 percent	10.3	13.4	32.4	36.4	51.0	51.3	57.5	60.0	65.6	63.5	69.1	68.8	70.3	71.7	70.9	74.2
134 percent to 199 percent	4.7	6.3	14.3	23.3	36.2	39.4	41.3	42.3	45.3	47.7	49.9	48.8	51.6	50.6	55.9	59.2
200 percent to 399 percent	1.0	*1.7	3.5	7.6	13.0	13.5	13.3	16.4	16.4	17.7	18.3	18.8	19.1	18.5	20.9	21.9
400 percent or more	*	*1.2	*	2.1	2.9	3.5	3.0	3.5	3.6	4.3	3.5	3.6	3.2	3.8	4.3	4.9

NOTE: The category Medicaid coverage includes persons who had any of the following at the time of interview: Medicaid, other public assistance (through 1996), state-sponsored health plan (starting in 1997), or Children's Health Insurance Program [(CHIP) starting in 1999]; it includes those who also had another type of coverage in addition to one of these. In 2016, 19.2% of persons under age 65 reported being covered by Medicaid, 0.8% by state-sponsored health plans, and 1.1% by CHIP. Estimates may not sum to total because of rounding. The number of persons with Medicaid coverage was calculated by multiplying the percentage with Medicaid coverage by the number of persons under age 65 in the civilian noninstitutionalized U.S. population, which was determined from the poststratification Census control total for each survey year. Percentages of persons with Medicaid coverage were calculated with unknown values excluded from denominators.
NA = Not available.
* = Estimates are considered unreliable. Starting with 2016 data, the reliability of survey percentage estimates was assessed using new multistep National Center for Health Statistics data presentation standards for proportions. Prior to 2016 data, the reliability of estimates for earlier years was evaluated based on relative standard errors (RSE). Data not shown have an RSE greater than 30%.
[1]Any private health insurance coverage (both individual and insurance obtained through the workplace) at the time of interview; includes those who had other types of coverage in addition to their private coverage.
[2]Data prior to 1997 are not strictly comparable with data for later years due to the 1997 questionnaire redesign.
[3]Beginning in quarter 3 of the 2004 NHIS, persons under age 65 with no reported coverage were asked explicitly about Medicaid coverage. Estimates were calculated without and with the additional information from this question in the columns labeled 2004(1) and 2004(2) (in spreadsheet version), respectively, and estimates were calculated with the additional information starting with 2005 data.
[4]Includes all other races not shown separately, those with unknown marital status, unknown disability status, and, in 1984 and 1989, persons with unknown poverty level.
[5]Includes persons 14 to 64 years of age.
[6]The race groups White, Black, American Indian or Alaska Native, Asian, Native Hawaiian or Other Pacific Islander, and 2 or more races include persons of Hispanic and non-Hispanic origin. Persons of Hispanic origin may be of any race. Starting with 1999 data, race-specific estimates are tabulated according to the 1997 Revisions to the Standards for the Classification of Federal Data on Race and Ethnicity and are not strictly comparable with estimates for earlier years. The five single-race categories and multiple-race categories shown in the table conform to the 1997 Standards. Starting with 1999 data, race-specific estimates are for persons who reported only one racial group; the category 2 or more races includes persons who reported more than one racial group. Prior to 1999, data were tabulated according to the 1977 Standards with four racial groups, and the Asian only category included Native Hawaiian or Other Pacific Islander. Estimates for single-race categories prior to 1999 included persons who reported one race, or if they reported more than one race, identified one race as best representing their race. Starting with 2003 data, race responses of other race and unspecified multiple race were treated as missing, and then race was imputed if these were the only race responses. Almost all persons with a race response of other race were of Hispanic origin.
[7]Percent of poverty level is based on family income and family size and composition using U.S. Census Bureau poverty thresholds. Poverty level was unknown for 10%–11% of persons under age 65 in 1984 and 1989. Missing family income data were imputed for 1995 and beyond.

Table 3-76. Medicaid Coverage Among Persons Under 65 Years of Age, by Selected Characteristics, Selected Years, 1984–2016—Continued

(Numbers in millions; percent; data are based on household interviews of a sample of the civilian noninstitutionalized population.)

Characteristic	1984¹	1989¹	1995¹	2000²	2005³	2006³	2007³	2008³	2009³	2010³	2011³	2012³	2013³	2014³	2015³	2016³
Under 18 years																
Below 100 percent	43.3	47.8	66.0	58.5	71.2	72.0	75.0	75.3	78.3	79.8	81.4	83.7	83.9	84.7	86.7	85.4
100 percent to 199 percent	6.6	8.7	21.6	28.4	42.5	44.7	48.1	49.5	53.5	54.3	57.6	57.3	60.1	60.0	62.6	65.3
100 percent to 133 percent	10.4	13.5	32.9	36.9	52.0	51.7	58.4	61.1	66.9	64.6	70.1	70.1	71.2	72.3	72.0	74.4
134 percent to 199 percent	4.8	6.4	14.4	23.8	36.9	40.1	42.2	43.2	45.9	48.2	50.6	49.6	52.9	51.6	56.5	59.9
200 percent to 399 percent	1.0	1.7	3.5	7.6	13.3	13.8	13.3	16.8	16.8	18.0	18.6	19.1	19.5	18.9	21.2	22.0
400 percent or more	*	*1.1	*	2.2	2.9	3.4	3.0	3.6	3.7	4.3	3.6	3.6	3.3	4.0	4.3	5.0
18 to 64 years																
Below 100 percent	25.3	29.1	34.8	24.9	29.6	28.9	30.6	33.0	33.6	32.4	33.0	34.0	35.4	39.7	44.8	44.6
100 percent to 199 percent	4.5	6.8	10.2	9.1	13.1	13.0	14.0	15.3	16.2	15.7	17.1	16.8	17.1	21.4	25.9	29.1
100 percent to 133 percent	7.6	10.8	16.3	13.2	17.9	17.8	20.2	21.9	23.7	21.0	22.7	21.8	22.0	28.3	34.2	35.8
134 percent to 199 percent	3.1	5.1	7.2	7.2	10.7	10.5	11.0	11.8	12.4	13.0	14.1	13.9	14.4	17.6	21.3	25.4
200 percent to 399 percent	0.7	1.1	1.7	2.4	3.8	4.2	4.0	4.1	4.6	4.8	5.2	5.1	5.1	6.7	7.6	9.2
400 percent or more	0.2	0.4	0.4	0.6	1.1	1.2	1.1	1.1	1.2	1.3	1.2	1.2	1.6	1.7	1.7	2.1
Level of Difficulty⁶																
18 to 64 years																
A lot of difficulty or cannot do at all	NA	NA	NA	NA	NA	NA	NA	NA	NA	27.3	30.3	29.7	30.3	33.1	36.1	34.8
Some difficulty	NA	NA	NA	NA	NA	NA	NA	NA	NA	9.4	14.2	12.5	12.4	13.7	14.7	16.6
No difficulty	NA	NA	NA	NA	NA	NA	NA	NA	NA	6.8	7.7	8.3	7.2	9.6	10.7	12.0
Geographic Region																
Northeast	8.6	6.6	11.7	10.6	13.3	16.8	15.4	16.1	17.3	17.9	19.6	19.3	20.8	21.4	21.6	22.7
Midwest	7.4	7.6	10.5	8.0	12.3	13.9	13.7	14.5	16.4	17.3	16.7	16.3	16.9	18.6	19.8	19.3
South	5.1	6.5	11.3	9.4	12.7	12.9	12.9	13.5	14.8	16.0	17.3	17.8	17.8	18.7	19.8	19.3
West	7.0	8.5	12.9	10.4	13.8	13.8	14.5	15.7	16.8	17.1	18.4	19.1	18.0	20.9	24.0	24.0
Location of Residence																
Within MSA⁹	7.1	7.0	11.3	8.9	12.4	13.3	13.3	14.2	15.2	16.1	17.0	17.4	17.4	18.9	19.8	20.4
Outside MSA⁹	6.1	7.9	12.3	11.9	15.5	17.7	17.1	17.2	20.8	21.4	22.1	21.4	22.5	24.4	25.4	25.5

NOTE: The category Medicaid coverage includes persons who had any of the following at the time of interview: Medicaid, other public assistance (through 1996), state-sponsored health plan (starting in 1997), or Children's Health Insurance Program [(CHIP) starting in 1999]; it includes those who also had another type of coverage in addition to one of these. In 2016, 19.2% of persons under age 65 reported being covered by Medicaid, 0.8% by state-sponsored health plans, and 1.1% by CHIP. Estimates may not sum to total because of rounding. The number of persons with Medicaid coverage was calculated by multiplying the percentage with Medicaid coverage by the number of persons under age 65 in the civilian noninstitutionalized U.S. population, which was determined from the poststratification Census control total for each survey year. Percentages of persons with Medicaid coverage were calculated with unknown values excluded from denominators.

NA = Not available.

* = Estimates are considered unreliable. Starting with 2016 data, the reliability of survey percentage estimates was assessed using new multistep National Center for Health Statistics data presentation standards for proportions. Prior to 2016 data, the reliability of estimates for earlier years was evaluated based on relative standard errors (RSE). Data not shown have an RSE greater than 30%.

¹Any private health insurance coverage (both individual and insurance obtained through the workplace) at the time of interview; includes those who had other types of coverage in addition to their private coverage.

²Data prior to 1997 are not strictly comparable with data for later years due to the 1997 questionnaire redesign.

³Beginning in quarter 3 of the 2004 NHIS, persons under age 65 with no reported coverage were asked explicitly about Medicaid coverage. Estimates were calculated without and with the additional information from this question in the columns labeled 2004(1) and 2004(2) (in spreadsheet version), respectively, and estimates were calculated with the additional information starting with 2005 data.

⁶Functional limitation is defined by the reported level of difficulty in six functioning domains: seeing (even if wearing glasses), hearing (even if wearing hearing aids), mobility (walking or climbing stairs), communication (understanding or being understood by others), cognition (remembering or concentrating), and self-care (such as washing all over or dressing). Respondents with answers to one or more of the six questions were included in one of three mutually exclusive categories. Those responding "A lot of difficulty" or "Cannot do at all/unable to do" to at least one question were classified in the "A lot of difficulty/cannot do" category. Of the remaining, those responding "Some difficulty" to at least one question were classified in the "Some difficulty" category, and those responding "No difficulty" to at least one question were classified in the "No difficulty" category. Those responding "Don't know" or "Refused" on all six questions were excluded. During 2010–2016, 1%–8% of respondents were missing data and excluded.

⁹MSA = metropolitan statistical area. Starting with 2016 data, MSA status is determined using 2010 Census data and the 2010 standards for defining MSAs.

Table 3-77. Medicaid Beneficiaries and Payments, by Basis of Eligibility, and Race and Hispanic Origin, Selected Fiscal Years, 1999–2013

(Number, percent, dollar.)

Characteristic	1999	2000	2005	2007	2008	2009	2010	2011[1]	2012[1]	2013[1]
Beneficiaries (Number in Millions)[2]										
All beneficiaries	40.1	42.8	57.7	56.8	58.8	62.6	65.7	71.4	71.6	73.7
Percent of Beneficiaries										
Basis of eligibility										
Aged (65 years and over)	9.4	8.7	7.6	7.1	7.1	6.7	6.5	5.7	5.7	5.6
Blind and disabled	16.7	16.1	14.2	14.8	14.8	14.4	14.3	13.1	13.2	13.0
Adults in families with dependent children[3]	18.7	20.5	21.8	21.8	22.0	23.1	23.7	18.9	19.5	19.0
Children under age 21[4]	46.9	46.1	47.2	48.4	47.8	47.7	48.3	40.5	40.6	40.4
Other Title XIX[5]	8.4	8.6	9.1	7.8	8.4	8.1	7.2	9.6	8.7	9.8
Separate CHIP[6]	NA	NA	NA	NA	NA	NA	NA	12.2	12.3	12.1
Race and Hispanic Origin[7]										
White	NA	NA	39.3	38.6	38.1	38.2	38.9	37.2	37.2	36.1
Black or African American	NA	NA	21.5	21.6	21.1	20.7	20.6	19.8	20.1	19.5
American Indian or Alaska Native	NA	NA	1.2	1.2	1.3	1.2	1.2	1.1	1.1	1.1
Asian or Pacific Islander	NA	NA	3.5	3.5	3.5	3.6	3.6	3.6	3.8	3.8
Asian	NA	NA	2.5	2.6	2.6	2.7	2.7	2.8	2.9	3.0
Pacific Islander	NA	NA	0.9	0.9	0.9	0.9	0.9	0.9	0.8	0.8
Hispanic or Latino	NA	NA	20.6	21.6	21.7	22.3	22.3	17.4	17.4	17.4
Multiple race or unknown	NA	NA	13.9	13.5	14.3	14.0	13.3	20.9	20.4	22.0
Payments (Billions of Dollars)[8]										
All payments	$153.5	$168.3	$274.9	$276.2	$296.8	$326.0	$339.0	$368.6	$363.9	$375.3
Percent Distribution	100.0	100.0	100.0	100.0	100.0	100.0	100.0	100.0	100.0	100.0
Basis of eligibility										
Aged (65 years and over)	27.7	26.4	23.1	20.7	20.6	19.7	19.4	16.6	16.7	16.7
Blind and disabled	42.9	43.2	43.4	43.3	43.5	43.4	43.4	40.8	41.2	41.0
Adults in families with dependent children[3]	10.3	10.6	11.8	12.4	12.7	13.9	14.2	12.6	13.3	13.1
Children under age 21[4]	15.7	15.9	17.2	19.4	19.2	19.6	19.8	18.1	18.2	18.4
Other Title XIX[5]	3.4	3.9	4.6	4.2	4.0	3.3	3.1	4.5	3.5	3.5
Separate CHIP[6]	NA	NA	NA	NA	NA	NA	NA	7.4	7.2	7.4
Race and Hispanic Origin[5]										
White	NA	NA	53.0	50.7	50.2	50.0	50.2	48.1	48.3	47.5
Black or African American	NA	NA	19.8	20.8	20.6	20.7	20.5	20.3	20.8	20.3
American Indian or Alaska Native	NA	NA	1.2	1.2	1.3	1.2	1.3	1.2	1.3	1.3
Asian or Pacific Islander	NA	NA	2.7	2.8	2.9	3.1	3.0	3.1	3.2	3.5
Asian	NA	NA	1.9	2.0	2.1	2.3	2.3	2.4	2.5	2.7
Pacific Islander	NA	NA	0.8	0.8	0.8	0.8	0.7	0.7	0.7	0.7
Hispanic or Latino	NA	NA	12.2	13.1	13.7	14.2	14.2	9.9	9.7	10.1
Multiple race or unknown	NA	NA	11.1	11.4	11.4	10.8	10.8	17.4	16.7	17.4
Payments per Beneficiary (Dollars)[6]										
All beneficiaries	$3,819	$3,936	$4,768	$4,862	$5,051	$5,209	$5,160	$5,159	$5,082	$5,094
Basis of eligibility										
Aged (65 years and over)	11,268	11,929	14,427	14,141	14,742	15,337	15,286	15,073	14,862	15,194
Blind and disabled	9,832	10,559	14,531	14,194	14,843	15,670	15,695	16,104	15,825	16,115
Adults in families with dependent children[3]	2,104	2,030	2,583	2,753	2,912	3,144	3,095	3,443	3,460	3,503
Children under age 21[4]	1,282	1,358	1,732	1,951	2,035	2,145	2,122	2,300	2,281	2,315
Other Title XIX[5]	1,532	1,778	2,380	2,622	2,407	2,104	2,219	2,402	2,030	1,803
Separate CHIP[6]	NA	NA	NA	NA	NA	NA	NA	3,125	2,979	3,083
Race and Hispanic Origin[7]										
White	NA	NA	6,422	6,390	6,657	6,809	6,663	6,677	6,598	6,691
Black or African American	NA	NA	4,397	4,669	4,928	5,216	5,142	5,308	5,266	5,314
American Indian or Alaska Native	NA	NA	4,626	4,826	5,218	5,382	5,421	5,461	5,649	5,824
Asian or Pacific Islander	NA	NA	3,710	3,863	4,133	4,402	4,300	4,483	4,365	4,585
Asian	NA	NA	3,624	3,847	4,123	4,386	4,307	4,482	4,383	4,575
Pacific Islander	NA	NA	3,947	3,907	4,161	4,448	4,275	4,484	4,302	4,624
Hispanic or Latino	NA	NA	2,822	2,960	3,175	3,322	3,276	2,944	2,821	2,958
Multiple race or unknown	NA	NA	3,816	4,106	4,014	4,025	4,173	4,298	4,161	4,025

NOTE: Data are for fiscal years ending September 30.
NA = Not available.
[1]Starting with 2011, a new tabular methodology was used. Therefore, estimates may not be comparable to earlier data and caution should be used with trend analysis.
[2]Beneficiaries include those who were enrolled or received services through Medicaid or the Children's Health Insurance Program (CHIP). Beneficiary counts for 2011 and subsequent years were derived from MSIS claims files. Separate CHIP beneficiaries are included for 2011 and subsequent years.
[3]Includes adults who meet the requirements for the Aid to Families with Dependent Children (AFDC) program that were in effect in their state on July 16, 1996, or, at state option, meet more liberal criteria (with some exceptions). Includes adults in the Temporary Assistance for Needy Families (TANF) program. Starting with 2001 data, includes women in the Breast and Cervical Cancer Prevention and Treatment Program and unemployed adults.
[4]Includes children (including those in the foster care system) in the TANF program.
[5]Includes some participants in the Supplemental Security Income program and other people deemed medically needy in participating states. Prior to 2001, includes unemployed adults. Excludes foster care children and includes unknown eligibility.
[6]CHIP is Children's Health Insurance Program. CHIP provides federal funds for states to provide health care coverage to eligible low-income, uninsured children who do not qualify for Medicaid. Some states use CHIP funds to expand Medicaid. For 2012 data, all states except Colorado and Idaho had separate CHIP benefciaries.
[7]Race and Hispanic origin are determined on initial Medicaid application. Categories are mutually exclusive. Starting with 2001 data, the Hispanic category included Hispanic persons, regardless of race. Persons indicating more than one race were included in the multiple race category.
[8]Medicaid payments exclude disproportionate share hospital (DSH) payments ($14.7 billion in FY2010) and DSH mental health facility payments ($2.9 billion in FY2010).

Table 3-78. Medicaid Beneficiaries and Payments, by Type of Service, Selected Fiscal Years, 1999–2013

(Number; percent.)

Type of service	1999	2000	2005	2007	2008	2009	2010	2011[1]	2012[1]	2013[1]
Beneficiaries (Number in Millions)[2]										
All beneficiaries	40.2	42.8	57.7	56.8	58.8	62.6	65.7	71.4	71.6	73.7
Percent										
Inpatient hospital	11.2	11.5	9.5	9.0	8.9	8.7	6.9	11.4	11.8	12.5
Mental health facility	0.2	0.2	0.2	0.2	0.2	0.2	0.2	0.2	0.2	0.2
Intermediate care facility for individuals with intellectual disabilities[3]	0.3	0.3	0.2	0.2	0.2	0.2	0.2	0.1	0.1	0.1
Nursing facility	4.0	4.0	3.0	2.9	2.7	2.6	2.4	2.5	2.3	2.3
Physician	45.7	44.7	42.0	38.8	36.9	36.9	36.9	62.6	64.4	65.5
Dental	14.0	13.8	16.2	16.8	16.7	17.8	19.1	26.6	27.4	28.3
Other practitioner	9.9	11.1	10.2	9.5	8.8	8.8	9.2	13.6	14.2	14.3
Outpatient hospital	30.9	30.9	28.2	26.2	25.2	26.4	24.2	38.8	39.5	40.1
Clinic	16.8	17.9	20.7	20.6	20.2	20.6	20.7	24.4	23.6	23.9
Laboratory and radiological	25.4	26.6	27.7	27.8	26.6	26.2	25.8	41.6	42.0	42.5
Home health	2.0	2.3	2.1	2.1	1.9	1.7	1.7	2.4	2.5	2.4
Prescribed drugs	49.4	48.0	49.2	42.1	41.8	42.6	44.7	56.8	57.2	57.5
Capitated care	51.5	49.7	58.1	64.5	64.9	66.6	70.8	93.6	86.9	88.4
Primary care case management	9.7	13.0	15.1	12.5	14.9	13.1	13.3	13.3	13.6	11.4
Personal support	10.1	10.6	11.8	11.6	10.8	10.7	11.0	1.7	1.7	1.6
Other care[4]	21.6	21.4	21.9	21.5	21.3	20.6	19.9	47.6	47.9	49.3
Payments (Billions of Dollars)[5]										
All payments	$153.5	$168.3	$274.9	$276.2	$296.8	$326.0	$339.0	$368.6	$363.9	$375.3
Percent Distribution	100.0	100.0	100.0	100.0	100.0	100.0	100.0	100.0	100.0	100.0
Inpatient hospital	14.5	14.4	12.8	13.4	12.5	11.8	9.9	10.7	10.3	9.5
Mental health facility	1.1	1.1	0.8	0.9	0.8	0.8	0.7	0.7	0.6	0.6
Intermediate care facility for individuals with intellectual disabilities[3]	6.1	5.6	4.3	4.3	4.2	3.9	3.7	3.6	3.3	3.1
Nursing facility	21.7	20.5	16.3	16.8	16.1	14.9	14.4	13.1	13.0	12.5
Physician	4.3	4.0	4.1	3.6	3.5	3.5	3.5	3.3	3.0	2.8
Dental	0.8	0.8	1.1	1.2	1.3	1.4	1.6	1.6	1.3	1.0
Other practitioner	0.3	0.4	0.4	0.3	0.3	0.3	0.3	0.5	0.5	0.5
Outpatient hospital	4.0	4.2	3.6	3.7	3.7	3.7	3.8	3.5	3.5	3.3
Clinic	3.8	3.7	3.2	3.1	3.1	3.1	3.2	3.4	3.2	3.3
Laboratory and radiological	0.8	0.8	1.1	1.1	1.0	1.0	1.0	1.0	0.8	0.8
Home health	1.9	1.9	2.0	2.3	2.2	2.2	2.1	2.0	1.8	1.7
Prescribed drugs	10.8	11.9	15.6	8.0	7.9	7.8	8.0	7.9	6.1	4.9
Capitated care	14.0	14.5	16.9	21.2	23.0	25.5	27.2	29.5	33.6	37.8
Primary care case management	0.3	0.1	0.1	0.1	0.1	0.1	0.1	0.1	0.1	0.1
Personal support	6.9	6.9	7.5	8.4	8.3	8.0	7.7	3.3	3.3	3.0
Other care[4]	8.6	8.8	10.2	11.6	12.0	11.9	12.7	15.9	15.6	15.0
Payments per Beneficiary (Dollars)[5]										
All beneficiaries	$3,819	$3,936	$4,768	$4,862	$5,051	$5,209	$5,160	$5,159	$5,082	$5,094
Inpatient hospital	4,943	4,919	6,411	7,191	7,083	7,070	7,347	4,858	4,437	3,885
Mental health facility	18,094	17,800	19,252	21,407	21,975	21,404	20,782	14,557	13,221	12,691
Intermediate care facility for individuals with intellectual disabilities[3]	76,443	79,330	107,028	113,735	123,053	127,837	125,851	129,806	119,903	120,995
Nursing facility	20,568	20,220	26,185	28,282	29,533	29,551	31,617	26,995	28,060	27,808
Physician	357	356	465	457	485	496	492	271	238	219
Dental	214	238	326	340	389	423	432	301	245	181
Other practitioner	118	139	200	170	171	171	190	186	183	173
Outpatient hospital	491	533	617	695	736	735	803	470	454	424
Clinic	860	805	749	741	772	792	791	712	680	709
Laboratory and radiological	114	113	183	185	188	198	205	119	102	91
Home health	3,571	3,135	4,487	5,334	5,789	6,628	6,375	4,286	3,565	3,581
Prescribed drugs	837	975	1,509	926	957	951	926	719	540	432
Capitated care	1,040	1,148	1,386	1,598	1,786	1,991	1,983	1,627	1,964	2,178
Primary care case management	119	30	27	33	32	41	49	45	47	50
Personal support	2,583	2,543	3,035	3,534	3,852	3,903	3,593	9,959	9,619	9,588
Other care[4]	1,508	1,600	2,228	2,611	2,856	3,015	3,289	1,724	1,653	1,554

[1]Starting with 2011, a new tabular methodology was used. Therefore, estimates may not be comparable to earlier data and caution should be used with trend analysis.
[2]Beneficiaries include those who were enrolled or received services through Medicaid or the Children's Health Insurance Program (CHIP). Separate CHIP beneficiaries are included for 2011 and subsequent years.
[3]This category was previously known as Intermediate care facility for the mentally retarded. This is a change in terminology only and not measurement.
[4]Estimates for 2010 and earlier include unknown services and payments with Other care.
[5]Medicaid payment data for 2010 and earlier exclude disproportionate share hospital (DSH)payments ($14.7 billion in FY2010) and DSH mental health facility payments ($2.9 billion in FY2010).

Table 3-79. Medicare Enrollees and Expenditures and Percent Distribution, by Medicare Program and Type of Service, Selected Years, 1970–2015

(Number; dollars; percent.)

Medicare program and type of service	1970	1980	1990	1995	2000	2005	2008	2009	2010	2011	2012	2013	2014	2015[1]
Enrollees (Numbers in Millions)														
Total Medicare[2]	20.4	28.4	34.3	37.6	39.7	42.6	45.5	46.6	47.7	48.9	50.9	52.5	54.1	55.3
Hospital insurance	20.1	28.0	33.7	37.2	39.3	42.2	45.1	46.3	47.4	48.5	50.5	52.1	53.7	54.9
Supplementary medical insurance (SMI)[3]	19.5	27.3	32.6	35.6	37.3	NA	NA	NA	NA	NA	NA	NA	NA	NA
Part B	19.5	27.3	32.6	35.6	37.3	39.8	42.0	42.9	43.9	44.9	46.5	48.0	49.4	50.7
Part D[4]	NA	NA	NA	NA	NA	1.8	32.6	33.6	34.8	35.7	37.4	39.1	40.5	41.8
Expenditures (Dollars in Billions)	$7.5	$36.8	$111.0	$184.2	$221.8	$336.4	$468.2	$509.0	$522.9	$549.1	$574.2	$582.9	$613.3	$647.6
Total Medicare	5.3	25.6	67.0	117.6	131.1	182.9	235.6	242.5	247.9	256.7	266.8	266.2	269.3	278.9
Total hospital insurance (HI)	NA	0.0	2.7	6.7	21.4	24.9	50.6	59.4	60.7	64.6	70.2	73.1	74.0	78.5
HI payments to managed care organizations[5]	5.1	25.0	63.4	109.5	105.1	156.6	172.8	179.5	183.3	186.9	189.2	184.7	186.4	191.5
HI payments for fee-for-service utilization	4.8	24.1	56.9	82.3	87.1	123.3	130.5	134.1	136.1	133.9	138.9	134.2	136.2	139.2
Inpatient hospital	0.2	0.4	2.5	9.1	11.1	19.3	24.3	26.1	27.0	31.9	28.4	28.4	28.5	29.7
Skilled nursing facility	0.1	0.5	3.7	16.2	4.0	6.0	6.6	7.0	7.1	7.1	6.8	6.8	6.5	6.6
Home health agency	NA	NA	0.3	1.9	2.9	8.0	11.4	12.3	13.1	14.0	15.0	15.2	15.2	15.9
Hospice	NA	NA	NA	NA	NA	NA	NA	NA	NA	0.9	2.8	3.5	3.7	2.6
Other programs[6]	NA	NA	NA	NA	1.7	NA	NA	NA	NA	NA	NA	NA	NA	NA
Home health agency transfer[7]	NA	NA	NA	NA	NA	NA	0.1	0.1	0.2	0.2	0.2	0.3	0.3	0.3
Medicare Advantage premiums[8]	NA	NA	NA	NA	NA	-1.9	8.5	NA	NA	NA	NA	NA	NA	NA
Accounting error (CY 2005-2008)[9]	0.2	0.5	0.9	1.4	2.9	3.3	3.6	3.5	3.8	4.0	4.3	4.7	4.9	5.9
Administrative expenses[10]	2.2	11.2	44.0	66.6	90.7	153.5	232.6	266.5	274.9	292.5	307.4	316.7	344.0	368.8
Total supplementary medical insurance (SMI)[3]														
Total Part B	2.2	11.2	44.0	66.6	90.7	152.4	183.3	205.7	212.9	225.3	240.5	247.1	265.9	279.0
Part B payments to managed care organizations[5]	0.0	0.2	2.8	6.6	18.4	22.0	48.1	53.4	55.2	59.1	66.0	72.7	85.7	93.8
Part B payments for fee-for-service utilization[11]	1.9	10.4	39.6	58.4	72.2	125.0	140.5	149.0	154.3	162.3	170.3	170.8	175.8	181.5
Physician/supplies[12]	1.8	8.2	29.6	NA	NA	NA	NA	NA	NA	NA	NA	NA	NA	NA
Outpatient hospital[13]	0.1	1.9	8.5	NA	NA	NA	NA	NA	NA	NA	NA	NA	NA	NA
Independent laboratory[14]	0.0	0.1	1.5	NA	NA	NA	NA	NA	NA	NA	NA	NA	NA	NA
Physician fee schedule	NA	NA	NA	31.7	37.0	57.7	60.6	61.8	63.9	67.5	69.5	68.6	69.2	70.3
Durable medical equipment	NA	NA	NA	3.7	4.7	8.0	8.6	8.2	8.3	8.2	8.2	7.2	6.3	6.8
Laboratory[15]	NA	NA	NA	4.3	4.4	6.9	7.9	8.2	8.4	8.4	9.2	9.1	8.2	8.5
Other[16]	NA	NA	NA	9.9	13.6	26.7	29.6	33.1	34.2	36.0	38.4	38.3	39.5	41.1
Hospital[17]	NA	NA	NA	8.7	8.1	18.7	23.6	26.0	27.6	30.2	33.6	36.2	41.5	43.7
Home health agency	0.0	0.2	0.1	0.2	4.5	7.1	10.3	11.7	12.0	12.1	11.4	11.4	11.1	11.1
Home health agency transfer[7]	NA	NA	NA	NA	-1.7	NA	NA	NA	NA	NA	NA	NA	NA	NA
Medicare Advantage premiums[8]	NA	NA	NA	NA	NA	NA	0.1	0.1	0.2	0.2	0.2	0.3	0.3	0.4
Accounting error (CY 2005-2008)[9]	NA	NA	NA	NA	NA	1.9	-8.5	NA	NA	NA	NA	NA	NA	NA
Administrative expenses[10]	0.2	0.6	1.5	1.6	1.8	2.8	3.1	3.2	3.2	3.7	4.0	3.4	4.1	3.3
Part D start-up costs[18]	NA	NA	NA	NA	NA	0.7	0.0	NA	NA	NA	NA	NA	NA	NA
Total Part D[4]	NA	NA	NA	NA	NA	1.1	49.3	60.8	62.1	67.1	66.9	69.7	78.1	89.8
Percent Distribution of Expenditures														
Total hospital insurance (HI)	100.0	100.0	100.0	100.0	100.0	100.0	100.0	100.0	100.0	100.0	100.0	100.0	100.0	100.0
HI payments to managed care organizations[5]	NA	0.0	4.0	5.7	16.3	13.6	21.5	24.5	24.5	25.2	26.3	27.5	27.5	28.2
HI payments for fee-for-service utilization	97.0	97.9	94.6	93.1	80.2	85.6	73.4	74.0	73.9	72.8	70.9	69.4	69.2	68.6
Inpatient hospital	91.4	94.3	85.0	70.0	66.4	67.4	55.4	55.3	54.9	52.2	52.1	50.4	50.6	49.9
Skilled nursing facility	4.7	1.5	3.7	7.8	8.5	10.6	10.3	10.8	10.9	12.4	10.7	10.7	10.6	10.7
Home health agency	1.0	2.1	5.5	13.8	3.1	3.3	2.8	2.9	2.9	2.8	2.6	2.6	2.4	2.4
Hospice	NA	NA	0.5	1.6	2.2	4.4	4.8	5.1	5.3	5.5	5.6	5.7	5.6	5.7
Other programs[6]	NA	NA	NA	NA	NA	NA	NA	NA	NA	0.3	1.1	1.3	1.4	0.9

NA = Not available.

0.0 = Quantity more than zero but less than 0.05.

[1]Preliminary estimates.

[2]Average number enrolled in the hospital insurance (HI) and/or supplementary medical insurance (SMI) programs for the period.

[3]Starting with 2004 data, the SMI trust fund consists of two separate accounts: Part B (which pays for a portion of the costs of physicians' services, outpatient hospital services, and other related medical and health services for voluntarily enrolled individuals) and Part D (Medicare Prescription Drug Account, which pays private plans to provide prescription drug coverage).

[4]The Medicare Modernization Act, enacted on December 8, 2003, established within SMI two Part D accounts related to prescription drug benefits: the Medicare Prescription Drug Account and the Transitional Assistance Account.

[5]Medicare-approved managed care organizations.

[6]Includes Community-Based Care Transitions Program ($0.1 billion in each of 2011–2015) and Electronic Health Records Incentive Program ($0.7 billion in 2011, $2.7 billion in 2012, $3.4 billion in 2013, $3.6 billion in 2014, and $2.5 billion in 2015).

[7]For 1998 to 2003 data, reflects annual home health HI to SMI transfer amounts.

[8]When a beneficiary chooses a Medicare Advantage plan whose monthly premium exceeds the benchmark amount, the additional premiums (that is, amounts beyond those paid by Medicare to the plan) are the responsibility of the beneficiary.

[9]Represents misallocation of benefit payments between the HI trust fund and the Part B account of the SMI trust fund from May 2005 to September 2007, and the transfer made in June 2008 to correct the misallocation.

[10]Includes expenditures for research, experiments and demonstration projects, peer review activity (performed by Peer Review Organizations from 1983 to 2001 and by Quality Review Organizations from 2002 to present), and to combat and prevent fraud and abuse.

[11]Type-of-service reporting categories for fee-for-service reimbursement differ before and after 1991.

[12]Includes payment for physicians, practitioners, durable medical equipment, and all suppliers other than independent laboratory through 1990. Starting with 1991 data, physician services subject to the physician fee schedule are shown. Payments for laboratory services paid under the laboratory fee schedule and performed in a physician office are included under Laboratory beginning in 1991.

[13]Includes payments for hospital outpatient department services, skilled nursing facility outpatient services, Part B services received as an inpatient in a hospital or skilled nursing facility setting, and other types of outpatient facilities.

[14]Starting with 1991 data, those independent laboratory services that were paid under the laboratory fee schedule (most of the independent laboratory category) are included in the Laboratory line; the remaining services are included in the Physician fee schedule and Other lines.

[15]Payments for laboratory services paid under the laboratory fee schedule performed in a physician office, independent laboratory, or in a hospital outpatient department.

[16]Includes payments for physician-administered drugs; freestanding ambulatory surgical center facility services; ambulance services; supplies; freestanding end-stage renal disease (ESRD) dialysis facility services; rural health clinics; outpatient rehabilitation facilities; psychiatric hospitals; and federally qualified health centers.

[17]Includes the hospital facility costs for Medicare Part B services that are predominantly in the outpatient department, with the exception of hospital outpatient laboratory services, which are included on the Laboratory line. Physician reimbursement is included on the Physician fee schedule line.

[18]Part D start-up costs were funded through the SMI Part B account in 2004-2008.

Table 3-79. Medicare Enrollees and Expenditures and Percent Distribution, by Medicare Program and Type of Service, Selected Years, 1970–2015—*Continued*

(Number; dollars; percent.)

Medicare program and type of service	1970	1980	1990	1995	2000	2005	2008	2009	2010	2011	2012	2013	2014	2015[1]
Home health agency transfer[7]	NA	NA	NA	NA	1.3	NA	NA	NA	NA	NA	NA	NA	NA	NA
Medicare Advantage premiums[8]	NA	NA	NA	NA	NA	NA	0.0	0.1	0.1	0.1	0.1	0.1	0.1	0.1
Accounting error (CY 2005-2008)[9]	NA	NA	NA	NA	NA	NA	3.6	NA	NA	NA	NA	NA	NA	NA
Administrative expenses[10]	3.0	2.1	1.4	1.2	2.2	1.8	1.5	1.4	1.5	1.6	1.6	1.8	1.8	2.1
Total supplementary medical insurance (SMI)[3]	100.0	100.0	100.0	100.0	100.0	100.0	100.0	100.0	100.0	100.0	100.0	100.0	100.0	100.0
Total Part B	100.0	100.0	100.0	100.0	100.0	99.3	78.8	77.2	77.4	77.1	78.2	78.0	77.3	75.6
Part B payments to managed care organizations[5]	1.2	1.8	6.4	9.9	20.2	14.3	20.7	20.0	20.1	20.2	21.5	22.9	24.9	25.4
Part B payments for fee-for-service utilization[11]	88.1	92.8	90.1	87.6	79.6	81.5	60.4	55.9	56.1	55.5	55.4	53.9	51.1	49.2
Physician/supplies[12]	80.9	72.8	67.3	NA	NA	NA	NA	NA	NA	NA	NA	NA	NA	NA
Outpatient hospital[13]	5.2	16.9	19.3	NA	NA	NA	NA	NA	NA	NA	NA	NA	NA	NA
Independent laboratory[14]	0.5	1.0	3.4	NA	NA	NA	NA	NA	NA	NA	NA	NA	NA	NA
Physician fee schedule	NA	NA	NA	47.5	40.8	37.6	26.0	23.2	23.2	23.1	22.6	21.7	20.1	19.1
Durable medical equipment	NA	NA	NA	5.5	5.2	5.2	3.7	3.1	3.0	2.8	2.7	2.3	1.8	1.8
Laboratory[15]	NA	NA	NA	6.4	4.8	4.5	3.4	3.1	3.1	2.9	3.0	2.9	2.4	2.3
Other[16]	NA	NA	NA	14.8	15.0	17.4	12.7	12.4	12.4	12.3	12.5	12.1	11.5	11.1
Hospital[17]	NA	NA	NA	13.0	8.9	12.2	10.1	9.7	10.0	10.3	10.9	11.4	12.1	11.9
Home health agency	1.5	2.1	0.2	0.3	4.9	4.6	4.4	4.4	4.4	4.1	3.7	3.6	3.2	3.0
Home health agency transfer[7]	NA	NA	NA	NA	-1.9	NA	NA	NA	NA	NA	NA	NA	NA	NA
Medicare Advantage premiums[8]	NA	NA	NA	NA	NA	NA	0.0	0.0	0.1	0.1	0.1	0.1	0.1	0.1
Accounting error (CY 2005-2008)[9]	NA	NA	NA	NA	NA	1.2	-3.6	NA	NA	NA	NA	NA	NA	NA
Administrative expenses[10]	10.7	5.4	3.5	2.4	2.0	1.8	1.3	1.2	1.2	1.3	1.3	1.1	1.2	0.9
Part D start-up costs[18]	NA	NA	NA	NA	NA	0.4	0.0	NA	NA	NA	NA	NA	NA	NA
Total Part D[4]	NA	NA	NA	NA	NA	0.7	21.2	22.8	22.6	22.9	21.8	22.0	22.7	24.4

NA = Not available.

0.0 = Quantity more than zero but less than 0.05.

[1]Preliminary estimates.

[3]Starting with 2004 data, the SMI trust fund consists of two separate accounts: Part B (which pays for a portion of the costs of physicians' services, outpatient hospital services, and other related medical and health services for voluntarily enrolled individuals) and Part D (Medicare Prescription Drug Account, which pays private plans to provide prescription drug coverage).

[4]The Medicare Modernization Act, enacted on December 8, 2003, established within SMI two Part D accounts related to prescription drug benefits: the Medicare Prescription Drug Account and the Transitional Assistance Account.

[5]Medicare-approved managed care organizations.

[7]For 1998 to 2003 data, reflects annual home health HI to SMI transfer amounts.

[8]When a beneficiary chooses a Medicare Advantage plan whose monthly premium exceeds the benchmark amount, the additional premiums (that is, amounts beyond those paid by Medicare to the plan) are the responsibility of the beneficiary.

[9]Represents misallocation of benefit payments between the HI trust fund and the Part B account of the SMI trust fund from May 2005 to September 2007, and the transfer made in June 2008 to correct the misallocation.

[10]Includes expenditures for research, experiments and demonstration projects, peer review activity (performed by Peer Review Organizations from 1983 to 2001 and by Quality Review Organizations from 2002 to present), and to combat and prevent fraud and abuse.

[11]Type-of-service reporting categories for fee-for-service reimbursement differ before and after 1991.

[12]Includes payment for physicians, practitioners, durable medical equipment, and all suppliers other than independent laboratory through 1990. Starting with 1991 data, physician services subject to the physician fee schedule are shown. Payments for laboratory services paid under the laboratory fee schedule and performed in a physician office are included under Laboratory beginning in 1991.

[13]Includes payments for hospital outpatient department services, skilled nursing facility outpatient services, Part B services received as an inpatient in a hospital or skilled nursing facility setting, and other types of outpatient facilities.

[14]Starting with 1991 data, those independent laboratory services that were paid under the laboratory fee schedule (most of the independent laboratory category) are included in the Laboratory line; the remaining services are included in the Physician fee schedule and Other lines.

[15]Payments for laboratory services paid under the laboratory fee schedule performed in a physician office, independent laboratory, or in a hospital outpatient department.

[16]Includes payments for physician-administered drugs; freestanding ambulatory surgical center facility services; ambulance services; supplies; freestanding end-stage renal disease (ESRD) dialysis facility services; rural health clinics; outpatient rehabilitation facilities; psychiatric hospitals; and federally qualified health centers.

[17]Includes the hospital facility costs for Medicare Part B services that are predominantly in the outpatient department, with the exception of hospital outpatient laboratory services, which are included on the Laboratory line. Physician reimbursement is included on the Physician fee schedule line.

[18]Part D start-up costs were funded through the SMI Part B account in 2004-2008.

Table 3-80. Medicare Enrollees, Enrollees in Managed Care, Payment Per Fee-for-Service Enrollee, and Short-Stay Hospital Utilization, by State, 1994 and 2015

(Number; percent; dollars; rate per 1,000 enrollees.)

State	Enrollment in thousands[1]		Percent of enrollees in managed care		Average payment per fee-for-service enrollee		Short-stay hospital utilization			
							Discharges per 1,000 enrollees[2]		Average length of stay in days[2]	
	1994	2015	1994	2015	1994	2015	1994	2015	1994	2015
United States[3]	36,190	54,286	7.9	31.3	$4,375	$9,635	345	282	7.5	5.3
Alabama	633	968	0.8	25.3	4,454	8,611	413	313	7.0	5.5
Alaska	33	84	0.6	1.0	3,687	8,301	269	181	6.3	6.0
Arizona	578	1,140	24.8	38.1	4,442	8,728	292	228	5.9	4.9
Arkansas	416	594	0.2	20.1	3,719	8,360	366	288	7.0	5.3
California	3,582	5,645	30.0	40.5	5,219	10,294	366	242	6.1	5.4
Colorado	413	786	17.2	36.9	3,935	7,914	302	218	6.0	4.7
Connecticut	497	630	2.6	25.6	4,426	10,636	287	293	8.1	5.7
Delaware	99	181	0.2	8.3	4,712	9,803	326	278	8.1	5.5
District of Columbia	80	88	3.9	13.1	5,655	10,058	376	320	10.1	6.3
Florida	2,584	4,040	13.8	39.8	5,027	10,715	326	324	7.1	5.3
Georgia	819	1,521	0.4	31.5	4,402	9,042	378	275	6.9	5.4
Hawaii	146	244	29.8	45.8	3,069	6,459	301	162	9.1	6.4
Idaho	146	283	2.5	32.6	3,045	7,706	274	181	5.2	4.6
Illinois	1,605	2,063	5.5	21.0	4,324	9,910	374	308	7.3	5.1
Indiana	805	1,151	2.6	23.8	3,945	9,332	345	293	6.9	5.1
Iowa	470	572	3.1	14.9	3,080	8,286	322	235	6.6	5.1
Kansas	378	487	3.3	13.7	3,847	8,652	348	261	6.5	4.9
Kentucky	578	863	2.3	26.2	3,862	9,012	396	315	7.2	5.2
Louisiana	572	793	0.4	30.1	5,468	10,047	399	301	7.2	5.4
Maine	198	306	0.1	22.9	3,464	8,232	322	218	7.6	5.3
Maryland	596	930	1.4	8.7	4,997	11,010	362	293	7.5	5.5
Massachusetts	924	1,217	6.1	20.9	5,147	10,394	350	295	7.6	5.2
Michigan	1,331	1,894	0.7	33.3	4,307	10,381	328	336	7.6	5.2
Minnesota	625	912	19.6	53.8	3,394	12,904	334	405	5.7	4.9
Mississippi	391	560	0.1	14.7	4,189	9,659	423	319	7.4	5.6
Missouri	821	1,136	3.4	28.3	4,191	9,042	349	306	7.3	5.1
Montana	128	201	0.4	18.3	3,114	7,277	306	185	5.9	4.9
Nebraska	247	314	2.2	12.3	2,926	8,948	281	239	6.3	5.0
Nevada	187	455	19.0	33.1	4,306	9,216	291	248	7.0	5.7
New Hampshire	152	266	0.2	7.5	3,414	8,374	281	218	7.6	5.4
New Jersey	1,158	1,489	2.6	15.4	4,531	10,898	354	294	10.2	5.8
New Mexico	205	373	13.6	31.7	3,110	7,680	301	208	6.0	5.0
New York	2,601	3,339	6.2	37.0	4,855	10,572	334	290	11.2	6.7
North Carolina	1,001	1,771	0.5	29.8	3,465	8,858	314	277	8.0	5.3
North Dakota	101	119	0.6	16.9	3,218	8,723	327	247	6.3	5.4
Ohio	1,649	2,153	2.4	41.0	3,982	9,613	350	309	7.1	5.0
Oklahoma	481	679	2.5	16.9	4,098	9,348	355	295	7.0	5.3
Oregon	469	756	27.7	43.8	3,285	7,842	305	191	5.2	4.8
Pennsylvania	2,053	2,531	3.3	39.9	5,212	9,687	379	304	8.0	5.3
Rhode Island	166	203	7.0	35.1	4,148	9,224	312	296	8.1	5.3
South Carolina	497	943	0.1	23.2	3,777	8,635	319	265	8.3	5.4
South Dakota	114	156	0.1	19.0	2,952	8,969	356	258	6.1	4.9
Tennessee	754	1,236	0.3	34.3	4,441	8,963	375	300	7.1	5.3
Texas	2,029	3,636	4.1	31.8	4,703	10,603	333	289	7.2	5.3
Utah	182	346	9.4	33.8	3,443	8,187	238	207	5.4	4.3
Vermont	82	131	0.1	7.5	3,182	7,917	283	179	7.6	5.5
Virginia	803	1,349	1.5	18.1	3,748	8,280	348	273	7.3	5.1
Washington	676	1,192	12.5	30.0	3,401	7,920	269	207	5.3	4.9
West Virginia	326	416	8.3	26.8	3,798	8,641	420	312	7.1	5.4
Wisconsin	752	1,050	2.0	37.9	3,246	8,746	310	253	6.8	4.9
Wyoming	58	95	3.3	3.9	3,537	8,235	315	205	5.6	4.8

[1] Total persons enrolled in hospital insurance, supplementary medical insurance, or both, as of July 1. Includes fee-for-service and managed care enrollees.
[2] Data are for fee-for-service enrollees only.
[3] Includes residents of any of the 50 states and the District of Columbia.

NOTES AND DEFINITIONS

Sources of Data

The principal source for data presented in this part is from National Center for Health Statistics. *Health, United States, 2017: With Special Feature on Mortality.* Hyattsville, MD. 2018, an annual report on trends in health statistics compiled by the National Center of Health Statistics (NCHS), a component of the Centers for Disease Control and Prevention (CDC).

The data for Tables 3-58 through 3-62 are from the Bureau of Labor Statistics (BLS), Occupational Employment Statistics. For more detailed information, see Occupational Employment and Wages news release. OES can be accessed at http://www.bls.gov/oes/.

Concepts and Definitions

Age-adjustment—used to compare risks of two or more populations at one point in time or one population at two or more points in time. Age-adjusted rates are computed by the direct method by applying age-specific rates in a population of interest to a standardized age distribution, to eliminate differences in observed rates that result from age differences in population composition. Age-adjusted rates should be viewed as relative indexes rather than actual measures of risk. Age-adjusted estimates from other age-adjusted estimates based on the same data and presented elsewhere if different age groups are used in the adjustment procedure.

Body mass index (BMI)—a measure that adjusts bodyweight for height. It is calculated as weight in kilograms divided by height in meters squared. Overweight for children and adolescents is defined as BMI at or above the sex- and age-specific 95th percentile BMI cut points from the 2000 CDC Growth Charts. Healthy weight for adults is defined as a BMI of 18.5 to less than 25; overweight, as greater than or equal to a BMI of 25; and obesity, as greater than or equal to a BMI of 30.

Cholesterol, serum—a measure of the total blood cholesterol. Elevated total blood cholesterol—a combination of high-density lipoproteins (HDL), low-density lipoproteins (LDL), and very-low density lipoproteins (VLDL)—is a risk factor for cardiovascular disease. According to the National Cholesterol Education Program, high serum cholesterol is defined as greater than or equal to 240 mg/dL (6.20 mmol/L). Borderline high serum cholesterol is defined as greater than or equal to 200 mg/dL and less than 240 mg/dL. Assessments of the components of total cholesterol or lower thresholds for high total cholesterol may be used for individuals with other risk factors for cardiovascular disease.

Condition—A health condition is a departure from a state of physical or mental well being. In the National Health interview Survey, each condition reported as a cause of an individual's activity limitation has been classified as chronic, not chronic, or unknown if chronic, based on the nature and duration of the condition.

Dental caries—evidence of tooth decay on any surface of the tooth. Untreated dental caries are determined by an oral examination conducted by a trained dentist.

Diagnosis—the act or process of identifying or determining the nature and cause of a disease or injury through evaluation of patient history, examination, and review of laboratory data.

Gross domestic product (GDP)—the market value of the goods and services produced by labor and property located in the United States. As long as the labor and property are located in the United States, the suppliers (i.e., the workers and, for property, the owners) may be U.S. residents or residents of other countries.

Health expenditures, national—estimated by the Centers for Medicare & Medicaid Services (CMS) it measures spending for health care in the United States by type of service delivered (e.g., hospital care, physician services, nursing home care) and source of funding for those services (e.g., private health insurance, Medicare, Medicaid, out-of-pocket spending). CMS produces both historical and projected estimates of health expenditures by category.

Health insurance coverage—broadly defined to include both public and private payers who cover medical expenditures incurred by a defined population in a variety of settings.

Health maintenance organization (HMO)—a health care system that assumes or shares both the financial risks and the delivery risks associated with providing comprehensive medical services to a voluntarily enrolled population in a particular geographic area, usually in return for a fixed, prepaid fee. Pure HMO enrollees use only the prepaid capitated health services of the HMO panel of medical care providers. Open-ended HMO enrollees use the prepaid HMO health services but, in addition, may receive medical care from providers who are not part of the HMO panel. There is usually a substantial deductible, co-payment, or co-insurance associated with use of non-panel providers.

Hispanic origin—includes persons of Mexican, Puerto Rican, Cuban, Central and South American, and other or unknown Latin American or Spanish origins. Persons of Hispanic origin may be of any race.

Hypertension—elevated blood pressure or hypertension is defined as having an average systolic blood pressure reading of at least 140mmHg or diastolic pressure of at least 90 mmHg, which is consistent with the Seventh Report of the Joint National Committee on Prevention, Detection, Evaluation, and Treatment of High Blood Pressure. People are also considered to have hypertension if they report that they are taking a prescription medicine for high blood pressure, even if their blood pressure readings are within normal range.

Incidence—the number of cases of disease having their onset during a prescribed period of time. It is often expressed as a rate (e.g., the incidence of measles per 1,000 children 5–15 years of age during a specified year). Incidence is a measure of morbidity or other events that occur within a specified period of time. Measuring incidence may be complicated because the population at risk for the disease may change during the period of interest, for example, due to births, deaths, or migration. In addition, determining that a case is new—that is, that its onset occurred during the prescribed period of time—may be difficult. Because of these difficulties in measuring incidence, many health statistics are measured using prevalence.

Instrumental activities of daily living (IADL)—activities related to independent living and include preparing meals, managing money, shopping for groceries or personal items, performing light or heavy housework, and using a telephone. In the National Health Interview Survey (NHIS) respondents are asked whether they or family members 18 years of age and over need the help of another person for handling routine IADL needs because of a physical, mental, or emotional problem. Persons are considered to have an IADL limitation in the NHIS if any causal condition is chronic.

Limitation of activity—may be defined different ways, depending on the conceptual framework. In the National Health Interview Survey, limitation of activity refers to a long-term reduction in a person's capacity to perform the usual kind or amount of activities associated with his or her age group as a result of a chronic condition. Limitation of activity is assessed by asking persons a series of questions about limitations in their or household members' ability to perform activities usual for their age group because of a physical, mental, or emotional problem. Persons are asked about limitations in activities of daily living, instrumental activities of daily living, play, school, work, difficulty walking or remembering, and any other activity limitations. For reported limitations, the causal health conditions are determined, and persons are considered limited if one or more of these conditions is chronic. Children under 18 years of age who receive special education or early intervention services are considered to have a limitation of activity.

Mammography—an x-ray image of the breast used to detect irregularities of the breast tissue.

Managed care—a term originally used to refer to the prepaid health care sector (health maintenance organizations or HMOs) where care is provided under a fixed budget and costs are therein capable of being managed. Increasingly, the term is being used to include preferred provider organizations (PPOs) and even forms of indemnity.

Medicare—the federal program which helps pay health care costs for people 65 and older and for certain people under 65 with long-term disabilities.

Medicaid—a program authorized by the Social Security Act in 1965 as a jointly funded cooperative venture between the federal and state governments to assist states in the provision of adequate medical care to eligible needy persons. Families with dependent children, the aged, blind, and disabled who are in financial need are eligible for Medicaid.

Notifiable disease—a disease, that when diagnosed, health providers are required, usually by law, to report to state or local public health officials. Notifiable diseases are those of public interest by reason of their contagiousness, severity, or frequency.

Pap smear—a microscopic examination of cells scraped from the cervix that is used to detect cancerous or precancerous conditions of the cervix or other medical conditions.

Physical activity, leisure-time—starting with 1998 data, leisure-time physical activity is assessed in the National Health Interview Survey by asking adults a series of questions about how often they do vigorous or light/moderate physical activity of at least 10 minutes duration and for about how long these sessions generally last. Vigorous physical activity is described as causing heavy sweating or a large increase in breathing or heart rate and light/moderate as causing light sweating or a slight to moderate increase in breathing or heart rate. Adults classified as inactive did not report any sessions of light/moderate or vigorous leisure-time physical activity of at least 10 minutes duration or reported they were unable to perform leisure-time physical activity. Adults classified with some leisure-time activity reported at least one session of light/moderate or vigorous activity of at least 10 minutes duration but did not meet the requirement for regular leisure-time activity. Adults classified with regular leisure-time activity reported at least three sessions per week of vigorous leisure-time physical activity lasting at least 20 minutes in duration or at least five sessions per week of light/moderate physical activity lasting at least 30 minutes in duration.

Poverty—based on definitions originally developed by the Social Security Administration. These include a set of money income thresholds that vary by family size and composition. Families or individuals with income below their appropriate thresholds are classified as below poverty. These thresholds are updated annually by the U.S. Census Bureau to reflect changes in the Consumer Price Index for all urban consumers (CPI-U). For example, the average poverty threshold for a family of four was $22,314 in 2010, $17,603 in 2000, and $13,359 in 1990.

Preferred provider organization (PPO)—a type of medical plan where coverage is provided to participants through a network of selected health care providers (such as hospitals and physicians). The enrollees may go outside the network, but they would pay a greater percentage of the cost of coverage than within the network.

Prevalence—the number of cases of a disease, infected persons, or persons with some other attribute present during a particular interval of time. It is often expressed as a rate (e.g., the prevalence of diabetes per 1,000 persons during a year).

Short-stay hospital—hospitals that provide general (rather than specialized) care and have an average length of stay of less than 30 days.

Specialty hospital—hospitals that provide a particular type of service to the majority of their patients such as psychiatric, tuberculosis, chronic disease, rehabilitation, maternity, and alcoholic or narcotic.

State Children's Health Insurance Program (SCHIP)—Title XXI of the Social Security Act, known as the State Children's Health Insurance Program (SCHIP), is a program initiated by the Balanced Budget Act of 1997 (BBA). SCHIP provides more federal funds for states to provide health care coverage to low-income, uninsured children. SCHIP gives states broad flexibility in program design while protecting beneficiaries through federal standards. Funds from SCHIP may be used to expand Medicaid or to provide medical assistance to children during a presumptive eligibility period for Medicaid. This is one of several options from which states may select to provide health care coverage for more children, as prescribed within the BBA's Title XXI program.

Substance use—the use of selected substances including alcohol, tobacco products, drugs, inhalants, and other substances that can be consumed, inhaled, injected, or otherwise absorbed into the body with possible detrimental effects.

Suicidal ideation—having thoughts of suicide or of taking action to end one's own life. Suicidal ideation includes all thoughts of suicide, both when the thoughts include a plan to commit suicide and when they do not include a plan. Suicidal ideation is measured in the Youth Risk Behavior Survey by the question "During the past 12 months, did you ever seriously consider attempting suicide?"

Uninsured—in the Current Population Survey (CPS) persons are considered uninsured if they do not have coverage through private health insurance, Medicare, Medicaid, State Children's Health Insurance Program, military or Veterans coverage, another government program, a plan of someone outside the household, or other insurance. Persons with only Indian Health Service coverage are considered uninsured. In addition, if the respondent has missing Medicaid information but has income from certain low-income public programs, then Medicaid coverage is imputed. The questions on health insurance are administered in March and refer to the previous calendar year.

PART IV:
MARRIAGE AND DIVORCE

PART IV: MARRIAGE AND DIVORCE

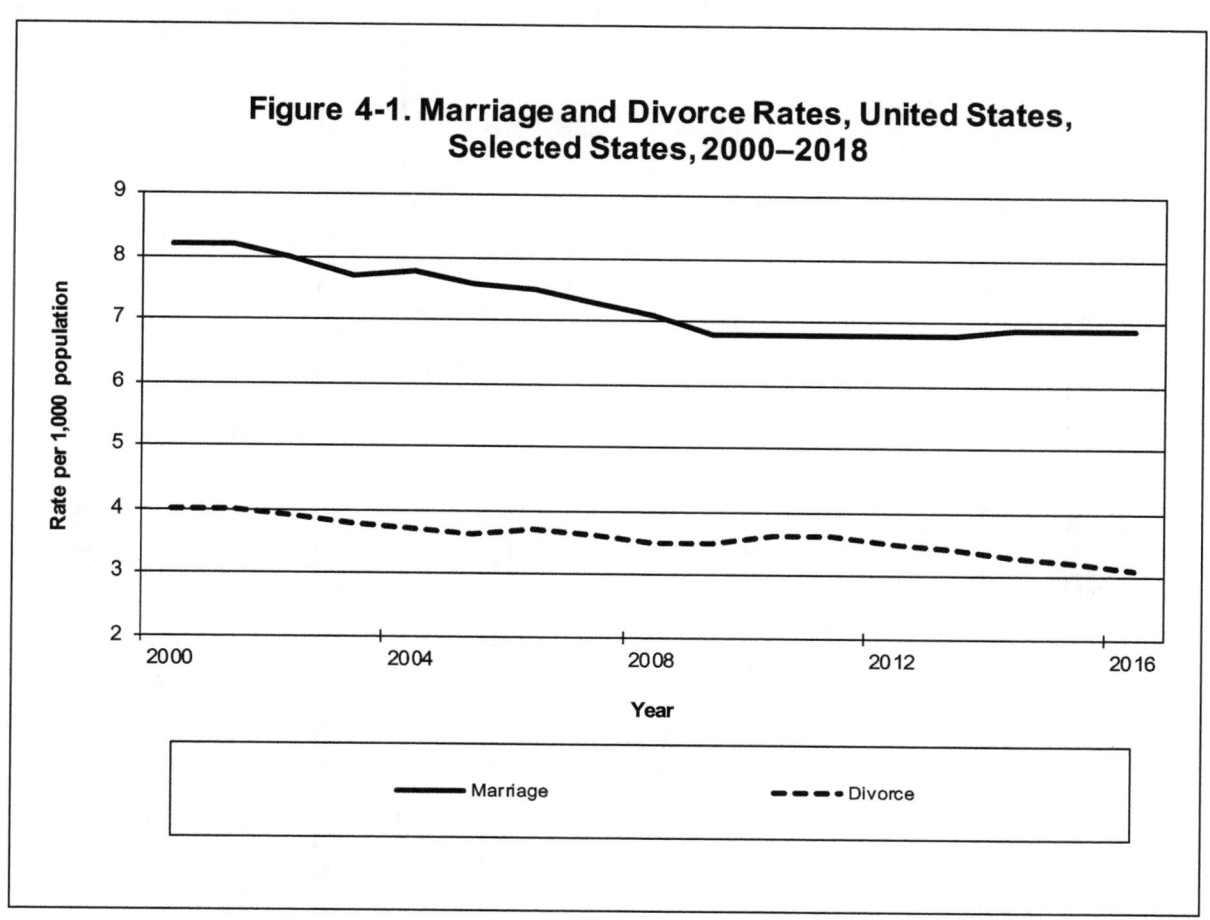

Figure 4-1. Marriage and Divorce Rates, United States, Selected States, 2000–2018

HIGHLIGHTS

- In 2018, Nevada had the highest rate of marriage per 1,000 resident population at 26.7, significantly greater than the next-highest states (Hawaii, 15.3; Arkansas, 8.9; and Utah, 8.4). Lousiana had the lowest marriage rate, at 5.1, followed by Delaware at 5.2, Connecticut and Minnesota at 5.3 each, and Kansas, New Jersey, and Wisconsin at 5.7 each.

- Among reporting states in 2018 (California, Hawaii, Indiana, Minnesota, and New Mexico did not have available data), Illinois had the lowest divorce rate, at 1.5 per 1,000 resident population, followed by Louisiana (1.7), Massachusetts (2.1), Iowa (2.2), and Kansas (2.3 each). Nevada (the state with the highest rate of marriage) had the highest divorce rate at 4.4, followed by Arkansas at 4.1 and Idaho, Oklahoma, Utah, and Wyoming, each at 3.8.

- The median age at first marriage for all races and origins in the United States was 29.9 years for males and 28.1 years for females in 2017. Male median ages ranged from 28.8 for Native Hawaiian and Other Pacific Islanders to 31.9 for Black or African American alone males. Ages for females ranged from 27.7 for Native Hawaiian and Other Pacific Islanders alone and Asian alone to 31.4 for Black or African American alone.

- In the United States, the median duration of current marriages was 19.7 years in 2017. The District of Columbia had the shortest median duration, at 10.6 years, while West Virginia had the longest median duration, at 22.6 years.

Table 4-1. Marriage Rates, by State, Selected Years, 2000–2018

(Rate per 1,000 total population residing in area.)

State	Marriage rate														
	2000	2005	2006	2007	2008	2009	2010	2011	2012	2013	2014	2015	2016	2017	2018
United States	8.2	7.6	7.5	7.3	7.1	6.8	6.8	6.8	6.8	6.8	6.9	6.9	7.0	6.9	6.5
Alabama......................	10.1	9.2	9.2	8.9	8.6	8.3	8.2	8.4	8.2	7.8	7.8	7.4	7.1	7.0	6.8
Alaska	8.9	8.2	8.2	8.5	8.4	7.8	8.0	7.8	7.2	7.3	7.5	7.4	7.1	6.9	6.7
Arizona......................	7.5	6.6	6.5	6.4	6.0	5.6	5.9	5.7	5.6	5.4	5.8	5.9	5.9	5.8	5.5
Arkansas	15.4	12.9	12.4	12.0	10.6	10.7	10.8	10.4	10.9	9.8	10.1	10.0	9.9	9.5	8.9
California[1]...................	5.8	6.4	6.3	6.2	6.7	5.8	5.8	5.8	6.0	6.5	6.4	6.2	6.5	6.3	6.0
Colorado	8.3	7.6	7.2	7.1	7.4	6.9	6.9	7.0	6.8	6.5	7.1	6.8	7.4	7.3	7.6
Connecticut................	5.7	5.8	5.5	5.5	5.4	5.9	5.6	5.5	5.2	5.0	5.4	5.3	5.6	5.6	5.3
Delaware	6.5	5.9	5.9	5.7	5.5	5.4	5.2	5.2	5.8	6.6	6.0	5.7	5.6	5.5	5.2
District of Columbia	4.9	4.1	4.0	4.2	4.1	4.7	7.6	8.7	8.4	10.8	11.8	8.2	8.1	8.2	7.8
Florida.......................	8.9	8.9	8.6	8.5	8.0	7.5	7.3	7.4	7.2	7.0	7.3	8.2	8.1	7.8	7.3
Georgia	6.8	7.0	7.3	6.8	6.0	6.6	7.3	6.6	6.5	---	---	6.2	6.8	6.9	6.4
Hawaii	20.6	22.6	21.9	20.8	19.1	17.2	17.6	17.6	17.5	16.3	17.7	15.9	15.6	15.3	15.3
Idaho	10.8	10.5	10.1	10.0	9.5	8.9	8.8	8.6	8.2	8.2	8.4	8.2	8.1	7.8	7.8
Illinois	6.9	5.9	6.2	6.1	5.9	5.7	5.7	5.6	5.8	5.4	6.2	5.9	5.8	6.0	5.5
Indiana......................	7.9	6.9	7.0	7.0	8.0	7.9	6.3	6.8	6.7	6.6	7.1	6.9	6.9	6.9	6.6
Iowa	6.9	6.9	6.7	6.6	6.5	7.0	6.9	6.7	6.8	7.4	6.9	6.3	6.1	6.2	5.7
Kansas	8.3	6.8	6.8	6.8	6.7	6.4	6.4	6.3	6.3	6.0	6.1	5.9	6.2	6.0	5.4
Kentucky	9.8	8.7	8.4	7.8	7.9	7.6	7.4	7.5	7.2	7.3	6.9	7.2	7.4	7.2	6.8
Louisiana	9.1	8.0	---	7.5	6.8	7.1	6.9	6.4	5.7	6.4	6.9	6.8	6.1	5.6	5.1
Maine........................	8.8	8.2	7.8	7.4	7.4	7.1	7.1	7.2	7.3	8.3	7.7	7.6	7.6	7.6	7.4
Maryland....................	7.5	6.9	6.6	6.5	5.9	5.8	5.7	5.8	5.6	6.8	6.5	6.2	6.3	6.3	5.9
Massachusetts............	5.8	6.2	5.9	5.9	5.7	5.6	5.6	5.5	5.5	5.5	5.6	5.5	5.8	5.7	6.3
Michigan	6.7	6.1	5.9	5.7	5.6	5.4	5.5	5.7	5.6	5.8	5.8	6.0	5.9	5.9	5.7
Minnesota	6.8	6.0	6.0	5.8	5.4	5.3	5.3	5.6	5.6	6.0	5.9	5.6	5.6	5.6	5.3
Mississippi.................	6.9	5.8	5.7	5.4	5.1	4.8	4.9	4.9	5.8	6.7	6.9	7.0	7.0	6.7	6.3
Missouri.....................	7.8	7.0	6.9	6.9	6.8	6.5	6.5	6.6	6.5	6.4	6.7	6.8	6.9	6.6	6.5
Montana.....................	7.3	7.4	7.4	7.5	7.6	7.3	7.4	7.8	7.8	7.4	7.9	8.0	7.8	8.0	7.7
Nebraska....................	7.6	7.0	6.8	6.8	6.9	6.6	6.6	6.6	6.7	6.3	6.4	6.4	6.5	6.3	6.0
Nevada......................	72.2	57.4	52.1	48.6	42.3	40.3	38.3	36.9	35.1	32.3	31.9	31.0	28.4	28.6	26.7
New Hampshire............	9.4	7.3	7.2	7.1	6.8	6.5	7.3	7.1	6.8	6.9	7.2	6.9	7.0	7.0	6.9
New Jersey	6.0	5.7	5.5	5.4	5.4	5.0	5.1	4.8	4.9	5.1	5.4	5.6	5.7	5.5	5.4
New Mexico	8.0	6.6	6.8	5.6	4.0	5.0	7.7	8.0	6.9	7.3	8.1	6.2	6.4	5.9	6.4
New York....................	7.1	6.8	6.9	6.8	6.6	6.5	6.5	6.9	7.0	6.9	6.7	7.1	7.5	7.3	7.1
North Carolina.............	8.2	7.3	7.3	7.0	6.9	6.6	6.6	6.7	6.6	6.5	6.9	7.0	7.0	6.8	6.4
North Dakota...............	7.2	6.8	6.7	6.6	6.5	6.4	6.5	6.7	6.6	6.3	6.3	6.2	6.0	5.8	5.7
Ohio	7.8	6.5	6.3	6.1	6.0	5.8	5.8	5.9	5.8	5.7	5.8	5.9	6.0	5.8	5.6
Oklahoma...................	---	7.3	7.3	7.3	7.1	6.9	7.2	6.9	6.9	7.1	7.1	7.4	6.7	6.8	6.4
Oregon	7.6	7.3	7.3	7.2	6.9	6.6	6.5	6.6	6.6	6.3	6.8	6.9	6.9	6.7	6.3
Pennsylvania..............	6.0	5.8	5.7	5.7	5.5	5.3	5.3	5.3	5.5	5.4	5.8	5.7	5.8	5.7	5.5
Rhode Island..............	7.6	7.0	6.6	6.4	6.1	5.9	5.8	6.0	6.1	6.2	6.7	6.4	6.7	6.8	6.3
South Carolina	10.6	8.3	7.8	7.9	7.3	7.3	7.4	7.2	7.4	7.1	7.6	7.5	6.6	7.0	6.6
South Dakota	9.4	8.4	8.0	7.8	7.7	7.3	7.3	7.5	7.5	7.0	7.1	7.2	7.2	6.7	6.5
Tennessee	15.5	10.9	10.6	10.1	9.4	8.4	8.8	9.0	8.8	8.4	8.4	8.5	8.6	8.2	8.0
Texas	9.4	7.8	7.6	7.4	7.3	7.1	7.1	7.1	7.3	7.0	6.9	7.2	7.1	7.1	6.1
Utah	10.8	9.8	9.2	9.6	9.0	8.4	8.5	8.6	8.4	7.5	7.3	8.1	9.0	8.7	8.4
Vermont.....................	10.0	8.9	8.6	8.5	7.9	8.7	9.3	8.3	8.2	9.2	8.7	8.1	8.3	7.9	7.9
Virginia......................	8.8	8.2	7.8	7.5	7.2	6.9	6.8	6.8	6.8	6.7	6.7	7.0	7.0	6.8	6.4
Washington................	6.9	6.5	6.5	6.4	6.3	6.0	6.0	6.1	6.3	7.1	7.0	6.2	6.2	6.2	6.0
West Virginia..............	8.7	7.4	7.3	7.3	7.1	6.7	6.7	7.2	7.0	6.6	6.7	6.6	6.4	6.3	6.1
Wisconsin	6.7	6.1	6.0	5.7	5.6	5.3	5.3	5.3	5.4	5.2	5.7	5.6	5.6	5.6	5.4
Wyoming	10.0	9.3	9.3	9.0	8.6	8.0	7.6	7.8	7.6	7.5	7.7	7.3	7.1	7.1	7.1

NA = Not available.

[1] Marriage data includes nonlicensed marriages registered.

Table 4-2. Divorce Rates, by State, Selected Years, 2000–2018

(Rate per 1,000 total population residing in area.)

State	Divorce rate[1]														
	2000	2005	2006	2007	2008	2009	2010	2011	2012	2013	2014	2015	2016	2017	2018
United States	4.0	3.6	3.7	3.6	3.5	3.5	3.6	3.6	3.4	3.3	3.2	3.1	3.0	2.9	2.9
Alabama	5.5	4.9	4.9	4.5	4.3	4.4	4.4	4.3	3.6	3.7	3.8	3.9	3.8	3.7	3.7
Alaska	3.9	4.3	4.2	4.3	4.4	4.4	4.7	4.8	4.5	4.5	4.0	4.1	3.9	3.6	3.7
Arizona	4.6	4.2	4.0	4.0	3.8	3.6	3.5	3.9	4.3	3.9	3.9	3.6	3.4	3.5	3.0
Arkansas	6.4	6.0	5.8	5.9	5.5	5.7	5.7	5.3	5.3	5.0	4.8	4.8	3.9	3.7	4.1
California	NA	NA	NA	NA	NA	NA	NA	NA	NA	NA	NA	NA	NA	NA	NA
Colorado	4.7	4.4	4.5	4.4	4.3	4.3	4.3	4.4	4.3	4.1	3.9	3.7	3.6	3.2	3.3
Connecticut	3.3	3.0	3.1	3.2	3.4	3.0	2.9	3.1	2.7	2.8	2.6	3.1	3.2	2.9	2.9
Delaware	3.9	3.8	3.8	3.7	3.5	3.6	3.5	3.6	3.5	3.4	3.3	3.1	3.1	3.0	2.8
District of Columbia .	3.2	2.0	2.1	1.7	2.7	2.7	2.8	2.9	2.9	2.8	2.6	2.8	2.7	2.5	2.5
Florida	5.1	4.6	4.7	4.6	4.3	4.2	4.4	4.5	4.2	4.1	4.0	4.0	3.9	3.6	3.6
Georgia	3.3	NA	NA	NA	NA	NA	NA	NA	NA	NA	NA	NA	NA	3.5	2.5
Hawaii	3.9	NA	NA	NA	NA	NA	NA	NA	NA	NA	NA	NA	NA	NA	NA
Idaho	5.5	5.0	5.0	4.9	4.8	5.0	5.2	4.9	4.7	4.5	4.2	4.1	4.0	3.9	3.8
Illinois	3.2	2.6	2.5	2.6	2.5	2.5	2.6	2.6	2.4	2.3	2.2	2.2	2.2	1.9	1.5
Indiana	NA	NA	NA	NA	NA	NA	NA	NA	NA	NA	NA	NA	NA	NA	NA
Iowa	3.3	2.7	2.7	2.5	2.6	2.4	2.4	2.4	2.2	1.9	1.5	1.2	1.3	2.0	2.2
Kansas	3.6	3.1	3.1	3.4	3.5	3.6	3.7	3.9	3.4	3.0	3.0	2.8	2.7	2.4	2.3
Kentucky	5.1	4.6	5.0	4.6	4.6	4.6	4.5	4.4	4.1	4.2	3.8	3.7	3.8	3.7	3.5
Louisiana	NA	NA	NA	NA	NA	NA	NA	NA	NA	2.2	2.3	2.8	2.0	1.9	1.7
Maine	5.0	4.1	4.2	4.2	4.2	4.1	4.2	4.2	3.9	4.0	3.6	3.4	3.4	3.2	3.2
Maryland	3.3	3.1	3.0	2.9	2.8	2.8	2.8	2.9	2.8	2.5	2.5	2.6	2.7	2.5	2.4
Massachusetts	2.5	2.2	2.3	2.3	2.0	2.2	2.5	2.7	2.7	2.6	2.7	2.6	2.3	2.2	2.1
Michigan	3.9	3.4	3.5	3.4	3.4	3.3	3.5	3.4	3.3	3.3	3.0	3.0	2.9	2.8	2.8
Minnesota	3.2	NA	NA	NA	NA	NA	NA	NA	NA	NA	NA	NA	NA	NA	NA
Mississippi	5.0	4.4	4.8	4.5	4.3	4.1	4.3	4.0	4.0	3.6	3.4	3.4	3.2	2.9	2.7
Missouri	4.5	3.6	3.8	3.8	3.7	3.8	3.9	3.9	3.7	3.4	3.3	3.2	3.3	3.1	3.0
Montana	4.2	4.5	4.4	4.0	4.1	4.0	3.9	4.0	3.9	3.4	3.4	3.4	3.1	3.1	3.0
Nebraska	3.7	3.3	3.4	3.4	3.3	3.4	3.6	3.5	3.4	3.3	3.1	3.2	3.1	3.0	2.9
Nevada	9.9	7.4	6.7	6.4	6.4	6.6	5.9	5.6	5.5	5.1	5.3	4.6	4.3	4.5	4.4
New Hampshire	4.8	3.9	4.1	3.8	3.9	3.7	3.8	3.8	3.6	3.7	3.5	3.3	3.4	3.1	3.1
New Jersey	3.0	2.9	3.0	3.0	3.0	2.7	3.0	2.9	2.8	2.8	2.8	2.8	2.7	2.6	2.7
New Mexico	5.1	4.6	4.3	4.2	4.1	3.9	4.0	3.3	3.0	3.4	3.6	3.3	NA	NA	NA
New York	3.0	2.9	3.1	2.9	2.8	2.6	2.9	2.9	2.9	2.7	2.8	2.7	2.7	2.7	2.8
North Carolina	4.5	4.1	4.0	4.0	3.8	3.8	3.8	3.7	3.7	3.4	3.4	3.1	3.2	3.1	3.1
North Dakota	3.4	2.9	3.0	2.9	2.9	2.8	3.1	2.7	3.1	2.9	2.8	2.8	2.6	2.5	2.6
Ohio	4.2	3.5	3.5	3.4	3.3	3.3	3.4	3.4	3.4	3.3	3.2	3.1	3.0	2.9	2.9
Oklahoma	NA	5.6	5.3	5.2	5.3	4.8	5.2	5.2	4.8	4.5	4.5	4.4	4.4	4.1	3.8
Oregon	4.8	4.2	4.0	3.9	3.9	3.9	4.0	3.8	3.8	3.6	3.4	3.4	3.4	3.4	3.4
Pennsylvania	3.1	2.3	2.8	2.8	2.7	2.7	2.7	2.8	2.8	2.7	2.7	2.6	2.6	2.6	2.6
Rhode Island	2.9	3.0	3.0	2.8	2.7	3.0	3.2	3.2	3.2	3.1	2.8	3.0	2.8	2.9	2.9
South Carolina	3.8	2.9	2.9	3.0	2.8	3.0	3.1	3.2	3.2	3.2	2.9	2.8	2.5	2.6	2.5
South Dakota	3.5	2.8	3.2	3.1	3.1	3.3	3.4	3.3	3.0	2.9	2.8	2.6	2.8	2.7	2.6
Tennessee	5.9	4.6	4.6	4.3	4.2	3.9	4.2	4.3	4.2	4.1	3.8	3.7	3.8	3.5	3.5
Texas	4.0	3.3	3.4	3.3	3.3	3.3	3.3	3.2	3.0	2.9	2.7	2.6	2.6	2.2	2.6
Utah	4.3	4.1	3.9	3.7	3.8	3.7	3.7	3.7	3.3	3.1	3.1	3.6	3.6	3.4	3.8
Vermont	4.1	3.6	3.8	3.6	3.6	3.6	3.5	3.8	3.6	3.5	3.5	3.1	3.1	2.9	3.1
Virginia	4.3	4.0	4.0	3.8	3.8	3.7	3.8	3.8	3.7	3.6	3.5	3.3	3.4	3.0	3.1
Washington	4.6	4.3	4.1	4.0	3.9	3.9	4.2	4.1	3.9	3.8	3.6	3.4	3.5	3.4	3.3
West Virginia	5.1	5.1	5.0	5.1	4.8	5.1	5.1	5.2	4.7	4.6	4.2	4.0	3.8	3.5	3.3
Wisconsin	3.2	2.9	3.0	2.9	3.0	2.9	3.0	2.9	2.9	2.8	2.7	2.6	2.6	2.4	2.5
Wyoming	5.8	5.2	5.1	4.9	4.9	5.1	5.1	4.8	4.4	4.3	4.6	4.1	4.2	4.0	3.8

NA = Not available.

[1] Includes annulments. Includes divorce petitions filed or legal separations for some counties or states.

Table 4-3. Marital Status, United States, American Community Survey 1-Year Estimates, by Age, Sex, Race and Hispanic Origin, Place of Birth, and Labor Force Status, 2017

(Number; percent.)

Characteristic	Total	Now married (except separated)	Widowed	Divorced	Separated	Never married
Total Population, 15 Years and Over..	259,992,659	48.2	5.8	10.9	2.0	33.1
Age and Sex						
Males, 15 years and over..	126,850,422	49.9	2.6	9.5	1.7	36.3
15 to 19 years..	10,859,638	0.9	0.0	0.0	0.1	99.0
20 to 34 years..	33,807,018	27.1	0.1	2.9	1.1	68.9
35 to 44 years..	20,243,714	61.4	0.4	10.5	2.5	25.2
45 to 54 years..	21,240,123	64.2	1.0	15.5	2.7	16.6
55 to 64 years..	19,644,621	67.3	2.5	16.5	2.3	11.4
65 years and over..	21,055,308	70.0	11.7	11.5	1.3	5.4
Females, 15 years and over..	133,142,237	46.6	8.9	12.1	2.3	30.1
15 to 19 years..	10,359,412	1.3	0.0	0.1	0.1	98.5
20 to 34 years..	32,739,120	34.0	0.2	4.1	1.9	59.7
35 to 44 years..	20,412,705	62.1	0.9	13.1	3.8	20.0
45 to 54 years..	21,851,020	62.2	2.7	18.4	3.6	13.0
55 to 64 years..	21,102,899	60.8	7.6	19.6	2.6	9.3
65 years and over..	26,677,081	43.6	35.2	14.7	1.2	5.3
Race and Hispanic Origin						
One race..	253,935,156	48.5	5.9	10.9	2.0	32.7
White..	193,470,962	51.5	6.2	11.3	1.7	29.2
Black or African American..	32,052,260	29.3	5.6	11.9	3.8	49.4
American Indian and Alaska Native..	2,037,202	36.7	5.1	12.9	2.8	42.5
Asian..	14,295,637	58.2	4.5	5.1	1.2	30.9
Native Hawaiian and Other Pacific Islander...............................	446,605	45.4	4.6	8.2	2.3	39.6
Some other race..	11,632,490	42.2	2.8	7.5	3.5	44.0
Two or more races...	6,057,503	33.8	3.1	9.9	2.3	50.9
Hispanic or Latino (of any race)...	41,196,019	43.2	3.4	8.4	3.2	41.8
White, not Hispanic or Latino...	166,301,970	52.7	6.7	11.7	1.5	27.5
Labor Force Participation						
Males, 16 years and over..	124,705,496	50.7	2.6	9.7	1.7	35.2
In labor force..	85,690,998	54.1	0.9	9.0	1.7	34.3
Females, 16 years and over..	131,092,196	47.3	9.0	12.3	2.4	29.0
In labor force..	76,493,327	48.1	2.8	13.4	2.7	33.0

Table 4-4. Marital Status, United States, American Community Survey 1-Year Estimates, by State, 2017

(Number; percent.)

State	Total population	Male							Female						
		Total population, 15 years and over	Now married (except separated)	Widowed	Divorced	Separated	Never married	Other	Total population, 15 years and over	Now married (except separated)	Widowed	Divorced	Separated	Never married	Other
Alabama	3,941,362	1,886,515	986,212	58,937	213,037	36,824	628,329	47,386	2,054,847	993,063	221,520	270,835	57,234	569,429	41,383
Alaska	582,153	305,887	151,197	5,870	31,990	4,561	116,830	14,867	276,266	143,579	15,837	35,344	5,595	81,506	8,899
Arizona	5,462,011	2,698,096	1,345,174	70,068	291,176	40,235	991,678	78,660	2,763,915	1,335,838	230,980	380,780	56,108	816,317	73,096
Arkansas	2,391,724	1,161,888	626,232	34,873	142,077	23,259	358,706	29,201	1,229,836	627,375	130,131	170,635	33,213	301,695	27,498
California	31,419,652	15,503,424	7,703,726	331,899	1,216,173	268,731	6,251,626	610,323	15,916,228	7,626,409	1,236,596	1,751,732	400,661	5,301,491	558,185
Colorado	4,391,535	2,196,515	1,150,363	46,441	228,316	27,151	771,395	58,811	2,195,020	1,145,338	145,092	294,681	36,582	609,909	52,358
Connecticut	2,975,923	1,437,690	735,738	37,582	126,522	15,328	537,848	35,692	1,538,233	728,155	136,380	189,607	22,577	484,091	31,075
Delaware	774,426	371,112	190,745	10,546	35,978	4,955	133,843	9,280	403,314	191,313	36,530	50,240	7,875	125,231	8,796
District of Columbia	569,884	267,371	89,085	5,121	21,248	5,908	151,917	9,062	302,513	85,735	20,184	30,509	6,731	166,085	9,474
Florida	16,886,151	8,181,890	4,142,286	262,121	922,622	163,495	2,854,861	287,849	8,704,261	4,082,733	915,535	1,262,610	233,794	2,443,383	269,489
Georgia	8,129,024	3,914,107	2,006,257	92,899	380,319	75,673	1,434,632	119,006	4,214,917	2,005,173	357,056	535,942	111,596	1,316,746	110,249
Hawaii	1,161,603	580,219	299,383	15,228	48,160	6,598	217,448	28,617	581,384	294,673	57,589	61,785	8,504	167,337	27,177
Idaho	1,295,350	645,531	364,474	16,428	69,890	7,001	194,739	17,293	649,819	361,720	49,885	85,669	8,624	152,545	15,229
Illinois	10,410,424	5,065,678	2,581,532	130,156	429,140	70,273	1,924,850	129,789	5,344,746	2,560,473	481,905	580,912	98,661	1,721,456	114,611
Indiana	5,309,479	2,590,623	1,347,327	69,825	296,442	31,329	877,029	53,592	2,718,856	1,346,122	247,362	369,542	42,423	755,830	49,634
Iowa	2,511,755	1,237,580	676,957	33,263	123,297	12,198	404,063	22,567	1,274,175	678,994	122,767	142,435	18,072	329,979	20,748
Kansas	2,304,149	1,139,682	622,315	31,433	115,847	13,119	370,087	26,173	1,164,467	617,273	105,753	142,544	17,507	298,897	22,840
Kentucky	3,584,178	1,747,324	928,985	53,548	210,032	31,760	554,759	41,753	1,836,854	932,122	184,164	258,554	45,241	462,014	35,310
Louisiana	3,734,802	1,808,152	863,184	55,665	192,713	39,911	696,590	49,766	1,926,650	860,494	192,231	250,070	56,078	623,855	40,182
Maine	1,120,835	543,491	289,970	15,690	69,002	4,434	168,829	9,461	577,344	293,320	53,525	86,388	6,721	144,111	9,290
Maryland	4,879,229	2,336,556	1,206,048	56,436	194,767	48,465	879,305	74,250	2,542,673	1,197,521	220,491	289,697	62,252	834,964	70,658
Massachusetts	5,656,501	2,715,300	1,364,705	66,047	213,328	38,118	1,071,220	72,781	2,941,201	1,372,651	249,802	319,351	60,721	999,397	67,903
Michigan	8,117,417	3,955,852	2,003,051	110,714	414,919	45,676	1,427,168	77,695	4,161,565	2,006,975	380,327	521,116	60,202	1,253,147	70,193
Minnesota	4,418,152	2,183,548	1,177,513	48,781	195,859	19,677	761,395	43,806	2,234,604	1,176,496	176,481	245,627	26,703	636,000	39,687
Mississippi	2,383,825	1,141,240	567,673	35,506	122,665	30,389	415,396	31,124	1,242,585	569,974	131,386	155,627	40,248	385,598	28,896
Missouri	4,924,498	2,392,153	1,262,429	68,980	266,619	38,342	794,125	50,229	2,532,345	1,262,911	244,719	330,204	50,559	694,511	48,179
Montana	841,483	421,163	225,733	12,369	48,902	4,954	134,159	9,294	420,320	224,381	36,759	55,135	5,694	104,045	7,884
Nebraska	1,499,899	741,576	409,072	18,357	69,815	7,715	244,332	16,262	758,323	405,418	67,023	85,319	10,956	200,563	13,580
Nevada	2,329,582	1,165,154	559,898	30,220	149,096	22,478	425,940	37,478	1,164,428	557,328	93,922	174,587	31,236	338,591	37,738
New Hampshire	1,118,047	550,259	301,043	13,747	58,602	5,693	176,867	10,338	567,788	297,359	47,541	74,198	7,404	148,690	8,864
New Jersey	7,314,415	3,532,645	1,875,603	91,194	241,649	55,491	1,324,199	107,721	3,781,770	1,851,495	357,457	380,253	84,362	1,192,565	94,526
New Mexico	1,670,789	821,168	392,672	24,712	93,771	12,651	310,013	23,610	849,621	387,253	76,622	120,880	17,502	264,866	22,789
New York	16,320,861	7,826,370	3,852,904	202,279	563,501	158,228	3,207,686	305,325	8,494,491	3,838,775	771,178	851,511	248,522	3,033,027	283,438
North Carolina	8,154,450	3,926,692	2,116,817	104,942	366,266	100,247	1,338,667	102,646	4,227,758	2,110,994	395,653	510,150	130,104	1,210,961	93,440
North Dakota	600,828	308,155	161,968	7,055	27,236	2,697	111,896	7,010	292,673	157,532	26,849	29,143	2,400	79,149	4,627
Ohio	9,445,755	4,579,414	2,345,389	135,095	497,221	69,641	1,601,709	91,125	4,866,341	2,354,051	468,399	631,375	90,628	1,412,516	81,895
Oklahoma	3,096,132	1,521,502	806,373	46,448	184,063	28,010	484,618	42,889	1,574,630	804,487	154,327	223,676	36,587	392,140	37,803
Oregon	3,308,259	1,626,907	848,628	40,786	185,146	23,889	552,347	39,745	1,681,352	848,894	136,666	243,080	33,156	452,712	37,954
Pennsylvania	10,579,008	5,129,266	2,664,609	156,544	441,330	96,153	1,866,783	110,416	5,449,742	2,651,783	562,176	571,583	125,408	1,664,200	94,775
Rhode Island	883,773	424,245	208,767	11,244	40,004	5,330	164,230	11,893	459,528	204,150	43,473	58,316	9,135	153,589	9,812
South Carolina	3,987,945	1,915,874	1,000,842	57,652	185,449	50,274	671,931	46,859	2,072,071	1,009,233	210,123	243,872	72,230	608,843	42,733
South Dakota	677,559	339,514	181,526	8,921	34,588	3,450	114,479	6,220	338,045	179,967	31,766	36,735	4,154	89,577	6,581
Tennessee	5,355,966	2,583,388	1,376,969	74,295	291,839	49,767	840,285	62,009	2,772,578	1,385,178	267,147	372,323	69,300	747,930	57,354
Texas	21,394,996	10,542,438	5,581,010	239,414	968,791	211,867	3,753,223	379,025	10,852,558	5,503,866	850,549	1,310,934	322,104	3,187,209	315,869
Utah	2,226,015	1,111,605	640,409	18,551	89,589	13,753	363,056	26,321	1,114,410	642,139	64,022	113,298	19,181	294,951	26,614
Vermont	527,332	257,778	133,871	6,751	28,773	2,778	88,383	4,109	269,554	134,303	23,022	36,882	3,111	75,347	4,179
Virginia	6,814,328	3,321,922	1,798,943	80,983	285,014	70,111	1,156,982	101,661	3,492,406	1,775,891	297,401	402,798	94,675	1,016,316	87,374
Washington	5,823,118	2,892,593	1,538,814	62,709	295,581	39,181	995,489	75,710	2,930,525	1,523,577	222,281	393,494	51,072	791,173	67,857
West Virginia	1,525,411	748,203	395,836	26,550	93,545	10,424	232,272	14,752	777,208	393,896	92,245	107,221	12,976	183,846	14,763
Wisconsin	4,693,889	2,317,063	1,219,216	58,982	228,803	20,247	810,062	38,576	2,376,826	1,214,752	204,555	273,022	26,984	684,497	35,461
Wyoming	466,777	238,104	130,209	6,070	29,112	3,170	72,713	5,168	228,673	126,150	19,011	30,192	3,193	53,320	3,825

Table 4-5. Median Age at First Marriage, American Community Survey 1-Year Estimates, by Sex and State, 2017

(Number.)

State	Male median age at first marriage	Female median age at first marriage
United States	29.9	28.1
Alabama	29.3	26.8
Alaska	28.6	26.1
Arizona	29.9	27.9
Arkansas	27.3	25.6
California	30.9	29.0
Colorado	29.9	28.2
Connecticut	30.9	29.7
Delaware	30.3	29.2
District of Columbia	30.7	30.4
Florida	30.6	29.0
Georgia	29.5	28.1
Hawaii	28.1	28.2
Idaho	26.7	25.2
Illinois	30.6	29.0
Indiana	29.0	27.0
Iowa	28.7	27.1
Kansas	28.3	26.0
Kentucky	28.0	26.4
Louisiana	29.8	28.3
Maine	30.1	28.3
Maryland	30.2	29.0
Massachusetts	31.2	30.1
Michigan	30.0	28.0
Minnesota	29.9	28.1
Mississippi	29.1	26.8
Missouri	28.9	27.3
Montana	29.8	26.9
Nebraska	28.5	26.4
Nevada	29.7	27.4
New Hampshire	30.7	29.1
New Jersey	30.7	29.1
New Mexico	29.8	27.9
New York	31.4	29.7
North Carolina	29.3	27.4
North Dakota	29.0	26.2
Ohio	29.6	27.9
Oklahoma	27.5	25.8
Oregon	30.0	27.8
Pennsylvania	30.4	28.9
Rhode Island	30.6	29.3
South Carolina	29.9	27.5
South Dakota	28.6	27.4
Tennessee	28.5	26.9
Texas	29.0	27.1
Utah	26.1	24.8
Vermont	30.5	28.0
Virginia	29.7	27.9
Washington	29.5	27.3
West Virginia	28.7	27.1
Wisconsin	29.9	27.9
Wyoming	28.5	25.0

Table 4-6. Median Age at First Marriage, American Community Survey 1-Year Estimates, by Sex and Race, United States, 2017

(Number.)

Race and origin	Male median age at first marriage	Female median age at first marriage
Median, Total, United States	29.9	28.1
White alone...	29.5	27.6
Black or African American alone	31.9	31.4
American Indian and Alaska Native alone...	30.2	29.7
Asian alone...	30.3	27.7
Native Hawaiian or Other Pacific Islander alone	28.8	27.7
Some other race alone	30.1	28.0
Two or more races	30.9	28.8
Hispanic or Latino (of any race)...	29.8	27.6
White alone, not Hispanic or Latino	29.5	27.6

Table 4-7. Marriages in the Last Year for the Population Age 15 Years and Over, American Community Survey 1-Year Estimates, by Sex and State, 2014

(Number.)

State	Total, age 15 years and over	Male					Female				
		Total	Never married	Ever married			Total	Never married	Ever married		
				Total, ever married	Married last year	Not married last year			Total, ever married	Married last year	Not married last year
United States	264,697,304	129,185,808	47,653,955	81,531,853	2,348,243	79,183,610	135,511,496	41,441,679	94,069,817	2,319,672	91,750,145
Alabama..................................	3,972,124	1,895,814	657,497	1,238,317	30,238	1,208,079	2,076,310	609,482	1,466,828	31,366	1,435,462
Alaska....................................	583,639	307,088	117,253	189,835	7,702	182,133	276,551	81,422	195,129	6,985	188,144
Arizona..................................	5,663,228	2,797,660	1,038,238	1,759,422	45,466	1,713,956	2,865,568	858,557	2,007,011	44,791	1,962,220
Arkansas................................	2,418,049	1,179,013	368,758	810,255	26,482	783,773	1,239,036	304,307	934,729	26,713	908,016
California................................	32,009,857	15,802,609	6,457,535	9,345,074	273,105	9,071,969	16,207,248	5,453,614	10,753,634	262,779	10,490,855
Colorado	4,558,575	2,281,955	819,807	1,462,148	50,942	1,411,206	2,276,620	647,734	1,628,886	50,143	1,578,743
Connecticut............................	2,986,837	1,442,504	550,228	892,276	23,512	868,764	1,544,333	497,398	1,046,935	20,367	1,026,568
Delaware................................	792,511	379,153	135,859	243,294	7,635	235,659	413,358	133,312	280,046	7,530	272,516
District of Columbia	585,161	274,333	161,791	112,542	6,586	105,956	310,828	172,944	137,884	6,337	131,547
Florida....................................	17,514,198	8,482,987	2,989,886	5,493,101	148,429	5,344,672	9,031,211	2,578,311	6,452,900	141,699	6,311,201
Georgia	8,349,724	4,009,958	1,489,940	2,520,018	76,816	2,443,202	4,339,766	1,382,082	2,957,684	74,997	2,882,687
Hawaii....................................	1,167,820	582,993	224,290	358,703	11,323	347,380	584,827	167,608	417,219	10,229	406,990
Idaho......................................	1,349,449	673,450	209,896	463,554	14,999	448,555	675,999	164,824	511,175	15,472	495,703
Illinois....................................	10,413,077	5,075,158	1,963,505	3,111,653	83,333	3,028,320	5,337,919	1,743,472	3,594,447	84,816	3,509,631
Indiana...................................	5,364,611	2,615,670	916,799	1,698,871	49,777	1,649,094	2,748,941	769,583	1,979,358	54,127	1,925,231
Iowa.......................................	2,537,862	1,252,885	420,617	832,268	22,748	809,520	1,284,977	338,142	946,835	22,644	924,191
Kansas...................................	2,318,621	1,148,850	380,487	768,363	23,789	744,574	1,169,771	297,144	872,627	24,283	848,344
Kentucky................................	3,612,529	1,761,269	567,973	1,193,296	39,309	1,153,987	1,851,260	471,878	1,379,382	39,326	1,340,056
Louisiana...............................	3,760,394	1,815,900	720,240	1,095,660	28,745	1,066,915	1,944,494	655,409	1,289,085	27,538	1,261,547
Maine.....................................	1,128,297	548,428	178,793	369,635	7,440	362,195	579,869	148,266	431,603	7,837	423,766
Maryland................................	4,936,544	2,365,357	893,377	1,471,980	44,791	1,427,189	2,571,187	847,453	1,723,734	44,612	1,679,122
Massachusetts........................	5,738,766	2,758,162	1,095,888	1,662,274	46,746	1,615,528	2,980,604	1,024,437	1,956,167	46,167	1,910,000
Michigan.................................	8,180,585	3,994,283	1,456,213	2,538,070	67,680	2,470,390	4,186,302	1,276,295	2,910,007	67,503	2,842,504
Minnesota..............................	4,493,286	2,226,162	785,172	1,440,990	34,662	1,406,328	2,267,124	657,960	1,609,164	35,016	1,574,148
Mississippi.............................	2,393,019	1,144,988	431,084	713,904	18,864	695,040	1,248,031	401,354	846,677	20,401	826,276
Missouri.................................	4,963,584	2,414,301	820,053	1,594,248	47,241	1,547,007	2,549,283	703,590	1,845,693	47,112	1,798,581
Montana.................................	859,328	428,973	138,775	290,198	6,933	283,265	430,355	107,702	322,653	7,540	315,113
Nebraska................................	1,521,245	753,862	250,410	503,452	13,326	490,126	767,383	208,681	558,702	12,469	546,233
Nevada...................................	2,429,800	1,214,411	449,027	765,384	24,773	740,611	1,215,389	358,076	857,313	22,659	834,654
New Hampshire.......................	1,133,744	557,566	180,342	377,224	9,908	367,316	576,178	154,991	421,187	9,055	412,132
New Jersey	7,377,448	3,566,444	1,343,357	2,223,087	52,350	2,170,737	3,811,004	1,205,625	2,605,379	52,582	2,552,797
New Mexico............................	1,681,966	826,549	323,388	503,161	11,256	491,905	855,417	274,047	581,370	12,962	568,408
New York................................	16,410,547	7,879,694	3,276,777	4,602,917	133,485	4,469,432	8,530,853	3,068,890	5,461,963	130,312	5,331,651
North Carolina........................	8,377,139	4,026,594	1,397,131	2,629,463	73,501	2,555,962	4,350,545	1,264,733	3,085,812	74,922	3,010,890
North Dakota..........................	606,716	311,799	115,490	196,309	6,746	189,563	294,917	79,553	215,364	6,774	208,590
Ohio.......................................	9,515,823	4,613,739	1,647,158	2,966,581	83,849	2,882,732	4,902,084	1,454,920	3,447,164	84,776	3,362,388
Oklahoma...............................	3,129,329	1,536,080	500,161	1,035,919	31,396	1,004,523	1,593,249	406,013	1,187,236	32,077	1,155,159
Oregon...................................	3,416,916	1,681,085	588,866	1,092,219	30,763	1,061,456	1,735,831	481,117	1,254,714	30,671	1,224,043
Pennsylvania..........................	10,611,437	5,148,815	1,908,802	3,240,013	85,287	3,154,726	5,462,622	1,701,934	3,760,688	85,831	3,674,857
Rhode Island..........................	890,333	426,468	166,848	259,620	6,121	253,499	463,865	162,729	301,136	5,075	296,061
South Carolina........................	4,110,098	1,971,172	723,315	1,247,857	32,506	1,215,351	2,138,926	646,109	1,492,817	34,628	1,458,189
South Dakota..........................	690,282	347,676	118,435	229,241	6,577	222,664	342,606	92,173	250,433	6,175	244,258
Tennessee..............................	5,466,987	2,637,308	874,661	1,762,647	53,954	1,708,693	2,829,679	785,847	2,043,832	55,517	1,988,315
Texas.....................................	22,164,607	10,923,789	3,952,095	6,971,694	229,661	6,742,033	11,240,818	3,372,702	7,868,116	224,915	7,643,201
Utah.......................................	2,327,933	1,164,596	388,566	776,030	32,506	743,524	1,163,337	317,723	845,614	31,711	813,903
Vermont..................................	526,751	257,783	91,627	166,156	3,981	162,175	268,968	77,049	191,919	4,008	187,911
Virginia...................................	6,919,620	3,370,061	1,179,996	2,190,065	65,344	2,124,721	3,549,559	1,060,259	2,489,300	63,509	2,425,791
Washington.............................	6,028,802	2,996,661	1,046,481	1,950,180	58,637	1,891,543	3,032,141	828,719	2,203,422	54,377	2,149,045
West Virginia..........................	1,505,831	736,517	235,076	501,441	12,306	489,135	769,314	190,630	578,684	12,127	566,557
Wisconsin...............................	4,739,661	2,341,660	832,075	1,509,585	39,469	1,470,116	2,398,001	702,077	1,695,924	38,717	1,657,207
Wyoming................................	462,614	235,576	73,917	161,659	5,248	156,411	227,038	52,802	174,236	5,493	168,743

Table 4-8. Marriages Ending in Widowhood for the Population Age 15 Years and Over, American Community Survey 1-Year Estimates, by Sex and State, 2017

(Number.)

State	Total, age 15 years and over	Male					Female				
		Total	Never married	Ever married			Total	Never married	Ever married		
				Total, ever married	Widowed last year	Not widowed last year			Total, ever married	Widowed last year	Not widowed last year
United States	264,697,304	129,185,808	47,653,955	81,531,853	451,848	81,080,005	135,511,496	41,441,679	94,069,817	987,293	93,082,524
Alabama........................	3,972,124	1,895,814	657,497	1,238,317	9,655	1,228,662	2,076,310	609,482	1,466,828	18,463	1,448,365
Alaska	583,639	307,088	117,253	189,835	530	189,305	276,551	81,422	195,129	1,362	193,767
Arizona.........................	5,663,228	2,797,660	1,038,238	1,759,422	10,539	1,748,883	2,865,568	858,557	2,007,011	19,926	1,987,085
Arkansas.......................	2,418,049	1,179,013	368,758	810,255	5,998	804,257	1,239,036	304,307	934,729	13,791	920,938
California.......................	32,009,857	15,802,609	6,457,535	9,345,074	43,384	9,301,690	16,207,248	5,453,614	10,753,634	108,294	10,645,340
Colorado	4,558,575	2,281,955	819,807	1,462,148	7,573	1,454,575	2,276,620	647,734	1,628,886	13,581	1,615,305
Connecticut...................	2,986,837	1,442,504	550,228	892,276	5,153	887,123	1,544,333	497,398	1,046,935	8,651	1,038,284
Delaware	792,511	379,153	135,859	243,294	1,044	242,250	413,358	133,312	280,046	3,571	276,475
District of Columbia	585,161	274,333	161,791	112,542	387	112,155	310,828	172,944	137,884	939	136,945
Florida..........................	17,514,198	8,482,987	2,989,886	5,493,101	31,675	5,461,426	9,031,211	2,578,311	6,452,900	72,617	6,380,283
Georgia	8,349,724	4,009,958	1,489,940	2,520,018	14,418	2,505,600	4,339,766	1,382,082	2,957,684	36,087	2,921,597
Hawaii..........................	1,167,820	582,993	224,290	358,703	1,414	357,289	584,827	167,608	417,219	5,696	411,523
Idaho............................	1,349,449	673,450	209,896	463,554	1,284	462,270	675,999	164,824	511,175	4,907	506,268
Illinois..........................	10,413,077	5,075,158	1,963,505	3,111,653	19,512	3,092,141	5,337,919	1,743,472	3,594,447	41,147	3,553,300
Indiana.........................	5,364,611	2,615,670	916,799	1,698,871	10,358	1,688,513	2,748,941	769,583	1,979,358	20,696	1,958,662
Iowa.............................	2,537,862	1,252,885	420,617	832,268	4,367	827,901	1,284,977	338,142	946,835	9,861	936,974
Kansas	2,318,621	1,148,850	380,487	768,363	4,612	763,751	1,169,771	297,144	872,627	7,067	865,560
Kentucky	3,612,529	1,761,269	567,973	1,193,296	7,758	1,185,538	1,851,260	471,878	1,379,382	14,488	1,364,894
Louisiana	3,760,394	1,815,900	720,240	1,095,660	9,950	1,085,710	1,944,494	655,409	1,289,085	15,522	1,273,563
Maine...........................	1,128,297	548,428	178,793	369,635	2,215	367,420	579,869	148,266	431,603	4,380	427,223
Maryland.......................	4,936,544	2,365,357	893,377	1,471,980	7,645	1,464,335	2,571,187	847,453	1,723,734	20,937	1,702,797
Massachusetts	5,738,766	2,758,162	1,095,888	1,662,274	7,970	1,654,304	2,980,604	1,024,437	1,956,167	18,603	1,937,564
Michigan.......................	8,180,585	3,994,283	1,456,213	2,538,070	16,125	2,521,945	4,186,302	1,276,295	2,910,007	29,974	2,880,033
Minnesota	4,493,286	2,226,162	785,172	1,440,990	6,406	1,434,584	2,267,124	657,960	1,609,164	13,709	1,595,455
Mississippi....................	2,393,019	1,144,988	431,084	713,904	3,367	710,537	1,248,031	401,354	846,677	11,675	835,002
Missouri........................	4,963,584	2,414,301	820,053	1,594,248	9,721	1,584,527	2,549,283	703,590	1,845,693	21,753	1,823,940
Montana........................	859,328	428,973	138,775	290,198	1,349	288,849	430,355	107,702	322,653	3,006	319,647
Nebraska.......................	1,521,245	753,862	250,410	503,452	2,434	501,018	767,383	208,681	558,702	4,941	553,761
Nevada.........................	2,429,800	1,214,411	449,027	765,384	3,746	761,638	1,215,389	358,076	857,313	8,835	848,478
New Hampshire..............	1,133,744	557,566	180,342	377,224	1,584	375,640	576,178	154,991	421,187	2,688	418,499
New Jersey	7,377,448	3,566,444	1,343,357	2,223,087	13,054	2,210,033	3,811,004	1,205,625	2,605,379	25,533	2,579,846
New Mexico	1,681,966	826,549	323,388	503,161	3,292	499,869	855,417	274,047	581,370	6,152	575,218
New York.......................	16,410,547	7,879,694	3,276,777	4,602,917	23,065	4,579,852	8,530,853	3,068,890	5,461,963	54,791	5,407,172
North Carolina................	8,377,139	4,026,594	1,397,131	2,629,463	14,321	2,615,142	4,350,545	1,264,733	3,085,812	30,366	3,055,446
North Dakota..................	606,716	311,799	115,490	196,309	770	195,539	294,917	79,553	215,364	1,773	213,591
Ohio.............................	9,515,823	4,613,739	1,647,158	2,966,581	21,178	2,945,403	4,902,084	1,454,920	3,447,164	38,909	3,408,255
Oklahoma......................	3,129,329	1,536,080	500,161	1,035,919	7,617	1,028,302	1,593,249	406,013	1,187,236	14,323	1,172,913
Oregon	3,416,916	1,681,085	588,866	1,092,219	5,271	1,086,948	1,735,831	481,117	1,254,714	12,497	1,242,217
Pennsylvania..................	10,611,437	5,148,815	1,908,802	3,240,013	21,999	3,218,014	5,462,622	1,701,934	3,760,688	44,723	3,715,965
Rhode Island..................	890,333	426,468	166,848	259,620	951	258,669	463,865	162,729	301,136	2,570	298,566
South Carolina	4,110,098	1,971,172	723,315	1,247,857	8,351	1,239,506	2,138,926	646,109	1,492,817	17,349	1,475,468
South Dakota	690,282	347,676	118,435	229,241	1,256	227,985	342,606	92,173	250,433	2,350	248,083
Tennessee	5,466,987	2,637,308	874,661	1,762,647	8,642	1,754,005	2,829,679	785,847	2,043,832	23,194	2,020,638
Texas............................	22,164,607	10,923,789	3,952,095	6,971,694	33,136	6,938,558	11,240,818	3,372,702	7,868,116	77,447	7,790,669
Utah	2,327,933	1,164,596	388,566	776,030	3,411	772,619	1,163,337	317,723	845,614	6,125	839,489
Vermont........................	526,751	257,783	91,627	166,156	1,103	165,053	268,968	77,049	191,919	935	190,984
Virginia.........................	6,919,620	3,370,061	1,179,996	2,190,065	10,521	2,179,544	3,549,559	1,060,259	2,489,300	24,721	2,464,579
Washington....................	6,028,802	2,996,661	1,046,481	1,950,180	8,417	1,941,763	3,032,141	828,719	2,203,422	19,052	2,184,370
West Virginia..................	1,505,831	736,517	235,076	501,441	4,171	497,270	769,314	190,630	578,684	7,521	571,163
Wisconsin......................	4,739,661	2,341,660	832,075	1,509,585	8,569	1,501,016	2,398,001	702,077	1,695,924	17,599	1,678,325
Wyoming	462,614	235,576	73,917	161,659	580	161,079	227,038	52,802	174,236	2,196	172,040

Table 4-9. Divorces in the Last Year for the Population Age 15 Years and Over, American Community Survey 1-Year Estimates, by Sex and State, 2017

(Number.)

State	Total, age 15 years and over	Male					Female				
		Total	Never married	Total, ever married	Divorced last year	Not divorced last year	Total	Never married	Total, ever married	Divorced last year	Not divorced last year
United States	264,697,304	129,185,808	47,653,955	81,531,853	974,618	80,557,235	135,511,496	41,441,679	94,069,817	1,075,500	92,994,317
Alabama......................	3,972,124	1,895,814	657,497	1,238,317	18,304	1,220,013	2,076,310	609,482	1,466,828	22,690	1,444,138
Alaska	583,639	307,088	117,253	189,835	2,780	187,055	276,551	81,422	195,129	2,142	192,987
Arizona.......................	5,663,228	2,797,660	1,038,238	1,759,422	25,544	1,733,878	2,865,568	858,557	2,007,011	24,076	1,982,935
Arkansas....................	2,418,049	1,179,013	368,758	810,255	13,388	796,867	1,239,036	304,307	934,729	16,520	918,209
California....................	32,009,857	15,802,609	6,457,535	9,345,074	97,315	9,247,759	16,207,248	5,453,614	10,753,634	112,111	10,641,523
Colorado	4,558,575	2,281,955	819,807	1,462,148	18,616	1,443,532	2,276,620	647,734	1,628,886	23,185	1,605,701
Connecticut.................	2,986,837	1,442,504	550,228	892,276	10,618	881,658	1,544,333	497,398	1,046,935	10,775	1,036,160
Delaware....................	792,511	379,153	135,859	243,294	2,035	241,259	413,358	133,312	280,046	4,730	275,316
District of Columbia	585,161	274,333	161,791	112,542	1,411	111,131	310,828	172,944	137,884	1,079	136,805
Florida.......................	17,514,198	8,482,987	2,989,886	5,493,101	67,752	5,425,349	9,031,211	2,578,311	6,452,900	74,210	6,378,690
Georgia	8,349,724	4,009,958	1,489,940	2,520,018	37,756	2,482,262	4,339,766	1,382,082	2,957,684	39,539	2,918,145
Hawaii	1,167,820	582,993	224,290	358,703	2,958	355,745	584,827	167,608	417,219	2,994	414,225
Idaho.........................	1,349,449	673,450	209,896	463,554	6,352	457,202	675,999	164,824	511,175	7,785	503,390
Illinois.......................	10,413,077	5,075,158	1,963,505	3,111,653	29,832	3,081,821	5,337,919	1,743,472	3,594,447	33,270	3,561,177
Indiana......................	5,364,611	2,615,670	916,799	1,698,871	23,863	1,675,008	2,748,941	769,583	1,979,358	24,510	1,954,848
Iowa..........................	2,537,862	1,252,885	420,617	832,268	8,527	823,741	1,284,977	338,142	946,835	10,044	936,791
Kansas.......................	2,318,621	1,148,850	380,487	768,363	9,455	758,908	1,169,771	297,144	872,627	8,811	863,816
Kentucky....................	3,612,529	1,761,269	567,973	1,193,296	16,881	1,176,415	1,851,260	471,878	1,379,382	21,685	1,357,697
Louisiana	3,760,394	1,815,900	720,240	1,095,660	14,448	1,081,212	1,944,494	655,409	1,289,085	15,549	1,273,536
Maine........................	1,128,297	548,428	178,793	369,635	4,740	364,895	579,869	148,266	431,603	5,860	425,743
Maryland....................	4,936,544	2,365,357	893,377	1,471,980	15,598	1,456,382	2,571,187	847,453	1,723,734	21,358	1,702,376
Massachusetts.............	5,738,766	2,758,162	1,095,888	1,662,274	15,987	1,646,287	2,980,604	1,024,437	1,956,167	23,792	1,932,375
Michigan....................	8,180,585	3,994,283	1,456,213	2,538,070	29,947	2,508,123	4,186,302	1,276,295	2,910,007	31,821	2,878,186
Minnesota..................	4,493,286	2,226,162	785,172	1,440,990	14,646	1,426,344	2,267,124	657,960	1,609,164	16,317	1,592,847
Mississippi.................	2,393,019	1,144,988	431,084	713,904	8,595	705,309	1,248,031	401,354	846,677	10,132	836,545
Missouri.....................	4,963,584	2,414,301	820,053	1,594,248	23,241	1,571,007	2,549,283	703,590	1,845,693	21,080	1,824,613
Montana.....................	859,328	428,973	138,775	290,198	3,501	286,697	430,355	107,702	322,653	2,794	319,859
Nebraska....................	1,521,245	753,862	250,410	503,452	5,630	497,822	767,383	208,681	558,702	6,454	552,248
Nevada.......................	2,429,800	1,214,411	449,027	765,384	9,382	756,002	1,215,389	358,076	857,313	11,640	845,673
New Hampshire............	1,133,744	557,566	180,342	377,224	3,865	373,359	576,178	154,991	421,187	5,488	415,699
New Jersey	7,377,448	3,566,444	1,343,357	2,223,087	22,944	2,200,143	3,811,004	1,205,625	2,605,379	23,708	2,581,671
New Mexico	1,681,966	826,549	323,388	503,161	7,709	495,452	855,417	274,047	581,370	6,774	574,596
New York....................	16,410,547	7,879,694	3,276,777	4,602,917	41,808	4,561,109	8,530,853	3,068,890	5,461,963	50,703	5,411,260
North Carolina.............	8,377,139	4,026,594	1,397,131	2,629,463	31,567	2,597,896	4,350,545	1,264,733	3,085,812	36,660	3,049,152
North Dakota...............	606,716	311,799	115,490	196,309	2,371	193,938	294,917	79,553	215,364	2,595	212,769
Ohio	9,515,823	4,613,739	1,647,158	2,966,581	32,434	2,934,147	4,902,084	1,454,920	3,447,164	37,475	3,409,689
Oklahoma...................	3,129,329	1,536,080	500,161	1,035,919	16,251	1,019,668	1,593,249	406,013	1,187,236	16,843	1,170,393
Oregon.......................	3,416,916	1,681,085	588,866	1,092,219	13,937	1,078,282	1,735,831	481,117	1,254,714	13,949	1,240,765
Pennsylvania...............	10,611,437	5,148,815	1,908,802	3,240,013	34,528	3,205,485	5,462,622	1,701,934	3,760,688	37,563	3,723,125
Rhode Island...............	890,333	426,468	166,848	259,620	2,294	257,326	463,865	162,729	301,136	3,321	297,815
South Carolina	4,110,098	1,971,172	723,315	1,247,857	16,013	1,231,844	2,138,926	646,109	1,492,817	18,612	1,474,205
South Dakota	690,282	347,676	118,435	229,241	3,847	225,394	342,606	92,173	250,433	2,670	247,763
Tennessee..................	5,466,987	2,637,308	874,661	1,762,647	24,776	1,737,871	2,829,679	785,847	2,043,832	28,847	2,014,985
Texas........................	22,164,607	10,923,789	3,952,095	6,971,694	88,612	6,883,082	11,240,818	3,372,702	7,868,116	92,008	7,776,108
Utah..........................	2,327,933	1,164,596	388,566	776,030	11,275	764,755	1,163,337	317,723	845,614	10,544	835,070
Vermont.....................	526,751	257,783	91,627	166,156	1,364	164,792	268,968	77,049	191,919	1,945	189,974
Virginia......................	6,919,620	3,370,061	1,179,996	2,190,065	27,878	2,162,187	3,549,559	1,060,259	2,489,300	28,481	2,460,819
Washington.................	6,028,802	2,996,661	1,046,481	1,950,180	24,541	1,925,639	3,032,141	828,719	2,203,422	25,563	2,177,859
West Virginia...............	1,505,831	736,517	235,076	501,441	8,397	493,044	769,314	190,630	578,684	6,888	571,796
Wisconsin	4,739,661	2,341,660	832,075	1,509,585	16,879	1,492,706	2,398,001	702,077	1,695,924	16,100	1,679,824
Wyoming	462,614	235,576	73,917	161,659	2,226	159,433	227,038	52,802	174,236	1,810	172,426

Table 4-10. Median Duration of Current Marriage in Years for the Population Age 15 Years and Over, American Community Survey 1-Year Estimates, by Sex, Marital Status, and State, 2017

(Years.)

State	Total, age 15 years and over	Male				Female			
		Total	Married, spouse present	Married, spouse absent	Separated	Total	Married, spouse present	Married, spouse absent	Separated
United States	19.7	`9.6	20.2	11.9	16.5	19.7	20.3	12.8	16.7
Alabama...........................	20.2	20.2	21.0	11.6	14.3	20.3	21.3	10.8	13.7
Alaska..............................	16.0	16.2	16.6	11.3	16.9	15.8	15.9	11.5	21.0
Arizona............................	19.9	19.9	20.5	11.5	16.4	20.0	20.5	13.4	17.1
Arkansas..........................	19.0	18.9	19.7	13.0	10.5	19.1	19.9	9.3	14.6
California..........................	18.8	18.6	19.2	12.2	18.0	19.0	19.3	13.4	19.3
Colorado	17.6	17.5	17.9	10.5	14.6	17.8	18.1	12.6	16.8
Connecticut......................	21.8	21.6	22.2	12.6	18.7	22.0	22.4	13.9	19.9
Delaware	21.2	20.9	22.1	12.1	14.5	21.4	22.3	17.2	16.4
District of Columbia	10.6	9.9	9.8	7.1	21.7	11.2	10.9	7.6	20.4
Florida.............................	20.3	20.3	21.0	12.4	16.8	20.3	21.2	13.8	16.4
Georgia	18.2	18.1	18.7	9.5	16.0	18.2	18.8	11.7	15.7
Hawaii..............................	18.8	18.6	19.5	9.5	18.8	19.0	19.7	11.9	13.3
Idaho...............................	18.7	18.7	19.5	12.8	10.0	18.7	18.9	13.6	18.3
Illinois.............................	20.7	20.7	21.2	14.0	17.1	20.8	21.2	15.0	17.8
Indiana............................	19.8	19.9	20.4	12.6	11.2	19.7	20.3	11.7	13.2
Iowa................................	21.8	21.7	22.1	18.2	12.7	21.9	22.4	14.8	13.8
Kansas............................	19.7	19.7	20.1	12.7	15.2	19.7	20.1	11.6	14.5
Kentucky	19.8	19.8	20.6	11.5	14.8	19.9	20.5	11.6	15.4
Louisiana	19.4	19.3	20.4	11.3	14.9	19.5	20.5	11.9	14.8
Maine...............................	22.6	22.9	23.0	22.4	22.2	22.3	22.8	13.9	20.0
Maryland..........................	18.9	18.8	19.5	10.9	16.7	19.0	19.5	12.5	17.1
Massachusetts.................	20.4	20.4	20.7	13.1	18.0	20.5	20.9	12.5	17.9
Michigan..........................	21.6	21.6	22.1	12.1	15.5	21.7	22.1	15.2	16.4
Minnesota	21.0	21.1	21.4	14.9	17.5	20.9	21.2	15.9	16.5
Mississippi.......................	19.6	19.7	20.7	9.8	15.3	19.5	20.4	11.8	17.5
Missouri...........................	20.3	20.3	20.7	14.3	14.0	20.4	20.9	15.0	14.7
Montana...........................	21.5	21.9	22.0	20.5	16.3	21.1	21.6	18.1	13.9
Nebraska..........................	20.4	20.3	20.8	12.2	14.8	20.5	21.0	14.1	12.6
Nevada	17.2	17.1	17.5	11.0	14.8	17.2	17.6	11.9	15.9
New Hampshire.................	22.1	21.9	22.2	17.2	19.2	22.4	22.6	19.1	18.5
New Jersey	20.5	20.4	20.9	11.9	17.5	20.7	21.1	12.3	18.1
New Mexico	20.8	21.0	21.9	11.4	18.8	20.5	21.5	11.6	15.7
New York..........................	20.0	19.8	20.5	11.6	18.6	20.2	20.8	13.2	19.5
North Carolina...................	19.5	19.6	20.1	12.6	16.2	19.5	20.1	11.9	15.7
North Dakota.....................	19.9	19.9	20.1	18.6	14.4	20.0	20.0	26.9	15.2
Ohio................................	21.2	21.1	21.7	11.8	15.9	21.2	21.8	13.3	14.9
Oklahoma.........................	18.0	18.1	18.9	10.4	12.3	18.0	18.8	11.5	12.6
Oregon.............................	19.4	19.6	20.0	14.0	16.0	19.3	19.8	13.2	16.1
Pennsylvania.....................	22.1	22.0	22.5	13.0	18.0	22.1	22.6	14.1	17.6
Rhode Island.....................	20.7	20.4	21.2	8.9	11.2	20.9	21.2	19.4	17.4
South Carolina	21.2	21.3	22.1	11.3	18.1	21.2	21.9	10.4	18.3
South Dakota	21.3	21.2	21.9	11.7	12.0	21.5	21.9	17.7	18.2
Tennessee.......................	19.3	19.3	19.9	13.8	12.4	19.2	20.0	11.5	13.1
Texas..............................	17.6	17.6	18.2	10.4	15.9	17.7	18.2	10.4	15.4
Utah................................	17.3	17.3	17.8	8.9	10.7	17.2	17.7	9.1	12.0
Vermont...........................	22.0	22.3	22.8	9.5	18.6	21.8	22.0	17.8	15.8
Virginia.............................	18.9	18.8	19.6	10.4	14.9	19.1	19.7	11.8	16.8
Washington......................	18.2	18.3	18.7	10.8	17.8	18.2	18.6	12.5	16.1
West Virginia....................	22.6	22.6	23.3	16.1	16.6	22.6	23.3	14.9	13.5
Wisconsin	22.3	22.3	22.5	17.8	17.8	22.3	22.5	17.8	15.3
Wyoming	19.1	19.0	19.5	16.5	6.5	19.2	19.2	22.3	16.8

Table 4-11. Number of Times Married for the Population Age 15 Years and Over, American Community Survey 1-Year Estimates, by Sex, Marital Status, and State, 2014

(Number.)

State	Total, age 15 years and over	Male						Female					
		Total	Never married	Ever married				Total	Never married	Ever married			
				Total	Once	Twice	Three or more times			Total	Once	Twice	Three or more times
United States ..	257,770,670	125,664,923	45,864,923	79,800,000	60,106,291	15,406,283	4,287,426	132,105,747	39,943,973	92,161,774	69,723,101	17,642,179	4,796,494
Alabama............	3,931,966	1,878,536	621,776	1,256,760	859,490	289,417	107,853	2,053,430	566,426	1,487,004	1,029,160	336,333	121,511
Alaska	579,778	305,440	117,205	188,235	136,624	40,581	11,030	274,338	83,733	190,605	133,026	43,802	13,777
Arizona.............	5,381,925	2,655,529	986,840	1,668,689	1,198,993	356,759	112,937	2,726,396	810,874	1,915,522	1,375,689	408,274	131,559
Arkansas	2,381,476	1,157,713	367,542	790,171	511,082	188,563	90,526	1,223,763	305,010	918,753	596,930	216,984	104,839
California...........	31,206,124	15,387,827	6,217,072	9,170,755	7,346,349	1,490,174	334,232	15,818,297	5,280,301	10,537,996	8,445,674	1,708,385	383,937
Colorado	4,309,301	2,153,568	760,603	1,392,965	1,043,063	280,636	69,266	2,155,733	601,891	1,553,842	1,152,664	319,438	81,740
Connecticut.......	2,967,896	1,433,554	539,976	893,578	714,395	154,838	24,345	1,534,342	485,371	1,048,971	851,633	171,556	25,782
Delaware	765,491	366,631	132,545	234,086	169,216	52,335	12,535	398,860	123,172	275,688	205,801	56,733	13,154
District of Columbia......	559,363	262,074	150,865	111,209	90,987	17,542	2,680	297,289	165,425	131,864	110,276	18,405	3,183
Florida..............	16,544,829	8,013,533	2,819,903	5,193,630	3,626,972	1,188,820	377,838	8,531,296	2,409,539	6,121,757	4,356,282	1,365,603	399,872
Georgia	8,019,982	3,862,111	1,444,653	2,417,458	1,733,764	516,889	166,805	4,157,871	1,315,258	2,842,613	2,071,177	585,702	185,734
Hawaii	1,158,752	583,110	220,895	362,215	292,541	58,181	11,493	575,642	166,862	408,780	328,573	68,481	11,726
Idaho................	1,274,423	632,611	194,809	437,802	311,663	92,634	33,505	641,812	148,957	492,855	344,780	107,545	40,530
Illinois..............	10,412,161	5,061,711	1,930,523	3,131,188	2,483,367	520,423	127,398	5,350,450	1,730,603	3,619,847	2,874,283	612,355	133,209
Indiana.............	5,284,811	2,572,431	865,086	1,707,345	1,215,895	366,392	125,058	2,712,380	751,182	1,961,198	1,386,327	430,774	144,097
Iowa.................	2,503,309	1,232,864	394,855	838,009	648,639	152,602	36,768	1,270,445	330,276	940,169	722,945	169,918	47,306
Kansas	2,299,146	1,136,728	370,573	766,155	568,242	148,932	48,981	1,162,418	299,323	863,095	630,216	172,907	59,972
Kentucky	3,569,190	1,740,854	555,037	1,185,817	818,693	266,085	101,039	1,828,336	457,294	1,371,042	937,230	323,402	110,410
Louisiana	3,716,740	1,797,076	694,903	1,102,173	793,708	235,565	72,900	1,919,664	625,735	1,293,929	945,800	269,825	78,304
Maine	1,119,690	541,803	170,892	370,911	265,317	83,207	22,387	577,887	150,136	427,751	311,872	91,991	23,888
Maryland...........	4,854,750	2,322,878	884,012	1,438,866	1,119,040	268,230	51,596	2,531,872	834,587	1,697,285	1,330,886	308,895	57,504
Massachusetts ..	5,604,860	2,687,387	1,074,332	1,613,055	1,329,819	248,537	34,699	2,917,473	1,004,940	1,912,533	1,593,711	281,019	37,803
Michigan...........	8,089,154	3,933,762	1,424,877	2,508,885	1,880,553	495,633	132,699	4,155,392	1,258,179	2,897,213	2,190,855	560,573	145,785
Minnesota	4,386,934	2,166,462	766,344	1,400,118	1,136,855	219,997	43,266	2,220,472	636,833	1,583,639	1,282,417	253,342	47,880
Mississippi........	2,383,607	1,141,338	415,131	726,207	504,819	162,196	59,192	1,242,269	385,898	856,371	594,936	192,931	68,504
Missouri...........	4,909,194	2,378,868	794,587	1,584,281	1,114,738	343,095	126,448	2,530,326	703,820	1,826,506	1,289,894	399,215	137,397
Montana...........	835,422	417,444	131,905	285,539	205,755	61,955	17,829	417,978	107,164	310,814	223,148	66,246	21,420
Nebraska	1,488,730	733,769	242,745	491,024	388,323	84,236	18,465	754,961	200,086	554,875	430,774	100,140	23,961
Nevada	2,287,984	1,144,209	429,417	714,792	496,052	159,412	59,328	1,143,775	342,521	801,254	558,049	178,586	64,619
New Hampshire.	1,111,188	545,435	177,905	367,530	279,399	73,648	14,483	565,753	151,360	414,393	313,158	83,693	17,542
New Jersey	7,282,046	3,518,889	1,328,240	2,190,649	1,820,834	324,452	45,363	3,763,157	1,196,420	2,566,737	2,167,880	354,751	44,106
New Mexico	1,667,854	820,542	308,918	511,624	373,786	104,193	33,645	847,312	265,986	581,326	427,048	120,554	33,724
New York........	16,248,072	7,787,815	3,207,375	4,580,440	3,775,941	689,953	114,546	8,460,257	3,045,518	5,414,739	4,542,921	765,085	106,733
North Carolina...	8,029,973	3,863,351	1,332,169	2,531,182	1,853,144	531,096	146,942	4,166,622	1,188,823	2,977,799	2,173,816	625,261	178,722
North Dakota.....	598,037	305,227	112,831	192,396	154,187	31,658	6,551	292,810	78,241	214,569	172,262	35,649	6,658
Ohio	9,422,595	4,562,386	1,610,302	2,952,084	2,172,296	611,220	168,568	4,860,209	1,417,330	3,442,879	2,549,988	691,610	201,281
Oklahoma.........	3,080,740	1,510,864	480,122	1,030,742	688,478	240,820	101,444	1,569,876	389,663	1,180,213	776,400	286,464	117,349
Oregon	3,258,094	1,601,320	547,721	1,053,599	751,074	225,596	76,929	1,656,774	452,271	1,204,503	829,439	277,575	97,489
Pennsylvania	10,562,571	5,117,508	1,878,338	3,239,170	2,549,066	583,686	106,418	5,445,063	1,675,810	3,769,253	3,006,800	645,668	116,785
Rhode Island.....	882,072	422,664	165,692	256,972	206,474	42,425	8,073	459,408	152,890	306,518	246,850	52,920	6,748
South Carolina ..	3,929,135	1,889,452	667,180	1,222,272	883,213	261,461	77,598	2,039,683	605,264	1,434,419	1,048,559	298,974	86,886
South Dakota	675,764	337,200	115,307	221,893	175,885	35,970	10,038	338,564	91,746	246,818	190,574	45,239	11,005
Tennessee	5,309,334	2,556,919	832,587	1,724,332	1,176,118	402,967	145,247	2,752,415	751,194	2,001,221	1,367,918	462,930	170,373
Texas	21,001,527	10,339,954	3,693,020	6,646,934	4,912,950	1,310,477	423,507	10,661,573	3,117,291	7,544,282	5,573,627	1,511,688	458,967
Utah	2,178,253	1,085,912	356,153	729,759	560,245	126,092	43,422	1,092,341	284,780	807,561	613,591	146,205	47,765
Vermont............	528,064	256,941	86,611	170,330	131,468	32,129	6,733	271,123	75,506	195,617	150,496	36,673	8,448
Virginia.............	6,772,134	3,297,416	1,144,868	2,152,548	1,610,202	435,493	106,853	3,474,718	1,019,938	2,454,780	1,870,370	471,874	112,536
Washington.......	5,722,255	2,845,066	982,876	1,862,190	1,373,097	373,280	115,813	2,877,189	784,563	2,092,626	1,529,938	427,574	135,114
West Virginia.....	1,532,355	751,800	240,214	511,586	353,442	123,013	35,131	780,555	184,876	595,679	413,515	138,130	44,034
Wisconsin	4,682,400	2,307,821	804,084	1,503,737	1,181,495	269,944	52,298	2,374,579	678,969	1,695,610	1,332,375	302,656	60,579
Wyoming	469,219	238,620	72,507	166,113	118,543	32,844	14,726	230,599	54,138	176,461	120,568	41,646	14,247

SOURCES OF DATA

Tables 4-1 and 4-2 are from the Centers for Disease Control and Prevention's National Vital Statistics System. Detailed state tables can be found at http://www.cdc.gov/nchs/mardiv.htm#state_tables. Rates for 2001 to 2009 have been revised and are based on intercensal population estimates from the 2000 and 2010 censuses.

Tables 4-3 through 4-11 are from the 1-year estimates from the 2017 American Community Survey, which is conducted by the U.S. Census Bureau. Although the American Community Survey (ACS) produces population, demographic and housing unit estimates, it is the Census Bureau's Population Estimates Program that produces and disseminates the official estimates of the population for the nation, states, counties, cities and towns and estimates of housing units for states and counties. At the time of publication, the U.S. Census Bureau was in the process of decommissioning the American FactFinder tool and moving the ACS data to data.census.gov.

NOTES AND DEFINITIONS

Accuracy of the data—Data are based on a sample and are subject to sampling variability. The degree of uncertainty for an estimate arising from sampling variability is represented through the use of a margin of error. The margin of error can be interpreted roughly as providing a 90 percent probability that the interval defined by the estimate minus the margin of error and the estimate plus the margin of error (the lower and upper confidence bounds) contains the true value. In addition to sampling variability, the ACS estimates are subject to nonsampling error. The effect of nonsampling error is not represented in these tables.

Foreign born—Foreign born excludes people born outside the United States to a parent who is a U.S. citizen.

Population—ACS population comprises individuals age 15 to 54 years.

Widowhood—Widowhood estimates may vary from the mortality data released by the National Center for Health Statistics (NCHS) because of differences in methodology and data collection. NCHS uses information collected on death certificates from each state that record the current marital status of the decedent at the time of death. From these administrative records, NCHS then publishes information about men and women who died in that calendar year by their marital status. By inference, people who were married at their time of death were survived by a widowed spouse. In contrast, the ACS collects survey-based reports from individuals as to whether or not they were widowed in the last 12 months. We recommend using caution when comparing the NCHS estimates to the ACS estimates of widowhood.

INDEX